NETTER'S PEDIATRICS

2nd EDITION

NETTER'S PEDIATRICS

Editors

Rebecca Tenney-Soeiro, MD, MSEd
Section Chief of Education, Division of General Pediatrics
Program Director, Pediatric Hospital Medicine Fellowship
Children's Hospital of Philadelphia
Advisory Dean
Associate Professor of Pediatrics
Perelman School of Medicine, University of Pennsylvania
Philadelphia, Pennsylvania

Erin Pete Devon, MD
Attending Physician, Pediatric Hospital Medicine, Division of General Pediatrics
Children's Hospital of Philadelphia
Pediatrics Clerkship Co-Director
Assistant Professor of Clinical Pediatrics
Perelman School of Medicine, University of Pennsylvania
Philadelphia, Pennsylvania

Illustrations **by Frank H. Netter, MD**

Contributing Illustrators
Carlos A.G. Machado, MD
John A. Craig, MD
DragonFly Media Group
Tiffany S. DaVanzo, MA, CMI
Anita Impagliazzo, MA, CMI
Kristen Wienandt Marzejon, MS, MFA
James A. Perkins, MS, MFA

ELSEVIER

Elsevier
1600 John F. Kennedy Blvd.
Ste 1800
Philadelphia, PA 19103-2899

NETTER'S PEDIATRICS, SECOND EDITION   ISBN-13: 978-0-323-79608-8
Copyright © 2023 by Elsevier Inc. All rights reserved.

Notice

Previous edition copyrighted 2011 by Saunders, an imprint of Elsevier Inc.

ISBN-13: 978-0-323-79608-8

Senior Content Strategist: Marybeth Thiel
Publishing Services Manager: Catherine Albright Jackson
Senior Project Manager: Doug Turner
Designer: Patrick Ferguson

Printed in India

Last digit is the print number: 9   8   7   6   5   4   3   2   1

Working together
to grow libraries in
developing countries

www.elsevier.com • www.bookaid.org

To my patients and their families, for always teaching me
To my colleagues, for always inspiring me
To Damon, Jamison, Devon, Lea, and Landon, for always grounding me
Rebecca Tenney-Soeiro

To my patients and their families, for the privilege of caring for you
To my colleagues, for your support and continual inspiration
To my family, for your unconditional love
Erin Pete Devon

Rebecca Tenney-Soeiro, MD, MSEd, is a hospitalist for general pediatrics and complex care patients at The Children's Hospital of Philadelphia. She is the Section Chief of Education for the Division of Pediatrics, Program Director for the Pediatric Hospital Medicine Fellowship, and an Advisory Dean for the Perelman School of Medicine at the University of Pennsylvania. Dr. Tenney-Soeiro graduated from Tufts University with a Bachelor of Science in Biology and received her medical degree from the Albert Einstein College of Medicine. She completed residency and chief residency in the Boston Combined Residency Program before moving to CHOP. While at the University of Pennsylvania, she completed a Master of Science in Medical Education to further her own skills in educational scholarship and leadership. Her scholarly interests include improving the feedback process and the promotion of autonomy for learners. She also enjoys mentoring learners and junior faculty at all stages. She is an active member of the Council on Medical Student Education in Pediatrics, serving previously as the Chair of the Research and Scholarship Collaborative, and is currently on the Executive Committee. Dr. Tenney-Soeiro lives in Swarthmore with her husband, four amazing children, and their two crazy labradoodles.

Erin Pete Devon, MD, is a pediatric hospitalist at the Children's Hospital of Philadelphia. Dr. Pete Devon grew up in central Pennsylvania and completed her undergraduate studies in Psychology at the University of Pennsylvania. After graduating from Drexel University College of Medicine, she completed her pediatric residency at the Children's Hospital of Philadelphia, where she has been practicing ever since. Dr. Pete Devon's academic focus is medical education, with a particular interest in undergraduate medical education. She is a Co-Director for the Pediatric Clerkship and created an intern preparatory course for graduating medical students. Her scholarship has centered around the pediatric pre-internship boot camp and undergraduate medical education learners. A student herself, Dr. Pete Devon is currently pursuing a master's degree in Medical Education. She lives in West Philadelphia with her husband, two energetic children, and a loveable goldendoodle.

Frank H. Netter, MD

Frank H. Netter was born in 1906 in New York City. He studied art at the Art Student's League and the National Academy of Design before entering medical school at New York University, where he received his MD degree in 1931. During his student years, Dr. Netter's notebook sketches attracted the attention of the medical faculty and other physicians, allowing him to augment his income by illustrating articles and textbooks. He continued illustrating as a sideline after establishing a surgical practice in 1933, but he ultimately opted to give up his practice in favor of a full-time commitment to art. After service in the United States Army during World War II, Dr. Netter began his long collaboration with the CIBA Pharmaceutical Company (now Novartis Pharmaceuticals). This 45-year partnership resulted in the production of the extraordinary collection of medical art so familiar to physicians and other medical professionals worldwide.

In 2005, Elsevier, Inc. purchased the Netter Collection and all publications from Icon Learning Systems. There are now more than 50 publications featuring the art of Dr. Netter available through Elsevier, Inc.

Dr. Netter's works are among the finest examples of the use of illustration in the teaching of medical concepts. The 13-book Netter Collection of Medical Illustrations, which includes the greater part of the more than 4000 paintings created by Dr. Netter, became and remains one of the most famous medical works ever published. *Netter's Atlas of Human Anatomy,* first published in 1989, presents the anatomical paintings from the Netter Collection. Now translated into 16 languages, it is the anatomy atlas of choice among medical and health professions students the world over.

The Netter illustrations are appreciated not only for their aesthetic qualities, but, more importantly, for their intellectual content. As Dr. Netter wrote in 1949, "…clarification of a subject is the aim and goal of illustration. No matter how beautifully painted, how delicately and subtly rendered a subject may be, it is of little value as a medical illustration if it does not serve to make clear some medical point." Dr. Netter's planning, conception, point of view, and approach are what inform his paintings and what makes them so intellectually valuable.

Frank H. Netter, MD, physician and artist, died in 1991.

Learn more about the physician-artist whose work has inspired the Netter Reference collection: https://netterimages.com/artist-frank-h-netter.html

Carlos A.G. Machado, MD

Carlos Machado was chosen by Novartis to be Dr. Netter's successor. He continues to be the main artist who contributes to the Netter collection of medical illustrations.

Self-taught in medical illustration, cardiologist Carlos Machado has contributed meticulous updates to some of Dr. Netter's original plates and has created many paintings of his own in the style of Netter as an extension of the Netter collection. Dr. Machado's photorealistic expertise and his keen insight into the physician/patient relationship inform his vivid and unforgettable visual style. His dedication to researching each topic and subject he paints places him among the premier medical illustrators at work today.

Learn more about his background and see more of his art at: https://netterimages.com/artist-carlos-a-g-machado.html

ACKNOWLEDGMENTS

We would like to thank Dr. Ludwig for believing in us and providing us the opportunity to edit the second edition of *Netter's Pediatrics*. We stand in awe of the many contributions he has made to the field of pediatrics and to the world of medical education. We also share our gratitude to the contributing authors and section editors for their hard work in updating or creating new chapters and their thoughtful approach to capturing the power of Netter's drawings in the teaching of medicine. We sincerely appreciate the diligence of the authors—residents, fellows, and faculty—whose passion and intellect never cease to amaze us. We are grateful to the section editors whose clinical expertise, dedication and commitment to mentorship, and passion for education are examples to each of us.

We thank our patients and their families for the privilege of being able to care for you. You continually provide inspiration, motivation, and are truly our best teachers. We hope this edition provides a foundation of knowledge to the next generation of pediatric providers as they strive to provide outstanding care to you and your families.

We would like to acknowledge the incredible images that Frank Netter created that made this book possible. We would like to thank the many talented artists who contributed their work to this volume with updated or newly created images: Carlos A.G. Machado, MD; John A. Craig, MD; DragonFly Media Group; Tiffany S. DaVanzo, MA, CMI; Anita Impagliazzo, MA, CMI; Kristen Wienandt Marzejon, MS, MFA; and James A. Perkins, MS, MFA.

A special thank you to our Elsevier editorial team. We would especially like to acknowledge Marybeth Thiel for her guidance in this large undertaking. Without their hard work, thoughtful feedback, and encouragement, we could not have done this.

We would also like to give our thanks to our work and home families. We could not have accomplished this without your support and mentorship. When things are crazy, whether due to a global pandemic or a busy service week, you keep us grounded. You remind us to smile, to laugh, and to celebrate small moments. We especially want to say thank you to our children, Jamison, Devon, Lea, Landon, Sam, and Eve; your patience, encouragement, and love remind us of why we chose pediatrics and of the importance of providing outstanding care to all children.

Drs. Ludwig, Florin, Aronson, and Werner were editors of the first *Netter's Pediatrics* 10 years ago. Their desire for that book to serve as a tribute to medical education and mentoring in all its forms continues in the second edition.

Most medical students rely on the incredible illustrations of Dr. Frank Netter to get through their anatomy and physiology courses. However, his work continues to be a warm and welcoming gateway to learn not only the anatomy, but also the pathogenesis, clinical signs, and symptoms of many disease processes. As Dr. Ludwig said in the first edition's preface, "The old adage that a picture is worth a thousand words was multiplied many times over by a Netter illustration." Our hope is that this edition will carry on the tradition of educating and inspiring the next generation of pediatricians.

Dr. Ludwig was and is an incredible mentor to many, including to each of us. His desire to have this book provide mentorship opportunities to trainees and young faculty was a tradition we wanted to continue. Each of the first authors is a medical student, resident, fellow, or young faculty member, for whom this may be their first publication. Section editors were chosen based on their clinical expertise and their desire to mentor these authors through writing and editing their chapters. We applaud all authors and section editors for their commitment to providing the highest quality educational content to share with each of you. These relationships remind us that, despite the advances in technology and changes in the provision of healthcare, the apprenticeship model is still at the center of our academic and educational process.

Our hope is that this updated edition will continue to aid you in the care of children. We hope these words and drawings will bring the subject matter alive and help you derive as much practical knowledge and pleasure from using *Netter's Pediatrics* as we experienced in bringing it to you.

Rebecca Tenney-Soeiro, MD, MSEd
Erin Pete Devon, MD
Philadelphia, Pennsylvania, 2021

CONTRIBUTORS

Editors

Rebecca Tenney-Soeiro, MD, MSEd
Section Chief of Education, Division of
  General Pediatrics
Program Director, Pediatric Hospital
  Medicine Fellowship
Children's Hospital of Philadelphia
Advisory Dean
Associate Professor of Pediatrics
Perelman School of Medicine, University of
  Pennsylvania
Philadelphia, Pennsylvania

Erin Pete Devon, MD
Attending Physician, Pediatric Hospital
  Medicine, Division of General
  Pediatrics
Children's Hospital of Philadelphia
Pediatrics Clerkship Co-Director
Assistant Professor of Clinical Pediatrics
Perelman School of Medicine, University of
  Pennsylvania
Philadelphia, Pennsylvania

Section Editors

Craig A. Alter, MD
Attending Physician; Director,
  Neuroendocrine Center
Children's Hospital of Philadelphia
Professor of Clinical Pediatrics,
  Endocrinology, and Diabetes
Perelman School of Medicine, University of
  Pennsylvania
Philadelphia, Pennsylvania

Terri F. Brown-Whitehorn, MD
Attending Physician, Allergy and
  Immunology
Children's Hospital of Philadelphia
Professor of Clinical Pediatrics, Allergy, and
  Immunology
Perelman School of Medicine, University of
  Pennsylvania
Philadelphia, Pennsylvania

Julianne E. Burns, MD, MSCE
Attending Physician, Pediatrics
Children's Hospital of Philadelphia
Philadelphia, Pennsylvania

Audrey Jacqueline Chan, MD
Assistant Professor, Pediatric Dermatology
Texas Children's Hospital
Assistant Professor of Dermatology
Baylor College of Medicine
Houston, Texas

Sanmati Rao Cuddapah, MD
Attending Physician, Human Genetics
Program Director, Medical Genetics
  Residency Program
Children's Hospital of Philadelphia
Assistant Professor of Clinical Pediatrics
Children's Hospital of Philadelphia
Philadelphia, Pennsylvania

Michelle Dunn, MD
Attending Physician, General Pediatrics
Children's Hospital of Philadelphia
Clinical Assistant Professor of Pediatrics
Perelman School of Medicine, University of
  Pennsylvania
Philadelphia, Pennsylvania

Matthew Elias, MD
Attending Physician, Division of Cardiology
Medical Director, Pennsylvania Cardiology
  Satellite Operations
Co-Medical Director, Cardiology Kawasaki
  Disease Program
Children's Hospital of Philadelphia
Clinical Assistant Professor of Pediatrics
Perelman School of Medicine, University of
  Pennsylvania
Philadelphia, Pennsylvania

Melissa Kennedy, MD
Attending Physician, Gastroenterology,
  Hepatology, and Nutrition
Children's Hospital of Philadelphia
Assistant Professor of Pediatric
  Gastroenterology, Hepatology, and
  Nutrition
Perelman School of Medicine, University of
  Pennsylvania
Philadelphia, Pennsylvania

Benjamin L. Laskin, MD
Attending Physician, Nephrology, The
  Kidney Transplant and Dialysis Program
Children's Hospital of Philadelphia
Assistant Professor of Nephrology
Perelman School of Medicine, University of
  Pennsylvania
Philadelphia, Pennsylvania

Katie K. Lockwood, MD, MEd
Attending Physician, Primary Care
Children's Hospital of Philadelphia
Assistant Professor of Pediatrics
Perelman School of Medicine, University of
  Pennsylvania
Philadelphia, Pennsylvania

Pamela Mazzeo, MD
Attending Physician, Pediatrics
Children's Hospital of Philadelphia
Assistant Professor of Pediatrics
Perelman School of Medicine, University of
  Pennsylvania
Philadelphia, Pennsylvania

Jennifer L. McGuire, MD, MSCE
Attending Physician, Neurology
Children's Hospital of Philadelphia
Assistant Professor of Neurology and
  Pediatrics
Perelman School of Medicine, University of
  Pennsylvania
Philadelphia, Pennsylvania

Joanna Parga-Belinke, MD
Attending Physician, Neonatology
Children's Hospital of Philadelphia
Clinical Assistant Professor of Pediatrics,
  Neonatology
Perelman School of Medicine, University of
  Pennsylvania
Philadelphia, Pennsylvania

Pelton A. Phinizy, MD
Attending Physician, Pulmonary Medicine
Children's Hospital of Philadelphia
Assistant Professor of Clinical Pediatrics,
  Pediatrics
Perelman School of Medicine, University of
  Pennsylvania
Philadelphia, Pennsylvania

Jonathan R. Pletcher, MD
Attending Physician, Adolescent Medicine
Medical Director for Inpatient Adolescent
  Medicine
Associate Professor of Clinical Pediatrics,
  Adolescent Medicine
Children's Hospital of Philadelphia
Philadelphia, Pennsylvania

Jennifer Robbins, MD, MPH, FAAP
Attending Physician, Healthy Weight
  Program
Children's Hospital of Philadelphia
Assistant Professor of Clinical Pediatrics
Perelman School of Medicine, University of
  Pennsylvania
Philadelphia, Pennsylvania

Anna K. Weiss, MD, MSEd
Attending Physician; Associate Director for
    Medical Education, Pediatric Emergency
    Medicine
Children's Hospital of Philadelphia
Assistant Professor of Clinical Pediatrics,
    Pediatrics
Perelman School of Medicine, University of
    Pennsylvania
Philadelphia, Pennsylvania

Pamela F. Weiss, MD, MSCE
Attending Physician, Rheumatology; Clinical
    Research Director
Children's Hospital of Philadelphia
Associate Professor of Pediatrics and
    Epidemiology
Perelman School of Medicine, University of
    Pennsylvania
Philadelphia, Pennsylvania

Char Witmer, MD, MSCE
Attending Physician; Assistant Director,
    Hemostasis and Thrombosis Center
Children's Hospital of Philadelphia
Clinical Associate Professor of Pediatrics
Perelman School of Medicine, University of
    Pennsylvania
Philadelphia, Pennsylvania

Lisa Wray, MD
Attending Physician, Cancer Center, Cancer
    Immunotherapy Program
Fellowship Director, Cancer
    Immunotherapy
Assistant Professor of Pediatrics
Perelman School of Medicine, University of
    Pennsylvania
Philadelphia, Pennsylvania

Contributing Authors

Amanda M. Ackermann, MD, PhD
Attending Physician, Pediatric
    Endocrinology and Diabetes
Associate Program Director, Pediatric
    Endocrinology Fellowship Program
Children's Hospital of Philadelphia
Assistant Professor of Pediatrics
Perelman School of Medicine, University of
    Pennsylvania
Philadelphia, Pennsylvania

Olufunke Afolabi-Brown, MBBS
Attending Physician, Pediatric Pulmonology
Children's Hospital of Philadelphia
Philadelphia, Pennsylvania

Atu Agawu, MD, MPH
Fellow, Gastroenterology, Hepatology, and
    Nutrition
Children's Hospital of Philadelphia
Philadelphia, Pennsylvania

Rebecca C. Ahrens-Nicklas, MD, PhD
Attending Physician, Genetics
Children's Hospital of Philadelphia
Assistant Professor, Human Genetics
Perelman School of Medicine, University of
    Pennsylvania
Philadelphia, Pennsylvania

Stamatia Alexiou, MD
Attending Physician, Pulmonary Medicine
Children's Hospital of Philadelphia
Assistant Professor of Clinical Pediatrics
Perelman School of Medicine, University of
    Pennsylvania
Philadelphia, Pennsylvania

Hana Alharbi, MD
Fellow, Biochemical Genetics
Children's Hospital of Philadelphia
Philadelphia, Pennsylvania

Jason B. Anari, MD
Pediatric Orthopaedic Surgeon,
    Orthopaedics
Children's Hospital of Philadelphia
Assistant Professor of Orthopedic Surgery
Perelman School of Medicine, University of
    Pennsylvania
Philadelphia, Pennsylvania

Marissa Anto, MD
Fellow, Pediatric Headache Medicine
Children's Hospital of Philadelphia
Philadelphia, Pennsylvania

Arvind Balaji, MD
Fellow, Primary Care Sports Medicine
Children's Hospital of Philadelphia
Philadelphia, Pennsylvania

H. Jorge Baluarte, MD
Emeritus Professor of Pediatrics,
    Nephrology
Children's Hospital of Philadelphia
Perelman School of Medicine, University of
    Pennsylvania
Philadelphia, Pennsylvania

Ulf H. Beier, MD
Attending Physician, Pediatric Nephrology
Children's Hospital of Philadelphia
Adjunct Associate Professor of Medicine
Perelman School of Medicine, University of
    Pennsylvania
Philadelphia, Pennsylvania

Holly Benz, MD
Attending Physician, Pediatrics
Children's Hospital of Philadelphia
Philadelphia, Pennsylvania

Lauren A. Beslow, MD, MSCE
Attending Physician, Pediatric Neurology
Children's Hospital of Philadelphia
Assistant Professor of Neurology and
    Pediatrics
Perelman School of Medicine, University of
    Pennsylvania
Philadelphia, Pennsylvania

Allison M. Blatz, MD
Fellow, Pediatric Infectious Diseases
Children's Hospital of Pennsylvania
Philadelphia, Pennsylvania

Aaron L. Bodansky, MD
Fellow, Critical Care Medicine–Pediatrics
University of California, San Francisco
San Francisco, California

Rahael Borchers, BA
Medical Student
Perelman School of Medicine, University of
    Pennsylvania
Philadelphia, Pennsylvania

Zoe M. Bouchelle, MD
Resident, Pediatrics
Children's Hospital of Philadelphia
Philadelphia, Pennsylvania

Aaron Briggs, MD
Resident, Pediatrics
Children's Hospital of Philadelphia
Philadelphia, Pennsylvania

Stephanie N. Brosius, MD, PhD
Fellow, Neuro-oncology
Children's Hospital of Philadelphia
Philadelphia, Pennsylvania

Terri Brown-Whitehorn, MD
Attending Physician, Allergy and
    Immunology
Children's Hospital of Philadelphia
Professor of Clinical Pediatrics, Allergy, and
    Immunology
Perelman School of Medicine, University of
    Pennsylvania
Philadelphia, Pennsylvania

Jefferson N. Brownell, MD
Attending Physician, Gastroenterology,
    Hepatology, and Nutrition
Children's Hospital of Philadelphia
Philadelphia, Pennsylvania

Rushelle Byfield, MD
Fellow, Pediatric Nephrology
Children's Hospital of Philadelphia
Philadelphia, Pennsylvania

Katharine Press Callahan, MD
Fellow, Neonatal-Perinatal Medicine
Children's Hospital of Philadelphia
Philadelphia, Pennsylvania

Sarah E. Capponi, MD
Resident, Pediatrics
Children's Hospital of Philadelphia
Philadelphia, Pennsylvania

Bryn Carroll, MD
Attending Physician, Pediatrics
Children's Hospital of Philadelphia
Clinical Assistant Professor of Pediatrics
Perelman School of Medicine, University of
    Pennsylvania
Philadelphia, Pennsylvania

Robin Chin, MD, MPP
Resident, Pediatrics
Children's Hospital of Philadelphia
Philadelphia, Pennsylvania

Winona D. Chua, MD
Attending Physician, Pediatrics
Children's Hospital of Philadelphia
Clinical Associate Professor of Pediatrics
Perelman School of Medicine, University of
    Pennsylvania
Philadelphia, Pennsylvania

Brian W. Coburn, MD, PhD
Resident, Internal Medicine–Pediatrics
Children's Hospital of Philadelphia
Hospital of the University of Pennsylvania
Philadelphia, Pennsylvania

R. Thomas Collins II, MD
Associate Professor of Pediatrics and
    Internal Medicine
Stanford University School of Medicine
Palo Alto, California

Morgan Congdon, MD, MPH
Attending Physician, Pediatrics
Children's Hospital of Philadelphia
Clinical Assistant Professor of Pediatrics
Perelman School of Medicine, University of
    Pennsylvania
Philadelphia, Pennsylvania

Hannah Connor, BA
Medical Student
Perelman School of Medicine, University of
    Pennsylvania
Philadelphia, Pennsylvania

Anna Costello, MD
Attending Physician, Pediatrics
Children's Hospital of Philadelphia
Clinical Assistant Professor of Pediatrics
Perelman School of Medicine, University of
    Pennsylvania
Philadelphia, Pennsylvania

Olivera Marsenic Couloures, MD
Physician, Pediatric Nephrology
Lucile Packard Children's Hospital
Palo Alto, California
Clinical Associate Professor of
    Pediatrics–Nephrology
Stanford University
Stanford, California

Megan Craddock, MD
Assistant Professor of Pediatric Dermatology
Texas Children's Hospital
Baylor College of Medicine
Houston, Texas

Evan Dalton, MD
Fellow, Pediatric Hospital Medicine
Children's Hospital of Philadelphia
Philadelphia, Pennsylvania

Bernard J. Danna, MD
Resident, Pediatrics
Baylor College of Medicine
Houston, Texas

Rahul Datta, MD, PhD
Attending Physician, Allergy and Immunology
Children's Hospital of Philadelphia
Assistant Professor of Clinical Pediatrics
Perelman School of Medicine, University of
    Pennsylvania
Philadelphia, Pennsylvania

Shelby Davies, MD
Fellow, Adolescent Medicine
Children's Hospital of Philadelphia
Philadelphia, Pennsylvania

Chiara Pandolfi de Rinaldis, BS
Medical Student
Perelman School of Medicine, University of
    Pennsylvania
Philadelphia, Pennsylvania

Andres Deik, MD, MSEd
Associate Professor of Clinical Neurology
Parkinson's Disease and Movement
    Disorders Center
University of Pennsylvania
Philadelphia, Pennsylvania

Kristine A. DellaBadia, MD, FAAP
Hospitalist, Pediatrics
Children's Hospital of Philadelphia
Clinical Assistant Professor of Pediatrics
Perelman School of Medicine, University of
    Pennsylvania
Philadelphia, Pennsylvania

Michelle Denburg, MD, MSCE
Attending Physician, Pediatric Nephrology
Children's Hospital of Philadelphia
Assistant Professor of Pediatrics
Perelman School of Medicine, University of
    Pennsylvania
Philadelphia, Pennsylvania

Kavita A. Desai, MD
Attending Physician, Neuro-oncology
    Pediatrics
Children's Hospital of Philadelphia
Assistant Professor of Oncology
Perelman School of Medicine, University
    of Pennsylvania
Philadelphia, Pennsylvania

Sandra Vazquez Diaz, MD
Fellow, Pediatric Endocrinology
Children's Hospital of Philadelphia
Philadelphia, Pennsylvania

Marissa DiGiovine, MD
Attending Physician, Pediatric Neurology
Children's Hospital of Philadelphia
Assistant Professor of Clinical Neurology
Perelman School of Medicine, University of
    Pennsylvania
Philadelphia, Pennsylvania

Caroline Diorio, MD
Fellow, Pediatric Hematology/Oncology
Children's Hospital of Philadelphia
Philadelphia, Pennsylvania

Leah Downey, MD
Resident, Pediatrics
Children's Hospital of Philadelphia
Philadelphia, Pennsylvania

Emily Echevarria, MD
Physician, Neonatology
NewYork-Presbyterian Komansky
    Children's Hospital
Assistant Professor of Clinical Pediatrics
Weill Cornell Medicine
New York, New York

Joshua D. Eisenberg, MD
Fellow, Gastroenterology, Hepatology, and
    Nutrition
Children's Hospital of Philadelphia
Philadelphia, Pennsylvania

Victoria C. Fairchild, MD
Emergency Department Pediatrician,
  Emergency Medicine
Children's Hospital of Philadelphia
Philadelphia, Pennsylvania

Yasaman Fatemi, MD
Fellow, Pediatric Infectious Diseases
Children's Hospital of Philadelphia
Philadelphia, Pennsylvania

Kristen Feemster, MD, MPH, MSHP
Director of Research, Vaccine Education
  Center
Children's Hospital of Philadelphia
Adjunct Associate Professor of Pediatrics
Perelman School of Medicine, University of
  Pennsylvania
Philadelphia, Pennsylvania

Julie L. Fierro, MD, MPH
Attending Physician, Pediatric Pulmonology
  and Sleep Medicine
Children's Hospital of Philadelphia
Assistant Professor of Clinical Pediatrics
Perelman School of Medicine, University of
  Pennsylvania
Philadelphia, Pennsylvania

David M. Finkelstein, MD, MS
Fellow, Pediatric Cardiology
Children's Hospital of Philadelphia
Philadelphia, Pennsylvania

Whitney Fitts, MD
Resident, Pediatric Neurology
Children's Hospital of Philadelphia
Philadelphia, Pennsylvania

Dustin D. Flannery, DO, MSCE
Attending Physician, Neonatology
Children's Hospital of Philadelphia
Assistant Professor of Pediatrics
Perelman School of Medicine, University of
  Pennsylvania
Philadelphia, Pennsylvania

Hannah R. Ford, MD
Resident, Pediatrics
Children's Hospital of Philadelphia
Philadelphia, Pennsylvania

Steven Fusillo, MD
Attending Physician, Gastroenterology,
  Hepatology, and Nutrition
Children's Hospital of Philadelphia
Assistant Professor of Clinical Pediatrics
Perelman School of Medicine, University of
  Pennsylvania
Philadelphia, Pennsylvania

Laurel Gabler, MD, MSc, DPhil
Resident, Pediatrics
Children's Hospital of Philadelphia
Philadelphia, Pennsylvania

Stanislaw J. Gabryszewski, MD, PhD
Fellow, Allergy and Immunology
Children's Hospital of Philadelphia
Philadelphia, Pennsylvania

Christopher E. Gaw, MD, MBE
Fellow, Pediatric Emergency Medicine
Children's Hospital of Philadelphia
Philadelphia, Pennsylvania

Jenna M. Gedminas, MD
Attending Physician, Pediatric Oncology
Children's Hospital of Philadelphia
Instructor, Pediatrics
Perelman School of Medicine, University of
  Pennsylvania
Philadelphia, Pennsylvania

Alisha George, MD
Fellow, Pediatric Pulmonology
University of Pennsylvania
Philadelphia, Pennsylvania

Laura Gober, MD
Attending Physician, Allergy and Immunology
Children's Hospital of Philadelphia
Philadelphia, Pennsylvania

Selasie Q. Goka, MD
Fellow, Pediatric Nephrology
Children's Hospital of Philadelphia
Philadelphia, Pennsylvania

Jessica I. Gold, MD, PhD
Fellow, Genetics
Children's Hospital of Philadelphia
Philadelphia, Pennsylvania

Laura B. Goldstein, MD
Fellow, Pediatric Hospital Medicine
Children's Hospital of Philadelphia
Philadelphia, Pennsylvania

Shubhi G. Goli, MD
Pediatrician, Emergency Medicine
Children's Hospital of Philadelphia
Philadelphia, Pennsylvania

Stephanie Green, MD
Fellow, Pediatric Endocrinology
Children's Hospital of Philadelphia
Philadelphia, Pennsylvania

Morgan E. Greenfield, MD
Attending Physician, Pediatrics
Children's Hospital of Philadelphia
Clinical Assistant Professor of Pediatrics
Perelman School of Medicine, University of
  Pennsylvania
Philadelphia, Pennsylvania

Jeremy M. Grenier, MD, PhD
Resident, Pediatrics
Children's Hospital of Philadelphia
Philadelphia, Pennsylvania

Adda Grimberg, MD
Attending Physician, Pediatric
  Endocrinology and Diabetes
Scientific Director of Diagnostic and
  Research Growth Center
Children's Hospital of Philadelphia
Professor of Pediatrics
Perelman School of Medicine, University of
  Pennsylvania
Philadelphia, Pennsylvania

Logan Grimes, MD
Resident, Pediatrics
Children's Hospital of Philadelphia
Philadelphia, Pennsylvania

Annie Laurie Gula, MD
Resident, Pediatrics
Children's Hospital of Philadelphia
Philadelphia, Pennsylvania

Rose Guo, DO
Fellow, Genetics
Children's Hospital of Philadelphia
Philadelphia, Pennsylvania

Herodes Guzman, MD, MPH
Fellow, Genetics, Metabolism, and Pediatric
  Endocrinology
Children's Hospital of Philadelphia
Philadelphia, Pennsylvania

Sara A. Hasan, MD
Attending Physician, Pediatrics
Children's Hospital of Philadelphia
Clinical Assistant Professor of Pediatrics
Perelman School of Medicine, University of
  Pennsylvania
Philadelphia, Pennsylvania

Sonia A. Havele, MD
Resident, Pediatrics
Children's Hospital of Philadelphia
Philadelphia, Pennsylvania

Daniel J. Herchline, MD
Fellow, Pediatric Hospital Medicine
Children's Hospital of Philadelphia
Philadelphia, Pennsylvania

Melissa Hewson, MD
Attending Physician, Pediatrics
Children's Hospital of Philadelphia
Philadelphia, Pennsylvania

Morgan Elise Hill, MD
Fellow, Neonatal Perinatal Medicine
Children's Hospital of Philadelphia
Philadelphia, Pennsylvania

Jessica Hills, MD
Hospitalist, Pediatrics
Children's Hospital of Philadelphia
Clinical Associate Professor of Pediatrics
Perelman School of Medicine, University of
    Pennsylvania
Philadelphia, Pennsylvania

Talia A. Hitt, MD, MPH, MSHP
Instructor, Pediatric Endocrinology
Johns Hopkins University
Baltimore, Maryland

Raegan D. Hunt, MD, PhD
Division Chief, Pediatric Dermatology
Texas Children's Hospital, Baylor College of
    Medicine
Houston, Texas

Rebecca N. Ichord, MD
Attending Physician, Pediatric Neurology
Children's Hospital of Philadelphia
Professor of Neurology and Pediatrics
Perelman School of Medicine, University of
    Pennsylvania
Philadelphia, Pennsylvania

Sarah Jaffar, MD
Resident, Pediatrics
Children's Hospital of Philadelphia
Philadelphia, Pennsylvania

Sonia Jarrett, MD
Fellow, Pediatric Emergency Medicine
Boston Children's Hospital
Boston, Massachusetts

Lillian Jin, MD, MPH
Resident, Pediatrics
Children's Hospital of Philadelphia
Philadelphia, Pennsylvania

Torsten A. Joerger, MD, MSCE
Fellow, Pediatric Infectious Diseases
Children's Hospital of Philadelphia
Philadelphia, Pennsylvania

Sandy Johng, MD
Fellow, Neonatal-Perinatal Medicine
Children's Hospital of Philadelphia
Philadelphia, Pennsylvania

Jeremy Jones, BA
Medical Student
Perelman School of Medicine, University of
    Pennsylvania
Philadelphia, Pennsylvania

Priyanka Joshi, MD
Resident, Pediatrics
Children's Hospital of Philadelphia
Philadelphia, Pennsylvania

Meena R. Julapalli, MD
Board-Certified Pediatric Dermatologist
Bluebird Dermatology
Spring, Texas

Soma C. Jyonouchi, MD
Attending Physician, Allergy and
    Immunology
Children's Hospital of Philadelphia
Associate Professor of Clinical Pediatrics
Perelman School of Medicine, University of
    Pennsylvania
Philadelphia, Pennsylvania

Eden Kahle, MD
Hospitalist, Pediatrics
Children's Hospital of Philadelphia
Philadelphia, Pennsylvania

Jennifer M. Kalish, MD, PhD
Attending Physician, Genetics
Children's Hospital of Philadelphia
Assistant Professor of Pediatrics and
    Genetics
Perelman School of Medicine, University of
    Pennsylvania
Philadelphia, Pennsylvania

Staci Kallish, DO
Associate Professor of Clinical Medicine
Department of Medicine, Division of
    Translational Medicine and Human
    Genetics
Department of Pediatrics, Division of
    Human Genetics
Perelman School of Medicine, University of
    Pennsylvania
Philadelphia, Pennsylvania

Camilia Kamoun, MD
Fellow, Pediatric Endocrinology and Diabetes
Children's Hospital of Philadelphia
Philadelphia, Pennsylvania

Alexis R. Karlin, MD
Fellow, Pediatric Neurology
Children's Hospital of Philadelphia
Philadelphia, Pennsylvania

Padmavathi V. Karri, BSW
Medical Student
McGovern Medical School
The University of Texas
Houston, Texas

Arthur J. Kastl Jr, MD
Attending Physician, Gastroenterology,
    Hepatology, and Nutrition
Children's Hospital of Philadelphia
Assistant Professor of Pediatrics
Perelman School of Medicine, University of
    Pennsylvania
Philadelphia, Pennsylvania

Katie Kennedy, MD
Attending Physician, Allergy and
    Immunology
Children's Hospital of Philadelphia
Philadelphia, Pennsylvania

Andrew S. Kern-Goldberger, MD
Fellow, Pediatric Hospital Medicine
Children's Hospital of Philadelphia
Philadelphia, Pennsylvania

Sudha Kilaru Kessler, MD, MSCE
Attending Physician, Neurology
Children's Hospital of Philadelphia
Assistant Professor of Neurology and
    Pediatrics
Perelman School of Medicine, University of
    Pennsylvania
Philadelphia, Pennsylvania

Bridget D. Kiernan, MD
Physician, Pediatric Gastroenterology
Hassenfeld Children's Hospital at NYU
    Langone Medical Center
New York University
New York, New York

Marissa J. Kilberg, MD, MSEd
Attending Physician, Endocrinology
Children's Hospital of Philadelphia
Philadelphia, Pennsylvania

Sara B. Kinsman, MD, PhD
Pediatrician and Adolescent Health
    Specialist
Philadelphia, Pennsylvania

Steven D. Klein, MD, PhD
Resident, Pediatrics and Genetics
Children's Hospital of Philadelphia
Philadelphia, Pennsylvania

Chelsea Kotch, MD, MSCE
Attending Physician, Oncology
Children's Hospital of Philadelphia
Philadelphia, Pennsylvania

Matthew R. Landrum, MD
Pediatric Orthopaedic Surgeon,
    Orthopaedics
The University of Texas Health Sciences
    Center at San Antonio
San Antonio, Texas

Ajibike Lapite, MD, MPHTM
Resident, Pediatrics
Children's Hospital of Philadelphia
Philadelphia, Pennsylvania

Benjamin L. Laskin, MD
Attending Physician, Nephrology, The
    Kidney Transplant and Dialysis Program
Children's Hospital of Philadelphia
Assistant Professor of Nephrology
Perelman School of Medicine, University of
    Pennsylvania
Philadelphia, Pennsylvania

Ilana S. Lavina, MD
Resident, Pediatrics
Children's Hospital of Philadelphia
Philadelphia, Pennsylvania

Katherine M. Laycock, MD
Fellow, Pediatric Infectious Diseases
Children's Hospital of Philadelphia
Philadelphia, Pennsylvania

Clement Lee, MD, MSc
Resident, Pediatrics
Children's Hospital of Philadelphia
Philadelphia, Pennsylvania

Grace L. Lee, MD
Pediatric Dermatologist
Texas Children's Hospital
Assistant Professor of Dermatology
Baylor College of Medicine
Houston, Texas

Kyle Lenz, MD
Resident, Pediatrics
Children's Hospital of Philadelphia
Philadelphia, Pennsylvania

Leora Lieberman, MD
Resident, Pediatrics
Children's Hospital of Philadelphia
Philadelphia, Pennsylvania

Jenny H. Lin, MD
Attending Physician, Pediatric Pulmonology
Children's Hospital of Philadelphia
Philadelphia, Pennsylvania

Alexandra R. Linn, MD
Resident, Pediatrics
Children's Hospital of Philadelphia
Philadelphia, Pennsylvania

Morgann Loaec, MD
Resident, Pediatric Critical Care Medicine
Children's Hospital of Philadelphia
Philadelphia, Pennsylvania

Katherine Lord, MD
Attending Physician, Endocrinology
Children's Hospital of Philadelphia
Assistant Professor of Pediatrics
Perelman School of Medicine, University of
    Pennsylvania
Philadelphia, Pennsylvania

Elizabeth D. Lowenthal, MD, MSCE
Attending Physician, Special Immunology
    Service
Research Director, CHOP Global Health
Children's Hospital of Philadelphia
Associate Professor of Pediatrics and
    Epidemiology
Perelman School of Medicine, University of
    Pennsylvania
Director of Developmental Core, Penn
    Center for AIDS Research
Philadelphia, Pennsylvania

Kristin D. Maletsky, MD
Fellow, Pediatric Hospital Medicine
Children's Hospital of Philadelphia
Philadelphia, Pennsylvania

Edna E. Mancilla, MD
Attending Physician, Endocrinology and
    Diabetes
Children's Hospital of Philadelphia
Assistant Professor of Pediatrics
Perelman School of Medicine, University of
    Pennsylvania
Philadelphia, Pennsylvania

Adam S. Mayer, MD
Resident, Internal Medicine–Pediatrics
Children's Hospital of Philadelphia
Hospital of the University of Pennsylvania
Philadelphia, Pennsylvania

Carolyn M. McGann, MD
Fellow, Neonatal-Perinatal Medicine
Children's Hospital of Philadelphia
Philadelphia, Pennsylvania

Laura M. McGarry, MD, PhD
Resident, Pediatric Neurology
Children's Hospital of Philadelphia
Philadelphia, Pennsylvania

Julianne McGlynn, MD
Resident, Pediatrics
Children's Hospital of Philadelphia
Philadelphia, Pennsylvania

Jennifer L. McGuire, MD, MSCE
Attending Physician, Neurology
Children's Hospital of Philadelphia
Assistant Professor of Neurology and
    Pediatrics
Perelman School of Medicine, University of
    Pennsylvania
Philadelphia, Pennsylvania

Jillian L. McKee, MD, PhD
Fellow, Epilepsy Neurogenetics
Children's Hospital of Philadelphia
Philadelphia, Pennsylvania

Kristin McKenna, MD, MPH
Attending Physician, Neonatology
Children's Hospital of Philadelphia
Assistant Professor of Clinical Pediatrics
Perelman School of Medicine, University of
    Pennsylvania
Philadelphia, Pennsylvania

Margaret Means, MD
Resident, Pediatric Neurology
Children's Hospital of Philadelphia
Philadelphia, Pennsylvania

Jamie E. Mehringer, MD
Fellow, Adolescent Medicine
Children's Hospital of Philadelphia
Philadelphia, Pennsylvania

Meghan K. Metcalf, MD
Fellow, Pediatric Cardiology
Children's Hospital of Philadelphia
Philadelphia, Pennsylvania

Aaron L. Misakian, MD, MFA
Resident, Pediatrics
Children's Hospital of Philadelphia
Philadelphia, Pennsylvania

Hannah K. Mitchell, BMBS, MSc, DTMH
Resident, Pediatrics
Children's Hospital of Philadelphia
Philadelphia, Pennsylvania

Papa Kwadwo Morgan-Asiedu, BS
Medical Student
Perelman School of Medicine, University of
    Pennsylvania
Philadelphia, Pennsylvania

Amanda B. Muir, MD, MTR
Attending Physician, Gastroenterology,
  Hepatology, and Nutrition
Children's Hospital of Philadelphia
Assistant Professor of Pediatrics
Perelman School of Medicine, University of
  Pennsylvania
Philadelphia, Pennsylvania

Deanna Nardella, MD
Resident, Pediatrics
Children's Hospital of Philadelphia
Philadelphia, Pennsylvania

Sona Narula, MD
Attending Physician, Pediatric Neurology
Children's Hospital of Philadelphia
Assistant Professor of Clinical Neurology
Perelman School of Medicine, University of
  Pennsylvania
Philadelphia, Pennsylvania

Dustin Nash, MD
Fellow, Pediatric Cardiology
Children's Hospital of Philadelphia
Philadelphia, Pennsylvania

Brittney Newby, MD, PhD
Resident, Pediatrics
Children's Hospital of Philadelphia
Philadelphia, Pennsylvania

Haley Newman, MD
Fellow, Pediatric Hematology/Oncology
Children's Hospital of Philadelphia
Philadelphia, Pennsylvania

Alexander Nguyen, BA
Department of Dermatology
Baylor College of Medicine
Houston, Texas

Michael L. O'Byrne, MD, MSCE
Attending Physician, Interventional
  Cardiology
Associate Director, Cardiac Center Clinical
  Research Core
Children's Hospital of Philadelphia
Assistant Professor of Pediatrics
Perelman School of Medicine, University of
  Pennsylvania
Philadelphia, Pennsylvania

William R. Otto, MD
Fellow, Pediatric Infectious Diseases
Children's Hospital of Philadelphia
Philadelphia, Pennsylvania

Melissa Patel, MD, MPH
Section Chief, Pediatric Hospital Medicine
Children's Hospital of Philadelphia
Associate Professor of Clinical Pediatrics
Perelman School of Medicine, University of
  Pennsylvania
Philadelphia, Pennsylvania

Trusha Patel, MD
Attending Physician, Gastroenterology,
  Hepatology, and Nutrition
Children's Hospital of Philadelphia
Assistant Professor of Pediatrics
Perelman School of Medicine, University of
  Pennsylvania
Philadelphia, Pennsylvania

Michelle-Marie Peña, MD
Fellow, Neonatal-Perinatal Medicine
Children's Hospital of Philadelphia
Philadelphia, Pennsylvania

Jessica Perfetto, MD
Resident, Pediatrics
Children's Hospital of Philadelphia
Philadelphia, Pennsylvania

Sara E. Pinney, MD, MS
Attending Physician, Endocrinology
Children's Hospital of Philadelphia
Assistant Professor of Pediatrics
Perelman School of Medicine, University of
  Pennsylvania
Philadelphia, Pennsylvania

Giulia S. Porcari, MD
Resident, Pediatric Neurology
Children's Hospital of Philadelphia
Philadelphia, Pennsylvania

Gayathri Prabhakar, MD
Resident, Pediatrics
Children's Hospital of Philadelphia
Philadelphia, Pennsylvania

Madhura Pradhan, MD
Attending Physician, Nephrology
Children's Hospital of Philadelphia
Professor of Clinical Pediatrics
Perelman School of Medicine, University of
  Pennsylvania
Philadelphia, Pennsylvania

Eric Pridgen, MD, PhD
Resident, Orthopedic Surgery
University of Pennsylvania
Philadelphia, Pennsylvania

Jessica R.C. Priestley, MD, PhD
Resident, Pediatrics and Genetics
Children's Hospital of Philadelphia
Philadelphia, Pennsylvania

Edward D. Re, MD
Attending Physician, Pediatric and
  Adolescent Sports Medicine
Children's Hospital of Philadelphia
Philadelphia, Pennsylvania

Whitney Reid, MD
Resident, Allergy and Immunology
Children's Hospital of Philadelphia
Philadelphia, Pennsylvania

Michaela B. Reinhart, MD
Resident, Pediatrics and Genetics
Children's Hospital of Philadelphia
Philadelphia, Pennsylvania

Kathryn Restaino, MD
Fellow, Pediatric Cardiology
Children's Hospital of Philadelphia
Philadelphia, Pennsylvania

Jennifer Robbins, MD, MPH, FAAP
Attending Physician, Healthy Weight
  Program
Children's Hospital of Philadelphia
Assistant Professor of Clinical Pediatrics
Perelman School of Medicine, University of
  Pennsylvania
Philadelphia, Pennsylvania

Ayelet Rosen, MD
Attending Physician, Pediatric Hospitalist
Children's Hospital of Philadelphia
Clinical Assistant Professor of Pediatrics
Perelman School of Medicine, University of
  Pennsylvania
Philadelphia, Pennsylvania

Elizabeth Rosenfeld, MD, MSCE
Fellow, Pediatric Endocrinology and
  Diabetes
Children's Hospital of Philadelphia
Philadelphia, Pennsylvania

Yoshi M. Rothman, MD
Resident, Pediatrics
Children's Hospital of Philadelphia
Philadelphia, Pennsylvania

David M. Rub, MD
Resident, Pediatrics
Children's Hospital of Philadelphia
Philadelphia, Pennsylvania

Kathryn M. Rubey, MD
Fellow, Neonatal-Perinatal Medicine
Children's Hospital of Philadelphia
Philadelphia, Pennsylvania

Jennifer Ruth, MD
Assistant Professor of Pediatric Dermatology
Dell Children's Medical Center
Dell Medical School, The University of Texas
    at Austin
Austin, Texas

Eloise C. Salmon, MD
Physician, Pediatric Nephrology
C.S. Mott Children's Hospital
Clinical Assistant Professor of Pediatric
    Nephrology
University of Michigan Health
Ann Arbor, Michigan

Yesenia Sanchez-Kleinberg, MD
Resident, Pediatrics
Children's Hospital of Philadelphia
Philadelphia, Pennsylvania

Katherine E. Schwartz, MD
Fellow, Neonatal-Perinatal Medicine
Children's Hospital of Philadelphia
Philadelphia, Pennsylvania

Rebecca R. Scobell, MD
Fellow, Pediatric Nephrology
Children's Hospital of Philadelphia
Philadelphia, Pennsylvania

Edward C. Shadiack III, DO, MPH
Fellow, Mitochondrial Medicine Frontier
    Program
Children's Hospital of Philadelphia
Philadelphia, Pennsylvania

Amish Shah, MD, PhD
Attending Physician, Neuro-oncology
    Pediatrics
Director, Neuro-oncology Fellowship
    Program
Children's Hospital of Philadelphia
Assistant Professor of Oncology
Perelman School of Medicine, University of
    Pennsylvania
Philadelphia, Pennsylvania

Amit A. Shah, MD, MSHP
Attending Physician, Gastroenterology,
    Hepatology, and Nutrition
Children's Hospital of Philadelphia
Philadelphia, Pennsylvania

Rachana Shah, MD
Attending Physician, Endocrinology and
    Diabetes
Children's Hospital of Philadelphia
Assistant Professor of Pediatrics
Perelman School of Medicine, University of
    Pennsylvania
Philadelphia, Pennsylvania

Mohammed A. Shaik, MD, PhD
Resident, Pediatrics
Children's Hospital of Philadelphia
Philadelphia, Pennsylvania

Michelle Shankar, MD
Resident, Pediatrics
Children's Hospital of Philadelphia
Philadelphia, Pennsylvania

Akhila V. Shapiro, MD, FAAP
Attending Physician, Pediatrics
Children's Hospital of Philadelphia
Philadelphia, Pennsylvania

Sarah E. Sheppard, MD, PhD
Attending Physician, Genetics
Children's Hospital of Philadelphia
Philadelphia, Pennsylvania

Maya R. Silver, MD
Resident, Pediatric Neurology
Children's Hospital of Philadelphia
Philadelphia, Pennsylvania

Timothy T. Spear, MD, PhD
Resident, Pediatric Oncology
Children's Hospital of Philadelphia
Philadelphia, Pennsylvania

Joshua H. Sperling, MD
Attending Physician, Pediatrics
Children's Hospital of Philadelphia
Philadelphia, Pennsylvania

Donna J. Stephenson, MD
Attending Physician, Pediatric Neurology
Medical Director of Operations and
    Outreach
Children's Hospital of Philadelphia
Associate Professor of Clinical Neurology
    and Pediatrics
Perelman School of Medicine, University of
    Pennsylvania
Philadelphia, Pennsylvania

Amy Strong, MD
Fellow, Pediatric Nephrology
Children's Hospital of Philadelphia
Philadelphia, Pennsylvania

Jennifer K. Sun, MD, PhD
Resident, Internal Medicine–Pediatrics
Children's Hospital of Philadelphia
Hospital of the University of Pennsylvania
Philadelphia, Pennsylvania

Rebecca M. Sutherland, MD
Attending Physician, Pediatrics
Children's Hospital of Philadelphia
Philadelphia, Pennsylvania

Sanjeev K. Swami, MD
Attending Physician, Pediatric Infectious
    Diseases
Children's Hospital of Philadelphia
Associate Professor of Clinical Pediatrics
Perelman School of Medicine, University of
    Pennsylvania
Philadelphia, Pennsylvania

Katherine M. Szigety, MD, PhD
Resident, Pediatrics and Genetics
Children's Hospital of Philadelphia
Philadelphia, Pennsylvania

Christina Lynch Szperka, MD, MSCE
Attending Physician, Pediatric Neurology
Director, Pediatric Headache Program
Children's Hospital of Philadelphia
Assistant Professor of Neurology and
    Pediatrics
Perelman School of Medicine, University of
    Pennsylvania
Philadelphia, Pennsylvania

Katherine S. Taub, MD
Attending Physician, Pediatric Neurology
Children's Hospital of Philadelphia
Associate Professor of Clinical Neurology
Perelman School of Medicine, University of
    Pennsylvania
Philadelphia, Pennsylvania

Jaclyn Tencer, MD
Fellow, Pediatric Neurology
Children's Hospital of Philadelphia
Philadelphia, Pennsylvania

Christopher Teng, MD
Resident, Pediatrics
Children's Hospital of Philadelphia
Philadelphia, Pennsylvania

Alyssa R. Thomas, MD
Resident, Pediatrics
Children's Hospital of Philadelphia
Philadelphia, Pennsylvania

Bruce L. Tjaden Jr, MD
Assistant Professor of Vascular and
    Endovascular Surgery
Cooper Medical School of Rowan University
Camden, New Jersey

Naomi E. Butler Tjaden, MD, PhD
Fellow, Gastroenterology, Hepatology, and
    Nutrition
Children's Hospital of Philadelphia
Philadelphia, Pennsylvania

Catherine E. Tomasulo, MD
Fellow, Pediatric Cardiology
Children's Hospital of Pennsylvania
Philadelphia, Pennsylvania

Oana Tomescu, MD, PhD
Associate Professor of Clinical Medicine and
    Pediatrics
Children's Hospital of Philadelphia
Hospital of the University of Pennsylvania
Philadelphia, Pennsylvania

Regina L. Toto, MD
Fellow, Pediatric Emergency Medicine
Children's Hospital of Philadelphia
Philadelphia, Pennsylvania

Linh Thi Tran, MD
Resident, Pediatrics
Children's Hospital of Philadelphia
Philadelphia, Pennsylvania

Michael Triebwasser, MD, PhD
Researcher, Hematology–Pediatrics
Children's Hospital of Philadelphia
Philadelphia, Pennsylvania

Roberto Alejandro Valdovinos, MD
Resident, Pediatrics
Children's Hospital of Philadelphia
Philadelphia, Pennsylvania

Brittany J. Van Remortel, MD, MPH
Resident, Pediatrics
Children's Hospital of Philadelphia
Philadelphia, Pennsylvania

Kanak Verma, MD, MPH
Resident, Pediatrics
Children's Hospital of Philadelphia
Philadelphia, Pennsylvania

Leonela Villegas, MD
Fellow, Pediatric Nephrology
Children's Hospital of Philadelphia
Philadelphia, Pennsylvania

Maria G. Vogiatzi, MD
Medical Director of Adrenal and Puberty
    Center
Children's Hospital of Philadelphia
Associate Professor of Endocrinology and
    Diabetes
Perelman School of Medicine, University of
    Pennsylvania
Philadelphia, Pennsylvania

Ethan S. Vorel, MD
Resident, Pediatrics
Children's Hospital of Philadelphia
Philadelphia, Pennsylvania

Amy T. Waldman, MD, MSCE
Attending Physician, Pediatric Neurology
Children's Hospital of Philadelphia
Assistant Professor of Neurology and
    Pediatrics
Perelman School of Medicine, University of
    Pennsylvania
Philadelphia, Pennsylvania

Evelyn Ruth Wang, MD
Resident, Pediatrics
Children's Hospital of Philadelphia
Philadelphia, Pennsylvania

Jennifer Webster, DO
Attending Physician, Gastroenterology,
    Hepatology, and Nutrition
Children's Hospital of Philadelphia
Assistant Professor of Clinical Pediatrics
Perelman School of Medicine, University of
    Pennsylvania
Philadelphia, Pennsylvania

Pamela F. Weiss, MD, MSCE
Attending Physician, Rheumatology
Clinical Research Director
Children's Hospital of Philadelphia
Associate Professor of Pediatrics and
    Epidemiology
Perelman School of Medicine, University of
    Pennsylvania
Philadelphia, Pennsylvania

Travus White, MD
Fellow, Pediatric Cardiology
Children's Hospital of Philadelphia
Philadelphia, Pennsylvania

Rebecca Whitmire, MD, MPH
Resident, Pediatrics
Children's Hospital of Philadelphia
Philadelphia, Pennsylvania

Deborah Whitney, MD
Attending Physician, Pediatrics
Children's Hospital of Philadelphia
Philadelphia, Pennsylvania

Wai Wong, MD
Attending Physician, Pediatric Pulmonology
Children's Hospital of Philadelphia
Assistant Professor of Clinical Pediatrics
Perelman School of Medicine, University of
    Pennsylvania
Philadelphia, Pennsylvania

Sabrina W. Yum, MD
Attending Physician, Pediatric Neurology
Children's Hospital of Philadelphia
Associate Professor of Clinical Neurology
    and Pediatrics
Perelman School of Medicine, University of
    Pennsylvania
Philadelphia, Pennsylvania

Wenjing Zong, MD
Attending Physician, Gastroenterology,
    Hepatology, and Nutrition
Children's Hospital of Philadelphia
Philadelphia, Pennsylvania

CONTENTS

ONLINE CONTENTS

Visit your ebook (see inside front cover for details) for the following printable patient education brochures from *Ferri's Netter Patient Advisor,* 3rd edition.

Care of the Acutely Ill Child

Anna K. Weiss

1

Assessment of the Acutely Ill Child

Ethan S. Vorel and Morgan E. Greenfield

✳ CLINICAL VIGNETTE

A 5-year-old unvaccinated boy who recently immigrated from Eastern Europe walks into a local primary care clinic with a complaint of "hard breathing." The patient is seen in triage and noted to be wheezing but is otherwise reasonably well-appearing; his vital signs are notable for fever to 102.2°F (39°C) and tachycardia. Thirty minutes after arrival, the pediatrician enters the room to find a profusely drooling child leaning forward with his hands on his knees. The patient's parents introduce themselves, noting the patient's voice is "getting funny." The physician remains calm in front of the patient and parents, discretely asking the nurse outside the doorway to call emergency medical services (EMS). The parents are informed about the presumptive diagnosis of epiglottitis and the need for emergent airway protection. EMS arrives 5 minutes later, and the patient is quickly transported to the regional pediatric intensive care unit for antibiotics and systemic steroids.

Increased care usage by children and their families has led to unprecedented patient volumes in primary care offices and urgent care centers, challenging pediatricians to balance workflow efficiency with meticulous care. In this context, providers must be proficient in confronting a wide range of illness, most often relatively benign but at times life-threatening. It is critical that providers recognize the often-subtle signs of early severe illness, which may necessitate quick intervention and patient transport to a higher level of care.

INITIAL ASSESSMENT

A sick visit begins by obtaining vital signs, which include temperature, heart rate, respiratory rate, oxygen saturation, and blood pressure. Children's vital signs vary significantly by age (Table 1.1). Grossly abnormal vital signs may call for postponement of the history and stabilization of the child, which may include ensuring airway patency, adequate breathing, and intact circulation.

Fever is defined as a core temperature of at least 100.4°F (38°C). Temperature is best recorded by an oral or rectal thermometer in otherwise healthy, nonimmunocompromised children. Although convenient, axillary and tympanic thermometers are less reliable.

Tachycardia is typically the result of the body's need for either increased cardiac output or oxygenation, which can occur during times of fever, exercise, or other physiologic stress. Worrisome causative factors of tachycardia include circulatory compromise from hypovolemia, anemia, significant pain or anxiety, or any other factor leading to metabolic stress. Must-not-miss causes of tachycardia include sepsis, tachyarrhythmias, and hemorrhage. In the office setting, tachycardia often resolves with appropriate antipyretic, analgesic, and oral rehydration therapies; however, persistent tachycardia warrants further investigation. **Bradycardia** is much rarer in the setting of the acutely ill child. Although physiologic asymptomatic bradycardia can be seen in sleeping children or athletes, pathologic bradycardia can be secondary to sepsis, arrythmias, and increased intracranial pressure (ICP), with the latter also being complicated by hypertension and irregular breathing (Cushing's triad).

Tachypnea is one of the most frequent findings among children with respiratory distress. Tachypnea may be caused by fever, hypoxemia, hypercarbia, metabolic acidosis, pain, or anxiety. Common causes include those of the respiratory (e.g., bronchiolitis, asthma, pneumonia) and cardiac systems (e.g., congenital cardiac disease, myocarditis, heart failure). Conditions causing metabolic acidosis result in compensatory tachypnea. A useful adjunct is **oxygen saturation** via pulse oximetry, with normal levels in healthy children typically greater than 95%. The hypoxic child should concern the provider and may warrant escalation of care. Like tachycardia, tachypnea precipitated by fever or pain will often resolve with antipyretic or analgesic therapy; however, persistent tachypnea—like persistent tachycardia—warrants further investigation. Of note, **bradypnea** may also occur in response to hypoxia in younger infants, or from respiratory fatigue, central nervous system (CNS) depression, or increased ICP. **Apnea,** or the cessation of spontaneous breathing, is a medical emergency.

Hypotension is an immediate cause of significant concern because of children's ability to compensate to greater extremes relative to adults. Children are often not hypotensive until approximately 50% of the circulating volume has been compromised, be it through volume loss, third spacing of fluids, vasodilation, or backup into the high-capacitance venous system. Therefore hypotension in a child should alert the provider that there is likely an underlying pathologic condition that requires investigation. **Hypertension** may be primary but also can be secondary to pathologic causes, including vascular and renal disorders, neuroendocrine tumors, and increased ICP.

HISTORY

A history of the presenting illness, including existing medical problems and events leading to the current presentation, provides important clues to the underlying diagnosis. Every history should explore the child's general well-being, specifically the patient's mood, activity level, feeding patterns, and urine output. Significant deviation from the child's baseline may shed light on the severity of the illness and on the possible need for more urgent intervention. For each chief complaint, practitioners should explore onset, duration, frequency, location, quality, severity, aggravating and alleviating factors, associated symptoms, self-treatment, and pertinent negative issues. In all sick visits, the child's medical history should be obtained, including underlying conditions, current medications, and vaccination history. Given the clinical scenario, family history may be relevant. Surgical history is often important in patients who may have undergone more intensive and invasive surgeries or medical device placement. A social history should cover ill contacts, daycare and/or school attendance, and recent travel. In adolescence, additional questions regarding substance use and sexual activity are necessary.

This chapter will cover several of the most common chief complaints of the ill child—that is, fever, respiratory distress, headache,

TABLE 1.1   Normal Vital Signs by Age

Age	Heart Rate (beats/min)	Blood Pressure (mm Hg)	Respiratory Rate (breaths/min)
0–3 months	100–150	55–75/35–45	40–70
3 months–1 year	80–120	70–100/50–65	25–45
1–6 years	65–110	90–110/55–75	20–30
6–12 years	60–95	100–120/60–75	14–22
12+ years	55–85	110–135/65–85	12–18

Adapted from Drayna PC, Gorelick MH. Evaluation of the sick child in the office and clinic. In: Kliegman RM, Stanton BS, St Geme III JW, Schor NF, Behrman RE, eds. *Nelson Textbook of Pediatrics*. Philadelphia: Elsevier; 2016.

BOX 1.1   Differential Diagnosis of Acute Pediatric Fever[a]

Common Viral Infections

Central Nervous System
- **Meningitis**
- **Encephalitis**
- Tumor
- Brain abscess

Head, Ears, Eyes, Nose, and Throat
- *Otitis media*
- *Pharyngitis*
- **Retropharyngeal abscess**
- Peritonsillar abscess
- Stomatitis
- *Influenza*
- Sinusitis
- Parotitis
- Cervical adenitis
- Periorbital cellulitis
- Orbital cellulitis

Respiratory System
- *Bronchiolitis*
- ***Croup***
- **Epiglottitis**
- ***Pneumonia***
- *Upper respiratory infection*

Cardiovascular System
- **Myocarditis**
- **Pericarditis**
- **Endocarditis**

Genitourinary System
- *Urinary tract infection*
- Tuboovarian abscess

Gastrointestinal Tract
- *Acute viral gastroenteritis*
- Bacterial enteritis
- ***Appendicitis***
- **Peritonitis**

Soft Tissue Infections
- *Cellulitis*
- **Necrotizing fasciitis**

Musculoskeletal System
- Osteomyelitis
- Septic arthritis

Rheumatologic Disorders
- **Acute rheumatic fever**
- Juvenile rheumatoid arthritis
- Henoch-Schönlein purpura

Vasculitis
- Behçet syndrome

Malignancy
- **Leukemia**
- **Lymphoma**

Systemic Illness
- *Bacteremia*
- *Viremia*
- ***Sepsis***
- ***Kawasaki disease***
- **Toxic shock syndrome**
- **Rocky Mountain spotted fever**
- **Meningococcemia**
- **Stevens-Johnson syndrome**

Toxicologic
- **Anticholinergic toxidromes**
- **Salicylate overdose**
- **Amphetamine**
- **Cocaine**

Endocrine
- **Thyrotoxicosis**

[a]Common causes are *italicized*; life-threatening causes are in **bold**.
Adapted from Anderson JL, Kiefer CS, Colletti JE. Child with fever. In: Adams JG, Barton ED, Collings J, DeBlieux PM, Gisondi MA, Nadel ES, eds. *Emergency Medicine*. Philadelphia, PA: Saunders; 2013.

abdominal pain, and altered mental status (AMS). The most common, as well as the "can't-miss," causes of these complaints will be discussed, acknowledging this list is not exhaustive.

Fever in infants younger than 56 days of age warrants evaluation in the emergency department (ED) given the elevated risk for a serious bacterial infection (SBI), which includes the growth of a bacterial pathogen in blood, urine, or cerebrospinal fluid. In older children, fever accounts for nearly a quarter of pediatric sick visits. Regardless of age, the most common cause of fever is a transient, self-resolving viral illness.

As noted, infants younger than 2 months of age are particularly vulnerable to infection given an immature immune system and the possibility of maternal-fetal transmission of disease, which may manifest in the form of bacteremia, urinary tract infections, sepsis, meningitis, or pneumonia. In the first month of life, the organisms most often implicated in SBIs are *Escherichia coli*, group B streptococcus (GBS), and *Listeria monocytogenes*. Viruses are also common culprits of serious disease, including herpes simplex virus (HSV). Details of the pregnancy, delivery, and postnatal course will be vital to identifying risk factors for sepsis. An infant suffering from an SBI may present with feeding issues, irritability, lethargy, and a number of infectious symptoms; however, some affected infants may appear well by history and examination.

In older children, the causes of fever are many, ranging from infections to rheumatologic disorders, vasculitides, malignancy, systemic illness, toxic ingestions, and endocrinologic disorders (Box 1.1). Fortunately, the most common causes of fever seen in pediatrics are rarely life-threatening. A history should elicit information regarding the fever itself (height, duration, pattern), antipyretic use, the patient's general well-being (activity levels, irritability, feeding), hydration status, and symptoms related to the ear/nose/throat, respiratory, gastrointestinal, genitourinary, and integumentary systems. Based on the organ system of concern, inquiry about "red flag" signs or symptoms may point toward an ongoing, underlying life-threatening process. A constellation of red flags should prompt the provider to transfer the patient to an ED or, if already there, to immediately proceed with appropriate interventions.

Respiratory distress can either be a manifestation of a primary respiratory problem or a secondary effect resulting from the disruption of another organ system (Fig. 1.1). In general, causes of respiratory distress may be classified as involving (1) the airway; (2) the lungs, chest wall, or both; (3) the CNS respiratory drive; or (4) the neuromuscular system. Alternatively, the respiratory system may be compromised by dysfunction in other organ systems (e.g., cardiovascular) that affect respiratory function or trigger respiratory compensatory mechanisms.

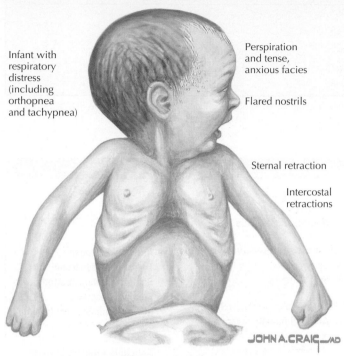

Fig. 1.1 Respiratory Distress in the Infant.

Infant with respiratory distress (including orthopnea and tachypnea)

Perspiration and tense, anxious facies

Flared nostrils

Sternal retraction

Intercostal retractions

The evaluation of a child with acute respiratory distress includes determining the severity and the underlying cause.

The initial approach will depend on whether the child is in respiratory arrest (Fig. 1.2) or in distress (Fig. 1.3), because the former will first necessitate stabilization. On history, the provider should inquire whether the onset of symptoms was acute or gradual. Alleviating factors may be relevant, such as postural change ("sniffing position" in upper airway obstruction) or medication (bronchodilators in asthma). Associated respiratory symptoms may narrow the differential—for example, cold symptoms (viral upper respiratory tract infection), cough and its quality ("barky" in croup), color change (cyanosis in low oxygen saturation states), respiratory effort (poor in neuromuscular disorders), and voice changes. Systemic symptoms such as fever or change in weight may suggest pathologic conditions such as infection or congestive heart failure, respectively. Respiratory distress red flags include decreased level of consciousness, resting or biphasic stridor, muffled voice, tripod positioning, diaphoresis, cyanosis, and significant work of breathing.

Headaches are common in children, affecting nearly half the pediatric population and increasing in prevalence with age. A detailed history is necessary to categorize headaches as primary or secondary (Box 1.2). The provider should inquire about the headache's temporality (time of day, duration, frequency, pattern, chronicity), location and laterality, and associated symptoms such as nausea, vomiting, or aura. The provider should pay close attention to focal neurologic abnormalities, including loss of sensation, numbness, tingling, tremors, weakness, paralysis, syncope, and seizure-like activity. Secondary headaches are typically most concerning, particularly those related to intracranial masses, vascular abnormalities, or infection. Relevant headache red flags

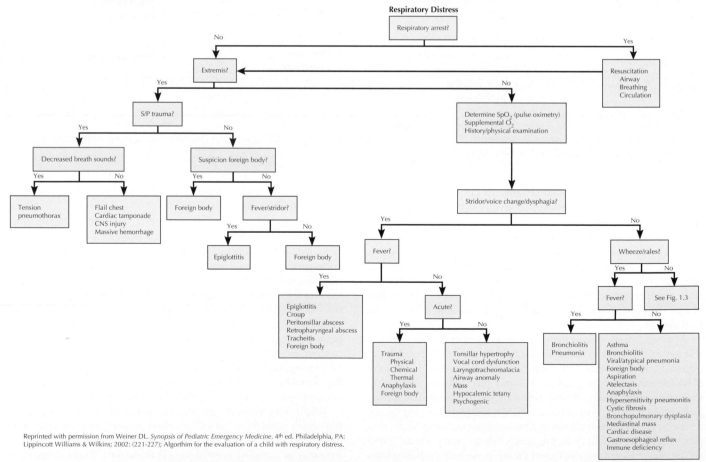

Reprinted with permission from Weiner DL. *Synopsis of Pediatric Emergency Medicine.* 4th ed. Philadelphia, PA: Lippincott Williams & Wilkins; 2002: (221-227); Algorthim for the evaluation of a child with respiratory distress.

Fig. 1.2 Approach to Respiratory Distress (Part I). *CNS,* Central nervous system; *S/P,* status post.

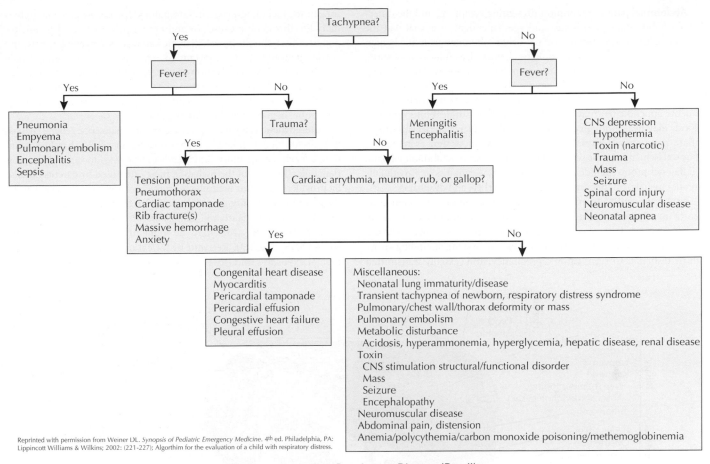

Reprinted with permission from Weiner DL. *Synopsis of Pediatric Emergency Medicine.* 4th ed. Philadelphia, PA: Lippincott Williams & Wilkins; 2002: (221-227); Algorthim for the evaluation of a child with respiratory distress.

Fig. 1.3 Approach to Respiratory Distress (Part II).

BOX 1.2 Common and Life-Threatening Headache Causes[a]

Primary
- *Cluster*
- *Migraine*
- *Tension-type*

Secondary
- *Trauma and concussion-related*
- Vascular
  - **Subarachnoid hemorrhage**
  - **Epidural or subdural hemorrhage**
  - **Intracerebral hemorrhage**
  - **Arteriovenous malformation**
  - **Aneurysm**
  - **Venous thrombosis**
  - **Stroke**
  - **Arterial dissection**
  - **Temporal arteritis**

- Infectious
  - **Meningitis**
  - **Encephalitis**
  - **Abscess or extension of extracranial infection (sinus, dental, ear)**
- Intracranial
  - **Tumor**
  - **Pseudotumor cerebri**
  - Cerebrospinal fluid leak
  - Hydrocephalus
- Other
  - Ophthalmologic (glaucoma, optic neuritis)
  - Pheochromocytoma
  - Hypercapnia, hypoxemia
  - Metabolic (hypoglycemia)
  - Postlumbar puncture
  - *Drug-induced*
  - Hypertension
  - Pregnancy-related

[a]Common causes are *italicized;* life-threatening causes are in **bold.**

may be remembered by the SNOOP mnemonic: **S**ystemic symptoms (fever, weight loss, joint pain, rash), **S**econdary risk factors (hypercoagulability, cancer, human immunodeficiency virus [HIV], various neurocutaneous/genetic/rheumatic disorders), **N**eurologic symptoms (AMS, focal neurologic deficits), **O**nset (sudden, awakening from sleep), **O**lder age of onset (not relevant in pediatrics), **P**revious headache history (first or worst headache, deviation from previous), **P**recipitated by Valsalva maneuvers, **P**ostural aggravation, and **P**apilledema.

Abdominal pain is a common presenting symptom, and the differential of abdominal pain is vast and age-dependent. It is vital that the provider differentiate the surgical or "acute" abdomen from the benign (Fig. 1.4). As always, the pain should be characterized fully as to location, severity, quality, and similarity to any previous episodes (Fig. 1.5). Reg flag symptoms such as bilious emesis (concerning for bowel obstruction) or peritoneal signs (suggestive of intraperitoneal infection, such as acute appendicitis) may indicate the need for surgical interventions. Bloody diarrhea, although commonly the result of a bacterial enteritis or inflammatory bowel disease, may be a more ominous sign, as in the case of bowel ischemia. In the setting of chronic or recurrent abdominal pain, red flag symptoms include unexplained fever, weight loss or growth failure, nocturnal pain, persistent emesis or diarrhea, and dysphagia.

In infants and toddlers, life-threatening diagnoses are often congenital or anatomic, including malrotation, volvulus, intussusception, and strangulated hernia. In adolescence, can't-miss causes expand to include those related to the reproductive system, including ovarian or testicular torsion, ectopic pregnancy, and sexually transmitted infections, including pelvic inflammatory disease. At any age, potentially life-threatening causes of abdominal pain include appendicitis, pancreatitis, ischemic bowel, diabetic ketoacidosis, pyelonephritis, and aortic aneurysm. It is important to remember that abdominal pain may be secondary to activation of visceral pain receptors found in the gastrointestinal tract or somatoparietal receptors of the peritoneum, muscle, and skin. In addition, pain may be secondary to pulmonary, metabolic, hematologic, and other causes.

Altered mental status (AMS) is a term used to describe general changes in brain function, manifested as abnormalities in a child's baseline cognition, behavior, or memory. AMS tends to lend itself to vague descriptors (lethargic, sleepy, "not themselves"), most often used by parents but also by providers. It is thus incumbent on the provider to better characterize the nature and extent of the child's deviation from baseline to communicate clearly with specialists and identify life-threatening diagnoses.

The causes of AMS may be remembered by the mnemonic VITAMINS (Box 1.3). Relevant historical questions include environmental exposures and drugs or medications in the home. It is worth

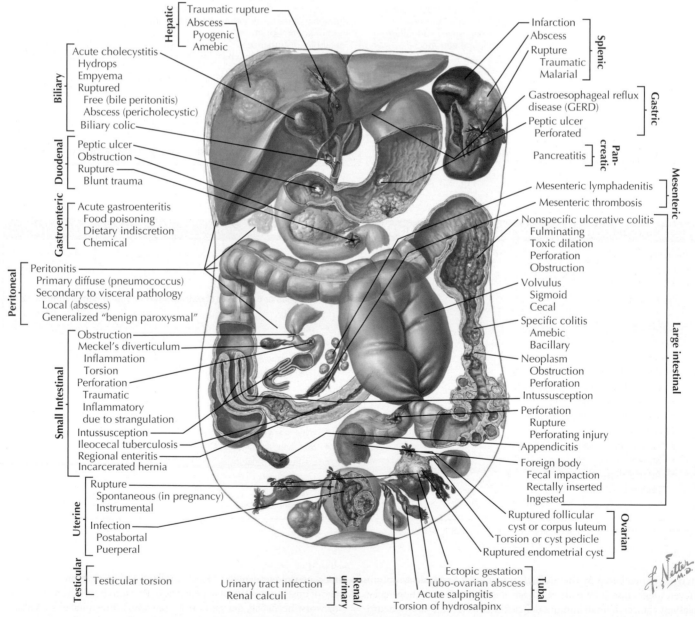

Fig. 1.4 Causes of Acute Abdominal Pain.

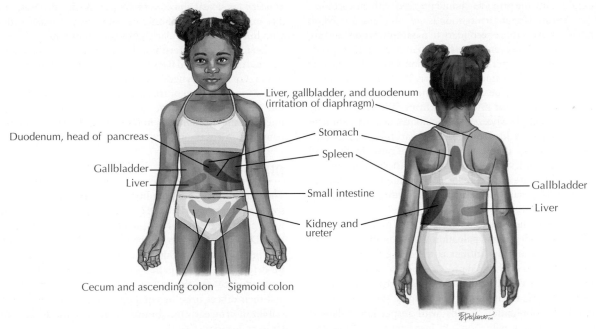

Fig. 1.5 Localization of Abdominal Pain.

Liver, gallbladder, and duodenum (irritation of diaphragm)

Duodenum, head of pancreas

Gallbladder

Liver

Stomach

Spleen

Small intestine

Kidney and ureter

Cecum and ascending colon

Sigmoid colon

Gallbladder

Liver

BOX 1.3 Common Causes of Altered Mental Status

Vascular
- Stroke
- Arteriovenous malformation
- Systemic vasculitis

Infection/**I**nflammatory
- Meningitis
- Encephalitis
- Sepsis

Toxins
- Environmental
- Medications
- Contaminated breast milk

Accidents/**A**buse
- Nonaccidental trauma
- Sequelae of previous trauma

Metabolic
- Hypoglycemia
- Diabetic ketoacidosis
- Thyroid disorders

Intussusception

Neoplasm

Seizure

---

noting here that children, particularly neonates and infants, may present with altered sensorium or abnormal behavior after nonaccidental trauma (NAT).

PHYSICAL EXAMINATION

The goal of the physical examination is to correlate and confirm details from the history, discover new findings, and monitor for clinical evolution over time or in response to interventions to ultimately arrive at a diagnosis.

The examination should begin with the child as exposed as possible. Parents should be encouraged to hold younger children in their lap to increase comfort. Initially, providers should maintain their distance to observe the patient unperturbed. Observation of the patient's interaction with both the environment and caregiver allows the provider to evaluate in part the child's level of energy, alertness, muscle tone, extremity use, exposed skin, and respiratory status.

The provider should proceed to conduct other noninvasive maneuvers, including the initial respiratory examination, observing the respiratory rate, oxygen saturation level, and any evidence of increased work of breathing. The provider may then inspect the patient's skin for lesions or rashes, noting all primary and secondary findings. Red flags on integumentary examination include nonblanching lesions such as petechiae or purpura, exquisite tenderness to palpation out of proportion to visual findings (necrotizing fasciitis), or bruising over nonbony prominences (possible NAT). The skin also may be evaluated for perfusion by assessing capillary refill, extremity warmth, and peripheral pulses. If indicated, the provider may also assess for extremity swelling, bony tenderness, and range of motion and/or swelling of joints. Abnormalities in these aspects of the examination could point toward infectious, vascular, or systemic processes. During the skin examination may be an ideal time to investigate for lymphadenopathy, which tends to be bilateral and shotty if infection-related versus unilateral and pronounced if ominous.

While calm, infants should have their anterior fontanelle assessed; a sunken fontanelle suggests dehydration, whereas a bulging fontanelle may suggest increased ICP and is always a red flag. The eye examination should evaluate pupillary size and reactivity, extraocular movements, and the conjunctiva. Red flags include asymmetric or unreactive pupils that may indicate an intracranial process, as well as pain with or limited extraocular movement (orbital cellulitis). Facial asymmetry and cranial nerve deficits are always red flags.

With the child calm, the provider should proceed with the cardiore-spiratory examination. Upper airway sounds are often auscultated on lung examination, such as those secondary to nasal congestion, and are usually benign. Stridor, however, is a red flag that may herald impending airway compromise. Proper lung auscultation allows the provider to assess for adequate and symmetric air entry. Unilateral, decreased, or absent breath sounds may be caused by pneumothorax or pulmonary fluid accumulations from infection or heart failure. Other lung sounds to listen for include wheezes (bronchiolitis, asthma), rhonchi (pneumonia), and rales/crackles (pneumonia, heart failure). Next, the provider should auscultate the heart, assessing the rate, rhythm, and heart sounds. Pericardial friction rubs, gallops, diastolic murmurs, or loud murmurs (>II/VI) are considered abnormal and warrant further evaluation for possible anatomic anomalies, infection, or inflammatory processes of the heart.

The provider should then proceed to evaluate the patient's neck for range of motion and tenderness to palpation. Limited range of motion attributed to neck pain and/or stiffness is a red flag for meningitis. Evaluating for midline cervical spinal process tenderness is also critical after head, neck, or high-velocity/impact injuries to explore for potential spinal cord injury and the need for cervical spine stabilization.

The abdominal examination begins with inspection, followed by auscultation, and finally palpation. On inspection, red flags after abdominal trauma include Cullen (bluish discoloration of the umbilicus) and Grey Turner (flank discoloration) signs that suggest retroperitoneal hemorrhage. Auscultation is very subjective, but absent sounds should concern the provider for a possible "acute" or surgical abdomen. If concerned for an acute abdomen, the provider should proceed with gentle palpation and assess for peritoneal signs such as rigidity, involuntary guarding, rebound tenderness, and positive cough test or heel drop sign.

The most commonly deferred portion of the physical examination is the genitourinary examination. It should be completed by the provider whenever the patient has a specific complaint relevant to the region, including dysuria, vaginal or urethral discharge, bleeding, or concern for sexual abuse, sexually transmitted diseases, or pregnancy. The examination also should be completed in males with abdominal pain to assess for testicular pathologic conditions.

Finally, the provider should inspect the ears, nose, and mouth. In the case of trauma, red flags include hemotympanum and septal hematomas. On oropharyngeal examination, worrisome signs include unilateral tonsil swelling or trismus, which may be found in the setting of retropharyngeal abscess, peritonsillar abscess, or other deep neck space infections. Frenulum tears in toddlers and infants without an accompanying story of trauma are concerning for NAT.

DISPOSITION

The acutely ill child is often first seen in the primary care office, which serves as the gateway into the emergency care system—an intricate network comprising out-of-hospital emergency medical services (EMS), the ED itself, and higher levels of care such as the intensive care unit. The primary care provider thus becomes the gatekeeper responsible for determining which patients are safe for discharge home and which must advance into this system of higher care. Primary care providers and their offices must be equipped for emergencies, enabling patient stabilization on early recognition of severe illness and also timely transfer to appropriate facilities.

Most acutely ill children presenting to the outpatient setting have reassuring vital signs and physical examinations, with responsible caretakers who will see to follow-up as prescribed. These patients may be safely discharged home. For the severely ill, however, transport to the ED by EMS may be necessary, particularly if the patient is unstable. It is the responsibility of the referring provider to not only choose an appropriate level of care and transport but also to provide necessary stabilizing care until the patient is officially transferred elsewhere.

SUGGESTED READINGS

Available online.

2

Resuscitation

Ethan S. Vorel

 CLINICAL VIGNETTE

A 9-month-old otherwise healthy male infant presents to the emergency department with fussiness, crying, and poor feeding for nearly 2 days. In triage, the patient's vital signs are notable for low-grade fever 100.6°F (38.1°C) and borderline hypotension (80/50 mm Hg); the nurse is unable to record a heart rate but feels that it is "very rapid." Concerned about the possibility of sepsis, the triage nurse alerts the attending physician and moves the patient to the resuscitation bay. A physician conducts the primary survey that shows a listless infant with a weak cry, regular tachycardia, no murmurs, and crackles at the lung bases; there is no other evidence of infection at this time. Intravenous access is obtained and 20 mL/kg of normal saline is given; however, there is no improvement in the tachycardia and the monitor is now showing a heart rate of 230 beats/min. An ECG is obtained, which shows narrow complex tachycardia, consistent with supraventricular tachycardia (SVT). Vagal maneuvers fail, so the patient is given adenosine without HR response; a second, larger dose of adenosine is given, with resumption of normal sinus rhythm at 110 beats/min. Laboratory test results are obtained showing an acute kidney injury and metabolic acidosis. The patient is consequently admitted to the intensive care unit.

The prevalence of SVT is estimated to be 1 in every 250 to 1000 pediatric patients. Prolonged SVT can lead to significant cardiac stress and eventual decompensation. If vagal maneuvers and medical management with adenosine fail or a patient becomes unstable, synchronized cardioversion is required. In this case it is imperative that a careful but efficient assessment occurs so as to not mistake such a presentation for sepsis and delay necessary care.

In 2015 some 30 million children—approximately 17% of all children living in the United States—were seen in a pediatric emergency department (ED), accounting for nearly 78.5 million pediatric ED visits. Less than 5% of those ED visits warranted hospital admission. It follows that most children do not present with severe illness or injury and even fewer require resuscitative measures. Nevertheless, pediatric physicians must be adept at identifying seriously ill children in order to provide necessary life-saving care. This is particularly true in recent years, as increasing numbers of children live with complex medical issues and rely on medical technology, which can complicate the identification of illness or injury.

In cases of dire cardiac and/or respiratory compromise, cardiopulmonary resuscitation (CPR) must be performed with the goal of restoring vital functions through optimization of cardiac output and tissue oxygen delivery. The two main components of CPR are external cardiac massage (chest compressions) and assisted respirations. Survival rates for children who require CPR from events that occur outside of the hospital setting are low, and those children who do survive often have residual neurologic deficits from the hypoxia and ischemia associated with the cardiopulmonary arrest. However, some children, especially those who experience cardiopulmonary arrest in a health care setting, do return to their premorbid function. This is likely the result of recognition and treatment of impending cardiorespiratory failure, early bystander CPR, and/or rapid correction of the life-threatening event. Thus all practitioners should know how to perform high-quality CPR so they can begin resuscitative efforts immediately for a child in extremis.

ETIOLOGY AND PATHOGENESIS

The signs and symptoms of the acutely ill child requiring immediate resuscitation are typically the result of failure of the delivery of two vital substrates—oxygen and glucose—to end organs. In most instances, the primary concern is oxygenation, which is primarily influenced by the respiratory and circulatory systems; however, derangement of the neurologic system can also affect oxygenation. Compromise of said systems can be the result of myriad severe illnesses or injuries. Most pediatric arrests occur after an initial respiratory arrest (rather than circulatory failure) and, if prolonged, result in terminal rhythms of bradycardia, pulseless electrical activity (PEA), and, finally, asystole. Recognition of these manifestations through a physical examination that focuses on airway, gas exchange, and cardiovascular stability allows for rapid resuscitation of children who have failure of substrate delivery and facilitates identification of those children whose substrate-delivery systems are at imminent risk.

INITIAL ASSESSMENT

It is important for providers, especially those not accustomed to pediatric care, to remember that children often display distress differently than do adults. Young children may not be able to communicate effectively or to localize pain, which makes a thorough and systematic examination crucial. It also follows that clinicians must rely heavily on the history provided by the family or caretaker.

Evaluation of a critically ill or injured child should begin with a *general assessment*. Vital signs should be obtained as quickly as possible, including heart rate, blood pressure, respiratory rate, temperature, and oxygen saturation. Vital sign changes in children may be related to multiple factors, including pain, fear, anxiety, and medications; however, significant deviation from age-specific norms may signal underlying illness or injury. It is critical to monitor vital sign trends throughout a resuscitation to evaluate clinical course and the effect of given interventions. Physical examination clues help the provider determine the extent of illness or injury and allows the identification of organ systems that require closer attention during the remainder of the assessment. The Pediatric Assessment Triangle of the Pediatric Advanced Life Support (PALS) course outlines the following components of the general assessment:

- *Appearance:* muscle tone, interaction, consolability, look or gaze, speech or cry;

- *Work of breathing:* increased work of breathing, decreased or absent respiratory effort, or abnormal sounds; and
- *Circulation:* abnormal skin color or bleeding.

The initial assessment can be done without laying hands on the patient and should take only a few seconds. If the patient's condition is life-threatening, immediately recruit additional support. After these rapid initial impressions, the clinician should aim to perform a swift yet careful primary assessment.

PRIMARY SURVEY

The primary assessment evaluates and addresses vital functions in a systematic way with priority to systems that are most crucial for sustaining life. The components of the primary survey can be remembered as the "ABCDEs": *airway, breathing, circulation, disability,* and *exposure* (Table 2.1). If a life-threatening abnormality is identified, the aberration should be addressed before moving on in the assessment (Table 2.2). Ideally, the primary survey is performed immediately upon ED arrival and takes no longer than 5 minutes. Of note, if there

is concern for cervical spine injury in the setting of trauma, the cervical spine should be immobilized as quickly as possible.

Airway

The patient's airway is the first priority. This is particularly true in the pediatric population given that cardiac instability is most often secondary to respiratory compromise. There are fundamental differences between the airway of a child and that of an adult. For instance, the pediatric airway (Fig. 2.1) is more anterior than the adult airway, requiring less manipulation to bring the oral, pharyngeal, and tracheal axes into alignment. In addition, the head-to-body proportion is larger in infants than in adults, and thus extreme hyperextension of the neck may exacerbate airway obstruction in younger children.

The provider should assess airway patency using the "look, listen, and feel" approach. The provider should *look* at the chest wall and *listen* to the mouth and nose to detect whether there is evidence of air

TABLE 2.1 Signs of a Life-Threatening Condition

System	Symptoms/Signs of Life-Threatening Injury
Airway	Complete or severe airway obstruction
Breathing	Apnea, significant work of breathing, bradypnea
Circulation	Absence of detectable pulses, poor perfusion, hypotension, bradycardia
Disability	Unresponsiveness, depressed consciousness
Exposure	Significant hypothermia, significant bleeding, petechiae or purpura consistent with septic shock, abdominal distention consistent with acute abdomen

Adapted from American Academy of Pediatrics and American Heart Association. *Pediatric Advanced Life Support.* Dallas, TX; American Heart Association; 2006.

TABLE 2.2 Life-Threatening Conditions Identified on Primary Survey

System	Life-Threatening Condition	Treatment
Airway	Airway obstruction	Endotracheal intubation; if not possible, consider cricothyroidotomy
Breathing	Tension pneumothorax	Needle decompression
	Open pneumothorax	Occlusive dressing (three sides secured)
	Massive hemothorax	Chest tube and hemodynamic support
	Flail chest	Respiratory support, fluids, analgesia
	Pulmonary contusion	Respiratory support
Circulation	Cardiac tamponade	Pericardiocentesis

Adapted from Fein DM, Fagan MJ. Overall approach to trauma in the emergency department. *Pediatr Rev.* 2018;39(10):479-489.

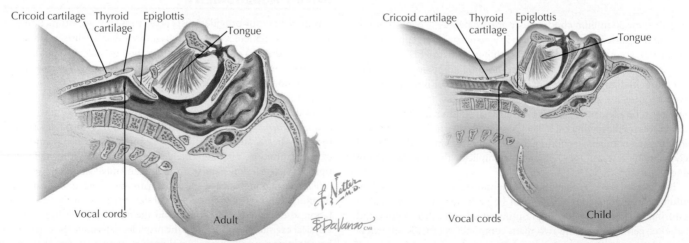

The pediatric airway is more anterior than an adult airway, requiring less manipulation to bring the oral, pharyngeal, and tracheal axes into alignment. The infant has a relatively large occiput, predisposing the neck to flexion and thus an increased propensity for airway obstruction when supine. Furthermore, extreme hyperextension may also result in airway obstruction in younger children as a result of the increased flexibility of the young airway. A child's airway is narrower and the tongue is relatively large compared to the jaw, increasing the risk of airway obstruction. The larynx is located more anteriorly and cephalad than the adult larynx, making the angle of entry into the trachea more acute.

Fig. 2.1 Pediatric and Adult Airway Anatomy.

movement. Findings suggesting airway obstruction include increased respiratory effort with retractions, abnormal inspiratory sounds, or episodes during which no airway or breath sounds are produced despite respiratory effort. If a child is speaking, crying, or otherwise verbalizing, the airway is intact. Attention should be paid to the quality of the sounds. A hoarse or high-pitched cry should alert the provider to the possibility of airway compromise.

The most effective maneuvers for opening an obstructed pediatric airway are the *head tilt–chin lift* or *jaw thrust* techniques (Fig. 2.2). In the head tilt–chin lift maneuver, the head is tilted back slightly (without overextending), and the chin is lifted gently with one finger on the bony prominence to avoid placing pressure on the soft tissues of the neck. If there is a risk for neck injury, it is critical to stabilize the cervical spine during evaluation of the airway and avoid extending the neck.

At any point, if it is determined that the patient is unable to independently maintain airway patency, the provider should open the airway to maintain adequate ventilation and protection from the aspiration of stomach contents. Simple suctioning should be attempted first because it may relieve an airway obstructed by secretions or foreign materials. Bag–valve–mask (BVM) ventilation (see later) may provide an open airway.

In an unconscious patient, an oropharyngeal airway can be used to help stent the mandibular block of tissue away from the posterior hypopharynx (Fig. 2.3). A nasopharyngeal airway is another option that is well tolerated in unconscious and semiconscious patients with upper airway obstruction. Laryngeal mask airways are supraglottic airway devices that are being increasingly used in resuscitation settings to help bypass the soft tissues of the anterior oropharynx.

When the patency of the airway cannot be maintained by other means, endotracheal intubation offers a relatively stable artificial airway. The following formula is used to determine the appropriate size (inner diameter) for an uncuffed endotracheal tube (ETT): (Age in years/4) + 4. Pharmacologic agents may be used to increase both chances of successful intubation and patient comfort and safety.

Direct laryngoscopy can be accomplished by positioning the patient's head and then using the right thumb and index finger to "scissor" open the mouth. The laryngoscope blade is inserted under direct vision toward the right corner of the mouth over the tongue and over the epiglottis (if using a straight blade) or into the vallecula (if using a curved blade). The tongue should be "swept" toward the left side the mouth while the laryngoscope handle is pulled upward at a 45-degree angle, taking care not to damage the teeth or gums (Fig. 2.4). The provider should maintain his or her view of the larynx and insert the ETT while watching it pass through the vocal cords. A projection for how deep to place the tube (centimeter mark at the teeth) can be calculated using the following formulas: (Age in years/2) + 12 or 3 × (External diameter of the ETT).

Primary confirmation of proper ETT insertion should always be confirmed by the detection of exhaled carbon dioxide (CO_2) through the use of a colorimetric CO_2 detector or use of inline capnography. Listening for symmetric breath sounds in bilateral lung fields, observing symmetric chest wall rise, and maintaining a good oxygen saturation are all secondary signs of appropriate tube placement. When time permits, a chest radiograph should be obtained to confirm placement.

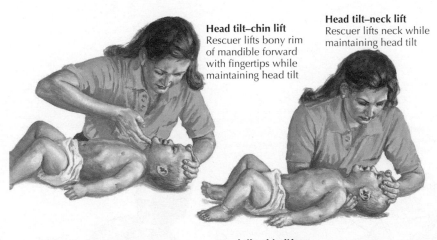

Head tilt–chin lift
Rescuer lifts bony rim of mandible forward with fingertips while maintaining head tilt

Head tilt–neck lift
Rescuer lifts neck while maintaining head tilt

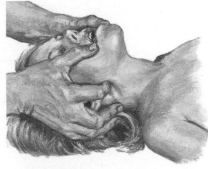

Neck extended, head tilted backward, jaw thrust forward

Head tilt–neck lift
Rescuer elevates neck at base of skull while tilting head backward

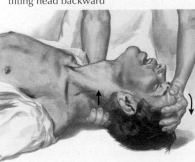

Head tilt–chin lift
With fingers under mandibular rim, rescuer lifts chin forward while tilting head backward

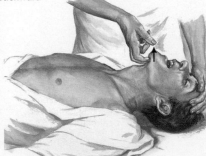

Jaw thrust (supplemental method)
Fingers of both hands grasp jaw behind mandibular angles and thrust mandible forward while head is tilted backward. Thumbs hold mouth open

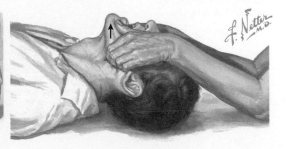

Fig. 2.2 Head Tilt–Chin Lift and Jaw Thrust Maneuvers.

Breathing

After the airway has been secured, assessment of ventilation and gas exchange should be initiated. Respiratory rate should again be noted; apnea, bradypnea, and tachypnea are all abnormal with bradypnea

and irregular breathing signaling the possibility of imminent respiratory failure. Observation of chest wall movement can provide clues regarding adequacy of respiratory effort. In infants, adequate chest wall movement is characterized by uniform expansion of the lower chest and upper abdomen. In older children and adolescents, observation should focus on upper chest expansion. Evidence of increased work of breathing includes but is not limited to grunting, retractions, and nasal flaring. Breath sounds should then be auscultated over the upper lung fields while focusing on adequacy of air movement and symmetry of breath sounds. Adequate gas exchange can be assessed using pulse oximetry, capnography, or direct measurement with either venous or arterial blood gas. Because hypoxia is the major initiator of pediatric cardiac arrest, supplemental oxygen should be given to all critically ill children to maximize oxygen delivery.

If the patient's efforts at ventilation or oxygenation are compromised, assisted ventilation with BVM should be initiated (Fig. 2.5). Masks of various sizes should be available, and the smallest mask that completely covers the mouth and nose should be selected. Airway patency is maximized when the patient's head is placed in the "sniffing position," with the neck slightly flexed while the head is rotated into extension.

When using the chin lift maneuver, the provider's nondominant hand should be used to hold the mask in place by forming a C around the connector with the thumb and index fingers while the remaining fingers maintain the chin lift along the angle of the mandible. Downward pressure on the mask should be used to provide countertraction against the upward force generated by the jaw maneuver, maintaining an adequate seal of the mask against the face. The provider should assess for an adequate seal and attempt to minimize air leaks.

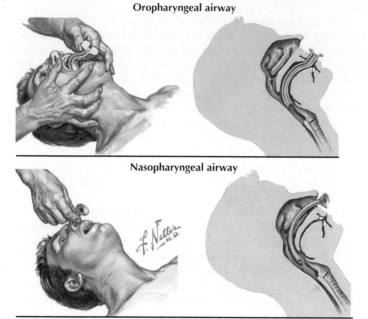

Oropharyngeal airway

Nasopharyngeal airway

Fig. 2.3 Oral and Nasopharyngeal Airways.

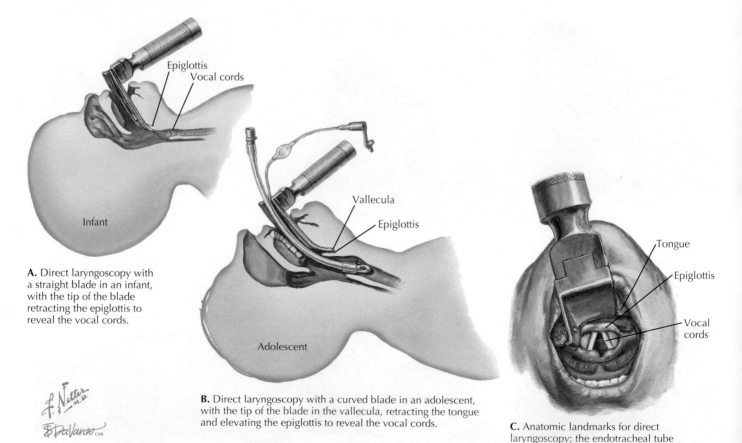

Epiglottis
Vocal cords

Infant

A. Direct laryngoscopy with a straight blade in an infant, with the tip of the blade retracting the epiglottis to reveal the vocal cords.

Vallecula

Epiglottis

Adolescent

B. Direct laryngoscopy with a curved blade in an adolescent, with the tip of the blade in the vallecula, retracting the tongue and elevating the epiglottis to reveal the vocal cords.

Tongue

Epiglottis

Vocal cords

C. Anatomic landmarks for direct laryngoscopy; the endotracheal tube is inserted from right of midline to keep the vocal cords in view at all times.

Fig. 2.4 Endotracheal Intubation.

After achievement of an adequate seal, ventilation can be accomplished by administering positive pressure via the resuscitation bag. A two-person technique is preferred, with one person holding the mask in place and the other providing breaths. The recommended number of respirations depends on age—infants and young children should receive 15 to 20 breaths/min; school-aged children and adolescents should receive 10 to 12 breaths/min.

Circulation

The goals of the circulatory assessment are to evaluate cardiovascular function and end organ perfusion. Cardiovascular dysfunction can be reflected by changes in skin color, temperature, heart rate, heart rhythm, blood pressure, pulses, and capillary refill time. End organ dysfunction can be reflected by changes in brain perfusion (manifesting as altered mental status), skin perfusion, and renal perfusion (manifesting as decreased urine output).

Heart rate should be appropriate for the child's age (Table 2.3) but may be affected by clinical conditions other than poor circulation (e.g., fever, dehydration, pain). Normal blood pressure is also age-dependent and also can be affected by associated clinical conditions. In children, compensatory mechanisms (tachycardia, increased stroke volume, and vasoconstriction) may cause blood pressure to be preserved even though there is inadequate tissue perfusion. This is termed *compensated shock*. However, hypotension should be treated as shock until proven otherwise in critically ill or injured children because it represents a state in which compensatory mechanisms have failed (uncompensated shock). Overall, it is critical to remember that hypotension in children is ominous, indicating that close to 50% of the circulating volume has been compromised.

Assessment of perfusion should include palpation of both central (most commonly femoral) and peripheral (radial and dorsalis pedis) pulses. Weak central pulses portend impending circulatory failure. Peripherally, prolonged capillary refill time is an indicator of inadequate perfusion.

Compromised circulation may be the result of a number of different factors, including blood loss, dehydration, neurologic injury, heart failure, and infection. Ideally, during the primary assessment, providers obtain vascular access. Large-bore intravenous (IV) lines are preferable; however, it may be difficult to establish venous access in a critically ill child who has compromised perfusion. In such instances, the intraosseous (IO) route is a quick and reliable technique. Fluid resuscitation is indicated in states of circulatory compromise. Isotonic fluid can be administered rapidly by the push-pull technique in aliquots of 20 mL/kg up to 60 mL/kg with continuous reassessment of vital signs, assessment of mental status, and physical examination for signs of improving perfusion. To date, there has been no benefit shown to albumin or synthetic colloids; glucose containing fluids should be avoided unless the patient is found to be hypoglycemic. Lack of response to fluid resuscitation should prompt providers to consider vasopressor use. Worsening respiratory status in the setting of large-volume fluid resuscitation should prompt providers to consider heart failure as a possible cause for the patient's condition. In trauma patients refractory to fluid resuscitation, early administration of blood should be considered.

Cardiac arrest is associated with the following arrest rhythms (Fig. 2.6): asystole, PEA, ventricular fibrillation (VF), and pulseless ventricular tachycardia (VT). Asystole is characterized by the absence of discernible electrical activity ("flatline"). PEA is a condition in which the patient has no palpable pulse despite showing electrical activity on cardiac monitoring (but excludes VF, VT, and asystole). For all of these rhythms, it is important to provide supplemental oxygen (100%) and to initiate CPR immediately.

Two-handed technique

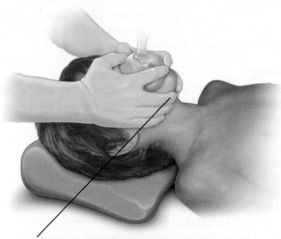

Three fingers are used to gently pull the mandible up into the mask using a gentle jaw thrust rather than pushing the mask down into the face.

One-handed technique

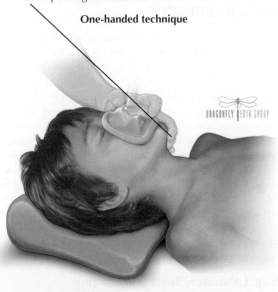

Fig. 2.5 Maintaining Airway Patency and Securing the Mask in Bag–Valve–Mask Ventilation.

TABLE 2.3 High-Risk Vital Signs by Age

Age	Heart Rate (beats/min)	Respiratory Rate (breaths/min)	Systolic Blood Pressure (mm Hg)
Infant (1 month–1 year)	>180	>34	<75
Toddler/preschool (1–5 years)	>140	>22	<74
School age (5–12 years)	>130	>18	<83
Adolescent (>12 years)	>120	>14	<90

Adapted from Farah MM, Tay Y, Lavelle J. A general approach to ill and injured children. In: Shaw KN, Bachur RG, eds. *Fleischer and Ludwig's Textbook of Pediatric Emergency Medicine.* Philadelphia, PA: Lippincott Williams & Wilkins; 2020.

Ventricular tachycardia

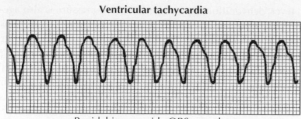

Rapid, bizarre, wide QRS complexes

Ventricular fibrillation

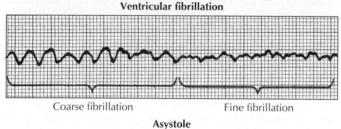

Coarse fibrillation   Fine fibrillation

Asystole

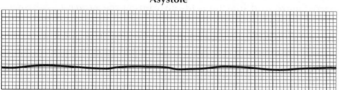

Fig. 2.6 Arrest Rhythms.

CPR (Fig. 2.7) is indicated for the management of cardiopulmonary arrest. Early initiation of adequate CPR both in and out of the hospital during cardiac arrest is shown to be the largest contributing factor to good outcomes. The mantra "push hard, push fast, minimize interruptions, allow full chest recoil, and do not overventilate" should guide the provider's efforts. In infants and children, the compression-to-ventilation ratio is different depending on whether there is a single rescuer or two rescuers performing CPR. A single rescuer should give 30 compressions for every 2 breaths, whereas two rescuers should perform CPR using the ratio of 15 compressions for every 2 breaths. In both scenarios, the goal is to provide at least 100 compressions per minute. After an artificial airway has been placed, continuous compressions at a rate of at least 100 compressions/min with ventilations at a rate of about 8 to 10 breaths/min should be performed.

Synchronized cardioversion is indicated for VT accompanied by a pulse. Defibrillation is indicated for VT without a pulse and VF. Although a full discussion of resuscitation medications is beyond the scope of this chapter, it is important to be familiar with the pharmacologic agents most commonly used during resuscitation. Epinephrine is used to promote vasoconstriction, which is important in increasing aortic diastolic pressure and coronary perfusion pressure. It is used as a first-line agent in pulseless arrest with nonshockable rhythms (i.e., asystole and PEA) and symptomatic bradycardia (heart rate <60 beats/min with poor perfusion despite CPR). It is also used for VF and pulseless VT that do not respond to defibrillation. CPR should be continued for at least one full cycle (2 minutes) of compressions after any intervention and until medications for the treatment of cardiorespiratory arrest have taken effect.

Disability

Disability assessment refers to evaluation of the two main components of the central nervous system: the cerebral cortex and the brainstem. Primary causes of neurologic abnormalities include increased intracranial pressure (ICP; secondary to a mass or hemorrhage), stroke, infection, and seizure activity. Secondary causes include any process that decreases oxygen delivery to the brain, most often from cardiorespiratory compromise. Lack of brain perfusion may manifest as any change in mental status, notably confusion, delirium, irritability, or somnolence.

A number of scales are used to assess neurologic function. The AVPU Pediatric Response Scale is quick and simple to apply. Level of consciousness is described as:

A—alert (child is awake, active, and appropriately responsive),
V—voice (child responds to voice),
P—pain (child responds only to painful stimulus), and
U—unresponsive (child does not respond to any stimulus).

A more detailed assessment for older children and adolescents, the Glasgow Coma Scale, is the most widely used method (Fig. 2.8). The patient's *best* responses in each of the categories (eye opening, verbal response, motor response) are added to produce a score out of 15.

In general, the primary means of addressing neurologic deterioration include hyperventilation and hypertonic fluids for increased ICP (surgical decompression in severe cases), antiepileptics for seizures, and antibiotics for infectious processes. While administering said therapies, it is critical to maintain brain perfusion through adequate mean arterial pressure and oxygen therapy.

An additional "D" that is included for a noninjured critical patient is a "D-stick" (fingerstick glucose measurement) because many medical conditions leading to critical illness are characterized or accompanied by disturbances in blood sugar.

Exposure

Critically ill or injured children should be completely exposed by undressing, ideally while the other components of the primary survey are being addressed. Complete exposure is important to facilitate a comprehensive physical examination as part of the secondary survey. Another important "E" is "environment." The provider should take care to institute warming measures (warm fluids and blankets, increased ambient temperature) for the exposed child. This is particularly important in pediatrics given the relatively larger body surface area in children that predisposes them to hypothermia. The environment should be free of contaminants that may exacerbate the child's clinical condition (e.g., a child with organophosphate poisoning should have contaminated clothing quickly removed and skin washed).

SECONDARY SURVEY

After completion of the primary assessment, including addressing any abnormalities found, the provider should initiate the *secondary survey*, which includes a focused history and physical examination. The secondary survey is a tool used to identify the cause of any respiratory, circulatory, and/or neurologic abnormalities that were revealed and/or treated during the primary survey. In the setting of trauma, the secondary survey identifies any further injuries that were not originally discovered on the primary survey. The SAMPLE mnemonic is helpful in addressing the important parts of the focused history: *signs and symptoms, allergies, medications, past medical history, last meal,* and *events* leading to current condition. A focused physical examination follows in a head-to-toe fashion. It is imperative to also maintain patient stability during the secondary survey, pausing, if necessary, to further stabilize the patient. If at any point in the secondary survey the patient's condition deteriorates, the provider should repeat the primary survey from the beginning to assess for changes in status.

Workup: Laboratory Tests and Imaging

A workup is initiated based in part on the findings of the primary and secondary surveys. In general, laboratory tests and imaging are ordered

Chest compressions: adult and child*

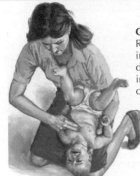

Central point of pressure area

Xiphoid

Liver

Posterior movement of xiphoid may lacerate liver. Lowest point of pressure on sternum must be at xiphisternal junction or slightly above

Patient horizontal on rigid surface

Rescuer palpates rib margin and follows medially to xiphisternal junction

With middle finger in xiphisternal junction, rescuer places index finger on lower end of sternum

Heel of other hand is placed on sternum next to index finger of palpating hand

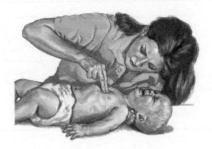

Heel of palpating hand is now placed on top of hand on sternum, and compression initiated. Fingers do not touch chest wall during compression

***Compression method for adult is 2 hands (heel of 1 hand, other hand on top); for child 2 hands (heel of 1 hand with second hand on top) OR 1 hand (heel of 1 hand); for infant 2 fingers.**

Chest compressions: infant (children younger than 12 months, excluding the newly born [see Chapter 92])

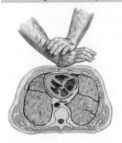

Chest thrusts
Rescuer holds infant on thigh in head-down position and delivers up to 4 chest thrusts in same manner as chest compressions (see next)

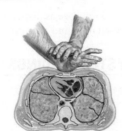

Compression and ventilation
Tips of index and middle fingers are used for compression over midsternum.
Compression rate in infants is 100 per minute. A single rescuer gives 2 ventilations after 30 compressions, while two rescuers should give 2 ventilations after every 15 compressions, observing closely for rise and fall of chest

Compression depth

Compression depth is at least 2 inches in an adult and at least ⅓ the depth of the chest in the infant and child (about 1½ inches [4 cm] in infants and 2 inches [5 cm] in most children)

Fig. 2.7 External Chest Compressions.

as clinically indicated. A complete blood count and basic metabolic panel are nearly always ordered. In trauma situations, additional laboratory tests to consider include a type and screen, prothrombin time/partial thromboplastin time, blood gas, hepatic function panel, amylase, lipase, and urinalysis. Based on patient age, a provider may consider a drug and alcohol serum screen, urine drug screen, and pregnancy test. Imaging, based on the clinical situation, may include plain films of the chest, pelvis, or extremities, head computed tomography without contrast, and neck imaging. Ultrasound is a valuable bedside modality to assess for bleeding or other fluid accumulation in the abdomen, pelvis, and pericardial sac.

OTHER CONSIDERATIONS: THE PATIENT'S FAMILY

In the organized chaos that is a resuscitation, it is important to not neglect the patient's family. By being present at the resuscitation, the family is able to comfort the patient at the bedside, increasing patient cooperation and thereby allowing clinicians to more easily proceed with management. The familial presence also enables improved bidirectional communication with the medical team. In situations in which resuscitation fails, familial presence at the end of life has been felt to be beneficial to both patient and family, enabling the latter to better navigate the grieving process. To date, studies have shown that familial presence neither hinders care nor negatively affects members of the medical team. The American Academy of Pediatrics thus currently recommends that all EDs have a system in place that accommodates family at bedside during pediatric resuscitations.

FUTURE DIRECTIONS

Current areas of research in resuscitation include therapeutic hypothermia, consideration of oxygen toxicity and reperfusion injury, the molecular genetics behind causes of cardiopulmonary arrest, and genetic polymorphisms and their implications in response to therapy.

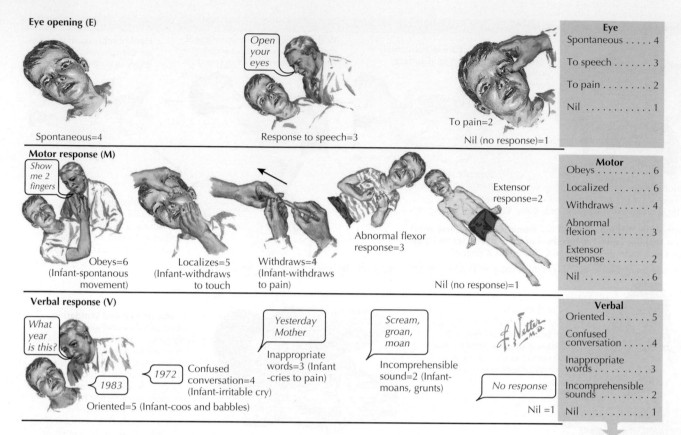

Fig. 2.8 Glasgow Coma Scale.

Preconditioning and postconditioning of the myocardium and brain epithelium, emergency preservation and resuscitation, postresuscitation myocardial support, mechanical circulatory support, quality CPR, and the epidemiology of CPR are also subjects of significant inquiry. Additional areas of research include improving resuscitation training for medical providers given the low frequency of these high-acuity situations. The once dismal prognosis of critically ill and injured children continues to improve as discoveries of therapeutic advances are made in preresuscitation and postresuscitation care.

SUGGESTED READINGS

Available online.

3

Shock and Sepsis

Daniel J. Herchline and Christopher E. Gaw

> ✳ **CLINICAL VIGNETTE**
>
> A 6-month-old female infant with short bowel syndrome and parenteral nutrition dependence by central line presented to the emergency department (ED) with a chief complaint of fever and lethargy for one day. Vital signs in the ED are temperature 102.9°F (39.4°C), pulse 130 beats/min, respiratory rate 30 breaths/min, blood pressure 75/40 mm Hg, and oxygen saturation 92% on room air. The patient's examination is notable for lethargy, weak pulses, and a capillary refill time of 5 seconds. Laboratories are notable for leukocytosis, elevated lactate, and elevated procalcitonin. The patient requires multiple crystalloid fluid boluses and initiation of vasoactive agents for persistent hypotension. She receives broad-spectrum antibiotics for presumed septic shock. The patient is transferred to the pediatric intensive care unit, where she rapidly improves and is weaned off of vasopressors. Blood cultures obtained in the ED grow methicillin-resistant *Staphylococcus aureus* 12 hours after inoculation. Her antimicrobial agents are narrowed based on susceptibility testing, and she is treated with a course of intravenous vancomycin before discharge.

Shock classically is defined as an acute clinical syndrome of circulatory dysfunction in which there is failure to deliver sufficient oxygen and substrate to meet metabolic demand. At the cellular level, scientific advances have highlighted the role of mitochondrial dysfunction and impaired cellular metabolism as contributors to the shock state. Patients who are in shock are at risk for developing end-organ damage, multisystem organ failure, and, ultimately, death. Therefore all providers who care for children must be capable of promptly identifying and initiating effective management for patients in shock.

ETIOLOGY AND PATHOGENESIS

Pathophysiology

The delivery of oxygen and nutrients is primarily governed by a combination of cardiac output (CO) and blood flow to organ tissues. CO is calculated by multiplying the stroke volume (SV) by the heart rate (HR). SV depends on the filling volume of the ventricle (preload), resistance against which the heart is pumping blood (afterload or systemic vascular resistance [SVR]), and myocardial contractility. Conditions such as intravascular volume depletion or impaired cardiovascular function can lead to decreased CO and development of a shock state.

CO and SVR are subject to neurohormonal regulation. A decrease in effective CO often leads to the compensatory activation of the sympathetic nervous system and renin-angiotensin system, as well as the release of cortisol. These are triggered in response to decreased SVR and renal perfusion. Activation of these mechanisms may temporarily counteract the clinical manifestations of shock.

Patients who sustain shock may continue to have end-organ damage even after correction of the shock state. Inflammatory cytokines released in response to infection or trauma can contribute to persistent microcirculatory dysfunction, characterized by ineffective distribution of capillary blood flow. Mitochondrial dysfunction and impaired cellular metabolism can lead to persistent energy deficits, perpetuating organ injury. Furthermore, restoration of effective CO may lead to oxidant stress and subsequent reperfusion injury. These pathophysiologic mechanisms likely underlie the development of multiorgan dysfunction syndrome in some children with shock.

Shock Continuum

Shock can be conceptualized as a continuum based on the body's ability to compensate for the shock state. Early in shock, neurohormonal mechanisms are activated in an effort to preserve CO and perfusion to vital organs. This *compensated shock* state is characterized by increases in HR, cardiac contractility, and SVR as a result of increased sympathetic tone and activation of the renin-angiotensin system. Of note, systolic blood pressure in compensated shock is often normal but tissue perfusion is suboptimal.

As shock continues, the body's compensatory mechanisms are unable to sustain effective CO. *Uncompensated shock* ensues and is characterized by a decrease in CO and hypotension. Tissue perfusion to vital organs, including the heart, brain, and kidneys, is compromised. End-organ damage and failure rapidly develops in uncompensated shock, and children are at risk for cardiovascular collapse and cardiac arrest. Even with appropriate management, some patients may develop *irreversible shock,* in which terminal damage to vital organs occurs, resulting in death.

Special Considerations in the Child

Children have faster HRs and smaller SVs than do adults. When faced with demands for increased CO, increasing HR, as opposed to SV, is the primary compensatory response in children. Pediatric patients also address circulatory insufficiency with increases in HR, SVR, and venous tone more effectively than adults. Therefore children can maintain normal blood pressures despite significantly compromised tissue perfusion before cardiovascular collapse. *For these reasons, it is especially important to recognize that hypotension is not part of the definition of shock in children.*

CLASSIFICATION OF SHOCK

Hypovolemic Shock

The most common type of shock in children is *hypovolemic shock,* which is characterized by decreased circulating blood volume. In hypovolemic shock, preload is decreased while HR and SVR are typically increased by compensatory mechanisms. The most common cause of hypovolemic shock is fluid loss associated with diarrhea and vomiting. Other causes include hemorrhage (e.g., trauma and postsurgical),

BOX 3.1   Systemic Inflammatory Response Syndrome Criteria

Identification of systemic inflammatory response syndrome must have two of the following criteria, one of which must be abnormal temperature or leukocyte count:

- Core **temperature** of >101.3°F (38.5°C) or <96.8°F (36°C)
- **Tachycardia** (mean HR >2 standard deviations above normal for age) in absence of external stimuli, chronic drugs or pain, or otherwise unexplained persistent elevation over a 0.5- to 4-hour time period *or* **bradycardia** for children younger than 12 months of age (mean HR <10th percentile for age) in the absence of external vagal stimuli, β-adrenergic blocker drugs, congenital heart disease, or otherwise unexplained persistent depression over a 0.5-hour period
- Mean **respiratory rate** >2 standard deviations above normal for age
- **Leukocyte count** elevated or depressed for age or >10% immature neutrophils

HR, Heart rate.
Adapted from American Academy of Pediatrics and American Heart Association. *Pediatric Advanced Life Support.* Dallas, TX: AHA; 2015.

plasma losses (burns, hypoproteinemia), and extra-gastrointestinal water losses (diuresis, heatstroke).

Distributive Shock

Distributive shock is the result of inappropriate vasodilatation and peripheral blood pooling, resulting in functional hypovolemia and inadequate tissue perfusion. The two most common causes of distributive shock in children are anaphylaxis and sepsis. In anaphylaxis, release of histamine, prostaglandins, and leukotrienes leads to a profound vasodilatory response that typically decreases SVR, leading to functional hypovolemia. CO is usually increased by compensatory neurohormonal responses.

Pediatric sepsis also can lead to a unique subtype of distributive shock—*septic shock.* Sepsis is defined as the presence of *systemic inflammatory response syndrome* (SIRS), caused by a presumed or confirmed infection (Box 3.1). Sepsis may occur as a result of infections by bacteria, fungi, or viruses. Septic shock is defined as sepsis with cardiovascular dysfunction and has traditionally been associated with hyperdynamic cardiac function and low SVR (i.e., "warm shock"). However, septic shock is gaining recognition as a complex and dynamic condition with the potential to present with a "mixed" shock picture. At least half of children in septic shock may present with low CO and elevated SVR (i.e., "cold shock").

Cardiogenic Shock

Myocardial dysfunction that comprises myocardial contractility can adversely affect CO, leading to *cardiogenic shock.* Causes of cardiogenic shock in children include viral myocarditis, arrhythmias, drug ingestions, trauma, and metabolic derangements. Shock related to congenital heart disease (CHD) is often colloquially referred to as cardiogenic shock, but some congenital heart lesions may have obstructive characteristics based on the underlying anatomy (see *obstructive shock*). Cardiogenic shock usually can be distinguished from other forms of shock because of the associated signs of congestive heart failure (e.g., crackles, gallop rhythm, hepatomegaly, jugular venous distension). A patient may exhibit increased HR and SVR and signs of decreased CO as a result of decreased myocardial contractility.

Obstructive Shock

Obstructive shock is the result of acute mechanical obstruction of cardiac outflow. Certain CHDs, such as critical coarctation of the aorta, are characterized by outflow obstruction, which can lead to a shock state. Other causes of obstruction include tension pneumothorax, cardiac tamponade, and massive pulmonary embolism. Patients experiencing obstructive shock exhibit hemodynamic parameters similar to those with cardiogenic shock, and some may also present with concurrent intrinsic cardiac disease.

Neurogenic Shock

Patients who sustain traumatic brain or central nervous system (CNS) injuries may develop *neurogenic shock.* CNS injury can disrupt sympathetic tone, leading to a decrease in SVR and hypotension. Unopposed vagal activity leads to hypotension without tachycardia, a hallmark of this shock type. Patients sustaining spinal injuries often have concurrent torso trauma. Therefore patients with known or suspected neurogenic shock should be treated concurrently for hypovolemia.

CLINICAL MANIFESTATIONS AND EVALUATION

In spite of scientific advances, shock remains a clinical diagnosis (Fig. 3.1). The clinical manifestations of shock are related to the pathophysiologic aberrations that underly the shock state. For example, inadequate perfusion of the brain and kidneys results in depressed mental status and decreased urine output, respectively. An increase in anaerobic metabolism due to tissue hypoxia leads to metabolic acidosis, which further interferes with cellular function. Inflammatory mediators can lead to microthrombi formation or worsening micro-ischemia. Multiple organs are often simultaneously affected, leading to a clinical presentation with systemic signs and symptoms.

Elements of the History

A targeted history should be performed in children with shock that is focused on identifying the type of shock and any reversible factors. A history of fluid loss—blood, gastrointestinal, or insensible—would suggest hypovolemic shock. Identifying a history of trauma may point to hemorrhagic shock (e.g., blunt abdominal trauma), neurogenic shock (CNS injury), or obstructive shock (tension pneumothorax). Exposure to an allergen, such as a food or an insect bite, could suggest distributive shock from anaphylaxis. A history of ingestion or medications should always be obtained, because shock may be attributable to toxin exposure. Patients' medical history should be reviewed; children who are immunocompromised are at risk for invasive infection and septic shock, and those with adrenal insufficiency can develop shock from adrenal crisis.

Physical Examination

Children in shock are often seriously or critically ill. Vital signs are crucial to the patient assessment and should be obtained immediately and continually monitored. Temperature is important, because a pediatric patient with fever or a neonate with hypothermia with shock features may suggest septic shock. Blood pressures in children may be normal in shock. The pulse pressure, however, may suggest a specific shock state if it is narrow (e.g., hypovolemic, cardiogenic) or wide (distributive shock). A child's weight should be obtained or estimated using a length-based tape system (e.g., Broselow tape) for future fluid or medication dosing.

Examination of the child should include rapid assessment of airway, breathing, and circulation (ABCs). The airway should be assessed to determine patency and the patient's ability to protect the airway. The presence, symmetry, and rate of respirations should be evaluated. Children in shock are often, but not always, tachypneic. Airway secretions or poor respiratory effort may suggest the need for airway protective interventions or respiratory support, respectively. Asymmetric breath sounds or chest rise may suggest pneumothorax.

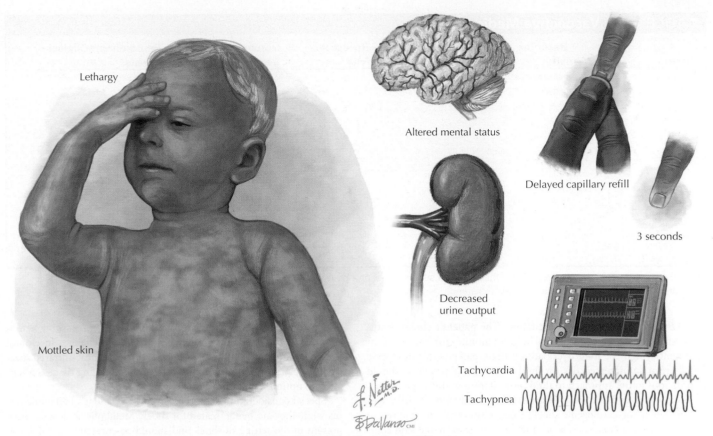

Lethargy

Altered mental status

Delayed capillary refill

3 seconds

Decreased urine output

Mottled skin

Tachycardia

Tachypnea

Fig. 3.1 Clinical Manifestations of Shock.

For children with suspected shock, assessing pulses is critical. Providers should palpate a child's pulses, focusing on rate, strength, and regularity. Both central (e.g., carotid, femoral, brachial in infants) and peripheral (radial, dorsalis pedis) should be assessed. Absent pulses suggest cardiovascular collapse or arrest and requires emergent resuscitation. Weak pulses raise concern for shock or severe hypovolemia. Rapid pulses are a nonspecific sign of distress. An irregular pulse may suggest cardiac dysrhythmia.

A child's skin can also provide information on perfusion. Normally, children have warm nail beds, mucous membranes, and extremities. As shock progresses and poor perfusion develops, the skin may become cool, pale, or mottled. Capillary refill time, assessed with light pressure to the fingernail bed, typically increases with worsening perfusion (normal: <2 seconds). However, flash (extremely rapid) capillary refill also can be an indicator of distributive shock. Note that capillary refill can be limited by clinician variability and by ambient temperature.

Mental status, including characterization of the Glasgow Coma Scale (GCS) score, is an essential part of the assessment of a child with shock. Changes in level of consciousness, including agitation, may suggest decreased cerebral oxygenation or perfusion. A depressed mental status may compromise other physiologic functions (e.g., airway protection) and should be recognized to inform management.

After the initial, rapid evaluation, a complete physical examination should be performed. This can help elucidate the type of shock or underlying cause of illness. For example, stridor, wheeze, and urticaria may suggest anaphylactic shock. Purpura or petechiae can be seen in children with septic shock. Bruises and abrasions can be seen with traumatic injury and may suggest underlying hemorrhagic shock.

MANAGEMENT

Initial Management

Early recognition and intervention are critical for reducing the morbidity and mortality associated with shock. Although mortality rates are lower in pediatric patients than in adults, any delays in care can potentially contribute to negative outcomes. This phenomenon has spurred efforts to create standardized care bundles that aim to expedite the provision of key interventions to patients with suspected or confirmed shock.

The initial management of shock should address airway, breathing, and circulation, guided by the American Heart Association's Pediatric Advanced Life Support (PALS) guidelines. Goal-directed care should attempt to normalize physiologic markers, including HR, urine output, capillary refill, and mental status. Additionally, respiratory support and placement of an artificial airway may be necessary to optimize oxygen delivery or if respiratory compromise is present.

Obtaining vascular access is a vital component of early resuscitation. Ideally, patients should have multiple large-bore peripheral intravenous (IV) lines in place to accommodate rapid fluid, medication, and blood product administration, if necessary. If providers are unable to obtain IV access, intraosseous (IO) access may be an acceptable alternative. Patients who require vasopressors or frequent blood draws or who have tenuous peripheral IV access may benefit from placement of a central venous catheter. Arterial lines may be placed to allow providers to continuously monitor hemodynamic status and achieve better goal-directed care.

Aggressive fluid resuscitation is important in managing most forms of shock. Isotonic crystalloid fluids should be given rapidly, either by rapid-infusers or push-pull delivery mechanisms, to increase the circulating volume and support organ perfusion. Boluses are typically given in aliquots of 20 mL/kg, with many patients requiring up to 60 to

TABLE 3.1 Vasoactive Medications

Agent	α-1 Receptor Activity	β-1 Receptor Activity	β-2 Receptor Activity	Dopaminergic Receptor Activity	Predominant Clinical Effects
Dopamine	Minimal; increases with dose	+	0	++	CO ↑ SVR ↑
Epinephrine	+++	+++	++	0	CO ↑ SVR ↓ (low dose) SVR ↑ (higher dose)
Dobutamine	0	+++	++	0	CO ↑ SVR ↓
Norepinephrine	+++	++	0	0	SVR ↑ CO ↔ or ↑
Phenylephrine	+++	0	0	0	SVR ↑
Milrinone[a]	0	0	0	0	CO ↑ SVR ↓

[a]Milrinone is a phosphodiesterase inhibitor that acts in a separate receptor pathway than catecholamines.
CO, Cardiac output; *SVR*, systemic vascular resistance.

80 mL/kg during the initial resuscitation. The patient's clinical status should be reassessed after each fluid bolus to monitor for improvement or potential signs of fluid overload. Of note, patients in cardiogenic shock are at an increased risk for fluid overload and providers should be judicious in the approach to fluid resuscitation in this population.

For patients with refractory distributive or hypovolemic shock, neurogenic shock, or cardiogenic shock, vasopressors may be required to maintain adequate organ perfusion. Table 3.1 lists some of the most commonly used vasoactive agents, their target receptors, and their physiologic mechanism of action. Vasopressor selection should be based on the type of shock present and the desired physiologic outcome. For example, epinephrine or dopamine may be preferred for refractory distributive shock to increase SVR and milrinone may be the agent of choice in cardiogenic shock because of its strong inotropic properties. If patients do not respond to appropriate fluid resuscitation and optimal vasopressors, use of extracorporeal membrane oxygenation may be considered.

Early administration of antibiotics is a key consideration for patients with suspected or confirmed septic shock. Although blood cultures ideally should be collected beforehand, providers should not delay administration of antibiotics given the increased morbidity and mortality associated with delays. Initial antibiotic selection should include broad-spectrum agents that provide coverage for both gram-negative and gram-positive organisms, including methicillin-resistant *Staphylococcus aureus* (MRSA). Additional considerations should include patient risk factors (e.g., immunosuppression, indwelling hardware, known exposure), clinical presentation, and local resistance patterns. Antibiotic coverage should be appropriately narrowed once the causal organism and its sensitivities have been identified.

Ultimately, identification and correction of the underlying cause of shock remains a mainstay of management. Initial laboratory evaluation should be tailored to the patient's clinical presentation and should also include markers of tissue perfusion such as serum lactate and base deficit. Imaging may be an important consideration in patients with obstructive shock caused by pneumothorax or pulmonary embolus or in patients with suspected neurogenic shock secondary to trauma, among others.

ADDITIONAL CONSIDERATIONS

The management of shock in pediatric patients often requires careful monitoring within an ICU setting. Cardiorespiratory and blood pressure monitoring provide important information regarding hemodynamic status that allows providers to identify changes in clinical status. Additionally, the use of technologies such as near-infrared spectroscopy can provide important information regarding tissue oxygenation to optimize goal-directed therapy.

Special consideration should be given to a patient's metabolic status while they are being treated for shock. Metabolic acidosis is often present in the setting of shock and should be corrected as quickly as possible through increased renal acid secretion and neutralization with sodium bicarbonate. Patients with shock are also at increased risk for hypoglycemia and electrolyte abnormalities such as hypocalcemia. These derangements should be addressed with IV dextrose and IV calcium supplementation, respectively.

Coagulopathies represent another frequent manifestation of shock, particularly in the setting of acidosis. For patients with bleeding, mainstays of therapy include vitamin K, fresh frozen plasma, and platelets. For patients in a hypercoagulable state, anticoagulation with an easily reversible agent, such as heparin, may be indicated.

Although steroids have not been proven to be impactful as a standard of care in pediatric shock, there are certain populations in which they may provide benefit. Patients with primary or secondary adrenal insufficiency due to chronic steroid use may require stress-dose steroids in the setting of shock.

Challenges in Neonates

Neonatal physiology poses special challenges in the diagnosis and management of shock. Septic shock in the neonatal period is often difficult to diagnose with vague signs and symptoms and requires consideration of additional causes, such as herpes simplex virus (HSV). Neonates with suspected sepsis should be treated with broad-spectrum antibiotics in addition to antivirals for HSV coverage. CHD represents another unique consideration for shock in the neonatal period. For more information regarding the diagnosis and management of CHD see Chapters 30 and 31.

FUTURE DIRECTIONS

Current research in pediatric shock aims to improve the diagnosis, management, and prevention of shock. Significant efforts are being made to enhance precision medicine in sepsis through the use of biomarkers and gene expression to improve diagnostic accuracy and targeted therapy. The approach to fluid resuscitation is evolving as clinicians strive to achieve optimal volume and acid-base status using patient-tailored strategies. Finally, as previously mentioned, care bundles are being explored as a means to provide faster, more equitable high-value care to pediatric patients with shock.

SUGGESTED READINGS

Available online.

4

Acute Abdominopelvic Emergencies

Priyanka Joshi and Regina L. Toto

 CLINICAL VIGNETTE

A fully immunized 8-year-old boy presents to the emergency department (ED) complaining of abdominal pain. The pain began 2 days ago around his umbilicus. It has intensified and has moved to his right lower abdomen. He has had three episodes of nonbloody, nonbilious emesis and does not feel hungry. There has been no documented fever, though he had chills the previous night. There are no sick contacts. He has no past medical history or surgical history.

On initial evaluation, he has a temperature of 100.4°F (38°C) and is mildly tachycardic for his age. His other vital signs are within normal limits. He is lying still and appears uncomfortable. His head, eyes, ears, nose, and throat, cardiac, and respiratory examinations are unremarkable. The abdomen is markedly tender to palpation of the right lower quadrant (RLQ). He does not have rebound tenderness or guarding. Genitourinary examination is unremarkable.

Screening laboratory studies and a focused RLQ ultrasound are obtained. He is kept on NPO status and receives acetaminophen for pain. Laboratory studies reveal a mildly elevated C-reactive protein and white blood cell count with a left shift. His ultrasound reveals an edematous, noncompressible tubular structure in the RLQ consistent with acute appendicitis.

This patient displays a classic presentation for pediatric acute appendicitis. His vomiting and anorexia, coupled with progressively worsening abdominal pain localizing to the RLQ, are common complaints of patients with appendicitis. Still, a thorough physical evaluation remains important, particularly to exclude other surgical pathologic conditions (e.g., testicular torsion in male patients or ovarian pathologic conditions in female patients).

Abdominal pain is a common chief complaint among children. Although typically minor and self-limited, acute abdominal pain may signify a process that requires immediate identification so treatment can be initiated and morbidity prevented.

ETIOLOGY AND PATHOGENESIS

Abdominal pain falls into three types: visceral, parietal (somatic), and referred pain. A general understanding of each type of pain helps determine its underlying cause.

Visceral pain is poorly localized and described as dull and aching. It results from stretching, distention, or ischemia of the viscera. *Parietal (somatic) pain* is well localized, discrete, and described as sharp and intense. It arises from stretching, inflammation, or ischemia of the parietal peritoneum. For example, pain due to appendicitis has features of both visceral and parietal pain. Initially, the patient experiences visceral pain: vague, poorly localized, and periumbilical. As the peritoneum becomes inflamed, the pain localizes in the RLQ at McBurney's point (Fig. 4.1).

Referred pain is perceived at sites distant from the affected organ and may be either sharp and localized or vague and aching. Examples include irritation of the parietal pleura of the lung perceived as abdominal pain and inflammation of the gallbladder perceived as scapular pain.

CLINICAL PRESENTATION

Differential Diagnosis

The differential diagnosis for abdominal pain in children is very broad. Certain conditions occur more commonly at specific ages; therefore it is also useful to classify causes of acute abdominal pain based on age (Table 4.1).

Life-threatening causes of abdominal pain include those related to trauma, intestinal obstruction, and peritoneal irritation. Examples of processes presenting with intestinal obstruction are intussusception, midgut volvulus, and extrinsic obstruction caused by adhesions from prior surgery or by intraabdominal masses. Peritoneal irritation may occur secondary to inflammation, bleeding, or perforated viscera.

Abdominal pain also can be classified based on location. The abdomen may be divided into four quadrants (Fig. 4.2); workup can then focus on the most common diagnoses based on the location of symptoms (see Fig. 1.4). For example, hepatic and gallbladder disease usually manifest with right upper quadrant (RUQ) pain (see Chapter 62). Gastritis may manifest with epigastric or left upper quadrant pain (see Chapter 56).

History

The evaluation of pediatric acute abdominal pain may prove challenging because children often cannot describe or localize symptoms. Children may be anxious, making it harder for the clinician to examine and identify positive findings. It is important to ask about feeding patterns, emesis, and stool pattern and character. Other pertinent history can include birth and perinatal history for neonates, potty training for toddlers and young children, menstrual history for girls over 9 years old, and sexual history for adolescents.

Pain Character

Acute abdominal pain caused by a medical or surgical emergency typically intensifies over time, may awaken the child at night, and interferes with activity. In addition to patient age (see Table 4.1) and pain location (see Fig. 4.2), other important features of the history include the onset, frequency and duration, pattern, radiation, associated symptoms, and pertinent medical history.

Infants and young children can seldom localize their pain, and parents often describe an inconsolable child who lays with legs drawn up to the chest. Pain that is intermittent or colicky, with paroxysms of pain alternating with return to normal, is characteristic of intussusception (Fig. 4.3). Peritoneal irritation is suggested by pain exacerbated by movement, such as a bumpy car ride or jumping. Pain that improves after vomiting or a bowel movement may reflect a small bowel or large bowel cause, respectively.

Associated Symptoms

Certain infections can cause abdominal pain. Abdominal pain associated with fever, headache, and sore throat suggests streptococcal pharyngitis.

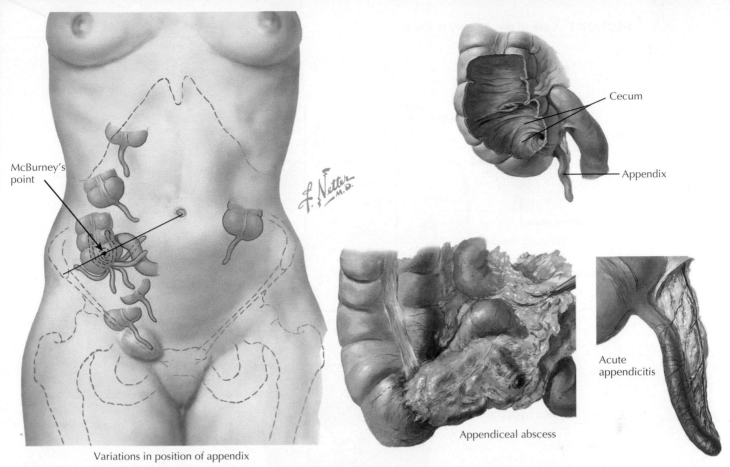

McBurney's point

Cecum

Appendix

Variations in position of appendix

Appendiceal abscess

Acute appendicitis

Fig. 4.1 Appendicitis.

TABLE 4.1	**Common Causes of Abdominal Pain**		
Neonate (0–1 month)	Colic Gastroesophageal reflux Milk-protein allergy **Necrotizing enterocolitis[a]** Neoplasm **Volvulus**	Adolescent (>12 years)	**Appendicitis** Cholecystitis Constipation **Diabetic ketoacidosis** Dysmenorrhea **Ectopic pregnancy** Endometriosis Functional abdominal pain Gastroenteritis **Hemolytic uremic syndrome** Inflammatory bowel disease Imperforate hymen **Incarcerated hernia** Lobar pneumonia **Ovarian torsion** Pancreatitis Pelvic inflammatory disease Renal stones **Ruptured ovarian cyst** Sexually transmitted infections Strep pharyngitis **Testicular torsion** Urinary tract infection
Infant (1 month–2 years)	Colic Gastroenteritis Gastroesophageal reflux Hirschsprung disease **Incarcerated hernia** **Intussusception** Neoplasm Urinary tract infection **Volvulus**		
Child (2–12 years)	**Appendicitis** Constipation **Diabetic ketoacidosis** Functional abdominal pain Foreign body ingestion Gastroenteritis **Hemolytic uremic syndrome** Inflammatory bowel disease **Incarcerated hernia** **Intussusception** Lobar pneumonia **Ovarian torsion** Renal stones Strep pharyngitis **Testicular torsion** Urinary tract infection		

[a]**Bolded diagnoses** may require emergent medical and/or surgical evaluation and management.

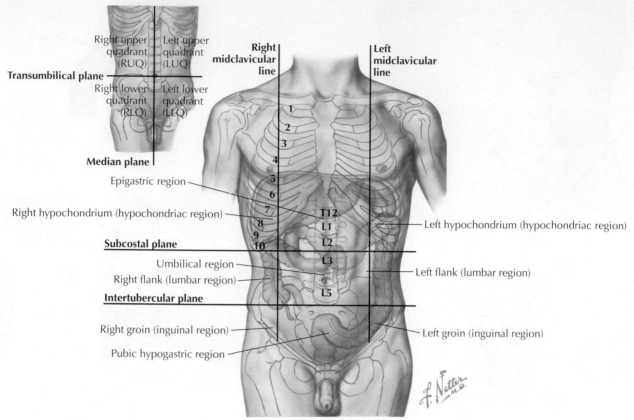

Fig. 4.2 Regions and Planes of the Abdomen.

Lower abdominal pain associated with dysuria may indicate urinary tract infection, whereas diffuse abdominal pain associated with tachypnea and cough may indicate lower lobar pneumonia. An associated rash may suggest vasculitis such as Henoch-Schönlein purpura as the cause of the abdominal pain (see Chapter 138). Bloody diarrhea could signal hemolytic uremic syndrome (see Chapter 104), inflammatory bowel disease (IBD) (see Chapter 57), or bacterial enteritis (see Chapter 63). Unusual sleepiness or altered mental status in a child may be a sign of intussusception. Abdominal pain accompanied by vomiting but not diarrhea should prompt an evaluation for potentially life-threatening conditions such as midgut volvulus, small bowel obstruction, or pancreatitis.

Pertinent Medical History

Certain chronic medical conditions are associated with abdominal complications. Patients with sickle cell disease are predisposed to cholecystitis, splenic sequestration, and abdominal vaso-occlusive crises (see Chapter 80). Patients with diabetic ketoacidosis often present with abdominal pain (see Chapter 50). Patients with oncologic disease are at risk for typhlitis. Those with IBD are at risk for toxic megacolon (see Chapter 57). Patients with a history of abdominal surgery are predisposed to adhesions, which may cause bowel obstruction. Trauma increases the risk for pancreatitis. Neonates born prematurely are at increased risk for necrotizing enterocolitis.

Physical Examination

Clinicians gain considerable information from the patient's general appearance. A child in severe pain may prefer to be curled up or to lie still. Vital signs should be attentively reviewed. Signs of poor perfusion may be seen with peritonitis or hypovolemia.

The abdominal examination is optimally performed when the child is calm and cooperative. Clinicians should consider examining young patients with the patient in the parent's lap. Evaluate for distention and

listen for bowel sounds. Parents can assist with the examination by palpating as instructed. It is helpful to start in the area away from reported pain. While palpating, feel for masses or focal tenderness; a palpable mass may indicate organomegaly, neoplasm, intussusception, or stool. Reproducible focal tenderness likely indicates an intraabdominal inflammatory process. Patients with peritoneal irritation present with involuntary guarding or rebound tenderness. Rebound is elicited by deep palpation followed by a sudden release. Pay attention to patients' faces when attempting these maneuvers, because younger children may not verbalize their discomfort. A rectal examination may be helpful: note the presence of hard stool in the rectal vault (constipation) or blood (intussusception, IBD, infection). A bimanual examination is indicated in sexually active females with abdominal pain to assess for pelvic inflammatory disease and other adnexal pathologic conditions.

Signs of an acute surgical abdomen include marked abdominal distention, rigidity, involuntary guarding, and rebound tenderness. Classic presentations of acute surgical conditions include a neonate with bilious vomiting (midgut volvulus), colicky abdominal pain (intussusception), and RLQ pain (appendicitis). Surgical subspecialists should be alerted early when a surgical cause is suspected. A delay in the diagnosis of appendicitis increases risk for perforation and postoperative complications.

EVALUATION AND MANAGEMENT

As always, the clinician should first identify and address any abnormalities of airway, breathing, and circulation. Abnormally weak pulses or delayed capillary refill may be signs of shock in children with abdominal crises. Following initial assessment, the clinician must identify potential abdominal processes requiring emergent surgical intervention. The patient's history and physical examination should guide the level of concern for such processes. Laboratory testing and imaging studies may help narrow the differential diagnosis.

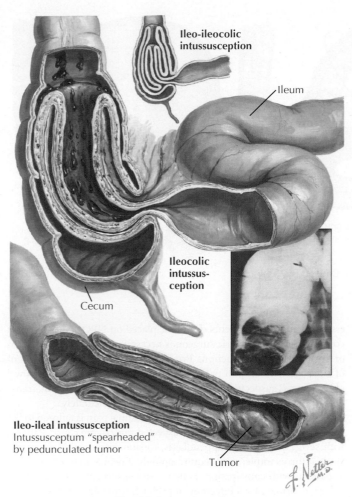

Ileo-ileocolic
intussusception

Ileum

Ileocolic
intussus-
ception

Cecum

Ileo-ileal intussusception
Intussusceptum "spearheaded"
by pedunculated tumor

Tumor

Fig. 4.3 Intussusception.

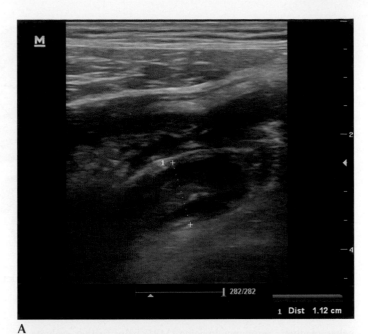

A

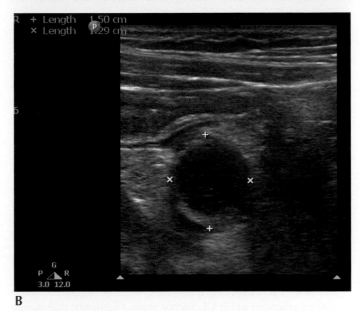

B

Fig. 4.4 (A) Longitudinal view of a dilated appendix. (B) Transverse view of a dilated appendix with a small amount of periappendiceal free fluid. (Reused with permission from Kimberly HH, Stone MB. Emergency ultrasound. In: Walls RM, Hockberger R, Gausche-Hill M, eds. *Rosen's Emergency Medicine: Concepts and Clinical Practice*. 9th ed. Philadelphia: 2017: Chapter e5, 2433-2433, e5.22, e5.23.)

Laboratory Testing

Most children with abdominal pain will not require laboratory testing as part of their evaluation. Any laboratory studies obtained should help narrow the differential diagnosis.

A complete blood count, and specifically the white blood cell (WBC) count, can help point toward or away from an infectious or inflammatory process. Likewise, C-reactive protein (CRP) may be useful as a marker of acute inflammation. Notably, neither WBC count nor CRP is specific for an infectious process.

A complete metabolic panel (CMP) may be useful in certain patients. This panel includes serum electrolytes, which may be abnormal in patients with gastrointestinal (GI) losses and signs of dehydration on examination. Of note, serum electrolyte evaluation is not necessary in the majority of pediatric patients with gastroenteritis. In addition to electrolytes, the CMP includes liver enzymes aspartate aminotransferase (ALT) and alanine aminotransferase (ALT), which may be elevated in viral illnesses, including hepatitis. Serum bilirubin may be elevated in cases of cholecystitis or cholangitis. Albumin may be low in children with IBD. A lipase value can be ordered separately and will be elevated in children with pancreatitis. It is essential to include a pregnancy test in the laboratory evaluation for any postpubertal female patient with abdominal pain.

Imaging Studies

Imaging studies should be performed judiciously, because most children presenting with abdominal pain will not require imaging and certain imaging modalities incur the risk for radiation exposure (e.g., for computed tomography [CT]) or sedation (e.g., for very young children).

Ultrasonography is a useful modality for diagnosing a variety of causes of pediatric acute abdominal pain. It is safe, does not expose children to radiation, is readily available, and often can be performed at the bedside. Ultrasound is the preferred imaging study for children with suspected appendicitis. A focused RLQ ultrasound may reveal a noncompressible tubular structure with increased bowel wall thickness, an enlarged diameter (>6 mm), and/or nearby free fluid (Fig. 4.4). Although its sensitivity is variable and highly operator-dependent, the specificity of ultrasound for diagnosing appendicitis in children is excellent (>95%). When ultrasound is inconclusive, focused

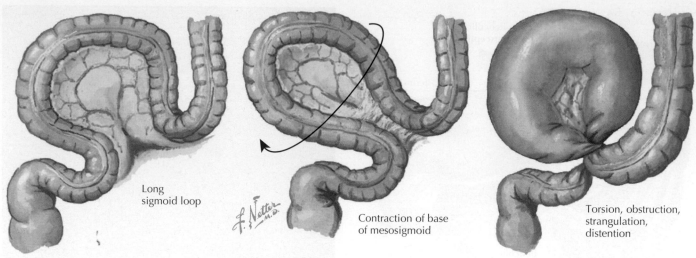

Long sigmoid loop

Contraction of base of mesosigmoid

Torsion, obstruction, strangulation, distention

Fig. 4.5 Bowel Obstruction Caused by Volvulus.

pelvic magnetic resonance imaging (MRI) helps further evaluate for appendicitis.

Ultrasound is also a useful diagnostic tool for many other causes of acute abdominal pain. A bowel ultrasound may be performed to exclude intussusception in young children with concerning symptoms. Testicular and pelvic ultrasound with Doppler are the ideal studies to diagnose testicular or ovarian torsion, respectively. In females with concern for pelvic inflammatory disease, a pelvic ultrasound evaluates for tubo-ovarian abscess. Renal bladder ultrasound is the preferred first imaging study for children with a suspected renal stone. Children with suspected biliary colic may undergo ultrasound of the RUQ to evaluate for cholelithiasis and signs of cholecystitis. In infants with concern for pyloric stenosis, a pylorus ultrasound is the diagnostic test of choice.

Abdominal radiography is useful in evaluating for obstruction or perforation. Supine and upright views of the abdomen are necessary to evaluate for air-fluid levels (bowel obstruction) or for free air (bowel perforation). Abdominal radiography is not useful for the assessment of stool burden; functional constipation may be diagnosed clinically. Plain films are not useful when evaluating for appendicitis or other causes of peritonitis.

Children with suspected malrotation with or without volvulus require an emergent upper GI contrast study. Classically, malrotation presents as bilious emesis in infancy. Volvulus (Fig. 4.5) is a complication of malrotation that can cause bowel infarction and can incur significant morbidity and mortality. Obtaining the upper GI study expediently is thus very important to facilitate early surgical correction.

CT may be necessary in some children with acute abdominal pain. It should be reserved to rule in or out significant pathologic conditions. Additionally, some children with abnormal anatomy and/or prior surgical histories may require CT to delineate the exact nature of their diagnoses. When considering obstruction, mass, or infectious or inflammatory etiologies, CT should be performed with contrast.

Management

The management of the pediatric patient with acute abdominal pain involves first triaging the overall illness of the patient. For patients who are critically ill and/or who display signs of an acute surgical emergency, early intravenous access and provision of crystalloid fluids are essential, and these patients should be placed on NPO status. Prompt consultation of a pediatric surgeon is necessary for patients with signs of peritonitis or obstruction. Providers should consider placement of a nasogastric sump in patients with bilious emesis in whom bowel obstruction is suspected. In settings without a pediatric surgeon, transfer to a higher level of care should be initiated immediately.

Medication management for acute abdominal pain is tailored to the type of pain, its severity, and the suspected underlying cause. Patients with severe pain due to appendicitis, torsion, pancreatitis, or cholecystitis, for example, may require opioids. Enemas may relieve pain in patients with constipation. Patients with suspected intraabdominal infection, urinary tract infection, or pyelonephritis should receive antibiotics tailored to probable causative organisms. Preoperative antibiotics are indicated for children with acute appendicitis.

Children with acute abdominal pain who have reassuring histories and examinations may be monitored at home with close follow-up. It is important to counsel families regarding the need to return to the ED for worsening pain or PO intolerance. Children who have concerning laboratory or imaging evaluation, without imminent concern for a surgical cause, may benefit from hospitalization and serial examination.

FUTURE DIRECTIONS

The efficacy and safety of nonoperative management of pediatric appendicitis is an area of ongoing research. Studies suggest that select low-risk children may be safely treated with antibiotics alone; more investigation is needed regarding the optimal antibiotic regimen. The use of MRI for the diagnosis of acute appendicitis is another area of research. MRI has shown promise in children over the age of 5 with very high sensitivity and specificity, safety, and tolerability without sedation. Currently the higher cost and limited availability of pediatric MRI at adult hospitals are barriers to widespread usage.

SUGGESTED READINGS

Available online.

5

Drowning in Children

Kyle Lenz

✳ CLINICAL VIGNETTE

A medic team arrives in the emergency department with an unconscious 10-year-old boy. He was on a boating trip with his family when he fell out of the boat and into the river. The boy struggled against the current and was ultimately dragged under the water for several minutes before he was pulled back into the vessel. At the time of his rescue, the boy was unresponsive without spontaneous respirations or a palpable pulse. Cardiopulmonary resuscitation was initiated by bystanders in the boat with return of spontaneous circulation before transport to the hospital.

Initial examination shows a minimally responsive boy with extensor posturing. His vital signs demonstrate a temperature of 96.1°F (35.6°C), a heart rate of 105 beats/min, a blood pressure of 80/45 mm Hg, and oxygen saturation of 91%. His pulses are diminished, and auscultation of the lungs reveals faint bibasilar crackles. An arterial blood gas demonstrates acidosis, and a complete blood count is normal. A chest radiograph illustrates basilar opacifications. He is intubated and transferred to the pediatric intensive care unit for continued close monitoring and management of his respiratory failure.

The child presenting after a drowning event requires immediate attention according to Pediatric Advanced Life Support (PALS) guidelines to ensure the best possible outcome. Special attention should be paid to the respiratory effort of children who have suffered a drowning injury, because they may lose the drive to breathe and may require intubation. Secondary injuries are also common, and a thorough examination should investigate other possible sources of trauma. Other important early steps include gastric decompression and strict temperature regulation.

EPIDEMIOLOGY

Drowning is the second leading cause of pediatric accidental death. The incidence of death by drowning is highest in children ages 1 to 4 years, followed by a second peak among adolescents. Males are at increased risk across all age groups. African American and Native American children have higher fatal drowning rates than do white or Asian American children. Other risk factors include history of seizures, alcohol use, proximity to bodies of water (especially pools and backyard lakes or streams), and reduced levels of adult supervision. Studies show that swimming lessons may confer a mortality-reduction benefit for children ages 1 to 4 years. However, such lessons only offer one layer of protection and may increase overestimation of abilities later in life.

The location of drownings varies across age groups. Bathtubs are the most common source for both *fatal* and *nonfatal* drowning in children younger than 1 year old. Swimming pools, particularly residential pools, become the most common location for *nonfatal* drowning in other age groups. Toddlers have large heads relative to their bodies, which predisposes them to losing balance or falling into tubs of water

(Fig. 5.1). In school-aged children, natural waterways such as rivers, lakes, or ponds constitute the most common sources for *fatal* drowning. In adolescents, most *fatal* drownings occur in open waterways.

PATHOPHYSIOLOGY

Hypoxemia secondary to aspiration is the primary driver of drowning-related morbidity and mortality. Children attempt to hold their breath during a drowning event. Small amounts of water are aspirated, which provokes involuntary laryngospasm (Fig. 5.2). The vocal cords then relax, and increasing quantities of water are swallowed and aspirated. Aspiration of water within the alveoli restricts oxygen diffusion across the alveolar/capillary membrane. It also damages the tissue endothelium, allowing the movement of fluid across the membrane and resulting in pulmonary edema. This causes an intrapulmonary shunt to occur, which in turn precipitates decreased blood oxyhemoglobin saturation.

As hypoxemia worsens, cardiac contractility and stroke volume decrease, worsening tissue perfusion. Prolonged hypoxemia can precipitate arrhythmias and eventually secondary cardiac arrest. As hypoxia and loss of cardiac output progress, metabolic disturbances cause additional downstream organ dysfunction. Vascular injury can result in third-spacing of fluid, hemolysis, and hypotension. Decreased renal and hepatic perfusion result in acute kidney injury and transaminitis, respectively.

ASSESSMENT AND MANAGEMENT

Initial Management

The initial evaluation of a drowned child should follow Basic Life Support and Pediatric Advanced Life Support algorithms to limit hypoxic damage. Unresponsive children who are either apneic or unable to protect their airways should be intubated. Not only is this important for ensuring adequate ventilation, but a secure airway also helps prevent aspiration of the gastric contents that are so often vomited during and after a drowning event. Supplemental oxygen also should be provided, with artificial ventilatory support as needed. A nasogastric or orogastric tube should be placed to decompress the stomach and remove gastric contents. Special attention should be paid to protecting or immobilizing the cervical spine if there is concern for injury, especially in cases of drowning associated with diving. Such precautions are particularly important if the event was unwitnessed. As part of the primary survey, remove all wet clothing and dry off any damp or wet skin.

Paradoxically, significant hypothermia during drowning (e.g., in winter) is one instance in which an abnormal decrease in body temperature may be protective against poor neurologic outcomes. Cold water submersion provokes the "diving reflex," or a set of physiologic

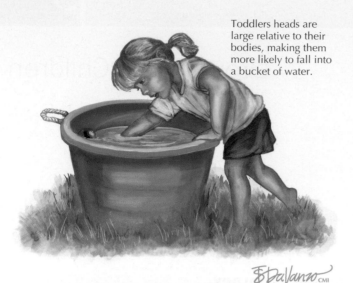

Toddlers heads are large relative to their bodies, making them more likely to fall into a bucket of water.

Fig. 5.1 Toddlers Have High Centers of Gravity.

responses that includes apnea and bradycardia. It is thought that this early apnea may protect against the gasping-related aspiration that often happens during the early phases of warm-water drowning. The diving reflex also causes selective vasoconstriction and decreases global metabolic demand, possibly offering both neuroprotective and tissue-protective effects compared to warm-water drownings.

Once children have been rescued from submersion and resuscitation is underway, severe hypothermia must be reversed to avoid the consequences of prolonged tissue hypoxia. Children with temperatures below 82.4°F (28°C) require active rewarming. Resuscitation teams should target a core temperature of 89.6° to 93.2°F (32° to 34°C); adjuncts for rewarming from least to most invasive include warm blankets and ambient warmers (e.g., heat packs in the groin and axillae), warmed intravenous fluids, thoracic lavage, and, if all else is unsuccessful, extracorporeal membrane oxygenation.

Secondary Management

After the initial resuscitation, cardiopulmonary status evolves rapidly and is most often managed in the intensive care unit. Aspirated water disrupts surfactant layers, damaging alveoli. Pulmonary edema and

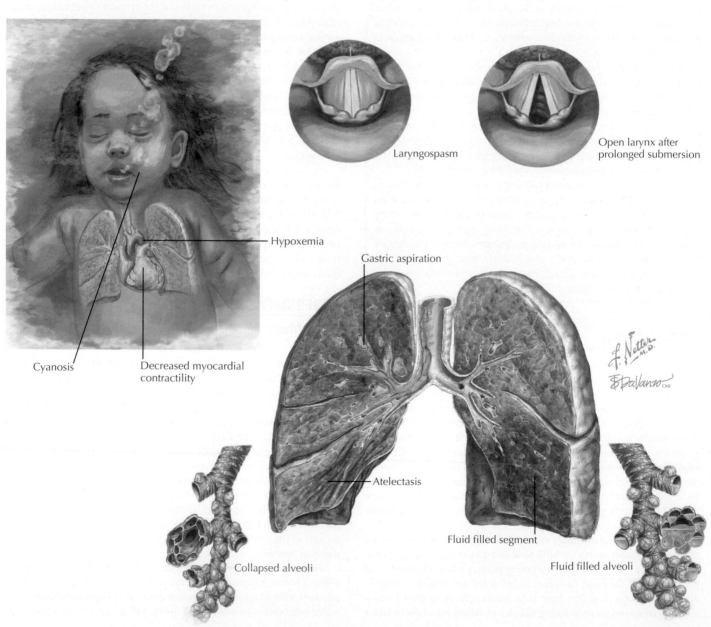

Laryngospasm

Open larynx after prolonged submersion

Hypoxemia

Cyanosis

Decreased myocardial contractility

Gastric aspiration

Atelectasis

Fluid filled segment

Collapsed alveoli

Fluid filled alveoli

Fig. 5.2 Pathophysiology of Drowning.

reduced lung compliance herald the development of acute respiratory distress syndrome (ARDS). ARDS frequently requires intubation and higher-than-usual ventilatory pressures to achieve adequate oxygenation. Bacterial pneumonia is a common occurrence in the setting of ARDS, with *Aeromonas* a frequently isolated organism.

In addition to pulmonary complications, drowned children can experience neurologic sequelae related to hypoxemic insult. Seizures frequently occur during both the initial and secondary stages of management. Administration of anticonvulsant medications is thought to reduce cerebral demand and may confer neuroprotective effects. Pediatric drowning victims are at high risk for cerebral edema and elevated intracranial pressure; therefore neurologic status must be closely monitored throughout all stages of resuscitative care.

PREVENTION

The prevention of drowning offers the best means of reducing morbidity and mortality related to submersion injury. Adult supervision has been shown to be the most effective means of protection against drowning. Parents and caregivers should be within arm's reach, especially when supervising young children. Additional precautions, such as gates and fencing offer additional barriers to access for children in homes with pools and other water sources. Anticipatory guidance and parent education on cardiopulmonary resuscitation also offers a means of rescue in the case of drowning.

School-aged children and adolescents should have swim lessons as a means of risk prevention. However, both they and their adult caregivers must remember that lessons do not make them immune to, or incapable of, drowning. Therefore even trained young swimmers should be supervised. Accessories such as floating devices can further shield children from swimming inexperience or fatigue, but care should be taken to ensure that such accessories are Coast Guard–approved for this purpose. Of note, most pool toys are not approved as safety devices and should not be used for drowning prevention. Lifeguards offer protection for swimmers of all ages, and families should preferentially swim in locations with lifeguards on duty. In addition to ordinary precautions, children with seizure disorders and known histories of cardiac arrhythmia should take extra care around water.

FUTURE DIRECTIONS

Currently, there are guidelines from the Society of Critical Care Medicine and the American College of Emergency Physicians for resuscitation of drowned children, but further studies to optimize care are ongoing. This is especially true with regard to techniques for optimizing patient temperature.

SUGGESTED READINGS

Available online.

6

Burns

Victoria C. Fairchild

 CLINICAL VIGNETTE

A previously healthy 4-year-old boy presents to the emergency department resuscitation bay after sustaining significant burns in the setting of a house fire. Initial vital signs are heart rate (HR) 167 beats/min, blood pressure (BP) 60/39 mm Hg, SpO$_2$ 92%, respiratory rate (RR) 30 breaths/min, and temperature 98°F (36.7°C). He has partial-thickness burns across an estimated 37% of his body surface area, including his face and neck. On primary survey, he does not have any stridor or wheezing and breath sounds are equal bilaterally; however, he has facial burns and there is soot in his nostrils and inside his mouth. Perfusion is poor, with delayed capillary refill and hypotension. Central venous access is obtained and fluid resuscitation initiated with two boluses of lactated Ringer's solution. Intubation is performed due to threat of airway compromise, and the patient receives 100% oxygen. After intubation and fluid resuscitation, vital signs are HR 123 beats/min, BP 80/57 mm Hg, SpO$_2$ 99%, RR 22 breaths/min, and temperature 98.2°F (36.8°C). Burns are cleansed with warm sterile saline, gently debrided, and covered with loose clean sheets. The patient is subsequently transferred to the burn unit for continued management of his severe burn injury and associated hypotensive shock and respiratory failure.

Burns are a significant source of both accidental and nonaccidental injury in the pediatric population, affecting millions of children worldwide. Categories of burns include thermal (due to fire, scalding, steam, or contact with a hot object), electrical, radiation, and chemical (Fig. 6.1). In developed countries, scald burns from kitchen and bathroom incidents are the major cause of injury among children younger than 5 years old. For children older than 5 years, flame-associated injury is most prominent. Child abuse accounts for 20% of burn injuries in young children and must be on the differential in cases with an inconsistent history or with patterns concerning for inflicted injury. A minority of burn injuries result in hospitalization, but those that do can lead to critical illness and require multidisciplinary coordinated care.

ETIOLOGY AND PATHOGENESIS

Burn injury can produce both local and systemic manifestations (Fig. 6.2), with systemic manifestations typically occurring in the setting of larger burns (>10% body surface area [BSA]). These clinical effects result from the loss of the protective skin barrier and its functions, including protection from infection, fluid regulation, and thermoregulation.

When a burn occurs, the heat radiates outward from the initial point of contact and forms a local response with three zones. The zone of coagulation is the central point of maximal damage in which

cell death, denaturation of proteins in the extracellular matrix, and disruption of the circulation occur. Surrounding the damaged circulation is the zone of stasis, which is characterized by vasoconstriction and thrombosis. The zone of hyperemia is the third peripheral zone and is characterized by increased circulation secondary to inflammatory mediators.

On a systemic level, the first days after injury are characterized by a state of decreased cardiac output and decreased metabolic rate. Vasoactive mediators, catecholamines, and inflammatory mediators are released, causing a capillary leak phenomenon that results in loss of protein and in development of interstitial edema and intravascular hypovolemia. Acute hemolysis can result from both direct heat damage and a subsequent microangiopathic hemolytic process. These systemic responses can result in renal and hepatic dysfunction, hypoxia, and mental status changes. After the initial hypodynamic state, a hypermetabolic and immunosuppressive physiologic condition arises, with increased cardiac output and energy expenditure. Disruption of the skin barrier, bacterial translocation from the gut and from nosocomial sources can lead to infection during this time. Malnutrition and multisystem organ failure can also result in the setting of increased energy expenditure during this phase.

CLINICAL PRESENTATION

The diagnosis of a burn is often evident from the history and physical examination. Differential diagnosis includes staphylococcal scalded skin syndrome, erythroderma, and toxic epidermal necrolysis/Stevens-Johnson syndrome. However, these entities typically can be distinguished with history and physical examination.

Prior classification of burns (first, second, and third degree) has been replaced by a classification system of superficial, superficial partial-thickness, deep partial-thickness, full-thickness, and fourth-degree (Fig. 6.3).

Superficial burns affect only the epidermis and are not included in body surface area calculations. Presentation typically consists of pain and blanching erythema without edema or blistering. Sunburns are a common example of a superficial burn. Partial-thickness burns can be further classified as superficial or deep and affect the entire epidermis and variable amounts of the dermis. Superficial partial-thickness burns extend through the epidermis and top half of the dermis, whereas deep partial-thickness burns extend beyond the top half of the dermis. Superficial partial-thickness burns typically form blisters within 24 hours and are characterized by pain, blanching erythema, and weeping from blistered areas. Fibrinous exudates and necrotic debris may accumulate on the surface, predisposing the wound to bacterial colonization and delayed healing. Deep partial-thickness

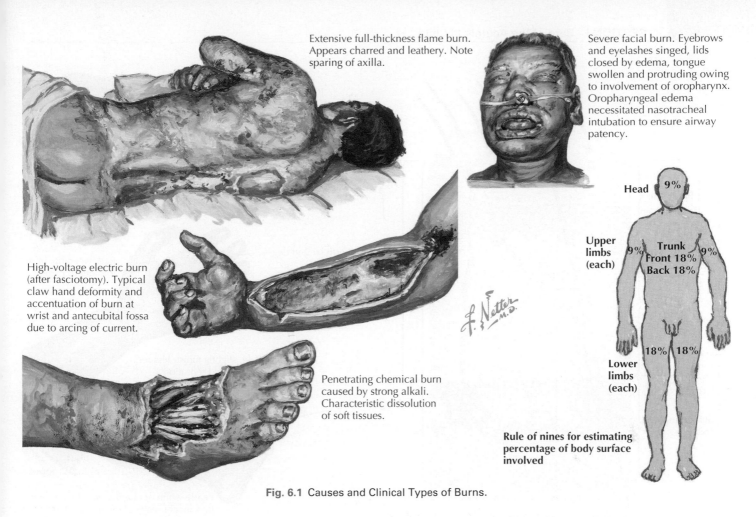

Extensive full-thickness flame burn. Appears charred and leathery. Note sparing of axilla.

Severe facial burn. Eyebrows and eyelashes singed, lids closed by edema, tongue swollen and protruding owing to involvement of oropharynx. Oropharyngeal edema necessitated nasotracheal intubation to ensure airway patency.

High-voltage electric burn (after fasciotomy). Typical claw hand deformity and accentuation of burn at wrist and antecubital fossa due to arcing of current.

Penetrating chemical burn caused by strong alkali. Characteristic dissolution of soft tissues.

Head 9%

Upper limbs (each) 9%

Trunk Front 18% Back 18% 9%

Lower limbs (each) 18% 18%

Rule of nines for estimating percentage of body surface involved

Fig. 6.1 Causes and Clinical Types of Burns.

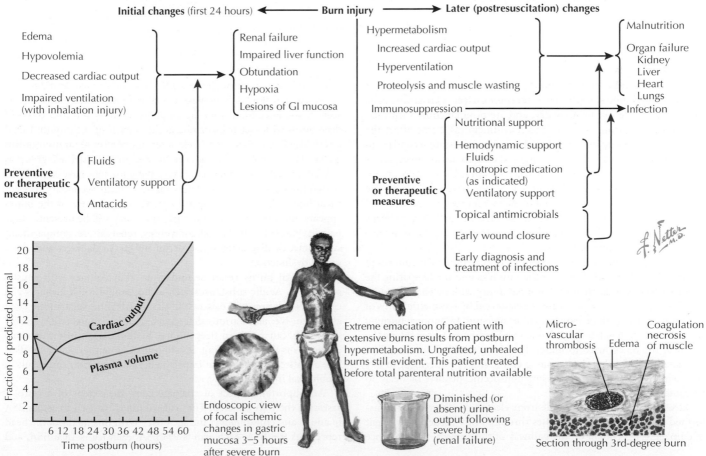

Initial changes (first 24 hours) ← **Burn injury** → **Later (postresuscitation) changes**

Edema
Hypovolemia
Decreased cardiac output
Impaired ventilation (with inhalation injury)

Renal failure
Impaired liver function
Obtundation
Hypoxia
Lesions of GI mucosa

Hypermetabolism
Increased cardiac output
Hyperventilation
Proteolysis and muscle wasting

Immunosuppression

Malnutrition
Organ failure
Kidney
Liver
Heart
Lungs

Infection

Preventive or therapeutic measures
Fluids
Ventilatory support
Antacids

Preventive or therapeutic measures
Nutritional support
Hemodynamic support
Fluids
Inotropic medication (as indicated)
Ventilatory support
Topical antimicrobials
Early wound closure
Early diagnosis and treatment of infections

Endoscopic view of focal ischemic changes in gastric mucosa 3–5 hours after severe burn

Extreme emaciation of patient with extensive burns results from postburn hypermetabolism. Ungrafted, unhealed burns still evident. This patient treated before total parenteral nutrition available

Diminished (or absent) urine output following severe burn (renal failure)

Micro-vascular thrombosis   Edema   Coagulation necrosis of muscle

Section through 3rd-degree burn

Fraction of predicted normal
Cardiac output
Plasma volume
6 12 18 24 30 36 42 48 54 60
Time postburn (hours)

Fig. 6.2 Metabolic and Systemic Effects of Burns.

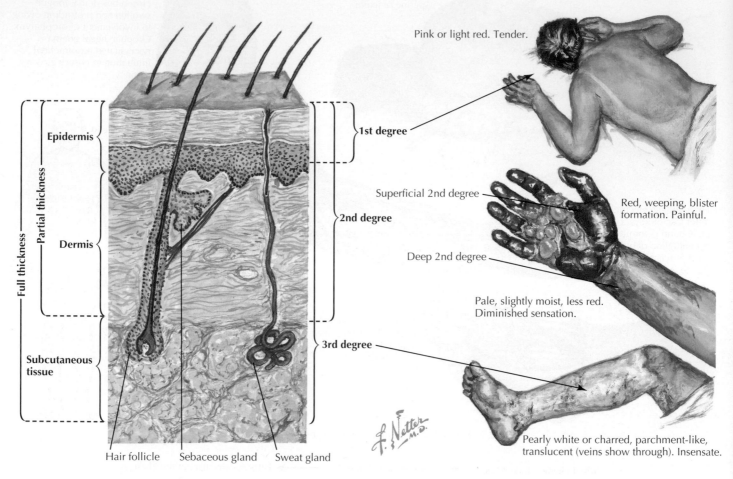

Fig. 6.3 Classification of Burns.

burns are typically only painful to pressure as a result of fewer exposed and viable sensory nerve receptors. Deep partial-thickness burns blister, are wet or waxy dry, and are nonblanching with variable coloration from white to red. Full-thickness burns affect the entire epidermis and dermis. These burns are insensate secondary to destruction of dermal cutaneous nerves, and any associated pain is typically caused by surrounding partial-thickness burns. Appearance can vary from waxy white to leathery gray to charred and black. The skin is inflexible, dry, and does not blanch with pressure. Vesicles and blisters do not develop in full-thickness burns. Fourth-degree burns extend through the skin and underlying soft tissue, and can involve the fascia, muscle, and bones.

Burn injuries due to child abuse often display particular patterns of injury (Fig. 6.4). Scald injuries of the buttocks and thighs sparing the flexor surfaces are classic for intentional injury with defensive posturing. Submersion burn injuries are characterized by symmetric burns of the hands or feet with defined lines of immersion. Intentional burning with objects often will be well-defined and geometric, often taking the shape of the object used to inflict the injury. Child abuse should be suspected in cases that display these classic injury patterns or in any case with inconsistent mechanism, nonspecific history, or delay to presentation.

Electrical burn injuries result from electrical energy being transformed into heat as current passes through body tissues. The extent of damage is dependent on the pathway of the current, the resistance to the current flow through the tissues, and the strength and duration of the current flow. Low-voltage (usually household) injuries can be seen in young children chewing on plugs or cords and may result in deep burns with eschar formation at the corners of the mouth. Labial artery bleeding can be seen weeks after injury after separation of this eschar. Higher voltage injuries can be seen in the older age group as risk-taking behaviors increase. These patients may have superficial, partial-thickness, or full-thickness thermal burns secondary to electrical injury. In cases in which the surface appearance of the injury appears minimal, extensive internal injury may still be present. These patients can suffer from rhabdomyolysis, renal failure, compartment syndrome, cardiac arrhythmia, peripheral nerve damage, and autonomic dysfunction.

Chemical burns result secondary to skin contact with caustic substances. Acidic substances such as household toilet cleaners can cause coagulation necrosis of the tissue. Alkaline substances, such as bleach, lye, and various detergents, generate liquefaction necrosis, which can result in deep injury. Systemic absorption of some chemicals is life-threatening. Splash injuries of either acidic or alkaline agents can cause visual impairment, and ingestion can result in esophageal injury.

An important aspect of characterizing the extent of a burn is assessing the BSA affected. The "rule of nines" is used to assess BSA in adults and children over the age of 15. With this method, the head represents 9% BSA, each arm is 9% BSA, each leg is 18% BSA, and

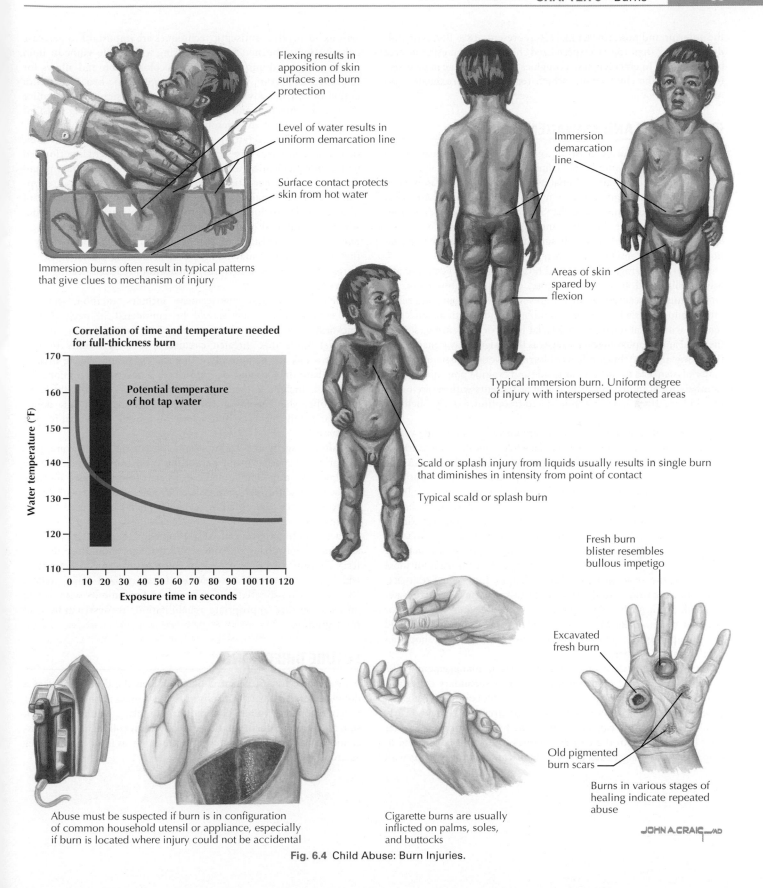

Flexing results in apposition of skin surfaces and burn protection

Level of water results in uniform demarcation line

Surface contact protects skin from hot water

Immersion burns often result in typical patterns that give clues to mechanism of injury

Immersion demarcation line

Areas of skin spared by flexion

Typical immersion burn. Uniform degree of injury with interspersed protected areas

Correlation of time and temperature needed for full-thickness burn

Potential temperature of hot tap water

Water temperature (°F)

Exposure time in seconds

Scald or splash injury from liquids usually results in single burn that diminishes in intensity from point of contact

Typical scald or splash burn

Fresh burn blister resembles bullous impetigo

Excavated fresh burn

Old pigmented burn scars

Burns in various stages of healing indicate repeated abuse

Abuse must be suspected if burn is in configuration of common household utensil or appliance, especially if burn is located where injury could not be accidental

Cigarette burns are usually inflicted on palms, soles, and buttocks

JOHN A. CRAIG—AD

Fig. 6.4 Child Abuse: Burn Injuries.

the anterior and posterior trunk each represents 18% BSA. For children younger than 15 years, specialized charts exist that estimate area based on age. In emergencies, a rough estimate of area can be determined using the child's palm, which represents approximately 1% of BSA.

EVALUATION AND MANAGEMENT

Management of a burn consists of four phases: initial evaluation and stabilization, initial wound care, definitive wound closure, and reconstruction and rehabilitation. Initial evaluation consists of assessment of airway, breathing, and circulation according to Pediatric Advanced Life Support algorithms. Burns that are deep-partial thickness or full-thickness and involve the face, hands, feet, or perineum or involve extensive or circumferential body surface area often require stabilization and more extensive management.

Stridor, wheezing, drooling, and hoarseness are indicative of airway swelling and airway compromise. In these circumstances, the airway must be secured rapidly to prevent airway closure and respiratory failure. Early intubation should be considered in patients presenting with facial burns, singed facial hairs, or evidence of soot in the nasal and oropharyngeal passages as these signs may signal potential airway damage. By-products of burning wood, plastic, and other materials can lead to carbon monoxide and cyanide poisoning as well as inhalational injury. As such, pediatric patients with severe burns should have 100% oxygen administered to optimize oxygen delivery to tissues.

Paramount to management of severe burns is establishing vascular access early and restoring euvolemia while avoiding fluid overload. The Parkland formula (4 mL/kg per percent of affected total BSA) is a calculation often used to estimate fluid requirements in burn patients. Half of the calculated fluid is given in the first 8 hours after the burn, and the remaining volume is given over the following 16 hours. However, the Parkland formula has been observed to underestimate required resuscitation volumes in children; thus it is necessary to monitor perfusion, blood pressure, and urine output (goal of maintenance of 1 to 2 mL/kg/h for children <30 kg and 0.5 to 1 mL/kg/h for those ≥30 kg) to ensure adequate fluid resuscitation. Initial fluid resuscitation should be with isotonic crystalloid to avoid extravasation of water and sodium through leaky capillaries. Dextrose should be added for children under 20 kg to avoid hypoglycemia. Monitoring of blood pressure, perfusion, and urine output is important because shock can develop in these patients.

After initial evaluation and stabilization, management shifts toward burn wound care and prevention of secondary complications. Burn wound management consists of cooling, cleansing, debridement, topical antimicrobials, and dressing changes. Early cooling of the burn can be accomplished by running cool water over the burn within the first 30 minutes to prevent edema and to stop thermal damage. Infection is a significant risk for patients with serious burns; thus antiseptic techniques are important to decrease colonization of burned areas. Cleansing with sterile saline or mild soap and water diminishes pathogen colonization and allows for improved inspection of the wound. Prophylactic broad-spectrum antibiotics are not advised, because they do not significantly reduce the risk for infection and increase the risk for developing resistant organisms. Topical antimicrobials (such as silver sulfadiazine, bacitracin, mafenide acetate) reduce bacterial colonization; however, there is no consensus on a superior agent. Debridement is performed with gentle mechanical techniques such as brushing or scraping and serves to remove necrotic tissue from the wound. Blisters are typically ruptured if painful, large, or likely to rupture. A variety of dressings exist, including standard fine mesh gauze, hydrocolloid, silver-containing dressings, biosynthetic, and biologic dressings. Some evidence exists that membranous dressings (both biosynthetic and biologic) may be favorable in treating partial-thickness burns due to better rates of reepithelization, reduced healing time, and reduced pain.

Definitive surgical management includes excision, grafting, and reconstruction, and should be considered in deep partial-thickness and full-thickness burns. For full-thickness circumferential burns that threaten circulation to an extremity or that present a risk for compromised thoracic expansion during breathing, escharotomy should be performed. Conventional options for skin grafts include full and split thickness (Fig. 6.5). Split-thickness grafts offer the benefit of covering large areas with less donor skin, and full-thickness grafts have improved skin texture and appearance.

Pain management is an important component of burn care, particularly in superficial and partial-thickness burns, which can be extremely painful. Opioid medications are commonly used to manage acute breakthrough pain, as well as pain associated with burn-care procedures. Ibuprofen or acetaminophen can be used for less severe pain.

Determining appropriate disposition for these patients is paramount in optimizing outcomes. Practitioners should use the criteria developed by The American Burn Association to determine which patients should be referred to specialized burn centers (Box 6.1). Coordinated care is required for patients with severe burns to ensure appropriate rehabilitation, reconstruction, and reintegration.

FUTURE DIRECTIONS

A future objective of pediatric burn injury is the development of a double-layered biologic skin substitute that mimics the normal barrier function of intact human skin and that stimulates wound repair and skin regeneration. Incorporation of intravenous colloid in early resuscitation is another area of interest and research, as is the use of honey as a topical antimicrobial adjunct.

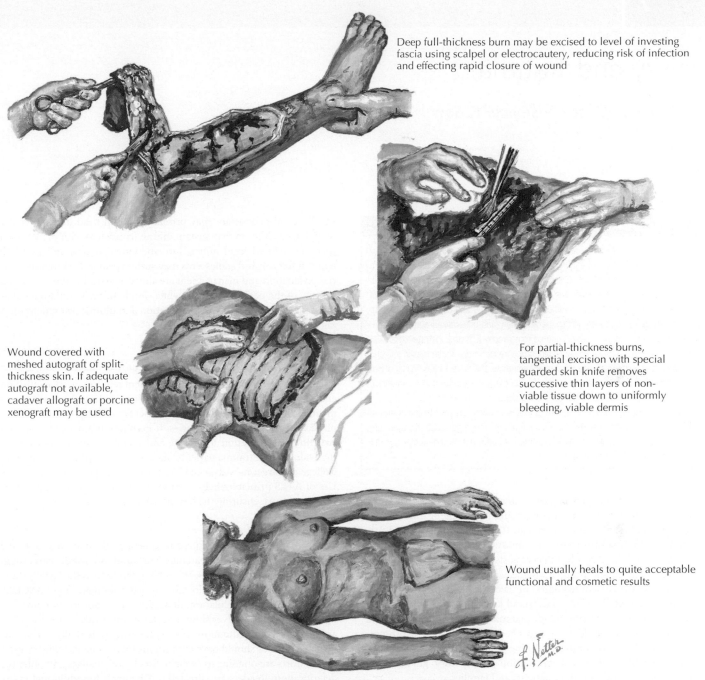

Deep full-thickness burn may be excised to level of investing fascia using scalpel or electrocautery, reducing risk of infection and effecting rapid closure of wound

Wound covered with meshed autograft of split-thickness skin. If adequate autograft not available, cadaver allograft or porcine xenograft may be used

For partial-thickness burns, tangential excision with special guarded skin knife removes successive thin layers of non-viable tissue down to uniformly bleeding, viable dermis

Wound usually heals to quite acceptable functional and cosmetic results

Fig. 6.5 Excision and Grafting for Burns.

BOX 6.1   **American Burn Association Criteria for Referral to a Burn Center**

1. Partial-thickness burns of greater than 10% of the total body surface area
2. Burns that involve the face, hands, feet, genitalia, perineum, or major joints
3. Third-degree burns in any age group
4. Electrical burns, including lightning injury
5. Chemical burns
6. Inhalation injury
7. Burn injury in patients with preexisting medical disorders that could complicate management, prolong recovery, or affect mortality
8. Any patients with burns and concomitant trauma (e.g., fractures) in which the burn injury poses the greatest risk for morbidity or mortality
9. Burned children in hospitals without qualified personnel or equipment for the care of children
10. Burn injury in patients who will require special social, emotional, or rehabilitative intervention

Excerpted from Committee on Trauma, American College of Surgeons. Guidelines for the Operation of Burn Centers. In: *Resources for Optimal Care of the Injured Patient 2006*. Chicago, IL: American College of Surgeons; 2014;79-86.

SUGGESTED READINGS

Available online.

7

Injury and Trauma

Shubhi G. Goli and Christopher E. Gaw

 CLINICAL VIGNETTE

A 13-year-old girl with no medical or surgical history presents to the emergency department (ED) after a head-on motor vehicle collision in which airbags were deployed. She was the front passenger and had her seatbelt securely fastened. On presentation, she is conscious and breathing spontaneously with stable vital signs. Initial examination is notable for scalp swelling and abrasions, a left arm deformity, a seatbelt sign across the abdomen, and generalized abdominal tenderness. Head and abdomen computed tomography (CT) demonstrate extra-axial hemorrhage and a grade II splenic laceration, respectively. Radiographic imaging of the left arm shows closed, displaced fractures of the distal radius and ulna. Her fracture is reduced and casted in the ED. The patient is admitted to the intensive care unit for close monitoring of her mental status and abdominal pain.

This patient is a classic example of one who might present to the pediatric ED after multisystem trauma. Her case highlights the importance of a thorough primary and secondary survey in guiding evaluation and management of the traumatically injured patient.

Traumatic injury is the leading cause of mortality in children ages 1 to 19 years in the United States, comprising over 30% of deaths in this age group and representing more than 10,000 annual pediatric deaths. Childhood trauma thus poses a significant burden on the health care system due to both direct health care costs and costs related to disability, rehabilitation, and occupational leave for family members. Given the high prevalence of injury and trauma in the pediatric population, it is imperative that clinicians understand key differences between child and adult anatomy and physiology that make pediatric trauma unique. Pediatric trauma should be approached systematically to promptly detect possible life- or limb-threatening injuries. Clinicians also should be comfortable with injury prevention anticipatory guidance and should emphasize this to their patients and families.

EPIDEMIOLOGY

The most common causes of injuries in the pediatric population are age-specific. In infants younger than 1 year of age, a high percentage of injuries are nonaccidental, and it is important to maintain a high index of suspicion for possible inflicted injuries (see Chapter 10) when evaluating an infant with traumatic injuries. In children ages 1 to 19 years, motor vehicle accidents and drowning account for the majority of fatal traumatic injuries, and falls and unintentional strikes by or against persons or objects make up the majority of nonfatal injuries. Burn injuries are the second most common cause of injuries in children ages 1 to 14 years, and firearm-related injuries are the second most common in children ages 15 to 19 years.

Patterns of injury are similarly age-specific and often can be predicted based on the mechanism of injury and on the size and age of the patient. For example, when struck by motor vehicles, younger and smaller child pedestrians may primarily sustain head injuries; young school-aged children may sustain injuries consistent with the Waddell triad (i.e., closed head injury, intraabdominal injury, and midshaft femur fracture); and adolescents may sustain primarily extremity injuries. Evaluation and management are aimed at assessing the nature and severity of the patient's injuries while simultaneously initiating medical management focused on stabilization and ultimately on determining patient disposition.

EVALUATION

Effective trauma resuscitation and treatment requires rapid acquisition and communication of large amounts of information about a patient's mental status, respiratory and cardiovascular stability, comprehensive physical examination, and injuries. It is common practice to follow a structured examination technique and management strategy during the evaluation of trauma patients, such as that taught in the American College of Surgeons' Advanced Trauma Life Support (ATLS) course. Use of ATLS principles helps minimize secondary injury in pediatric trauma victims, ensuring the best possible outcomes.

Primary Survey

The primary survey is structured to generate information vital to the rapid recognition of life-threatening issues and to assist the clinician in initiating resuscitative efforts. It is often referred to as the "ABCs" (airway, breathing, and circulation) but is better thought of as "ABCDE" (airway, breathing, circulation, disability, and exposure and environment) The primary survey should be started immediately after a child's arrival to medical attention. Any child with potentially serious or unstable injuries should have continuous reassessments while resuscitative efforts are ongoing to evaluate for clinical changes and potential deterioration. Readers are directed to Chapter 2 for additional information on the primary survey.

Airway

A child who can phonate normally has a patent airway. In children with hoarseness, stertor, or stridor, or in the unconscious child, inspection for airway compromise should occur immediately. Foreign bodies, blood or secretions, bony facial injuries, or crepitus over the tracheal cartilage are all potential causes for airway compromise that require intervention. Simultaneously, a provider should also consider restricting cervical spinal (c-spine) motion in patients with a mechanism of injury concerning for spinal trauma, with neurologic or multisystem injury, or with midline c-spine tenderness.

After these areas have been examined, the physician should quickly move to secure the airway if it is compromised. Head lift–chin tilt and jaw thrust maneuvers can help improve airway patency and can provide direct access to the airway (see Fig. 2.2). Suctioning of the oropharynx may be warranted based on a clinician's findings, especially if secretions are contributing to airway obstruction. Once the airway is determined to be patent or secured, the provider may move on to assessment of ventilatory efficacy.

Breathing

Providers should next take note of the patient's respiratory rate, quality of breath sounds, and symmetry of chest rise. The patient should be connected to a pulse oximeter for close monitoring of oxyhemoglobin saturation while a provider auscultates and palpates the chest, paying special attention to symmetry of breath sounds and identifying any areas of crepitus or injury. Additional signs of respiratory distress may include bradypnea or tachypnea, accessory muscle use, stridor, grunting, paradoxical breathing, or cyanosis. Asymmetric chest rise or asymmetric breath sounds suggest the possibility of pneumothorax, hemothorax, flail chest, or an open chest wound. Radiographs often can be obtained quickly to determine the presence and amount of air or blood in the pleural space, air trapping, or lung collapse.

If respiratory distress or hypoxemia is identified, the patient should be placed on high-concentration oxygen using a nonrebreather device. The use of bag–valve–mask (BVM) ventilation or the placement of an artificial airway may be needed to ensure adequate oxygenation and ventilation, depending on the extent and cause of respiratory compromise.

Circulation

After the respiratory assessment, circulatory status should be assessed. This involves an evaluation of a patient's overall mental status, which can be a proxy of perfusion, followed by auscultation of heart sounds, palpation of central pulses (e.g., carotid, brachial, or femoral), and evaluation of skin color and capillary refill. Shock in a pediatric trauma patient is often due to hemorrhage (see Chapter 3). Because most pediatric trauma victims have sustained blunt trauma, hemorrhage is often related to internal injuries such as splenic or hepatic lacerations, which are not readily visualized. If hemorrhage is not present or is adequately controlled, shock may be due to other causes. Cardiac tamponade may lead to cardiogenic shock if thoracic trauma is present. Hypotension with an inappropriately normal heart rate or bradycardia may suggest neurogenic shock and should be correlated with the injury mechanism.

In patients presenting with significant trauma and suspected shock, the provider should next obtain access, ideally with two large-bore intravenous (IV) catheters or intraosseous (IO) access if peripheral access cannot be obtained quickly. Prompt administration of isotonic fluids and/or O-negative packed red blood cells is the mainstay for shock reversal. Administration of blood should be prioritized if hemorrhagic shock is suspected or known to be present. Any obvious area of external hemorrhage should be identified and addressed with pressure or occlusion. In patients not responding to medical therapy, operative management may be required to locate and control sources of internal bleeding.

Disability

After the patient's hemodynamic status has been stabilized, the neurologic status is evaluated. Numerical scales such as the Glasgow Coma Scale (GCS; see Fig. 2.8) or the simplified Awake, Verbal, Pain, Unresponsive (AVPU) system allow for rapid assessment of the patient's neurologic status and can be repeated as part of reassessments over time (see Chapter 2).

In patients who are alert and can cooperate with the examination, strength and sensation should be assessed in all four extremities. Tenderness and deformities of the cervical, thoracic, and lumbar spine also should be assessed, a task that can be challenging in younger

---

BOX 7.1   AMPLE History Elements

Allergies: Assess for any food, medication, or environmental allergies the patient may have.
Medications: Include both medications the patient takes regularly and medications administered before arrival.
Past medical history: Review medical conditions and prior surgeries.
Last meal: Identify the last time the patient took anything by mouth.
Events leading to injury: Summarize the events preceding the injury or trauma with a focus on injury mechanism and any interventions that occurred before arrival.

---

children. Observation of spontaneous movement, watching for how the patient reaches for objects, and the patient's response to touch or painful stimulus should be assessed, particularly in very young or less responsive children.

Exposure and Environment

The final step in the primary survey is to ensure that all clothing has been removed from the patient so that all areas of the body can be visually inspected for missed injuries. In this step, the patient's core temperature also should be evaluated with the understanding that trauma patients are often hypothermic because of the environment and significant blood loss. Children are at heightened risk for hypothermia because they lose a significant amount of heat through their skin because of their relatively large surface area to body ratio. Rewarming should be undertaken as well as the prevention of further heat loss. The ambient temperature of the resuscitation area should be kept warm, and when inspection for injury is completed, warm blankets should be used to cover the patient to prevent heat loss.

Secondary Survey

After completion of the primary survey, stabilization of the patient, and initial management of life-threatening injuries, the provider may proceed to the secondary survey. The goal of the secondary survey is to perform a thorough, systematic head-to-toe physical examination as well as a targeted history (see Chapter 2). Of note, the genitourinary examination should not be deferred, and a digital rectal examination can be considered if there is concern for perineal or spinal cord trauma. Pertinent history elements are encapsulated by the mnemonic *AMPLE* (see Box 7.1).

General Management and Injury-Based Diagnostics

Fortunately, the majority of pediatric trauma is not life-threatening. In stable children, further evaluation and management can proceed, often without additional laboratory studies or radiographic imaging. For significant or major trauma, management includes continuous monitoring of vital signs, pain, and urine output. Analgesics, antibiotics, and tetanus immunization should be administered as clinically indicated. If an endotracheal airway has been secured, sedation of the patient is required. If head injury is present, frequent neurologic assessments should be performed. In severe trauma, a more extensive laboratory workup is often warranted to assess for hemorrhage, coagulopathy, metabolic or electrolyte derangements, and intoxication. Trauma-related laboratories often include a complete blood count, electrolytes, coagulation profile, type and screen, urinalysis, drug screen, blood gas, and lactate. Of importance, blood glucose should be obtained in all pediatric patients because hypoglycemia is a frequent contributor to altered mental status.

Although CT is the definitive imaging test for diagnosing many traumatic injuries, especially those involving the abdomen, it is used

BOX 7.2   Factors Associated With Positive Findings on Computed Tomography Scans in Children With Seemingly Mild Head Injuries

Children Younger Than 2 Years
- Altered mental status
- Occipital, parietal, or temporal scalp hematomas
- Loss of consciousness longer than 5 seconds
- Severe mechanism of injury
- Palpable or possible skull fracture
- Not acting normally per parent

Children 2 Years Old or Older
- Altered mental status
- Loss of consciousness
- History of vomiting
- Severe mechanism of injury
- Signs of basilar skull fracture
- Severe headache

Adapted from Kuppermann N, Holmes JF, Dayan PS, et al. Identification of children at very low risk of clinically-important brain injuries after head trauma: a prospective cohort study. *Lancet.* 2009;374:1160-1170.

judiciously in pediatrics. Young children are particularly at risk for the development of secondary cancers caused by ionizing radiation due to a combination of increased susceptibility and longer postexposure life-expectancy compared to adults. Therefore imaging in children is typically directed by positive findings on the primary and secondary survey and by mechanism of injury. Although focused assessment sonography in trauma (FAST) examination has become a standard of care in adult traumas for identifying free fluid in the abdomen, the FAST examination has not been validated in children and is not recommended for pediatric trauma. In the sections that follow, anatomic and physiologic considerations in children, key physical examination findings, and evaluation and management are discussed with respect to specific types of injury.

HEAD TRAUMA

Approach to Care

Traumatic brain injury (TBI) is a significant health care burden in the pediatric population, accounting for over 500,000 ED visits and 60,000 hospitalizations in the United States annually. Falls, sports injuries, and motor vehicle accidents are frequent contributors to pediatric TBI. Nonaccidental trauma (NAT) also should be considered in all ages. Children have important anatomic variations that should be considered when approaching TBI. A larger cranial vault and higher water-to-myelin ratio in children compared to that in adults predisposes children to higher degrees of internal torque and shearing forces, which can lead to more severe parenchymal injury and posttraumatic seizures.

Initial evaluation of mental status and documentation of all hematomas, lacerations, abrasions, skull depressions, and points of tenderness are of the utmost importance. Most children with TBI have seemingly mild injuries and look well on initial presentation. In these children, the relatively low risk for significant intracranial injuries must be weighed against the radiation risk involved in imaging the brain. A decision rule based on a large, multicenter, prospective study has identified historical and physical findings associated with intracranial injuries on CT scans in children (Box 7.2). All children with a decreased level of consciousness or other neurologic abnormalities after head injury should undergo CT of the brain to identify any intracranial injuries and to guide both their immediate and subsequent care.

Diffuse Axonal Injury and Hematomas

Diffuse axonal injury (DAI) and epidural and subdural hematomas are often seen after significant TBI. Swelling, hematomas, and other signs of injury near the temporal skull raise concern for an underlying epidural hematoma because the middle meningeal artery courses through this area of the skull and is subject to tearing with injuries to the temporal and parietal skull. Epidural hematomas often manifest with a lucid interval, followed by a rapid deterioration in mental status when the volume of blood filling the epidural space reaches the threshold to cause significant mass effect. Significant epidural hematomas are a neurosurgical emergency because evacuation before herniation can be lifesaving. Subdural hematomas are due to rupture of bridging veins between the cortex and dura mater. In infants and young children, these should prompt further evaluation for NAT. Subdural hematomas are more likely to lead to gradual neurologic deterioration compared to epidural hematomas.

On CT, DAI is characterized by diffuse edema and small, punctate hemorrhages on CT. Epidural hematomas (Fig. 7.1) are seen as a convex fluid collection between the skull and brain while subdural hematomas (Fig. 7.2) are seen as concave fluid collections. When there is concern for increased intracranial pressure, additional management may include securing the airway, gentle hyperventilation, hypertonic fluids, and surgical decompression of the hematoma.

Skull Fractures

Linear, nondisplaced skull fractures are the most common type of skull fracture in children. These rarely require intervention and are associated with a relatively good prognosis. Skull fractures that are diastatic or extend into preexisting suture lines are more likely to require correction to prevent future development of leptomeningeal cysts at these sites. Skull fractures with significant depression causing risk to underlying brain tissue may also require surgical correction.

Basilar skull fractures should be suspected in the presence of "raccoon eyes," (periorbital ecchymosis), the "Battle sign," (periauricular ecchymosis), hemotympanum, or cerebrospinal fluid leakage resulting in clear rhinorrhea or otorrhea (Fig. 7.3). It is important to note that the absence of these symptoms does not exclude basilar skull fractures; signs can take hours or days to develop. These fractures require additional evaluation, because they may herald late intracranial hemorrhages, carotid artery dissections, and intracranial infections. Neurosurgical input should be obtained early in management.

Contusions and Concussions

Both contusions and concussions occur when an injury with or without loss of consciousness results in the brain shaking within the cranial vault. Children often demonstrate transient altered mental status, headache, nausea, vomiting, focal neurologic deficits, and other somatic, cognitive, behavioral, and sleep symptoms. A CT brain can be considered for severe symptoms and may show bruising if contusions are present. Brain imaging is normal in concussions except in cases in which additional intracranial or extra-axial injuries have been sustained. Treatment for both contusions and concussions generally involves physical and cognitive rest with gradual return to activity as tolerated.

FACIAL TRAUMA

Approach to Care

A thorough examination for facial trauma includes assessment of the stability of the facial bones and oral structures, including nares and ear canals, eyes and extraocular movements, and dental integrity. Injuries to the facial bones, including the maxilla and mandible, may lead to airway compromise, secondary infections, and cosmetic deformities

Temporal fossa hematoma

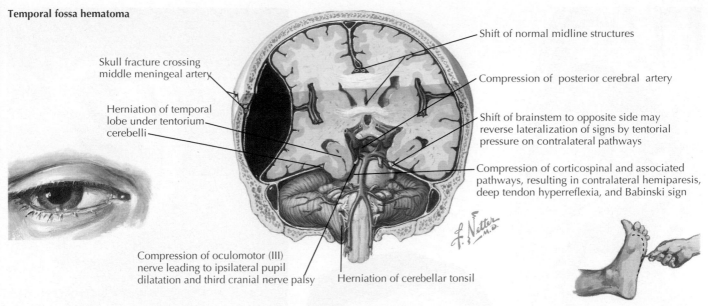

Shift of normal midline structures

Skull fracture crossing middle meningeal artery

Compression of posterior cerebral artery

Herniation of temporal lobe under tentorium cerebelli

Shift of brainstem to opposite side may reverse lateralization of signs by tentorial pressure on contralateral pathways

Compression of corticospinal and associated pathways, resulting in contralateral hemiparesis, deep tendon hyperreflexia, and Babinski sign

Compression of oculomotor (III) nerve leading to ipsilateral pupil dilatation and third cranial nerve palsy

Herniation of cerebellar tonsil

Fig. 7.1 Epidural Hematoma.

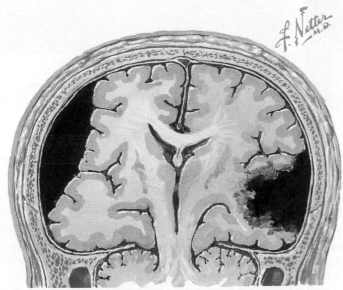

Section showing acute subdural hematoma on right side and subdural hematoma associated with temporal lobe intracerebral hematoma ("burst" temporal lobe) on left

Fig. 7.2 Subdural Hematoma.

if not recognized promptly and treated appropriately. Any concern for penetrating trauma to the globe, hyphema, or other serious ocular injury necessitates emergent evaluation by an ophthalmologist. In children in whom extraocular movements are decreased, facial CT scans should be performed to assess for orbital fractures and possible entrapment of the extraocular muscles or other injury affecting the ophthalmic nerve. Clear fluid from the nares or ear canals may suggest intracranial trauma and presence of cerebrospinal fluid leakage.

NECK TRAUMA

Approach to Care

Initial evaluation of the neck should involve thorough examination for blunt and penetrating injuries. Subtle clues suggesting the presence of neck or upper airway trauma includes tracheal deviation, changes in voice, dysphagia, odynophagia, hemoptysis, stridor, crepitus, or obscuration of cartilaginous landmarks. Patients with neck trauma also should be evaluated for spinal cord injuries. In conscious patients, this may involve palpation for midline cervical spine tenderness and assessment of neck range of motion.

Any child who has sustained a severe head injury should be assumed to have a c-spine injury and should remain in spinal immobilization until there is clear clinical or radiologic evidence that there is no spinal injury. Plain radiographs, CT scans, and magnetic resonance imaging (MRI) may aid in evaluation of the spinal column. As long as immobilization is maintained, MRI may be delayed until the child has been stabilized and other major traumatic injuries have been addressed.

Spinal Cord Injury

The relatively large head size, ligamentous laxity, and lack of calcification of cartilaginous structures in pediatric patients predisposes children to flexion and extension injuries of the spine. These features also set the spinal fulcrum closer to C2 to C3 in toddlers, predisposing this age group to fractures and spinal cord injury without radiologic abnormalities (SCIWORA) above the C3 level. In this age group, plain radiographs and CT scans may be normal; MRIs often are needed to identify the spinal injury. As children develop, the fulcrum gradually migrates downward to C5 to C6 in children under age 8 and approaches adult patterns around age 15. Detailed discussion of spinal injuries can be found in Chapter 115.

THORACIC TRAUMA

Approach to Care

A child's thorax has unique anatomic and physiologic features that have an impact on children's patterns of thoracic injury. The pediatric chest wall has increased compliance and elasticity compared to that of adults. Thus, blunt forces may be less obviously injurious to the chest wall, and internal thoracic injury may be masked. The pediatric mediastinum is also more mobile and therefore less resistant to pressure from air or fluid, placing children at greater risk for cardiorespiratory collapse from pleural space compromise. Thoracic trauma rarely occurs in isolation, and providers should consider trauma to other

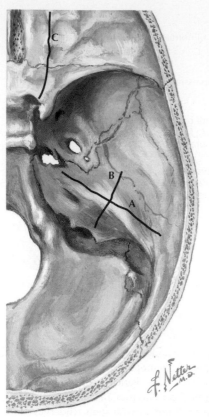

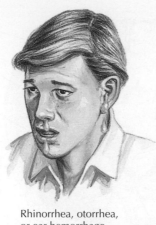

Rhinorrhea, otorrhea,
or ear hemorrhage

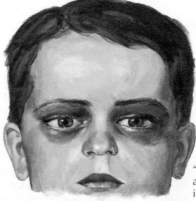

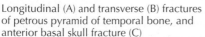

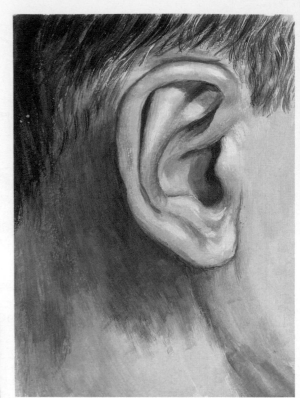

Battle's sign: postauricular hematoma

Longitudinal (A) and transverse (B) fractures
of petrous pyramid of temporal bone, and
anterior basal skull fracture (C)

"Panda bear" or "raccoon" sign due to leakage of blood from
anterior fossa into periorbital tissues. Note absence of conjunctival
injection, an important differential from direct eye trauma

Fig. 7.3 Physical Findings in Basilar Skull Fractures.

body regions when chest trauma is present. Attention to the primary survey and associated management is crucial in thoracic injury given the proximity of life-sustaining organs.

Pneumothorax and Hemothorax

Asymmetric chest rise or breath sounds may signify the presence of a pneumothorax or hemothorax. Additional symptoms or signs include chest pain, respiratory distress, and hypoxemia. A pneumothorax typically occurs due to disruption of the lung parenchyma, tracheobronchial tree, or esophagus, leading to air entry into the pleural space. An absence of breath sounds, especially in conjunction with tachycardia, hypotension, or tracheal deviation should alert the clinician to possible tension pneumothorax (Fig. 7.4). All pneumothoraces, regardless of size, are at risk for converting to tension physiology. BVM ventilation and endotracheal intubation can further increase this risk by introducing positive pressure.

A hemothorax typically arises due to injury to the intercostal or mammary arteries, though intrapulmonary and great vessel disruption are also possible. If bleeding is significant, lung collapse and mediastinal deviation can occur, resulting in compromise of oxygenation, ventilation, and venous return. Hypotension can also occur due to substantial loss of blood volume.

Radiographs can be used to determine the presence and amount of air or blood in the pleural space. In a clinically stable patient, a small pneumothorax may be treated noninvasively with inpatient monitoring, oxygen therapy, and serial chest radiography. Larger pneumothoraces or hemothoraces should be managed with chest tube drainage. A child with tension physiology is especially at risk for cardiovascular

collapse due to a mobile mediastinum, and emergent needle decompression followed by chest tube placement should be performed.

Pulmonary Contusion

Pulmonary contusions occur when the capillary or vascular network of the lung is damaged. Patients typically present with chest pain, difficulty breathing, or hypoxemia related to ventilation-perfusion mismatch from fluid in the lung parenchyma. Radiographs can identify contusions, though they may not be visible until several hours after the injury. Treatment is focused on maintaining appropriate oxygenation and fluid balance.

Chest Wall Injury

Chest wall injuries are less common in children due to their compliant chest wall; therefore, the presence of visible injuries to the chest wall should raise suspicion of concurrent intrathoracic injury. Simple rib fractures typically occur from direct trauma or anterior-posterior compression of the chest wall. They can be painful and may cause children to splint or cause hypoventilation, leading to atelectasis. Pain control and respiratory monitoring remain foundations of care for rib fractures. Posterior rib fractures or multiple rib fractures at different stages of healing should raise suspicion of NAT.

Fractures to multiple ribs on the same side may predispose to the development of flail chest, where a segment of the chest wall becomes discontinuous with the rest of the thorax. Findings include asymmetric chest rise, tenderness and crepitus on palpation, and a history of a high-velocity mechanism. Management of flail chest depends on the severity of respiratory compromise and ranges from pain control and

Pathophysiology

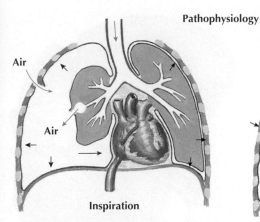

Air

Air

Inspiration

Air enters pleural cavity through lung wound or ruptured bleb (or occasionally via pene- trating chest wound) with valve-like opening. Ipsilateral lung collapses, and mediastinum shifts to opposite side, compressing contra- lateral lung and impairing its ventilating capacity

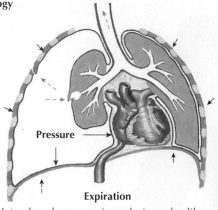

Pressure

Expiration

Intrapleural pressure rises, closing valve-like opening, preventing escape of pleural air. Pressure is thus progressively increased with each breath. Mediastinal and tracheal shifts are augmented, diaphragm is depressed, and venous return is impaired by increased pressure and vena caval distortion

Clinical manifestations

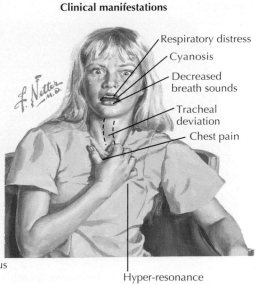

Respiratory distress

Cyanosis

Decreased breath sounds

Tracheal deviation

Chest pain

Hyper-resonance

Fig. 7.4 Tension Pneumothorax.

monitoring to intubation for positive pressure ventilation to counter- act the flail segment.

Cardiac and Great Vessel Injury

Myocardial contusions are the most common blunt cardiac injury in children and can manifest as chest pain or tachycardia. Children with myocardial contusions are at risk for arrhythmias and should be evaluated with a 12-lead electrocardiograph and continuously moni- tored. Cardiac enzymes and echocardiography are helpful adjuncts in ascertaining the severity of the cardiac injury. Other traumatic cardiac injuries include myocardial tears or rupture and valvular disruption. These injuries are life-threatening and often rapidly fatal due to circu- latory compromise from diminished function or development of car- diac tamponade. Emergent pericardiocentesis should be performed if tamponade is confirmed on ultrasound (Fig. 7.5).

Aortic disruption may occur in blunt trauma, especially those asso- ciated with rapid deceleration. Patients with aortic injury who reach the hospital tend to have incomplete lacerations, often located near the liga- mentum arteriosum. Radiographs demonstrating widened mediastinum, an obliterated aortic knob, or tracheal deviation are suggestive of aortic or other great vessel injury. Hemodynamic stability should be maintained for these patients while awaiting transfer for definitive surgical management.

Diaphragmatic Injury

Diaphragmatic injury may occur due to abrupt, compressive forces to the abdomen from blunt injury (e.g., motor vehicle collision) or pene- trating injuries. Often, these lead to diaphragmatic hernia and protrusion of abdominal contents into the thorax. Respiratory distress or scaphoid abdomen may be the presenting sign, though this is not always present. Chest radiographs and chest CT can assist in confirming the diagno- sis. Chest tubes should be placed cautiously if diaphragmatic injury is present given the risk for abdominal organ injury with tube placement. Surgical correction of diaphragmatic hernias is typically required.

ABDOMINOPELVIC TRAUMA

Approach to Care

Abdominal injuries are relatively common in children due to the large size of their abdomens relative to the rest of their bodies. Additionally,

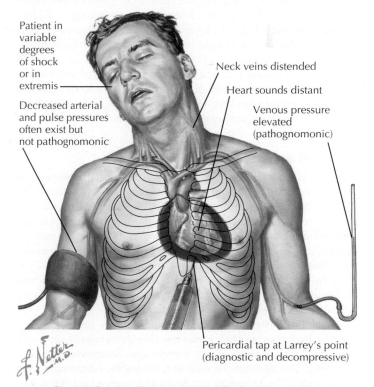

Patient in variable degrees of shock or in extremis

Decreased arterial and pulse pressures often exist but not pathognomonic

Neck veins distended

Heart sounds distant

Venous pressure elevated (pathognomonic)

Pericardial tap at Larrey's point (diagnostic and decompressive)

Fig. 7.5 Cardiac Tamponade and Pericardiocentesis.

their abdominal organs are less protected than those of adults by their rib cage and abdominal musculature. Abdominal bruising, tender- ness, rigidity, or distension should raise suspicion for intraabdominal injury. Perforation or bleeding of abdominal organs has the potential to be severe and may lead to a shock state. Clinicians should maintain a high index of suspicion for occult but clinically significant abdominal trauma, which is often missed during the initial patient assessment.

Spleen and Liver Injury

The spleen is the most commonly injured abdominal organ (Fig. 7.6). Patients with splenic lacerations may present with left upper quadrant

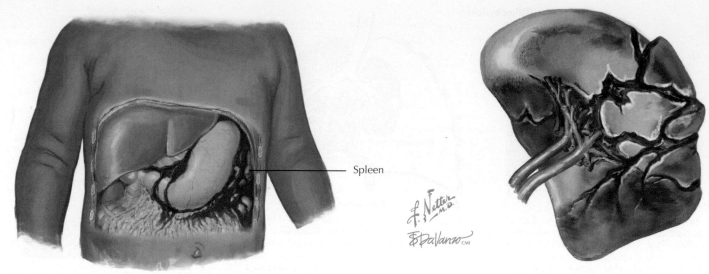

Blood surrounding spleen and spreading throughout abdominal cavity

Multiple lacerations in spleen

Fig. 7.6 Splenic Laceration.

pain that radiates to the left shoulder (Kehr sign) with or without signs of peritoneal irritation. The liver is also commonly injured in children sustaining trauma (Fig. 7.7). Liver lacerations after blunt abdominal trauma may manifest with right upper quadrant tenderness that may radiate to the right shoulder. Hemodynamically stable children with spleen or liver lacerations can be conservatively managed with bed rest and close monitoring of vital signs and hematocrit levels. Children with unstable vital signs that do not improve with aggressive volume resuscitation may require operative intervention or embolization of bleeding vessels.

Pancreas and Kidney Injury

Injury to the pancreas is less common in the pediatric population given its protected position in the abdomen compared to other organs. Thus, presence of pancreatic injury should raise suspicion of additional intraabdominal trauma. Nonspecific complaints of pain and minimal examination findings are common, and CT imaging may not capture early pancreatic trauma. Pancreatic injuries typically evolve over time—pseudocyst formation is a common complication seen in children. Rarely, children may present with peritonitis, hypovolemia, and shock from severe pancreatic injury with enzyme spillage into the intraabdominal cavity.

Renal injury should be suspected in children presenting with flank or back pain or gross hematuria (Fig. 7.8). Injuries can range from renal lacerations to kidney rupture with disruption of the urinary tract. Urinalysis can be used as screening for subtle injury, and CT or renal ultrasonography can be used to confirm and detail injuries. Management is supportive for mild injuries and operative in cases of hemodynamic instability, vasculature rupture, or urinary extravasation.

Bowel Injury

Injury to the bowel is difficult to diagnose, requiring a high degree of suspicion. Persistent abdominal pain, tenderness, or vomiting may be the only symptoms. A history of handlebar injury or the presence of a seatbelt sign (i.e., abdominal wall contusion at the location of seatbelt placement) should raise clinician suspicion of bowel involvement. Injuries to the intestines include perforation, hematomas, and mesenteric injuries. Initial radiographs may demonstrate subdiaphragmatic air, and CT scans may show pneumoperitoneum or extravasation of

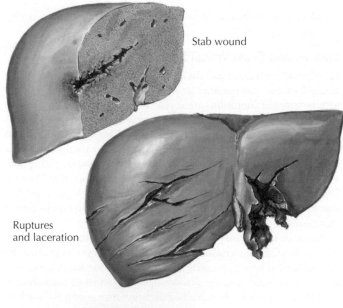

Stab wound

Ruptures and laceration

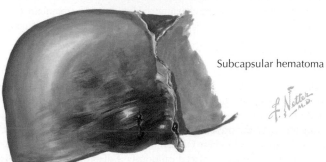

Subcapsular hematoma

Fig. 7.7 Types of Liver Injury.

contrast, but often they are normal or depict nonspecific bowel wall edema. Bowel injuries typically require surgical intervention to fully evaluate the extent of the injury and allow for repair. Late diagnosis of bowel injuries may be associated with the development of bowel necrosis and peritonitis.

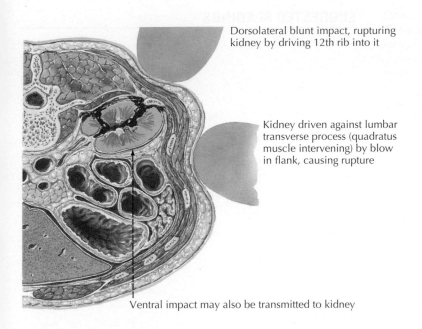

Dorsolateral blunt impact, rupturing kidney by driving 12th rib into it

Kidney driven against lumbar transverse process (quadratus muscle intervening) by blow in flank, causing rupture

Ventral impact may also be transmitted to kidney

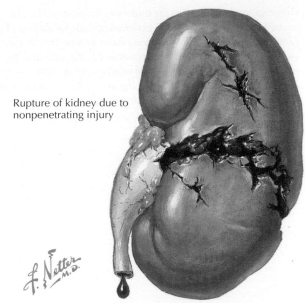

Rupture of kidney due to nonpenetrating injury

Fig. 7.8 Nonpenetrating Renal Trauma.

Pelvic Injury

Pelvic instability or focal tenderness on clinical examination suggests the possibility of open-book fractures of the pelvis. These injuries should be treated with placement of a pelvic splint to decrease the pelvic volume and the likelihood of severe hemorrhage into the pelvis. Lateral compression pelvic fractures, in contrast, are less often associated with significant blood loss and are more frequently associated with injury to the bladder and urethra. Pelvic fractures are associated with other high-impact abdominal and retroperitoneal injuries that should be considered in the full evaluation of trauma patients.

EXTREMITY TRAUMA

The extremities are at risk for musculoskeletal and neurovascular injury from trauma. Tenderness to palpation and/or visible deformity of an extremity should prompt radiologic evaluation. Further discussion of common pediatric fractures can be found in Chapter 26. Neurologic deficits may suggest either peripheral nerve injury or possible spinal or intracranial injury. Vascular disruption, especially of an artery, can lead to rapid and life-threatening blood loss that may require immediate direct pressure or tourniquet application.

BURNS

Patients presenting with traumatic injuries may be found to have burns or vice versa. For example, children sustaining thermal burns from a house fire also may have head injury from loss of consciousness related to smoke inhalation, or hypoxemia related to carbon monoxide inhalation. A thorough primary and secondary survey and simultaneous management of burns with other traumatic injuries is warranted. The management of burns is discussed further in Chapter 6.

PREVENTION

Prevention of injury should be a priority of all health care providers involved in the care of children. Opportunities exist to educate children and their families during health supervision visits as well as after minor injuries. Mixed methods can be considered, including traditional counseling, demonstration of safety techniques, and referral to available community resources. Given the breadth of injury causes and mechanisms, prevention efforts should be focused on injuries with the greatest incidence or risk for morbidity and mortality.

Motor vehicle safety has been a focus of injury prevention, and advances in child passenger safety research have led to the refinement of evidence-based child safety seat (CSS) recommendations. Current CSS recommendations are weight- and height-based, as opposed to age-based. Young children should be restrained in a rear-facing car safety seat until they reach the highest weight or height limit specified by the car seat manufacturer (in many cases for as long as 4 years). They should subsequently transition to a forward-facing CSS with an appropriate five-point harness restraint. Once they exceed the weight or height limit for a forward-facing CSS, children should transition to a belt-positioning booster seat until they can wear a vehicle's lap and shoulder belt (typically at a height of 4 feet, 9 inches or between 8 and 12 years of age). Children should ride in the vehicle's rear seat until at least 13 years of age.

Head injuries are common in the pediatric population, and appropriate safety measures should be used to reduce injury frequency and severity. Helmets should be worn during the use of bicycles, skateboards, and scooters. Organized contact sports, such as lacrosse or football, should use helmets and other associated safety equipment to protect areas of likely trauma from injury. Enactment and enforcement of rules that promote safe play should be promoted, and coaches should be educated in injury prevention.

Consumer product safety is an additional area of emphasis in injury prevention. Safety-proofing based on a child's developmental stage, such as the installation of cabinet-locking devices and stair safety gates or the removal of window blind cords, should be encouraged. Parents should be made aware of recent recalls of consumer products that pose a danger to children. Appropriate fences on all four sides with locking gates should isolate swimming pools and hot tubs.

FUTURE DIRECTIONS

Research related to pediatric trauma traditionally has been limited due to multiple factors, such as the relatively lower incidence of severe traumatic injury in children compared to adults and ethical considerations.

However, multiple studies are underway to improve the care of acutely injured children. Areas being explored include validation of point-of-care ultrasound in pediatric trauma and prospective characterization of children receiving massive transfusions. Physical and psychosocial outcomes after trauma is another emphasis of current research. There is also growing interest in analyzing and linking federal and hospital data to improve injury surveillance and epidemiologic risk assessments.

SUGGESTED READINGS

Available online.

8

Poisoning and Ingestion

Gayathri Prabhakar and Shubhi G. Goli

 CLINICAL VIGNETTE

A 6-year-old previously healthy boy is brought to the emergency department by his father for vomiting and fatigue. On history, his father notes that earlier in the week, he had high fevers and diarrhea, for which he was treated with acetaminophen every 3 hours. His father is unsure of the exact dose of acetaminophen. He has had no further fevers, and his vomiting and diarrhea improved initially, but started again today. His vital signs are normal. On examination, the patient appears tired but does stir with examination. He has right upper quadrant tenderness. He is also noted to have a petechial rash on his abdomen. Given the father's uncertainty about acetaminophen dosing, a level of the medication is sent and is found to be greater than the toxicity limit of 150 mg/dL. The child is also found to have elevations of his transaminases and of his coagulation markers. Administration of N-acetylcysteine is initiated, and the child is transferred to the intensive care unit for further management.

Poisoning is one of the most common medical emergencies in young children and adolescents. Based on the Centers for Disease Control and Prevention Childhood Injury Report, poisoning represented 5% of the unintentional injury deaths among children 0 to 19 years of age. According to the American Association of Poison Control Centers (AAPCC), there were almost 2.1 million total human exposures in 2018, of which 44% were in children younger than 5 years of age. Of these exposures, 77% were unintentional and approximately 13% to 19% were intentional and included suicide attempts.

ETIOLOGY AND PATHOGENESIS

Although there are many causes of pediatric poisoning, the most frequent causes, especially in young children, are ingestions of readily accessible household products such as cosmetics, hair products, cleaning substances, and analgesics. The incidence of adolescents participating in recreational drug use with alcohol, vaping products, opioids, and marijuana is also increasing, with associated increases in morbidity and mortality. The most lethal or potentially lethal poisonings, however, are most commonly related to pharmaceuticals, including acetaminophen, β-blockers, calcium channel blockers, oral hypoglycemics, salicylates, and tricyclic antidepressants (TCAs). The mechanism of toxicity varies from one agent to another, yet there are some classic presentations that can be seen with particular ingestions (Table 8.1). Specific ingestions are reviewed in more depth here.

Medications
Acetaminophen
Acetaminophen (or paracetamol) is the most commonly used analgesic and antipyretic in the United States. It is very safe when used at therapeutic doses, but is a very common cause of overdose, whether accidental or intentional. The primary risk from acetaminophen overdose is hepatotoxicity from the by-products of acetaminophen metabolism, which in large quantities can lead to hepatocellular damage. With acute exposures, children may be asymptomatic but may also present with nausea and vomiting, right upper quadrant pain, or lethargy and encephalopathy. Over the first day, laboratory test results may show an elevation in liver enzymes and coagulation markers, with the eventual development of liver failure over 72 to 96 hours. After obtaining a history involving timing and quantity of ingestion and examining the patient, laboratory evaluation should include performing liver and kidney function tests and obtaining electrolyte levels. Treatment involves gastric decontamination and N-acetylcysteine when the serum acetaminophen level is above threshold based on the Rumack-Matthew nomogram.

Antihypertensive Medications
Calcium channel blockers are most often used to treat hypertension, angina, migraines, and glaucoma, and they work by antagonizing L-type voltage-gated calcium channels in vascular smooth muscle and cardiac tissue. By preventing calcium influx into these cells, calcium antagonists cause vasodilatation and depression of both myocardial conduction and contractility. In large doses, this can lead to life-threatening bradycardia, heart block, and hypotension. Of note, patients may present with normal mental status, with rapid decline as cerebral perfusion decreases. After assessment of airway, breathing, and circulation (ABCs), treatment involves stabilization with fluids, glucagon, pressors, and the administration of calcium.

β-Adrenergic antagonists (or β-blockers) similarly act on receptors found on cardiomyocytes and bronchial and peripheral vasculature. Ingestion at supratherapeutic doses can lead to reduced cardiac contractility, inappropriate vasodilation, and bronchoconstriction. Patients may present with bradycardia, hypotension, altered mental status, hypoglycemia, seizures, and bronchospasm. Treatment involves stabilization with atropine for bradycardia, dextrose for hypoglycemia, pressor therapy for hypotension, and supportive care.

Salicylates
Aspirin, oil of wintergreen, and Pepto-Bismol all contain various quantities of salicylates. Salicylates work at multiple locations, including the respiratory center, the chemoreceptor trigger zone in the medulla, and the cellular level. Symptoms of salicylate poisoning include nausea, vomiting, and altered mental status. Additionally, there is often a classic laboratory finding of anion gap metabolic acidosis with respiratory alkalosis. In severe cases, patients may exhibit agitation, delirium, seizures, pulmonary edema, coma, and cardiovascular collapse. Treatment involves alkalinization with sodium bicarbonate to allow for rapid renal excretion of the salicylates and supportive care.

TABLE 8.1   Clinical Manifestations of Selected Toxic Ingestions

Ingestion	Clinical Findings
Acetaminophen	Nausea, vomiting, anorexia early in course; late findings of jaundice and liver failure
Antihistamines	Initially CNS depression but stimulation in higher doses (hyperactivity, tremors, hallucinations, seizures)
β-Blockers	Bradycardia, hypotension, coma or convulsions, hypoglycemia, bronchospasm
Calcium channel blockers	Bradycardia, hypotension, junctional arrhythmias, hyperglycemia, metabolic acidosis
Caustics	Coagulation necrosis (acid) or liquefaction necrosis (alkali), scarring, strictures, burning, dysphagia, glottic edema
Digoxin	Nausea, vomiting, visual disturbances, lethargy, electrolyte disturbances, hyperkalemia, prolonged atrioventricular dissociation and heart block, arrhythmias
Ethanol	Nausea, vomiting, stupor, anorexia; late toxicity: triad of coma, hypothermia, and hypoglycemia (especially in young children)
Ethylene glycol	CNS depression, metabolic acidosis, convulsions and coma, hypocalcemia, renal failure *Laboratory findings:* Anion gap metabolic acidosis, osmolal gap, urine oxalate crystals
Hypoglycemic agents	Hypoglycemia, coma, seizures
Iron	Hemorrhagic necrosis of GI mucosa, hypotension, hepatotoxicity, metabolic acidosis, coma, seizure, shock
Isopropyl alcohol	Altered mental status, gastritis, hypotension *Laboratory findings:* Elevated osmolal gap, ketonuria (no metabolic acidosis or hypoglycemia)
Lead	Abdominal pain, constipation, anorexia, listlessness, encephalopathy (peripheral neuropathy; rare in children), microcytic anemia
Methanol	CNS depression, delayed metabolic acidosis, optic disturbances *Laboratory findings:* Anion gap metabolic acidosis, osmolal gap
Salicylates	Tachypnea, respiratory alkalosis, metabolic acidosis, tinnitus, coagulopathy, slurred speech, seizures
Tricyclic antidepressants	Lethargy, disorientation, ataxia, urinary retention, decreased GI motility, coma, seizures *Cardiovascular alterations:* Sinus tachycardia, widened QRS complex; may progress to hypotension, ventricular dysrhythmias, cardiovascular collapse

CNS, Central nervous system; *GI,* gastrointestinal.
Compiled from Eldridge DL, Van Eyk J, Kornegay C. Pediatric toxicology. *Emerg Med Clin North Am.* 2007;15:283-308; and O'Donnell KA, Oster-houdt KC, Burns MM, Calello DP, Henretig FM, eds. *Textbook of Pediatric Emergency Medicine.* 7th ed. Philadelphia, PA: Lippincott Williams & Wilkins; 2016:1064-1111.

Oral Hypoglycemic Agents

Oral hypoglycemic agents, including sulfonylureas and metformin, stimulate insulin secretion or sensitivity. Oral hypoglycemic agents are dangerous because patients may present with a delayed clinical onset of hypoglycemia accompanied by behavior changes, irritability, seizures, weakness, and eventually coma. Toxicity can occur from ingestions of even one or two sulfonylurea pills, and therefore overnight (fasting) observation and glucose monitoring are recommended after ingestion of most sulfonylureas, in addition to treatment with dextrose-containing fluids.

Psychiatric Medications

Psychiatric medications, specifically antidepressants such as selective serotonin reuptake inhibitors (SSRIs) or TCAs, contribute to a large number of ingestions, particularly intentional ingestions. TCAs in particular have a potent anticholinergic effect that can manifest as mydriasis, urinary retention, and gastroparesis. Patients can also present with seizures. Death most often occurs from cardiotoxicity, specifically arrhythmias and hypotension. TCAs have a dose-dependent response in that ingestions less than 5 mg/kg are often asymptomatic, but fatalities can be seen with doses of 15 mg/kg and most often with doses greater than 30 mg/kg. Treatment involves gastric decontamination, cardiac stabilization with sodium bicarbonate, and seizure treatment with benzodiazepines. In comparison, SSRIs lead to significantly less morbidity unless they are involved in co-ingestions, but have the risk for precipitating serotonin syndrome or dysrhythmias.

Metals
Iron

Iron ingestions and overdose are primarily unintentional. The amount of iron in pediatric vitamins is an unlikely cause, and overdoses tend to be from exploratory ingestion by young children of prenatal vitamins and iron tablets. Toxicity depends on the concentration of elemental iron in the tablet, and ingestions of more than 60 mg/kg can be associated with toxicity. Patients may present with gastrointestinal (GI) upset, hematemesis, hepatotoxicity, metabolic acidosis, and shock. Eventually, GI scarring can lead to bowel obstruction. Treatment involves gastric decontamination and chelation with deferoxamine.

Lead

Lead can be found in paint chips, especially in American homes built before 1978, plumbing, and, in some countries, gasoline. The American Academy of Pediatrics has stated that there is no safe blood lead level. Lead interferes with multiple signal transduction pathways, leading to cell death in the central nervous system (CNS), decreased hemoglobin synthesis, and renal injury. Children may present with neurocognitive deficits (speech delay, behavioral dysregulation), abdominal pain, fatigue, or encephalopathy. After initial evaluation, treatment for low lead levels may be primarily supportive and close monitoring of lead levels but at higher concentrations may necessitate chelation therapy.

Substances of Abuse
Alcohols

Alcohols are especially dangerous toxins given how commonplace they are in household products. Although best known as the active ingredient in adult beverages such as beer, wine, and liquor, alcohols such as ethanol are also found in topical antiseptics and mouthwash. Other alcohols such as methanol and isopropyl alcohol, are commonly found in antifreeze and as a household solvent or in rubbing alcohol, respectively. Toxic effects result from the production of by-product metabolites by liver enzymes. Presentation after ingestion typically involves altered mental status, nausea, vomiting, and gait disturbance. Hypoglycemia can be seen in cases of significant ingestion, particularly in young children, given their lower glycogen stores. Anion-gap metabolic acidosis is seen with ethanol and methanol ingestion, and an osmolar gap without metabolic acidosis is seen with isopropyl alcohol. Methanol ingestion also predisposes patients to permanent blindness. Coma and death may result from all in cases of significant consumption. Treatment involves supportive care and, in severe cases, inhibition of toxic metabolite production and elimination enhancement.

Marijuana

Marijuana (THC) is the second-most commonly ingested psychoactive drug after ethanol. Recent decriminalization and legalization of the drug in many states has led to a rise in unintentional exposures in children. THC can be absorbed via the lungs with inhalation and absorbed systemically by the gut on ingestion, though the latter results in decreased bioavailability but more prolonged effects. Its clinical effects result from binding of the drug to CNS receptors. Commonly, presenting symptoms include a sense of well-being and relaxation in small quantities and hallucinations and delusions in large quantities. Patients may also report an increased appetite and demonstrate altered mood, memory, motor coordination, and perception. Physical examination often reveals conjunctival injection, tachycardia, and hypertension. Care is largely supportive.

Nicotine and E-Cigarettes

Pediatric exposure to nicotine, by both ingestion and noningestion routes, has been rising because of the recent introduction of e-cigarettes. This new method gives children, especially adolescents, an appealing, reusable, and easy-to-hide mechanism for drug intake. Clever marketing and a variety of flavors also contributes to this appeal. Given a significant lack of regulation of these products, the "per milliliter" dose of ingestion is highly variable and lethal quantities are still undetermined and can vary by product. Children may present with a variety of findings based on activation of both the sympathetic and parasympathetic nervous systems. Management involves supportive care, monitoring for seizures, and administration of atropine or scopolamine for significant cholinergic symptoms. Increasingly, the phenomenon of vaping-associated lung injury has been described; studies of this entity are ongoing, because it is unclear exactly which component of the vaping delivery mechanism is responsible.

Opioids

Opioids (e.g., codeine, morphine, oxycodone, hydrocodone, and fentanyl) are an increasingly common cause of pediatric poisoning, largely because of the ongoing opioid epidemic. Longer-acting partial opioid agonist/antagonist medications such as methadone and buprenorphine, commonly used as treatments for opioid addiction, also have become more available to children as their parents and caregivers enter medication-assisted treatment for opiate use disorder. In addition to analgesics, opioids also can be found in cough suppressants and antidiarrheal medications. Ingestions present with a classic triad of respiratory depression, miosis, and CNS depression. Management involves evaluation and securing of the ABCs and rapid administration of naloxone—an opioid antagonist—especially in cases of respiratory and CNS depression.

Household Products
Ethylene Glycol

Ethylene glycol, a common ingredient in antifreeze, is best known as the ingredient that lends a sweet taste to the product that is appealing to young children. As with other toxic alcohols, toxicity results from the production of dangerous metabolites that produce profound metabolic acidosis and calcium oxalate crystals that then deposit throughout the body. The clinical syndrome of ethylene glycol poisoning involves three stages: (1) altered mental status, nausea, vomiting, hypocalcemia, and metabolic acidosis; (2) coma and cardiopulmonary failure resulting from the metabolic acidosis; and (3) renal failure resulting from deposition of crystals. Management involves supportive care, inhibition of metabolite production, and elimination enhancement.

Household Cleaners and Caustics

Household cleaners, such as detergents, disinfectants, bleaches, and ammonia, have immense corrosive potential when they come into contact with body tissue given their acidic or alkaline nature. The recent development of single-use detergent or dishwashing pods has made these products especially appealing to young children. Acidic chemicals are often found in mineral acids and dish and drain cleaners. Histopathologic examination of the exposed tissue demonstrates superficial coagulation. On the other hand, alkalis, such as those in laundry and dishwasher detergents and drain cleaners, produce deep, penetrating liquefaction necrosis that can predispose to tissue perforation and eventual scarring and stricture formation. Patients typically present with significant dysphagia and asphyxia. Providers should have a low threshold for a diagnosis of esophageal or gastric perforation. Immediate management involves evaluation of the ABCs and ensuring airway stability, followed by evaluation of the upper GI tract.

CLINICAL PRESENTATION

Patients with poisonings may present with a wide array of clinical signs and symptoms. Most often, children present with nonspecific signs such as nausea, vomiting, and altered mental status. Depending on the exposure, patients may also have burns or rashes, alterations in their respiration, and metabolic changes that are not typically seen in more common illnesses. Nevertheless, there are characteristic clinical features, representing altered central and autonomic nervous system findings, which have been termed "toxidromes" (Table 8.2).

Several key differences in the physiology of children versus that of adults, far more than can be covered in this text, can explain why children are especially susceptible to toxins and ingestions:

- A larger ratio of surface area to body in children increases risk for dermal absorption from skin exposures.
- An increased respiratory rate and minute ventilation in children predisposes them to seeing higher doses of toxins such as carbon monoxide in a shorter time period.
- A relative lack of glycogen stores puts children at greater risk for severe hypoglycemia from drugs and medications altering glucose homeostasis such as ethanol and β-receptor antagonists.

EVALUATION

Calello and Henretig's 2014 publication summarizes the overall approach to evaluation and management of the poisoned child. As with the management of any patient, the care of the patient with suspected poisoning begins with primary and secondary surveys (Chapters 2 and 7), followed by stabilization of the ABCs and consideration of emergent therapies such as supplemental oxygen, dextrose, and naloxone. Disability, including neurologic status and pupil size and reactivity, should then be quickly evaluated. Decontamination of any ocular or skin exposures also should be performed. GI decontamination can be considered in certain cases, although this has grossly fallen out of favor given the risk for adverse effects. Once the patient has been stabilized,

TABLE 8.2	**Common Pediatric Toxidromes**	
Toxidrome	**Examples**	**Significant Clinical Findings**
Anticholinergic	Atropine Antihistamines Cyclic antidepressants	VS: ↑ T, ↑ HR, ↑ BP (↓ BP, dysrhythmias with CAs) CNS: Delirium, coma, seizures Eyes: Mydriasis (sluggishly reactive), blurred vision Skin: Flushed, hot, dry Miscellaneous: Ileus, urinary retention
Cholinergic	Organophosphorus and carbamate pesticides Military nerve agents	VS: ↑ or ↓ HR, ↑ RR (with pulmonary effects) CNS: Confusion/drowsiness to coma, seizures Eyes: Miosis, blurry vision, lacrimation Skin: Diaphoresis Miscellaneous: SLUDGE; bronchorrhea, bronchospasm, pulmonary edema; muscle fasciculations, weakness to paralysis
Sympathomimetic	ADHD medications Amphetamines Cathinones Cocaine	VS: ↑ T, ↑ HR, ↑ BP CNS: Agitation, delirium, psychosis Eyes: Mydriasis (normally reactive) Skin: Diaphoresis Miscellaneous: Tremor, myoclonus
Opioid	Prescription analgesics Antitussives Antidiarrheals Antihypertensives (clonidine) ADHD medication	VS: ↓ T, ↓ HR, ↓ BP, ↓ RR CNS: Euphoria to coma Eyes: Miosis (pinpoint pupils) Skin: Normal Miscellaneous: Hyporeflexia
Sedative-hypnotic	Anxiolytics Antiepileptics Barbiturates Benzodiazepines Muscle relaxants	VS: ↓ T, ↓ HR, ↓ BP, ↓ ↓RR CNS: Somnolence, coma Eyes: No change Skin: Normal or dry Miscellaneous: Normal or ileus

↑, Increased; ↓, decreased; *ADHD,* attention-deficit/hyperactivity disorder; *BP,* blood pressure; *CA,* cyclic antidepressants; *HR,* heart rate; *RR,* respiratory rate; *SLUDGE,* salivation, lacrimation, urination, defecation, gastric cramping, emesis; *T,* temperature; *VS,* vital signs.
Adapted from Calello DP, Henretig FM. Pediatric toxicology: specialized approach to the poisoned child. *Emerg Med Clin North Am.* 2014;32(1):29-52. https://doi.org/10.1016/j.emc.2013.09.008. PMID: 24275168.

poisonings or suspected poisonings should be reported to the local poison control center (1-800-222-1222) so they can assist with appropriate treatment and monitoring on a case-by-case basis.

Attention can then be turned to discerning what the ingestion may have been by a focused history and physical examination. Some patients may not present with a clear history of poisoning, but rather with an acute illness that does not quite fit with the history. The concern for ingestion should be raised in any child who presents with a suspicious clinical picture, particularly if the child is a toddler or adolescent. For observed or highly suspected poisonings, gathering information with respect to who, what, where, and when the incident or illness onset occurred may lead to uncovering the cause of the poisoning. It is also important to determine a patient's weight, what medications or chemicals are in the house, the timing of the incident, how much of the toxin was potentially ingested, and where the exposure took place, in terms of both where the patient was at the time and the body part(s) exposed. Adolescents with intentional ingestions should be assumed to have ingested multiple toxins—regardless of what they report—and testing should be directed accordingly. Attention also must be paid to a patient's coexisting medical conditions so they can be concurrently managed. When possible, caretakers should be asked to bring the containers of the culprit ingestion so that approximate quantity and dose can be assessed.

In addition to the history, the physical examination of a patient with a poisoning can be extremely revealing because many ingestions manifest with well-defined toxidromes (see Table 8.2). Close attention to heart rate, respiratory pattern, pupillary response, mental status,

abdominal examination, and reflexes can uncover clues to particular exposures. The laboratory workup should begin with a bedside test for blood glucose, complete blood count, electrolytes, liver function testing, and urinalysis. Studies have shown that urine and serum toxicologic studies are less important emergently but are still often part of a patient's initial evaluation. Additionally, if agents such as salicylates, acetaminophen, ethanol, methanol, ethylene glycol, digoxin, iron, lithium, or anticonvulsants are suspected, serum drug levels can be helpful for instituting the appropriate therapeutic management of the ingestion. Electrocardiography is essential for patients with cardiotoxic drug ingestion and for children with significant electrolyte or metabolic derangements that might predispose them to arrhythmias. Radiography may be helpful in patients who have or are at risk for developing aspiration or pulmonary edema.

MANAGEMENT

Treatment of a poisoning is fourfold: supportive care and stabilization, minimizing toxin exposure and absorption, enhancing elimination (when possible), and managing the sequelae of the exposure.

Supportive Care

Most pediatric poisonings, even when symptomatic, can be managed with supportive care. The provider should observe for continued stability of the ABCs and vital signs and should provide cardiac and pulse oximetry monitoring as needed. There are several methods of minimizing topical and inhaled toxin exposure, including irrigation

TABLE 8.3 Common Antidotes

Drug or Toxin	Antidote
Acetaminophen	N-Acetylcysteine
Anticholinergics	Physostigmine
Benzodiazepines	Flumazenil
β-Adrenergic blockers	Glucagon[a]
Calcium channel blockers	Calcium[a]
	High-dose insulin euglycemia (insulin and glucose)[a]
	Intravenous lipid emulsion[a]
Carbon monoxide	100% oxygen
Cholinesterase inhibitors	Atropine, pralidoxime
Cyanide	Hydroxocobalamin (preferred)
	Sodium nitrite and sodium thiosulfate
Digoxin	Digoxin immune Fab
Ethylene glycol and methanol	Fomepizole (preferred)
	Ethanol[a]
Iron	Deferoxamine
Lead	Dimercaprol (British anti-Lewisite)
	CaNa$_2$ EDTA (versenate)
	Succimer (dimercaptosuccinic acid)
Methemoglobinemic agents	Methylene blue
Opioids	Naloxone
Organophosphates and nerve agents (cholinergics)	Atropine
	Pralidoxime
Salicylates	Sodium bicarbonate
Sulfonylureas	Dextrose
	Octreotide
Tricyclic antidepressants	Sodium bicarbonate
	Intravenous lipid emulsion[a]
Warfarin (and other rodenticides)	Vitamin K$_1$

[a]Without specific U.S. Food and Drug Administration approval for this indication.

Adapted from Calello DP, Henretig FM. Pediatric toxicology: specialized approach to the poisoned child. *Emerg Med Clin North Am.* 2014;32(1):29-52. https://doi.org/10.1016/j.emc.2013.09.008. PMID: 24275168.

of exposed eyes, removal of soiled clothing followed by washing of the skin and hair, and movement of the patient to fresh air, as appropriate. Many ingestions, such as of acetaminophen, digoxin, lithium, and salicylates, also require frequent drug levels or close monitoring of organ system function. Care can and should be initiated when the child first presents to medical attention and continues through the remainder of the hospitalization. A child presenting without symptoms can likely be discharged from medical care only after the ingestion has been determined to be of negligible quantity and toxicity *and* the child has been observed for a period that accounts for the exposure's pharmacokinetics to avoid a delayed toxidrome.

Antidotes

As in cases of adult poisonings and ingestions, specific antidotes (Table 8.3) can be life-saving for the pediatric patient. These antidotes act by countering the toxin itself or its dangerous metabolites or by assisting in the toxin's removal from the body. As mentioned previously, some treatments—specifically supplemental oxygen (for patients with hypoxia, carbon monoxide exposure, or cyanide toxicity), dextrose (for hypoglycemia resulting from insulin, oral hypoglycemics, ethanol), naloxone (for opioid-induced respiratory depression), and

atropine/pralidoxime (for organophosphate poisoning)—should be considered empirically and emergently when a specific ingestion is suspected given that benefits of treatment outweigh the risk for toxicity from the antidote itself. The local poison control center is another valuable resource to help ensure adequate patient management regardless of the exposure.

Gastrointestinal Decontamination

GI decontaminants (e.g., activated charcoal, gastric lavage, dilution, syrup of ipecac, cathartics, and whole bowel irrigation) were previously the mainstay of toxic ingestions. Their mechanism entails adsorption of toxins in the gut lumen (as with activated charcoal) or elimination of toxins from the upper and lower GI tracts. Over time, these agents have fallen out of favor given the short window for administration after the exposure and possible life-threatening side effects, most notably aspiration, oxygen desaturation, arrhythmias, and electrolyte disturbances.

Excretion Enhancement and Removal

When a relatively acidic drug such as a salicylate or TCA has been ingested, sodium bicarbonate can be used to alkalinize urine, thereby increasing excretion of the drug in the urine. Urinary alkalinization also has been shown to be helpful in the excretion of barbiturates, carbamazepine, and theophylline. In patients with significant serum drug concentrations or in those who are unstable or at risk for end-organ damage and severe metabolic derangements, extracorporeal toxin removal may be considered. Hemodialysis (HD) clears toxins and their metabolites by diffusion, and convection across a permeable membrane. HD is particularly effective for removal of lithium, salicylates, and toxic alcohols. In cases in which a patient may not tolerate HD, continuous renal replacement therapy is an option. Peritoneal dialysis, exchange transfusions, and plasmapheresis are significantly less effective in the amount and rate of toxin removal.

Prevention

The majority of unintentional ingestions occur in the child's home at times when caretakers are present but there are lapses in supervision. The Poisoning Prevention Act of 1970 requires manufacturers of medications, household chemicals and other hazardous substances to ensure that all packaging and containers are child resistant. However, it is important for providers to note that "child resistant" does not mean "child proof." Box 8.1 reviews some of the most common measures on which providers can educate families to prevent household poisoning incidents, especially those in younger patients. Providers should also encourage parents and caretakers to be knowledgeable of and monitor medications and drugs accessible to adolescents. The local poison control center can and should be called for specific recommendations. Other exposure-specific advice providers may give caretakers includes:

- For exposures to the eye, rinse the eye immediately in room temperature water. Taking the child into the shower is often easiest;
- For skin exposures, any contaminated clothing must be removed and the skin should be rinsed immediately; and,
- For inhaled exposures, providers should advise the exposed to move to fresh air immediately.

FUTURE DIRECTIONS

Childhood poisonings lead to significant morbidity and mortality each year. Trends in adolescent substance abuse, especially an increase in use of opioids, marijuana, and e-cigarettes/vaping devices, have led to changes in the demographics of pediatric poisoning. If each exposure

---

BOX 8.1   **Poisoning Prevention Tips**

DO

- Buy products in child-resistant packaging when possible.
- Keep medicines and other hazardous substances out of sight and reach from children. Ensure children cannot use chairs or stack items to reach these items.
- Install safety latches on cabinets and other storage used for medicines and other household substances.
- Turn the light on and check the dose before administering medications.
- Monitor the use of prescription and nonprescription medications by children and teenagers, such as those for attention-deficit disorders, mental health illness, painkillers, antihistamines, and cold/cough medications.
- Keep the toll-free Poison Help number (1-800-222-1222) on hand and encourage families and other caretakers to program it into their phones.

NEVER

- Transfer medicines and substances to an easy-to-open container.
- Store food and medications and household substances in the same location.
- Leave medicines and hazardous substance containers open or unattended during interrupted use or at a child's bedside.
- Use household utensils to measure medication. Instead, use the device included with the medication.
- "Borrow" friends' medications or take old medications.

Adapted from Poison Prevention Week Council 2015 poster, part of Health Resources & Services Administration. http://www.poisonprevention.org/50plusWaysToPreventPoisonings.pdf.

or possible exposure is called into the local poison control center, public health measures can be focused on the areas that currently lead to the most morbidity and mortality with respect to pediatric poisonings. Efforts then can be aimed at reducing such exposures by instituting safety mechanisms on potentially dangerous substances. One such effective innovation was the creation of child-resistant pill bottle caps, which are difficult for young children to open. Additional interventions need to be made to further reduce exposure to the more common household products, including cosmetics, household cleaners, and personal care products, because these currently make up the majority of pediatric poisonings. Furthermore, there exists quite a bit of gray area around issues such as optimal gastric decontamination or antidote therapy.

For example, a new life-saving intervention being studied includes intravenous lipid emulsion, which has shown success with the clearance of lipophilic drugs such as anesthetics, calcium channel blockers, and TCAs. More data are needed to better define when this intervention should be considered and to characterize side effects in acute use. Additional basic and clinical research, combined with public health efforts, can work to help minimize the morbidity and mortality that currently surround pediatric poisonings.

SUGGESTED READINGS

Available online.

9

Brief Resolved Unexplained Event and Sudden Infant Death Syndrome

Andrew S. Kern-Goldberger

✳ CLINICAL VIGNETTE

A 3-month-old male infant born at 38 weeks' gestation and with no prior medical issues is brought to the emergency department (ED) by emergency medical services (EMS) because he "turned blue" and had "slow breathing" for approximately 20 seconds at home. He was lying supine in his crib but awake at the time of the event and had last breastfed 1 hour before. His mother witnessed the episode and reports that her son was "out of it" and she "thought he was dying" during this time, prompting her to call 911. After crying for approximately 1 minute, the infant was "back to himself," displaying his baseline color and breathing, so no intervention was required when EMS arrived at his home. He has experienced no recent illnesses, and his mother describes his home environment as safe with no other caregivers aside from herself and the infant's father.

In the ED, the infant is well-appearing with age-appropriate vital signs. On history, the physician does not elicit any clear explanation for the event, and there are no concerning features on physical examination.

This infant would meet criteria for a low-risk, brief resolved unexplained event (BRUE) according to the American Academy of Pediatrics guidelines. The team caring for this infant may consider performing a 12-lead electrocardiogram, testing for pertussis infection, and briefly monitoring the infant with visual observation and continuous pulse oximetry. Clinicians should provide education about BRUEs and cardiopulmonary resuscitation training resources to the caregivers of infants who experience BRUE and should arrange close follow-up with primary care pediatricians.

BRIEF RESOLVED UNEXPLAINED EVENT

In 2016 the American Academy of Pediatrics (AAP) created a clinical practice guideline that defined, risk-stratified, and provided management recommendations for the clinical presentation newly described as a brief resolved unexplained event (BRUE). This nomenclature replaced a clinical presentation previously referred to as an Apparent Life-Threatening Event (ALTE), which encompassed a broad range of frightening events of sudden onset affecting infants of unspecified age. The criteria for ALTE relied on the subjective description of the caregiver and were frequently thought to reflect near-missed deadly events. In contrast, BRUE is a more narrowly and objectively defined term, consisting of "an event occurring in infants younger than 12 months of age that is described by the observer as brief (lasting less than one minute, but typically <20 to 30 seconds), resolved (meaning the patient returned to baseline state of health after the event), and with a reassuring history, physical examination, and vital signs at the time of clinical evaluation by trained medical providers."

Although epidemiologic measures of BRUE are lacking due to the recent establishment of this definition, the incidence of ALTE has been reported as ranging from 0.6 to 5.0 per 1000 live births, and 0.6% to 1.7% of emergency department (ED) visits by infants. The post-ALTE mortality has been estimated as 1 in 800 infants, and the mortality rate is anticipated to be lower in infants presenting with a BRUE, given its narrower definition.

Etiology and Pathogenesis

By definition, an event is characterized as a BRUE only if there is no identifiable explanation. The most frequently identified problems, which must be excluded before characterizing an event as a BRUE, include gastroesophageal reflux, lower respiratory tract infections, urinary tract infections, seizures, nonaccidental head trauma, and inborn errors of metabolism. The diagnosis of child abuse, in particular, is very difficult to make and is highly consequential, because a growing body of evidence suggests that victims of child abuse are likely to present with unexplained events and higher-than-expected mortality. It is therefore essential for providers to consider the possibility of nonaccidental trauma before labeling an event as a BRUE, including maintaining awareness of any inconsistencies between the history and the infant's developmental stage.

Clinical Presentation

As an infant presenting with BRUE is, by definition, asymptomatic at the time of presentation, a detailed history and physical examination are essential to understanding the nature of the event. For instance, a history of fever or rhinorrhea may suggest an upper respiratory tract infection, which would disqualify the event as a BRUE and would prompt evaluation and management for the specific cause under consideration. Normal infant behaviors such as irregular breathing during rapid eye movement (REM) sleep, periodic breathing, respiratory pauses (5 to 15 seconds), and transient coughing or gagging during feeding also may be misinterpreted as abnormal and may be presented by caregivers as the primary cause of concern. Historical features to elicit from the caregiver include:

- **General description.**
- **Who reported and witnessed the event.** Are the historian(s) reliable?
- **Infant's state immediately before the event.** Awake or asleep? Feeding? In what position (supine, prone, upright, sitting)? Playing with any objects?
- **Infant's state during the event.** Was the infant choking or gagging? Active or quiet? Conscious? Were there any movements or changes in breathing, muscle tone, skin color, or lip color?
- **End of the event.** How long did the event last? How did it stop? What treatment if any was provided by the caregiver? Was 911 called?

- **Infant's state after event.** Is the infant back to baseline? Before return to baseline, what did the infant look like?
- **Recent history.** Were there any preceding illnesses or injuries?
- **Medical history.**
- **Family history.** Any history of sudden unexplained death in first- or second-degree family members before age 35, BRUE in sibling, family member(s) with long QT syndrome, arrhythmia, inborn errors of metabolism, or developmental delay?
- **Environmental history.** What type of housing does the family live in; is there exposure to tobacco smoke or other environmental hazards?
- **Social history.** Any recent family changes or stressors? Any history of child protective services or law enforcement involvement? What support systems do the family have in place?

As stated previously, to be defined as a BRUE, the unexplained event must last less than 1 minute, be resolved on arrival to care, and have a reassuring history. The infant must have normal examination findings and normal vital signs on presentation. In addition, the episode should be characterized by one or more of the following:

- **Cyanosis or pallor.** Redness is specifically excluded because it may be associated with normal behaviors such as coughing, crying, and straining.
- **Absent, decreased, or irregular breathing.** This should be differentiated from choking or gagging, which may suggest gastroesophageal reflux as a cause.
- **Marked change in tone.** This may include hypertonia (e.g., the infant appears rigid) or hypotonia (e.g., the infant appears limp).
- **Altered responsiveness.**

Evaluation and Management

Once it is determined that an infant has experienced a BRUE, it is important to differentiate whether the infant meets the lower risk guidelines established by the AAP or is at higher risk. An event can be classified as lower risk if there are no concerning findings after a full history and physical examination; if the infant is older than 60 days, 32 weeks or older gestational age, and 45 weeks or older corrected gestational age; if the infant did not receive cardiopulmonary resuscitation (CPR) by a trained medical provider; and the event occurred for the first time with a duration of less than 1 minute (Box 9.1). Infants meeting all these criteria are less likely to have a serious underlying condition or to have recurrent episodes that would place them at risk for morbidity or mortality. Accordingly, the AAP guidelines recommend minimal further evaluation for infants with lower-risk BRUEs. For infants at lower risk, the guidelines state that providers should (1) educate caregivers about BRUEs and engage in shared decision-making to guide evaluation, disposition, and follow-up and (2) offer resources for CPR training to the caregiver, providing critical skills for families to respond to emergent events at home. The guidelines do suggest considering testing for pertussis infection based on potential exposures, vaccine history, community prevalence, and testing availability and to consider performing a

Data from Tieder J, Bonkowsky J, Etzel R, et al. Brief resolved unexplained events (formerly apparent life-threatening events) and evaluation of lower-risk infants. *Pediatrics.* 2016;137(5):e1-32, Fig. 1.

12-lead electrocardiogram (ECG) because of the noninvasive nature of this test and the risks associated with undiagnosed cardiac disease. Per the guidelines, providers also may consider a brief period of monitoring (1 to 4 hours) with continuous pulse oximetry and close observation. However, the guidelines discourage hospitalization of infants with lower-risk BRUEs solely for cardiorespiratory monitoring (Box 9.2).

In contrast, a patient at higher risk—one who does not meet all criteria for the lower-risk classification—may warrant a more extensive evaluation. Although no society-endorsed guidelines exist that standardize the management of these patients, an expert panel published a framework for the evaluation of high-risk BRUEs in 2019. The panel suggests that an initial evaluation include at least 4 hours of continuous pulse-oximetry monitoring and bedside feeding evaluations; an ECG, respiratory viral panel, and pertussis testing (especially if the infant is underimmunized and/or has potential exposures); and blood hematocrit, glucose, venous blood gas, and lactate. If child maltreatment is suspected, additional workup may include social work assessment, child abuse expert consultation, and imaging. If this evaluation is unavailable in the setting where the child presents, or if the evaluation takes place without an explanation for the event, hospital admission is warranted to facilitate completion of the workup. Inpatient evaluation may include:

- Videofluoroscopic swallowing study to detect silent dysphagia not detected on bedside feeding evaluation;
- Prolonged electroencephalogram (at least 12 to 24 hours); and
- Comprehensive polysomnography, which can detect and differentiate central and obstructive apnea.

If there is no pathologic explanation for the event found within 24 hours of admission and there are no repeat events while admitted, the patient may be discharged home with close primary care follow-up and caregiver guidance.

Future Directions

Additional research is needed to define the pathophysiology of BRUE. Large multicenter, prospective studies are needed to better delineate the characteristics of the small subgroup of infants with higher-risk BRUEs who may have an associated serious condition, so that invasive testing can be better targeted. Additionally, larger studies are needed to validate the specific evaluation for infants with higher-risk BRUEs to determine which are most predictive of an underlying condition.

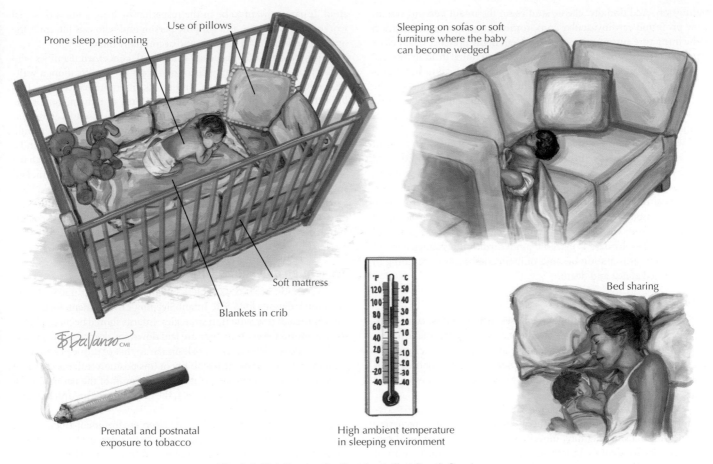

Fig. 9.1 Risk Factors for Sudden Infant Death Syndrome.

SUDDEN INFANT DEATH SYNDROME

Sudden unexpected infant death (SUID) is defined as a sudden, unexpected death occurring during infancy. Sudden infant death syndrome, or SIDS, is a subcategory of these cases in which the cause of death remains unexplained despite a complete investigation, including history, examination, autopsy, and death scene investigation. SIDS accounts for approximately half of SUID cases; other common causes include suffocation, asphyxia, and trauma.

SIDS is the leading cause of infant mortality between 1 month and 1 year of age in the United States and is responsible for over 1900 US infant deaths annually. In a study by the National Institute of Child Health and Development, the median age for SIDS deaths was 11 weeks; the peak incidence was between 2 and 4 months, and 90% occurred before 6 months of age. The SIDS rate in industrialized countries varies from 0.1 to 0.8 per 1000 infants. Preterm infants are at higher risk for SIDS than term infants, with the postmenstrual age of peak vulnerability for SIDS occurring 4 to 6 weeks earlier among preterm than term infants. The risk for SIDS is also over twice as high among non-Hispanic African American and American Indian/Alaskan Native infants compared to non-Hispanic white infants. The risk for SIDS is also higher in infants born to women who smoked during pregnancy and in infants born to very young mothers.

Etiology and Pathogenesis

The most recent research suggests that SIDS is a multifactorial condition that includes genetic, environmental, behavioral, and sociocultural factors. Well-established modifiable risk factors for SIDS include prone sleep positioning; use of pillows, soft mattresses, or blankets in cribs; sleeping on sofas or other soft furniture in which the infant could become wedged; bed sharing; high ambient temperature in the sleeping environment; and prenatal and postnatal exposure to tobacco (Fig. 9.1).

For many years, an ALTE was thought to be the predecessor of SIDS. However, several factors argue against a causal relationship between ALTE/BRUE and SIDS. Most notably, the timing of ALTE events versus SIDS deaths is distinctly different. Of SIDS deaths, 80% occur between midnight and 6 AM, whereas 82% of ALTE episodes occur between 8 AM and 8 PM. Additionally, in a prospective study that enrolled 300 infants with ALTE, no infant died during hospital stay or within 72 hours of discharge and none was diagnosed with serious bacterial infection (bacterial meningitis, bacteremia, or urinary tract infection). Furthermore, on review of effective preventive measures, interventions proven to reduce the incidence of SIDS by 30% to 50% (most notably supine sleep position) have not decreased the incidence of ALTE. In fact, the vast majority of SIDS victims do not experience ALTE before death. Further analysis reveals that prior ALTE episodes were reported in only 5% of SIDS victims.

Because SIDS does not appear to occur beyond infancy, emerging evidence suggests that underlying brain immaturity may play a role in its pathogenesis. As noted earlier, the highest incidence of SIDS occurs between the second and fourth months of life, a period of intensive developmental changes in ventilatory, cardiac, and sleep–wake patterns in normal infants. The coincidence of timing suggests that infants are vulnerable to sudden death during a critical period of autonomic maturation. Additionally, classic studies on the infant nervous system show profound cardiovascular compromise in infants on stimulation of the immature autonomic nervous system in the presence of apnea or hypoxia during sleep. This compromise was not noted in adult models. Currently, abnormalities in neurologic serotonin signaling and brainstem functioning, genetic polymorphisms interacting with specific environmental risk factors, and alterations in inflammatory cytokines due to recent viral infections and/or bacterial colonization are focuses of ongoing research.

The final common pathway that seems to explain most cases of SIDS involves (1) a life-threatening event that causes asphyxia and brain hypoperfusion (e.g., rebreathing exhaled gases in prone position, gastroesophageal regurgitation causing obstructive apnea or activation of laryngeal receptors causing reflex apnea), (2) failure of arousal in response to asphyxia so that the infant does not turn his or her head and recover from the apnea, (3) hypoxic coma as a consequence of the continued asphyxia, (4) extreme bradycardia and gasping, and (5) failure of autoresuscitation because of ineffectual gasping, resulting in uninterrupted apnea and death.

Clinical Presentation

SIDS is a diagnosis of exclusion. Diagnoses that should be considered in suspected SIDS cases include accidental or nonaccidental trauma, congenital adrenal hyperplasia, cardiac arrhythmia, prolonged QT syndrome, cardiomyopathy, congenital heart defects, inherited metabolic disorders (e.g., fatty acid oxidation disorders), pneumonia, and sepsis.

A family that has experienced one SIDS death has a 2% to 6% risk of another SIDS death in a subsequent child. In the case of recurrent SIDS deaths in a single family, inherited disorders must be ruled out. Although nonaccidental trauma and homicide are rare, they must remain on the differential when evaluating the cause of infant death, particularly with a subsequent sudden unexpected death in a family or with a single caregiver (see Chapter 10).

Evaluation and Management

First-response teams should be trained to make observations at the scene, including the position of the infant, any marks on the body, body temperature and rigor, type of bed and position of clothing and bedding, room temperature, type of ventilation and heating, and reactions of caregivers.

An infant coming to the ED in cardiopulmonary arrest should be managed as per the principles of Pediatric Advanced Life Support (PALS) with a period of well-executed CPR. During this period, the patient's history should be reviewed with emergency medical services and with the parent, if they are available; the infant should be examined thoroughly with a primary and secondary survey. The examination should include evaluation for signs of prolonged death such as rigor mortis, corneal clouding, and dependent lividity. The infant should be transferred to the pediatric intensive care unit if resuscitative efforts achieve cardiorespiratory stability. Infants who arrive in the ED in asystolic arrest have a poor prognosis. Prolonged resuscitation efforts lasting beyond 20 minutes without return of spontaneous circulation are usually futile in the absence of treatable problems such as hypothermia, drug overdose, or shockable cardiac dysrhythmia. The team leader should make the diagnosis of death and should decide about discontinuation of resuscitative efforts based on the previously mentioned factors.

Family presence in the resuscitation room is becoming the norm in pediatric EDs. Many parents want to be with their children during what may be the last moments of life, and it is often meaningful for them to observe that ED staff have done all that is possible to resuscitate their child. If parents want to be in the resuscitation area, a nurse or social worker who can serve as a support person and who can interpret the ongoing resuscitative efforts should accompany them.

The loss of an infant is devastating for all concerned. Families who suffer a loss from SIDS may encounter a police investigation, a waiting period for autopsy results, and a lack of emotional closure. It is important for the professional response teams to remain supportive, empathic, and nonjudgmental while obtaining essential information surrounding the death of the infant. Emotional support should be offered to the caregivers in the ED by both the medical staff and a social worker or a grief counselor. The parents may be informed that a SIDS death happens quickly and silently without causing any pain and suffering to the infant. Additionally, a well-prepared ED should have a plan in place for issues such as bereavement measures, postmortem care, support for surviving siblings, and notification of medicolegal authorities, the infant's pediatrician, and any referring physicians and consultants.

Prevention and Future Directions

The prevention of SIDS, as outlined by the AAP in their updated 2016 Recommendations for a Safe Infant Sleeping Environment, focuses on environmental risk reduction strategies. Infants should be placed in the supine position every time they are laid down for sleep. Placing infants on their side for sleep carries a risk similar to that of prone positioning, presumably because of the instability of this position (infants are more likely to roll into the prone position). As a result of the national Back to Sleep campaign launched in 1994, the SIDS rate in the United States has fallen by more than 50%.

In addition to sleep position, the sleep environment (inclusive of sleep surface, sleepwear, bedding, and the incidence of co-sleeping) affects the risk for SIDS. It is recommended that infants sleep on a firm surface that abides by Consumer Product Safety Commission (CPSC) standards, such as on a crib mattress covered with a fitted sheet. It is imperative to avoid loose bedding (including blankets and nonfitted sheets) or soft objects (including pillows and toys) in the bassinet or crib, because these increase the risk for suffocation, strangulation, and entrapment. Ideally for the first year of life—but at least for the first 6 months of life—infants should sleep in a shared room, but on a separate surface designed for infants. Bed sharing has benefits such as bonding and promoting breastfeeding, but it has been linked to higher rates of both SIDS, especially if the infant is younger than 4 months of age or is born with prematurity or low birth weight and if either parent smokes, drinks alcohol before bedtime, or is using prescription or illicit drugs. Additionally, sharing a sofa or armchair confers a particularly high risk for SIDS.

Studies have demonstrated a protective effect of pacifier use in infants against SIDS, even when the pacifier falls out of the infant's mouth while sleeping. The mechanism has not been confirmed, but it is hypothesized that it may lower the arousal threshold and improve autonomic control in sleeping infants. The AAP therefore recommends that caregivers consider offering a pacifier at naptime and at bedtime, though this may be delayed for breastfed infants until breastfeeding is firmly established. Overheating the infant's sleep room should be avoided because it increases the SIDS risk; however, there is insufficient evidence to suggest that use of a fan in the room is an effective risk-reduction strategy. The AAP also recommends avoidance of maternal smoking and alcohol and illicit drug use before and after pregnancy; conversely, the AAP recommends breastfeeding or giving expressed breast milk for as much and as long as possible and ensuring administration of routine childhood immunizations. Finally, the updated 2016 AAP recommendations advise that home cardiorespiratory monitoring should not be prescribed to prevent SIDS in infants, including infants born preterm and those with a sibling who died of SIDS, because there is no evidence suggesting that monitor use reduces the risk for SIDS. These devices may lead to false reassurance or, conversely, false alarms that lead to unnecessary anxiety and health care usage.

Future Directions

Additional research is needed to further elucidate the underlying pathophysiology of SIDS, which can help identify infants most at-risk and target effective preventive measures. Because there has been no decrease in the SIDS rate since 2006 and racial and ethnic disparities persist, future work also must be directed toward optimizing educational efforts for SIDS prevention.

SUGGESTED READINGS

Available online.

10

Child Abuse and Neglect

Annie Laurie Gula

 CLINICAL VIGNETTE

An 11-month-old girl is brought to the emergency department with a chief complaint of crying. She was noted to be crying more than usual after being picked up from her grandparents' home today, where she stays when her parents are at work. On examination, she is fussy but consolable by her mother, cruising and crawling around the room, and drinking her bottle. There are three bruises: one on her left ear, one on her left upper arm, and one on her left chest. She undergoes a skeletal survey, where a left humerus fracture and two healing rib fractures are diagnosed. Parathyroid hormone, 25-OH vitamin D, transaminases, amylase, and lipase are all within normal limits. A report is filed with child protective services because of concern for physical child abuse.

Child maltreatment may present with subtle findings or complaints, as with this patient with increased fussiness and crying. Health care providers must maintain a high index of suspicion for child abuse or maltreatment and should include these in the differential diagnosis. Particularly for young infants who cannot communicate effectively, evaluation should look for acute and chronic injuries, including skin lesions, fractures, intraabdominal trauma, and neurologic complications. Health care providers are mandated reporters of concerns for child maltreatment. Early diagnosis and referral are important to prevent further injury and connect children and families with resources to support their safety.

Child maltreatment is defined as any act or failure to act on the part of a parent or caregiver that results in death, serious physical or emotional harm, or sexual abuse or exploitation of a child or as an act or failure to act that presents an imminent risk for serious harm to a child. In the most recent U.S. Department of Health and Human Services report, 4.3 million reports were filed involving 7.8 million children in the United States in 2018. The annual rate of confirmed child abuse and/or neglect is approximately 9.2 cases per 1000 children in the United States. Rates of child abuse and neglect are likely higher than this reported number, because of the difficulty of diagnosis and the tendency to underreport. Notably, 17% of US adults report a history of abuse in their own childhoods, and 20% of children who present with abusive fractures have seen at least one provider before being diagnosed with nonaccidental trauma.

The consequences of child maltreatment are significant and may include death, injury, and poor long-term health outcomes related to adverse childhood experiences. In 2018 there were 1770 deaths resulting from child abuse and/or neglect. Additionally, it is important to note that the diagnosis of child abuse and neglect is inherently influenced by bias. Despite the majority of perpetrators being white, children of color are more likely to be referred for evaluation than white children. To ensure that health care providers are advocating for and protecting children and their families in an equitable fashion, it is important to have a standardized approach to evaluating children for maltreatment.

TYPES OF MALTREATMENT

Several different types of child maltreatment have been defined. In the United States, each state has specific laws defining each type of maltreatment (Table 10.1). It is important for providers to be familiar with the law of the state(s) in which they practice, because they may vary slightly.

RISK FACTORS

Any child of any socioeconomic status, race, ethnicity, or gender may be a victim of child maltreatment. However, several risk factors have been defined that are associated with child abuse and neglect (Table 10.2). These risk factors should be used in identifying patients that may benefit from support services; however, they should not be used for screening or risk stratification. As earlier, it is important to be aware of how bias may be implicated in child abuse reporting.

DIAGNOSIS

The diagnosis of child maltreatment relies on a comprehensive history and physical examination and an appropriate index of suspicion because presentations are often nonspecific. Laboratory studies and imaging are helpful in supporting the diagnosis and ruling out other pathologic conditions.

History

Child maltreatment often presents with vague complaints. Common presenting symptoms for all types of child maltreatment include difficulties with school performance, behavior changes and/or developmental regression, or sleep disturbances. Additionally, caregivers may note that the child acts fearful around or attempts to avoid certain adults. Child victims of sexual abuse may present with genitourinary complaints; caregivers may note encopresis, dysuria, or other genital pain or symptoms.

There are several historical details that can serve as "red flags" for child maltreatment. Concerning findings on history include an inappropriate delay in seeking care for an injury or illness, as well as details of the history that change with multiple retellings. Alternatively, a history of seeking care from many different providers or of portraying a child as more ill than the child is perceived to be by the provider may be concerning, especially if the behavior is recurrent. Similarly, a caregiver insisting that a child's illness does not respond to typical

TABLE 10.1   Types of Child Maltreatment Defined

Type of Maltreatment	Definition
Physical abuse	Nonaccidental injury to child by caregiver act or omission
Sexual abuse	Exposure to sexual stimulation inappropriate for age, cognitive development, or position in relationship (includes nonconsensual sexual contact, incest, and rape)
Psychological abuse	Injury to the psychological capacity or emotional stability of a child with resulting change in behavior, cognition, or mental health
Neglect	Inadequate provision of food, medical care, housing, clothing, hygiene, and/or educational support; abandonment is the most extreme form
Medical abuse	Inappropriate use of medical care in a way that harms the child: "Factitious disorder imposed on another," in which caregivers invent, exaggerate, or cause symptoms in children to seek unnecessary medical treatment *OR* "Medical neglect," in which caregivers either do not seek care or do not follow medical advice
Human trafficking	Exploitation for sex, labor, or other services; does not necessitate that a child is physically moved from one location to another

TABLE 10.2   Risk Factors for Child Maltreatment

Child-Related Factor	Parent-Related Factor	Environment (Community and Society)
Emotional/behavioral difficulties	Low self-esteem	Social isolation
Chronic illness	Poor impulse control	Poverty
Physical disabilities	Substance abuse/alcohol abuse	Unemployment
Preterm birth	Young maternal or paternal age	Low educational achievement
Unwanted	Abused as a child	Single-parent home
Unplanned	Depression or other mental illness	Non–biologically related male living in the home
	Poor knowledge of child development or unrealistic expectations for child	Family or intimate partner violence
	Negative perceptions of normal child behavior	

Reused with permission from Flaherty EG, Stirling J Jr; American Academy of Pediatrics, Committee on Child Abuse and Neglect. Clinical report: the pediatrician's role in child maltreatment prevention. *Pediatrics.* 2010;126(4):833-841Table 1, page 834. https://doi.org/10.1542/peds.2010-2087. PMID: 20945525.

therapies and/or insisting that a child should undergo multiple painful or unnecessary procedures is concerning for medical child abuse. Importantly, health care providers should be aware of history that is not compatible with physical findings. Examples include "mysterious" injuries that appear without an inciting event, significant injuries with a relatively minor inciting event, or a reported mechanism of injury that is not physiologically consistent with physical examination findings or with the child's developmental capabilities.

In cases in which there is concern for child maltreatment, it is important to elicit the history with care. When possible, health care providers should partner with members of an interdisciplinary team who can provide support to the child and family. Providers also should be conscious of ensuring privacy and providing reassurance. In collecting the history, providers should avoid repeated and extensive questioning to minimize child distress. As a means to prevent bias and to protect the child, the interdisciplinary team should include a professional who has experience with forensic interviewing. A forensic interview is a structured discussion with a child with the goal of eliciting details about something that the child may have experienced or witnessed. The goals of forensic interviewing are to ensure the safety of the child and to gather information that may contribute to a criminal investigation. Professionals trained in forensic interviewing have skills that allow them to talk with children in developmentally appropriate language while introducing as little bias or influence as possible.

Providers should work with forensic interviewers to determine the details of the abuse that are necessary for acute management and safety. Important details to determine include:

- last contact with the alleged perpetrator, and
- other minors to whom the alleged perpetrator may have access.

If there is concern for sexual abuse:

- if the child has showered, bathed, and/or changed clothes since the last contact with the alleged perpetrator; and
- if the child has urinated or defecated since the last contact with the alleged perpetrator.

Of note, the forensic interview process often takes several sessions and occurs over the course of weeks to months.

Physical Examination

Often, signs of child maltreatment will be identified on physical examination. Particularly in children younger than 5 years, it is important to perform a full physical examination (including an examination of the skin) at each encounter, regardless of the chief complaint. With every patient encounter, it is important to partner with the patient and the patient's caregiver(s) and to ensure that the examination is private and respectful. When examining a child with concern for maltreatment, minimizing the number of examinations can help minimize the risk for further traumatizing the child. Providers should be conscious and precise in their documentation, because notes may be used in criminal investigations. Injuries should be described carefully, and, whenever possible, photos should be taken with a ruler for size.

As with the history, there are several findings on physical examination that are "red flags" for child maltreatment. Injury with severity that is out of proportion to the described mechanism and injury with an unknown or "magical" mechanism are concerning for nonaccidental trauma. Injuries in different stages of healing, such as cuts, bruises, or burns, could be

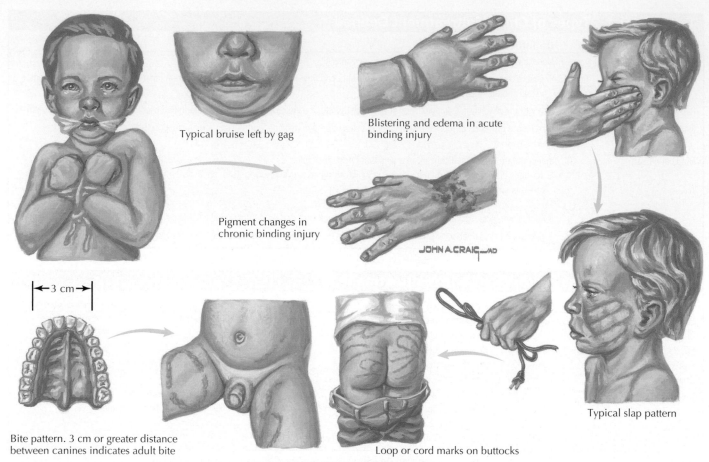

Typical bruise left by gag

Blistering and edema in acute binding injury

Pigment changes in chronic binding injury

JOHN A. CRAIG—MD

|← 3 cm →|

Bite pattern. 3 cm or greater distance between canines indicates adult bite

Loop or cord marks on buttocks

Typical slap pattern

Fig. 10.1 Child Abuse Injury Patterns.

concerning for multiple inflicted injuries over time. Injuries that do not fit with a patient's stage of development are also concerning. For example, any bruises in a child who is not yet walking or cruising would be inconsistent with normal development. Once a child becomes more mobile, bruises from accidental injuries are often on bony prominences such as the shins or glabella, whereas bruises from inflicted injuries may be found on the trunk, ears, neck, or fleshy parts of the extremities. Geographic patterns of injuries, such as circular burns from cigarettes, handprints from a slap, bite marks, or "glove and stocking" burns from hands and feet being dipped in scalding water, are cause for further investigation for inflicted injury (Fig. 10.1). Additionally, tattoos may be a sign that a patient has been marked as property by a trafficker, pimp, or madame.

When there is concern for sexual abuse, it is particularly important that the examination is conducted in a sensitive and private manner. Whenever possible, a provider who is specialized in the management of sexual abuse, rape, and trauma should assist in performing and documenting the physical examination. A careful perineal-genital examination should be completed with the child in the frog-legged, supine, or knees-to-chest position. Providers should be sure to carefully examine the introitus, hymenal ring, and labia in girls and the scrotum and penis in boys for bruises, lacerations, abrasions, scars, or other injuries. The anus also should be examined for fissures, scarring, and loss of tone (Fig. 10.2). Invasive examinations, such as anoscopy or speculum examinations, are rarely indicated. If such examinations are indicated because of pelvic injury or severe anal injury or pain, they should take place under anesthesia with a trained specialist.

Typical findings on physical examination by system are listed in Table 10.3.

MANAGEMENT

Further Evaluation

Once a concern for child maltreatment is raised, further evaluation with laboratory studies and imaging is often indicated to identify complications of maltreatment, to evaluate for occult injury, and to rule out underlying pathologic conditions that may masquerade as abuse (e.g., metabolic bone disease in the case of a child with multiple fractures).

With signs of abuse, a skeletal survey is indicated in all children under the age of 2 years. Skeletal injuries are often the strongest radiologic indicators of abuse. Fractures with high specificity for physical abuse include metaphyseal, rib, scapular, spinous process, and sternum fractures. Other concerning findings include epiphyseal separations, vertebral body fractures and subluxations, digital fractures, complex skull fractures, the presence of multiple fractures, or of fractures of varying ages and/or stages of healing (Fig. 10.3).

Children under the age of 7 years should undergo additional workup to evaluate for intraabdominal trauma with complete blood count, complete metabolic panel, pancreatic enzymes, and urinalysis. In children older than 7 years of age, these additional tests are indicated if the child reports abdominal pain, dysuria, or having experienced trauma to the abdomen or trunk (Fig. 10.4).

Additional workup may be pursued specific to the patient's presentation. For example, if a fracture is discovered, the patient should undergo evaluation for disorders of bone metabolism, including measurements of calcium, magnesium, phosphorus, alkaline phosphatase, intact parathyroid hormone, and 25-OH vitamin D. If bruising or intracranial hemorrhage are discovered, the patient should undergo

Signs of sexual abuse

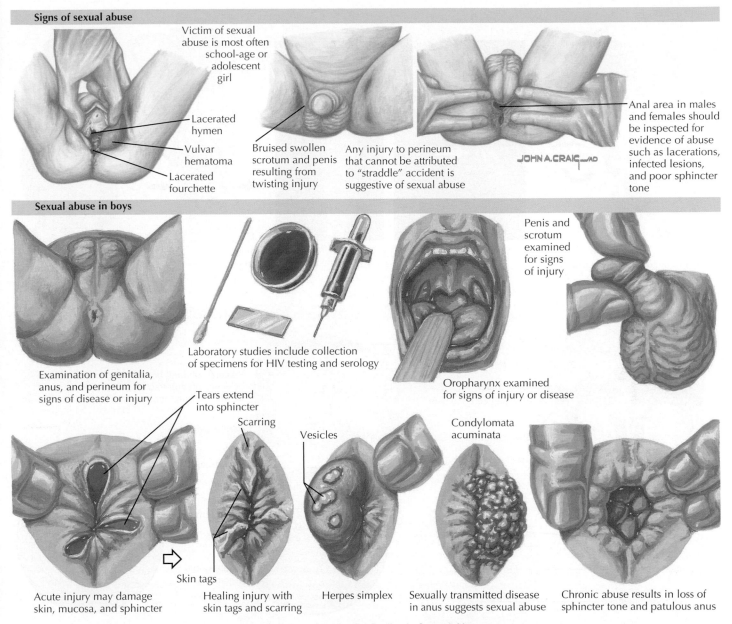

Fig. 10.2 Examination for Pediatric Sexual Abuse.

TABLE 10.3	Physical Examination Findings by System Concerning for Maltreatment
Body System	**Findings on Physical Examination**
General	Behavior disturbances, fear of parent, developmentally inappropriate affection with examiner, parental aloofness
Neurologic	Irritability, seizure, altered mental status
Oral	Frenulum tear
Skin	Bruises (especially those not over bony prominences), scars, lacerations, abrasions, burns
Musculoskeletal	Refusal to bear weight, deformity
Abdominal	Evidence of malnutrition with scaphoid or protuberant abdomen, acute abdomen
Genitourinary	Labial, introital, hymenal, or vaginal lacerations; labial, scrotal, or penile bruising; anal fissures; loss of anal sphincter tone; anal scarring
Ophthalmologic	Subconjunctival and/or retinal hemorrhages

Fractures

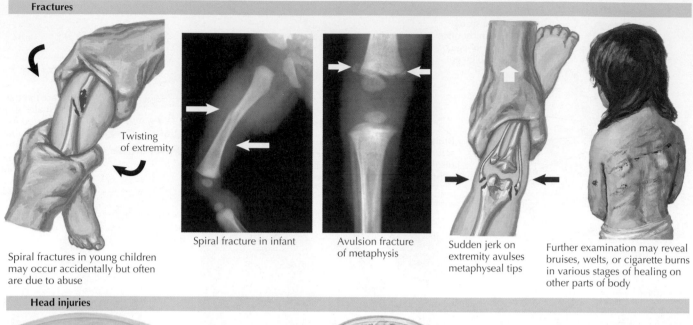

Spiral fractures in young children may occur accidentally but often are due to abuse

Spiral fracture in infant

Avulsion fracture of metaphysis

Sudden jerk on extremity avulses metaphyseal tips

Further examination may reveal bruises, welts, or cigarette burns in various stages of healing on other parts of body

Head injuries

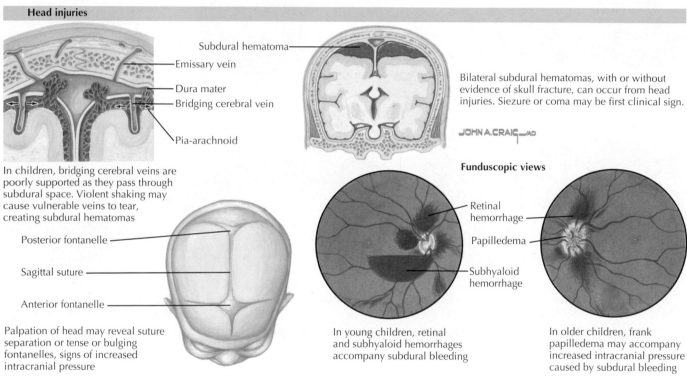

Subdural hematoma
Emissary vein
Dura mater
Bridging cerebral vein
Pia-arachnoid

Bilateral subdural hematomas, with or without evidence of skull fracture, can occur from head injuries. Siezure or coma may be first clinical sign.

JOHN A.CRAIG—AD

In children, bridging cerebral veins are poorly supported as they pass through subdural space. Violent shaking may cause vulnerable veins to tear, creating subdural hematomas

Funduscopic views

Posterior fontanelle

Sagittal suture

Anterior fontanelle

Retinal hemorrhage
Papilledema
Subhyaloid hemorrhage

Palpation of head may reveal suture separation or tense or bulging fontanelles, signs of increased intracranial pressure

In young children, retinal and subhyaloid hemorrhages accompany subdural bleeding

In older children, frank papilledema may accompany increased intracranial pressure caused by subdural bleeding

Fig. 10.3 Fractures and Head Injuries in Child Abuse.

evaluation for coagulopathy with measured prothrombin time and partial thromboplastin time. If there is concern for drug ingestion, urine or serum drug screens should be sent. If there is concern for neglect, providers should consider evaluating for causes contributing to malnutrition and complications of malnutrition by reviewing a complete blood count, basic metabolic panel, magnesium, phosphorus, methylmalonic acid, and 25-OH vitamin D_2 and by reviewing the newborn screen in infants.

Additional workup is indicated if there is concern for sexual abuse. In many cases, forensic evidence should be collected. It is important for a trained provider to assist with the collection of evidence. If the patient has not changed clothes since the alleged sexual activity, have him or her undress on a sheet and save all removed clothing for legal evidence. If the child has changed but not bathed, collect only the underwear. If the child has pubic hair, comb it onto a paper towel and seal the towel, combings, one plucked pubic hair, and the comb in a labeled envelope.

Screening for sexually transmitted infections should be completed if the child is postpubertal, if the child is prepubertal with symptoms or evidence of genital trauma, or if the perpetrator was known to have a sexually transmitted infection. Urine sample should be sent for *Chlamydia trachomatis, Neisseria gonorrhoeae,* and *Trichomonas vaginalis* testing. Swabs of mucous membranes should be sent for herpes simplex virus testing. Serum testing should be ordered for human immunodeficiency virus (HIV), syphilis, and hepatitis B. If there is concern that the child is a victim of human trafficking, hepatitis C

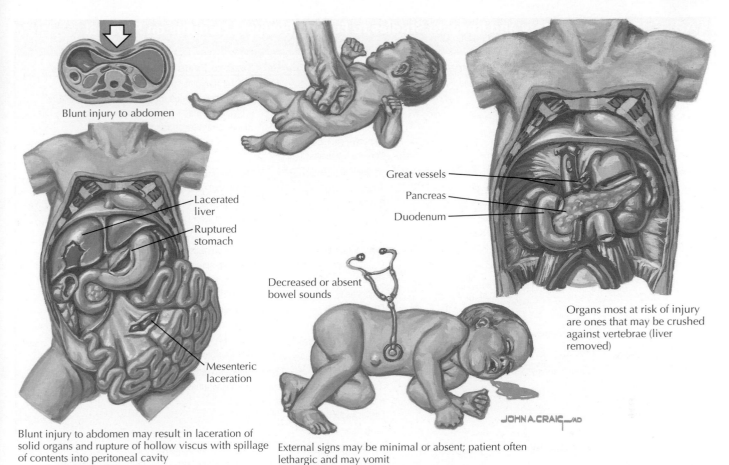

Blunt injury to abdomen

Lacerated liver

Ruptured stomach

Mesenteric laceration

Great vessels

Pancreas

Duodenum

Organs most at risk of injury are ones that may be crushed against vertebrae (liver removed)

Decreased or absent bowel sounds

JOHN A. CRAIG—AD

Blunt injury to abdomen may result in laceration of solid organs and rupture of hollow viscus with spillage of contents into peritoneal cavity

External signs may be minimal or absent; patient often lethargic and may vomit

Fig. 10.4 Abdominal Injuries in Child Abuse.

testing also should be performed on the serum. Additionally, postpubertal females should be screened for pregnancy by urine testing.

Notably, many other underlying disorders may manifest with similar findings on physical examination. See Table 10.4 for other diagnoses to consider in the differential and distinguishing features.

Treatment

The initial mainstay in therapy is stabilization and management of acute trauma. See Chapter 7 for a complete discussion of the management of acute traumatic injuries.

Postexposure prophylaxis is indicated for many patients after sexual abuse to prevent sexually transmitted infections and pregnancy. Postexposure prophylaxis or treatment is indicated in all postpubertal patients. Therapy is indicated for prepubertal patients if they are experiencing symptoms; if they have oral, anal, or vaginal injuries; if there is evidence of perpetrator ejaculation on examination; or if the perpetrator has a confirmed sexually transmitted infection. Recommendations for therapy are described in Table 10.5.

Notably, postexposure prophylaxis for HIV may be indicated if the patient presents less than 72 hours after alleged assault that was considered a high-risk exposure. Contributing factors to exposure risk include the perpetrator's HIV status and a history of mucous membranes or nonintact skin exposure to blood, semen, or other body fluids contaminated with blood. Postexposure prophylaxis for HIV is highly nuanced; if indicated, health care providers should provide highly active antiretroviral therapy (HAART) in consultation with a specialist and with close follow-up ensured.

After initial stabilization, workup, and therapy in the ambulatory setting, it is important to determine a safe disposition plan. In many cases, the child is able to be discharged into the care of a safe and reliable relative. If that is not possible, the child may need to be admitted to the hospital for observation until a safe disposition plan to a relative or to a foster family can be determined.

Reporting

Health care providers are required to report their **suspicion** of abuse to child protective services; importantly, they need not have definitive proof of an abusive incident or knowledge of a perpetrator's identity to make a report to child protective services. The reporting process may be completed in partnership with the interdisciplinary team. After a report is filed, immediate risk stratification is completed to ensure that the child and any other children who have contact with the alleged perpetrator are safe. If one child in the household has experienced maltreatment, all of the children in the household are considered at risk until they can be evaluated. In many cases, other children are brought from home for evaluation for signs of maltreatment. As mentioned earlier, the children may be discharged with a responsible family member, admitted to the hospital for observation, or discharged with a foster family. Soon after, the report will be reviewed and either dismissed or investigated further. Investigation may result in providing the family with resources and/or criminal investigation.

Child maltreatment is a challenging topic to discuss with all families. It is imperative to take a nonjudgmental approach and to partner with caregivers as much as possible; when communicating concerns and next steps, the focus should be on mutual concern for the child. It is also imperative to be clear and honest in communicating with the caregiver. Take care to explain the roles of each member of the care team. Ensure to clearly voice the obligation and plan to report the

TABLE 10.4	Laboratory and Imaging Studies to Further Evaluate Findings on Physical Examination		
Findings	**Tests to Determine Extent of Injury**	**Differential Diagnosis**	**Tests to Evaluate for Organic Disease**
Bruising (extensive or deep)	CBC for severe bleeding/anemia	Accidental trauma ITP Hemophilia Von Willebrand disease Henoch-Schönlein purpura Purpura fulminans	CBC for thrombocytopenia Tests of coagulation for prolonged PT, PTT, and/or bleeding time Blood culture for sepsis if ill appearing
Abdominal pain	Abdominal ultrasonography for free fluid (FAST examination) CMP for liver injury Amylase, lipase for pancreatic injury Urinalysis for bladder, kidney injury	Accidental trauma Tumor Infection	Urinalysis for hematuria Abdominal ultrasonography CMP for liver inflammation CBC, ESR for inflammation
Fractures (multiple or in stages of healing)	Skeletal survey	Accidental trauma Osteogenesis imperfecta Rickets Malignancy Osteomyelitis	Dedicated radiographs Measurements of bone density Calcium, phosphorus, and alkaline phosphatase for abnormalities in calcium metabolism Peripheral smear for blasts or atypical cells Biopsy of lesion for malignancy CBC, ESR, CRP to evaluate for inflammation Blood culture for infection
Metaphyseal or epiphyseal lesions	Skeletal survey	Accidental trauma Scurvy Rickets Little Leaguer's elbow Birth trauma	Dedicated radiographs Specific vitamin levels for nutritional deficiency
Subperiosteal ossification	Skeletal survey	Accidental trauma Osteogenic malignancy Osteoid osteoma Scurvy	Dedicated radiographs Specific vitamin levels for nutritional deficiency
CNS injury	CT for acute hemorrhage Retinal examination by Ophthalmology	Accidental trauma Aneurism Tumor	CT brain for acute hemorrhage MRI brain for parenchymal anomalies and/or chronic hemorrhage Angiogram for vascular anomalies
Dehydration	BMP for electrolytes Urinalysis for specific gravity	Renal Prerenal	BMP for creatinine, BUN Urinalysis for specific gravity
Malnutrition	CBC for inflammation, anemia BMP, magnesium, phosphorus, for electrolytes Methylmalonic acid, 25-OH vitamin D_2 for nutritional deficiencies Review the newborn screen in infants, metabolic disorders	Inadequate intake Malabsorption Increased metabolic demand	CMP for electrolytes, albumin Stool studies for osmolytes, fecal fat

BMP, Basic metabolic panel; *BUN*, blood urea nitrogen; *CBC*, complete blood count; *CMP*, complete metabolic panel; *CNS*, central nervous system; *CT*, computed tomography; *ESR*, erythrocyte sedimentation rate; *MRI*, magnetic resonance imaging; *PT*, prothrombin time; *PTT*, partial thromboplastin time; *WBC*, white blood cell.

concern to child protective services. Finally, work with the caregiver to determine a plan for follow-up so that the family and health care team can continue to partner to promote the health and safety of the child.

OUTCOMES

Immediate and long-term outcomes should ensure that the safety and development of the child are prioritized. Whenever possible, the goal is to provide support to families to create safer living spaces for children and to support eventual reunification in cases in which children have been removed from the home of their primary caregiver(s). Children

may be placed into foster care temporarily or permanently. However, despite efforts at intervention, children who have experienced maltreatment have by definition suffered at least one adverse childhood experience. Adverse childhood experiences, or ACEs, are traumatic events in childhood such as abuse, neglect, and household dysfunction such as mental illness, domestic violence, substance abuse, divorce, or an incarcerated family member. The detrimental effects of ACEs are cumulative, and children experiencing more traumatic events have worse outcomes. ACEs are associated with adverse outcomes in adulthood, including decreased overall health and increased likelihood of participating in violent or criminal activity. Prior history of

TABLE 10.5	Management of Select Complications of Sexual Abuse	
Condition Treated	**Prepubertal Patients**	**Postpubertal Patients**
Gonorrhea, *Chlamydia, Trichomonas* and bacterial vaginosis	*If <45 kg:* Ceftriaxone 25–50 mg/kg, with a maximum dose of 125 mg IV or IM once Erythromycin base (tablet) or ethylsuccinate base (liquid) 50 mg/kg/DAY divided every 6 hours with a maximum dose of 2000 mg/DAY for 14 days Metronidazole 15 mg/kg/dose three times/day for 7 days; maximum dose 2000 mg/day *If ≥45 kg:* Ceftriaxone 500 mg IV or IM Azithromycin 1 g PO Metronidazole 2 g PO or 500 mg twice daily for 7 days	Ceftriaxone 500 mg IV or IM Azithromycin 1 g PO Metronidazole 2 g PO or 500 mg twice daily for 7 days
Human papillomavirus	Vaccine indicated for patients ≥9 years of age who have not received their first dose	
Hepatitis B	*If unimmunized:* First dose in hepatitis B vaccine series *If perpetrator positive for hepatitis B surface antigen:* Hepatitis B immunoglobulin Hepatitis B Vaccine	
Human immunodeficiency virus	Consult with special immunology or infectious diseases specialists	
Pregnancy	N/A	*If presenting within 120 hours of assault:* 1.5 mg levonorgestrel
Side effects of therapy	Antiemetic of choice	

IV, Intravenously; *IM,* intramuscularly; *N/A,* not applicable; *PO,* by mouth.

trauma—specifically child abuse, sexual abuse, or domestic violence—is also associated with higher potential for becoming a perpetrator of child abuse.

FUTURE DIRECTIONS AND CAUTIONS

Considering the detrimental effects of child maltreatment and other ACEs, it is important to recognize and manage child maltreatment as early as possible. Many of the negative effects of ACEs can be mitigated by the child forming a consistent, supportive relationship with a trusted adult. Early recognition of child maltreatment must result in the provision of safety, resources, and mentorship such that children can form these supportive bonds with their caregivers on reunification or with their foster families if reunification is not possible. Preventing future child maltreatment involves breaking the cycle of generational trauma and ensuring that all families have the necessary supports in place for safe growth and development.

Providers should also take caution to ensure that they are aware of and challenging their biases in diagnosing and reporting child maltreatment. Particularly in the United States where structural racism affects both access to resources and the perception of people of color, it is important to approach all children with a consistent framework. Biases that lead to an underreporting of concern for child maltreatment in white children and an overreporting of concern for child maltreatment in black children can be devastating because of both unrecognized maltreatment and disruption of the family structure.

SUGGESTED READINGS

Available online.

Care of the Complex Child

Pamela Mazzeo

11

Symptom Evaluation and Management in Children With Medical Complexity

Sara A. Hasan and Ayelet Rosen

 CLINICAL VIGNETTE

Joshua is an 8-year-old boy with severe neurologic impairment as a result of traumatic brain injury (TBI), with associated complex medical problems, including oropharyngeal dysphagia with gastrojejunostomy (GJ) dependence and obstructive sleep apnea with continuous positive airway pressure dependence. He has no verbal skills but communicates with his parents by eye contact and facial expressions. He was brought to the hospital by his family for tachycardia and episodes of extremity stiffening, back arching, and grimacing. He has been acting withdrawn and seeking comfort but is difficult to console. His family has not noticed correlation of the episodes with feeds, and he is having regular bowel movements while using his usual bowel regimen. His parents think that he has been having a harder time voiding on his own. He has been requiring warm packs and abdominal massage to void, and despite this is voiding smaller amounts than usual.

Before his TBI, he was healthy, with mild asthma. Computed tomography scan at the time of his TBI showed diffuse axonal injury. His current medications include levetiracetam, diazepam, omeprazole, famotidine, metoclopramide, glycopyrrolate, polyethylene glycol, sennosides, and, when needed, a glycerin suppository.

On examination he is tachycardic, hypertensive, and afebrile, with normal oxygen saturation level on room air. He is diaphoretic and having intermittent extensor posturing. His pupils react to light symmetrically. He has moist mucous membranes with pooled secretions in his mouth. His cardiac and respiratory examinations are normal. His abdomen is soft without organomegaly, and his GJ tube site is clean, dry, and intact. His extremities are hypertonic.

The initial workup includes a complete blood count, basic metabolic panel, erythrocyte sedimentation rate, and C-reactive protein, all of which are reassuring. Urinalysis shows an increase in white blood cells, leukocyte esterase, and nitrites. A chest radiograph is similar to his prior images. An abdominal radiograph shows increased stool burden. A point-of-care ultrasonographic bladder scan shows 450 mL of retained urine, even though he recently voided.

He is given a dose of clonidine through his gastrojejunostomy tube, and his heart rate and blood pressure improve. Bladder catheterization produces a large volume of urine, and after these two interventions his posturing and diaphoresis improve. He is admitted to the hospital with concern for exacerbation of parasympathetic hyperstimulation, which may be secondary to a urinary tract infection (UTI), urinary retention, constipation, or a combination of all three factors. The goals of hospitalization will be to establish bladder volumes and devise an appropriate regimen for home clean intermittent catheterization under the guidance of the pediatric urology consultants. He will receive antibiotics for his UTI. He will also need supportive care and treatment of this exacerbation of paroxysmal sympathetic hyperactivity.

Children with medical complexity (CMC) may present with signs and symptoms when ill that are different from those of typically developing children. Challenges of symptom management for CMC include difficulty in communicating because of developmental delay or severe neurologic impairment (SNI), interrelatedness of disease processes, variability in goals of care, and the need for clear communication among multidisciplinary teams. Varying degrees of neurologic impairment lead to different communication abilities, as well as atypical perceptions and expressions of pain. A thorough history and inclusion of input from parents and caretakers can uncover important patterns and alterations from baseline. An individual child's many chronic conditions can affect each other and lead to cycles of worsening symptoms. For example, a patient can present with worsening spasticity because of pain as a result of worsening gastroesophageal reflux symptoms. Treating the reflux may break the cycle of pain and spasticity.

A multidisciplinary approach often offers patients the best symptom management. This can include the involvement of physical, occupational, and speech therapists, along with subspecialists in physiatry, orthopedics, neurology, and neurosurgery. Providers are encouraged to verbally acknowledge the child's pain or discomfort, verbalize the steps of the physical examination, and allow the child time to relax after uncomfortable parts of the physical examination.

PAIN

Definitions of Pain

Pain is most commonly defined as an unpleasant sensory and emotional experience associated with actual or potential tissue damage. In CMC, particularly those with SNI, this sensation can be exacerbated by dysregulation of the central nervous system (CNS). CMC often experience increased stimuli for pain, such as with phlebotomy, surgeries, and other procedures, starting at a young age.

Nociceptive pain, also referred to as somatic pain, arises from damage to nonneural tissue that activates the nociceptors. It is usually acute and resolves with treatment of the injury. Examples of nociceptive pain include a bone fracture or skin laceration. As with less medically complex children, typical treatment is with acetaminophen, nonsteroidal antiinflammatory drugs, and opioids if needed. **Neuropathic pain** is caused by a lesion or disease of the somatosensory nervous system and can manifest in children with SNI as chronic pain with acute exacerbations. Chronic neuropathic pain may be treated with physical therapy, occupational therapy, behavioral health interventions, and medications. **Allodynia** is a specific type of neuropathic pain caused by a stimulus that would not typically cause pain, such as gently touching the skin. **Visceral pain** is that which results from internal organ

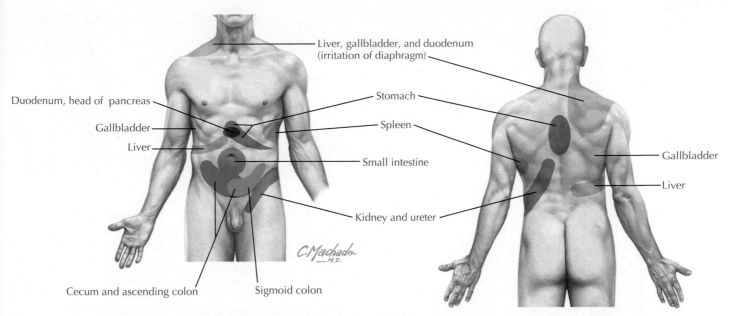

Fig. 11.1 Visceral Referred Pain.

inflammation or injury. It may be poorly localized or can be referred to distant locations (Fig. 11.1). **Hyperalgesia,** including visceral hyperalgesia, is a type of neuropathic pain in which the child may have an altered pain threshold in response to a painful or uncomfortable stimulus.

Challenges of Assessing Pain in Children With Medical Complexity

Common manifestations of pain in children with neurologic impairment can include increased vocalization, tachycardia, hypertension, respiratory distress, or any change from baseline behaviors and vital signs. Dysregulation of the CNS causes a variety of manifestations of pain, which can be similar to those of typically developing children, such as grimacing or crying. However, some children with SNI have worsening dystonia, posturing, or even laughing with pain. This highlights the importance of asking caregivers about the child's baseline behavior and usual signs of pain. Pain scales modified for children with neurologic impairment can be helpful in assessment. In addition to focusing on the patient's history as a guide for assessing causes of pain, it is imperative to also consider other age-appropriate diagnoses.

Minimizing Procedural Pain

For painful procedures, sedation or anesthesia should be considered when appropriate. Various administration routes are available for analgesic medications, including topical, oral, intranasal, enteral, intramuscular, and intravenous options. Calming and distraction techniques should be used whenever possible.

AN ORGAN SYSTEM-BASED APPROACH TO SYMPTOM EVALUATION AND MANAGEMENT

There are innumerable diagnoses to consider for CMC, particularly those with neurologic impairment, who present with symptoms of agitation or possible pain or with any alteration from baseline behavior. It is helpful to use a systematic approach in assessing a patient whose behavior is not at baseline. In addition to considering the diagnoses discussed later, medication review is imperative because certain medications may cause or worsen symptoms.

Neuromuscular and Musculoskeletal

Disturbances in muscle tone can cause acute distress, as well as chronic growth-related musculoskeletal deformities such as joint contractures.

Hypertonia is abnormally increased resistance to externally imposed movement (on physical examination) around a joint. **Spasticity** is a type of velocity-dependent hypertonia in which muscles stiffen or tighten, preventing normal fluid movement. This differs from a muscle spasm, which is a sudden contraction of a muscle or group of muscles. It also differs from rigidity, which is bidirectional resistance throughout the range of motion, independent of velocity. Spasticity itself is not painful; pain comes from the resulting muscle injury. Untreated spasticity can result in permanent contractures, which contribute to chronic pain because of stretching and pressure on nerves, muscles, and bones (Fig. 11.2). Contractures significantly decrease a child's ability to function and participate in activities of daily living and can make physically caring for CMC much more difficult. Physical and occupational therapy, braces, splinting, and adaptive devices are important for the prevention and treatment of contractures associated with spasticity. Medical treatment of spasticity can include oral or intrathecal baclofen, diazepam (or other benzodiazepines), clonidine, tizanidine, or gabapentin. Intramuscular botulinum toxin and phenol injections can be useful for localized spasticity. Surgical adjuncts may be considered, including intrathecal baclofen pump placement, tendon/soft tissue release, dorsal root rhizotomy, and selected peripheral neurotomy.

Dystonia is a movement disorder in which involuntary muscle contractions involving one or many muscle groups cause repetitive movements, abnormal posturing, or both. Dystonia can be painful, and this pain in turn may trigger further spasticity and dystonia in a cyclical fashion. It can be a primary movement disorder or secondary to CNS insult. Like spasticity, dystonia treatment often involves a multimodal approach using therapies and medical and surgical options such as deep brain stimulation (Fig. 11.3). Treating dystonia often involves the same medications as those for spasticity, as well as dystonia-specific medications including carbidopa/levodopa and trihexyphenidyl.

Joint subluxation and occult fractures can be common in children with SNI as a result of poor bone health and hypertonia. For example,

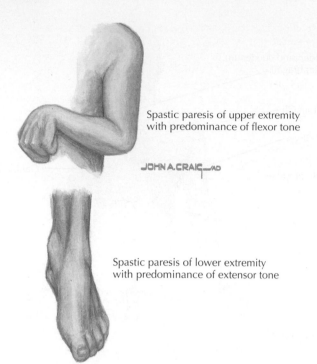

Spastic paresis of upper extremity with predominance of flexor tone

JOHN A. CRAIG. MD

Spastic paresis of lower extremity with predominance of extensor tone

Fig. 11.2 Contractures.

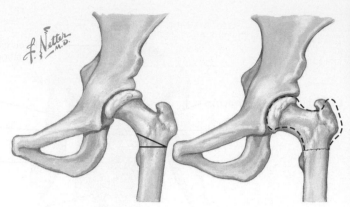

Preoperative view

Femoral head flattened and subluxated, protruding well outside lateral margin of acetabulum. Red lines indicate proposed osteotomy and wedge of bone to be resected.

Postoperative view

Resection of bone wedge has abducted neck and head of femur so that epiphysis is well covered within acetabulum. Broken red line indicates original position. Procedure accentuates limb-length discrepancy.

Fig. 11.4 Femoral Varus Derotational Osteotomy.

Central Nervous System

Possible CNS causes of pain or altered behavior include headache, seizures, ventriculoperitoneal (VP) shunt malfunction, and paroxysmal sympathetic hyperactivity. A thorough physical examination is necessary, along with a history and discussion with caregivers of the patient's baseline status. If headaches are suspected, a trial dose of an analgesic could be a first step. Electroencephalogram and blood levels of antiepileptic medications should be considered when seizure is a possibility. For patients with a VP shunt, a low threshold should be maintained to evaluate for evidence of shunt malfunction with a shunt radiography series and neuroimaging such as computed tomography (CT) of the head. Consultation with a pediatric neurosurgeon is important, because shunt revision or other intervention may be indicated (Fig. 11.5).

Autonomic instability or dysfunction is a broad term applied to the symptoms brought on by damage to the autonomic nervous system. This condition may manifest as alterations in heart rate and blood pressure, temperature changes, flushing, pallor, sweating, tone changes, grimacing, or in some cases vocalization or laughter. It may also manifest as gastrointestinal (GI) dysmotility, which can lead to constipation, retching, and abdominal pain. A mainstay of management is ensuring a predictable environment with a schedule and minimal external stimuli, especially during times of sleep or rest. Additional pharmacologic interventions include clonidine (an α-2 adrenergic agonist) and benzodiazepines.

Paroxysmal sympathetic hyperactivity (PSH) also has been referred to as "autonomic storming" or "sympathetic storming." It is a specific type of autonomic instability seen in patients who have suffered brain injury. Lesions within the diencephalon, midbrain, pons, posterior limb of the internal capsule, periventricular white matter, corpus callosum, and deep gray nuclei increase a child's risk for developing PSH. Treatment options include a low-stimulation environment, adherence to a daily routine for medical care, and medications such as clonidine, benzodiazepines, propranolol (β-blocker), or baclofen (gamma aminobutyric acid [GABA]-B agonist). Prognosis is variable, but episodes can improve over months to years.

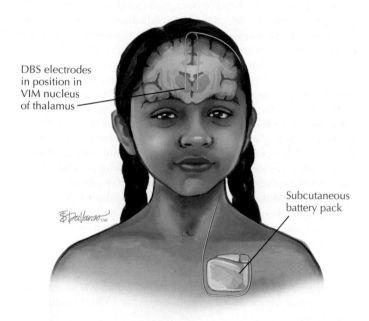

DBS electrodes in position in VIM nucleus of thalamus

Subcutaneous battery pack

B. DaVanzo CMI

High-frequency deep brain stimulation (DBS) of VIM region of thalamus is the predominant treatment of medically refractory tremor. Globus pallidus and substantia nigra sites provide relief for Parkinson disease and dystonia. DBS electrodes are implanted and connected to subclavicular battery pack.

Fig. 11.3 Deep Brain Stimulator. *VIM,* Ventral intermediate nucleus.

spasticity can lead to progressive hip dislocation, for which femoral varus derotational osteotomy, performed by an experienced pediatric orthopedic surgeon, may be indicated (Fig. 11.4). Consultation with pediatric nutrition and endocrinology specialists can be helpful to optimize bone health.

Gastrointestinal

GI causes such as gastroesophageal reflux (GERD), constipation, gallstones, and intestinal dysmotility should be considered when trying to elicit the cause of pain or discomfort in CMC. Children may have increased retching or vomiting, worsening reflux, or behaviors suggestive to caregivers of abdominal pain. Obtaining a thorough GI history is imperative, along with evaluation of a symptom diary if possible. Consideration may be given to temporarily pausing oral or tube feedings and switching to enteral rehydration solution or IV hydration; maximizing GERD treatment, including reflux precautions and medications; and starting or optimizing a bowel regimen when there is concern for constipation, which can be a major driver of discomfort in CMC. A simple history along with an abdominal radiograph to assess stool burden can help make this diagnosis. Ensuring the child has the appropriate diet and adequate hydration is the first step in ameliorating this discomfort. If needed, laxative medications such as polyethylene glycol and sennosides may be started, along with more aggressive measures such as enemas and suppositories.

Many CMC have underlying diagnoses or use medications that make them vulnerable to hepatitis, pancreatitis, and cholecystitis. Appendicitis and other diagnoses that would be considered in a typical child should be similarly considered and evaluated in CMC. Abnormal innervation or anatomy in CMC may increase the risk for acute bowel obstruction or volvulus (Fig. 11.6). Abdominal radiography or ultrasound studies can aid in evaluation for enteric tube malfunction, dislodgement, or associated intussusception.

A low threshold should be maintained for consulting a pediatric gastroenterologist for suspected or evident feeding intolerance or for GI symptoms.

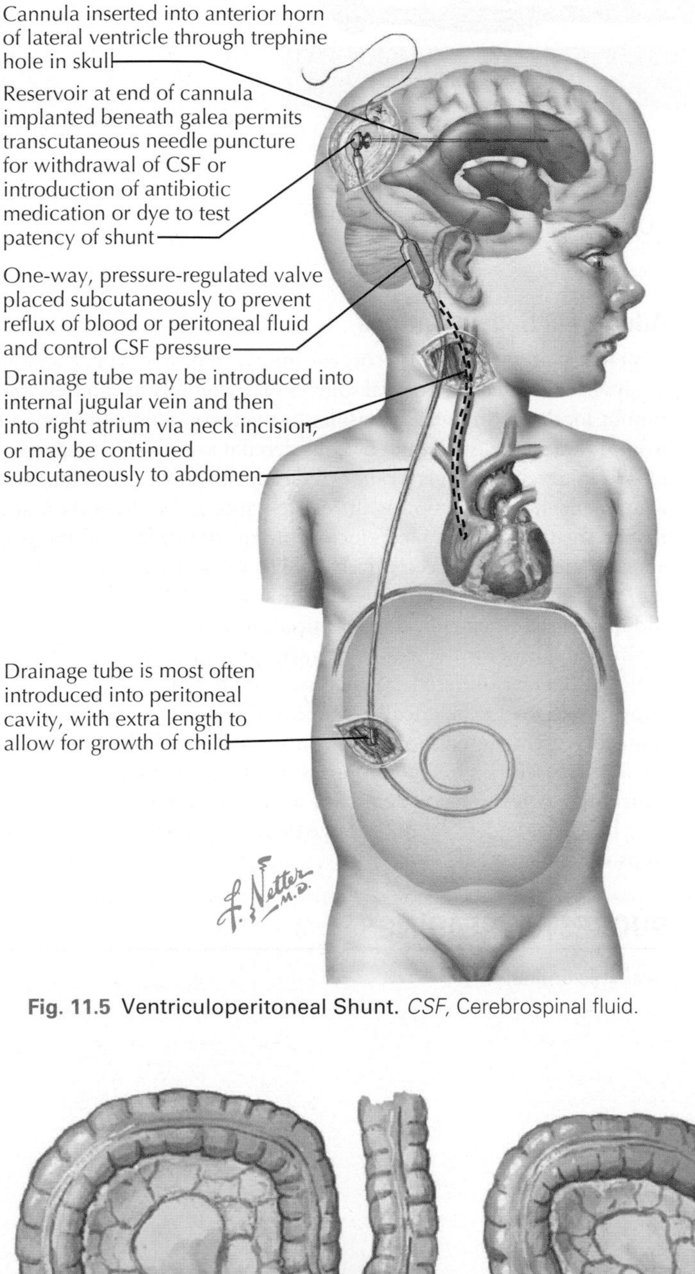

Respiratory

Cough and dyspnea can be a significant source of distress for CMC. As for any typical child with such symptoms, a thorough history and physical examination help guide next steps. Diagnoses to be considered in CMC include community-acquired or aspiration pneumonia, difficulty managing increased respiratory or oral secretions, malfunction of or complication associated with respiratory equipment such as noninvasive positive pressure ventilation or ventilator, or, especially in older children with limited mobility, pulmonary embolism. Workup may include chest radiograph, tracheal respiratory culture, and/or a respiratory viral polymerase chain reaction panel. A CT angiogram is the gold standard for diagnosis of pulmonary embolism. Consultation with a pediatric pulmonologist for acute or chronic respiratory symptom management should be considered.

Cannula inserted into anterior horn of lateral ventricle through trephine hole in skull

Reservoir at end of cannula implanted beneath galea permits transcutaneous needle puncture for withdrawal of CSF or introduction of antibiotic medication or dye to test patency of shunt

One-way, pressure-regulated valve placed subcutaneously to prevent reflux of blood or peritoneal fluid and control CSF pressure

Drainage tube may be introduced into internal jugular vein and then into right atrium via neck incision, or may be continued subcutaneously to abdomen

Drainage tube is most often introduced into peritoneal cavity, with extra length to allow for growth of child

Fig. 11.5 Ventriculoperitoneal Shunt. *CSF,* Cerebrospinal fluid.

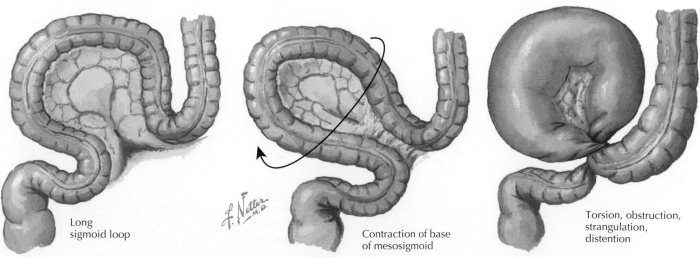

Long sigmoid loop

Contraction of base of mesosigmoid

Torsion, obstruction, strangulation, distention

Fig. 11.6 Volvulus.

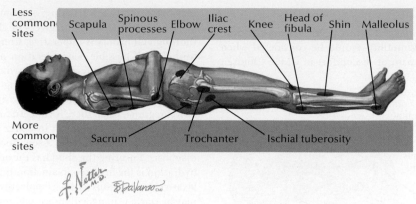

Fig. 11.7 Pressure Ulcer Sites.

Managing airway secretions and supporting the patient with appropriate oxygenation and ventilation is further discussed in Chapter 12.

Urologic

Bladder dysfunction can be common in children with neurologic impairment. This can lead to uncomfortable bladder distention, incomplete emptying, or urinary tract infection (UTI). If the patient has temperature derangements or is in any distress, a low threshold should be maintained to collect a urinalysis and clean catch or catheterized specimen for urine culture to evaluate for UTI. To assess whether bladder dysfunction is a cause of discomfort, in some health care settings, point-of-care bladder ultrasound can be used to assess for proper emptying. Some patients with bladder dysfunction routinely undergo clean intermittent catheterization at baseline, often under the guidance of a pediatric urologist. For persistent symptoms, next steps may include increasing catheterization frequency, obtaining further imaging, or initiation of prophylactic antibiotics to prevent UTI.

Nephrolithiasis should be considered as a potential source of pain, especially in nonverbal patients. A renal-bladder ultrasound may help identify the stone or secondary signs such as ureteral dilation, and radiography of the pelvis may show radiopaque stones. Urinalysis to evaluate for microscopic hematuria and urine studies to assess the calcium-to-creatinine ratio can assist with diagnosis. As with many of the conditions discussed, seeking specialist input on management is often indicated.

Additional Considerations

Dental or intraoral lesions, corneal injury, and skin injury should always be evaluated as potential sources of discomfort in children who cannot localize symptoms. Consults to dentistry, ophthalmology, or wound care specialists should be considered if available. Management of skin injury, in particular, can include adjusting invasive or adaptive equipment in coordination with relevant specialists. Prevention and management of pressure ulcers includes frequent turning and applying appropriate dressings preemptively in high-friction areas or at the first sign of erythema to prevent pressure injuries (Fig. 11.7). Antibiotics should be used when indicated for infection.

In evaluating for the causes of symptoms in CMC, it is important to consider differential diagnoses that would also be age-appropriate for less medically complex children. The possibility of nonaccidental trauma should be considered as well, because CMC are at increased risk for such injuries. For children with progressive neurologic conditions, progression of disease can be a source of a new baseline, and reframing the goals of care is pertinent to next steps in management.

SUGGESTED READINGS

Available online.

12

Respiratory Considerations in Children With Medical Complexity

Annie Laurie Gula and Akhila V. Shapiro

 CLINICAL VIGNETTE

A 10-month-old boy born at 24 weeks' gestation presents to the primary care office for a routine well child visit. His caregiver reports that he has been well. He has been diagnosed with chronic lung disease and is prescribed a diuretic by his pulmonologist, but he does not require any supplemental oxygen or other respiratory support at baseline. His caregiver notes that the patient still has difficulty sitting up independently, snores, and appears to have pauses in breathing during sleep. His caregiver asks if it is normal for infants to snore at his age.

On physical examination, the patient is well appearing and active. His caregiver states that the mild tachypnea and subcostal retractions observed are consistent with his baseline. It is also observed that he has poor head control and cannot sit unassisted. Given the concern for obstructive sleep apnea based on history and neurologic examination, the patient is referred to his pulmonologist for evaluation with polysomnogram and consideration of therapy with continuous positive airway pressure (CPAP) and to his neurologist for evaluation of hypotonia.

Although occasional snoring occurs in approximately 12% of healthy infants, frequent snoring associated with pauses in breathing and/or other risk factors for obstructive sleep apnea (including hypotonia, as seen in this patient) should elevate concern for a pathologic condition. Children with medical complexity are at high risk for respiratory problems as a result of abnormalities in neurologic function, airway anatomy, and/or pulmonary parenchyma. This patient is at risk for respiratory dysfunction given his truncal hypotonia and pulmonary parenchymal abnormalities related to chronic lung disease of prematurity or bronchopulmonary dysplasia (see Fig. 12.4).

Many children with medical complexity (CMC) have respiratory problems related to their underlying disease processes. These children often require intensive resource usage and/or technologic assistance to achieve optimal health outcomes. This population of children is likely increasing in prevalence because of increased survival rates of infants born prematurely and born with various congenital anomalies and chronic conditions, as well as improved treatments for acute illnesses in fields such as intensive care. There are many underlying disease processes that cause respiratory compromise in this patient population (Box 12.1).

PATHOPHYSIOLOGY

The respiratory system consists of a pumping mechanism (the respiratory muscles, the chest wall, and the conducting airways), a membrane gas exchanger (the interface between the air spaces and the pulmonary circulation), and a central neural control connected to a network of chemical and mechanical sensors distributed throughout the system. Children, particularly young children and infants, are at increased risk for respiratory failure compared with adults because of developmental and anatomic differences. Premature infants, in particular, have incompletely developed intrapulmonary air spaces at birth, reducing the available surface area for gas exchange and compromising their ability to compensate when stress is placed on the respiratory system (Figs. 12.1 and 12.2).

A fully functioning respiratory system requires adequate ventilation via the respiratory pump and sufficiently patent airways to support ventilation. Minute ventilation describes the volume of air breathed per minute and is defined as:

$$(\text{Tidal volume}) \times (\text{Respiratory rate})$$

A pathologic condition that decreases the tidal volume of each breath is likely to decrease minute ventilation. Obstructive pathologic conditions and restrictive chest wall pathologic conditions decrease tidal volume (Table 12.1). Young children are at particularly high risk for obstructive pathologic conditions; they have narrow airways in general, particularly in the subglottic region. Should already narrow airways become inflamed, filled with secretions, or stenotic, resistance to flow increases significantly.

Pathologic conditions that decrease the respiratory rate, including dysfunctional central control of breathing, may also decrease minute ventilation. Immature respiratory centers in the brain can result in pauses or irregular breathing (Fig. 12.3).

Additionally, easy fatigability may contribute to decreased minute ventilation by affecting both respiratory rate and tidal volume. Children are more vulnerable to fatigue because of more flattened diaphragmatic domes and less fatigue-resistant type 1 muscle fibers in the diaphragm. When lung compliance decreases as a result of inflammation or infection, children use accessory muscles to maintain lung capacity and can fatigue quickly.

A fully functioning respiratory system also requires a mechanism for gas exchange. Gas exchange entails absorbing oxygen and removing carbon dioxide. Pulmonary characteristics that contribute to adequate gas exchange include sufficient diffusion of gases across the alveolar/vascular interface and appropriate matching of blood flow to airspace ventilation. Fibrosis, pulmonary edema, and/or inflammation may affect gas diffusion and exchange.

Inappropriate matching of blood flow and ventilation (V/Q mismatch) is a common contributor to respiratory failure and may be related to atelectasis, consolidation, increased respiratory secretions causing obstruction of large airways with mucus plugs, and/or tracheobronchial tree anomalies. These conditions are especially common in CMC with severe neurologic impairment; these children, for example, may have diminished neuromuscular capacity to clear airway secretions or may be at risk for aspiration events. In general, children under the age of 3 years are more likely to experience difficulty related to atelectasis or collapse of the alveoli and small airways, because of a decreased number of alveoli and overall underdevelopment.

BOX 12.1   Common Etiologies Resulting in Respiratory Problems

Anatomic Causes
- Craniofacial anomalies
- Congenital diaphragmatic hernia
- Vascular rings/slings
- Thoracic insufficiency
- Tracheomalacia
- Bronchomalacia
- Obstructive sleep apnea

Congenital Causes
- Chronic lung disease or bronchopulmonary dysplasia
- Pulmonary fibrosis
- Cystic fibrosis
- Cardiomyopathy
- Mucopolysaccharidoses
- Mitochondrial disease

Neurologic Causes
- Neuromuscular weakness
- Central hypoventilation syndromes
- Hypoxic ischemic encephalopathy
- Hypotonia
- Cerebral palsy

MANAGEMENT OF CHRONIC RESPIRATORY DYSFUNCTION

Goals of managing chronic respiratory dysfunction in CMC should include maintaining adequate oxygenation and ventilation, decreasing work of breathing to promote growth and development, and preventing worsening respiratory impairment.

Modalities of Respiratory and Ventilatory Support

Many patients with chronic respiratory failure will require invasive or noninvasive ventilation (NIV) to manage their oxygenation, work of breathing, and/or hypoventilation. Please see Chapter 14 for more specifics regarding technologic devices that provide support of ventilation.

For patients with impairment of oxygenation alone (e.g., those with bronchopulmonary dysplasia/chronic lung disease [BPD/CLD]), supplemental oxygen by nasal cannula may be sufficient support. Patients may use supplemental oxygen by nasal cannula at all times, during activity, during sleep, and/or during illness.

Children with chronic hypoventilation, on the other hand, may have advanced pulmonary disease, neuromuscular disease, or defects in respiratory drive, resulting in insufficient minute ventilation to maintain normocapnia and/or adequate oxygen saturations. They can range in severity from children who have inadequate respiration solely during sleep, hence requiring nocturnal respiratory assistance alone, to those who require supported ventilation at all times for survival.

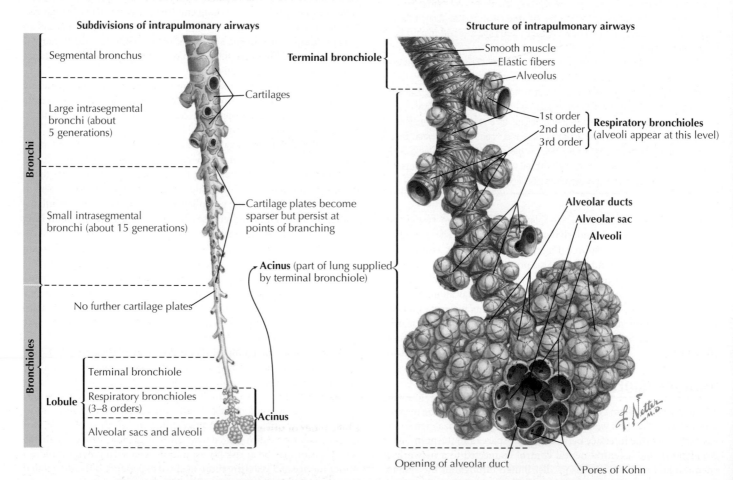

Subdivisions of intrapulmonary airways

Bronchi
- Segmental bronchus
- Large intrasegmental bronchi (about 5 generations)
- Small intrasegmental bronchi (about 15 generations)
  - Cartilages
  - Cartilage plates become sparser but persist at points of branching
  - No further cartilage plates

Bronchioles
- Lobule
  - Terminal bronchiole
  - Respiratory bronchioles (3–8 orders)
  - Alveolar sacs and alveoli
  - Acinus

Acinus (part of lung supplied by terminal bronchiole)

Structure of intrapulmonary airways

Terminal bronchiole
- Smooth muscle
- Elastic fibers
- Alveolus

1st order
2nd order
3rd order
Respiratory bronchioles (alveoli appear at this level)

Alveolar ducts
Alveolar sac
Alveoli

Opening of alveolar duct
Pores of Kohn

Fig. 12.1 Development of Bronchioles and Alveoli Intrapulmonary Airways: Schema Subdivisions and Structure of Intrapulmonary Airways.

Hypoventilation may be central, obstructive (Fig. 12.4), or restrictive. In deciding on a management strategy, it is important to identify the main cause for hypoventilation. Whereas patients with a restrictive or obstructive pathologic condition or thoracic insufficiency may benefit from continuous positive airway pressure (CPAP) alone, those with central hypoventilation, or anomalies in the respiratory center of the brain, often require bilevel positive airway pressure (BLPAP) support that can provide breaths independent of patient effort.

CPAP, which provides a consistent flow of air/pressure, increases the positive end-expiratory pressure (PEEP). Increased PEEP results in an increased mean airway pressure (MAP), which helps prevent airway collapse in upper and lower airways. In addition to maintaining open alveoli, increased PEEP helps support flexible or floppy areas of the airway such that they remain open rather than collapsing and causing obstruction.

BLPAP is similar in that it provides a flow of air that increases MAP. However, in addition to increasing PEEP by providing expiratory positive airway pressure (EPAP), it also further augments inspiratory efforts by providing inspiratory positive airway pressure (IPAP). BLPAP provides IPAP to a patient in either a spontaneous (triggered by the patient taking a breath) or timed (at a specified rate or interval) fashion. BLPAP augments respiration such that both ventilation and work of breathing are improved.

Complications of NIV can occur. The interfaces that are used to deliver NIV are often poorly tolerated in children. Skin breakdown can occur with long-term use, especially if the same interface is used continuously. NIV airflow can also fill the stomach with air, which can cause bloating, discomfort, feeding intolerance, and increased risk for tracheal aspiration of gastric contents. Additionally, high pressures can cause trauma to the lung tissue itself and result in blebs or pneumothorax. It is often difficult to eat or speak while using NIV, which can affect the ability of CMC to participate in therapies that are vital to their development.

For certain patients, better airway control with tracheostomy is indicated. Common indications for tracheostomy in CMC include severe upper airway obstruction, prolonged need for mechanical ventilation, and need for improved suctioning. The decision to provide respiratory support by tracheostomy is quite nuanced; ventilator settings must be optimized to meet ventilatory needs, a patient's caregivers must undergo extensive training, and a patient must be cared for in an environment that can safely support such technology. Other challenges to note include the need for meticulous stoma care and the increased risk for infection with an invasive airway.

Supportive Therapies

Optimization of secretion management, both oral and respiratory, is imperative. Oral secretions may be difficult to control in some CMC because of medication side effects or impaired swallowing mechanisms. Management of oral secretions includes frequent suctioning and/or the use of anticholinergic medications to decrease production of secretions. In some cases, patients will undergo modification of the salivary glands by duct ligation or botulinum toxin injection to directly decrease production of secretions. Respiratory secretions may be difficult to control in some CMC because of inflammation of the respiratory system and poor cough or mobilization of secretions. Tenets of management of respiratory secretions include decreasing bronchospasm, managing viscosity of

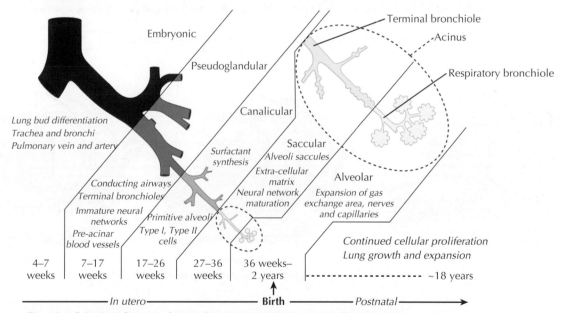

Fig. 12.2 Principal Stages of Lung Development in Humans. (Reused with permission from Kajekar R. Environmental factors and developmental outcomes in the lung. *Pharmacol Ther.* 2007;114[2]:129-145. https://doi.org/10.1016/j.pharmthera.2007.01.011. PMID: 17408750, Fig. 1.)

TABLE 12.1   Respiratory Pathophysiology Classified

OBSTRUCTIVE RESPIRATORY DISEASE		RESTRICTIVE RESPIRATORY DISEASE	
Anatomic	Functional	Alteration in Elastic Properties	Restrictive Chest Wall Disease
Craniofacial anomalies	Airway hypotonia	Chronic lung disease	Scoliosis
Tracheomalacia and laryngomalacia		Lung tissue disease (pulmonary fibrosis and pulmonary edema)	Neuromuscular disease

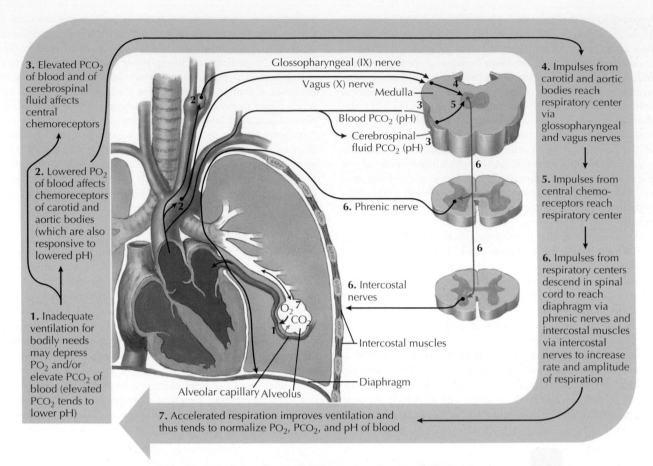

3. Elevated PCO$_2$ of blood and of cerebrospinal fluid affects central chemoreceptors

2. Lowered PO$_2$ of blood affects chemoreceptors of carotid and aortic bodies (which are also responsive to lowered pH)

1. Inadequate ventilation for bodily needs may depress PO$_2$ and/or elevate PCO$_2$ of blood (elevated PCO$_2$ tends to lower pH)

Glossopharyngeal (IX) nerve

Vagus (X) nerve
Medulla

Blood PCO$_2$ (pH)

Cerebrospinal fluid PCO$_2$ (pH)

6. Phrenic nerve

6. Intercostal nerves

Intercostal muscles

Diaphragm

Alveolar capillary   Alveolus

O$_2$ CO$_2$

4. Impulses from carotid and aortic bodies reach respiratory center via glossopharyngeal and vagus nerves

5. Impulses from central chemoreceptors reach respiratory center

6. Impulses from respiratory centers descend in spinal cord to reach diaphragm via phrenic nerves and intercostal muscles via intercostal nerves to increase rate and amplitude of respiration

7. Accelerated respiration improves ventilation and thus tends to normalize PO$_2$, PCO$_2$, and pH of blood

Fig. 12.3 Chemical Control of Respiration (Feedback Mechanism).

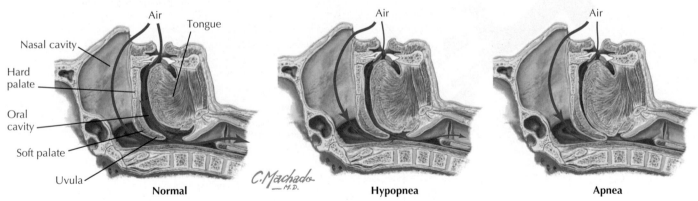

Air   Tongue

Nasal cavity

Hard palate

Oral cavity

Soft palate

Uvula

Air

Air

C. Machado — M.D.

Normal   **Hypopnea**   **Apnea**

Fig. 12.4 Anatomic Representation of Sleep Apnea.

secretions, and improving clearance of secretions. See Chapter 14 for further discussion regarding technology that is used to assist with clearance of secretions, including suction, cough assist device, and percussive devices.

It is critical to optimize patients' overall physical status to optimize their respiratory status and minimize risk for further damage to the respiratory system. In infants and children whose lungs are still developing, it is important to ensure adequate nutrition to support growth and development. Physical therapy, occupational therapy, and speech/feeding therapy can all help patients strengthen and coordinate respiratory muscles and control secretions. Acute exacerbations of respiratory illness, discussed further below, are often related to infection

or aspiration events. Appropriate nutrition, good muscular control, and optimized swallowing skills all help minimize risks associated with infection and aspiration-related inflammation and ensure that patients have improved reserve for recovery.

Of note, technology to support patients' respiratory mechanics continues to evolve. Select patients with thoracic insufficiency can undergo surgical procedures to reconstruct and stabilize the thorax, such as placement of a vertical expandable prosthetic titanium rib (VEPTR), which is then surgically lengthened at regular intervals with the goal of less restricted respiration (Fig. 12.5). The primary goal is to gradually correct the chest wall deformity to improve pulmonary function, and a secondary goal is correction of an associated spinal deformity.

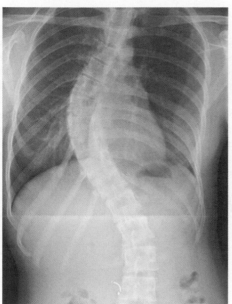

A. Frontal view of the spine demonstrates an S-shaped scoliosis, which indicates an idiopathic form of scoliosis. However, a search for vertebral body anomalies as a cause is always indicated. Worth noting is that spine surgeons hang these films in an opposite manner from radiologists -as if patient's back were to them. The curvilinear metallic density in the abdomen is a navel ring in this teenager.

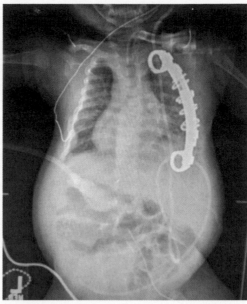

B. A postoperative posteroanterior radiograph of a patient with Jeune syndrome after placement of a right rib-to-rib VEPTR

Fig. 12.5 Radiologic Imaging of Therapies. *VEPTR*, Vertical expandable titanium prosthetic rib. (A, Reused with permission from Major NM. *A Practical Approach to Radiology.* Philadelphia, PA: Saunders; 2006; and B, Mistovich RJ, Spiegel DA. The spine. In: Kliegman RM, Geme JS, eds. *Nelson Textbook of Pediatrics.* 21st ed. Elsevier; 2020:3633-3646.e3, Fig. 699.4.)

ACUTE EXACERBATIONS OF RESPIRATORY ILLNESS

Although respiratory tract symptoms such as cough, wheeze, and stridor can occur in all children, in CMC they are more likely to persist for longer periods or be associated with more extensive respiratory disease. CMC may also develop persistent or recurring lung infiltrates with or without symptoms. These are commonly the result of upper or lower respiratory tract infections or aspiration events. Initially, clinicians must assess whether the symptoms are the manifestation of a minor or easily treatable condition or a life-threatening process, determine the most likely underlying pathogenic mechanism, select the simplest effective therapy for the underlying process, and carefully evaluate the therapeutic effect.

Evaluation of Acute Exacerbations

Diagnosis of the child's condition includes taking a thorough history, including evaluation for fever, limitation of activity, and shortness of breath. History of fever, change in secretions, or sick contacts may suggest an infectious cause, whereas the history of vomiting and/or altered mental status may raise concern for an aspiration event. Initial physical examination should identify any tachypnea, tachycardia, use of accessory muscles to support ventilation, and mental status changes. Laboratory workup should be targeted to the clinical presentation. In many cases, venous or arterial blood gas testing may be useful; identification of severe hypoxemia or hypercarbia may serve as an indicator of severity and acuity of illness. Chest radiographs may be useful, especially when compared to a patient's prior films, to support clinical diagnoses of pneumonia, bronchiolitis, atelectasis, or effusions. More specific testing, such as viral testing, blood culture, complete blood count, and advanced imaging, may be pursued as indicated by the clinical presentation and local epidemiology.

Management of Acute Exacerbations

Management of an acute exacerbation of respiratory illness involves determining the underlying cause, as mentioned previously, and optimizing respiratory support. Although increased respiratory support may be integral in supporting a medically complex patient through an acute respiratory exacerbation, optimizing pulmonary clearance, treating infection, and preventing aspiration will help optimize lung function and minimize further damage.

Many patients experiencing respiratory exacerbations will benefit from assisted clearance of airway secretions, which may be increased with illness. Increased secretions may compound respiratory compromise by decreasing lung compliance, worsening obstructive physiology, and obstructing large airways with mucus plugs. An assisted airway clearance regimen may include increased frequency of therapies from the baseline regimen and/or additional modalities of clearance. In addition, if bacterial infection is presumed to be present, an appropriate antibiotic regimen should be initiated. Of note, although the majority of infectious respiratory exacerbations will be secondary to viral illness, CMC are at higher risk for bacterial infections such as pneumonia or tracheitis than children with typical respiratory physiology.

Finally, it is critical to prevent further worsening of respiratory pathologic conditions by minimizing the risk for aspiration of oral or gastric contents. Techniques to minimize risk for aspiration include positioning and restricting oral and gastric intake *(nil per os)* if the child is unable to adequately coordinate swallowing because of altered mental status or tachypnea.

In many cases, patients will require increased respiratory support by NIV or invasive ventilation. Increased support may be provided in the form of increased CPAP or BLPAP pressures, increased duration of ventilatory support over the course of the day, or a change in modality from baseline. For example, a patient who requires CPAP overnight may require BLPAP at all times to achieve adequate ventilation during an illness.

PROGNOSIS

The overall prognosis of respiratory pathologic conditions in CMC depends on the underlying diagnosis and management. Children with underlying lung disease (e.g., BPD/CLD) may be able to wean off of respiratory support as they grow. However, patients with neuromuscular pathologic conditions often develop the need for increased support as their disease progresses with time. Clinicians should consider the patient as a whole and consider respiratory support needs in the context of the child's overall growth, development, and activity level. An appropriate baseline pulmonary clearance and ventilatory support regimen, as well as guidance for escalation during acute illnesses, is optimally developed under the guidance of and with ongoing support from a pediatric pulmonologist.

The need for life-sustaining technology can expose many inequities in the health care system because of requirements for safe storage of materials, temperature control, and a consistent power source. Moreover, the demand on families can be quite high. Caring for CMC can lead to increased stress, decreased flexibility, and decreased ability to make spontaneous decisions. It is imperative that the health care team be sensitive, patient, and supportive with families and caregivers.

As a means of providing appropriate support, the health care team should involve other services (i.e., social work and case management) as available. The medical home model, with the primary care physician as the central hub for care coordination, has been espoused as ideal for the care of CMC. However, implementation of the medical home model has been limited, likely because of time restrictions, inadequate reimbursement, and lack of decision-making support for primary care providers. Shared decision-making aids are another potentially useful tool that can help patients and families make value-based, informed choices among relevant health care options.

SUGGESTED READINGS

Available online.

13

Feeding and Nutrition in Children With Medical Complexity

Ilana S. Lavina and Winona D. Chua

 CLINICAL VIGNETTE

Michael, a 4-month-old infant boy born at 26 weeks' gestational age, is transferred out of the neonatal intensive care unit (NICU) to the complex care service. He has a history of chronic lung disease and is currently receiving respiratory support by high-flow nasal cannula. Initially, in the NICU he received total parenteral nutrition (TPN), but tolerated advancement to continuous enteral feeds by nasogastric (NG) tube. His feeds were gradually condensed, and at the time of transfer he is receiving bolus feeds of breast milk and a premature infant formula, fortified to 24 kcal/oz, run over 90 minutes eight times daily. Attempts to condense his feeds further have been limited by increased reflux symptoms and hypoglycemia. His family is eager to introduce breastfeeding, and the speech-language pathology team plans to evaluate his swallowing function when his respiratory support is decreased.

DEFINING NUTRITIONAL STATUS AND REQUIREMENTS IN PEDIATRIC PATIENTS

Appropriate nutrition helps children with medical complexity (CMC) attain optimal growth and development. Anthropometric measurements, including weight, length, head circumference, weight-for-length (in children younger than 2 years), and body mass index (BMI) (in children older than 2 years) are monitored in children because these parameters reflect growth and development. These measurements are plotted on standardized growth charts to allow comparisons to a reference population. Specialized growth curves exist for unique subpopulations who may have different growth trajectories because of a medical condition, such as the Fenton growth charts for infants with prematurity and the Centers for Disease Control and Prevention growth charts for children with Down syndrome. Using these references to evaluate a patient's anthropometric measurements allows for identification of abnormal growth parameters, such as underweight (below 5th percentile for weight or BMI), overweight/obesity (85th to 95th percentile/above 95th percentile for weight or BMI), or failure to thrive (weight for age <5th percentile, weight-for-length or BMI <5th percentile, or weight decreasing across two major percentiles over approximately 6 months).

To optimize a patient's feeding regimen, pediatricians and registered dietitians calculate the patient's estimated energy needs taking several factors into account. A child's metabolic expenditure includes the basal metabolic rate, which is defined as the energy needed to maintain physiologic function in an awake person at rest; the thermic effect of food, which is the energy required to carry out digestive function; the physical activity coefficient, which accounts for energy spent during exercise; and energy deposition, which is the energy required for growth (the deposition of new body tissues) in pediatric patients.

UNIQUE NUTRITIONAL CHALLENGES IN CHILDREN WITH MEDICAL COMPLEXITY

Disease processes or congenital defects in CMC may increase their total metabolic expenditure above the reference value for a typical child of the same age. For example, in Clinical Vignette, baby Michael experienced poor weight gain and required fortification (increasing the caloric density) of his formula. His underlying pulmonary illness (bronchopulmonary dysplasia) contributes to this increased caloric need because he expends additional energy to breathe. In general, premature babies need about 120 to 130 kcal/kg/day, compared to term infants who need 100 to 110 kcal/kg/day. Other conditions that similarly lead to increased caloric expenditure include congenital cardiac disease, anatomic/structural defects such as severe laryngomalacia, malignancy, immunodeficiency, and recurrent or chronic infections. Metabolic and mitochondrial diseases similarly may change the way the body absorbs, processes, and uses energy, leading to unique nutritional needs in this subpopulation. Children who have severe neurologic disease that diminishes their motor function, such as spinal muscular atrophy, may have a decreased total energy expenditure because of decreased movement and activity.

Published nutrition recommendations must be interpreted with thoughtful consideration of each child's unique constellation of health challenges. In creating a feeding plan, emphasis should be placed on a child's specific medical condition(s) and on monitoring the child's growth parameters, although measuring an accurate body length and calculating weight-for-length or BMI in children who have limb deformities or contractures may be challenging.

Medical complexity does not just influence the overall caloric needs of patients; it also may play a role in how and what they are fed. Some children may be able to eat regular table food but may have specific micronutrient or macronutrient needs. Others may have nutritional options limited by swallowing dysfunction (dysphagia), which is common among CMC as a result of prematurity, cerebral palsy, neuromuscular disorders, congenital defects such as cleft palate, and numerous other conditions. To ensure safe feeding practices and minimize the risk for choking and aspiration events, dietary alterations such as slow-flow bottle nipples or texture modification may be necessary. In some children, there may be no safe option for feeding by mouth because of severe dysphagia and the associated risk for tracheal aspiration.

Feeding can be a dynamic process that evolves over the child's life and illness course. For example, baby Michael may ultimately achieve full oral feeding after intensive feeding therapy. Some children may have adequate oropharyngeal skills to feed by mouth without complication, but may require supplemental feedings by an alternative route because their caloric needs are so great that they cannot be sustained with oral

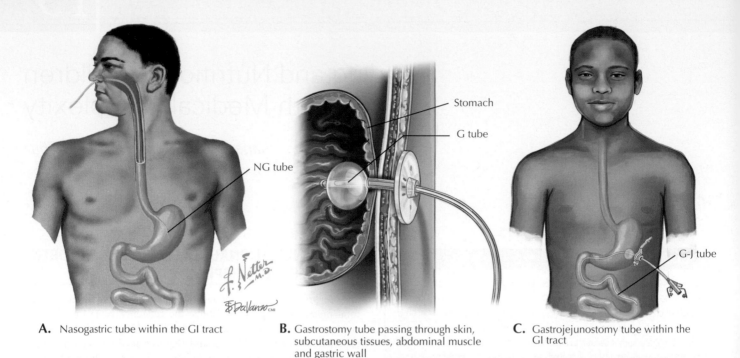

A. Nasogastric tube within the GI tract

B. Gastrostomy tube passing through skin, subcutaneous tissues, abdominal muscle and gastric wall

C. Gastrojejunostomy tube within the GI tract

Fig. 13.1 Anatomic Placement of Nasogastric, Gastric, and Gastrojejunal Tubes.

feeding alone. Others may be able to eat purees or solid foods safely but cannot safely consume enough liquid to maintain adequate hydration.

ALTERNATIVES TO ORAL FEEDING

Alternative feeding methods for children who cannot eat or drink by mouth include enteral tube feedings and total parenteral nutrition (TPN). Fig. 13.1 demonstrates the anatomic placement of enteral feeding tubes. TPN, a solution of macronutrients and micronutrients that is administered intravenously, is an option for children with disorders of the gastrointestinal (GI) tract that preclude enteral feeding.

Enteral Tube Feeding
Gastric Feeding

Children who require enteral nutrition are most commonly fed into the stomach, because this best simulates natural feeding. Tube feeding into the stomach can be delivered by nasogastric (NG), orogastric, or gastrostomy (GT) tubes.

An NG tube is a flexible, thin tube placed through the nare, extending through the nasopharynx into the esophagus and terminating in the stomach. This tube can be placed at the bedside by a nurse, physician, or caregiver who has training in this noninvasive, relatively simple procedure. Although patients may experience some minor discomfort as the tube is inserted, the procedure is generally well-tolerated with no sedation or anesthesia requirement. NG tubes are an ideal choice in patients who may need only a short course of enteral tube feeding. However, dislodgement or displacement can occur frequently, making NG tubes challenging for long-term use.

A GT should be considered if the patient requires tube feeding for more than 6 months and has exhibited tolerance of gastric feeding by NG tube. The placement of a GT is an invasive procedure in which a tube is placed in the stomach, extending through the abdominal wall and terminating outside the body. This creates a more stable, long-term route for nutrition. Low-profile GT "button" devices lie flat against the skin surface and are intermittently connected to extension tubing during a feed. Long tube devices contain a flexible tube that extends beyond the skin surface. These devices are further described in Chapter 14.

Postpyloric Feeding

Some patients cannot tolerate a gastric route of feeding because of anatomic or physiologic constraints. For these patients, postpyloric feeding, in which enteral nutrition is administered through a tube that terminates in the small intestine and bypasses the stomach, may be a successful alternative. For example, severe gastroesophageal reflux disease (GERD) affecting a patient's growth or respiratory status is a common indication for postpyloric feeding. There are numerous medical options (histamine-2 blockers, proton pump inhibitors, prokinetic agents) and surgical options (fundoplication) for managing GERD; however, some children may not be appropriate candidates for these therapies or they may have severe disease that persists despite exhausting these therapies. In such cases, postpyloric feeding may be an appropriate option.

Options for postpyloric enteral access are similar to those for gastric access (see Fig. 14.3). However, nasoduodenal (ND) or nasojejunal (NJ) tubes are not typically placed at the bedside but rather usually require radiographic guidance. Like NG tubes, ND and NJ tubes are appropriate for children who may require a short-term course of enteral feeding. A nasoenteral tube is also indicated in children in whom tolerance of postpyloric feeding is being assessed before a surgical procedure to establish longer-term postpyloric feeding access.

A combination gastrojejunostomy (GJ) tube has two external ports, one that connects to a tube terminating in the stomach and one that connects to a longer tube that extends into the jejunum. The gastric port is commonly used for venting and for medication administration, because many medications are most efficacious when administered into the stomach. The jejunal port can then be used for feeding and hydration. Jejunal tubes are smaller in caliber than gastric tubes because they must course through the narrower small intestines. Therefore these tubes are at increased risk for clogging. They also carry a risk for intussusception, with the tube acting as a lead point. Direct jejunostomy tubes that extend from the skin surface into the jejunum are sometimes placed in children with gastric outlet obstruction or gastric dysmotility.

Tube Feeding Regimens

After a route of access is established in a child who cannot adequately eat by mouth, the volume, rate, and schedule of feed administration is determined. The total daily required volume is based on both calorie and hydration needs. The total volume can be administered in multiple intermittent boluses throughout the day or can be run at a continuous rate.

Like most aspects of the care of CMC, the feeding regimen will be guided by the child's specific conditions and needs. For example, children with endocrine or metabolic disorders that predispose to hypoglycemia may require continuous feeds, because long periods between meals may predispose to dangerously low glucose levels. Children with severe GERD may better tolerate continuous feeding, because a large-volume bolus feed administered rapidly might worsen reflux. A feeding pump is used to deliver a specific volume over a given amount of time at a consistent rate.

Comparatively, a regimen of intermittent boluses simulates physiologic feeding more closely. The volume, frequency, and duration of each bolus feed is determined by the child's tolerance. Bolus feeds can be administered "by gravity," in which the formula passively enters the stomach when the feed reservoir (usually a special bag or an enteral feeding syringe) is suspended above the child. Each gravity feeding usually lasts 20 to 30 minutes. Boluses also can be given by a feeding pump. Bolus feedings allow the child to have periods of time detached from the feeding apparatus, minimizing restriction of activities and mobility.

Some families and clinicians may opt for a mixed regimen with bolus feeds during the day and continuous feeding overnight. Children who require enteral nutrition as a supplement to oral feeding may opt for eating by mouth during the day with continuous overnight feeding.

Retching, vomiting, discomfort, distension, or abnormal stools may suggest that a child is not tolerating the current regimen, prompting alterations such as lengthening the duration of a bolus feed; dividing the total daily volume into smaller, more frequent boluses; converting from bolus to continuous feeds; or changing the formula itself. When tube feedings are first initiated, it is customary to start at a slow rate or small volume, with gradual advancement toward the goal feeding regimen as the child demonstrates tolerance at each intermediate step.

Many medications interact with food, so the timing of medication administration must be taken into account when establishing a feeding regimen. Children may become bloated during or after a feed, and it may be useful to "vent" the GT. This is accomplished by connecting an empty feeding syringe to the GT and gently massaging the abdomen to push the air out.

For children with NJ or GJ tubes, bolus feeds are typically not given directly into the jejunum, because doing so may cause discomfort or diarrhea. If the child requires postpyloric feeding, the total volume required for the day should be given continuously over a number of hours, with the rate and duration usually determined by the child's size, tolerance, and activity level.

Formulas

Most nutritional formulas provide complete balanced nutrition; however, formulas for particular dietary restrictions and medical conditions are available. For example, children with renal dysfunction require "renal formulas" that are low in phosphorous and potassium. Other formulas contain hydrolyzed proteins or free amino acids for children with allergies, intolerances, malabsorption disorders, or short bowel syndrome.

Calorie content of standard infant formulas are 20 kilocalories per ounce (kcal/oz). Formulas designed for premature babies are usually 22 kcal/oz. Pediatric formulas for children older than 12 months of age are usually 1 kilocalorie per milliliter (kcal/mL), although reduced-calorie and calorie-dense versions (1.5 kcal/mL) exist for patients with different caloric needs. Standard formulas can be diluted or concentrated by altering the amount of water mixed in, providing a method for titration of caloric density. Fortifiers can be added to increase the caloric content of enteral nutrition.

Parenteral Nutrition

Some patients' nutritional needs cannot be met with enteral nutrition. This includes children who cannot tolerate any enteral feedings and those who may tolerate a limited amount but require additional supplementation. In these cases, parenteral nutrition (PN) may be indicated to provide the child with the necessary calories, macronutrients, and micronutrients. PN is an intravenous infusion of dextrose, amino acids, lipids, electrolytes, and minerals that provides nutrition while bypassing the GI tract. PN can be administered through a peripheral intravenous line in some cases, such as when it is first initiated or when it is only required for a short time. This subtype of PN is often referred to as peripheral or partial PN, because this less-concentrated solution can be administered safely through a more distal vein. Comparatively, TPN is higher in osmolality and concentration and requires central access for safe administration. Therefore most patients who receive PN will require a central venous catheter.

PN is used in a variety of clinical situations, such as prematurity, critical illness, and disorders of the GI tract such as dysmotility and malabsorption. Children with short bowel syndrome resulting from genetic syndromes, in-utero ischemic insults, necrotizing enterocolitis, or other causes are a subpopulation of medically complex patients who may require long-term PN.

When initiating PN, standardized reference ranges for carbohydrates (dextrose), protein (amino acids), fat (lipids), and electrolytes exist to guide initial formulations. Children on PN require frequent laboratory monitoring, including electrolytes, renal function, transaminases, liver function, triglycerides, essential fatty acids, iron, zinc, and selenium. Transaminases and other hepatic function tests such as conjugated bilirubin are trended to evaluate for development of intestinal failure–associated liver disease (IFALD), which unfortunately develops in a large proportion of patients receiving long-term parenteral nutrition.

MULTIDISCIPLINARY APPROACH

It is not unusual for CMC to have a team of clinicians involved in their care. A pediatric gastroenterologist may be helpful in managing dysmotility or malabsorption. The involvement of a registered dietitian is ideal in optimizing nutrition. The involvement of a speech-language pathologist and/or an occupational therapist to address oromotor skills can maximize safe oral feeding opportunities for CMC, even while they are on enteral or PN. Some children with oral aversion may benefit from a behavior specialist to increase food acceptance.

FUTURE DIRECTIONS

Improving the efficacy and convenience of home nutrition for patients and their caregivers is a major priority. To that end, feeding pump manufacturers have made the devices increasingly portable, and hospitals have created formalized training programs that teach parents and caregivers how to operate these devices. Developments such as smartphone integration and virtual simulations and trainings could streamline home enteral nutrition even further. In the realm of PN, novel intravenous lipid formulations have been introduced to mitigate liver toxicities. As these innovations undergo more widespread adoption, future research is required to evaluate their long-term clinical outcomes.

SUGGESTED READINGS

Available online.

14

Devices and Technology for Children With Medical Complexity

Ilana S. Lavina and Morgan E. Greenfield

 CLINICAL VIGNETTE

Rosie is a 3-year-old girl with a complex medical history presenting for a well-child visit. Rosie was born prematurely at 28 weeks' gestation and had a neonatal intensive care unit course complicated by grade III intraventricular hemorrhage and posthemorrhagic obstructive hydrocephalus requiring a ventriculoperitoneal shunt. She also developed necrotizing enterocolitis at 1 month of age, requiring surgical resection and leaving only 30 cm of small bowel remaining. Rosie is dependent on total parenteral nutrition, which she receives through a tunneled central venous catheter. She receives medications and small-volume enteral feeds through a gastrostomy tube (GT). On examination, she is well-appearing, smiling, and interactive. The skin entry sites of her central line and her GT have no surrounding erythema, tenderness, or swelling to suggest infection. Her neurologic examination is notable for mild hypertonia of all extremities.

As illustrated in the preceding vignette, devices and technologies are used routinely in the care of children with medical complexity (CMC). These include respiratory support devices, feeding tubes and pumps, vascular access catheters, cerebrospinal fluid (CSF) shunts, and implantable medication pumps. Pediatric subspecialists in fields such as pulmonology, gastroenterology, and neurosurgery play an integral role in guiding the selection and implementation of these devices. Multidisciplinary team members such as case managers, nurses, and dietitians ensure that families have the supplies and support required to use these devices effectively to meet a child's needs. In this chapter, we will review indications, use, and complications for devices and technologies used frequently by CMC.

RESPIRATORY EQUIPMENT

Because of a variety of underlying conditions, CMC are at increased risk for developing respiratory dysfunction and often rely on mechanical devices to ensure appropriate oxygenation and ventilation and to assist with clearance of respiratory secretions.

Noninvasive Positive Pressure Ventilation

Noninvasive positive pressure ventilation (NIV) devices are frequently used by CMC in the acute and chronic settings. Such devices allow for delivery of positive pressure ventilation by external interfaces without requiring endotracheal intubation. CMC may require chronic NIV for a variety of indications, including primary pulmonary diseases, congenital airway anomalies, and neurologic and neuromuscular disorders. There are two main types of NIV: continuous positive airway pressure (CPAP) and bilevel positive airway pressure (BLPAP). CPAP delivers a consistent baseline pressure throughout the respiratory cycle, whereas BLPAP delivers a higher pressure during inspiration and

a lower pressure during expiration. See Chapter 12 for further discussion of modes of NIV and rationale for its use for CMC.

Polysomnography, typically performed in a sleep laboratory, is a diagnostic tool used to evaluate apneas, hypopneas, and oxyhemoglobin desaturation events throughout the various stages of sleep, revealing which patients could benefit from NIV. Many patients with chronic respiratory insufficiency primarily use NIV during sleep to support ventilation Additionally, in the setting of acute illness or worsening respiratory decompensation, some patients may also temporarily require escalation of their NIV use to include waking hours as well. In these cases, patients are generally weaned back to their baseline settings or to a new baseline as their acute illness resolves.

Typically, NIV is first initiated while a patient is in the hospital, to allow for identification of optimal pressures and interface, close monitoring of respiratory status, and titration of device settings as needed. Several types of mask interfaces are commercially available, including nasal prongs, nasal masks, or full-face masks. Once a patient's most appropriate mask interface and pressure parameters are finalized, NIV can be delivered at home through a compact, portable machine. Polysomnography may be repeated in the future to further titrate machine settings, because the optimal parameters may change as a child grows and develops or with disease progression. Ongoing management is usually performed by a pediatric pulmonologist.

Invasive Mechanical Ventilation and Tracheostomy

In contrast to NIV, some patients may require long-term invasive ventilation. These patients will require a tracheostomy, which is a surgical procedure that creates an artificial airway by cannulating the cervical trachea (Fig. 14.1). However, although a tracheostomy tube allows for continuous delivery of mechanical ventilation, it is important to note that not all patients with a tracheostomy will need mechanical ventilation. Infants and children with anatomic airway abnormalities that compromise their natural airway may also undergo tracheostomy with or without accompanying mechanical ventilation.

Pediatric tracheostomy tubes are typically made from polyvinyl chloride or silicone. Tracheostomy tube sizes are based on parameters including inner diameter, outer diameter, and length. Customized tubes are also available, especially for children with complex anatomic airway anomalies. A horizontal flange anchors the tube against the skin surface on the neck, and an adjustable collar further stabilizes the tube. Tracheostomy tubes are available with and without inflatable balloon cuffs; inflatable cuffs allow for occlusion of the airway around the tracheostomy to prevent air from leaking above the device. Because of the potential for irritation or trauma to the airway mucosa if it is in constant contact with an inflated cuff, uncuffed tubes are preferred in many cases.

A multitude of complications can occur with tracheostomy tubes. One frequent issue is mucus plugging, in which the tube becomes obstructed by tracheal secretions and airflow is blocked. If the plug cannot be dislodged by suctioning through the tracheostomy, the tracheostomy tube will need to be changed (Fig. 14.2). Inadvertent decannulation, in which the device is accidentally displaced from the ostomy site, is another potentially life-threatening complication that requires swift tube replacement. Caregivers typically carry extra devices at all times in the event of such issues. Other complications include stomal granulation tissue, which often can be treated with steroid and antibiotic ointments or silver nitrate cautery by an experienced provider. Children with tracheostomies are more susceptible to bacterial tracheitis. Maintaining excellent hygiene at the tracheostomy site with frequent routine device changes can mitigate the risk for these complications. Long-term complications may include structural airway damage such as subglottic stenosis or suprastomal collapse, which may require a surgical intervention such as tracheoplasty before consideration of decannulation in these patients.

Adjunctive Airway Clearance Devices

In addition to the respiratory support devices described previously, there are many adjunctive devices that assist with mobilization and removal of mucus and secretions from the respiratory tract, a process colloquially known as "airway clearance." A cough assist device, also called a mechanical insufflator-exsufflator, delivers positive pressure to instill a large volume of gas into the lungs, then rapidly switches to negative pressure, generating a high expiratory flow rate that simulates

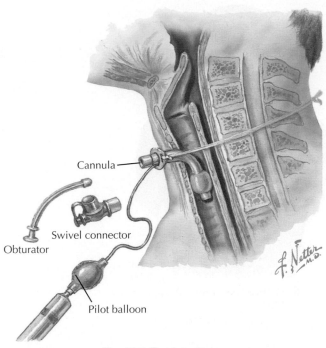

Cannula

Swivel connector

Obturator

Pilot balloon

Fig. 14.1 Tracheostomy.

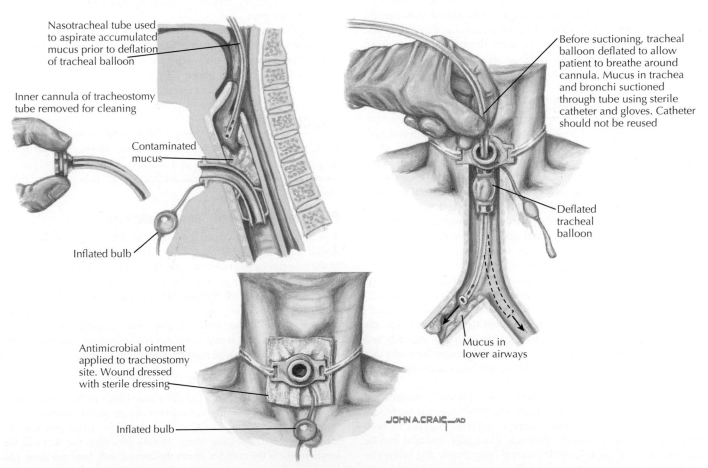

Nasotracheal tube used to aspirate accumulated mucus prior to deflation of tracheal balloon

Inner cannula of tracheostomy tube removed for cleaning

Contaminated mucus

Inflated bulb

Before suctioning, tracheal balloon deflated to allow patient to breathe around cannula. Mucus in trachea and bronchi suctioned through tube using sterile catheter and gloves. Catheter should not be reused

Deflated tracheal balloon

Mucus in lower airways

Antimicrobial ointment applied to tracheostomy site. Wound dressed with sterile dressing

Inflated bulb

JOHN A. CRAIG—AD

Fig. 14.2 Tracheostomy Care.

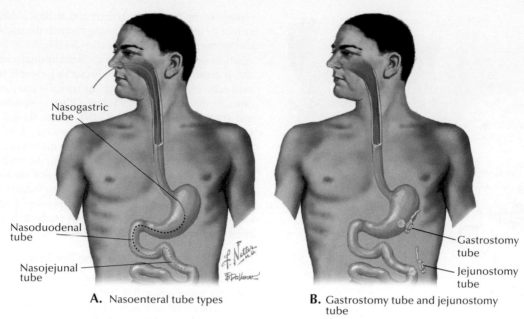

Nasogastric
tube

Nasoduodenal
tube

Nasojejunal
tube

A. Nasoenteral tube types

Gastrostomy
tube

Jejunostomy
tube

B. Gastrostomy tube and jejunostomy
tube

Fig. 14.3 (A) Nasoenteral tube types. (B) Gastrostomy tube and jejunostomy tube.

a strong cough. An intrapulmonary percussive ventilator is a machine that delivers small volumes of air at a high frequency, creating percussive bursts inside the respiratory tract that loosen secretions. These therapies can be delivered through a patient's existing NIV interface or through a separate mouthpiece, based on patient preference.

During the use of each of these devices, inhaled bronchodilators such as albuterol or ipratropium may be administered concurrently, providing pharmacologic dilation of the airways so that mucus and secretions have a larger conduit to move through as the mechanical devices work to physically mobilize the secretions so they can be coughed or suctioned out of the patient's oropharynx.

DEVICES FOR FEEDING AND NUTRITION

As discussed in Chapter 13, CMC may require alternatives to oral feeding. The least invasive type of feeding tube is a nasoenteral tube, which is a thin, flexible tube made from silicone or polyurethane that terminates in either the stomach (nasogastric) or small intestine (nasoduodenal or nasojejunal; Fig. 14.3A). Whereas nasogastric tubes can be placed at the bedside by a trained clinician or caregiver, tubes that pass into the small intestine are usually placed under fluoroscopic guidance. The position of the tube can be confirmed on a plain radiograph or, for tubes that terminate in the stomach, by testing the pH of aspirate or by other means according to local protocol.

In children who require long-term enteral feeds, a gastrostomy tube (GT; Fig. 14.3B) or gastrojejunostomy tube (GJT) may be indicated. A GT will have one port for administration of feeds and medications directly into the stomach. A GJT has two ports, one typically used for administration of medications through the stomach and one for administration of feeds into the small intestine by a tube that extends from the device past the pylorus and into the jejunum (see Fig. 13.1B).

Both long tubes and low-profile (or "button") devices are available. Long tube devices contain a flexible tube that protrudes beyond the skin surface. These have an internal bumper to hold the device in place within the stomach. Externally, the tube may be held in place with an adjustable external cross-bar or disc or may be used in conjunction with a special skin dressing to anchor the tube (see Fig. 13.1 C).

Button devices lie flat against the skin surface and are intermittently connected to extension tubing during a feed (Fig. 14.4). These tubes are less conspicuous than long tubes, increasing their aesthetic appeal and decreasing the risk for displacement by pulling or snagging of the tube when it is not in use. Button tubes may have a balloon or nonballoon internal bolster. Balloon bolsters are filled with water through a small external port.

Caregivers can be taught to replace a GT at home. A GJT, on the other hand, cannot be replaced at home, because fluoroscopy is needed to direct replacement of the postpyloric component.

For select patients in whom GT and GJT are not feasible, jejunal access can be placed by a direct jejunostomy tube (JT; Fig. 14.3B).

VASCULAR ACCESS

CMC may require stable, long-term vascular access. The particular device chosen depends on the indication, the duration of use, the frequency with which intravascular therapeutics are delivered, and other case-specific factors.

Peripherally Inserted Central Catheters

A peripherally inserted central catheter, or PICC, is a vascular access device that is inserted through a distal peripheral vein and terminates in the superior or inferior vena cava (Fig. 14.5A). PICC lines are indicated when a patient is projected to require an intermediate-term, temporary course of intravenous therapy. They can be safely used for weeks to months after placement. PICCs also offer the advantage of access for blood draws; however, given the risk profile of indwelling venous catheters, this is rarely a primary indication for placement if the patient does not otherwise require intravenous therapies.

Central Venous Catheters

Central venous catheters (CVCs) differ from PICCs in that a more proximal central vein is used for the initial site of cannulation. There are both tunneled and nontunneled CVCs. Tunneling refers to the physical distance between the location where the catheter enters the skin and the location where the catheter enters the central vein. Between these two locations, the catheter travels in a "tunnel" through the subcutaneous tissue (Fig. 14.5B). The tunneled approach offers several advantages,

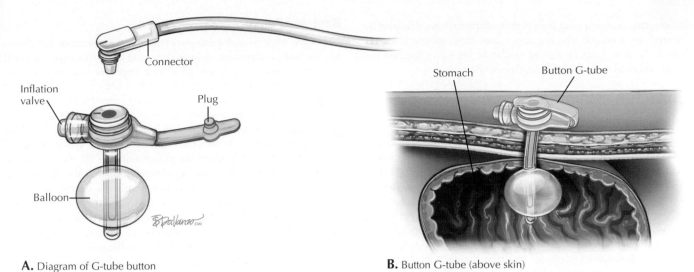

A. Diagram of G-tube button

B. Button G-tube (above skin)

Fig. 14.4 Button Gastrostomy Tube (G-tube).

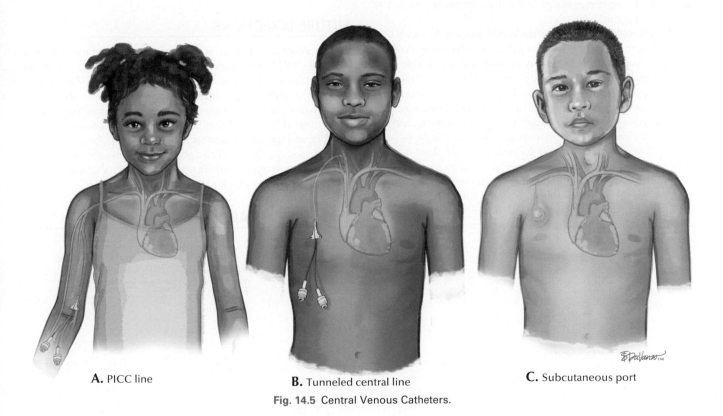

A. PICC line

B. Tunneled central line

C. Subcutaneous port

Fig. 14.5 Central Venous Catheters.

including increased stability of the catheter and decreased risk of infection. Common indications for these catheters include chronic total parenteral nutrition (TPN) or daily intravenous medication administration.

Nontunneled catheters, in which the skin exit site closely overlies the venous cannulation site, are typically reserved for temporary use in emergency settings in which central access must be achieved quickly to administer resuscitative medications and fluids. If longer-term access is required, nontunneled catheters will typically be converted to a more stable option.

Implanted Port

An implanted port is a vascular access device that is placed completely beneath the skin and intermittently connected to external infusion tubing for medication administration and blood draws. The device consists of a small chamber placed subcutaneously and a catheter that extends from this chamber, accesses a large vein, and terminates at the junction of the superior vena cava and the right atrium (Fig. 14.5C). The port chamber is about the size of a quarter and is covered on its anterior surface with a septum made of a self-sealing silicone rubber material. When the port needs to be used or "accessed," a special needle is placed through the skin overlying the chamber and through the silicone septum. When the port is not accessed, the entire device lies beneath the skin surface, with no connection between the body and the external environment.

Implanted ports are an ideal choice for patients who require intermittent intravenous therapies. For example, a patient with an oncologic condition may receive a port for chemotherapy that is given weekly. Comparatively, a patient who requires a daily large-volume infusion, such as TPN, would not be a good candidate for a port because the device would need to be accessed nearly continuously.

DEVICES FOR NEUROLOGIC CONDITIONS

Cerebrospinal Fluid Shunts

CSF shunting is a mainstay of treatment for hydrocephalus, an excessive accumulation of CSF in the cerebral ventricles that causes ventricular dilation and increased intracranial pressure (Fig. 11.5). The most commonly encountered type of shunt is a ventriculoperitoneal (VP) shunt. A VP shunt consists of a catheter with one end placed in one of the lateral ventricles and the other end placed in the peritoneal space. A one-way valve, located between the two ends, opens when the intracranial pressure rises above a certain threshold, allowing CSF to drain through the catheter and into the peritoneal space. If the peritoneal space is not amenable to catheter placement, such as in patients with prior abdominal surgeries and scarring, the distal end of the catheter is sometimes placed in the right atrium of the heart or in the pleural space of the lungs.

Complications of CSF shunts include malfunction, in which CSF cannot drain from the ventricles, and infection, which may manifest as meningitis or peritonitis. Both may present with nonspecific signs and symptoms, such as altered mental status, nausea, vomiting, and headache. Shunt infection may also manifest with fever, whereas peritonitis may manifest with abdominal pain and tenderness. Infections are most common within several months of shunt placement, and the most frequently involved pathogens are skin flora and *Staphylococcus aureus*. To allow for recovery of CSF for evaluation, the shunt features a small subcutaneous reservoir that can be accessed by a trained provider. Shunt malfunctions can occur at any time and may be due to a break or kink in the catheter or abnormal valve function. Head computed tomography to evaluate for evidence of ventricular dilation and shunt series radiographs are typically the first steps in the workup of a suspected shunt malfunction.

Baclofen Pumps

CMC may have neurologic disorders that cause spasticity and dystonia. Baclofen is a gamma aminobutyric acid (GABA) receptor agonist that modulates neurotransmission and improves abnormal muscle contraction. Baclofen given enterally is a first-line treatment option for spasticity or dystonia; however, patients may experience adverse effects such as sedation at the doses needed to achieve symptomatic relief. In these patients, an intrathecal baclofen pump may be indicated. This device is inserted in the subcutaneous tissue of the abdomen, and a small catheter extends from the pump reservoir to the intrathecal space. Because the medication is delivered locally to the spinal cord, the dose needed for efficacious symptom relief is significantly lower than when the medication is given enterally, and the risk for systemic adverse effects is minimized. The pump rate can be programmed using an external wand, and the pump must be refilled every few months by injection of the medication through the overlying skin into the reservoir port. Complications associated with intrathecal baclofen pumps include infection, seroma or hematoma at the port site, CSF leak, and device malfunction.

FUTURE DIRECTIONS

As technology continues to evolve, improvements in medical devices used by CMC can be expected. For example, feeding pumps have become highly portable and easy to use, allowing children who rely on them to participate in activities outside the home. As clinicians who care for CMC await these developments, it is imperative that they ensure that patients and families have all of the necessary support, supplies, and training to successfully operate their current devices and technologies. A strong interdisciplinary team consisting of physicians, nurses, case managers, dietitians, and respiratory therapists can work together to optimize care for CMC.

SUGGESTED READINGS

Available online.

SECTION III

Adolescent Medicine

Jonathan R. Pletcher

15

Behavioral Health Conditions

Evan Dalton

 CLINICAL VIGNETTE

A 15-year-old patient presents for a well-child check. The mother reports that the patient has a history of anxiety without a formal diagnosis. She also expresses that the patient has shown increased irritability over the past few months and seems to be spending more time alone. The patient describes feelings of sadness and notes troubles in school resulting in falling grades and strained relationships. The patient's appetite has decreased sharply, with a loss of 10 lb over the past month. There is a strong family history of alcoholism, and a paternal uncle attempted suicide. During a confidential interview, the patient reports a history of physical trauma from the father, personal daily alcohol use, intermittent suicidal ideation, and attempted suicide by acetaminophen ingestion 1 week ago that is not known to the mother.

Physical examination reveals a thin, sullen, and tearful teenager who makes poor eye contact. During the integumentary examination, countless linear forearm lacerations at various stages of healing are noted. The patient discloses the presence of numerous others on the inner thighs. The patient is diagnosed with depressive disorder and active suicidal ideation. Treatment options are discussed with the patient and the mother. They agree to immediately check in to the local children's hospital emergency department for further assessment. Urgent initiation of behavioral health counseling in the community and safety planning are discussed before the patient and the mother leave for the emergency department by private vehicle.

Behavioral health problems have become increasingly prevalent among children and adolescents over the past two decades, affecting approximately 1 in 5 children under 18 years of age. Nearly half of these children lack a formal diagnosis or care. This need for pediatric and adolescent behavioral health care has overwhelmed available resources, contributing to a doubling in visits to children's hospitals for suicidal ideation and suicide attempts over the past decade. Pediatric clinicians have taken on an increased role in the assessment and care of children affected by behavioral health problems. This has been amplified by societal and family disruptions caused by the COVID pandemic. Although depression, anxiety, and suicidal ideation are highly recognizable and treatable, suicide is the second leading cause of death for adolescents and young adults. Death by suicide is far more likely when there is ready availability to lethal means, with firearms being one of the most common methods of self-inflicted death in the United States.

The economic impact of pediatric behavioral health conditions is profound. Prior studies have valued the total annual cost to be over $240 billion. Untreated behavioral health conditions lead to considerable medical and social costs to society. Children afflicted by behavioral health conditions struggle at home, at school and in their interpersonal relationships, which leads to future losses in productivity and quality of life. Costly medical admissions can result from the sequelae of untreated behavioral health conditions, including ingestions, suicide attempts, and the development of eating or substance use disorders. Although behavioral health disorders are among the most expensive conditions to treat in children, their reimbursement rates are far less than the reimbursement for medical conditions.

Certain subpopulations of children have shown a proclivity to develop behavioral health conditions. Half of all children with chronic medical conditions will develop a comorbid behavioral health condition. Children of minority race and ethnicity experience health inequities, disparities, and racism that predispose them to developing behavioral health conditions. LGBTQIA+ individuals and children with family histories of behavioral health conditions are also at higher risk than the general population.

ETIOLOGY AND PATHOGENESIS

The etiology of behavioral health conditions in children is multifactorial. There is undoubtedly a neurobiological susceptibility stemming from genetic and epigenetic factors. Environmental factors provide a significant influence in the forms of adverse childhood experiences, timing of significant events, and the cumulative impact of adverse childhood experiences. Acute and chronic stressors during childhood and adolescence can alter the hypothalamic-pituitary-adrenal axis, affect brain development, and affect future responses to stress. For example, perinatal drug exposure, childhood trauma, social discrimination, and lack of family support have been shown to contribute to the development of behavioral health conditions in children.

The meteoric rise in pediatric behavioral health conditions over the past two decades can be explained through various theories. Studies have linked the rise in social media and smartphones with increasing behavioral health conditions. Children may also be affected by increasing stressors at schools lacking in appropriate resources. Studies have shown a pattern of presentation for behavioral health conditions based on the timing in the school year cycle—decreasing during summer months and peaking at the end of the school semesters. Finally, the high rate of untreated behavioral health conditions may contribute to households with multiple family members afflicted by their own behavioral health conditions.

Behavioral health conditions present, and often can be diagnosed, as children reach different stages of their development. Autism tends to manifest earlier in childhood because the characteristic delay in social-emotional interaction often manifests in the early preschool years. Attention-deficit hyperactive disorder (ADHD) is more commonly diagnosed in school-age children after deficiencies in concentration and impulse control are noted by teachers. Anxiety disorders tend to manifest in older children as they near adolescence (Fig. 15.1). However, their presentation can be delayed because of the development

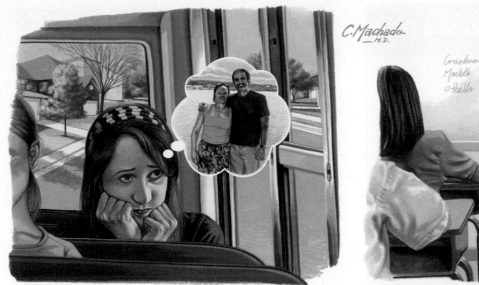

Generalized anxiety disorder (many worries and fears)

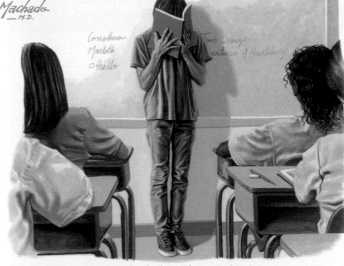

Social anxiety disorder (afraid of social interactions)

Fig. 15.1 Anxiety disorders are characterized by excessive and pathologic worrying and are prevalent in older children and adolescents. They may manifest with internalizing symptoms rather than externalizing. Uncontrolled anxiety can lead to the development of depression and substance use disorders.

of coping mechanisms and diagnostic challenge given the internalizing nature of anxiety. Depression, obsessive compulsive disorder, and bipolar disease present most often in adolescence (Fig. 15.2).

When uncontrolled, behavioral health conditions may become further complicated by maladaptive coping mechanisms. For instance, children and adolescents presenting with substance use and eating disorders often have preexisting behavioral health conditions. Children and adolescents with untreated behavioral health conditions are at high risk for suicide.

CLINICAL PRESENTATION

In large part because of societal stigma resulting in feelings of shame and guilt, clinical signs of behavioral health problems can be difficult to assess. Furthermore, children and adolescents suffering from behavioral health conditions often present with few physical examination findings, leading clinicians to rely primarily on the history for diagnosis. Children may even hide pertinent physical examination findings that, on discovery, could act as clues to the diagnosis. There is a constellation of physical examination findings that can be indicative of an underlying behavioral health condition, as seen in Table 15.1.

When taking a behavioral health history, pediatricians should focus on family and social histories for evidence of biological and environmental influences. Particular attention should be provided for unexplained changes in function, quality of life, and achievement, including declines in grades, school attendance, or participation in social and family activities. For adolescents, individual interviews should be performed after a discussion of confidentiality. Pediatricians should provide both adolescents and their parents with clear limits to the confidentiality of the interview. Keeping within statutory limits, adolescents should be informed that their history will be kept in confidence unless they give permission to disclose. The confidentiality of certain sensitive topics, including sexually transmitted infections, pregnancy, substance abuse, and suicidality, are governed by specific state and federal laws.

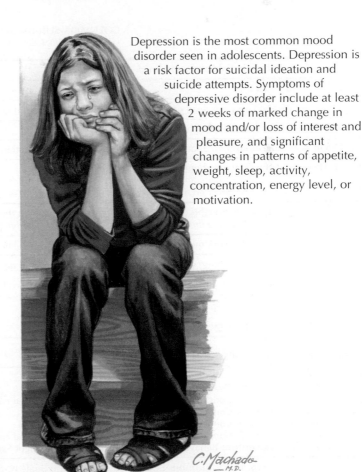

Depression is the most common mood disorder seen in adolescents. Depression is a risk factor for suicidal ideation and suicide attempts. Symptoms of depressive disorder include at least 2 weeks of marked change in mood and/or loss of interest and pleasure, and significant changes in patterns of appetite, weight, sleep, activity, concentration, energy level, or motivation.

Fig. 15.2 Depression.

TABLE 15.1   Correlation of Physical Examination Findings With Underlying Behavioral Health Conditions

Clinical Presentation	Physical Examination Findings	Behavioral Health Conditions
Self-injurious behavior	Lacerations, bruises, abrasions, burns, scars, petechiae	Autism spectrum disorder Depression Obsessive compulsive disorder
Substance use disorder	Pupillary changes, altered mental status, hypertension, weight loss, tachycardia, conjunctival injection, nystagmus, recurrent abscesses, ulcerated nasal mucosa	Depression Attention-deficit hyperactivity disorder Anxiety Bipolar disorder
Eating disorder	Bradycardia, weight loss, hypothermia, thinning scalp hair, dry skin, Russell sign (calluses on the dorsum of the fingers), acrocyanosis, parotid gland hypertrophy, dental enamel erosions	Anxiety Depression Obsessive compulsive disorder

If suicidal ideation is disclosed, pediatricians should be competent in performing a suicide risk assessment. Multiple screening tools exist to aid clinicians, including the Ask Suicide-Screening Questions, Suicide Assessment Five-Step Evaluation and Triage, and the Columbia-Suicide Severity Rating Scale (Fig. 15.3). Key components of suicide screening include prior planning and suicide attempts, access to lethal means and pharmaceuticals, and social structure, including the support of family and friends.

DIFFERENTIAL DIAGNOSIS

Pediatricians need to carefully exclude the presentation of a primary medical condition when assessing a child with a suspected behavioral health condition. Table 15.2 displays subtle symptoms of behavioral health conditions that can be indicative of uncommon primary medical conditions. Alternatively, children with primary behavioral health conditions may present with physical or somatic symptoms, as summarized in Table 15.3.

EVALUATION AND MANAGEMENT

After identifying the presence of a behavioral health condition in a child, pediatricians should perform a risk assessment by identifying the severity of the condition and the appropriate level of treatment. Multiple modalities for the treatment of pediatric behavioral health

COLUMBIA-SUICIDE SEVERITY RATING SCALE
*Screen with Triage Points for **Primary Care***

Ask questions that are in bold and underlined.		Past month	
Ask Questions 1 and 2		Yes	No
1) Have you wished you were dead or wished you could go to sleep and not wake up?			
2) Have you had any actual thoughts of killing yourself?			
If YES to 2, ask questions 3, 4, 5, and 6. If NO to 2, go directly to question 6.			
3) Have you been thinking about how you might do this? e.g. *"I thought about taking an overdose but I never made a specific plan as to when, where, or how I would actually do it....and I would never go through with it."*			
4) Have you had these thoughts and had some intention of acting on them? as opposed to *"I have the thoughts but I definitely will not do anything about them."*			
5) Have you started to work out or worked out the details of how to kill yourself? Do you intend to carry out this plan?			
6) Have you ever done anything, started to do anything, or prepared to do anything to end your life?		**Lifetime**	
Examples: Collected pills, obtained a gun, gave away valuables, wrote a will or suicide note, took out pills but didn't swallow any, held a gun but changed your mind or it was grabbed from your hand, went to the roof but didn't jump; or actually took pills, tried to shoot yourself, cut yourself, tried to hang yourself, etc.			
If YES, ask: **Was this within the past 3 months?**		**Past 3 Months**	

Response Protocol to C-SSRS Screening

Item 1 Behavioral Health Referral
Item 2 Behavioral Health Referral
Item 3 Behavioral Health Consult (Psychiatric Nurse/Social Worker) and consider Patient Safety Precautions
Item 4 Behavioral Health Consultation and Patient Safety Precautions
Item 5 Behavioral Health Consultation and Patient Safety Precautions
Item 6 Behavioral Health Consult (Psychiatric Nurse/Social Worker) and consider Patient Safety Precautions
Item 6 3 months ago or less: Behavioral Health Consultation and Patient Safety Precautions

Fig. 15.3 Columbia-Suicide Severity Rating Scale (C-SSRS) for Primary Care. The C-SSRS is an evidence-based tool that uses a series of concise questions to assess the risk for suicide. The responses to this scale can assist pediatricians in identifying the severity and contiguity of suicide risk. The associated response protocol is a tool that can aid providers on the next steps based on positive answers to the C-SSRS. (Reused from The Columbia Lighthouse Project, Kelly Posner Gertenhaber PhD, Founder and Director, https://cssrs.columbia.edu/.)

TABLE 15.2 Behavioral Health Symptoms Associated With Primary Medical Conditions

Behavioral Health Symptoms	Primary Medical Conditions
Depressed mood	Thyroid disorders, Addison disease, inflammatory bowel disease, hypopituitarism
Elevated mood	anti-NMDA receptor encephalitis, intoxication, systemic lupus erythematosus
Obsessive compulsive	PANDAS
Psychosis	Porphyria, systemic lupus erythematosus, Wilson disease, thyrotoxicosis, central nervous system abnormality, drug toxicity
Self-injurious behavior	Child abuse

PANDAS, Pediatric autoimmune neuropsychiatric disorders associated with streptococcal infections.

TABLE 15.3 Physical Symptoms of Primary Behavioral Health Conditions

Behavioral Health Condition	Physical Symptoms
Autism spectrum disorder	Speech delay, encopresis, self-harm
Attention-deficit hyperactivity disorder	Anger problems, disciplinary action at school
Anxiety	Headaches, shortness of breath, chest pain, globus sensation
Depression	Weight loss, insomnia, fatigue
Suicidal ideation or attempt	Lacerations, bruising, petechiae, bleeding diathesis, burns
Psychosis	Hyperactivity, changes in speech

TABLE 15.4 Diagnostic Tools and First-Line Treatments for Behavioral Health Conditions

Behavioral Health Condition	Diagnostic Tool	First-Line Treatments
Autism spectrum disorder	MCHAT	Applied behavior analysis therapy, risperidone, aripiprazole
Attention-deficit hyperactivity disorder	NICHQ Vanderbilt Assessment Scale	Methylphenidates, amphetamines, guanfacine, atomoxetine, counseling
Anxiety	SCARED	Cognitive behavioral therapy, fluoxetine, escitalopram, sertraline
Depression	PHQ-9	Cognitive behavioral therapy, fluoxetine, escitalopram

MCHAT, Modified Checklist for Autism in Toddlers; *NICHQ*, National Institute for Children's Health Quality; *PHQ-9*, Patient Health Questionnaire; *SCARED*, Screen for Child Anxiety Related Disorders.

conditions exist. Outpatient treatment, through a trained primary care provider, psychologist, or psychiatrist, is the least restrictive level of care. Children can be seen on an intermittent basis with scheduled therapy sessions and medication management. More acute and severe presentations of behavioral health conditions may be appropriate for intensive outpatient or partial hospitalization. Partial hospitalization is most appropriate for children who require immediate intervention, but do not pose a risk for harm to themselves or others. Most partial hospitalization programs involve multiple types of therapy and medication management through a psychiatrist. Inpatient psychiatric hospitalization is the most intensive level of care and is recommended for children at high risk for, or who have a recent history of, harming themselves or others. In this setting, children are admitted to a locked unit and work with a multidisciplinary team daily to optimize their medical and therapeutic treatment.

If a child with a behavioral health condition presents to an outpatient facility with active suicidal or homicidal ideation or evidence of a recent suicide attempt such as an ingestion, they should be directed to an emergency department, either by private vehicle or ambulance, depending on their risk assessment and medical stability. Children with passive suicidal ideation can collaborate with their pediatrician and family to create a safety plan if they are to be discharged home. Important components to a safety plan include contact information for a health professional if suicidal ideation recurs, counseling on restriction of lethal means such as toxic medicines or firearms, and a follow-up plan for timely behavioral health assessment and linkage to care.

Laboratory monitoring in children with behavioral health conditions should be tailored to each clinical presentation. A urine drug screen should be strongly considered for children presenting to a hospital with behavioral health concerns, especially if altered mental status is present. A urine pregnancy test should be obtained for female patients of childbearing age. If an ingestion is suspected, multiple additional tests may be indicated, including acetaminophen, salicylate, and ethanol levels, electrocardiogram, and abdominal or chest radiography. Screening for endocrine and autoimmune dysfunction also may be indicated, because disorders ranging from thyroid disease to systemic lupus erythematosus commonly manifest with altered mood and behaviors.

Pediatricians can develop their skills in diagnosing and treating common behavioral health conditions with first-line therapies. Table 15.4 lists commonly diagnosed behavioral health conditions, their associated diagnostic scales, and first-line treatments.

FUTURE DIRECTIONS

The future of care for behavioral health conditions in children is promising. Technological and social advances have allowed for the rise of telehealth, which has proved to be a useful care model for expanding access to behavioral health care at a low cost. Digital therapeutics may become an adjunctive therapy, particularly considering the influence of technology on younger generations. However, the resources allocated to treating behavioral health conditions remain scarce compared to those allocated for medical conditions. The potential economic benefit of improved pediatric behavioral health treatment gives pediatricians an important advocacy avenue.

SUGGESTED READINGS

Available online.

16

Dysmenorrhea and Abnormal Uterine Bleeding

Michelle Shankar

 CLINICAL VIGNETTE

During a routine well visit, a 13-year-old girl reports a history of heavy and irregular menstrual bleeding since menarche 1 year previously. Menses occur every 4 to 8 weeks and last 4 to 7 days, and she changes tampons every 4 hours when they are completely soaked with blood. She has to change her pad in the middle of the night or it will soak through her clothes, and she has missed several days of school because of fear of bleeding through her clothes. She denies pain or cramps with menses, but has also limited her participation on the swim team. Her parent reports she is more irritable and generally stays in her room during menses. She denies sexual activity and substance use. She is otherwise healthy and does not take medications. Her physical examination is notable for normal vital signs for her age, mild conjunctival pallor, benign abdominal examination, and Sexual Maturity Rating (SMR) of stage 4 for breast and 5 for pubic hair on visual genital examination. The patient is started on oral iron supplementation, and she is encouraged to maintain a menstrual calendar, with follow-up scheduled in 3 months.

Dysmenorrhea and abnormal uterine bleeding (AUB) are two of the most common concerns that pediatricians address with their adolescent cis-female and trans-male patients. Perimenstrual symptoms can have a significant impact on quality of life for patients, interfering with participation in school, extracurricular activities, and important family and social activities. Despite the prevalence of these complaints, few patients seek medical advice from their primary care doctor; therefore it is important for clinicians to take a complete menstrual history in all adolescents at risk for symptoms and to be familiar with management strategies.

Primary dysmenorrhea refers to recurrent crampy lower abdominal pain that occurs during menstruation in the absence of pelvic pathologic conditions. Associated symptoms can be premenstrual and include nausea, vomiting, diarrhea, constipation, headache, dizziness, fatigue, back pain, and mood disturbance. Primary dysmenorrhea is thought to be mediated by prostaglandins released by myometrial tissue causing local and systemic symptoms.

AUB is menstrual bleeding that is outside of regular menstrual cycle length, frequency, or flow. AUB can vary widely in presentation, but typically includes bleeding that lasts longer than 8 days or occurs more frequently than every 3 weeks. Assessment of blood flow by history is notoriously difficult; however, bleeding through clothes, particularly when high-absorbency menstrual products are employed, and associated symptoms of fatigue, pallor, or dizziness, are cause for clinical concern. AUB most commonly occurs within 5 to 7 years after menarche, especially in the first 2 years, when more than 50% of cycles are anovulatory and therefore lacking the stabilizing effects of progesterone on endometrial tissue.

Diagnosis and management of both dysmenorrhea and AUB are focused on excluding secondary causes, educating patients and parents on preventive and mitigating strategies, and selecting treatment appropriate to the patient's individual characteristics and symptom severity.

ETIOLOGY AND PATHOGENESIS

An adult menstrual cycle is driven by increases and periodic drops in ovarian estrogen manufactured by granulosa cells of ovarian follicles. As estrogen levels increase during the first phase of the menstrual cycle, endometrial tissue growth and proliferation occurs during the follicular stage. Estrogen provides positive feedback centrally to the hypothalamus and pituitary gland, causing a mid-cycle surge in luteinizing hormone (LH). The LH surge results in ovulation. Ovulation results in formation of the corpus luteum (CL), and estrogen levels decrease as the CL produces progesterone during the luteal stage. Progesterone promotes the stabilization and glandular changes within the endometrial mucosa to provide an environment for implantation of a fertilized ovum. Without implantation, the CL cannot maintain the production of progesterone, leading to sloughing of the endometrial lining as estrogen and progesterone levels decrease 14 days after ovulation.

Menstrual cycle length, duration, and flow vary considerably during the first few years after menarche because of immaturity of the hypothalamic-pituitary-ovarian (HPO) axis, resulting in anovulation and inconsistent ovulation. Anovulatory cycles typically occur during the first 2 years after menarche and can last longer with later onset and slower progression through puberty. Anovulation occurs when the increase in estrogen during the follicular stage does not result in a surge of LH. Once regular ovulation is established, the majority of cycles in adolescents last 21 to 45 days with 2 to 7 days of menstrual bleeding, and the median blood loss per cycle is 20 to 80 mL.

The most common cause of AUB in adolescents is anovulatory cycles, which is often associated with severe blood loss. Because the endometrium is exposed to estrogen without progesterone, it can become highly thickened and friable, resulting in heavy, prolonged, or unsynchronized sloughing of the endometrial lining with submucosal arterioles open to the uterine cavity (Fig. 16.1). When AUB occurs in an adolescent who has established regular ovulatory cycles, bleeding may be less severe; however, the differential diagnosis expands greatly.

Dysmenorrhea generally does not occur until ovulatory menstrual cycles are established and appears to be caused by excess production of endometrial prostaglandin F2 alpha (PGF2 alpha), which can cause dysrhythmic uterine contractions, hypercontractility, and increased uterine muscle tone leading to uterine ischemia. This also accounts for nausea, vomiting, and diarrhea by stimulation of the gastrointestinal

Hypothalamic regulation of pituitary gonadotropin production and release

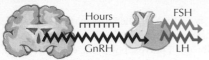

Pulsed release of GnRH by hypothalamus (1 pulse /1–2 hr) permits anterior pituitary production and release of FSH and LH (normal)

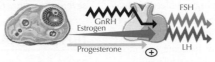

Continuous, excessive, absent, or more frequent GnRH release inhibits FSH and LH production and release (downloading)

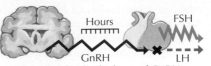

Decreased pulsed release of GnRH decreases LH secretion but increases FSH secretion (slow-pulsing model)

Ovarian feedback modulation of pituitary gonadotropin production and release

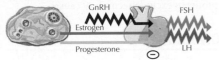

Pulsed GnRH and low estrogen and progesterone levels result in increased levels of pulsed LH and FSH (negative feedback)

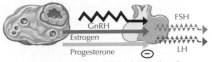

Pulsed GnRH, rapidly increasing levels of estrogen, and small amounts of progesterone result in high pulsed LH and moderately increased pulsed FSH levels (positive feedback)

Pulsed GnRH and high levels of estrogen and progesterone result in decreased LH and FSH levels (negative feedback)

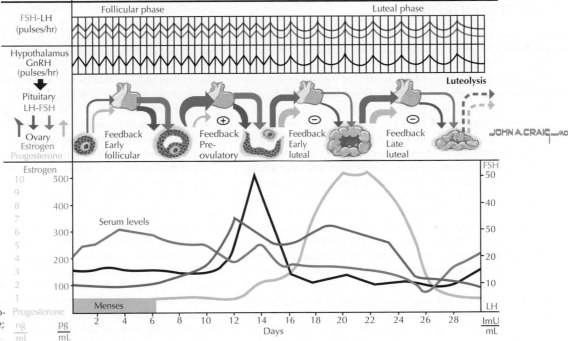

Correlation of serum gonadotrophic and ovarian hormone levels and feedback mechanisms

FSH, follicle-stimulating hormone; GnRH, gonadotropin-releasing hormone; LH, luteinizing hormone.

Fig. 16.1 Neuroendocrine Regulation of Menstrual Cycle.

(GI) tract and contributes to systemic effects mediated by pelvic muscles and possibly circulating prostaglandins crossing the blood-brain barrier.

HISTORY

A complete history should be obtained both with and without the adolescent's caregiver present. A thorough menstrual history includes the age of menarche, menstrual pattern, associated symptoms, and events that coincided with any changes in the menstrual pattern. It is helpful to ask patients to maintain a menstrual calendar, and smartphone apps are readily available. To quantify the volume of menstrual blood flow, the history should include the type and size of pad or tampons used, the number used per day or the hours each item is worn, and an estimate of the degree to which it is soaked. Indirect indicators of heavy flow include passing blood clots larger than 1 inch in diameter, bleeding through clothes, the need to change sanitary protection during the night, and symptoms of volume depletion.

History related to dysmenorrhea should include presence of cramping, nausea, vomiting, diarrhea, back pain, dizziness, fatigue, and headache around the time of menstruation. It is important to note initial onset of symptoms and progression over time, relation of symptoms to periods, impact of symptoms on daily activities (e.g., school attendance and sports participation), factors that worsen symptoms, and the impact of measures taken to relieve symptoms.

A confidential sexual and social history should be obtained, including contraceptive and condom use, number of lifetime partners, new partners in the past few months, history of sexually transmitted infections (STIs), current symptoms (e.g., vaginal discharge, pelvic pain, bleeding with intercourse), previous pregnancy or abortion, and history of sexual abuse or assault. Social history should include information about stressors, substance use, and intensity of exercise. Questions about school engagement and achievement or decreased participation in recreational activities can provide valuable information about the effects on quality of life.

The medical history should include information about hematologic or renal disease, GI bleeding, cervical polyps, and current or recent medications that may interfere with ovulation or bleeding. The family history should include information about bleeding disorders, infertility, menstrual disorders, thyroid disease, polycystic ovary syndrome (PCOS), diabetes, lipid disorders, and leukemia or other types of cancer.

A complete review of systems should include symptoms of acute or chronic anemia, such as lightheadedness, fatigue, syncope, weakness, and headaches. Easy bruising, epistaxis, and/or gingival bleeding may be suggestive of a bleeding disorder. Weight loss or gain, disordered eating behaviors, palpitations, heat or cold intolerance, hirsutism, acne, and/or changes in hair, skin, or nails may indicate endocrine abnormalities. Visual changes, headaches, and galactorrhea may suggest hyperprolactinemia secondary to pituitary adenoma. Bleeding that occurs solely with urination or defecation suggests a urinary or GI source.

CLINICAL PRESENTATION

In a patient with primary dysmenorrhea, the abdominal examination is usually benign when the patient is not menstruating or it reveals generalized lower abdominal tenderness during menses. A finding of highly localized reproducible tenderness, with or without a mass, suggests a diagnosis other than primary dysmenorrhea. The abdominal examination is often normal in patients with AUB.

Physical examination findings in the setting of AUB are essential for triage and clinical decision making. Signs of severe acute volume loss include symptomatic or abnormal orthostatic vital signs, markedly elevated heart rate at rest, cool or clammy skin, and acute anxiety or agitation. Signs of anemia include skin or mucosal pallor, elevated heart rate, or flow murmur. Petechiae, bruising, epistaxis, or gingival bleeding may be evidence of an underlying bleeding disorder. It is also important to evaluate for signs of thyroid dysfunction, androgen excess (hirsutism, acne), and pituitary mass (bitemporal hemianopsia).

The external breast examination can identify sexual maturity rating (SMR) staging; menarche usually does not occur before SMR stage 3, so bleeding before this stage suggests a nonmenstrual source of bleeding. The external genital examination can reveal clitoromegaly, signs of trauma, hymenal integrity, and retained foreign body. With wide availability of nucleic acid amplification testing, a pelvic examination is rarely indicated regardless of history of sexual activity, with the exception of a history of trauma. For sexually active adolescents, a bimanual examination may reveal cervical motion tenderness or pelvic fullness, raising suspicion for pelvic inflammatory disease (PID).

DIAGNOSTIC EVALUATION

Laboratory evaluation is not required to confirm anovulation or immaturity of the HPO axis. It is important to obtain a urine pregnancy test in all adolescents who present with vaginal bleeding, regardless of the sexual history. If anemia or an underlying bleeding disorder is suspected, workup may include a complete blood count, peripheral blood smear, iron studies, coagulation studies, and von Willebrand panel. If infection or sexual abuse is suspected, evaluate for STIs such as *Chlamydia trachomatis* and *Neisseria gonorrhea* (see Chapter 19).

Endocrine workup should include thyroid function tests, prolactin levels, and/or androgen levels (total and free testosterone, dehydroepiandrosterone sulfate [DHEA-S], and androstenedione). Follicle-stimulating hormone (FSH) level obtained in the first week of menstruation can help identify ovarian insufficiency if elevated. Laboratory studies may include evaluation for autoimmune disease, or

medication-related bleeding as warranted by the history and physical examination.

Pelvic ultrasonography is indicated when pregnancy is possible and to assess for structural causes of bleeding such as uterine anomalies, uterine leiomyomas (fibroids), polyps, polycystic ovaries, ovarian tumors, and/or adrenal masses. Magnetic resonance imaging (MRI) of the pelvis may be indicated for patients with a suspected pelvic or adrenal mass when ultrasonography does not clearly define the anatomy. Pelvic ultrasound or MRI should be considered in all females with severe dysmenorrhea symptoms to exclude secondary causes.

DIFFERENTIAL DIAGNOSIS

The presence of pelvic pain between menses suggests secondary dysmenorrhea, including anatomic abnormalities such as incomplete fenestration of the hymen or developmental anomalies of the müllerian duct. Menstrual pain that has become progressively worse over time is characteristic of endometriosis, which may manifest as cyclic or noncyclic pain. Adolescents with a history of PID may develop adhesions resulting in chronic pelvic pain that worsens during menstruation. Similarly, chronic recurrent pelvic pain from the GI system can also worsen during menses, including inflammatory bowel diseases, irritable bowel syndrome, or chronic constipation. A complete psychosocial history may suggest other causes or exacerbating factors of abdominal pain such as depression, substance abuse, or stress.

The bleeding pattern of AUB can help guide the differential diagnosis and diagnostic workup. Normal cyclic intervals with prolonged (>7 days) or heavy bleeding during each cycle may suggest a bleeding disorder such as von Willebrand disease, immune thrombocytopenia, platelet dysfunction, and thrombocytopenia. It also can be caused by a systemic illness that affects ovarian or liver function, causing abnormalities in ovulation or coagulation. Structural lesions such as polyps or uterine leiomyomas can manifest with heavy menstrual bleeding. Medications that affect coagulation can exacerbate bleeding.

Irregular menstrual cycles may suggest anovulatory cycles, which can be physiologic in the first 2 or more years after menarche but also can occur as a result of endocrinopathies such as PCOS, thyroid dysfunction, hyperprolactinemia, or HPO axis suppression as a result of stress, exercise, malnutrition, weight loss, obesity, regular use of marijuana, or autoimmune or other chronic systemic illness. Medications that affect ovulation can also contribute to AUB.

Intermenstrual bleeding can be caused by pregnancy, abortion, or infection. It is also a common side effect of hormonal contraceptives. Less common causes include trauma, retained foreign body, and vascular or anatomic abnormalities.

TREATMENT

Hydration, homeopathic interventions, and nonsteroidal antiinflammatory drugs (NSAIDs) are first-line treatment for primary dysmenorrhea. NSAIDs should be started at or before the onset of menses and continued for the first 1 to 2 days of the menstrual cycle. NSAIDS are most effective when begun early in the course of symptoms because of their effects on prostaglandin synthetase. Estrogen-containing hormonal contraceptives prevent menstrual pain by suppressing ovulation, thereby decreasing uterine prostaglandin levels. Hormonal contraceptives are appropriate as second-line therapy, although they may be appropriate for first-line therapy in patients who are sexually active. Patients should be followed closely for the first few months after treatment is initiated; those who fail to respond to first- or second-line treatments, have recurrent pain, or have symptoms that worsen should be reevaluated for other causes.

A positive pregnancy test in the setting of AUB warrants urgent evaluation by an obstetrician/gynecologist, typically in an emergency department. If pregnancy can be ruled out, severe AUB is defined in any adolescent who exhibits signs or symptoms of hemodynamic instability, hemoglobin less than 7 g/dL, or a hemoglobin less than 10 g/dL with active bleeding. For severe AUB, patients may benefit from hormonal therapy using combined oral contraceptive pill (OCP) containing higher doses of estrogen. If severe anemia (hemoglobin <7 to 8 g/dL) or hemodynamic instability is present, blood transfusion is indicated, as well as combination hormonal therapy. When estrogen is contraindicated, progestin-only methods can be provided orally or intramuscularly. In extreme circumstances, intrauterine tamponade or surgical dilation and curettage can be considered with appropriate consultation.

Adolescents who are not pregnant and are hemodynamically stable can be triaged to mild (normal hemoglobin [Hgb]) or moderate (Hgb >10 g/dL, or >7 g/dL without active bleeding) AUB. The underlying cause of AUB determines the treatment. For mild AUB, treatment largely involves reassurance until the ovulatory cycles resume.

Menstrual calendar and iron supplementation are helpful. If the problem persists, or in moderate AUB, consider hormonal therapy with a daily combined OCP. If estrogen is contraindicated, a progesterone-only pill or intrauterine device will result in less overall bleeding but resolution may take longer.

SUMMARY

Dysmenorrhea and AUB are two of the most common concerns that pediatricians address with their adolescent female patients. Both can have a significant impact on quality of life, be the presenting symptoms of underlying chronic disease, or indicate a life-threatening process. A thorough history, review of systems, and physical examination can help guide diagnostic workup and effective management.

SUGGESTED READINGS

Available online.

17

Polycystic Ovarian Syndrome in Adolescents

Shelby Davies and Jennifer K. Sun

 CLINICAL VIGNETTE

A 15-year-old girl presents to her pediatrician for amenorrhea and weight gain. She had normal puberty with menarche at age 12, and her cycles had been regular until her last menstrual period 4 months ago. She is concerned about weight gain and has started to restrict her diet. She has never been sexually active, and a urine pregnancy test is negative. Physical examination reveals a body mass index above the 95th percentile, whereas she had been growing around the 75th percentile. She has new findings of hyperpigmented and velvety appearing skin on her neck and axilla, and moderate inflammatory acne on her face, back, and chest. No facial hirsutism is evident, but she reports using depilatory measures on her upper lip and chin. Coarse dark hair is noted growing on her lower abdomen and chest. Laboratory evaluation reveals an elevated free testosterone; normal follicle-stimulating hormone, luteinizing hormone, and 17-OH progesterone; and an unremarkable ovarian ultrasound. She is diagnosed with polycystic ovary syndrome, counseled on appropriate lifestyle changes, and started on a combined oral contraceptive pill. At her 6-month follow-up, she had return of regular menstrual cycles, and a reduction in her free testosterone level, although she notes no significant difference in facial or body hair growth.

Polycystic ovary syndrome (PCOS) is the most common endocrine disorder of reproductive age women, frequently manifesting between menarche and early adulthood. In this age group, PCOS is characterized by anovulatory menstrual dysfunction, hyperandrogenism, and metabolic disturbances. In adolescents, persistent oligo/anovulation for 2 years in the setting of hyperandrogenic phenotypic changes are needed to distinguish PCOS from physiologic anovulation. Early identification is recommended, even if making a provisional diagnosis, so that clinicians are able to address immediate health concerns, prevent or mitigate psychosocial pathologic conditions, and reduce likelihood of long-term cardiovascular and metabolic sequelae. If unrecognized and untreated, morbidity includes impaired reproductive health, including potential for infertility, psychosocial dysfunction, metabolic syndrome characterized by insulin resistance, cardiovascular disease, and increased cancer risk.

Many sets of diagnostic criteria for PCOS exist for adult women (Table 17.1). In 2015, the American Association of Clinical Endocrinologists, American College of Endocrinology, and the Androgen Excess and PCOS Society summarized current best practices for clinicians. Briefly stated, the diagnosis of PCOS can be made when two of three criteria are established: oligo/anovulation, clinical or biochemical evidence of hyperandrogenism, and polycystic ovarian morphology.

ETIOLOGY AND PATHOGENESIS

PCOS results from an interaction of genetic and environmental factors that disrupt metabolic pathways, including disrupted neuroendocrinologic gonadotropic secretion, ovarian androgen production, and insulin resistance. Insulin resistance and compensatory hyperinsulinemia synergizes with luteinizing hormone (LH) to increase ovarian androgen secretion. Hyperandrogenism contributes to abnormal hypothalamic gonadotropin-releasing hormone (GnRH) secretion, resulting in anovulation (Fig. 17.1). Elevated insulin levels both stimulate ovarian androgen production and simultaneously inhibit liver synthesis of sex hormone binding globulin (SHBG), which increases the fraction of bioavailable free testosterone.

CLINICAL PRESENTATION

Although menstrual irregularities are very common during adolescence (Chapter 16), the combination of oligomenorrhea or abnormal uterine bleeding with clinical signs of hyperandrogenism should raise suspicion for PCOS. Oligomenorrhea is defined as cycle length persistently longer than 32 days and is associated with endometrial hyperplasia that can result in AUB. Clinical signs of hyperandrogenism include hirsutism, inflammatory acne, and alopecia. The Ferriman-Gallwey score is used to grade the degree of hirsutism in androgen-sensitive areas (Fig. 17.2). Adolescents with inflammatory acne that is resistant to oral or topical agents should be assessed for hyperandrogenism and may have an increased risk for PCOS up to 40% over that of the general population. Severe hirsutism or virilization is rarely seen with PCOS and may be indicative of nonclassic congenital adrenal hyperplasia, exogenous anabolic steroids, or other hyperandrogenic states. Excessive weight gain can result from hyperandrogenism and insulin resistance; however, this is not a universal finding. Because most adolescents experience physiologic anovulatory cycles for up to 2 years after menarche, and because of the high degree of genetic variability resulting in mild hirsutism, potential delays in diagnosis are to be expected. Thus it is important to closely follow young women suspected to be at risk for developing PCOS for early diagnosis and intervention.

Differential Diagnosis

Although PCOS is the most common reason that adolescent females present with androgen excess, other rare causes must be excluded, including nonclassic congenital adrenal hyperplasia (NC-CAH), androgen-secreting neoplasms (ASNs), other endocrinopathies, and exposure to drugs or medications. ASNs are the only life-threatening disorder on the differential diagnosis and should be considered if clinical findings are suggestive of virilization, including clitoromegaly, deepening of the voice, and male pattern baldness. Several other endocrine disorders that can disrupt the menstrual cycle but rarely present with hyperandrogenism include thyroid disease, hyperprolactinemia, and premature ovarian failure. Exogenous anabolic steroids and antiepileptic medications may also result in clinical signs of hyperandrogenism.

TABLE 17.1	Polycystic Ovarian Syndrome Phenotypes Included in Specific Diagnostic Criteria		
NIH 1990	**Rotterdam 2003/2006**	**Androgen Excess-PCOS Society**	**NIH 2012**
Chronic anovulation	Oligo/anovulation	Ovarian dysfunction (defined by oligo/anovulation or polycystic morphology or both)	Oligo/anovulation
Clinical and/or biochemical signs of hyperandrogenism	Clinical and/or biochemical signs of hyperandrogenism Polycystic ovarian morphology	Clinical and/or biochemical signs of hyperandrogenism	Clinical and/or biochemical signs of hyperandrogenism Polycystic ovarian morphology
Both criteria needed	**Two of three criteria needed**	**Both criteria needed**	**Two of three criteria needed**

All four criteria require the exclusion of other endocrinopathies.
NIH, National Institutes of Health; *PCOS*, polycystic ovarian syndrome.
From *International Journal of Women's Health*, 2014;6:613–621. Originally published by and used with permission from Dove Medical Press Ltd.

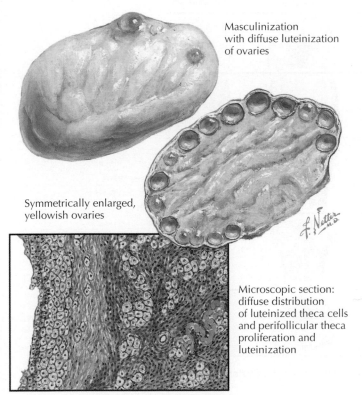

Masculinization with diffuse luteinization of ovaries

Symmetrically enlarged, yellowish ovaries

Microscopic section: diffuse distribution of luteinized theca cells and perifollicular theca proliferation and luteinization

Fig. 17.1 Polycystic Ovarian Disease.

SCREENING AND EVALUATION

The most sensitive test for hyperandrogenism is serum free testosterone, which is the bioactive fraction of testosterone that is not bound to SHBG. Elevations in weaker androgens from the adrenal gland, including androstenedione or DHEA-S, may account for hyperandrogenism in 10% of patients with PCOS. Elevated levels of 17-hydroxyprogesterone may suggest the diagnosis of NC-CAH in patients with enough clinical suspicion. Obtaining thyroid function tests, prolactin, LH, FSH, random serum cortisol, and estradiol levels will help to exclude other endocrinopathies and premature ovarian failure. Ultrasound can be used to evaluate for polycystic ovaries and exclude rare ovarian tumors or other pelvic pathologic conditions. Multifollicular ovaries and larger ovarian volume, however, can be a normal variant in youth and unrelated to androgen excess. Most experts recommend that adolescents with PCOS be routinely screened for dyslipidemias. Acanthosis nigricans and weight gain can result from insulin resistance, which can be determined with an oral glucose tolerance test, even when fasting blood glucose and insulin levels are normal.

MANAGEMENT

Management should focus on the clinical concerns and the long-term health outcomes of the patient. Lifestyle modifications are considered first-line management for overweight adolescents with PCOS. A modest amount of weight loss can help achieve menstrual regularity, decrease cardiovascular and metabolic risks, and lessen androgen excess.

Combined oral contraceptives (COCs) are the first-line pharmacologic treatment for adolescents. The combination of estrogen and progesterone suppresses the endogenous gonadal axis and interrupts the pathophysiologic mechanism of PCOS. Estrogen increases the concentration of SHBG, which decreases bioactive free testosterone. In addition to normalizing menstrual cycles, progesterone prevents unopposed estrogen from causing endometrial hyperplasia and AUB. In patients with contraindications to COCs, progesterone monotherapy can be used to normalize endometrial cycling, but circulating androgens may not be as well suppressed. Menstrual irregularities are generally expected to improve within the first 2 to 3 months of treatment.

COCs may also help improve acne and stop progression of hirsutism, although this may take 6 months or more. Testosterone levels typically improve by the third month of therapy. Spironolactone, an antiandrogen agent, may be used as an adjunct to improve menstrual irregularities and cutaneous manifestations of hirsutism but not metabolic abnormalities. Metformin is commonly used when weight gain from insulin resistance is prevalent, and it suppresses appetite, enhances weight loss, and reduces hyperinsulinemia. Metformin has about a 50% probability of restoring menstrual cycles but has minimal effect on hirsutism.

There are agents that exist to help induce ovulation in adolescents, and patients should be assured that when they plan to get pregnant their physician will recommend treatment if needed to enhance fertility. In older adolescents with a provisional diagnosis of PCOS, it is recommended to withhold COCs for about 3 months to determine whether hyperandrogenic oligo/anovulation returns. However, the benefits of withholding COCs must be weighed against the potential risk for pregnancy.

FUTURE DIRECTIONS

While the diagnostic criteria for PCOS in adolescents continues to evolve, PCOS should be considered in any female adolescent who presents with

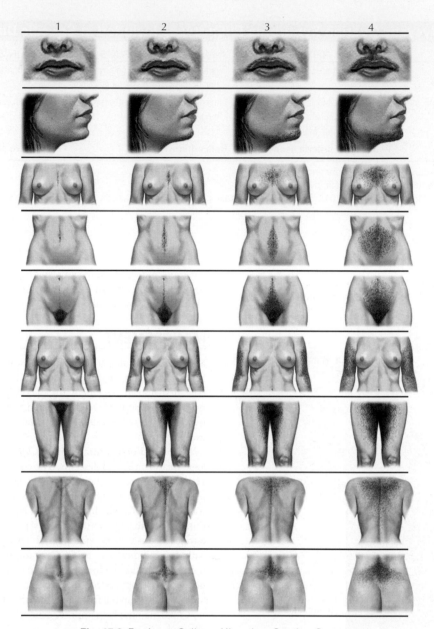

Fig. 17.2 Ferriman-Gallwey Hirsutism Scoring System.

unexplained persistent hyperandrogenic oligo/anovulation. Effective strategies to manage symptoms and reduce health risks can significantly improve the immediate and long-term well-being of adolescents with PCOS.

ACKNOWLEDGMENT

The authors would like to acknowledge the work of Oana Tomescu, MD, and Sara B. Kinsman, MD, on the previous edition.

SUGGESTED READINGS

Available online.

18

Transgender and Gender Diverse Youth

Aaron L. Misakian and Jamie E. Mehringer

 CLINICAL VIGNETTE

A 14-year-old youth assigned male at birth presents for routine well-child care. The youth's mother is very concerned about her child's mood and reports poor academic performance at school, which is unusual given the patient used to be an excellent student. The patient does not make eye contact and speaks in a quiet voice using four- to five-word sentences. The forearms are notable for several scars in various stages of healing.

When the mother steps out of the room for the confidential portion of the examination, the youth takes a large sigh of relief. The youth says she prefers to go by the name Natalie and identifies as a girl. She reports fighting with her parents over her preference for long hair and more feminine clothing. She is upset by her deepening voice and rapidly developing facial hair. She wants to know if there is anything to make these body changes stop. When asked about the scars on her arms, she says cutting helps her deal with feeling sad and hopeless.

Thank Natalie for sharing this important information about who she is and how she's feeling. If she is okay with it, let her know of the intention to start referring to her by her affirmed name and pronouns.

Natalie's presentation is concerning for depression. It is critical to assess for suicide risk, develop a safety plan, and get her connected with an affirming mental health provider. Align with Natalie's mother over the shared desire to see Natalie thrive. Provide Natalie and her mother with information on supportive local and online resources. Finally, it is important to connect Natalie with a provider who can offer gender-affirming medical care such as puberty blockers to halt the progression of the further masculinization that Natalie has found so distressing.

When children are born they are assigned a sex (typically male or female) based on external genitalia. *Gender identity* is an individual's innate sense of being male, female, both, somewhere in between, or neither. *Gender expression* refers to the outward way that individuals express their gender, such as through clothing, hairstyle, or behaviors. Most people have concordance between their assigned sex, gender identity, and gender expression. Individuals with a discordance among any of these three dimensions are referred to as *gender diverse*. *Transgender* refers to an individual for whom there is discordance between the assigned sex and gender identity. Natalie, in the Clinical Vignette, would be referred to as a transgender female because she was assigned male sex at birth but identifies as female. *Cisgender* refers to an individual for whom there is concordance between assigned sex and gender identity. Gender identity should not be confused with *sexual orientation* because these are independent dimensions of a person's identity. Given that gender identity is a highly individualized and sensitive process, one can avoid further stigmatization and unnecessary distress by simply asking what a person prefers to be called and how they identify.

GENDER DEVELOPMENT

The evolution of gender identity begins early in life. By the time they are 2 years old, toddlers begin to use gender stereotypes by showing preference for objects or people of the same gender. By age 3 they will typically be able to state whether they are a boy or girl and can label other children as such. Between ages 3 and 5, gender stereotypes deepen. Most, but not all, children will show some degree of inclination for clothes and toys that are culturally associated with their assigned sex (e.g., boys preferring trucks, girls preferring dolls). It is also during this time that gender constancy typically develops. This is when children typically come to understand gender as fixed and unchanging.

The timeline of gender development is generally the same for gender diverse and cisgender children. For example, a trans boy may show preference for culturally appropriated male objects around the same time as a cisgender boy. There are individuals, too, who are not able to articulate their gender identity at such a young age. It may take years before they have developed the language or self-understanding to articulate their gender identity. Others may not be able to express their feelings around gender until they are in a safe and supportive environment. Finally, there are individuals who do not experience discomfort with their assigned sex until puberty begins. Only then do changes in their body trigger an awareness that such features do not align with their gender identity.

EPIDEMIOLOGY

It is difficult to determine prevalence of transgender youth because these data are not consistently captured in population-level studies. Additionally, individuals may choose not to disclose this information because of societal stigma, fear of discrimination or violence, or personal preference. Studies that have attempted to quantify transgender prevalence have published widely varying results. In the US, studies have reported prevalence of approximately 0.5% in adults and approximately 1.8% in adolescents. Regardless of published data, the number of children presenting to gender centers for appropriate care is increasing. All pediatric providers at some point will encounter transgender children, whether they are aware of the patient's gender identity or not.

HEALTH DISPARITIES FACING TRANS YOUTH

Transgender and gender diverse (TGGD) individuals face significant health disparities; 30% to 50% report a past suicide attempt. Others suffer increased rates of depression, anxiety, homelessness, and trauma. Around 10% of TGGD individuals are living with human immunodeficiency virus (HIV), including one in five trans women.

These health inequities are not the result of an individual's gender identity, but rather the result of *minority stress:* chronic stress resulting from marginalization, victimization, and lack of access to appropriate care and resources because of belonging to a stigmatized group. The disparities are even greater for TGGD individuals with multiple minority identities, especially transgender women of color who face staggering rates of violence, victimization, poverty, and HIV. Violence is a major threat to transgender individuals worldwide. In the United States, many 30 transgender individuals die of hate-driven homicide annually and a disproportionate number are trans women of color.

Access to appropriate and necessary medical care is an issue for many transgender individuals. This is due to the limited number of providers offering gender affirming medical care, high rates of uninsured, insurer denial of coverage for gender affirming services, lack of caregiver consent for gender affirming medical care, or avoidance of medical care because of concerns about confidentiality and mistreatment. Such concerns are not unfounded, with many transgender individuals having reported harassment in the medical setting and/or refusal of care.

Despite these inequities, there is much that we can do to protect TGGD youth and help them thrive. The importance of caregiver support and acceptance cannot be understated. Transgender youth whose parents are strongly supportive have been found to be 10-fold less likely to attempt suicide. Support from other adults, such as teachers, also can have protective effects. The gender affirming care model is another way that we can help TGGD youth thrive.

THE GENDER AFFIRMING CARE MODEL

Gender affirming care is a comprehensive and evidence-based treatment model that supports, validates, and assists children in accepting and/or expressing their gender identities. Endorsed by the American Academy of Pediatrics (AAP) and other professional societies, it leads to better, long-term mental health outcomes and decreased rates of the previously mentioned health disparities. It is important to note that other treatment modalities, notably reparative therapy, do not work in the treatment of trans youth but instead lead to poorer health care outcomes. The AAP and numerous other professional organizations stand against conversion therapy. To date, 20 US states have legally banned its use for gender identity or sexual orientation.

The gender affirming care model is an approach to care, not a preset "treatment" regimen. The process is tailored to each youth based on their individual feelings, goals, and circumstances. It is multidisciplinary and integrates mental health, medical treatment, and social services to deliver youth- and family-centered care. Elements of gender affirming care may include social affirmation, medical affirmation, and/or surgical affirmation.

Research has repeatedly shown that transgender youth who are cared for in the gender affirming care model have better mental health outcomes, including decreased rates of suicidal behavior and improved quality of life. Although well-meaning adults may ask whether care can be postponed until the youth is "older" or a legal adult, delaying gender affirming interventions when they are clinically indicated is *not* a neutral option and may put the youth in danger.

Social Affirmation

Social affirmation is the process by which an individual asserts their gender identity through reversible nonmedical means such as clothing, hairstyle, pronouns, or name. It may involve body modifications such as binding or padding the chest area or using garments or prostheses to hide or create the contour of male genitalia. In situations that are often gender-segregated (e.g., public restrooms, locker rooms, sports teams), youth are free to choose the space that aligns with their asserted gender

identity. Social affirmation can be initiated at any age because it is safe and fully reversible.

Medical Affirmation

Medical affirmation is the use of medication to help an individual's body better align with their asserted gender identity. It may include a gonadotropin-releasing hormone (GnRH) agonist to halt pubertal progression, gender affirming hormones (i.e., estrogen or testosterone) to induce secondary sex characteristics, antiandrogens, or hormonal contraceptives for menstrual suppression.

Puberty Blockade With Gonadotropin-Releasing Hormone Agonists

GnRH agonists (e.g., leuprolide, histrelin) function to suppress hypothalamic gonadotropin (LH, FSH) release and in turn stop the progression of puberty. For youth with gender dysphoria, this prevents the development of unwanted and distressing pubertal body changes while affording the youth more time to explore gender identity, build psychosocial support, and decide on further steps in gender affirming care.

Treatment with GnRH agonists can be initiated as early as Tanner stage 2. For youth experiencing worsening gender dysphoria with the onset of pubertal changes, it is advisable to begin pubertal blockade as soon as puberty starts to prevent unwanted irreversible changes that may otherwise require surgery or cause lifelong distress. If GnRH agonist therapy is stopped, endogenous puberty resumes where it left off unless the youth begins gender-affirming hormonal therapy. The main risk of GnRH agonist therapy is adverse effects on bone health. Thus it can be used for only a limited number of years unless combined with gender affirming hormones. To mitigate the effects on bone health, DEXA scans are monitored and vitamin D and calcium intake are optimized.

It is important for youth and caregivers to discuss fertility before initiating treatment, including long-term goals and options for fertility preservation. GnRH agonists do not affect long-term fertility on their own. When youth begin GnRH agonist therapy before the reproductive organs have completed maturation, these organs are paused in an immature state. If youth then begin treatment with gender affirming hormones without first discontinuing the GnRH agonist and completing endogenous puberty, they may have irreversible infertility.

Gender Affirming Hormonal Therapy

Gender affirming hormonal therapy refers to the use of estrogen or testosterone to induce the development of secondary sex characteristics that are more aligned with the individual's asserted gender. See Table 18.1 for an overview of available routes of delivery, anticipated effects, and potential risks. Individuals receiving gender affirming hormone therapy require regular follow-up to ensure that hormone levels are within physiologic ranges and to monitor for adverse effects. Although there are potential risks associated with gender affirming hormone therapy, serious complications are very rare when the hormones are prescribed at physiologic doses, especially in otherwise healthy individuals. These potential risks must be carefully weighed with the known risks of withholding treatment for gender dysphoria (e.g., suicidal behavior and depression).

As with GnRH agonist therapy, fertility goals should be discussed before starting gender affirming hormones. Estrogen therapy can have an impact on semen parameters and may result in irreversible infertility. The long-term fertility effects of testosterone are not known. There are reports of individuals becoming pregnant during or shortly after stopping long-term testosterone therapy. Testosterone should never be considered a contraceptive, regardless of whether menses are suppressed. Testosterone is teratogenic and contraindicated during pregnancy. All youth on testosterone should be counseled on pregnancy prevention and offered an effective contraceptive method if interested.

TABLE 18.1 Gender Affirming Hormonal Therapy

Hormone	Route of Delivery	Effects	Potential Risks
Testosterone	• Subcutaneous or intramuscular injection • Transdermal gel/patch • Subcutaneous pellet	• Growth of facial/body hair • Increased muscle mass/strength • Voice deepening • Clitoral enlargement • Adam's apple enlargement • Menstrual suppression	• Acne • Male pattern baldness • Hypertension • Dyslipidemia • Polycythemia • Uncertain effects on fertility
Estrogen	• Oral or sublingual tablet • Transdermal patch • Intramuscular injection	• Breast development • Nipple enlargement • Fat redistribution to hips and buttocks • Skin softening • Decreased facial/body hair growth • Decreased sperm production, testicular volume, erections	• Irreversible infertility • Thromboembolism • Cardiovascular disease • Macro-prolactinoma • Breast cancer

BOX 18.1 Commonly Used Hormonal Contraceptive Regimens for Menstrual Suppression

• Depo medroxyprogesterone acetate (injection)
• Extended- or continuous-cycling combined hormonal contraceptives
• Norethindrone acetate (2.5 to 10 mg daily)[a]
• 52 mg levonorgestrel IUD (Mirena, Liletta)

[a] Note: Norethindrone has been approved for contraception only when dosed at 0.35 mg daily ("the mini pill"). However, this seldom suppresses menses. Norethindrone acetate (dosed at 2.5 to 10 mg daily) is often effective for menstrual suppression but should not be considered contraception.

All hormonal contraceptives, the copper IUD, and emergency contraception are safe to use concurrently with testosterone therapy.

Estrogen therapy inhibits endogenous testosterone production but is rarely sufficient to keep testosterone adequately suppressed and prevent masculinizing effects on its own. As a result, estrogen therapy is often used in conjunction with either GnRH agonists or antiandrogens such as spironolactone or bicalutamide. In some situations, an antiandrogen may be used as monotherapy.

Menstrual Suppression

For many gender diverse youth, menses may be a major trigger of dysphoria. Hormonal contraceptives can be a useful option for menstrual suppression, especially in situations in which a youth desires amenorrhea yet lacks access to or is not a candidate for GnRH agonist or testosterone therapy (see Box 18.1 for commonly used regimens).

Surgical Affirmation

Surgical affirmation is the process of undergoing surgery to help an individual's body better align with their asserted gender identity. Not all gender diverse individuals pursue surgical affirmation. Those who do may seek various procedures depending on their individual goals, priorities, body, and experience of dysphoria.

Surgical affirmation is typically deferred until age 18, although it may be considered earlier on a case-by-case basis with involvement of the youth, the family, and the care team. It is becoming increasingly common for transmasculine minors to undergo masculinizing chest surgery (involving removal of the breasts and creation of a flatter chest contour); current evidence shows good outcomes and lack of regret when performed during adolescence.

BOX 18.2 First Steps Toward Supporting Gender Diverse Youth in A Practice

• Ask youth about what name and pronouns they go by and refer to them as such (unless requested otherwise for confidentiality reasons).
• Summon youth from waiting areas using preferred name or a number.
• When asking questions about sexuality or reproductive health, explain to the youth why this information is relevant.
• Offer use of drapes and gowns whenever a youth must disrobe.
• When examining sensitive body areas, explain why this portion of the examination is pertinent and allow the youth to remain in control.
• Familiarize self with local and online resources for referral of youth or their families for further support.
• Whenever possible, avoid unnecessary gendering of items and spaces.
• Intake forms should allow youth to assert their identified gender rather than requiring choice of a binary check box. If necessary to obtain information on a youth's sex assigned at birth, it should be asked in a separate question.
• All providers and staff should receive training to ensure a basic understanding of gender diversity and importance of providing a gender affirmative care environment.
• Display flyers or pamphlets with information on LGBTQIA+ resources and signage that indicates that youth and families of all identities are welcomed.

FUTURE DIRECTIONS

The health inequities facing transgender and gender diverse youth are tremendous, and we cannot underestimate the power that caring adult figures can have in a young person's life. A thoughtful and compassionate provider who offers a safe and affirming space while facilitating connections to necessary resources can have a life-changing—and even life-saving—effect. Primary care providers play a key role in the gender affirming care model because they are often the first contact for youth and families, a trusted source of information, and an ongoing source of care and support throughout a young person's development. Although it is not necessary for every provider to be an expert, one should strive to have a basic familiarity with gender diversity and practice in a way that is welcoming and supportive to youth of all genders and identities (see Box 18.2 for examples).

SUGGESTED READINGS

Available online.

19

Adolescent Sexual Health

Michelle Shankar and Kristen Feemster

 CLINICAL VIGNETTE

A 16-year-old boy presents to a primary care clinic with his parent for a sports preparticipation physical examination. During the routine confidential interview for adolescent visits, he reports sexual activity for a year, and three female partners during this time. He reports condom use "most of the time" and that he has never been tested for sexually transmitted infections (STIs). On review of systems, he discloses an abnormal sensation on the tip of his penis with urination for the past few weeks. Physical examination reveals scant urethral discharge, with no evidence of vesicles, ulcers, or inguinal lymphadenopathy. Urine and blood testing is ordered for gonorrhea, chlamydia, human immunodeficiency virus, and syphilis. The patient is treated empirically for gonorrhea and chlamydia coinfection, and asked to follow up in 3 months for repeat testing.

Sexually transmitted infections (STIs) are a significant source of morbidity among adolescents and young adults (15 to 24 years), disproportionately affecting young women, as well as sexual, gender, and ethnic minorities. In 2018 the Centers for Disease Control and Prevention (CDC) estimates of the incidence and prevalence suggested that young people aged 15 to 24 years acquire half of all new STIs, although representing only a quarter of the sexually active population. Adolescents, particularly minority youth, are more likely to experience delays in diagnosis and treatment, and may be more likely to experience short-term and long-term sequelae of STIs.

Systemic barriers contributing to educational, economic, and health disparities in the United States also play a large role in disparate rates of STI acquisition. Risk factors for acquiring STIs include younger age at first sexual intercourse, placement in juvenile justice or adult detention facilities, injection drug use, and young men who have sex with men (YMSM). Behavioral risk factors include having multiple sexual partners concurrently or during a short period of time, and inconsistent or incorrect use of barrier protection. Young women have increased biological susceptibility to chlamydial and other infections because of increased cervical ectopy, referring to columnar cells (which are typically found within the cervical canal in adults) located on the outer surface of the cervix. The higher incidence and prevalence of STIs in recent years among adolescents may reflect improved screening methods; however, they are likely driven by barriers to accessing health care, including cost, transportation, school conflicts, social pressures, and concerns about confidentiality.

Regular screening is a necessity among adolescents and young adults, because STIs may manifest with a wide range of symptoms and physical findings and most commonly are asymptomatic. Because of the high rates of STIs among adolescents, pediatric providers should perform a thorough sexual health history, prevention and risk-reduction counseling, and STI screening. Effective clinical programs involve routine screening during extended clinic hours in a private setting using urine-based nucleic acid amplification techniques (NAATs). This chapter focuses on counseling and prevention of STIs and the most common clinical presentations associated with STIs in adolescents.

COUNSELING AND PREVENTION

The prevention of STIs is based on effective risk assessment, education, and counseling; preexposure vaccination or prophylaxis when possible; effective diagnosis, treatment, and follow-up of infected individuals; and evaluation, treatment, and counseling of sex partners.

Clinicians should conduct a sexual history on all adolescent patients without a caregiver present. Sensitive, nonjudgmental, and thorough counseling is vital for adolescents who may not feel comfortable discussing sexual behaviors, especially those that place them at high risk for STIs. Effective communication techniques include the use of open-ended questions and developmentally appropriate, nonjudgmental language that normalizes sexual identity and behaviors as a part of routine preventive health care for teens and adults.

The "Five Ps" approach to obtaining a sexual history is one strategy for eliciting information concerning risk factors for STIs:
- Partners, including number and gender of partners
- Practices, including receptive or donor oral, anal, and/or vaginal sex and sex under the influence of substances
- Prevention of pregnancy
- Protection from STIs
- History of STIs

Risk increases with more lifetime partners (particularly new partners within the prior several months), receptive anal and vaginal intercourse, and inconsistent or improper use of barrier contraception. STIs are biological markers of risk for reinfection and acquisition of additional STIs.

Clinicians need to incorporate sexual education on risk factors for STIs, mechanisms of transmission, and strategies for prevention and risk reduction. These strategies include preexposure vaccination (human papillomavirus [HPV]), abstinence and reduction of the number of new sex partners, and consistent male condom use. The use of female condoms can prevent the acquisition and transmission of STIs, although data are limited. Interactive counseling approaches, such as high-intensity behavioral counseling and motivational interviewing, are effective in supporting behavior change. Clinicians should ask all sexually active adolescents if they intend pregnancy and provide counseling regarding family planning and contraception options.

VAGINITIS, CERVICITIS, AND URETHRITIS

Inflammation of the lower genital tract is among the most common physical complaints among adolescents. Inflammatory symptoms typically include increased or new vaginal or urethral discharge that may or may not be malodorous, as well as erythema, pruritus, burning, dysuria, vaginal spotting, or local edema (Fig. 19.1). Although chemical or mechanical irritants are frequently the cause of lower genital tract inflammation, any disruption of local immunologic and environmental factors places adolescents at increased risk for acquiring STIs. In postpubertal females, protective factors, including acidic vaginal pH, cervical immunoglobulin A, and mucus are altered by chemicals, *Candida* species, or bacterial vaginosis (overgrowth of *Gardnerella vaginalis*, genital mycoplasmas, anaerobic bacteria). STI causes of vaginitis include *Trichomonas vaginalis;* however, the risk for vaginal overgrowth with *Candida* or organisms associated with bacterial vaginitis increases with sexual activity.

Urethritis in males and females, and cervicitis, are most often caused by *Neisseria gonorrhoeae* and *Chlamydia trachomatis,* but also can be caused by HPV, *Mycoplasma genitalium,* and herpes simplex virus (HSV). The signs, symptoms, diagnostic criteria, and treatments for each infection are shown in Tables 19.1 and 19.2.

PELVIC INFLAMMATORY DISEASE

Pelvic inflammatory disease (PID) is a polymicrobial infection of the upper genital tract, encompassing endometritis, salpingitis, oophoritis, pelvic peritonitis, and perihepatitis. The presenting symptoms of patients with PID are described in Table 19.1. Recurrent PID can lead to chronic pelvic pain, ectopic pregnancy, and infertility. Subclinical infection can be discovered when evaluation for infertility reveals fallopian tube scarring. Treatment for PID should be initiated if, on examination, patients have lower abdominal tenderness without other explanation, cervical motion or adnexal tenderness with bimanual vaginal examination, or an adnexal mass is detected. PID is typically preceded by cervicitis, most commonly caused by *N. gonorrhoeae* and *C. trachomatis.* With a weakened cervical barrier, *N. gonorrhoeae, C. trachomatis,* and other vaginal organisms may ascend into the uterus and fallopian tubes. Infected material in the fallopian tubes may result in a tubo-ovarian abscess, and overflow may lead to peritonitis or perihepatitis. The risk for PID is associated with young age at first intercourse,

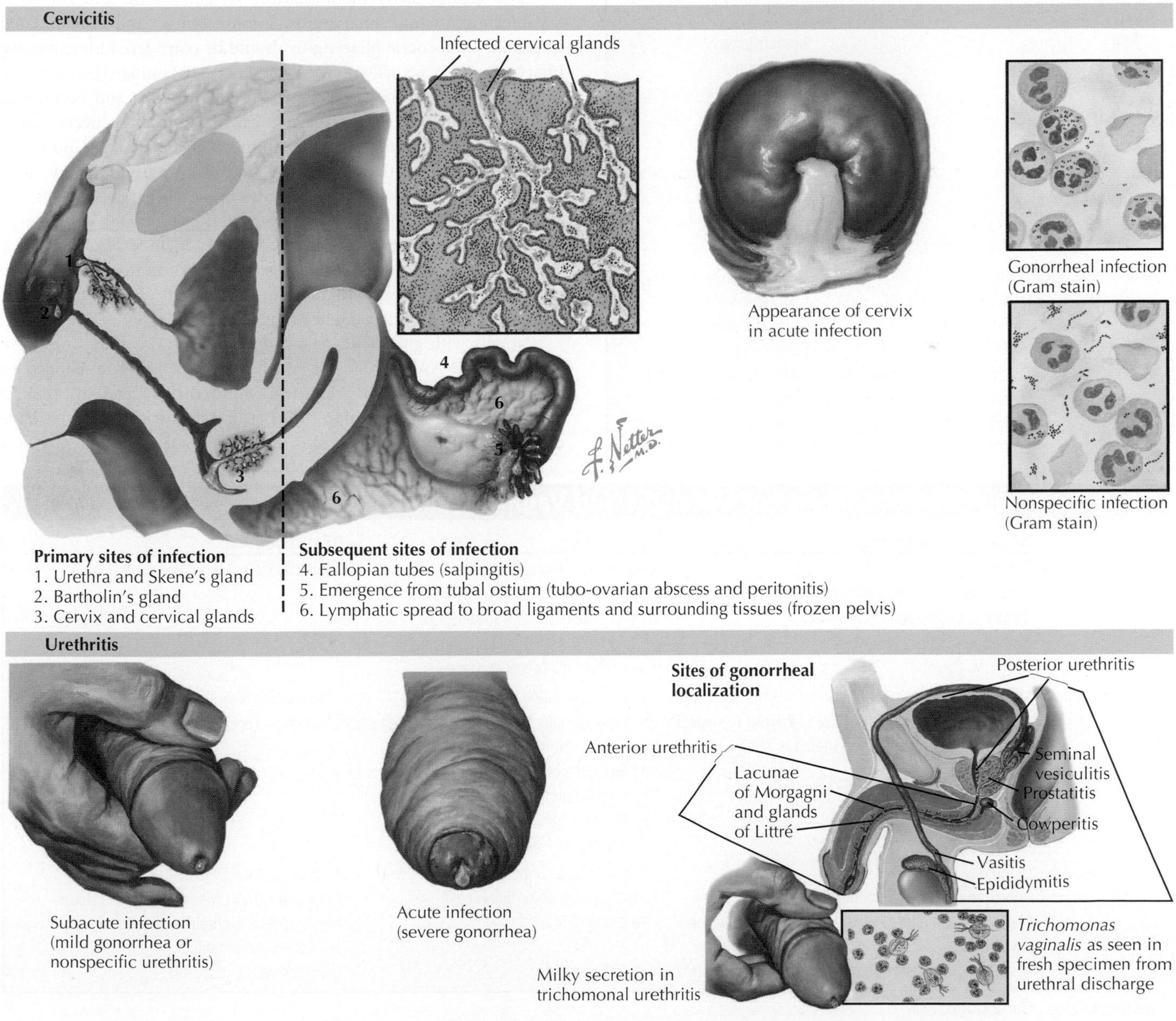

Cervicitis

Infected cervical glands

Appearance of cervix in acute infection

Gonorrheal infection (Gram stain)

Nonspecific infection (Gram stain)

Primary sites of infection
1. Urethra and Skene's gland
2. Bartholin's gland
3. Cervix and cervical glands

Subsequent sites of infection
4. Fallopian tubes (salpingitis)
5. Emergence from tubal ostium (tubo-ovarian abscess and peritonitis)
6. Lymphatic spread to broad ligaments and surrounding tissues (frozen pelvis)

Urethritis

Subacute infection (mild gonorrhea or nonspecific urethritis)

Acute infection (severe gonorrhea)

Sites of gonorrheal localization

Posterior urethritis

Anterior urethritis

Lacunae of Morgagni and glands of Littré

Seminal vesiculitis
Prostatitis
Cowperitis

Vasitis
Epididymitis

Milky secretion in trichomonal urethritis

Trichomonas vaginalis as seen in fresh specimen from urethral discharge

Fig. 19.1 Cervicitis and Urethritis.

TABLE 19.1 Signs and Symptoms of Urethritis, Cervicitis, and Associated Syndromes

Syndrome	Men	Women
Urethritis	Dysuria Purulent urethral discharge	Dysuria Urinary frequency Urethral discharge Suprapubic pain
Epididymitis	Urethral discharge Dysuria Scrotal pain, swelling, erythema Inguinal or flank pain Pain or swelling of epididymis or spermatic cord	
Endocervicitis		Increased vaginal discharge Cervical erythema, edema, friability
Pelvic inflammatory disease (PID)		Abdominal pain Intermenstrual bleeding Menorrhagia Dyspareunia Cervical motion or adnexal tenderness Adnexal mass
Perihepatitis (Fitz-Hugh-Curtis syndrome)		Exquisite right upper quadrant abdominal pain Nausea or vomiting
Anorectal gonorrhea	Proctitis Rectal bleeding Anorectal pain Purulent exudate Erythema or edema of rectal mucosa Tenesmus or constipation	Usually asymptomatic Rectal bleeding Anorectal pain Purulent exudate Erythema or edema of rectal mucosa Tenesmus or constipation

multiple partners, and vaginal douching. Timely diagnosis and treatment of PID are important to prevent infertility. Because the signs and symptoms of infection are not specific, the CDC developed criteria to guide diagnosis and empiric treatment (Box 19.1). The fulfillment of minimal criteria (uterine, adnexal, or cervical tenderness) should prompt presumptive treatment.

Gonorrhea and Chlamydia

Gonorrhea and chlamydia are the most common reportable bacterial STIs in the United States. Incidence and prevalence are particularly high among adolescents and young adults: in 2018, 61.8% of all reported chlamydia cases in the United States occurred in individuals aged 15 to 24 years and rates of reported gonorrhea cases were highest among adolescents and young adults (women aged 15 to 24 and men aged 20 to 29).

Transmission occurs by oral, vaginal, or anal sexual contact. The transmission rate for each pathogen is much higher from males to females. Each organism may be transmitted vertically to a newborn via passage through an infected birth canal (Chapter 99).

Extra-genitourinary manifestations of gonococcal and chlamydial infection include pharyngitis, conjunctivitis, and disseminated infection. Gonococcal pharyngitis should be considered for exudative pharyngitis in a sexually active adolescent. Disseminated gonococcal infection often manifests as arthritis, tenosynovitis, and dermatitis. Chlamydia is associated with reactive arthritis that can co-occur in susceptible individuals with urethritis, spondylitis, and uveitis. Gonorrhea can be diagnosed by Gram stain and culture from urethral and endocervical swabs. Chlamydia, as an intracellular organism, is difficult to grow in culture and has therefore been more difficult to diagnose. Newer and more rapid diagnostic methods include NAATs, which have greatly increased the ease and sensitivity of testing. They can be performed on urine samples in addition to urethral, endocervical, or self-administered blind vaginal swabs.

Patients with gonorrhea or chlamydia are at risk for coinfection; therefore, if NAAT results are not available, it is recommended to cover for both pathogens when treating urethritis, cervicitis, or PID (Table 19.3). This is critical in PID, because the inciting STI may have cleared by the time the diagnosis of PID is made. Recommendations

TABLE 19.2 Infectious Causes of Urethritis and Vaginitis

	Signs and Symptoms	Diagnosis	Treatment
Trichomonas vaginalis	Pruritus, dysuria Frothy cream or green-colored discharge Dyspareunia, postcoital bleeding Strawberry cervix, vulvovaginal edema, erythema Urethritis (men)	Wet mount: trichomonads Vaginal pH >4.5 Culture (sensitive but expensive) Rapid test (OSOM Trichomonas Rapid Test[a] or Affirm nucleic acid probe[b])	Metronidazole, tinidazole
Bacterial vaginosis	Most common cause of abnormal vaginal discharge: grayish white with fishy odor, adherent to vaginal walls, no vulvovaginal erythema or edema	Three of the following: • Homogenous, white or watery discharge exuding from vaginal walls • Presence of >50% clue cells on wet prep • Vaginal pH >4.5 • Positive "whiff test" (fishy odor after adding 10% KOH)	Metronidazole oral or topical gel Clindamycin oral or topical gel
Candida species	Burning and pruritus Vulvar edema and erythema Thick "cottage cheese–like" discharge with no odor Dysuria or dyspareunia May have satellite lesions on thighs and in skinfolds	Pseudohyphae or budding yeast on wet mount and white blood cells Vaginal pH <4.5	Butoconazole 2% cream Clotrimazole 1% cream or vaginal tablets Miconazole 2% cream or vaginal suppository Nystatin vaginal tablets Oral regimen: fluconazole

[a]Genzyme Corp., Cambridge, MA.
[b]BD, Franklin Lakes, NJ.
KOH, Potassium hydroxide.

BOX 19.1 Signs and Symptoms of Pelvic Inflammatory Disease

Minimal Criteria
- Uterine tenderness, *or*
- Adnexal tenderness, *or*
- Cervical motion tenderness

Additional Criteria Improving Specificity
- Temperature 101°F (38.3°C)
- Abnormal cervical or vaginal discharge
- White blood cells on microscopic evaluation of vaginal discharge
- Elevated erythrocyte sedimentation rate and C-reactive protein
- Laboratory documentation of gonorrhea or chlamydial infection

Definitive Criteria
- Evidence of endometritis from endometrial biopsy
- Transvaginal sonography or other imaging showing thickened fluid-filled tubes, free pelvic fluid, or tubo-ovarian complex
- Laparoscopic abnormalities

for PID also include broad-spectrum anaerobic coverage because of the polymicrobial nature of the infection. Given the prevalence of gonorrhea and chlamydia, particularly among adolescents, routine screening on an annual basis is recommended for all sexually active females younger than 25 years.

ANOGENITAL ULCERS AND WARTS

The most common causes of anogenital lesions in adolescents include HSV, HPV, and *Treponema palladium* (syphilis). The differential diagnosis should also include chancroid caused by *Haemophilus ducreyi*. In general, painful ulcerative lesions are associated with herpes genitalis and chancroid, whereas painless ulcers (chancres) are associated with syphilis. HPV can cause painless anogenital growths.

Herpes Simplex Virus

HSV is among the most prevalent of all STIs. HSV-1 is primarily associated with herpes labialis, and HSV-2 is primarily associated with herpes genitalis; however, an increasing proportion of anogenital infections have been attributed to HSV-1. Genital herpes infections are transmitted through contact with lesions, mucosal surfaces, genital secretions, or oral secretions, and may be transmitted from asymptomatic individuals.

In primary infection, the virus replicates in the skin or mucosal cells and then spreads by sensory nerves. The virus then becomes latent, remaining in sacral dorsal root ganglia until reactivation. During reactivation, the virus spreads along peripheral sensory nerves back to the skin or mucosal surfaces, resulting in the recrudescence of skin lesions.

Viral shedding is highest in the presence of lesions, but asymptomatic shedding also occurs, especially within the first 3 months after primary infection. Shedding occurs in salivary, cervical, and seminal secretions. Many individuals have mild or unrecognized infections but shed the virus intermittently in the anogenital area; therefore most transmission occurs by individuals who are asymptomatic and unaware that they are infected.

Primary infection usually presents with a burning sensation in the genital area, followed by the development of small (1 to 2 mm) vesicular lesions with an erythematous base that erode and become ulcers. The distribution of lesions can be extensive, involving the labia, vagina, perineum, cervix, and penis (Fig. 19.2). The lesions are almost always painful. In primary infection, regional tender lymphadenopathy, fever,

and malaise occur. Patients also may have dysuria, urinary retention, or dyspareunia. Lesions typically last from 4 to 15 days before crusting, and systemic symptoms usually peak in the first 3 to 4 days and then resolve.

Recurrences and subclinical shedding are much more frequent for genital HSV-2 infection than for genital HSV-1 infection. Recurrent episodes are usually less severe and involve fewer lesions. Overall, the episodes last approximately 1 week, and the virus sheds for 2 to 7 days. There may be paresthesias or pain in the anogenital region before the appearance of ulcers, and mild systemic symptoms can occur. The likelihood and frequency of recurrence vary; recurrences are more frequent in the first year after infection. Although herpes results in chronic infection, episodes are usually self-limited. Complications can occur, including secondary bacterial infection of lesions, labial adhesions, sacral radiculopathy, proctitis, encephalitis, and meningitis. Another important complication is neonatal herpes (see Chapter 99).

The clinical diagnosis of genital herpes can be difficult, because many infected individuals have mild or no symptoms. Polymerase chain reaction (PCR) and cell culture are the preferred HSV tests. NAATs, including PCR assays for HSV DNA, are more sensitive and are increasingly available. The sensitivity of viral culture is low, especially for recurrent and healing lesions. Failure to detect HSV by culture or PCR does not indicate an absence of HSV infection because viral shedding is intermittent. Cytologic detection of cellular changes associated with HSV infection is an insensitive and nonspecific method of diagnosing genital lesions (i.e., Tzanck smear).

Management of genital HSV should address the chronic nature of the disease. Counseling regarding the natural history of genital herpes and methods to reduce transmission is integral to clinical management. Systemic antiviral drugs can partially control symptoms of genital herpes but will not eradicate latent virus nor affect the risk, frequency, or severity of recurrences after they are discontinued. All patients with first episodes of genital herpes should receive oral antiviral therapy for 7 to 10 days; for recurrent genital herpes oral antiviral therapy can be administered either as suppressive therapy to reduce the frequency of recurrences or episodically to ameliorate or shorten the duration of lesions. Intravenous acyclovir therapy should be provided for patients who have severe HSV disease, complications that necessitate hospitalization (e.g., disseminated infection, pneumonitis, or hepatitis), or central nervous system involvement.

Syphilis

Syphilis is a systemic infection caused by the spirochete *T. palladium*. According to surveillance data, rates of reported syphilis cases increased 28.6% and 7.2% during 2017 and 2018 and increased 100.0% and 44.6% during 2014 through 2018 for females and males aged 15 to 24 years, respectively. These rates have been consistently higher among adolescent and young adult males than among females; however, the largest increase in cases has been observed in females aged 15 to 24 years.

The agent is usually transmitted by sexual contact but also can be transmitted in utero, through blood transfusions, or by direct contact with infectious lesions. After the organism enters the body, the infection spreads through the blood and lymphatic systems, infiltrating cells and causing granuloma formation and endarteritis. If left untreated, the infection is chronic and can be transmitted for up to 4 years.

The clinical manifestations of syphilis depend on the stage of infection, as shown in Table 19.4 and Fig. 19.3. The diagnosis of syphilis should be considered in the presence of any ulcerative anogenital or oral lesion. Breasts and fingers also can be affected. Latent syphilis is defined as syphilis characterized by seroreactivity without other evidence of primary, secondary, or tertiary disease. Because latent syphilis is not transmitted sexually, the objective of

TABLE 19.3   Treatment Recommendations for Urethritis, Cervicitis, and Pelvic Inflammatory Disease

	Treatment	Special Considerations
Chlamydial urethritis or cervicitis	Doxycycline 100 mg PO twice a day for 7 days Alternative regimens: • Levofloxacin 500 mg PO once daily for 7 days • Ofloxacin 300 mg PO twice a day for 7 days • Azithromycin 1 g PO × 1	Patients should abstain from sexual intercourse for 7 days from starting treatment. Partners should be notified and treated.
Gonococcal urethritis or cervicitis	Ceftriaxone 500 mg IM × 1 *or* cefixime 800 mg PO × 1 *or* gentamicin 240 mg IM × 1 *plus* azithromycin 2 g PO × 1	CDC treatment recommendations updated 2021
Pelvic inflammatory disease	*Parenteral regimen:* Ceftriaxone 1 G IV every 24 hours *plus* doxycycline 100mg PO or IV every 12 hours *plus* metronidazole 500mg PO or IV every 12 hours *or* cefoxitin 2g IV every 6 hours plus doxycycline *or* cefotetan 2g IV every 12 hours *plus* doxycycline *Outpatient regimen:* Ceftriaxone 500 mg IM x1 *or* cefoxitin 2 g IM x 1 IM + probenecid 1 g PO x 1 PO *plus* doxycycline 100 mg twice per day PO for 14 days + metronidazole 500 mg PO twice per day	IV antibiotics until 24 h after improvement; then continue PO doxycycline to complete 14-day course. As earlier, patients should abstain from sexual intercourse for 7 days from initiation of treatment. Partners should be evaluated and treated.
Epididymitis	Ceftriaxone 500 mg IM × 1 *plus* doxycycline 100 mg PO twice a day for 10 days	For men who have sex with men, ceftriaxone plus levofloxacin or ofloxacin is recommended because of presence of enteric organisms

CDC, Centers for Disease Control and Prevention; *IM,* intramuscular; *IV,* intravenous; *PO,* oral.

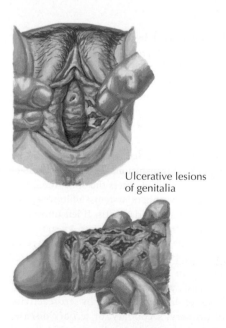

Ulcerative lesions of genitalia

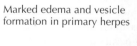

Regional lymphadenopathy, common in genital herpes

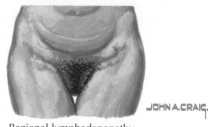

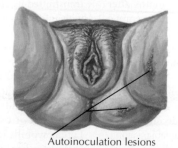

Autoinoculation lesions

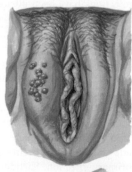

Marked edema and vesicle formation in primary herpes

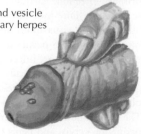

Fig. 19.2 Lesions of Herpes Simplex.

TABLE 19.4   Clinical Manifestations and Treatment of Syphilis

	Timing	Clinical Manifestations	Treatment
Primary syphilis	9–90 days after exposure	1- to 2-cm *painless* chancre or ulcerative lesion on external genitalia Typically single lesion but can have multiple Heals in 3–6 weeks	Benzathine penicillin G 2.4 million units IM x 1 If penicillin allergy, doxycycline or tetracycline can be used.
Secondary syphilis	6–8 weeks (after exposure) 4–10 weeks (after chancre)	Generalized macular, papular, or papulosquamous rash of trunk and extremities, including palms and soles, bilateral and symmetric, follows line of cleavage, and can involve mucous membranes. Rash lasts few weeks to 12 months General or regional painless lymphadenopathy. Flulike syndrome with malaise, sore throat, fever, and so on.	Benzathine penicillin G IM If penicillin allergy, doxycycline or tetracycline can be used.
Latent syphilis	Early (within first year) vs. late (after first year)	No clinical signs or symptoms of syphilis Persistently positive serologic test results (VDRL and FTA-ABS) Negative syphilis test results from CSF	Benzathine penicillin G *Alternative:* Doxycycline *Late:* LP should be performed to look for neurosyphilis
Late syphilis	2–10 years after infection	Gummas (hypersensitivity reaction) Cardiovascular syphilis *Has not* been reported in adolescents	Benzathine penicillin G 2.4 million units IM weekly x 3 doses (total 7.2 million units) LP should be performed to look for neurosyphilis
Neurosyphilis	Within 2 years	Asymptomatic: CSF pleocytosis, increased protein, and positive CSF VDRL results Acute meningitis with cranial nerve palsies Meningovascular syphilis: local infarction resulting in headache, memory loss, hemiparesis, Argyll-Robertson pupils, tabes dorsalis; rare in adolescents	Aqueous crystalline penicillin G 18-24 million units per day x 10-14 days *or* Procaine penicillin + probenecid LP should be repeated every 6 months until pleocytosis has resolved

CSF, Cerebrospinal fluid; *FTA-ABS,* fluorescent treponemal antibody absorption test; *IM,* intramuscular; *LP,* lumbar puncture; VDRL, Venereal Disease Research Laboratory.

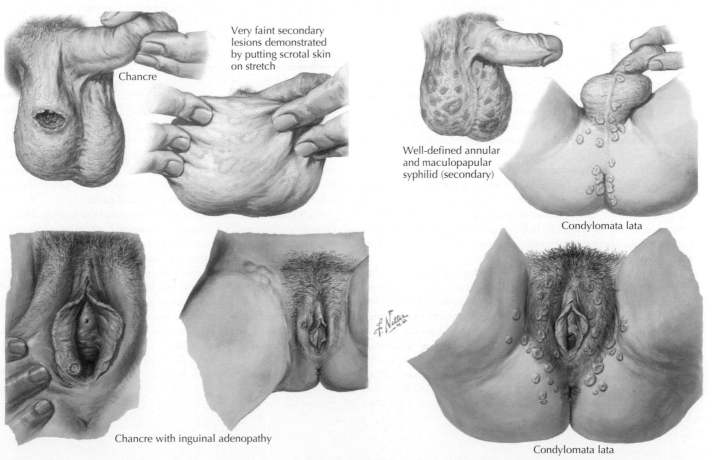

Very faint secondary lesions demonstrated by putting scrotal skin on stretch

Chancre

Well-defined annular and maculopapular syphilid (secondary)

Condylomata lata

Chancre with inguinal adenopathy

Condylomata lata

Fig. 19.3 Syphilis.

treating persons in this stage of the disease is to prevent complications and transmission from a pregnant woman to her fetus (see Chapter 99).

The diagnosis uses screening nontreponemal antibody tests (rapid plasma reagin [RPR] and Venereal Disease Research Laboratory [VDRL]) and confirmatory specific treponemal antibody tests (fluorescent treponemal antibody absorption [FTA-ABS]). The RPR is a qualitative test that requires confirmation by the FTA-ABS. The VDRL is a quantitative test used to monitor treatment. The treponemal-specific antibody test also yields antibody titers, but levels do not change in response to treatment; the FTA-ABS result will remain positive for life. The sensitivity of these tests depends on the timing after infection: they are most sensitive 4 weeks after infection but before the onset of late syphilis. There is also a high likelihood of false-positive results, particularly for the nontreponemal tests. False-positive results can occur with viral, spirochetal, mycoplasmal, other bacterial infections, and autoimmune vasculitides. Although screening test results are confirmed with the FTA-ABS, definitive diagnosis is made through darkfield examination of transudate from lesions or through direct fluorescent antibody.

The mainstay of treatment for syphilis is penicillin. Although other regimens are available to treat primary and secondary syphilis for patients who are allergic to penicillin, data to support their use are limited. The treatment regimens are shown in Table 19.4. Follow-up should include repeat nontreponemal quantitative antibodies (VDRL) at 6, 12, and 24 months after completion of therapy. If initially high titers have not decreased fourfold or if the titers have increased, treatment should be repeated. Regular screening for syphilis is recommended for pregnant women and YMSM.

Human Papillomavirus

HPV is perhaps the most common STI in the United States. Similar to other STIs, adolescent and young adult women are most likely to be affected. HPV is usually acquired shortly after sexual initiation, and the number of partners is the most important risk factor for HPV infection.

HPV is a double-stranded DNA virus of which there are 130 known genotypes. Approximately 40 of these genotypes infect the anogenital region and are divided into low- and high-risk types based on their association with dysplastic changes. Although most HPV infections are asymptomatic and self-resolve, infection with low-risk types can cause anogenital warts and high-risk types can cause precancerous anogenital lesions (i.e., cervical dysplasia) and anogenital cancers.

Transmission of HPV is primarily through sexual contact; however, genital lesions also can be caused by autoinoculation from skin warts. There is also evidence that HPV types that cause skin warts are transmissible by fomites, although such evidence does not exist for genital HPV types. HPV infects rapidly dividing basal epithelial cells that predominate in the cervical transformation zone and genital areas during sexual intercourse (Fig. 19.4).

Low-risk HPV types 6 and 11 cause approximately 90% of anogenital warts. Four different types of genital warts include condyloma acuminata, papular warts, keratotic warts, and flat-topped warts (Fig. 19.5). The lesions are usually painless, but they also can be associated with burning, itching, or bleeding. The diagnosis of genital warts is generally made by visual inspection. If external genital lesions are

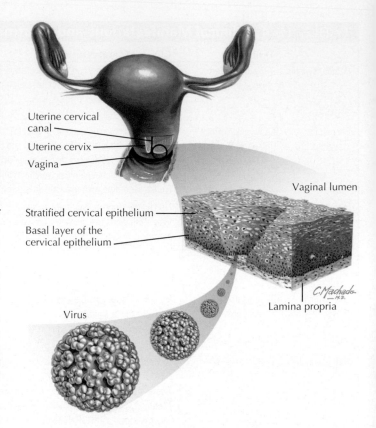

Uterine cervical canal

Uterine cervix

Vagina

Vaginal lumen

Stratified cervical epithelium

Basal layer of the cervical epithelium

Lamina propria

Virus

Fig. 19.4 Human Papillomavirus.

found in women, an internal examination of the genital tract is warranted. Anoscopy and urethroscopy may be indicated. If left untreated, anogenital warts can resolve spontaneously, remain unchanged, or increase in size or number. Patient-applied therapies include imiquimod, podofilox, or sinecatechins. Provider-administered therapies include cryotherapy, surgical removal, and trichloroacetic acid or bichloroacetic acid solution.

High-risk types 16 and 18 cause approximately 25% of low-grade cervical dysplasia, 50% of high-grade cervical dysplasia, and 66% of cervical cancers. Cervical dysplasia is either low- or high-grade squamous intraepithelial dysplasia (LSIL and HSIL) or cervical intraepithelial neoplasia (CIN). Although most are LSIL that spontaneously regress, some young women develop HSIL or CIN, which are considered precancerous, requiring more aggressive intervention. Although the cervix is the most affected anogenital region, HPV can also cause vulvar or vaginal intraepithelial neoplasia and cancer.

Cervical dysplasia is diagnosed by Papanicolaou testing. The US Preventive Services Task Force recommends cervical cancer screening every 3 years with cervical cytologic examination in women aged 21 to 29 years. Treatment of an abnormal Papanicolaou test depends on the degree of cervical dysplasia. A highly effective ninevalent HPV vaccine was approved in 2015 for the prevention of genital lesions and cervical cancers caused by nine different HPV types. The vaccine is recommended for routine administration to 11- and 12-year-olds, and as early as age 9, with catch-up vaccination recommended up to age 26.

Clinical presentation of genital warts

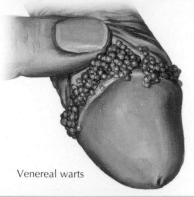

Venereal warts

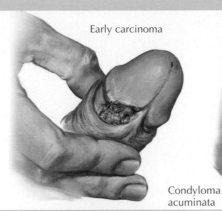

Early carcinoma

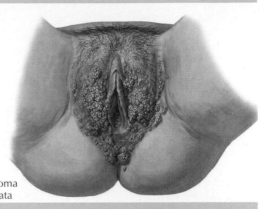

Condyloma acuminata

Colposcopic views of abnormal cervical changes

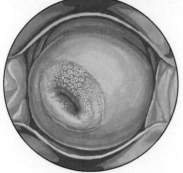

Coarse mosaicism and punctation in transformation zone

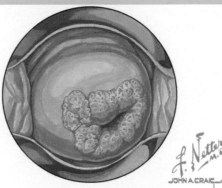

Papilloma of cervix. Some papillomas may predispose to cervical malignancy

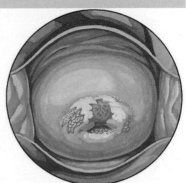

Changes suggestive of carcinoma in situ. Abnormal vasculature with leukoplakia, mosaicism, and punctation

Fig. 19.5 Genital Warts.

SUMMARY

STIs are an important part of adolescent health care. In a population that may have limited access to STI services, it is important for pediatric providers to take a thorough sexual history for every adolescent and to incorporate sexual health education and strategies for prevention and harm reduction, including routine STI screening.

SUGGESTED READINGS

Available online.

Allergy and Immunology

Terri Brown-Whitehorn

20

Anaphylaxis

Lillian Jin, Katie Kennedy, and Terri Brown-Whitehorn

> **CLINICAL VIGNETTE**
>
> A 12-month-old girl with a history of eczema presents to the emergency department with hives, coughing, and vomiting after eating a few bites of scrambled eggs. She is diagnosed with anaphylaxis and treated with epinephrine and diphenhydramine with improvement. Eggs are added to her allergy list, avoidance recommended, an epinephrine autoinjector is prescribed, and she is referred to an allergist.

ETIOLOGY AND PATHOGENESIS

Immunoglobulin E (IgE)-mediated anaphylaxis, a type I hypersensitivity reaction, is the most understood form of anaphylaxis (Fig. 20.1). A person is exposed to an antigen, and, on re-exposure, cross-linkage of IgE occurs, followed by an immediate release of potent mediators from tissue mast cells and peripheral basophils. These mediators include histamine, leukotrienes, nitric oxide, and neutral proteases, which all lead to vasodilatation, increased vascular permeability, bronchoconstriction, and additional inflammation. At times, the reaction occurs with the first known exposure.

Other mechanisms include direct stimulation of mast cells and basophils, as is observed with morphine, exercise, and cold-induced anaphylaxis. Blood products and radiocontrast media may lead to activation of complement and subsequent reactions. Anaphylaxis to aspirin and nonsteroidal antiinflammatory drugs (NSAIDs) may result from the interference of the arachidonic acid pathway. In scombroid poisoning, ingestion of fish containing high levels of histamine (because of improper packaging or storage) can lead to symptoms.

Food is the leading cause of anaphylaxis in children. In the United States, the most common foods implicated in anaphylactic reactions include milk, eggs, soy, wheat, peanuts, tree nuts, fish, and shellfish. Of patients allergic to milk and egg, 70% may tolerate baked milk or baked egg. Over time, some children outgrow their food allergy, "developing tolerance." This occurs more commonly in those allergic to milk, egg, soy, and wheat. Although peanut allergy is often feared the most, fatalities can occur from any food.

Other causes of anaphylaxis include medications (most commonly penicillin), routine immunizations, venom, allergy immunotherapy, blood products, latex, and radiocontrast media. Latex reactions (seen in patients with spina bifida and health care workers) have stabilized as a result of awareness, latex-free gloves, and latex precautions.

Exercise-induced anaphylaxis may be associated with a food trigger. In some cases, it may be due to specific foods (e.g., wheat or celery), but in other cases, any food will trigger a reaction. For those with a food trigger, symptoms occur when patients exercise within 4 hours of ingestion.

More recently reported is an IgE-mediated response to the mammalian oligosaccharide epitope galactose-alpha-1,3-galactose, also known as alpha-gal, that is associated with both immediate and delayed-onset anaphylaxis. The most common triggers of "alpha-gal syndrome" are mammalian food products (e.g., beef and pork) causing delayed-onset anaphylaxis with symptoms occurring 3 to 6 hours after ingestion. It is theorized that Lone Star tick bites are a key mechanism of alpha-gal sensitization, because alpha-gal has been detected in Lone Star tick saliva. Therefore a history of Lone Star tick bite is often obtained.

Finally, there is a small group of patients in whom there is no known cause of anaphylaxis, thus classifying them as idiopathic.

Clinical Presentation

Patients with anaphylaxis may have different clinical manifestations (Table 20.1). Anaphylaxis is often underdiagnosed or misdiagnosed because of clinicians' failure to recognize symptoms. Standardization of diagnostic criteria has been established to help clinicians better recognize anaphylaxis (Box 20.1 and Fig. 20.2). Approximately 90% of children with allergic reactions have skin manifestations, most commonly hives and angioedema. In those who do not, their reactions may be more severe. Respiratory tract symptoms, divided into upper and lower airway, are described in Table 20.1. Gastrointestinal symptoms, including abdominal pain and vomiting, are frequent in food-induced anaphylaxis. Lethargy, change in behavior, and sense of "impending doom" are quite worrisome.

Symptoms can develop within minutes of exposure, although most occur within 30 to 60 minutes depending on the route of exposure (i.e., an intravenous medication reaction will occur quicker than an oral medication reaction). Most anaphylactic reactions are uniphasic, in which the patient has a reaction, is treated, and improves. A biphasic response also may occur, in which a patient becomes asymptomatic after the initial reaction and treatment, and then develops a second reaction that may be the same or more severe than the initial reaction. Protracted anaphylaxis also has been described in which patients have symptoms that persist for days. Both biphasic and protracted reactions seem to occur less frequently in the pediatric population.

DIFFERENTIAL DIAGNOSIS

Given the involvement of multiple organ systems in anaphylaxis, many other diagnoses can present similarly (Table 20.2). A good history may help distinguish these diagnoses from anaphylactic reactions. More commonly seen conditions include vocal cord dysfunction (VCD), viral-induced hives, and hereditary angioedema (HAE). Patients presenting with VCD have difficulty inhaling air. Patients with asthma triggered by viral illnesses may present with both hives and wheezing. HAE can present with isolated swelling of various parts of the body,

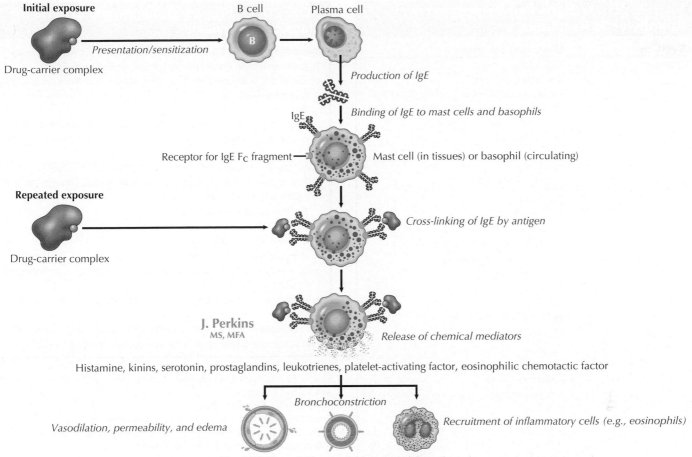

Initial exposure   B cell   Plasma cell

Presentation/sensitization

Drug-carrier complex

Production of IgE

IgE   *Binding of IgE to mast cells and basophils*

Receptor for IgE F$_C$ fragment —— Mast cell (in tissues) or basophil (circulating)

Repeated exposure

Drug-carrier complex   *Cross-linking of IgE by antigen*

J. Perkins
MS, MFA

Release of chemical mediators

Histamine, kinins, serotonin, prostaglandins, leukotrienes, platelet-activating factor, eosinophilic chemotactic factor

Bronchoconstriction

Vasodilation, permeability, and edema   *Recruitment of inflammatory cells (e.g., eosinophils)*

Fig. 20.1 Type 1 (Acute, Anaphylactic) Reactions.

including the face, hands, feet, or airway. Patients often suffer from concurrent bouts of severe abdominal pain caused by swelling in the intestinal wall. The edema is not histamine-mediated, making treatments for anaphylaxis unhelpful for these patients.

EVALUATION

The diagnosis and treatment of anaphylaxis are based on the history of event, clinical manifestations, and examination. No diagnostic tests are available that will help guide management in the immediate setting. However, if performed judiciously and expeditiously, some diagnostic tests, such as serum histamine, urinary histamine, and serum tryptase (Table 20.3) can prove useful in supporting the clinical diagnosis of anaphylaxis after the event. Positive results are helpful, but a patient may still have had an anaphylactic reaction if results are negative, particularly if the concerning trigger is a food.

After someone has a reaction, the cause can be pursued at a later date. However, if the cause is known, clinicians must add it to a patient's allergy list and recommend strict avoidance. Referral to an allergy specialist is recommended. Knowledge of positive and negative predictive values and sensitivity and specificity of various tests are important. False-positive and false-negative testing can occur; therefore, *specific* skin prick testing and radioallergosorbent testing (RAST) are often useful to confirm one's suspicion (Fig. 20.3). Of note, intradermal testing should *never* be used for food allergy testing because of anaphylaxis concerns. The authors do not recommend broad panels of testing; however, if there is a suspicion for a specific food, the clinician should test accordingly. Targeted skin prick testing is most accurate

at least 4 weeks after an episode of anaphylaxis given the possibility of diffuse mast cell degranulation and false-negative testing if performed in close proximity to the event.

MANAGEMENT

For patients who have already had an anaphylactic reaction, prevention of future reactions is of highest priority. Ideally, avoidance of the inciting agent is the best prevention. However, accidental exposures may occur, so knowledge of appropriate management of allergic reactions is essential. An anaphylaxis management plan should be developed and should contain the following: name of patient, known allergen, type of reaction, corresponding dose and type of medication for each clinical scenario, and when to seek additional medical care. For example, a child who develops facial hives from ingestion of milk, a known allergen, should be given a proper dose of diphenhydramine or cetirizine for his weight. He may not need to seek immediate medical attention if the reaction does not progress. Another child, with the same allergy and exposure, develops a wheeze and angioedema. Because the reaction is more severe, this child should be given epinephrine and emergency services (911) called.

In addition to the anaphylaxis plan, food allergy education and awareness are important. School staff and nurses should be made aware of a child's allergens and provided an anaphylaxis management plan and epinephrine autoinjector. Food allergy awareness, symptom recognition, and anaphylaxis treatment instruction are more helpful than removing particular allergens from the school itself (i.e., peanut-free daycare).

TABLE 20.1 Signs and Symptoms of Anaphylactic Reactions

Systems	Signs and Symptoms
Cutaneous	Angioedema
	Conjunctival erythema
	Edema or pruritus of lips, tongue, and uvula
	Flushing
	Periorbital edema and erythema
	Periorbital pruritus
	Urticaria
	Pale skin
Respiratory: Upper	Dysphagia
	Dysphonia
	Hoarseness
	Nasal congestion
	Pruritus of nose, throat, or both
	Pruritus of external auditory canals
	Rhinorrhea
	Sneezing
	Stridor
	Throat tightness or choking
Respiratory: Lower	Bronchospasm
	Coughing
	Chest tightness
	Dyspnea
	Shortness of breath
	Wheezing
Cardiovascular	Arrhythmia
	Chest pain
	Hypotension
	Syncope
	Tachycardia
Gastrointestinal	Abdominal pain
	Diarrhea
	Nausea
	Vomiting
	Incontinence
Neurologic	Altered mental status
	Headache
	Hypotonia
	Sense of impending doom
	Dizziness

BOX 20.1 Proposed Diagnostic Criteria for Classic Anaphylaxis

Need Any One of Three Criteria to Qualify as Anaphylaxis

1. Acute onset of an illness (minutes to hours) with involvement of:
   Skin or mucosal tissue (e.g., hives; generalized itch or flush; swollen lips, tongue, or uvula)
   and
   Respiratory compromise (e.g., dyspnea, wheeze or bronchospasm, stridor, reduced peak expiratory flow)
   or
   Hypotension or associated symptoms (e.g., hypotonia, syncope)
2. Two or more of the following after exposure to known allergen for that patient (minutes to hours):
   a. History of severe allergic reaction
   b. Skin or mucosal tissue involvement
   c. Respiratory compromise
   d. Hypotension or associated symptoms
   e. In suspected food allergy: gastrointestinal symptoms (e.g., abdominal pain, vomiting)
3. Hypotension after exposure to known allergen for that patient (minutes to hours)
   Infants and children: low SBP (age specific) or >30% decrease in SBP[a]
   Adults: SBP 90 mm Hg or >30% decrease from baseline

[a] Low SBP for children is defined as <70 mm Hg from 1 month to 1 year; <70 mm Hg + (2× age) from 1 to 10 years; and <90 mm Hg from age 11 to 17 years.
SBP, Systolic blood pressure.
From Sampson HA, Munoz-Furlong A, Bock SA, et al. Symposium of the definition and management of anaphylaxis: summary report. *J Allergy Clin Immunol.* 2005;115:584-591.

Emergency Management

Managing an anaphylactic reaction begins like any other emergent clinical scenario, with the assessment of airway, breathing, and circulation. Supplemental oxygen should be administered as needed, and the Trendelenburg position is recommended when possible. The treatment of choice in a patient with anaphylaxis is epinephrine (1:1000 solution) given in a dose of 0.01 mL/kg up to a maximum of 0.3 mL/dose for children and 0.5 mL/dose for adults. The dose should be given intramuscularly (IM) because absorption of epinephrine is faster if given IM compared with the subcutaneous route. Epinephrine can be readministered every 5 minutes, with a maximum of three doses before an infusion is started. Epinephrine infusions, along with other vasopressors, such as dopamine, have been used in severe cases. At some institutions, epinephrine autoinjectors are available to improve accuracy and speed of administration. For severe reactions, an intravenous line must be placed to aid with fluid replacement because patients with severe reactions, such as anaphylactic shock, require rapid administration of large volumes of fluids.

Antihistamines, including histamine-1 (H1) and H2 blockers, have been used for the treatment of anaphylaxis. Medications such as diphenhydramine (1 to 2 mg/kg; maximum, 50 mg) can be given orally (PO) or intravenously (IV) depending on the severity of the reaction. Cetirizine also can be given PO. H2 blockers, such as famotidine (0.25 mg/kg; maximum 20 mg), have been used in combination with H1 blockers in those with persistent hives, abdominal pain, or severe reactions. For those with a history of asthma or who have persistent wheezing despite epinephrine, β-2 adrenergic agents, such as albuterol, should be used. The exact role of corticosteroids in the management of anaphylaxis is unclear, but they may prevent or ameliorate the late phase reaction. Prednisone or prednisolone can be given PO (1 to 2 mg/kg; maximum 60 mg/day), or methylprednisolone can be given IV (1 to 2 mg/kg; maximum 60 mg). In addition, once symptoms subside, long courses of oral antihistamines and oral steroids do not appear to be needed.

Hospital Management

Anaphylaxis in a hospitalized patient is treated the same way. The offending agent, if known and applicable (e.g., an antibiotic infusion), should be stopped (and added to allergy list). If the antigen has been injected, as with allergy immunotherapy, use of a tourniquet proximal to the injection site is recommended. For patients with a previous reaction to intravenous radiocontrast media, future premedication with corticosteroid and diphenhydramine is recommended. If one has a known reaction to a drug, and there are no other alternatives,

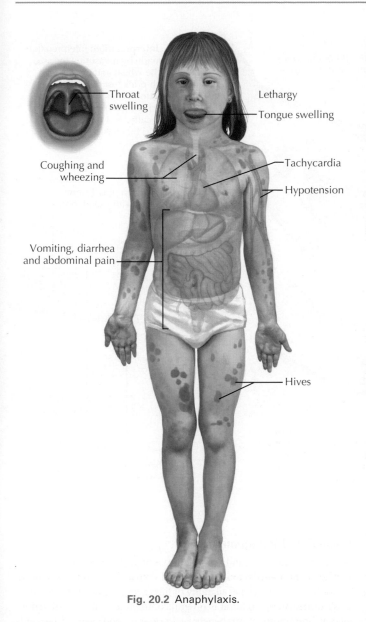

Throat swelling

Lethargy

Tongue swelling

Coughing and wheezing

Tachycardia

Hypotension

Vomiting, diarrhea and abdominal pain

Hives

Fig. 20.2 Anaphylaxis.

TABLE 20.2 Differential Diagnosis by Symptoms

System	Diagnosis
Circulatory	Shock
	Systemic inflammatory response syndrome
	Vasovagal reaction
	Dysrhythmia
	Myocardial infarction
Cutaneous	Carcinoid syndrome
	Monosodium glutamate ingestion
	Red man syndrome
	Scombroid fish poisoning
	Sulfite ingestion
	Urticarial dermatitis
	Drug eruption
	Bullous pemphigoid
	Autonomic epilepsy
	Alcohol consumption
	Menopause
	Medullary carcinoma of thyroid
Respiratory	Airway foreign body
	Asthma exacerbation
	Oral allergy
	Vocal cord dysfunction
	Pulmonary embolism
	Pneumothorax
	Epiglottitis
Other/Mixed	Capillary leak syndrome
	Hereditary angioedema
	Munchausen syndrome
	Panic attack
	Systemic mastocytosis
	Hereditary periodic fever syndromes
Gastrointestinal	Scombroidosis
	Pollen-food allergy syndrome
	Food poisoning
	Caustic ingestion
	Anisakiasis
Neurologic	Seizure
	Stroke

TABLE 20.3 Laboratory Evaluation

Tests	Marker	Time
Histamine	Released by mast cells	Serum: Within 1 h of event Urine: Methylhistamine can be collected up to 24 h after event
Tryptase (although prefer beta tryptase)	Released by mast cells	Serum or plasma: Within 15 min to 6 h of event (within 3 h of symptom onset is ideal)
Skin prick testing	IgE-mediated skin response to specific allergen (only test to a specific allergen)	After exposure (may need to perform 4 weeks after event)
ImmunoCAP	Measures IgE levels in patient's blood (only test to a specific allergen) Component testing may be useful	After exposure (may need to perform 4 weeks after event)

IgE, Immunoglobulin E.

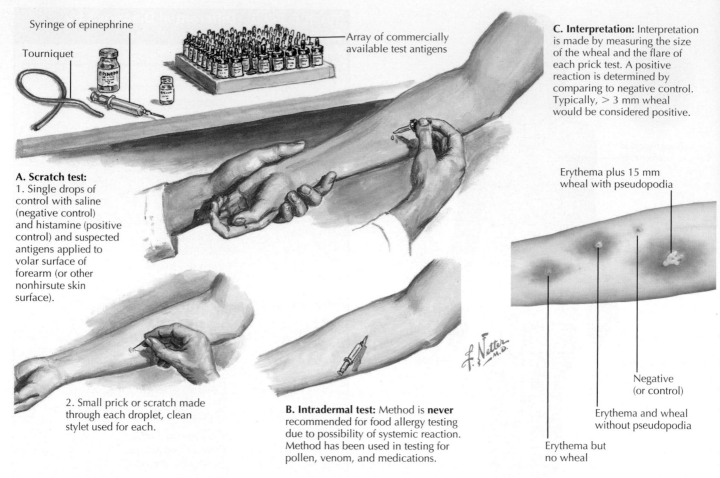

Syringe of epinephrine

Tourniquet

Array of commercially available test antigens

A. Scratch test:
1. Single drops of control with saline (negative control) and histamine (positive control) and suspected antigens applied to volar surface of forearm (or other nonhirsute skin surface).

2. Small prick or scratch made through each droplet, clean stylet used for each.

B. Intradermal test: Method is **never** recommended for food allergy testing due to possibility of systemic reaction. Method has been used in testing for pollen, venom, and medications.

C. Interpretation: Interpretation is made by measuring the size of the wheal and the flare of each prick test. A positive reaction is determined by comparing to negative control. Typically, > 3 mm wheal would be considered positive.

Erythema plus 15 mm wheal with pseudopodia

Negative (or control)

Erythema and wheal without pseudopodia

Erythema but no wheal

Fig. 20.3 Skin Testing for Allergy.

consultation with an allergist is warranted. Antibiotic desensitization protocols have been established and successful in many patients with IgE-mediated reactions. Patients taking beta-blocker therapy present a special challenge to anaphylaxis treatment, although the drug of choice remains epinephrine. If persistence of hypotension and bradycardia occurs, glucagon is recommended because it has both inotropic and chronotropic effects on the heart. Atropine is useful only for patients with bradycardia.

Disposition

There is no standardized observation period after an anaphylactic reaction. Not all patients with anaphylactic reactions require hospitalization. For reactions with symptom resolution or improvement, 4 hours of observation may be appropriate. Indications for inpatient care include patients with a severe reaction, such as respiratory or circulatory compromise at time of presentation, concomitant asthma exacerbation at time of reaction, history of severe prior reaction, need for more than 1 dose of epinephrine, need for fluid bolus, or any concern in which the patient needs reevaluation.

Upon discharge, patients must be prescribed an epinephrine autoinjector and trained in how and when to use it (depending on cause of the reaction). If treatment is needed, patients and families should call 911 (or emergency responder) and be seen in the emergency department. Calling emergency services is recommended in the event of persistent or worsening symptoms.

Outpatient Management

Avoidance, education, and an anaphylaxis plan are important aspects of management. Patients must understand their risk for future reactions. In addition, immediate availability of life-saving medications is a must at all times. Allergy referral is often recommended. In cases of venom allergy, immunotherapy is beneficial. In cases of food allergy, label reading and avoidance are important. In addition, desensitization protocols such as oral immunotherapy directed at food may be offered either in a research or clinical setting. In cases of drug allergy, alternative medications and possible desensitization protocols may be helpful.

FUTURE DIRECTIONS

Anaphylaxis is a medical emergency with a host of potential causes, most commonly, foods and medications. We do not know why patients develop anaphylaxis, why some outgrow their allergies and others do not, or why some develop new reactions to things they once tolerated. This poses many questions and research opportunities. Although the treatment of anaphylaxis is often successful, patients still die from anaphylaxis. Ways to improve awareness, prevention, and treatment are also of great importance.

SUGGESTED READINGS

Available online.

21

Urticaria and Angioedema

Whitney Reid Fink and Laura Gober

CLINICAL VIGNETTE

A 15-year-old girl with a history of mild persistent asthma and atopic dermatitis presents with hives. The first episode of hives occurred 2 years ago on her arm after direct skin contact for 5 minutes with a cold water bottle. This self-resolved after 20 minutes without medications. Hives were then episodic with increasing frequency over the past year, always triggered by cold exposures such as exposed fingers and ears in cold weather or swimming in the cold ocean. On a recent swim in the ocean, she developed generalized hives within a few minutes of exiting the water. She denied associated respiratory or gastrointestinal symptoms.

On examination, she was well-appearing without rash or edema. After placing a cool pack on the volar surface of her forearm for 5 minutes, she developed well-circumscribed wheals with surrounding erythema within 3 minutes of cool pack removal. Her clinical presentation was consistent with cold urticaria, and she was prescribed a second-generation antihistamine and advised to avoid contact with extreme cold. A set of epinephrine autoinjectors were prescribed because of the potential for anaphylaxis with extensive cold exposure; in particular, she was warned about swimming in cold bodies of water and to never go swimming alone.

Urticaria is a mast cell–driven process causing the rapid onset of transient, pruritic hives and/or angioedema, often without an identifiable trigger. Acute urticaria is relatively common, occurring in 20% of the population, in comparison to chronic urticaria, which occurs in less than 5% of the general population. Hives, or wheals, are described as areas of well-demarcated edema of the epidermis with surrounding erythema and intense, histamine-driven itch (Fig. 21.1). Hives typically resolve within 24 hours of onset, although new lesions often appear. Angioedema is edema of the deep skin or mucous membranes involving the dermis and subcutaneous tissue and is typically less well-circumscribed than hives. Unlike hives, angioedema is described as painful or burning and can last several days. Urticaria is classified into acute urticaria and chronic urticaria based on duration of symptoms. Chronic urticaria is defined as recurring episodes of wheals with or without angioedema lasting longer than 6 weeks, whereas acute urticaria lasts less than 6 weeks. Chronic urticaria is further subdivided into chronic spontaneous urticaria (CSU) and chronic inducible urticaria (CIndU), with the latter having specific, identifiable triggers for hives onset such as cold or vibration.

Chronic urticaria is uncommon in the pediatric population, occurring in 0.1% to 0.3%, but can have a significant social and financial impact. Urticaria can be a frustrating disease for patients because there is often no identifiable trigger for exacerbations and relapses are unpredictable. The pruritus, which is a hallmark of urticaria, leads to high disease burden with effects on sleep, daily activities, and school and work life. It can also lead to mood disorders such as depression and anxiety. Patients with chronic urticaria often take multiple medications and have multiple medical visits, including to acute care settings such as the emergency department, and frequent absences from work and school, all factors that contribute to the economic burden of the disease.

ETIOLOGY AND PATHOGENESIS

Although urticaria is quite common, the pathogenesis of the disease remains relatively poorly understood. The waxing and waning wheals characteristic of urticaria result from the activation of dermal mast cells after crosslinking of the high-affinity receptor for immunoglobulin (Ig) E. This mast cell activation triggers the release of a collection of vasoactive substances, including histamine, and leads to skin vasodilation with an increase in vascular permeability and leakage of fluid into surrounding tissues and to the stimulation of sensory nerve endings, manifesting clinically as superficial swelling, erythema, and pruritus. Histologically, urticarial lesions consist of a mixed, lymphocyte-predominant perivascular infiltrate made up of monocytes, eosinophils, basophils, rarely neutrophils, and CD4$^+$ T cells with evidence of a mixed T helper cell type 1/type2 (T_H1/T_H2) immune response.

Acute Urticaria

There are several potential causes of acute urticaria, though a trigger is not identifiable in many cases. Viral infections are the most common cause in children, accounting for up to 60% of pediatric cases of acute urticaria. Hives typically occur a few days after the start of viral symptoms; however, they may also occur after symptom resolution, making it hard to associate the infection as a trigger. Other potential triggers can be attributed to either IgE-mediated or non–IgE-mediated processes. IgE-mediated urticaria in children can be caused by immediate reaction to medications, insects bites/stings, and foods. Non–IgE-mediated causes of acute urticaria may include immune responses such as serum sickness or reactions to pseudoallergens such as aspirin and other salicylates. Vasoactive amines found in cheeses, beer, and wine can also elicit urticaria. In general, IgE-mediated food allergies, such as to milk or peanut, cause symptoms most commonly within a few minutes to a few hours after ingestion (most often within 30 minutes of ingestion). In addition, for children with drug allergy, hives typically occur after the first dose of medication, most often having previously tolerated a first course. Hives in the context of an allergic reaction to a food either escalate to involve other symptoms (e.g., gastrointestinal or respiratory symptoms) or resolve either spontaneously or with medications given to treat allergic reaction (e.g., antihistamines) without recurrence.

Chronic Spontaneous Urticaria

CSU is the more common form of chronic urticaria in children with mean age at presentation of 6.7 years. CSU is defined as spontaneous

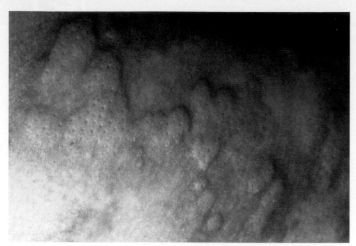

Fig. 21.1 Urticaria.

development of itchy wheals and sometimes angioedema, at least 3 days per week with disease duration lasting more than 6 weeks without an identifiable trigger. Much of the pathogenesis of CSU remains to be elucidated, but it is considered a mast cell–driven disease and is more common in females. Up to 40% of patients with CSU have autoantibodies directed against IgE (10%) or the high-affinity IgE receptor (90%), FcεRI. These autoantibodies have been hypothesized to be pathogenic, although this remains controversial because they also can be found in healthy individuals and in the context of other autoimmune diseases. The autologous serum skin test, which involves intradermal injection of a patient's own serum with elicitation of a wheal-and-flare response, is more common in patients with CSU compared with healthy controls and atopic patients but is no longer available. Chronic urticaria may occur in the context of autoimmune disease, most commonly in the hypothyroid or hyperthyroid state but has been described in other autoimmune diseases, such as celiac disease, Sjögren disease, systemic lupus erythematosus, rheumatoid arthritis, and type 1 diabetes mellitus.

The role of mast cells and basophils has been investigated in CSU. Skin biopsies of patients with CSU demonstrate mast cell degranulation accompanied by increased mast cell releasability that reverses with disease remission. Basophils, which typically are not present in the skin, are observed in both lesional and nonlesional CSU skin biopsies. Peripheral blood basopenia and altered basophil FcεRI function also have been shown in CSU, with improved disease severity leading to an increase in peripheral blood basophils and IgE-mediated histamine release. Furthermore, basophil activation markers have been shown to be enhanced in patients with CSU and may contribute to basophil chemotaxis and reactivity.

Chronic Inducible Urticaria

CIndUs have a specific trigger that directly induces hives within minutes, typically lasting minutes to a few hours. CIndUs are further classified by physical and nonphysical causes, each having a different trigger and individuals potentially having more than one subtype. Mast cell degranulation is included in the pathogenesis of most subtypes of CIndUs, including symptomatic dermatographism and cold, solar, and cholinergic urticaria, but serum immunoglobulin also may be involved as demonstrated by passive transfer experiments.

ANGIOEDEMA

Angioedema, which is nonpitting swelling of the deep dermis, subcutaneous, and submucosal tissues, coexists with urticaria in approximately

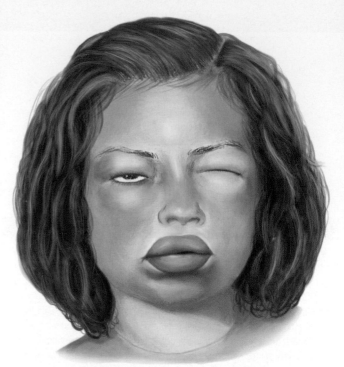

Fig. 21.2 Angioedema.

40% of cases but typically persists past 24 hours (Fig. 21.2). Angioedema is typically asymmetric, nondependent, and described as a painful or burning sensation rather than pruritic. Angioedema that accompanies urticaria is thought to be caused by mast cells and histamine-mediated, although up to 10% of patients with mast cell–driven disease will not have hives. Angioedema without urticaria also can be kinin-mediated with activation of the bradykinin pathway, as is seen with patients taking angiotensin-converting enzyme (ACE) inhibitors.

CLINICAL PRESENTATION

Urticarial lesions are intensely pruritic and can affect any location on the body. They are typically transient, lasting less than 24 hours and leaving no residual scarring or bruising on the skin on resolution. Unlike atopic dermatitis, excoriation is not a typical examination finding in urticaria, regardless of the degree of pruritus experienced, although scratches may be noted if dermatographism is present. Lesions can vary in size and can become confluent. Similar to urticaria, angioedema can occur anywhere on the body, frequently involving the face, lips, and extremities; but unlike urticaria, it commonly involves mucous membranes. Cold urticaria is the exception because it may involve swelling of the tongue or palate.

Patients with long-lasting lesions or the presence of other systemic symptoms should be evaluated for other diseases (Box 21.1). *Urticarial vasculitis* is classified by painful and/or pruritic lesions lasting longer than 48 hours and may leave residual skin changes unrelated to excoriation. Concurrent systemic complaints or abnormal laboratory findings indicative of an inflammatory process, such as an elevated erythrocyte sedimentation rate (ESR), elevated C-reactive protein (CRP), or low complement levels, are typically seen. A skin biopsy is required to rule out urticarial vasculitis. *Urticaria pigmentosa*, a form of cutaneous mastocytosis, may mimic urticaria, although these lesions are typically pigmented and stationary and urticate when rubbed (Darier sign). The presence of fever with urticaria can occur in Schnitzler syndrome and Muckle-Wells syndrome.

BOX 21.1 Differential Diagnosis of Urticaria and Angioedema

Acute Urticaria

IgE Mediated
- Food allergy
- Drug allergy
- Stinging insect allergy

Non–IgE Mediated
- Papular urticaria secondary to insect bite
- Urticaria multiforme
- Transfusion reaction
- Infections

Chronic Urticaria or Angioedema

With Urticaria
- Spontaneous urticaria
- Inducible urticarias
- Urticarial vasculitis
- Urticaria pigmentosa
- Serum sickness
- Infection
- Muckle-Wells syndrome
- Schnitzler syndrome

Without Urticaria
- Idiopathic angioedema
- Hereditary angioedema
- Malignancy

IgE, Immunoglobulin E.

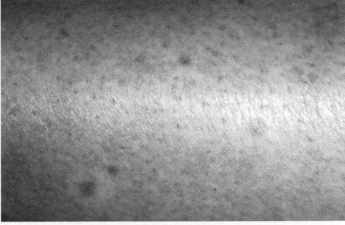

Fig. 21.3 Cholinergic Urticaria.

Schnitzler syndrome is described as recurrent urticaria with arthralgia, fever, elevated IgM, and elevation in inflammatory markers (ESR). *Muckle-Wells syndrome* is a periodic fever syndrome with urticaria associated with periodic, unexplained fevers.

History

In diagnosing either acute or chronic urticaria, a thorough history and detailed physical examination are the most important elements. The history should elicit the time of onset of hives, because some patients may experience diurnal variation and may point to certain triggers, duration of hives, and frequency of episodes. A description of the lesions, including their shape, size, distribution, color, pigmentation, and quality of pain or itch, is important in confirming the diagnosis of urticaria. Itch must be present to diagnose urticaria and must respond to antihistamines. To identify acute triggers, the history should elicit recent use of medications (e.g., antibiotics, nonsteroidal anti-inflammatory drugs [NSAIDs], aspirin), food ingested shortly before symptom onset (i.e., no longer than 2 hours before), implanted surgical devices, insect stings, and changes in environment. It is important to ask about recent infections. A good review of systems is also key in ruling out autoimmune disease, most commonly thyroid disease, as a cause of chronic urticaria. For female patients, it is important to investigate if there is a variation of hives in relation to hormonal changes observed with menses or pregnancy because progesterone can play a role in urticaria. Asking about physical triggers is important for defining CIndUs. Further evaluation of life stressors may assist in understanding the timing of episodes or worsening disease. It is also important to evaluate how the patient is coping and what therapeutics, including nonprescription medications or dietary

changes, are being used and if they are providing any relief. Some patients with chronic urticaria are on restricted diets, which are often unnecessary and may lead to nutritional deficits. Medication side effects also should be evaluated, with sedation from antihistamines being the leading side effect contributing to disease burden in patients with chronic urticaria.

For patients with angioedema without a history of urticaria, it is important to ask about family history of angioedema. Hereditary angioedema (HAE), an autosomal dominant disease involving decreased levels or decreased function of C1 esterase inhibitor, manifests with isolated angioedema that sometimes can be disfiguring and life-threatening because the airway can be involved. HAE typically manifests in late childhood or early adolescence, with 50% of patients having their first attack by the age of 10 years. It is important to ask about episodic abdominal pain and abdominal surgeries in these patients and their families because many times their sole presenting symptoms are abdominal pain and vomiting.

Physical Examination

The physical examination is important in solidifying the diagnosis of urticaria, but cannot distinguish between acute and chronic urticaria. The examination should focus on the size, distribution, and color of the lesions. Whereas wheals are characteristically pink or red because of histamine-induced vasodilation in the skin and are easily blanched, vasculitic lesions have a darker red or purple appearance resulting from vascular damage and are typically nonblanching. Cholinergic urticaria has a characteristic "fried egg" appearance with a small wheal and surrounding large flare (Fig. 21.3). The physical examination should include testing for dermatographism, which can be elicited by applying linear pressure to the skin using a blunt object, such as a tongue depressor. In some types of CIndU, eliciting urticaria with additional maneuvers is diagnostic, as in the ice cube test for cold urticaria. The physical examination should include thyroid palpation to assess for thyroid gland abnormalities.

EVALUATION AND MANAGEMENT

Laboratory Testing

No routine laboratory testing is indicated in urticaria unless the patient has an atypical clinical presentation and/or the clinician has high suspicion for an underlying cause such as thyroid disease or food allergy. For patients with acute urticaria suspected of having a food allergy, history-guided specific skin testing and specific IgE measurements may be helpful. There is a high percentage of false-positive test results in skin testing to foods, so testing should be carried out only to foods of concern. Skin testing is difficult to perform in patients with chronic urticaria because of the high prevalence of dermatographism and delayed pressure features in this group, as well as their dependence on antihistamines, but it still may be a valuable tool. Patients with physical urticaria do not need laboratory testing.

In CSU, laboratory testing may act as an adjunct to history and examination, especially in patients who fail to respond to conventional therapies or who have uncharacteristic lesions. Laboratory screening tests, such as a complete blood count with differential, complete metabolic panel, ESR, and/or CRP, should be obtained if there are concerns for systemic disease. If there are concerns for vasculitis or autoimmune disorders, an antinuclear antibody (ANA) and complement levels, specifically C3 and C4, should be considered. Patients with significant angioedema without urticaria also should have C1 esterase inhibitor function testing. C4 levels are typically low in patients with HAE during acute episodes. Symptoms consistent with thyroid disease warrant thyroid screening with a thyroid-stimulating hormone (TSH) level.

Although viral infections, particularly viral upper respiratory tract infections, are the most common cause of acute urticaria in children, viral testing has little impact on therapy or outcomes. Other infectious etiologies have been implicated in urticaria, and testing for these should be guided by the history and examination. Hepatitis, especially hepatitis C, has been reported to manifest as chronic urticaria; thus screening studies for hepatitis B and C should be considered in patients with risk factors or abnormalities on physical examination. In patients with CSU with symptoms of gastroesophageal reflux or gastritis, *Helicobacter pylori* serology may be indicated because this organism may contribute to urticaria. If there is peripheral eosinophilia, the stool should be tested for ova and parasites. Bacterial and fungal cultures do not need to be ordered for urticaria because these are unusual triggers of hives.

Management

The treatment of CSU often poses a greater challenge than that of acute and CIndUs. For all types of urticaria with a clearly identified trigger, such as in confirmed food allergy or physical urticaria, the trigger should be avoided as much as possible. For all patients with urticaria, avoidance of aspirin and salicylate-containing medications, as well as NSAIDs, is advisable. Both aspirin and NSAIDs can aggravate urticaria and angioedema by inhibition of prostaglandin synthesis; thus patients should switch to alternative NSAIDs that do not inhibit cyclooxygenase-1 inhibitory activity if a chronic analgesic agent is needed. Of note, use of cyclooxygenase-2 inhibitors is discouraged for children younger than 16 years. For patients with angioedema, ACE inhibitors should be avoided. All patients should avoid morphine and codeine-containing products, which can directly stimulate dermal mast cells.

The mainstay of treatment for acute or chronic urticaria is antihistamines (H1-blockers). Nonsedating, second-generation H1-blockers, including cetirizine, levocetirizine, loratadine, and fexofenadine, are first-line treatment, whereas the more sedating, older generation H1-blockers, such as diphenhydramine and hydroxyzine, are reserved for use on an as-needed basis or to aid with sleep. Different H1-blockers may be trialed because one may work better per individual. For chronic urticaria in pediatric patients (ages 1 to 17 years), the dose of nonsedating antihistamines may need to be increased up to four times the standard dose to be effective, although this dosing is not approved by the US Food and Drug Administration and risks and benefits should be considered and discussed with the patient/family. H2-blockers can provide an added benefit in combination with H1-blockade and may even increase serum concentration of the H1-blocker. Leukotriene antagonists also can be used as an adjunct to H1- and H2-blockade if the patient's symptoms are still not controlled, although they should be used with caution in children with mood disorders.

In severe cases of chronic urticaria not responsive to the previously mentioned regimens, subcutaneous injection of omalizumab has been shown to be effective. Omalizumab is a monoclonal antibody that targets IgE, decreasing free IgE serum levels, limiting binding of IgE to high-affinity IgE receptors on mast cells, and resulting in downregulation of the IgE receptor. Omalizumab has been shown to improve symptoms and patient quality of life in chronic urticaria, including physical urticaria (cold-induced and delayed pressure), which typically responds poorly to antihistamines. It is important to keep in mind the natural history of chronic urticaria with remissions in 19%, 54%, and 68% of pediatric cases at 1, 3, and 5 years, respectively, because symptoms tend to return when omalizumab treatment is discontinued. Another biologic drug, ligelizumab, also targeting IgE, may be available in the future for children failing omalizumab. Cyclosporine has been shown to improve symptoms of chronic urticaria; however, this off-label use should be reserved for patients failing other regimens described earlier given its potential adverse effects and need for routine blood testing to monitor for end-organ damage.

Unlike in HAE, angioedema associated with acute or chronic urticaria is rarely life-threatening and epinephrine autoinjector is not indicated, except in the case of cold urticaria in which extensive cold exposure, such as with water submersion, can potentially lead to anaphylaxis. Patients with cold urticaria should be prescribed a set of two epinephrine autoinjectors, trained in use of the device, and given an anaphylaxis plan in addition to counseling to never swim alone and wear appropriate clothing in cold weather months. Topical corticosteroids play no role in the treatment of patients with urticaria, with the exception of perhaps some minimal benefit in localized delayed pressure urticaria. Systemic steroids can be used to treat hives in certain settings to provide temporary relief, but use should be avoided especially in chronic urticaria because they have a high side effect profile, the benefit is transient, and patients may have rebound effect.

Referral to an allergist and/or dermatologist knowledgeable in the care of pediatric patients is helpful in terms of management and medications, although families and patients should be made aware and have reasonable expectations that a cause is often not found.

Patients with CSU have a higher incidence of thyroid autoantibodies compared with the general population, but use of thyroid hormone replacement is indicated only in patients who have active thyroid disease and not those with a euthyroid state regardless of the presence of thyroid autoantibodies.

FUTURE DIRECTIONS

Chronic urticaria is a frustrating and burdensome disease that is often difficult to control, requiring trial of multiple treatment regimens. Although antihistamines are sufficient treatment for the majority of patients with acute urticaria, higher than usual doses are often required and may lead to significant sedation, thus altering quality of life and perhaps interfering with school/work attendance. Studies of omalizumab treatment for chronic urticaria have shown the safety and efficacy of dosing at 150 mg or 300 mg subcutaneously every 4 weeks for 6 months in children aged 12 years and older, though clinical experience suggests that perhaps longer duration and more frequent dosing could be effective in more resistant cases. This highlights the need for large, well-designed, double-blind, and placebo-controlled randomized trials to investigate the use of omalizumab in children with CSU, especially those younger than 12 years.

Overall, urticaria remains a frustrating, difficult-to-control disease associated with significant morbidity. A better understanding of underlying disease mechanisms is essential to the development of new, targeted therapeutics.

SUGGESTED READINGS

Available online.

22

Allergic Rhinitis

Stanislaw J. Gabryszewski and Rahul Datta

Allergic rhinitis refers to allergy-associated inflammation of the nasal mucosa. Nasal symptoms include congestion, rhinorrhea, and sneezing. The term *allergic rhinoconjunctivitis* accounts for concomitant ocular symptoms, such as itching, tearing, and conjunctival erythema. Allergic rhinitis is a late member of the atopic march (Fig. 22.1) and affects about 20% of children, primarily during school-age years. It is associated with reduced quality of life, negative effects on school and work performance, and significant economic costs. Affected patients report fatigue, irritability, inability to focus, and poor sleep. Asthma occurs in approximately 40% of patients with allergic rhinitis. The prevalence of these comorbid diseases has increased over the last half-century, suggesting an important role for environmental factors. Allergic rhinitis–associated inflammation may compromise eustachian tube function and sinus drainage, predisposing to otitis media and rhinosinusitis, respectively.

ETIOLOGY AND PATHOGENESIS

Allergic rhinitis is a type I immunoglobulin E (IgE)-mediated hypersensitivity and consists of two phases, immediate and late. In predisposed individuals, allergen exposure initially stimulates allergen-specific IgE production by plasma cells. IgE molecules bind to Fcε receptors on the surface of mast cells and basophils. The immediate phase, which occurs within 15 minutes, is caused by crosslinking of receptor-bound IgE molecules. This stimulates degranulation and release of preformed and newly formed mediators, including histamine, prostaglandins, and leukotrienes, causing itching, sneezing, and rhinorrhea. Eosinophils, macrophages, and neutrophils are subsequently recruited, and additional release of vasoactive mediators occurs approximately 6 hours after the inciting exposure, causing mucous production and congestion. This is referred to as the late phase. T helper type 2 (T_H2) cells promote inflammation through their expression of the cytokines interleukin-4 (IL-4), IL-5, and IL-13, which stimulate IgE production, eosinophil recruitment, and mucous hypersecretion.

The most common triggers of allergic rhinitis are airborne environmental allergens. Seasonal symptoms are associated with tree, grass, and weed pollens in the spring, summer, and fall, respectively. Perennial symptoms are associated with dust mites, cockroaches, and animal (e.g., cat, dog, mouse) dander. Mold may cause both seasonal and perennial allergic rhinitis. Seasonal allergens can vary among geographic regions and depend on the local flora. Many patients in the United States are sensitized to multiple allergens, and seasonality of symptoms may evolve with age. Toddlers may initially have year-long symptoms caused by perennial allergens (e.g., dust or pets) and, with time, progress to exhibit seasonal symptoms related to seasonal allergens (e.g., pollens).

Predisposition to allergic rhinitis is thought to result from complex interactions between genetic and environmental factors. The heritability of allergic rhinitis is supported by studies in monozygotic and dizygotic twins, which demonstrate concordances of approximately 50% and 25%, respectively. Functions of gene variants associated with allergic rhinitis include type I hypersensitivity, T_H2 signaling, antigen presentation, and pathogen recognition. In addition to history of atopic disease, risk factors for development of allergic rhinitis include air pollution, male sex (in early childhood), and limited early-life exposure to microbes. Some studies have suggested protective effects for breastfeeding and consumption of a Mediterranean-type diet; studies further exploring these relationships are ongoing.

CLINICAL PRESENTATION

Nasal symptoms are the predominant manifestations of allergic rhinitis. Patients complain of nasal itching, sniffing, sneezing, clear rhinorrhea, and congestion. Postnasal discharge may stimulate coughing. If coughing persists despite treatment, patients should be evaluated for possible comorbid asthma. Significant congestion may cause mouth breathing, which also may be attributed to concomitant tonsillar and/or adenoidal hypertrophy. Accompanying ocular symptoms may include conjunctival erythema, itching, tearing, and crusting. The presence of nasal symptoms, with or without ocular symptoms, for

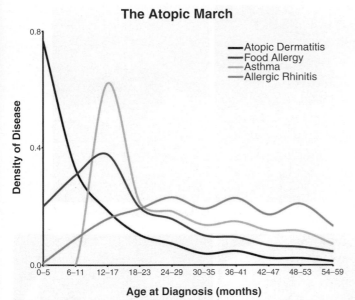

The Atopic March

Fig. 22.1 Age Distribution of Allergic Rhinitis and Other Diseases Composing the Atopic March. The atopic march refers to the prototypical sequence of atopic dermatitis, immunoglobulin E–mediated food allergy, asthma, and allergic rhinitis that occurs over the course of life in patients predisposed to allergic disease. Allergic rhinitis is typically a late manifestation of atopy. Shown are age distributions at time of diagnosis for each allergic disease. (Adapted from Hill DA, Spergel JM. The atopic march: critical evidence and clinical relevance. *Ann Allergy Asthma Immunol.* 2018;120[2]:131-137. https://doi.org/10.1016/j.anai.2017.10.037. Erratum in: *Ann Allergy Asthma Immunol.* 2018; PMID: 29413336; PMCID: PMC5806141, Fig. 1)

over 1 hour on most days is consistent with the diagnosis of allergic rhinitis.

Patients with pollen-associated allergic rhinitis may also suffer from oral allergy syndrome. Manifestations include mouth itching after ingestion of certain uncooked foods, such as pitted fruits, apples, and certain vegetables. This occurs as a result of cross-sensitization between pollens and food allergens and is managed by avoidance of uncooked culprit foods. Patients typically tolerate cooked forms of the food, because cooking denatures the allergenic proteins. Oral food allergy is rarely life-threatening.

EVALUATION

A comprehensive history and physical examination are typically sufficient to diagnose allergic rhinitis. The examiner should perform close examinations of the head, eyes, ears, nose, mouth, neck, lungs, and skin. Physical manifestations of allergic rhinitis (Fig. 22.2) may include periorbital congestion with darkening of the skin under the eyes, also referred to as allergic shiners. Patients may have characteristic folds of skin below the lower eyelids, termed Dennie-Morgan folds. There may be a crease on the nasal bridge as a result of frequent nose rubbing. Other associated findings include conjunctival erythema, rhinorrhea, pale mucosa, engorged turbinates, and cobblestoning of the posterior pharynx (Fig. 22.3). The tympanic membranes may be dull, and concomitant serous otitis media may be identified. In some instances, the palate is high-arched, and there may be an appreciable overbite. Rhinoscopy, typically performed in the specialist setting for adolescents and adults, may assist in identifying nasal polyps, deviated septum, or other anatomic abnormalities. In a patient with underlying atopy, concurrent conditions may be identified. For instance, cough

and prolonged expiratory phase are suggestive of asthma (Chapter 131), while xerotic skin with erythematous and pruritic patches may be a sign of atopic dermatitis (Chapter 39).

The frequency and severity of symptoms should be assessed to determine the burden of disease. A cutoff of 4 days per week or 4 weeks per year distinguishes between intermittent and persistent allergic rhinitis. Mild disease is characterized by absence of intolerable symptoms along with no effects on daily functioning, academic or work performance, or sleep. Presence of any of these criteria is characteristic of moderate-to-severe disease. The clinician should inquire about seasonality of symptoms and frequency of direct exposures to common environmental allergens, including pollen, grass, weed, dust, cockroach, animals (e.g., cat, dog, mouse), and mold. History may reveal a culprit allergen in only some instances, because many patients are sensitized to multiple allergens. Assessment of home living conditions should include questions about the frequency of cleaning (e.g., washing bedding, cleaning floors) and the presence of pets, carpets, ventilation, and pest infestations. In addition, asking about open windows or use of air conditioning may be helpful.

The efficacy of prior trials of medications, such as antihistamines or intranasal corticosteroids, should be assessed. Adherence and technique of medication administration, often incorrect in the case of intranasal corticosteroids, should be reviewed. The clinician should inquire about medications known to precipitate rhinitis-type symptoms, such as nonsteroidal anti-inflammatory drugs (NSAIDs). It is essential that a thorough atopic history be obtained, because patients with allergic rhinitis may have personal and/or family history of IgE-mediated disease, such as atopic dermatitis, food allergy, asthma, or eosinophilic esophagitis. Patients with significant history of atopy should be referred to an allergist for coordinated medical management. Additionally, the clinician should question about recurrent infections, because patients with immunodeficiency (Chapter 23) may have concomitant allergic rhinitis.

In the setting of a convincing history and examination and positive response to medications, diagnostic studies are not necessary for diagnosis. However, environmental allergen–specific skin testing is helpful for patients with ongoing symptoms and can be performed with relative ease by an allergist. Knowledge of specific triggers may confirm suspicions about inciting allergens, guide avoidance measures, and direct timing of medications. Environmental allergen skin testing entails skin prick testing and, more infrequently, intradermal testing. Results should be correlated with clinical history. In toddlers, allergy testing may be falsely negative because of immaturity of the immune system. In older children and adolescents, false positive results are occasionally observed; negative results in this age group strongly suggest against a causal relationship. Serum allergen-specific IgE testing also may be performed and would be expected to be elevated for a causal allergen. Imaging of the nasal and paranasal cavities is rarely done in the pediatric setting, though it may be performed in select cases (e.g., anatomic defects, recurrent sinusitis, or severe chronic rhinosinusitis). At times, a lateral neck radiograph is obtained to assess for adenoidal hypertrophy.

DIFFERENTIAL DIAGNOSIS

Rhinitis may occur in the setting of anaphylaxis, such as in the case of IgE-mediated food allergy. Allergic rhinitis can be distinguished from anaphylaxis by the absence of multisystemic manifestations, including hives, angioedema, wheezing, and hypotension.

There is overlap in the clinical manifestations of allergic rhinitis and nonallergic, or vasomotor, rhinitis, which occurs as a result of aberrant neuronal signaling at the nasal mucosa. Ocular symptoms

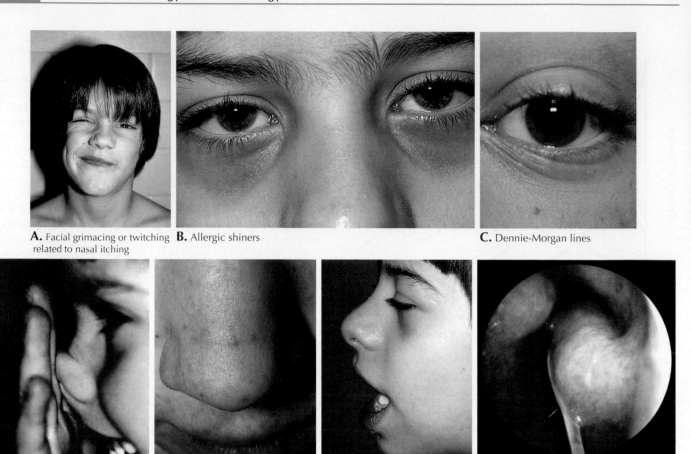

A. Facial grimacing or twitching related to nasal itching   **B.** Allergic shiners   **C.** Dennie-Morgan lines

D. The allergic salute   **E.** Nasal creasing related to the allergic salute   **F.** Allergic facies   **G.** Edematous, boggy mucosa

Fig. 22.2 Clinical Features of Allergic Rhinitis. The pathophysiologic processes of allergic rhinitis result in the typical examination findings illustrated here. See text for full descriptions. (A) Facial grimacing or twitching related to nasal itching. (B) Allergic shiners. (C) Dennie-Morgan lines. (D) The allergic salute. (E) Nasal creasing related to the allergic salute. (F) Allergic facies. (G) Edematous, boggy mucosa. (From Chong H, Green T, Larkin A. Allergy and immunology. In: Zitelli B, McIntire S, Nowalk A. *Zitelli and Davis' Atlas of Pediatric Physical Diagnosis.* Philadelphia, PA: Elsevier; 2018:108-109, Figs. 4.11-4.18; with permission.)

are typically absent. Triggers of nonallergic rhinitis include irritants (e.g., smoke, aerosols, fragrances, preservatives), drugs (e.g., NSAIDs, prolonged use of topical decongestants), hormonal changes, weather changes, strong emotions, and infections. Difficult-to-treat symptoms may represent a combination of nonallergic and allergic rhinitis. Differentiating between the two may not be possible without allergy testing.

Allergic rhinitis should be distinguished from acute infectious rhinosinusitis, which may be caused by viruses, bacteria, and, less commonly, fungi. Associated features include fever, facial tenderness, purulent discharge, and other systemic signs of infection. Another comorbid condition, chronic rhinosinusitis, is characterized by nasal obstruction, purulent drainage, hyposomia, and recurrent bouts of sinusitis. Management of chronic rhinosinusitis overlaps with that of allergic rhinitis and also includes roles for antibiotics and, in some cases, surgical intervention. Patients with frequent sinus and/or ear infections may have compromised humoral immunity and should be evaluated for underlying immunodeficiency.

Anatomic abnormalities must be considered in the differential diagnosis of allergic rhinitis, particularly in children younger than 2 years of age and those with atypical presentations, such as asymmetry of symptoms. Causes include deviated nasal septum, choanal atresia, adenoidal hypertrophy, and nasal polyps. The presence of

nasal polyps with or without allergy should raise suspicion for cystic fibrosis. A foreign body may, over time, cause the formation of a rhinolith, filling the nasal cavity and causing obstruction and nasal discharge.

MANAGEMENT

The primary approach to allergic rhinitis is avoidance of allergic triggers to prevent exacerbation of underlying inflammation. Recommendations for environmental modifications should be tailored to an individual's allergen profile and particular circumstances and should aim to balance control of symptoms with improving overall quality of life. In the case of dust mite allergy, mattresses and pillows should be covered with dust mite–proof protectors, and sheets should be washed weekly with hot water. If possible, carpets may be replaced with hardwood flooring. A dehumidifier and high-efficiency particulate air (HEPA) filters should be used. For allergy to animals, such as cats and dogs, exposure should be minimized (e.g., keeping the animal outside the bedroom), and hands should be washed after any physical interactions. In some cases, removal of the inciting animal from the home may be needed. Cockroach exposure may be minimized by removing potential food sources, washing floors, and using appropriate pesticides or engaging an exterminator

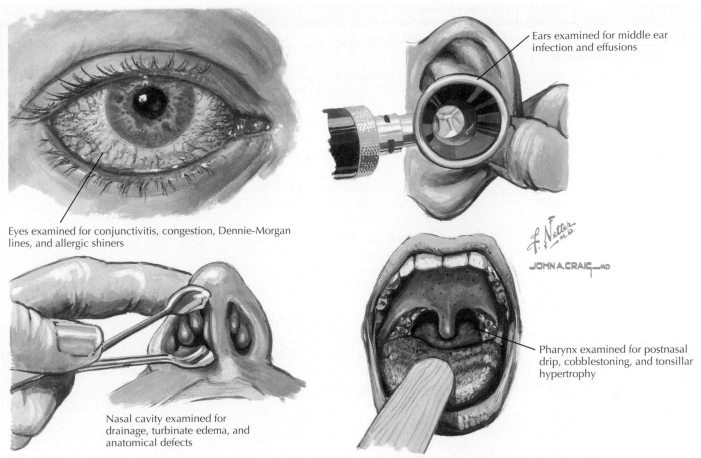

Ears examined for middle ear infection and effusions

Eyes examined for conjunctivitis, congestion, Dennie-Morgan lines, and allergic shiners

Pharynx examined for postnasal drip, cobblestoning, and tonsillar hypertrophy

Nasal cavity examined for drainage, turbinate edema, and anatomical defects

Fig. 22.3 Components of Physical Examination in Allergic Rhinitis. A comprehensive physical examination includes examination of the eyes, ears, nasal cavity, and throat. Characteristic physical examination features are illustrated in Fig. 22.2.

if necessary. Although staying indoors during high-pollen days or during certain times of the day may be helpful, this recommendation is not always practical or possible. Shutting windows, turning on air conditioning, and taking nightly showers may reduce symptom severity.

Intranasal corticosteroids and oral antihistamines form the mainstay of pharmacologic therapy and are supplemented with adjunctive therapies for persisting symptoms (Table 22.1). Through multiple antiinflammatory mechanisms, intranasal corticosteroids (e.g., fluticasone, mometasone) provide significant relief of nasal and ocular symptoms. Because full effect may not be appreciated until 2 weeks after initiation, patients and caregivers may assume lack of efficacy prematurely. This is often exacerbated by incorrect administration technique. Families should be instructed to have the patient hold the head upright, aim the nasal spray away from the nasal septum, and inhale while holding the opposite nostril closed. Side effects include nasal dryness, epistaxis, and headaches. In the absence of use of corticosteroids for other indications, intranasal corticosteroids are generally not associated with stunted growth.

Oral antihistamines targeting the H1 receptor also reduce rhinitis symptoms, providing relief within the first few hours of use. First-generation antihistamines (e.g., diphenhydramine) readily cross the blood-brain barrier and should be avoided because of their sedating properties. They may be considered in certain settings. Second-generation antihistamines (e.g., cetirizine, loratadine, levocetirizine, and fexofenadine) are commonly used, well tolerated, and nonsedating.

Rare additional side effects may include dryness of mucous membranes and irritability.

Persistent ocular symptoms in patients with allergic rhinoconjunctivitis can be relieved with ocular antihistamines and mast cell stabilizers (e.g., ketotifen, olopatadine). Topical steroid eye drops may be used in those with severe ocular disease. Supervision by an ophthalmologist is indicated, because of the risk for increased intraocular pressure. Patients with concomitant asthma may benefit from the leukotriene receptor antagonist montelukast, which reduces both rhinitis and asthma symptoms. The potential clinical benefits of montelukast should be weighed with its known risk for neuropsychiatric side effects. Oral decongestants, which may be helpful for short-term use, should not be used long-term because of concerns for increased blood pressure and increased side effects.

Patients with significant congestion and rhinorrhea may benefit from a trial of second-line intranasal antihistamines (e.g., azelastine, olopatadine) along with intranasal corticosteroids. Intranasal anticholinergics (e.g., ipratropium) may be trialed for persistent rhinorrhea or with upper respiratory tract infections. Nasal decongestants (e.g., oxymetazoline, phenylephrine) are generally discouraged because of their rebound side effects. Cautious use for a few days as a bridging agent may be considered for patients with severe rhinorrhea and congestion. Intranasal cromolyn, a mast cell–stabilizing agent, may provide relief of rhinitis. Its efficacy depends on consistent administration multiple times a day for at least 2 to 4 weeks. Nasal saline drops and nasal saline irrigations also may be helpful.

TABLE 22.1 Allergic Rhinitis Pharmacotherapy

Medication	Minimum Age	Common Dosage(s)	Side Effects
Intranasal Corticosteroids			
Beclomethasone (Qnasl 40 mcg or 80 mcg)	4 years	4–11 years: 1 spray (40 mcg) per nostril daily; ≥12 years: 2 sprays (160 mcg) per nostril daily	Bitterness, burning, dryness, epistaxis, headache
Budesonide	6 years	6-11 years: 1–2 sprays (32–64 mcg) per nostril daily; ≥12 years: 1–4 sprays (32–128 mcg) per nostril daily	
Ciclesonide (Omnaris)	6 years	2 sprays (100 mcg) per nostril daily	
Flunisolide	6 years	6–14 years: 1 spray (25 mcg) per nostril 3 times daily or 2 sprays (50 mcg) per nostril twice daily; ≥15 years: 2 sprays (50 mcg) per nostril 2–4 times daily	
Fluticasone furoate	2 years	2–11 years: 1–2 sprays (27.5–55 mcg) per nostril daily; ≥12 years: 2 sprays (55 mcg) per nostril daily	
Fluticasone propionate	4 years	4-11 years: 1–2 sprays (50–100 mcg) per nostril daily; ≥12 years: 2 sprays (100 mcg) per nostril 1–2 times daily	
Mometasone	2 years	2–11 years: 1 spray (50 mcg) per nostril daily; ≥12 years: 2 sprays (100 mcg) per nostril daily	
Triamcinolone	2 years	2–5 years: 1 spray (55 mcg) per nostril daily; 6–11 years: 1–2 sprays (55–110 mcg) per nostril daily; ≥12 years: 2 sprays (110 mcg) per nostril daily	
Oral Antihistamines			
Cetirizine	6 months	6–11 months: 2.5 mg daily; 1–5 years: 2.5 mg 1–2 times daily; 6–11 years: 5–10 mg daily; ≥12 years: 10 mg daily	Dry mouth, irritability, sedation (particularly diphenhydramine)
Desloratadine	6 months	6–11 months: 1 mg daily; 1–5 years: 1.25 mg daily; 6–11 years: 2.5 mg daily; ≥12 years: 5 mg daily	
Diphenhydramine	2 years	1 mg/kg/dose every 6–8 hours, maximum 50 mg/dose	
Fexofenadine	2 years	2–11 years: 30 mg twice daily; ≥12 years: 60 mg twice daily or 180 mg daily	
Levocetirizine	6 years	6–11 years: 2.5 mg daily; ≥12 years: 5 mg daily	
Loratadine	2 years	2–5 years: 5 mg daily; ≥6 years: 10 mg daily	
Ocular Mast Cell Stabilizers/Antihistamines			
Cromolyn	4 years	1–2 drops per eye 4–6 times daily	Irritation, dryness, blurred vision, headache
Ketotifen	3 years	1 drop per eye twice daily	
Olopatadine	2 years	1 drop per eye 1–2 times daily	
Leukotriene Receptor Antagonists			
Montelukast	6 months	6 months to 4 years: 4 mg daily; 5–14 years: 5 mg daily; ≥15 years: 10 mg daily	Flu-like symptoms, neuropsychiatric symptoms
Intranasal Antihistamines			
Azelastine	6 months	6 months to 11 years: 1 spray per nostril twice daily; ≥12 years: 1–2 sprays per nostril twice daily	Bitterness, burning, dryness, epistaxis, headache, sedation
Intranasal Anticholinergics			
Ipratropium	5 years	2 sprays (42 mcg) per nostril 2–3 times daily	Burning, dryness, epistaxis, headache
Intranasal Mast Cell Stabilizers			
Cromolyn	2 years	1 spray per nostril 3–4 times daily	Burning, epistaxis

The latter is a mainstay in the treatment of patients who suffer from chronic rhinosinusitis.

Typically reserved for moderate-to-severe allergic rhinitis refractory to pharmacologic therapy, allergen immunotherapy, either subcutaneous immunotherapy (SCIT) or sublingual immunotherapy (SLIT), has the potential to provide significant relief of symptoms through desensitization to specific allergen triggers. SCIT is more commonly employed in the United States and can be particularly effective in the case of severe pollen, dust, and animal allergies. The underlying mechanism, induction of immunologic tolerance, requires multiple administrations. The ideal candidate will be able to commit to at least 3 to 5 years of consecutive clinic visits for injections, initially weekly during the buildup phase and then monthly during the maintenance phase. Anaphylaxis is a rare side effect, and patients require close clinical monitoring for 30 minutes after administration. Poorly controlled asthma is a contraindication to allergen immunotherapy, which may otherwise confer improvement of asthma symptoms in patients with concurrent stable, persistent asthma.

FUTURE DIRECTIONS

Despite the availability of effective therapies, allergic rhinitis continues to adversely affect the quality of life of many children and adolescents. SLIT (approved in tablet form for grasses, ragweed, and dust mites) poses an attractive alternative to SCIT for some. Various SLIT investigations are underway, including efficacy-focused evaluations of unapproved environmental allergens, mixtures of multiple allergens, and liquid drop formulations. Given the efficacy of the monoclonal anti-IgE antibody omalizumab in reducing rhinitis symptoms in children with severe persistent allergic asthma, there has been increasing interest in exploring the role of biologic therapies in the treatment of severe allergic rhinitis. Finally, further elucidation of the genetic and environmental factors contributing to the pathophysiology of allergic rhinitis and overlapping diseases will inform future discussions about disease risk, diagnosis, and management.

SUGGESTED READINGS

Available online.

23

Immune Deficiency

Aaron L. Bodansky and Soma C. Jyonouchi

 CLINICAL VIGNETTE

A previously healthy 15-year-old girl has had difficulty with recurrent monthly sinus infections for 2 years and three episodes of pneumonia. She has also been treated for autoimmune hemolytic anemia. Laboratory testing revealed very low immunoglobulin (Ig) G (296 mg/dL), IgA (14 mg/dL), and IgM (6 mg/dL) levels and low pneumococcal vaccine titers (0/23 serotypes protective). She received a pneumococcal vaccine booster and demonstrated minimal response (2/23 serotypes protective). These findings were consistent with a diagnosis of common variable immunodeficiency (CVID). The patient was started on monthly intravenous immunoglobulin therapy (IVIG) with marked improvement in infections.

Primary immunodeficiency disorders (PIDDs) are a diverse and expanding group of inborn errors of the immune system, currently encompassing more than 400 diseases. Although many secondary disease states (e.g., chemotherapy, human immunodeficiency virus [HIV] infection, medication) can weaken or dysregulate the immune system, this chapter focuses only on PIDDs.

The immune system must be able to quickly and efficiently respond to and fight against any invading pathogen (while demonstrating tolerance to the host). PIDDs commonly manifest with increased infection susceptibility, and many are also associated with autoimmune disease or autoinflammatory disease resulting from immune dysregulation. For the majority of these conditions, the primary care clinician works closely with an immunologist in the care of these patients.

ANTIBODY IMMUNE DEFICIENCY

Background

Antibody immunodeficiency (also referred to as humoral immune deficiency) is the most common category of primary immune deficiency, accounting for more than 60% of PIDD diagnoses.

Antibodies (also referred to as immunoglobulins) are important for clearance of a wide range of pathogens but are particularly important to defend against encapsulated bacteria. They also represent a key component of immune memory (vaccines are designed to generate long-lasting protective antibody responses in the body).

The most severe form of antibody deficiency is agammaglobulinemia (complete absence of B cells and all antibodies). Common variable immune deficiency (CVID) refers to patients who have low immunoglobulin (Ig) G, often with low IgA and IgM, and low or absent vaccine responses. CVID can be diagnosed at any age, with infections starting for the first time when a patient is older. Importantly, 25% of patients with CVID suffer from autoimmune disease such as autoimmune hemolytic anemia (AIHA), immune thrombocytopenia (ITP), and Sjögren disease. In some patients, autoimmunity can precede the development of recurrent infections. Specific antibody deficiency refers

to patients who have normal IgG, IgA, and IgM levels but impaired responses to vaccines. Transient hypogammaglobulinemia of infancy is noted when infants/toddlers have low immunoglobulin levels but normal vaccine responses that improve with age. Selective IgA deficiency, noted by absence of IgA, is the most common PIDD, affecting 1 in 400 Caucasians.

Clinical Presentation

Patients with antibody deficiency present with recurrent or severe sinopulmonary infections, most commonly from encapsulated organisms such as *Streptococcus pneumoniae* and *Haemophilus influenzae*. Invasive infections, including bacteremia, osteomyelitis, and meningitis, can occur. Gastrointestinal infections from *Giardia lamblia*, *Salmonella enterica*, and *Campylobacter jejuni* can also occur.

Because of the presence of protective maternally derived antibodies, patients with antibody deficiency often present with infections after 6 months of age. The absence of tonsillar and palpable lymphoid tissue is a pathognomonic finding in boys with X-linked agammaglobulinemia.

Laboratory Evaluation

Measurement of IgG, IgA, and IgM levels and responses to common childhood vaccinations (e.g., tetanus, diphtheria, pneumococcus) represents the cornerstone of screening for antibody deficiency. Patients who have low vaccine responses should receive appropriate booster immunizations and have repeat vaccine titers checked 4 to 6 weeks later. Absence of B cells by flow cytometry is useful for diagnosis of agammaglobulinemia.

Management

The standard of care for severe antibody deficiencies is uninterrupted immunoglobulin replacement therapy (monthly intravenous immunoglobulin [IVIG] or weekly subcutaneous immunoglobulin therapy). Prophylactic antibiotics (e.g., amoxicillin 20 mg/kg divided twice daily) are commonly used in symptomatic patients with milder antibody deficiencies.

T CELL AND COMBINED IMMUNE DEFICIENCY

Background

T cell (cellular) and combined immune deficiency (CID) is the second most common type of PIDD. This category includes the most severe forms of immune deficiency, severe combined immune deficiency (SCID), which is fatal during infancy without a hematopoietic stem cell transplant (HSCT). Cellular immunity is needed to combat intracellular pathogens or cancer cells. Defects in cellular immunity typically arise from a genetic insult leading to defective T cell development and function. CID refers to any PIDD that impairs both T cell immunity and antibody immunity (natural killer [NK] cells also may be affected).

The traditional categorization system for severe T cell defects, such as SCID or CID, is based on which cell types are most affected. The severity of disease is primarily determined by the degree of T cell involvement, measured both quantitatively (T cell count) and qualitatively (T cell function by mitogen response). Patients with classic SCID have CD3 T cell count less than 300 cells/mm^3 and T cell function less than 10% of control.

Clinical Presentation

There is a clinical spectrum of disease caused by mutations in known genes for SCID. Different mutations within a gene that causes SCID can result in various clinical manifestations. Patients with typical SCID present during early infancy with severe (often fatal) infections from otherwise common viruses (e.g., respiratory syncytial virus [RSV], parainfluenza) or after administration of live viral vaccines (e.g., rotavirus), persistent mucocutaneous candidiasis, failure to thrive, and *Pneumocystis jiroveci* pneumonia. Patients with Omenn syndrome present with lymphadenopathy, skin erythroderma, and hepatosplenomegaly. Children with SCID in the United States most commonly present through abnormal results on the newborn screen (this is still uncommon internationally).

Patients with CIDs may present with recurrent bacterial and viral infections and pathogens, but unlike SCID, typically survive into childhood.

Laboratory Evaluation

In addition to the newborn screen, patients with SCID typically have a low absolute lymphocyte count (<2500 cells/µL). Testing includes flow cytometry to assess lymphocyte populations, including CD3, CD4, naïve and memory CD8 T cells, B cell, and NK cell counts. Testing of T cell function is achieved by measuring their ability to proliferate in response to mitogens (mitogen response <10% of control in SCID; 10% to 30% control in leaky SCID or CID). Chest radiograph evaluation that reveals an absent thymus in an infant should raise concern about underlying SCID.

Management

Any child with an abnormal SCID newborn screen should be immediately referred to an immunologist and kept in protective isolation, either in a hospital or at home. The patient must avoid live viral vaccines, and close contacts should be given inactivated vaccines. If SCID is confirmed, treatment with antibiotics and immunoglobulin replacement are started to reduce infection risk. Antibiotics prophylaxis includes trimethoprim-sulfamethoxazole (TMP-SMX) prophylaxis for pneumocystis and fluconazole prophylaxis for candida. Breastfeeding should be avoided if a mother is positive for cytomegalovirus (CMV) given the risk for fatal CMV infection. If needed, irradiated blood products should be given.

The most common and readily available definitive treatment for SCID remains HSCT. Gene therapy is an option for certain types of SCID and is available in the United States on a limited basis as part of clinical trials.

PHAGOCYTE DISORDERS

Background

Phagocytic disorders are the third most common category of PIDD. Phagocytes collectively serve as an essential component of the innate immune response. Neutrophils are the most common type of phagocyte and will be a focus in this section. Neutrophils are produced in the bone marrow, travel to the site of infection, and then successfully ingest and destroy pathogens. Genetic defects impairing any of these steps can lead to a phagocyte PIDD. Phagocytic disorders can be due to a defect in neutrophil production (i.e., congenital neutropenia), migration (i.e., leukocyte adhesion deficiency [LAD]), or function (i.e., chronic granulomatous disease [CGD]). Because of their short half-life in circulation compared with that of many other immune cells, granulocytes are particularly susceptible to extrinsic factors such as viruses and medications, but only intrinsic genetic defects are considered to be PIDDs.

Clinical Presentation

Patients with a primary phagocytic deficiency classically present with severe and persistent bacterial (*Staphylococcus aureus*, *Pseudomonas aeruginosa*, *Nocardia*, *Serratia*, *Burkholderia*, and *Cepacia*) and fungal (*Candida* and *Aspergillus*) infections. Patients present with skin infections, visceral abscesses (e.g., liver abscess), pneumonia, lymphadenitis, and sepsis.

In addition, patients with CGD can have difficulty with nontuberculous mycobacterial (NTM) infections. They can also develop sterile inflammatory granulomas (which can obstruct the gastrointestinal or genitourinary tract) and develop severe inflammatory bowel disease (IBD). Patients with LAD may present with delayed umbilical cord separation, gingivitis, and poor wound healing.

Laboratory Evaluation

A complete blood count with differential is an important starting point to determine if there is neutropenia (severe, <500 cells/mm^3; moderate, 500 to 1000 cells/mm^3; mild, 1000 to 1500 cells/mm^3). Functional defects can be more difficult to determine. Neutrophil oxidative burst can be measured using the dihydrorhodamine-123 (DHR) assay. Patients with LAD have a markedly elevated resting white blood cell count (neutrophils are trapped in the vasculature, unable to migrate to sites of infection). Flow cytometry for CD11b/18 cell surface markers is useful for the diagnosis of LAD type I. Gene sequencing is useful for a definitive diagnosis of specific neutrophil disorders.

Management

Patients with severe congenital neutropenia may be treated with prophylactic antibiotics and granulocyte colony-stimulating factor (GCSF). Patients with CGD require antibacterial (TMP-SMX) and antifungal (itraconazole) prophylaxis. Interferon-γ is also commonly used for CGD. Patients with LAD also receive antimicrobial prophylaxis. In the setting of acute infection, identification and aggressive, targeted treatment of infections are critical. Stem cell transplantation is a curative therapy that is indicated for severe forms of congenital neutropenia, CGD, and LAD.

SYNDROMIC IMMUNODEFICIENCY

Background

Many syndromic diseases are also associated with PIDDs. When evaluating a child with dysmorphisms or other concerning features of syndromic disease, it is important to consider immune system involvement in addition to some of the more classic organ systems. Beyond this general consideration, certain well-characterized syndromes have specific associated immune defects; these disorders will be the focus in the following section.

Trisomy 21 (Down Syndrome)

Although immune dysfunction has not historically been discussed as a major feature of trisomy 21, it is becoming increasingly appreciated as a major source of morbidity and mortality. Overall, children with trisomy 21 have higher rates of severe infection and poor outcomes, even when taking into account other organ comorbidities. The immune defects associated with trisomy 21 are multiple and may include abnormal T cell number and function, increased autoimmunity (e.g., celiac disease, type 1 diabetes mellitus, hypothyroidism), decreased B cell numbers, hypogammaglobulinemia, poor vaccine responses, and abnormal neutrophil chemotaxis and function. In addition, certain anatomic differences also contribute to infection, such as shortened eustachian tubes leading to recurrent otitis media and relative macroglossia increasing risk for aspiration and pneumonia. It is important for practitioners to consider immune deficiency to be part of trisomy 21 and to be vigilant given the increased risk for severe and recurrent infections. Patients diagnosed with immune abnormalities may benefit from treatments such as prophylactic antibiotics or immunoglobulin replacement therapy.

22q11.2 Deletion Syndrome (DiGeorge Syndrome)

Patients with 22q11.2 deletion syndrome can have dysmorphic facial features, cardiac abnormalities, developmental delay, and hypocalcemia. Thymic hypoplasia can result in variable T cell lymphopenia in 80% of patients. Patients with 22q11.2 deletion syndrome are commonly identified by newborn screen (as a result of low T cells on SCID screen). Most patients do not have complete absence of T cells because of the presence of residual thymic tissue (mild-to-moderate T cell lymphopenia is present with normal T cell function). There is an increased risk for autoimmunity in patients. Approximately 10% to 20% of patients develop antibody immune deficiency and may require immunoglobulin replacement therapy. Patients with complete athymia (approximately 0.5% to 1.5% of patients) will have a profound T cell immune deficiency. Curative treatment for these children requires thymic transplantation.

Hyper–Immunoglobulin E Syndromes

Although there are many common causes of elevated IgE levels, such as allergic conditions, patients with true autosomal dominant hyper-IgE syndrome (a result in mutations in *STAT3*) are clinically characterized by coarse facial features, eczema, newborn rash, delayed shedding of primary teeth (often requiring extraction), minimal trauma fractures, scoliosis, and hyperextensibility. The immunologic characteristics include skin abscesses, recurrent pneumonias complicated by pneumatoceles, mucocutaneous candidiasis, elevated IgE, and reduced Th17 T cell population. Patients are treated with antibacterial prophylaxis (TMP-SMX), skin hydration, and reduction of skin bacterial colonization (e.g., bleach baths, chlorhexidine).

INNATE IMMUNE DEFECTS

Background

The innate immune system is the first line of defense of the body and is armed and ready to immediately respond to infection. NK cells, toll-like receptors (TLRs) and complement proteins are key examples of the innate immune system.

NK cells are innate lymphocytes that protect against herpesvirus infections (herpes simplex virus [HSV], Epstein-Barr virus [EBV], CMV, and varicella-zoster virus [VZV]) and destroy tumor cells. TLRs recognize unique microbial structures and trigger production of various inflammatory cytokines (tumor necrosis factor-alpha [TNF-α], IL-1, and IL-6). Complement proteins function to opsonize bacteria and form membrane attack complex (MAC), which causes lysis of bacteria.

Presentation

Patients with NK cell deficiency present with severe or recurrent herpesvirus infections and increased risk for malignancy. Patients with TLR pathway defects (e.g., MyD88 or IRAK4 deficiency) present with recurrent invasive bacterial infections (e.g., sepsis, meningitis) with *S. pneumoniae, S. aureus,* and *P. aeruginosa.* A key TLR defect hallmark is that patients lack associated fever and elevated inflammatory markers with infections (because of the impaired inflammatory response).

Patients with early complement deficiencies (C1q, C1r, C1s, C2, C4, C3) present with severe recurrent infections with encapsulated bacteria and systemic lupus erythematosus. Patients with terminal complement deficiencies (C5, C6, C7, C8, C9) present with recurrent *Neisseria meningitidis* infections. Alternative complement defects can manifest with recurrent meningitis (properdin and factor D deficiency) or atypical hemolytic uremic syndrome (factor H and factor I deficiency).

Laboratory Evaluation

NK cell deficiency can be evaluated for by enumeration of cell counts by flow cytometry and NK cell cytotoxicity assay (to assess NK cell killing). TLR deficiency is characterized by an inappropriately low C-reactive protein (CRP) and erythrocyte sedimentation rate (ESR) in the setting of serious bacterial infection and reduced TLR assay test. The CH50 and AH50 (to test the classic and alternative complement pathways, respectively) are screening tools to evaluate for complement deficiency.

Treatment

Patients with NK cell deficiency may benefit from antiviral prophylaxis (e.g., acyclovir or valacyclovir for HSV). Patients should avoid the live varicella vaccine (because of the risk for vaccine strain infection) and instead receive the non-live recombinant zoster vaccine. The human papillomavirus (HPV) vaccine is also recommended for both male and female patients. Providers should be aware of increased risk for malignancy in patients.

Patients with TLR deficiency require antibiotic prophylaxis with amoxicillin or TMP-SMX. Optimizing pneumococcal vaccine responses is critical. Patients with impaired vaccine response may benefit from immunoglobulin replacement.

Patients with early and terminal complement deficiency require antibiotic prophylaxis. Patients with terminal complement deficiency require optimization of meningococcal (A, B, C, Y, W-135) vaccine responses.

IMMUNE DYSREGULATION

Diseases of immune dysregulation are a relatively new category of PIDD and are characterized by severe autoimmunity resulting from abnormalities in central and/or peripheral tolerance (recurrent infections may or may not be associated).

Regulatory T-cells (Tregs) play an essential role in suppressing autoreactive T-cells in the periphery, thereby preventing autoimmune disease. IPEX (immune dysregulation, polyendocrinopathy, enteropathy, X-linked) is a severe immune deficiency caused by a mutation in *FOXP3*, which is a protein required for Treg development. Patients with IPEX syndrome have severe infant-onset autoimmune disease, including severe eczema, enteropathy, lymphadenopathy, thyroiditis, and type 1 diabetes mellitus. IPEX is often fatal in infancy if not aggressively managed with immunosuppression, total parenteral nutrition (TPN), and HSCT.

CTLA4 is an inhibitory receptor expressed on T cells, including Tregs, that plays a role in suppressing autoimmune inflammation. The intracellular protein LRBA is required for proper CTLA4 expression on the cell surface. CTLA4-induced inhibition acts as a counter balance to the T cell stimulatory receptor CD28. Patients with CTLA4 and LRBA deficiency present with antibody deficiency similar to CVID but also suffer from severe autoimmune disease, including psoriasis, IBD, autoimmune cytopenias, and thyroid disease.

In contrast to the diseases previously characterized by severe autoimmunity, other immune dysregulation disorders are characterized by immune deficiency and severe hyperinflammatory response. One particularly notable example would be the group of diseases that comprise the familial hemophagocytic lymphohistiocytosis (fHLH) syndromes (Chapter 130).

AUTOINFLAMMATORY (PERIODIC FEVER SYNDROMES)

Background

The inflammatory cytokine response is an integral component of the immune system, which is typically activated in response to specific triggers such as pathogens or tissue injury. However, in individuals with periodic fever syndromes, this inflammatory response is activated in the absence of an appropriate physiologic trigger, leading to excessive release of proinflammatory cytokines and recurrent fever. This category is distinct from autoimmune disorders in that it does not involve any autoreactive T cells or autoantibodies but rather is limited to activation of the innate immune system.

Clinical Presentation

Patients with periodic fever syndromes present with recurrent fever (typically occurring every few weeks) in the absence of an identifiable source such as infection, rheumatologic disease, or malignancy. In addition, patients may have rash, abdominal pain, joint pain and swelling, and lymphadenopathy. The two most common periodic fever syndromes are familial Mediterranean fever (FMF) and periodic fever with aphthous stomatitis, pharyngitis, and adenitis (PFAPA) syndrome.

Laboratory Evaluation

Patients present with classic laboratory indications of inflammation such as elevated white blood cell count, CRP, and ESR. Genetic testing can be useful to confirm a specific periodic fever syndrome (however, there is no known gene involved in PFAPA).

Management

Oral steroids are useful for treatment of attacks in PFAPA. FMF is responsive to colchicine therapy. Targeted cytokine blockade (e.g., anti–IL-1 therapy) is effective for a number of periodic fever syndromes.

SUGGESTED READINGS

Available online.

Bone and Joint Disorders

Katie K. Lockwood

24

Disorders of the Neck and Spine

Matthew R. Landrum and Jason B. Anari

 CLINICAL VIGNETTE

A 17-year-old male patient presents to clinic with a 1-month history of atraumatic lower back pain. He has a remote history of back pain from a football injury that completely resolved with a course of physical therapy. He is active and involved in football, basketball, and baseball. He denies lower extremity numbness, tingling, weakness, or bowel or bladder symptoms.

On physical examination, he has normal strength, sensation, and reflexes. He denies any tenderness to palpation over his entire spine; however, he does have pain with forward bending and hyperextension of his lower back.

Oblique and lateral radiographs reveal an L4 spondylolysis with a grade 1 spondylolisthesis (Fig. 24.1). Complete symptom resolution and return to sports occurred after 6 weeks of rest and physical therapy focusing on core strengthening and stretching.

Pediatric disorders of the neck and spine are rare. The majority of these conditions can be treated with rest, nonsteroidal antiinflammatory drugs (NSAIDs), physical therapy, and orthotics. Operative management is typically reserved for severe or refractory pathologic conditions and symptoms.

CONGENITAL MUSCULAR TORTICOLLIS

Torticollis, from the Latin words "twisted neck," is a head tilt toward and chin rotation away from the affected side (Fig. 24.2). Although the majority of torticollis cases result from sternocleidomastoid muscle (SCM) contracture, other causes include neurologic conditions, cervical spine abnormalities, and vision or hearing deficits.

Congenital muscular torticollis (CMT) occurs in 0.3% to 2% of newborns. Although the cause is unknown, intrauterine crowding or birth trauma may cause muscle damage. Risk factors include breech position and difficult delivery. Magnetic resonance imaging (MRI) and surgical histopathologic examination have demonstrated muscle atrophy and fibrosis similar to that in compartment syndrome. Abnormal head positioning in CMT can cause plagiocephaly and facial asymmetry.

Evaluation of CMT should include a thorough birth history. The physical examination classically demonstrates an infant with the head tilted toward the side of SCM contraction with the chin rotated toward the opposite shoulder (see Fig. 24.2). A nontender mass may be palpable in the body of the SCM. Visual tracking, hearing, and neurologic function also should be assessed to rule out nonmuscular causes. CMT can be secondary to intrauterine crowding; therefore a thorough hip and lower extremity examination should be performed for developmental dysplasia of the hip and metatarsus adductus.

Initial treatment should consist of massage and physical therapy for stretching. Ultrasound may be performed, which typically shows a hyperechogenic intramuscular mass. For infants who do not respond to stretching, cervical spine radiographs should be obtained to rule out osseous abnormalities. These include congenital fusions (Klippel-Feil

syndrome), hemivertebrae, or rotational abnormalities (atlantoaxial instability). Advanced imaging (computed tomography [CT] or MRI) can be performed to further define neurologic or osseous causes. In refractory cases, surgery in the form of lengthening or release may be performed by an orthopedic surgeon.

SCOLIOSIS

Scoliosis is a three-dimensional deformity of the spine affecting the coronal, sagittal, and axial planes (Fig. 24.3). Scoliosis can be idiopathic, congenital, neuromuscular, or syndromic in cause.

Idiopathic disease accounts for 80% of all scoliosis cases and is divided by age into infantile (0–3 years), juvenile (3–10 years), and adolescent (older than 10 years) groups. Infantile idiopathic scoliosis is rare and unique in that it is more common in boys, has left-sided curvature, and can spontaneously resolve. Juvenile idiopathic scoliosis is similar to the adolescent type; girls are predominantly affected, and the thoracic curvature is typically right sided. Although juvenile idiopathic scoliosis does not occur during a period of rapid spine growth, there is a high risk for progression. Idiopathic scoliosis most commonly manifests in adolescence (70%). Although the cause and pathogenesis of idiopathic scoliosis are largely unknown, there are multiple theories that include genetic, muscular, or neurologic factors.

The evaluation of scoliosis should include a careful history and physical examination. Patients are screened for thoracolumbar asymmetry with an Adam forward bend test and scoliometer (see Fig. 24.3). Girls should be screened twice at ages 10 and 12, and boys should be screened once at age 13 or 14. The physical examination should be performed without a shirt and with the patient in a gown. This facilitates comparison of the shoulders, scapulae, trunk, pelvis, and legs and allows appropriate visualization for skin abnormalities, including café au lait spots, neurofibromas, dermal sinus tracts, or a midline tuft of hair. Because idiopathic scoliosis is a diagnosis of exclusion, a careful assessment of neurologic function, reflexes (including abdominal) and signs of associated orthopedic disorders should be assessed. Congenital scoliosis should not be mistaken for infantile idiopathic scoliosis because the former is associated with other osseous and visceral anomalies. Definitive diagnosis and disease severity are determined by measuring the angle between the two most tilted vertebrae (Cobb angle) on a posteroanterior spinal radiograph, with any curvature of more than 10 degrees being diagnostic. MRI should be performed in the setting of focal neurologic findings.

Treatment of patients with idiopathic scoliosis depends on the age of onset and degree of curvature. Children with mild-to-moderate curves (<25 degrees), especially in the skeletally mature, can be observed clinically and with serial radiographs. Patients with more severe curves, particularly younger children, may require bracing to minimize curve progression and prevent potential surgical correction. Surgical correction is reserved for patients with severe curvatures

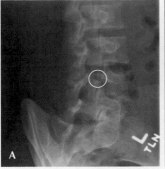
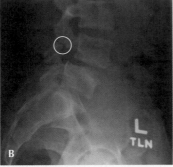

Fig. 24.1 Oblique (A) and lateral (B) images of the lumbar spine showing spondylolysis *(white circle)* with grade I spondylolisthesis.

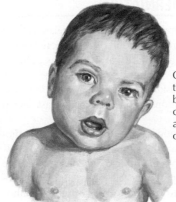

Child with muscular torticollis. Head tilted to left with chin turned to right because of contracture of left sternocleidomastoid muscle. Note facial asymmetry (flattening of left side of face)

Fig. 24.2 Torticollis.

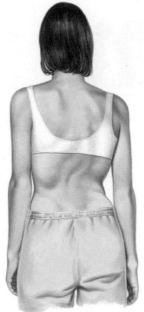

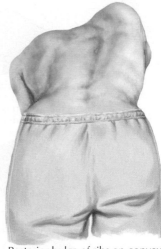

Posterior bulge of ribs on convex side forming characteristic rib hump in thoracic scoliosis

Note waist and shoulder asymmetry

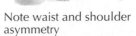
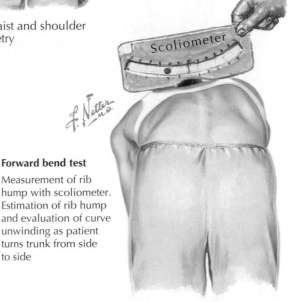

Forward bend test

Measurement of rib hump with scoliometer. Estimation of rib hump and evaluation of curve unwinding as patient turns trunk from side to side

Fig. 24.3 Scoliosis.

(>50 degrees) or progressive disease that could compromise pulmonary or musculoskeletal function. Surgery can improve both the physical and psychological sequelae of idiopathic scoliosis. Patients and their parents should be cautioned that although operative management can provide permanent structural correction, there are risks for complications or persistent symptoms.

KYPHOSIS

Normal sagittal plane alignment for the thoracic spine is 10 to 40 degrees of kyphosis. Larger angles are pathologic and result in a rounding of the upper back or "hunchback deformity." The most common causes are postural kyphosis and Scheuermann disease (Fig. 24.4). Rare causes of sagittal plane malalignment include congenital anomalies, infection, malignancy, and other neuromuscular or osseous disorders.

Postural kyphosis is mostly seen in adolescent boys as a result of slouching. There is typically no back pain nor any radiographic abnormality. Treatment consists of positional exercises.

Scheuermann disease is a rigid hyperkyphotic alignment of the thoracic spine defined by anterior vertebral wedging of greater than 5 degrees in three adjacent vertebrae. Physical therapy and orthotics may be beneficial for smaller curves (45–60 degrees); however, surgery is indicated for larger angles (>75 degrees), progressive deformity, neurologic deficits, or pain.

SPONDYLOLYSIS AND SPONDYLOLISTHESIS

Spondylolysis is a defect of the pars interarticularis, whereas spondylolisthesis is the displacement of one vertebral segment in relation to the

adjacent segment. This can be caused by trauma, degenerative disease, dysplasia, or neoplasms.

Spondylolysis is a common cause of back pain in children and adolescents. A higher prevalence is seen in certain athletes (e.g., football, gymnastics, wrestling). Patients may present with lumbar back pain, radiated buttock pain, or hamstring spasms. Physical examination may be normal or may reveal tenderness, limited lumbar flexibility, or, rarely, neurologic symptoms.

Oblique vertebral radiographs in an unaffected patient demonstrate a "Scottie dog" with the transverse process as the head, the superior articular process as the ear, the spinous process and lamina as the body, and the inferior articular process as the front leg. In spondylolysis, the dog has a fracture line through the neck (Fig. 24.5). In spondylolisthesis, the entire head of the dog is displaced, with or without spondylolysis, on a scale graded from I (<25% slip) to V (complete spondyloptosis) (see Fig. 24.5). Spondylolysis and spondylolisthesis most commonly occur at L5 on S1, which can be seen on anteroposterior and lateral

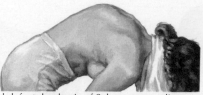

Unlike postural defect, kyphosis of Scheuermann disease persists when patient is prone and thoracic spine extended or hyperextended and accentuated when patient bends forward (above)

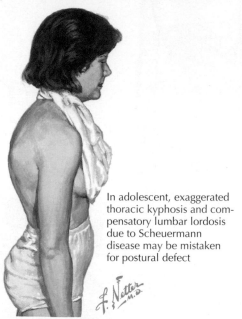

In adolescent, exaggerated thoracic kyphosis and compensatory lumbar lordosis due to Scheuermann disease may be mistaken for postural defect

Fig. 24.4 Scheuermann Disease.

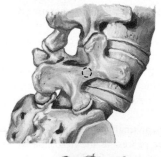

- Superior articular process (ear of Scottie dog)
- Pedicle (eye)
- Transverse process (head)
- Isthmus (neck)
- Lamina and spinous process (body)
- Inferior articular process (foreleg)
- Opposite inferior articular process (hindleg)

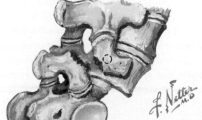

radiographs. CT and MRI are helpful if there is an atypical presentation, if the degree of slip is severe, or for preoperative planning. MRI has become the modality of choice to evaluate the lumbar spine for spondylolysis and spondylolisthesis as a result of gonadal tissue radiation levels from a lumbar spine CT scan.

Medical treatment of spondylolysis and spondylolisthesis includes rest, NSAIDs, and physical therapy. Rehabilitation should focus on reduction of the lumbar lordosis and hamstring stretching. For more symptomatic patients with spondylolysis, orthotics may be useful to reduce lumbar lordosis. The majority of lesions heal with medical therapy alone. Surgery is usually reserved for chronic spondylolysis unchanged with nonoperative management, severe spondylolisthesis (greater than grade III), or dysplastic spondylolisthesis with neurologic symptoms.

INTERVERTEBRAL DISK HERNIATION

Symptomatic pediatric intervertebral disk herniation is a relatively rare condition, especially when compared with adults. This typically causes a significant delay in diagnosis. The majority of herniations occur in the lumbar spine (90% L4-5 or L5-S1), but they can also rarely occur in the thoracic or cervical spine. Risk factors include heavy lifting and sports participation. Disk herniations frequently can be associated with apophyseal fracture.

The typical chief complaint includes acute onset of pain and radiculopathy. Physical examination can show postural or gait abnormalities, limited back motion, pain, or neurologic deficit. Pain may be exacerbated by back extension or straight leg raise. Although spine radiographs should be obtained to rule out other sources of pathologic conditions, MRI is the imaging modality of choice. Reactive scoliosis can be present but typically resolves with treatment of the herniation.

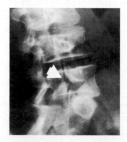

Spondylolysis without spondylolisthesis. Posterolateral view demonstrates formation of radiographic Scottie dog. On lateral radiograph, dog appears to be wearing a collar

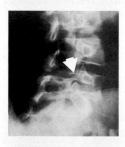

Dysplastic (congenital) spondylolisthesis. Luxation of L5 on sacrum. Dog's neck (isthmus) appears elongated

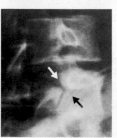

Isthmic type spondylolisthesis. Anterior luxation of L5 on sacrum due to fracture of isthmus. Note that gap is wider and dog appears decapitated

Fig. 24.5 Spondylolysis and Spondylolisthesis.

Initial treatment consists of rest, pain control, and physical therapy. An epidural steroid injection may be considered. Disk herniations in the pediatric population can be persistent, especially in the setting of an apophyseal fracture. Operative treatment should be pursued in cases refractory to nonoperative modalities and expedited in the cases of debilitating neurologic deficits. Herniations associated with an apophyseal fracture have higher rates of requiring operative intervention.

SUMMARY

Disorders of the neck and spine are uncommon in children but are potentially debilitating. Although many disorders are benign and self-limiting, patients must be adequately assessed for comorbidities, persistent pathologic conditions, or symptoms that affect cosmesis and quality of life and appropriately referred to a pediatric orthopedic surgeon for evaluation.

SUGGESTED READINGS

Available online.

25

Disorders of the Hip and Lower Extremity

Edward D. Re and Joshua H. Sperling

Upright mobility has an enormous impact on the functional capacity of pediatric patients, and disorders of the hip and lower extremities are numerous and highly varied. The care of these patients is interprofessional; orthopedic surgeons, physical therapists, occupational therapists, physiatrists, and pediatricians must work together to provide optimal musculoskeletal care. Pediatricians must accurately refine their differential diagnoses to provide appropriate reassurance in some cases and mobilize function-saving interventions in others. They are uniquely positioned to appreciate and emphasize the long-lasting developmental harm that can be caused by lower extremity abnormalities, particularly those that affect the very young. We divide several common disorders of the hips and lower extremities into one of three categories: congenital, developmental, and acquired.

CONGENITAL

Dysmorphology can appear congenitally, secondary to a variety of mechanisms. A vast array of genetic syndromes present with lower limb anomalies at birth, including polydactyly and syndactyly, with various degrees of functional implications. In utero teratogen exposure—such as exposure to thalidomide, illicit drugs, or alcohol—can lead to limb malformations. Amniotic bands can also disrupt limb formation, leading to full or partial amputation.

Clubfoot

Clubfoot, or talipes equinovarus, affects 1 in 1000 live births and is often diagnosed in utero. This example of congenital deformation is characterized by a smaller foot on the affected side, rigidity to plantar flexion, adductus of the forefoot, and inward angulation of the hindfoot (Fig. 25.1). Half of the cases are bilateral. Although many cases are idiopathic, maternal smoking, certain ethnic backgrounds, and genes affecting both the musculoskeletal and nervous systems have been identified as risk factors. Some think that disordered development of the talus in utero causes the disorder.

Management of clubfoot has trended away from immediate surgical reconstruction because of the need for multiple corrective procedures and resultant muscle weakness or stiffening in favor of progressive treatments. Commonly used is the Ponseti method, which begins with tenotomy in most cases and is followed by serial casting and manipulation procedures. This is best started early in the neonatal period, so early referral to a pediatric orthopedist is necessary. Clubfeet that do not respond to conservative measures necessitate operative management.

DEVELOPMENTAL

In utero packaging causes some expected changes in every infant; some of these variations may take 3 to 4 years to resolve. The more common disorders associated with packaging include rotational problems of the lower extremities such as in-toeing and out-toeing, which are often noted when a child begins to walk.

Developmental Dysplasia of the Hip

Developmental dysplasia of the hip (DDH) bears special mention because it must be diagnosed promptly and does not resolve without intervention. DDH represents a spectrum of disorders ranging from mild ligamentous laxity of the hip joint to a fully displaced femoral head. Diagnosis is made by physical examination of the neonate; finding a hip clunk on the Barlow or Ortolani maneuvers warrants immediate orthopedics referral. The Barlow test can identify a dislocatable hip, and the Ortolani test attempts to reduce a dislocation (Fig. 25.2). After the first few months of life, limitation or asymmetry of hip abduction is a more reliable examination finding.

Babies who are in the breech position during the third trimester have additional stress placed on the developing hip joint and are therefore at higher risk for the disorder. The American Academy of Pediatrics (AAP) recommends screening these patients with hip ultrasounds at 6 weeks (adjusted for prematurity). Further risk factors include female sex, family history of DDH, and high birth weight. Plain radiographs

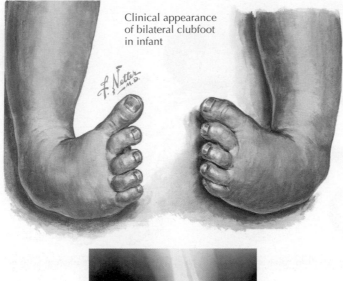

Clinical appearance
of bilateral clubfoot
in infant

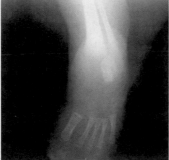

Anteroposterior (above) and
lateral (below) radiographs show
congenital clubfoot in newborn.

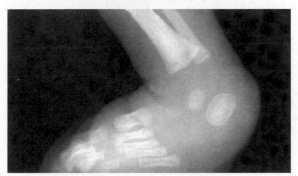

Fig. 25.1 Congenital Clubfoot.

are more accurate as ossification centers form and are the imaging modality of choice when the infant is older than 4 to 6 months of age.

Very mild abnormalities of the hip joint often resolve spontaneously in the first few months of life. When a true dislocation is diagnosed before 6 months of age, the Pavlik harness is the treatment of choice. It is a splint that prevents hip extension and adduction, which can be adjusted as the child grows (see Fig. 25.2). Triple diapering or other measures to force the hip into place are no longer seen as effective treatment measures. Diagnosis after age 6 months usually requires surgical repair. When DDH is not diagnosed in infancy, parents or pediatricians may notice that the affected child has a waddling or Trendelenburg gait when beginning to walk (see Fig. 25.2).

In-Toeing

Some degree of in-toeing is expected in children until the lower limbs externally rotate over time; adult walking patterns are not observed until about 7 or 8 years of age. The cause of in-toeing varies by age and is classically caused by metatarsus adductus in infants, internal tibial torsion in toddlers, and excessive femoral anteversion in preschool-aged children.

Metatarsus Adductus

Metatarsus adductus is the medial deviation of the tarsometatarsal joints in the transverse plane. This variant is detected in 1% to 2% of infants. Metatarsus adductus is observed in infants who were crowded in utero, such as with oligohydramnios or twin gestation, and soon self-corrects, with 85% to 90% resolving by 1 year of age. Indeed, the majority of children with metatarsus adductus have no long-term functional impairment and do not require surgical repair. Severe cases can increase development of bunions and hammertoes, so serial casting or bracing is helpful when the deformity does not resolve on its own.

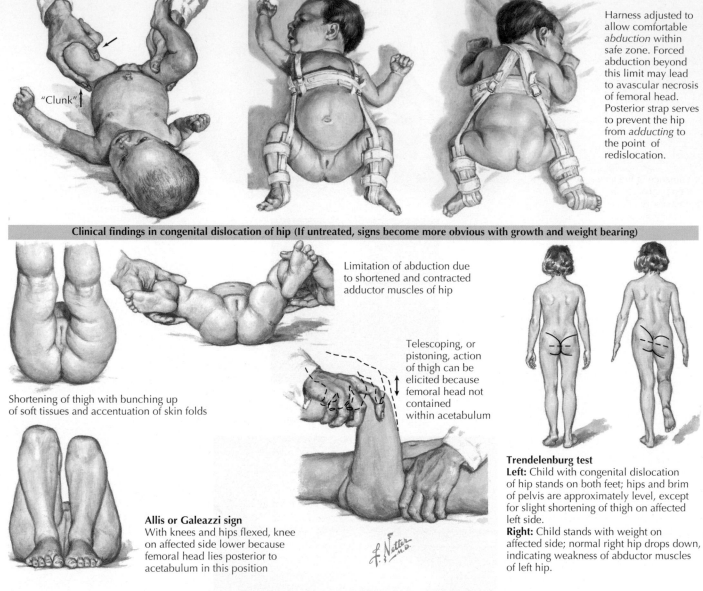

Barlow and Ortolani maneuvers

"Clunk"

Pavlik harness

Harness adjusted to allow comfortable *abduction* within safe zone. Forced abduction beyond this limit may lead to avascular necrosis of femoral head. Posterior strap serves to prevent the hip from *adducting* to the point of redislocation.

Clinical findings in congenital dislocation of hip (If untreated, signs become more obvious with growth and weight bearing)

Limitation of abduction due to shortened and contracted adductor muscles of hip

Telescoping, or pistoning, action of thigh can be elicited because femoral head not contained within acetabulum

Shortening of thigh with bunching up of soft tissues and accentuation of skin folds

Allis or Galeazzi sign
With knees and hips flexed, knee on affected side lower because femoral head lies posterior to acetabulum in this position

Trendelenburg test
Left: Child with congenital dislocation of hip stands on both feet; hips and brim of pelvis are approximately level, except for slight shortening of thigh on affected left side.
Right: Child stands with weight on affected side; normal right hip drops down, indicating weakness of abductor muscles of left hip.

Fig. 25.2 Developmental Dysplasia of the Hip.

Internal Tibial Torsion

Internal tibial torsion is the most common cause of in-toeing and can be associated with metatarsus adductus. It is usually noted in toddlerhood when children begin to walk. It affects boys and girls equally and is bilateral in about two-thirds of cases. On examination, the knee remains in neutral position while the foot is medially rotated (Fig. 25.3). Most cases self-resolve as children begin to walk independently, with normal alignment noted as early as 4 years or as late as 10 years of age.

Femoral Anteversion

Excessive femoral anteversion is seen in preschool-aged children and is thought to be either a remnant of in utero positioning or increased ligamentous laxity. It is more common in girls and is almost universally bilateral. On physical examination, the knees are medially rotated, distinguishing this entity from internal tibial torsion. Normal growth usually leads to resolution by 8 to 10 years of age.

For all causes of in-toeing, surgery is rarely warranted but may be considered for persistent cases or those causing functional impairment.

Bowlegs

Bowlegs, or genu varum, is noted when children begin walking and can be considered normal until about 3 years of age. Beyond this age group, however, bowing of the legs is pathologic, and other causes must be considered to establish proper treatment plans.

Blount Disease and Adolescent Tibia Vara

Blount disease, also known as osteochondrosis deformans tibia or tibia vara, is an abnormality seen most frequently in obese African American girls younger than 3 years of age and can be inherited in an autosomal recessive fashion. A less aggressive cause of progressive bowing is adolescent tibia vara, seen in boys older than 8 years of age. Similar to Blount disease, adolescent tibia vara is observed more commonly in obese African Americans. Both disorders are associated with

Child seated with knees flexed 90°. Patellae point directly forward, indicating that femurs are in neutral position, but feet point inward, suggesting tibial torsion. Measure tibial torsion by positioning the thigh in neutral rotation, then placing the thumb of one hand over the tibial tuberosity and with the other hand placing the thumb over the prominence of the medial malleolus and the long finger over the prominence of the lateral malleolus. The degree of tibial torsion is the estimate of the angle made by the transmalleolar axis and the axis of the coronal plane of the proximal tibia.

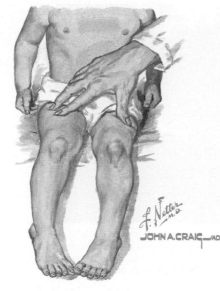

Fig. 25.3 Internal Tibial Torsion.

early walking. Starting corrective bracing early may prevent progressive deformity, and this additional support is especially crucial while walking. Tibial osteotomy may be considered for correction of bowlegs based on symptoms such as pain or asymmetry despite proper bracing for 1 year.

Rickets

Rickets is a correctable cause of bowlegs that can be differentiated from tibia vara by family history, radiographic stigmata, and laboratory assessment. Rickets is an anomaly of bone mineralization that develops gradually in growing children because of calcium, phosphate, or vitamin D deficiency or resistance (Chapter 48). Bowing of the legs, metaphyseal flaring, and "rachitic rosary" deformity of the ribs may be seen on physical examination or plain films. The AAP recommends 400 IU of vitamin D supplementation for all infants receiving less than 1 L of formula daily to prevent rickets. Metabolic bowing usually resolves with metabolic control and rarely requires surgical correction.

ACQUIRED

Most acquired lower extremity disorders are traumatic in origin. Atraumatic lower extremity pain and limp can be the source of much doubt for pediatricians, because the differential diagnosis for these findings is broad and includes infectious, oncologic, rheumatologic, metabolic, and inflammatory processes. We focus here on acquired processes not covered elsewhere in this textbook.

Slipped Capital Femoral Epiphysis

Slipped capital femoral epiphysis (SCFE) refers to an instability of the proximal femoral growth plate resulting in the femoral head slipping posteriorly and inferiorly relative to the neck of the femur (Fig. 25.4). SCFE demands urgent surgical attention, and any delay in diagnosis and surgical correction can lead to avascular necrosis and permanent functional impairment. A causal relationship has been found between SCFE and obesity in children in their preadolescent and early adolescent years. The incidence of SCFE is higher in boys than girls and in African Americans than Whites.

One of the greatest challenges in the diagnosis of SCFE is its varied presentation, because patients may complain of hip, knee, thigh, or groin pain. It is imperative to examine the hip in children with complaints of isolated knee pain, because hip pain can refer to the knee via the obturator nerve. SCFE presents most typically as insidious pain over weeks or months but presents acutely as well, often in the setting of minor trauma.

On physical examination, patients with SCFE may refuse to bear weight, hold the affected limb in passive external rotation, and resist internal rotation because of pain. Additionally, about 20% of SCFEs are bilateral at the time of presentation and another 20% develop bilateral slips if not prevented. The risk for developing a contralateral slip over time increases for patients diagnosed with SCFE at younger ages.

Diagnosis is made on anteroposterior (AP) and frog-leg radiographs of the pelvis. The AP view can show widening of the physis and misalignment of the femoral capital epiphysis. On the AP view, the lack of intersection of a line drawn along the femoral neck (Klein line) and the femoral epiphysis can confirm the diagnosis. On the frog-leg view, the posterior portion of the femoral head becomes medial, making the slippage more apparent and giving a slipped "ice cream cone" appearance (see Fig. 25.4). Patients diagnosed with SCFE should be made non–weight bearing and seen by an orthopedist emergently. Treatment consists of internal fixation using a single cannulated screw, which prevents further slippage and provides symptom relief.

Legg-Calvé-Perthes Disease

Legg-Calvé-Perthes (LCP) is the eponym given to idiopathic osteonecrosis of the femoral head. LCP affects children aged 3 to 12 years, and it peaks in the early school years. As with SCFE, there is a male predominance, with males afflicted four times as often as females. Unlike SCFE, however, White children are far more likely to have LCP.

Patients with LCP usually have an insidious onset of mild pain worsened by activity that may refer to the thigh or knee. On examination, patients may have a Trendelenburg gait, pain, or decreased range of motion with internal rotation and abduction. In advanced disease, radiographs can be helpful and may show fragmentation of the femoral head (Fig. 25.5). In early cases, however, radiographic changes can be subtle or nonexistent. A significant concern for LCP may mandate further imaging such as a bone scan or magnetic resonance imaging.

As in SCFE, patients with LCP should be made non–weight bearing and referred to an orthopedic surgeon. Treatment consists of conservative management, including administration of nonsteroidal antiinflammatory drugs (NSAIDs), crutches, and immobilization, with the goal of containing the femoral head within the acetabulum. Older children with LCP have a worse prognosis because of the decreased potential for bone remodeling and may experience disabling osteoarthritis in the adult years.

Transient Synovitis

Transient synovitis (TS) is the most common cause of acute hip pain in young children, characterized by inflammation of the hip synovium. Children with TS are generally well appearing but have hip pain, a limp, or both. They often have low-grade fevers as well. TS typically presents at 3 to 8 years of age, and boys are affected twice as often as girls. It is often attributed to an infectious cause because many children have a history of a preceding upper respiratory tract infection. The principal concern with TS is distinguishing it from septic arthritis (Chapter 28), which can result in significant morbidity if not promptly

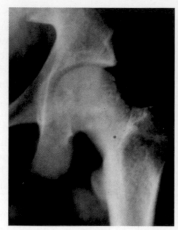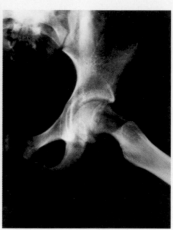

Slipped capital femoral epiphysis not readily apparent on antero-posterior radiograph because slip is usually posterior

Frog-leg radiograph, which demonstrates slipped epiphysis more clearly, always indicated when disorder is suspected

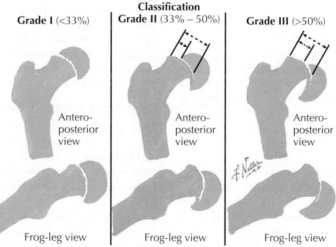

Classification

Grade I (<33%)   **Grade II** (33% – 50%)   **Grade III** (>50%)

Antero-posterior view

Antero-posterior view

Antero-posterior view

Frog-leg view   Frog-leg view   Frog-leg view

Fig. 25.4 Slipped Capital Femoral Epiphysis.

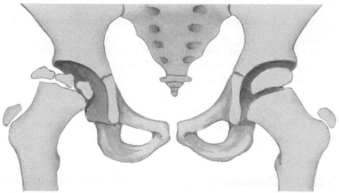

Fig. 25.5 Legg-Calvé-Perthes Disease: Ancillary Prognostic Indicators.

diagnosed and treated. To this end, inflammatory markers can be helpful. Children with high fevers or elevated inflammatory markers often require hip ultrasonography and aspiration of hip fluid if effusion is identified. TS is self-limited, but NSAIDs have been shown to shorten the duration of symptoms.

Osteoid Osteoma

Osteoid osteoma is a relatively common benign skeletal neoplasm that typically occurs in the femur, although it can occur anywhere. Most cases of osteoid osteoma occur in children and young adults, and males are affected twice as often as females. They typically manifests with localized pain at the site of the lesion that is worse at night and responds well to NSAIDs. A limp may be observed as well. Osteoid osteomas usually appear as a dense central nidus smaller than 2 cm surrounded by a well-circumscribed lucency on plain radiographs or computed tomography. Osteoid osteomas have no malignancy potential and usually regress or become dormant spontaneously. If pain persists, the lesion can be surgically excised or ablated.

FUTURE DIRECTIONS

The lower extremity disorders explored here are best managed after prompt recognition and diagnosis. Although advanced imaging modalities have proven useful in the evaluation of these conditions, a targeted history and thorough physical examination remain critical skills of any pediatrician. Several of the disorders discussed here merit further study of treatment outcomes in randomized controlled trials to determine optimal medical or surgical management.

SUGGESTED READINGS

Available online.

26

Common Fractures

Arvind Balaji and Sonia Jarrett

 CLINICAL VIGNETTE

A 20-month-old girl presents to the emergency department with her parents after falling down four steps at home. After falling, she cried and favored her right leg. Soon after, she was unwilling to put weight on that leg. Concerned, her parents brought her in for evaluation.

Examination of the right lower extremity shows no signs of swelling or erythema. Palpation along the right femur elicits no pain, but palpation along the distal tibia appears to cause discomfort. Radiographs of the tibia and fibula reveal no abnormalities.

She receives a long leg cast, and her family is instructed to follow up with her pediatrician. Two weeks later, repeat radiographs show new bone formation along the distal tibia. The patient remains in her cast for 2 more weeks, and, upon removal, she returns to full, painless use of the right leg.

Trauma to patients at this age, such as falls or being dropped from carrying height, can cause fractures of the tibia called *toddler's fracture*. The pain can cause a limp or refusal to bear weight on the affected extremity. Evaluation consists of radiographic imaging of the tibia and fibula. The classic spiral or oblique pattern of injury seen with this fracture may not be visible on initial radiographs. Based on clinical suspicion, it is appropriate to immobilize the affected leg in a long leg cast and to follow the patient over 4 to 6 weeks to treat the fracture. Repeat radiographs looking for new bone formation would be appropriate if the diagnosis is in doubt, because the presence of new bone formation along the tibia would support the diagnosis of toddler's fracture.

EPIDEMIOLOGY

Pediatric fractures represent a significant portion of emergency room visits each year in the United States. Almost half of all children will sustain a fracture during childhood. These injuries can result in significant morbidity for the patient and have an impact on the daily life of caregivers. Despite ongoing public health initiatives, the incidence of pediatric fractures continues to rise, possibly as a result of increased sports participation.

ETIOLOGY AND PATHOGENESIS

There are key differences between pediatric and adult bone with respect to patterns of injury. First, pediatric bones are more porous, which leads to increased susceptibility to fracture. Additionally, the physis, or growth plate, which distinguishes pediatric bone from adult bone, is vulnerable to injury, and damage to it can carry long-term growth consequences.

Moreover, the thicker periosteum of pediatric bone decreases the likelihood of significant displacement of fracture fragments in pediatric

orthopedic injury. The remodeling potential of pediatric bone is high, which can allow for nonsurgical healing of even significantly displaced fractures.

FRACTURE TYPES AND DESCRIPTIONS

Using appropriate fracture nomenclature is important for discussing management with orthopedic consultants and health care providers. Table 26.1 gives an overview of essential terminology when describing fractures. Figs. 26.1 and 26.2 illustrate the location and appearance of specific fractures.

Physeal Fractures

The physis is an area of pediatric bone that is particularly vulnerable to fracture. The patterns of injury involving the physis of long bones are most commonly described using the Salter-Harris classification system. This system, published in 1963 by Dr. Robert Salter and Dr. William Harris, is used to describe the degree of involvement of the physis, the epiphysis, and the metaphysis in pediatric long bone fractures (Fig. 26.3). The different classifications carry prognostic and therapeutic consequences.

Salter-Harris Type I Fracture

A Salter-Harris type I fracture involves separation of the epiphysis and most of the physis from the metaphysis. Diagnosis can be difficult if displacement is minimal because radiographs often appear normal. This type of fracture should be suspected clinically when there is swelling and tenderness over a growth plate. Management consists of immobilization and orthopedic follow-up. Healing usually occurs over 4 weeks, and complications are rare. These fractures rarely result in growth disturbance.

Salter-Harris Type II Fracture

Salter-Harris type II fractures are the most common type of pediatric physeal fractures. These fractures extend through the physis into the metaphysis. Similar to Salter-Harris type I fractures, these fractures rarely result in growth disturbance, and management consists of immobilization and orthopedic follow-up.

Salter-Harris Type III Fracture

Salter-Harris type III fractures extend through the physis and then propagate through the epiphysis into the intraarticular space. Growth disturbance may occur if anatomic position is not reestablished. Therefore these fractures require prompt orthopedic consultation and may need surgical reduction.

Salter-Harris Type IV Fracture

Salter-Harris type IV fractures involve the metaphysis, physis, articular surface, and epiphysis. These fractures may also result in growth arrest

TABLE 26.1 Fracture Descriptors

Element	Terminology
Name of fractured bone	Use anatomical name to identify injured bone
Location of injury	Anatomic aspect: that is, "medial" or "ulnar," "lateral" or "radial," "dorsal," or "palmar" for forearm and hand *Long bone fractures:* Identify location along metaphysis, diaphysis, epiphysis (Fig. 26.1) *Physeal fractures:* Use Salter-Harris terminology *Joint involvement:* Intraarticular or extraarticular
Extent of fracture	*Complete:* Extends across width of bone *Incomplete:* Involves partial width of bone
Fracture orientation	*Transverse:* Perpendicular to long axis of bone *Oblique:* Diagonally crosses long axis of bone *Spiral:* Helical break
Position and alignment	*Displaced:* Fracture fragments moved apart *Angulated:* Degree of malalignment relative to the affected bone's long axis
Fragments	*Comminuted:* More than two fracture fragments from the same bone *Segmented:* Two fracture lines divide a bone into three pieces
Overlying skin integrity	*Open:* Exposure of fractured bone to environment (i.e., obvious bone protrusion or subtle laceration) *Closed:* Intact skin overlying fracture

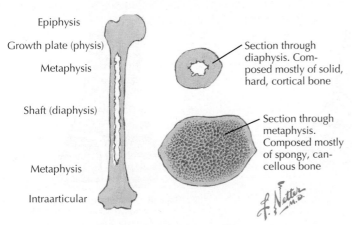

Epiphysis

Growth plate (physis)

Metaphysis

Shaft (diaphysis)

Metaphysis

Intraarticular

Section through diaphysis. Composed mostly of solid, hard, cortical bone

Section through metaphysis. Composed mostly of spongy, cancellous bone

Fig. 26.1 Basic Science of Bone.

and deformity if anatomic position is not reestablished, often through surgical repair. Thus emergent orthopedic consultation is required.

Salter-Harris Type V Fracture

Salter-Harris type V fractures result from a crush injury with resultant disruption of the growth plate. Similar to Salter-Harris type I fractures, these fractures can be difficult to diagnose because radiographs may be normal, and the diagnosis is often made in hindsight. Because these fractures disrupt the germinal matrix, they can cause severe injury with growth arrest and can have a poor prognosis. When recognized, these fractures merit emergent orthopedic consultation.

Greenstick Fractures

Greenstick fractures are the most common fracture pattern in children and occur in long bones in pediatric patients. They are a partial

thickness fracture that breaches the cortex and periosteum on one side of bone, but does not extend completely through the width of the bone. Depending on the degree of angulation, closed reduction may be necessary to facilitate healing in proper alignment (Fig. 26.4).

Torus Fractures

Torus, or buckle, fractures are common in young children. They result from a compressive load causing metaphyseal compaction of trabecular bone and buckling of cortical bone without breaching the periosteum. The porosity of pediatric bone along with increased strength of pediatric periosteum leaves pediatric patients at particular risk for this type of injury. These fractures often occur in the distal radius after a fall onto an outstretched hand. As a child matures, the metaphysis stiffens, and the incidence of torus fractures decreases. These fractures are stable and can be managed with immobilization for 4 weeks (see Fig. 26.4).

Bowing Fractures

Bowing fractures represent a plastic deformity of bone and are unique to children. They occur when a longitudinal force exceeds the bone's ability to recoil to its normal position and results in a bend without a fracture. These injuries most commonly involve the radius and ulna. Bowing fractures can be subtle, and comparison views of the contralateral arm may be necessary. If the deformity occurs in a child younger than 4 years, or if the deformation is less than 20 degrees, the angulation usually corrects with growth. However, open reduction may be required if the bowing is greater than 20 degrees and the patient is older than 6 years of age (see Fig. 26.4).

UPPER EXTREMITY FRACTURES

Clavicle Fractures

The clavicle is the most commonly fractured bone in childhood. In neonates, these fractures can occur during traumatic birth and can manifest with pseudoparalysis. Clavicle fractures in older children may be caused by a direct blow to the clavicle or indirect forces transmitted to the clavicle from a fall. Most fractures involve the distal two-thirds of the clavicle. Diagnosis often can be made on physical examination because patients typically have swelling, tenderness, and occasionally crepitus at the fracture site. Although neurovascular injury is rare, it is important to assess for any associated brachial plexus injury.

Most clavicle fractures heal well without complication, and management consists of immobilization in a figure-of-8 clavicle strap or sling and swathe (Fig. 26.5). Patients with open fractures, neurovascular or respiratory compromise, significantly displaced midshaft fractures, or grossly unstable distal injuries need orthopedic consultation because closed reduction may be indicated. The vast majority of clavicle fractures heal quickly, usually within 3 to 6 weeks. A bony callus appears during the healing process, and a remnant may persist permanently.

Humerus Fractures

Fractures of the humerus include supracondylar fractures (discussed later), proximal humerus fractures, and midshaft fractures. The latter two fractures are relatively rare. Consider child abuse when a patient younger than 3 years of age presents with a spiral fracture of the humerus.

The proximal humeral growth plate is responsible for the majority of growth of the humerus, giving these fractures a remarkable ability to remodel and avoid nonunion. Most of these fractures can be managed with a shoulder immobilizer or sling and swathe with orthopedic referral.

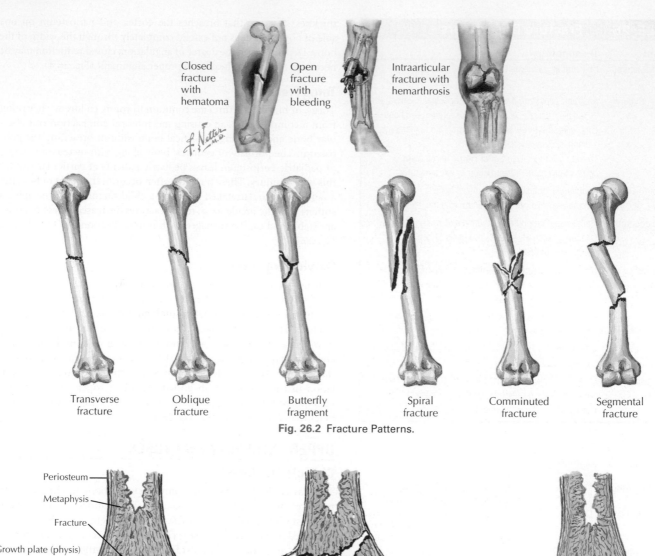

Closed fracture with hematoma

Open fracture with bleeding

Intraarticular fracture with hemarthrosis

| Transverse fracture | Oblique fracture | Butterfly fragment | Spiral fracture | Comminuted fracture | Segmental fracture |

Fig. 26.2 Fracture Patterns.

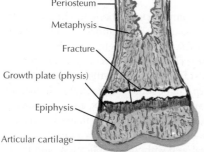

Periosteum
Metaphysis
Fracture
Growth plate (physis)
Epiphysis
Articular cartilage

Type I. Complete separation of epiphysis from shaft through calcified cartilage (growth zone) of growth plate. No bone actually fractured; periosteum may remain intact. Most common in newborns and young children

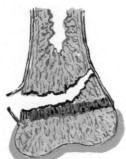

Type II. Most common. Line of separation extends partially across deep layer of growth plate and extends through metaphysis, leaving triangular portion of metaphysis attached to epiphyseal fragment

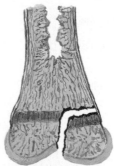

Type III. Uncommon. Intra-articular fracture through epiphysis, across deep zone of growth plate to periphery. Open reduction and fixation often necessary

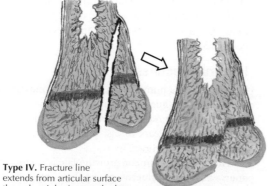

Type IV. Fracture line extends from articular surface through epiphysis, growth plate, and metaphysis. If fractured segment not perfectly realigned with open reduction, osseous bridge across growth plate may occur resulting in partial growth arrest and joint angulation

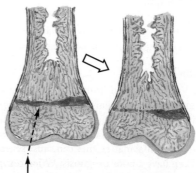

Type V. Severe crushing force transmitted across epiphysis to portion of growth plate by abduction or adduction stress or axial load. Minimal or no displacement makes radiographic diagnosis difficult; growth plate may nevertheless be damaged, resulting in partial growth arrest or shortening and angular deformity

Fig. 26.3 Injury to Growth Plate (Salter-Harris Classification).

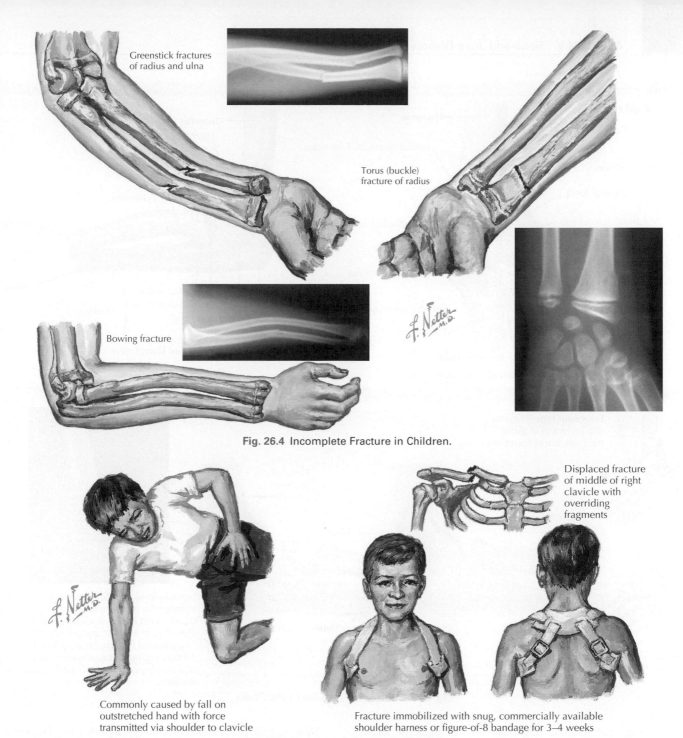

Greenstick fractures
of radius and ulna

Torus (buckle)
fracture of radius

Bowing fracture

Fig. 26.4 Incomplete Fracture in Children.

Displaced fracture
of middle of right
clavicle with
overriding
fragments

Commonly caused by fall on
outstretched hand with force
transmitted via shoulder to clavicle

Fracture immobilized with snug, commercially available
shoulder harness or figure-of-8 bandage for 3–4 weeks

Fig. 26.5 Fracture of Clavicle in Children.

Supracondylar Fractures

Supracondylar fractures make up more than half of all elbow fractures in pediatric patients. These fractures often require surgical management and can result in neurovascular compromise or joint malunion if treated inappropriately.

Supracondylar fractures involve injury or displacement of the distal humerus. This fracture risks injury to multiple neurovascular structures: the brachial artery running superficial to the brachialis muscle along the anteromedial aspect of the humerus, the median and radial nerves crossing the elbow anteriorly, and the ulnar nerve crossing the elbow posteriorly to the medial epicondyle (Fig. 26.6).

The most common mechanism of injury is a fall onto an outstretched hand with hyperextension of the elbow and subsequent posteriorly displaced fracture. Less commonly, a direct blow to the posterior elbow in flexion can result in an anteriorly displaced fracture.

Typically, patients have significant elbow pain and swelling with limited range of motion. Evaluate for lacerations or wounds that would be concerning for open fracture. Elbow movement should not be assessed or encouraged until radiography excludes a displaced fracture. A thorough neurovascular assessment is critical for suspected supracondylar fractures. Analgesia may be required for better assessment.

Diagnosis requires an anteroposterior view of the elbow joint in extension and a lateral view with the elbow flexed at 90 degrees (Fig. 26.6). Look for abnormalities of the fat pads overlying the joint capsule of the distal humerus and any altered alignment among the humerus, radius, and ulna. Normally, the anterior fat pad is visible on lateral radiography, whereas the posterior fat pad does not show because it sits deep in the olecranon fossa. Fracture of the elbow can cause hemarthrosis resulting in fluid in the joint space displacing the fat pads, accentuating the anterior fat pad, and making the posterior fat pad visible.

Bones of the elbow

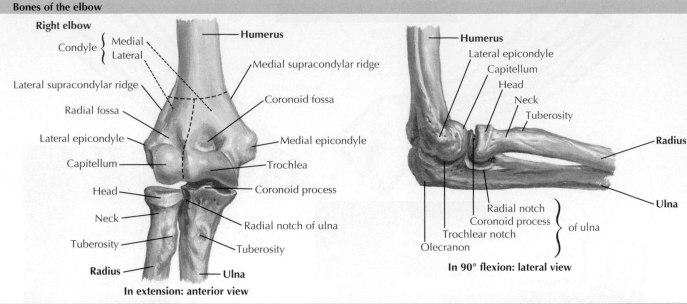

Right elbow

Condyle { Medial / Lateral

Humerus

Medial supracondylar ridge

Lateral supracondylar ridge

Coronoid fossa

Radial fossa

Lateral epicondyle

Medial epicondyle

Capitellum

Trochlea

Head

Coronoid process

Neck

Radial notch of ulna

Tuberosity

Tuberosity

Radius

Ulna

In extension: anterior view

Humerus

Lateral epicondyle

Capitellum

Head

Neck

Tuberosity

Radius

Radial notch

Coronoid process

} of ulna

Trochlear notch

Ulna

Olecranon

In 90° flexion: lateral view

Supracondylar fractures

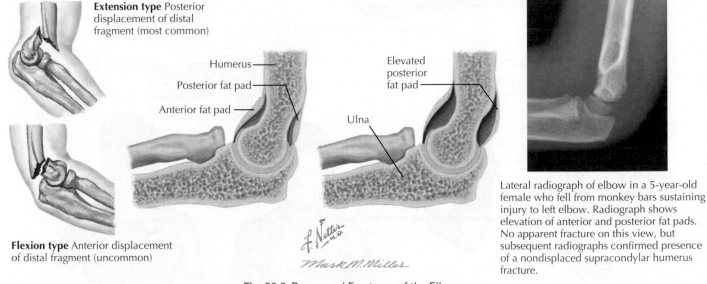

Extension type Posterior displacement of distal fragment (most common)

Humerus

Posterior fat pad

Anterior fat pad

Elevated posterior fat pad

Ulna

Flexion type Anterior displacement of distal fragment (uncommon)

Lateral radiograph of elbow in a 5-year-old female who fell from monkey bars sustaining injury to left elbow. Radiograph shows elevation of anterior and posterior fat pads. No apparent fracture on this view, but subsequent radiographs confirmed presence of a nondisplaced supracondylar humerus fracture.

Fig. 26.6 Bones and Fractures of the Elbow.

Appropriate radiographic alignment of the humerus allows a line drawn along the anterior cortex of the distal humerus on a true lateral view to intersect the middle third of the capitellum. A radiocapitellar line drawn down the radius should bisect the capitellum. Displacement of either of these lines suggests supracondylar fracture or an occult radial neck fracture or radial head dislocation, respectively.

When evaluating elbow radiography, pediatric-specific ossification centers that change with age may be mistaken for a fracture on radiography. The mnemonic aid CRITOE serves as a way to remember the appearance of ossification centers: capitellum, age 1 year; radial head, age 3 years; internal (medial) condyle, age 5 years; trochlea, age 7 years; olecranon, age 9 years; external (lateral) condyle, age 11 years.

Immobilization and analgesia are key in the initial phases of supracondylar fracture management. Supracondylar fractures generally require realignment. Closed reduction with percutaneous fixation is preferred. Open reduction is indicated if there is vascular compromise, an open fracture, or if the fracture cannot be reduced by closed method.

Neurovascular injury is the most common complication of supracondylar fractures. Brachial artery compression, contusion, or vasospasm at the fracture site can lead to distal ischemia or vascular insufficiency. A displaced supracondylar fracture risks injury to the median, radial, or ulnar nerve that may result in transient nerve palsies or neuropraxias and may take months to recover. Forearm compartment syndrome can also result in Volkmann ischemic contracture, which is characterized by loss of function in the hand and wrist (Fig. 26.6).

Forearm Fractures

Fractures of the forearm and wrist comprise nearly half of all fractures seen in pediatric patients. Forearm fractures involve the radius or ulna, often with concomitant injury to the paired bone. These fractures usually involve the metaphysis and distal portion of these bones, with the majority being torus or greenstick morphology. The most common mechanism of injury is a fall onto an outstretched hand.

Examination of forearm fractures typically reveals point tenderness, swelling, ecchymosis, and decreased grip strength. With any

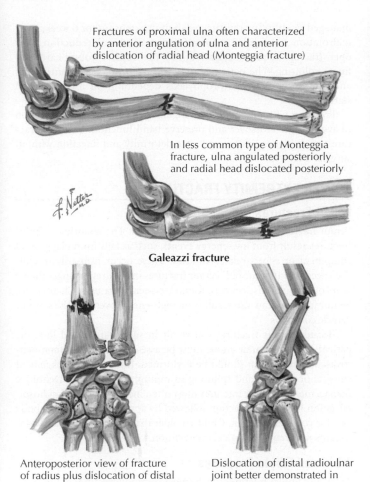

Fractures of proximal ulna often characterized by anterior angulation of ulna and anterior dislocation of radial head (Monteggia fracture)

In less common type of Monteggia fracture, ulna angulated posteriorly and radial head dislocated posteriorly

Galeazzi fracture

Anteroposterior view of fracture of radius plus dislocation of distal radioulnar joint (Galeazzi fracture)

Dislocation of distal radioulnar joint better demonstrated in lateral view

Fig. 26.7 Monteggia Fracture.

TABLE 26.2	**Radiograph Views for Fracture Evaluation**
Type of Fracture	**Radiograph Views**
Upper Extremity	
Clavicle fracture	2 View (AP and cephalic tilt)
Proximal humerus fracture	2 View of humerus (AP and lateral); consider 2 view of shoulder (AP and lateral or Y-view)
Elbow fracture	3 View elbow (AP, lateral, and external oblique), consider addition of forearm views if clinical concern warrants
Forearm fracture	2 View forearm (AP and lateral), consider including elbow and wrist views if clinical concern warrants
Wrist fracture	3 View wrist (PA, lateral, oblique)
Metacarpal fracture	3 View hand (PA, lateral, oblique)
Phalangeal fracture	3 View (PA, lateral, oblique) of affected phalanx or thumb
Lower Extremity	
Femur fracture	2 View (AP and lateral) of the femur, consider 2 view (AP and lateral) of knee and hip
Tibia/fibula fracture	2 View (AP and lateral) of the tibia and fibula 2 View (AP and lateral) knee and ankle
Ankle fracture	3 View (AP, mortise, lateral) of ankle, consider full-length tibia radiograph to rule out Maisonneuve fracture
Foot fracture	3 View (AP, lateral, and oblique) of foot

AP, Anteroposterior; *PA,* posteroanterior.

fracture examination, neurovascular assessment is necessary to evaluate for signs of compartment syndrome.

Radiography of the forearm should include both the wrist and elbow joints to exclude an associated fracture at the opposite end. For example, a fracture at the distal third of the radius can be associated with distal radioulnar joint dislocation, also known as a Galeazzi fracture (Fig. 26.7). A fracture of the proximal ulna associated with concomitant dislocation of the radial head is known as a Monteggia fracture (Fig. 26.7). Proximal radius fractures usually result in Salter-Harris type I and type II fractures of the radial neck. These fractures can occur in conjunction with elbow dislocations and are associated with medial epicondyle, olecranon, and coronoid process fractures.

Nondisplaced or minimally displaced fractures of the radial head and neck often can be treated with splinting and orthopedic follow-up. Displaced and angulated fractures require manipulative closed reduction under sedation or surgical repair.

Rotational abnormalities of forearm fractures must be corrected to prevent permanent loss of pronation and supination functions. Forearm fracture complications are uncommon, but vascular compromise or compartment syndrome can still occur.

Wrist Fractures

Fractures of the distal radius are the most common fracture in children and adolescents. These fractures typically occur as a result of falling on an outstretched hand. Carpal bones are infrequently fractured in childhood, but if they are affected, the scaphoid is most commonly involved, especially in adolescents.

Any evaluation of a wrist injury should assess for scaphoid fracture. Palpation along the anatomic snuffbox will elicit tenderness. Wrist extension, flexion, forced supination, and longitudinal compression of the thumb will also cause pain.

On plain radiographs, scaphoid fractures can be best visualized with the anteroposterior scaphoid view with ulnar deviation. Often, plain radiographs may not reveal an acute fracture immediately after injury. See Table 26.2 for a list of suggested radiograph views that correspond to extremity injuries.

Clinical findings are sufficient to diagnose suspected scaphoid fracture even if initial radiography does not show acute fracture. For suspected nondisplaced fractures, immobilize the wrist in a thumb spica splint. The patient should have a close orthopedic follow-up for repeat radiography or advanced imaging to better evaluate the fracture. Although rare in pediatric patients, scaphoid fractures have a risk for nonunion if immobilization is delayed.

Metacarpal Fractures

The most common metacarpal fracture in children is the fractured distal fifth metacarpal, accounting for 30% to 40% of all hand fractures. Metacarpal neck fractures often result from direct trauma, such as a strike against a closed fist, hence the name *boxer's fracture.*

Examination may show a swollen dorsal surface of the hand over the affected metacarpal with focal bony tenderness. Extension of the fingers should be evaluated because of angulation of the fracture that can pull on interosseous muscles. Three radiographic views of the hand can adequately assess angulation of metacarpal neck fractures.

Metacarpal fractures with angulation more than 30 to 40 degrees require closed reduction followed by immobilization and orthopedic

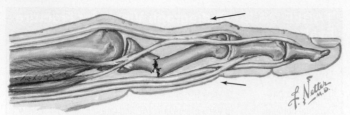

Transverse fractures of proximal phalanx tend to angulate volarly because of pull of interosseous muscles on base of proximal phalanx and collapsing action of long extensor and flexor tendons.

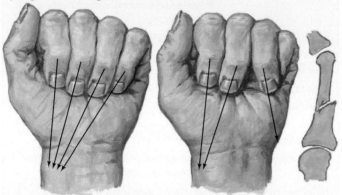

Reduction of fractures of phalanges or metacarpals requires correct rotational as well as longitudinal alignment. In normal hand, tips of flexed fingers point toward tuberosity of scaphoid, as in hand at left. Hand at right shows result of healing of ring finger in rotational malalignment. Rotational malalignment, usually discernible clinically, may also be evidenced on radiographs by discrepancy in cross-sectional diameter of fragments, as shown at extreme right. Discrepancy in diameter is most apparent in true lateral radiograph but is visible to some extent in anteroposterior view.

Fig. 26.8 Fracture of the Proximal Phalanx.

follow-up. Nondisplaced or minimally displaced metacarpal fractures should be immobilized for 2 to 4 weeks.

Phalanges Fractures

Finger fractures occur commonly in children with multiple phalangeal fracture patterns. These patterns include physeal, diaphyseal, and tuft fractures being the most common involving the distal phalanx.

Phalangeal fractures often occur as a result of a crush injury, such as a door closing onto a finger, or a direct blow. These fractures are often complicated by nail bed and soft tissue injuries, including lacerations, which are considered open fractures. Other mechanisms of injury include hyperflexion resulting in a mallet finger deformity due to avulsion fracture of the physis of the distal phalanx and inability to extend the distal finger. Abduction injuries can cause physeal finger fractures.

Evaluation for phalangeal fractures requires examination of the nail bed, tendon function, and rotational alignment. All patients should be asked to flex their fingers to assess for angular or rotational deformity. Normally, the fingers should all point toward the scaphoid (Fig. 26.8).

Anteroposterior and lateral views of the affected finger are required at minimum for diagnosis. Look for evidence of a Seymour fracture, which is an open physeal fracture of the distal phalanx with possible involvement of the nail matrix. Middle and proximal phalangeal fractures usually occur at the physis and are Salter-Harris type II fractures.

Physeal injuries of the proximal and middle phalanx are treated with cast immobilization. Mallet finger distal phalanx fractures are

managed by splinting the affected digit in extension for 6 weeks. Any malrotation or angular deformity requires closed reduction. Any open fracture requires irrigation, nail bed repair, wound care, and finger splinting. The patient should receive prophylactic antibiotics and appropriate tetanus prophylaxis depending on immunization status.

Fractures with malrotation or angular deformity require reduction to avoid finger crossover and preserve hand function. Seymour fractures are at higher risk for nail plate deformity and infection without surgical treatment.

LOWER EXTREMITY FRACTURES

Femur Fractures

Femur fractures occur commonly in children. The majority of femur fractures result from low-energy events, such as falls from playground equipment or sports-related injuries. These occur primarily in children aged 5 to 10 years old. Femur fractures in children younger than 2 years old should raise concern for nonaccidental trauma (Chapter 10). Femur fractures can also result from high-energy events such as motor vehicle collisions.

Because femur fractures can result in significant blood loss, the patient's hemodynamic status must be assessed and a thorough neurovascular evaluation should be performed. Immediate management consists of traction and splinting to minimize blood loss. Definitive management of femur fractures most often includes a period of hospitalization for skeletal traction followed by application of a spica body cast for younger children. Children older than 6 years of age and adolescents may require surgical intervention.

Tibia and Fibula Fractures

Tibial and fibular fractures are the most common fractures of the lower extremity in children. Both low-energy and high-energy traumatic events can cause these types of injuries.

Patients with lower leg injuries may present with pain, swelling, deformity, and inability to bear weight on the affected limb. Evaluation of these injuries includes performing a thorough neurovascular examination. Diagnosis is confirmed with radiographs. Most of these injuries can be managed with immobilization and orthopedic referral as long as the neurovascular status is normal. Orthopedic consultation is often indicated to determine whether emergent reduction is necessary. Patients with significant tibial and fibular fractures are also at risk for compartment syndrome, which mandates an emergent orthopedic consultation.

Ankle Fractures

Ankle fractures are among the most common fractures of the lower extremity in older children. Two types of ankle fractures, Tillaux and Triplane, occur in adolescents who are nearing skeletal maturity, usually between ages 11 to 15 years.

Ankle fractures typically result from inversion and eversion injuries. Children have stronger ankle ligaments, which makes injury to the distal tibial and fibular epiphysis more likely than ligamentous disruption. Because of the inherent weakness of the distal tibial epiphysis, fractures of the distal tibia are the most common ankle fracture. Examination reveals swelling, pain, and deformity of the ankle with limited ability to bear weight. Distal neurovascular examination is important to evaluate for signs of compartment syndrome.

Tillaux fracture is an avulsion fracture of the anterolateral tibial epiphysis due to forced external rotation of the foot (Fig. 26.9). This injury typically occurs with low-energy trauma such as skateboarding or baseball sliding injuries. Triplane fracture is a Salter-Harris type IV fracture with three fragments involving a break that

Fracture of tibia in children

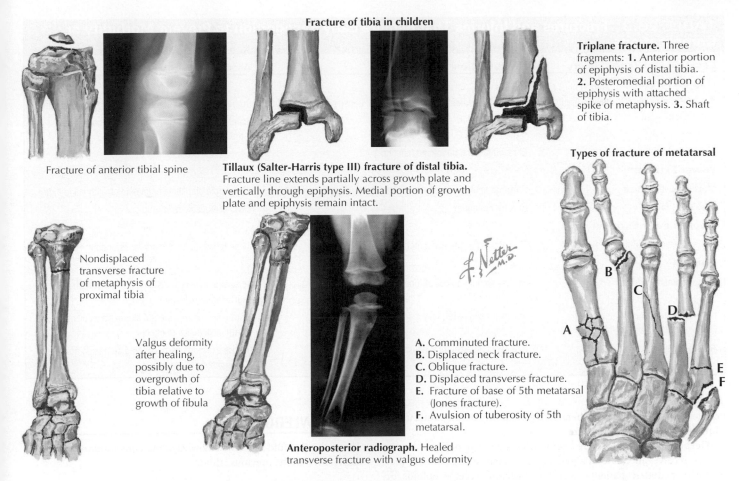

Fracture of anterior tibial spine

Tillaux (Salter-Harris type III) fracture of distal tibia. Fracture line extends partially across growth plate and vertically through epiphysis. Medial portion of growth plate and epiphysis remain intact.

Triplane fracture. Three fragments: **1.** Anterior portion of epiphysis of distal tibia. **2.** Posteromedial portion of epiphysis with attached spike of metaphysis. **3.** Shaft of tibia.

Types of fracture of metatarsal

Nondisplaced transverse fracture of metaphysis of proximal tibia

Valgus deformity after healing, possibly due to overgrowth of tibia relative to growth of fibula

A. Comminuted fracture.
B. Displaced neck fracture.
C. Oblique fracture.
D. Displaced transverse fracture.
E. Fracture of base of 5th metatarsal (Jones fracture).
F. Avulsion of tuberosity of 5th metatarsal.

Anteroposterior radiograph. Healed transverse fracture with valgus deformity

Fig. 26.9 Fractures of the Ankle and Foot.

extends through the transverse, sagittal, and coronal planes affecting the growth plate, epiphysis, and distal tibial metaphysis respectively (Fig. 26.9).

Examination of the entire length of the lower leg is important to evaluate for more proximal injury. Eversion ankle injuries may disrupt the tibiofibular syndesmosis, resulting in fracture of the proximal fibula, also known as a Maisonneuve fracture.

Radiography with anteroposterior, lateral, and mortise views can characterize ankle fractures. Include the knee joint if clinically indicated. Findings of Tillaux and Triplane fractures on plain radiography warrants cross-sectional imaging to better characterize fracture geometry and delineate displacement.

Fractures of the distal tibia and fibula without significant displacement require splinting followed by orthopedic referral for casting. Tillaux fractures are usually treated by closed reduction. Premature growth arrest, joint pain, and stiffness may be long-term sequelae of Triplane and Tillaux fractures.

Foot Fractures

Foot fractures involve injury to the metatarsals and phalanges. In children younger than 5 years, the first metatarsal is most commonly injured. In older children, fracture of the base of the fifth metatarsal is more common.

Metatarsal and toe fractures usually result from direct trauma, commonly when the patient is barefoot. Proximal avulsion fractures of the tuberosity at the base of the fifth metatarsal are usually associated with lateral ankle sprains. Any bleeding suggests the possibility of an open fracture. Evaluation requires anteroposterior, lateral, and oblique radiograph views of the foot.

Fractures of the lesser toes do not usually require closed reduction unless significantly displaced. Buddy taping of the fractured toe to an adjacent toe provides sufficient alignment and support. Nondisplaced metatarsal fractures can be treated with a closed below-knee cast, stiff-soled shoe, or boot. Jones fracture, a transverse fracture of the fifth metatarsal, although uncommon, is associated with a high rate of nonunion and need for bone grafting or internal fixation. It requires non–weight bearing in a short leg cast. Displaced metatarsal fractures generally require closed or open reduction with internal fixation. Table 26.3 provides a list of complications related to many fractures discussed previously.

FUTURE DIRECTIONS

Newer evidence indicates that simple torus fractures of the wrist can be safely treated with a removable brace in cooperative patients. No follow-up is required if the patient has normal, pain-free use of the extremity after immobilization. Future research may indicate similar, minimally restrictive types of immobilization devices can be employed successfully for other types of fractures.

The role of ultrasound in diagnosis of fractures also appears to be expanding. The lack of radiation exposure and point-of-care nature presents clear benefits for diagnostic purposes in pediatric fractures.

TABLE 26.3   Fractures and Injuries That Require Early Recognition to Prevent Morbidity or Complications

Location and Type of Injury	Complication	Assessment
Upper Extremity		
Brachial plexus injury in clavicle fracture	Residual weakness and sensory loss of upper extremity	Strength and sensation evaluation distal to fracture
Scaphoid fracture	Risk of nonunion	Scaphoid view imaging, clinical diagnosis with thumb immobilization
Malrotated phalangeal fracture	Crossed fingers, poor hand function	Closed hand evaluation
Lower Extremity		
Maisonneuve fracture	Proximal fibula fracture with tibiofibular ligamentous instability	Image tibia and fibula or knee joint with ankle injury
Jones fracture	Risk for nonunion	Close orthopedic follow-up
Upper/Lower Extremity		
Seymour fracture of fingers or toes	Nail bed deformity and infection	Close follow-up to monitor for infection
General		
Compartment syndrome	Muscle ischemia, loss of function or limb amputation	Assess neurovascular status and sensation, particularly forearm, lower leg
Nonaccidental trauma	Recurrent and potentially more severe injury	History and developmental stage are inconsistent with mechanism of injury
Appropriate cast sizing	Risk for compartment syndrome	Assess extremity perfusion and sensation after cast placement

Further research may better characterize the utility of diagnostic ultrasound for pediatric fracture care.

Despite the painful nature of fractures, pediatric patients do not always receive adequate analgesia. One recent study showed that minority pediatric patients were less likely to receive opioids or achieve optimal pain reduction. Health care providers must increase awareness of their own implicit biases and strive to standardize fracture care.

ACKNOWLEDGMENT

The authors would like to acknowledge the contribution of Monika Goyal, MD, to the previous edition.

SUGGESTED READINGS

Available online.

27

Pediatric Sports Medicine

Eric Pridgen and Melissa Hewson

 CLINICAL VIGNETTE

A 16-year-old girl presents to her pediatrician with 5 months of left knee pain and no known injury. She endorses anterior knee pain that is exacerbated by running, ascending and descending stairs, and squatting. She is a competitive dancer and started soccer last season. Recently she also has been complaining of stiffness in her left knee after prolonged periods of sitting. Her examination in clinic is notable for minimal tenderness over the patella exacerbated by squatting, and mild pes pronatus is noted. Conservative management is recommended with rest, ice, a short course of nonsteroidal antiinflammatory drugs, bracing, and return precautions are reviewed. However, 2 months later, she returns to clinic with persistent knee pain despite following recommendations. To rule out an alternative cause of knee pain, plain radiographs are ordered, which return normal. She is referred to physical therapy, which focuses on quadriceps and hip strengthening. After 3 months of physical therapy, the patient's father reports significant improvement in her pain and upcoming plans for a gradual return to sports.

This case represents a classic presentation of patellofemoral pain syndrome (PFPS), which is among the most common causes of adolescent anterior knee pain encountered in the outpatient setting. Physical therapy represents the most beneficial treatment option for patients with PFPS.

National surveillance of US youth sports participation estimates that nearly 6 in 10 high school students have participated in a sports activity. Participation in sports among children and adolescents could increase further because several recent national initiatives have focused on increasing participation, especially in the setting of obesity trends. In addition to the physical benefits of sports participation such as bone health, weight status, and cardiopulmonary fitness, there are psychosocial benefits, including improved confidence and self-esteem, reduced risk for depression, and improved cognitive functioning. However, participation in sports starting at the youth level also exposes participants to increased risk for injuries, some of which are unique to the pediatric population. In addition, recent trends in sports participation such as early specialization, increased competitiveness, and year-round participation without much diversity in the type of sports played, places participants at greater risk for both acute injuries and chronic overuse injuries. Many of these injuries initially present to primary care physicians who should be prepared to manage these injuries and counsel families on prevention, rehabilitation, and return to play. This chapter will provide a brief overview of common sports-related injuries.

PATHOGENESIS

The pediatric musculoskeletal system has several differences compared with that in adults that make them susceptible to different types of injuries. Pediatric bones are less brittle with thicker periosteum and a more robust blood supply. In addition, the physis (growth plate) at the ends of long bones is cartilaginous, making it more susceptible to injury than surrounding structures. Ligaments in children are stronger than bone, making avulsion fractures more common than ligamentous injuries. Bone also grows faster than muscle and tendons predisposing children to overuse injuries and tendinopathies. Fortunately, the increased blood supply and physis provide a greater capacity for remodeling and faster healing than in adults.

SHOULDER

The shoulder girdle is composed of three joints: the sternoclavicular joint, acromioclavicular (AC) joint, and the glenohumeral joint. The shoulder is the most mobile joint in the human body, but mobility comes at the expense of stability. The humeral head and the glenoid fossa can be thought of as a golf ball sitting on top of a tee (Fig. 27.1). With little bony support, the joint relies on the labrum, rotator cuff, and the long head of the biceps to provide dynamic stability. This puts the shoulder at increased risk for acute traumatic and chronic injuries in pediatric athletes.

Acromioclavicular Separation

AC joint separation, or shoulder separation, is a traumatic injury to the AC joint. The joint comprises the acromion and distal clavicle bones and is stabilized by the acromioclavicular and coracoclavicular ligaments. The injury is caused by a direct blow to the shoulder, usually sustained while falling. Patients present with pain localized to the AC joint and a visible change in contour of the shoulder relative to the contralateral side. Plain radiographs are necessary for diagnosis and to assess the degree of separation. Most separations are treated nonoperatively with sling immobilization, while the less common severe separations require surgical repair. Other injuries to consider in the differential with similar mechanism of injury include clavicle fractures, medial and lateral clavicle physeal injuries, and sternoclavicular joint separations.

Shoulder Dislocation

Traumatic anterior shoulder dislocations are one of the most common shoulder injuries. It is typically caused by an anteriorly directed force on the arm while the shoulder is abducted and externally rotated, such as falling on an outstretched hand or making contact with another player. Patients often complain of a popping sensation, and examination reveals shoulder deformity and limited range of motion with pain. Initial evaluation should include a thorough neurovascular examination, particularly of the axillary and musculocutaneous nerves. An acute shoulder dislocation is an orthopedic emergency and requires closed reduction. Traction-countertraction and the Stimson maneuver are the most common techniques for closed reduction and should be

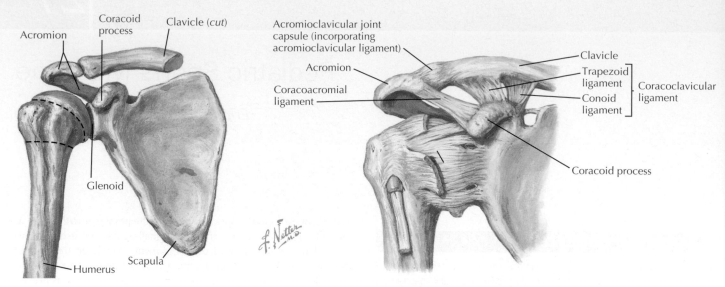

Fig. 27.1 Anterior View Scapula and Proximal Humerus.

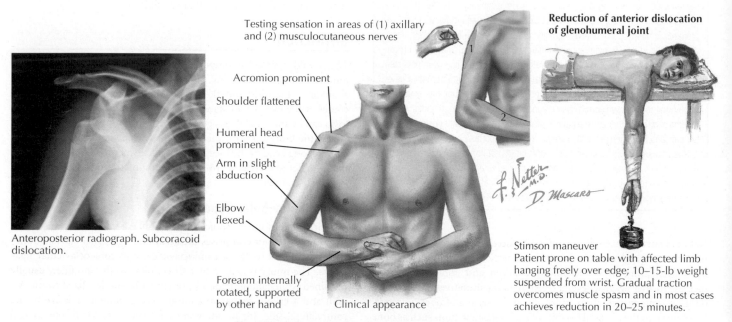

Anteroposterior radiograph. Subcoracoid dislocation.

Testing sensation in areas of (1) axillary and (2) musculocutaneous nerves

Acromion prominent

Shoulder flattened

Humeral head prominent

Arm in slight abduction

Elbow flexed

Forearm internally rotated, supported by other hand

Clinical appearance

Reduction of anterior dislocation of glenohumeral joint

Stimson maneuver
Patient prone on table with affected limb hanging freely over edge; 10–15-lb weight suspended from wrist. Gradual traction overcomes muscle spasm and in most cases achieves reduction in 20–25 minutes.

Fig. 27.2 Anterior Dislocation of Glenohumeral Joint.

followed by a repeat neurovascular examination (Fig. 27.2). Patients can be managed in a sling for 1 week, followed by gradual increases in range-of-motion activities. Patients with a traumatic anterior shoulder dislocation who are younger than 20 years of age have a 90% chance of recurrence. Patients with persistent pain, feelings of instability, or subsequent subluxations/dislocations warrant magnetic resonance imaging (MRI) to evaluate for labral and rotator cuff tears, glenoid fractures, and humeral head impaction injuries.

Little League Shoulder

"Little League shoulder" is an overuse injury seen in skeletally immature overhead athletes resulting in injury to the proximal humerus physis. Patients, often pitchers, present with pain over the lateral proximal humerus. Plain radiographs may show widening of the proximal humerus physis, although they also may be normal. Treatment is rest from throwing for 3 months followed by physical therapy and a progressive throwing program once symptoms resolve.

ELBOW

The elbow joint comprises the humerus, ulna, and radius bones. Articulations between these bones allow for flexion and extension of the elbow, as well as supination and pronation. Medial and lateral collateral ligaments (i.e., the MCL and LCL) provide stability to varus and valgus stresses. Many of the flexor and extensor muscles of the wrist and hand originate at the elbow.

Elbow Dislocation

Pediatric elbow dislocations account for 3% to 6% of all elbow injuries and are most common in 10- to 15-year-old children. They are typically posterior because of the relatively small coronoid process in children (Fig. 27.3). The mechanism is usually hyperextension with valgus stress while the forearm is supinated, typically sustained when falling backward on an outstretched hand. Patients present with pain and swelling at the elbow with limited range of motion and obvious

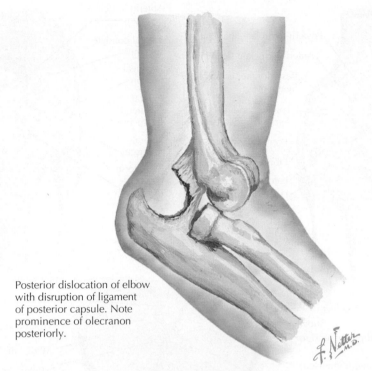

Posterior dislocation of elbow with disruption of ligament of posterior capsule. Note prominence of olecranon posteriorly.

Fig. 27.3 Elbow Dislocation.

deformity. A thorough neurovascular examination is critical to evaluate for brachial artery, median, and ulnar nerve injuries. Plain radiographs are necessary to determine the direction of dislocation and associated fractures. In particular, medial epicondyle avulsion fractures are commonly seen and may necessitate surgical intervention. Treatment is closed reduction and brief sling immobilization for 1 to 2 weeks.

Little League Elbow

"Little League elbow" is an overuse injury seen in adolescent overhead athletes, particularly in throwing sports, that encompasses a range of medial elbow injuries, including medial epicondyle stress fractures, MCL injuries, and forearm flexor-pronator muscle strains. Patients present with medial elbow pain, pain with valgus stress of the elbow, possible instability, and decreased sport performance. Plain radiographs might show avulsion of the medial epicondyle, but if there is clinical suspicion, MRI can visualize stress fractures, MCL injuries, and muscle strains. Most patients respond to rest followed by activity modification with limited pitch counts. For fractures or elbow instability because of MCL injuries, surgical intervention may be necessary.

Lateral Epicondylitis

Lateral epicondylitis or "tennis elbow" is an overuse injury resulting from repetitive wrist extension as seen in tennis players and is due to overload of the wrist extensors that originate at the lateral epicondyle of the humerus. Patients present with pain over the lateral elbow with resisted wrist extension and decreased grip strength. Most patients improve with rest and activity modification.

Osteochondritis Dissecans of the Elbow

Osteochondritis dissecans (OCD) lesions of the elbow are injuries to the articular cartilage and underlying subchondral bone typically seen in adolescent athletes participating in upper extremity weight-bearing activities such as gymnastics. The lesions typically occur on the capitellum and are thought to be due to repetitive compression. Patients present with insidious elbow pain and sometimes loss of elbow extension and catching or locking if loose bodies are present in the joint. Lesions may present on plain radiographs, but MRI is more useful for assessing the size of lesion, extent of involvement of the cartilage and bone, and presence of loose bodies. Treatment ranges from rest with gradual return to play for stable lesions to arthroscopic surgery.

HIP

The hip joint is a ball-and-socket joint providing articulation between the femur and acetabulum. However, the muscles associated with hip flexion, extension, abduction, and adduction originate from the pelvis. Forces through the femur can reach three to five times the body's weight during running and jumping activities. In high school athletes, hip injuries account for 5% to 10% of all sports injuries. They consist of acute injuries such as avulsion fractures or muscle strains and chronic overuse injures such as stress fractures.

Avulsion Injuries

Avulsion injuries of the hip and pelvis are due to apophyseal avulsions that occur with strong muscle contractions causing a disruption in the tendon's origin. They are typically seen in sports activities with explosive movements such as jumping, sprinting, and kicking. Common sites of injury include ischial avulsions resulting from hamstring and adductor contractions, anterior inferior iliac spine avulsions resulting from rectus femoris contractions, and anterior superior iliac spine avulsions resulting from sartorius contractions. Patients present with pain with palpation of the site of injury. Most injuries are seen on plain radiographs. Treatment is protected weight bearing with gradual return to activity. Patients with significant displacement of the avulsion or elite athletes may need surgical intervention.

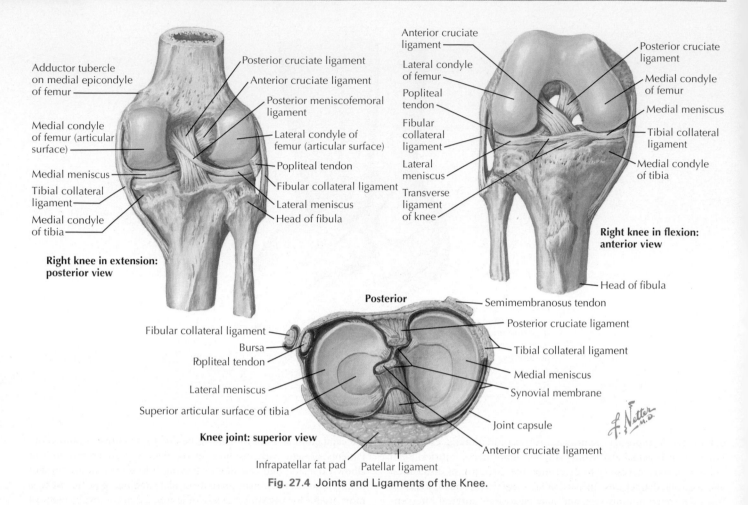

Fig. 27.4 Joints and Ligaments of the Knee.

Femoral Neck Stress Fractures

Stress fractures in the femoral neck are an overuse injury common in runners. Patients present with insidious onset of groin pain or anterior thigh pain worse with activity and associated with a change in training regimen. It is commonly associated with the "female athlete triad" so questions about menstrual cycle and diet must be included in the history for any females with a stress fracture. Plain radiographs are typically normal, so MRI is used to detect changes in the bone. For inferior neck stress fractures, conservative management consisting of non–weight bearing followed by activity modification may be appropriate depending on the extent. For superior neck stress fractures, operative management is necessary to avoid a complete femoral neck fracture.

KNEE

The knee is a common site of sports-related injuries. The knee joint comprises the femur, tibia, and patella bones. Articulations between the tibia and femur allow for flexion and extension of the knee. The patella is part of the extensor mechanism, which also includes the quadriceps muscles, quadriceps tendon, and patella tendon. Several ligaments contribute to knee stability, including the MCL, LCL, anterior cruciate ligament (ACL), and posterior cruciate ligament (PCL). The medial and lateral menisci provide stability and optimize force transmission across the knee (Fig. 27.4).

Anterior Cruciate Ligament Injuries

ACL ruptures are a common sports injury that occur in adolescent athletes, particularly females (4.5:1 ratio), participating in soccer, football,

skiing, and basketball. The mechanism is usually noncontact pivoting. Patients often feel a pop in the knee at the time of injury with immediate swelling because of hemarthrosis, instability, and limited range of motion as a result of pain. The most sensitive examination maneuver is the Lachman test. Plain radiographs are often normal, although a Segond fracture (avulsion of the lateral proximal tibia) is pathognomonic for an ACL tear. MRI is the best imaging modality to assess the integrity of the ACL and rule out other injuries, including meniscus tears, collateral ligament sprains, and chondral injuries. Treatment entails surgical reconstruction of the ACL. In pediatric athletes, it is also important to consider as part of the differential diagnoses tibial spine avulsion fractures that occur by the same mechanism with similar presentation. The fracture usually can be seen on plain radiographs, and treatment may be nonoperative versus operative based on the displacement of the fracture fragment.

Patella Instability

Patella dislocations in pediatric athletes occur when the patella dislocates, usually laterally out of the trochlear groove, from a direct blow to the knee or after a noncontact twisting injury with the knee extended and foot externally rotated. Most will reduce immediately when the player reacts by flexing the quadricep, but, if the patient presents dislocated, reduction should be performed promptly with the knee extended and hip flexed. Patients present with anterior knee pain, effusion from hemarthrosis, medial knee tenderness because of medial patellofemoral ligament (MPFL) disruption, and instability of the patella (Fig. 27.5). Plain radiographs can be used to assess for patellar dislocation and large loose bodies in the joint. MRI is more sensitive

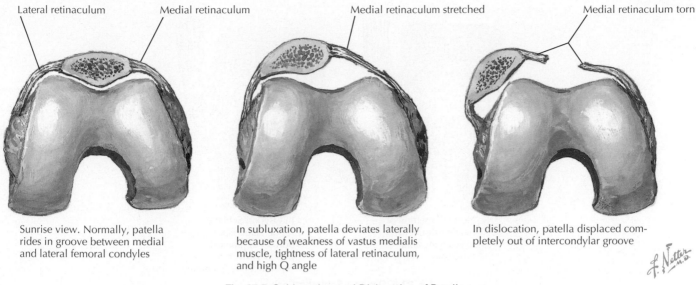

Lateral retinaculum   Medial retinaculum

Sunrise view. Normally, patella rides in groove between medial and lateral femoral condyles

Medial retinaculum stretched

In subluxation, patella deviates laterally because of weakness of vastus medialis muscle, tightness of lateral retinaculum, and high Q angle

Medial retinaculum torn

In dislocation, patella displaced completely out of intercondylar groove

Fig. 27.5 Subluxation and Dislocation of Patella.

to assess for MPFL disruption and osteochondral fractures that can occur when the patella reduces. If there is no history of dislocation and no loose bodies or articular damage, treatment entails immobilization followed by gradual increase in range of motion. Surgical intervention is appropriate if there are osteochondral fragments present or multiple dislocations.

Osteochondritis Dissecans of the Knee

Similar to OCD lesions of the elbow, these are lesions of the articular cartilage and subchondral bone. The knee is the most common location for OCD lesions, usually on the medial femoral condyle. The cause can be hereditary versus traumatic and results in cartilage loosening with eventual separation of chondral or osteochondral fragments. Younger patients with an open physis tend to have a better prognosis. Patients present with insidious knee pain with possible swelling and stiffness. Mechanical symptoms such as locking or catching likely indicate loose bodies in the joint. The lesions may be visible on plain radiographs, but MRI is much more useful for characterizing the size and location of the lesion, status of the cartilage and subchondral bone involvement, and presence of loose bodies. For stable lesions, patients can be treated with restricted weight bearing and for more advanced lesions, arthroscopic surgery is necessary.

Patellofemoral Pain Syndrome

PFPS is a common cause of anterior knee pain in adolescents. The cause is multifactorial and can include limb malalignment, muscle weakness, and patella malalignment. It tends to affect females more than males. Patients present with insidious anterior or generalized knee pain exacerbated by prolonged sitting (theater sign), squatting, kneeling, and ascending or descending stairs. Examination may show quadricep muscle weakness as well as patella maltracking. Plain radiographs can be used to rule out other causes of knee pain, but the diagnosis is often based on clinical assessment. Most patients respond to activity modification and physical therapy.

Osgood Schlatter Disease

Osgood Schlatter is an overuse traction apophysitis of the patella tendon insertion at the tibial tubercle. It is common in adolescent males, can be bilateral in up to 30% of patients, and is associated with explosive movements such as jumping and sprinting.

Patients present with anterior knee pain exacerbated by kneeling. Examination often reveals a prominent tibial tubercle with tenderness to palpation and pain with resisted knee extension (Fig. 27.6). Plain radiographs show irregularity or fragmentation of the tibial tubercle on the lateral view. The majority improve after conservative management with rest and activity modification. Straps or sleeves along with quadriceps stretching to decrease tension on the tibial tubercle may also help. Pain usually does not resolve entirely until after cessation of growth.

LEG, ANKLE, AND FOOT

Shin Splints

Shin splints are an overuse injury causing pain in the tibia. Typically seen in runners, risk factors include sudden increases in training, improper shock absorption on cement, running more than 20 miles per week, and hill training. Patients present with vague diffuse pain over the tibia and on examination typically have tenderness to palpation of the tibia and pain with resisted foot plantarflexion. Plain radiographs will exclude stress fractures, but bone scan or MRI may be necessary for definitive diagnosis. Treatment entails activity modification and physical therapy. Differential diagnoses should include tibial stress fractures and exertional compartment syndrome. Shin splints are also associated with the female athlete triad, which places patients at increased risk for progression to stress fractures.

Ankle Sprains

Ankle injuries are extremely common in athletes. Although these injuries are usually ankle sprains, physeal fractures are actually more common in pediatric patients than sprains. The mechanism is variable, but ankle inversion is most common. Patients present with either localized or general ankle pain with weight bearing. Swelling and ecchymosis also may be present. The anterior drawer test and talar tilt test can be used to assess the most commonly injured ligaments (anterior talofibular ligament and calcaneofibular ligament). Plain radiographs are helpful to assess for fractures, but physeal fractures may not be visible. Treatment includes immobilization followed by early functional rehabilitation to allow for return to play.

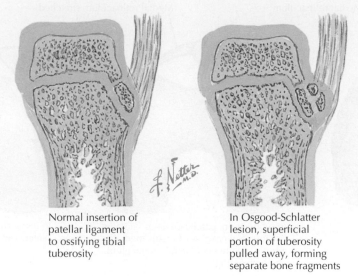

Normal insertion of
patellar ligament
to ossifying tibial
tuberosity

In Osgood-Schlatter
lesion, superficial
portion of tuberosity
pulled away, forming
separate bone fragments

Fig. 27.6 Osgood-Schlatter Lesion.

Sever Disease

Sever disease is an overuse injury affecting the calcaneal apophysis in adolescents causing heel pain. It is commonly seen in athletes of sports that require running and jumping. Patients present with pain over the posterior heel exacerbated by activity, and on examination demonstrate tenderness over the calcaneal apophysis with tight Achilles tendons. The diagnosis is clinical, so imaging would only allow rule out of other causes of heel pain such as fractures or bone cysts. Treatment is rest, activity modification, stretching, and shoe modifications. Recurrence is common but tends to resolve with cessation of growth.

FUTURE DIRECTIONS

Future directions should focus on prevention of sports injury with attention to educating those involved in youth sports, including coaches, trainers, families, and patients. Physician education and experience in the realm of sports medicine should likewise be enhanced to ensure appropriate recognition and management of injuries.

SUGGESTED READINGS

Available online.

28

Osteomyelitis and Other Bone and Joint Infections

Brian W. Coburn and Sanjeev Swami

✳ CLINICAL VIGNETTE

A previously healthy 4-year-old boy presented to the emergency department (ED) with left knee pain for 7 days. He saw his primary care physician on day 3 of illness and reported mild leg trauma a week previously. He was instructed to take ibuprofen, which provided initial improvement in the pain. However, a few days later he was unable to walk so his parents took him to the ED. On evaluation, he had a fever to 103.1°F (39.5°C) and tenderness just proximal to the left patella. His white blood cell count was 17,000 cells/μL, his erythrocyte sedimentation rate (ESR) was 71 mm/h and his C-reactive protein (CRP) was 15 mg/dL. A blood culture was obtained. Magnetic resonance imaging showed left distal femur bone marrow edema and a small subperiosteal abscess without septic arthritis. His abscess was too small to drain, so he was started empirically on intravenous clindamycin. His fever and pain improved over the next 36 hours, and he was transitioned to oral clindamycin. His blood cultures remained negative, and his CRP was lower compared with the day of admission. He was discharged with 4 weeks of oral clindamycin and follow-up with an infectious disease doctor. He completed his antibiotic course successfully and had no recurrence or long-term consequences.

Over 50% of osteomyelitis cases will have a positive blood or bone culture that will guide therapy, and the remainder of cases are typically treated empirically for a bacterial infection. Empiric antibiotics should include treatment for methicillin-resistant *Staphylococcus aureus* (MRSA) in areas with high rates (>20%) of MRSA osteomyelitis. Concomitant septic arthritis should be considered in young (<5 years) patients and arthrocentesis pursued if clinical suspicion is high.

OSTEOMYELITIS

Osteomyelitis is a localized infection of the bone caused by microorganisms. In children, it is most often caused by hematogenous spread of bacteria to the bone, but can also be caused by trauma, surgery, or contiguous spread (Fig. 28.1). In high-income countries, approximately 7 to 13 per 100,000 children will develop osteomyelitis. Low-income and low to middle–income countries can have rates up to 10-fold greater. Males are affected twice as often as females, and the median age affected is 10 years, with 25% occurring in those younger than 5 years. Most cases occur at a single site. Untreated, osteomyelitis can acutely lead to sepsis and over the long term cause bone growth arrest and limb deformity.

Etiology and Pathogenesis

The most common cause of osteomyelitis is bacteria. The most common pathogen is *Staphylococcus aureus,* representing up to 65% of cases, and the second most common is *Streptococcus pyogenes* (see Fig. 28.1). Vaccination programs have nearly eliminated *Haemophilus influenzae* type b (Hib) osteomyelitis, and most cases of *Streptococcus pneumoniae* are now caused by nonvaccination serotypes.

The likelihood of infection with each pathogen depends on the patient's age and other risk factors. For children younger than 3 months of age, common causes include group B streptococci and gram-negative bacilli such as *Escherichia coli*. In children between 6 and 48 months, *Kingella kingae* is increasingly identified as the cause of osteomyelitis. It typically has a subacute presentation after an upper respiratory tract infection and is difficult to culture in the laboratory, making it a more challenging diagnosis. *Salmonella* species are more commonly isolated from patients with sickle cell disease. *Pseudomonas aeruginosa* has been reported in patients with puncture wounds of the foot through shoes. *Actinomyces* species are associated with facial osteomyelitis. *Bartonella henselae* is associated with cat exposure and multifocal disease involving the vertebrae and pelvis. *Mycobacterium tuberculosis* should be considered in patients with known high-risk exposures or time spent in higher risk regions.

Fungal causes of osteomyelitis are rare, but *Coccidioides* can be considered in endemic areas. *Aspergillus* also has been reported, especially in patients with chronic granulomatous disease.

Osteomyelitis is thought to be more common in children because of rich vascular supply at the metaphysis of long bones where slow blood flow occurs in the sinusoids (Fig. 28.2). Epidemiologic studies suggest minor preceding injuries may be associated with osteomyelitis. The injuries are thought to cause damage to the sinusoids, leading to microhematomas that act as a nidus for infection. As children age, the bone cortex and periosteum become thicker and metaphyseal capillaries atrophy, decreasing areas of slow blood flow. These changes limit the effect of minor injuries and extension of infections from the bone to nearby joint and soft tissue spaces.

Clinical Presentation

Most patients with osteomyelitis present with localized pain that developed within the preceding 2 weeks. Up to 50% will also have a fever or decreased use of the affected area. In neonates and young children, symptoms are less specific and include irritability, decreased appetite, or decreased activity. Systemic symptoms beyond fever are uncommon unless the patient also has sepsis. On physical examination, the patient will often have point tenderness over the affected area and may have limited range of motion of the joint(s) nearest the affected bone, although micromotion joint pain is uncommon unless there is concomitant septic arthritis. Swelling, erythema, and warmth may also be present.

The most common sites of acute hematogenous osteomyelitis are long tubular bones, with the femur being most common. Pelvic osteomyelitis pain tends to localize to the hip, gluteal region, groin, or lower abdomen. There is often point tenderness, but pain may be primarily

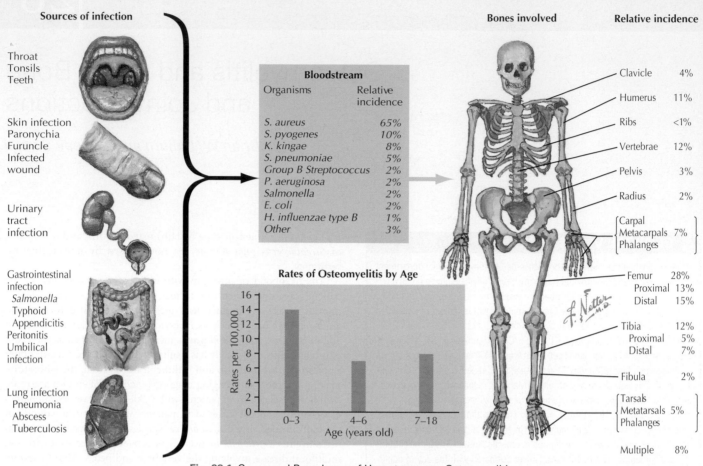

Sources of infection

Throat
Tonsils
Teeth

Skin infection
Paronychia
Furuncle
Infected
wound

Urinary
tract
infection

Gastrointestinal
infection
Salmonella
Typhoid
Appendicitis
Peritonitis
Umbilical
infection

Lung infection
Pneumonia
Abscess
Tuberculosis

Bloodstream	
Organisms	Relative incidence
S. aureus	65%
S. pyogenes	10%
K. kingae	8%
S. pneumoniae	5%
Group B Streptococcus	2%
P. aeruginosa	2%
Salmonella	2%
E. coli	2%
H. influenzae type B	1%
Other	3%

Rates of Osteomyelitis by Age

Bones involved   **Relative incidence**

Clavicle	4%
Humerus	11%
Ribs	<1%
Vertebrae	12%
Pelvis	3%
Radius	2%
Carpal Metacarpals Phalanges	7%
Femur	28%
Proximal	13%
Distal	15%
Tibia	12%
Proximal	5%
Distal	7%
Fibula	2%
Tarsals Metatarsals Phalanges	5%
Multiple	8%

Fig. 28.1 Cause and Prevalence of Hematogenous Osteomyelitis.

Terminal branches of
metaphyseal arteries form
loops at growth plate and
enter irregular afferent
venous sinusoids. Blood
flow slowed and turbulent,
predisposing to bacterial
seeding. In addition, lining
cells have little or no
phagocytic activity. Area is
catch basin for bacteria,
and abscess may form.

As abscess spreads, segment
of devitalized bone
(sequestrum) remains within
it. Elevated periosteum may
also lay down bone to form
encasing shell (involucrum).
Occasionally, abscess is
walled off by fibrosis and
bone sclerosis to form
Brodie abscess.

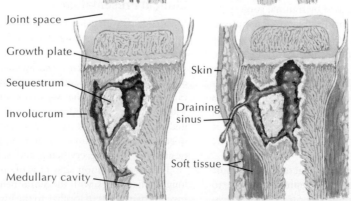

Epiphysis
Looped
capillaries
Venous
sinusoids
Abscess
Metaphyseal
arteries
Nutrient artery

Growth
plate
Periosteum

Joint space
Growth plate
Sequestrum
Involucrum
Medullary cavity

Skin
Draining
sinus
Soft tissue

Abscess, limited by growth plate,
spreads transversely along Volkmann
canals and elevates periosteum; extends
subperiosteally and may invade shaft. In
infants under 1 year of age, some
metaphyseal arterial branches pass
through growth plate, and infection
may invade epiphysis and joint.

Infectious process may erode
periosteum and form sinus
through soft tissues and
skin to drain externally. Process
influenced by virulence of
organism, resistance of host,
administration of antibiotics, and
fibrotic and sclerotic responses.

Fig. 28.2 Pathogenesis of Hematogenous Osteomyelitis.

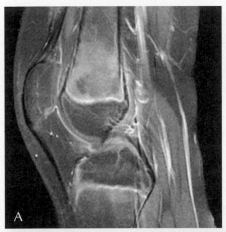

(A) Lateral T2-weighted MRI of distal femur with early acute osteomyelitis. 10-year-old female with progressive pain in left knee region and difficulty walking. Plain radiographs normal. MRI showed signal changes of distal femur metaphyseal region consistent with osteomyelitis.

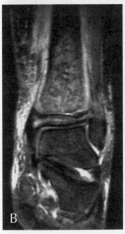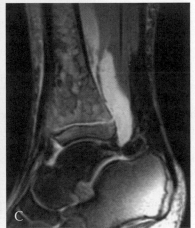

AP (B) and lateral (C) of T2-weighted MRI of the distal tibia with late acute osteomyelitis. Note the inflammatory changes in the distal tibia metaphysis, the signal changes beneath the elevated periosteum, and the large posterior abscess from pus breaking through the periosteum.

Fig. 28.3 Magnetic Resonance Imaging Findings in Early and Late Acute Osteomyelitis.

elicited with hip movement or walking, which makes distinction from septic arthritis challenging.

Vertebral osteomyelitis is similarly challenging because pain may be localized to the back, abdomen, or chest, and there may not be point tenderness over the involved vertebra.

Subacute osteomyelitis tends to manifest with intermittent pain or decreased use of the affected area and rarely with fever. Diagnosis is usually made because of recurrent presentations or progressive symptoms. Chronic osteomyelitis is characterized by a prolonged course of localized pain over months to years and may not resolve completely with antibiotics. Chronic recurrent multifocal osteomyelitis (also known as chronic nonbacterial osteomyelitis) is a sterile inflammatory process of the bone and beyond the scope of this chapter.

Diagnosis

Diagnosis typically begins with laboratory evaluation, which may show elevated white blood cell (WBC) count, erythrocyte sedimentation rate (ESR), and C-reactive protein (CRP). In 95% of cases either ESR or CRP will be elevated, but these are nonspecific findings and imaging is required before making a diagnosis. If ESR and CRP are normal, high clinical suspicion may lead to repeat testing in 2 days or proceeding directly to imaging. Radiographs are obtained first and are most useful to exclude other causes of focal pain such as fractures or tumors. Radiographs may show soft tissue swelling and/or periosteal

reaction 3 to 14 days after symptom onset but are frequently normal in patients with acute osteomyelitis. Magnetic resonance imaging (MRI), the preferred imaging modality, has a sensitivity of over 90%, avoids radiation, and best characterizes any extension of the infection to nearby structures, including the joint space (Fig. 28.3). Bone scintigraphy and computed tomography (CT) scans are less sensitive and specific than MRI. Ultrasound is not used because of poor sensitivity and specificity.

Cultures, drawn before antibiotics, can provide important information to guide antibiotic management. Tissue cultures may be pursued and have been shown to increase microbiologic identification relative to blood cultures alone. However, the relative cost and benefits of tissue cultures have not been well studied and patients generally have good outcomes on empiric antibiotics.

Management

Treatment of osteomyelitis includes empiric parenteral antibiotics and surgical intervention if indicated. Often blood cultures, imaging, and surgical intervention can be completed before starting empiric antibiotics. However, if a patient presents with concomitant sepsis, antibiotics should not be delayed. Empiric antibiotics for osteomyelitis require good bone penetration and are guided by the patient's age and risk factors, as well as local antibiotic resistance patterns. In most of the United States, clindamycin has replaced beta-lactams as empiric

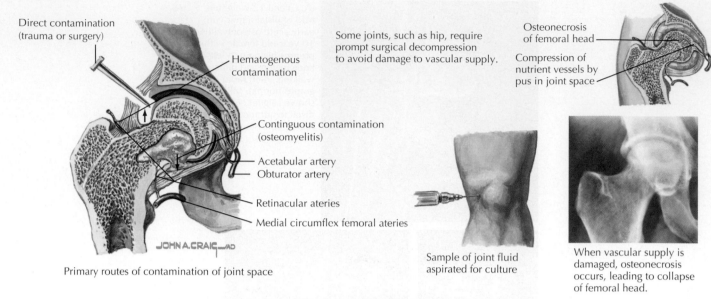

Direct contamination
(trauma or surgery)

Hematogenous
contamination

Some joints, such as hip, require
prompt surgical decompression
to avoid damage to vascular supply.

Osteonecrosis
of femoral head

Compression of
nutrient vessels by
pus in joint space

Continguous contamination
(osteomyelitis)

Acetabular artery
Obturator artery

Retinacular ateries

Medial circumflex femoral ateries

JOHN A. CRAIG___MD

Primary routes of contamination of joint space

Sample of joint fluid
aspirated for culture

When vascular supply is
damaged, osteonecrosis
occurs, leading to collapse
of femoral head.

Fig. 28.4 Septic Arthritis.

therapy because of high rates of MRSA infections. Patients in areas with high rates of clindamycin resistance or with severe infections should initially receive vancomycin.

Among neonates, empiric therapy should cover for group B streptococci and enteric gram-negative rods in addition to MRSA if indicated by screening results or local epidemiology. Empiric monotherapy with an intravenous third-generation cephalosporin is appropriate if MRSA is not suspected. For children 3 years and younger with concern only for *K. kingae*, empiric therapy includes penicillin, ampicillin, or a cephalosporin. If *S. aureus, S. pyogenes,* and *K. kingae* are all considerations, management options include (1) combined coverage with vancomycin or clindamycin and an agent active against *K. kingae*; (2) starting vancomycin or clindamycin before adding *K. kingae* coverage if cultures provide no guidance after 24 hours or the child fails to improve; or (3) cefazolin as empiric monotherapy for subacute presentations when MRSA is not suspected (MRSA coverage should be added if the patient worsens or fails to improve).

Good clinical outcomes have been demonstrated with conversion from parenteral to oral antibiotics once the patient is afebrile and has shown clinical improvement. Transition to oral antibiotics should be guided by culture results if available. Over two-thirds of patients convert to oral antibiotics by day 4. Typical dosing of oral antibiotics for osteomyelitis is higher than for most other infections. Repeat laboratory testing can be guided by clinical response, with many patients needing only one or two additional tests if improving. Further antibiotic treatment should be considered at follow-up if inflammatory markers such as CRP or ESR remain elevated. Antibiotics are typically continued for 4 weeks. Shorter courses of 3 weeks have been successfully studied, but only in areas with low MRSA prevalence. Courses 6 weeks or longer may be necessary in severe cases of osteomyelitis. Home parenteral therapy can be considered in certain circumstances but is usually unnecessary and central line–associated complications limit prolonged parenteral therapy. Neonatal osteomyelitis is often treated with parenteral antibiotics for the entire course.

Surgical intervention should be considered in patients presenting with abscesses, necrotic bone, sinus tracts, or severe disease, including signs of sepsis. Prolonged symptoms, persistent inflammatory marker elevation, or persistent bacteremia despite appropriate antibiotic therapy are additional surgical indications. Complications of osteomyelitis

include adjacent septic arthritis, bone growth arrest, chronic osteomyelitis, and pathologic fractures.

Active areas of research include shortening antibiotic duration and the effect of antibiotic initiation before surgical intervention on tissue culture yield.

SEPTIC ARTHRITIS

Septic arthritis is a microbial infection, typically bacterial, of the joint space. It is less common than osteomyelitis, with an incidence of 3 to 8 cases per 100,000 children depending on age and study population. Most cases involve a single joint, and concomitant osteomyelitis occurs in less than 20% of cases. The incidence of septic arthritis decreases approximately 35% after 3 to 4 years of age and is twice as common among males than females.

Etiology and Pathogenesis

Two-thirds of patients with septic arthritis will have an organism identified on blood or synovial fluid cultures. Bacterial causes of septic arthritis have age and risk group profiles similar to those of osteomyelitis; *S. aureus* represents more than 50% of positive cultures. Additional organisms of interest for septic arthritis include *Neisseria gonorrhea* and *Neisseria meningitidis*. *N. gonorrhea* tends to occur in newborns and sexually active patients. *N. meningitidis* can cause a septic arthritis in association with disseminated disease, although it more frequently causes a reactive arthritis.

The pathogenesis of septic arthritis is typically by hematogenous spread (Fig. 28.4). Transient bacteremia can seed the synovium because of high blood flow around the synovium and the lack of synovial basement membrane. Direct inoculation by puncture wounds or direct extension from nearby infections such as osteomyelitis can also lead to septic arthritis. Extension from osteomyelitis to the joint is more often seen in hip and shoulder septic arthritis because of the intracapsular location of the proximal femur and humerus. This is most often seen in infants and toddlers.

Clinical Presentation

Septic arthritis is characterized by rapid onset of joint pain over hours to days. Older children often present with a limp, refusal to

TABLE 28.1	Differential Diagnosis for Osteomyelitis and Septic Arthritis	
Condition	**Typical Illness Description**	**Differential**
Appendicitis	Abdominal pain with psoas muscle irritation may result in pain with hip movement	O, SA
Bone contusion/fracture	History of injury with pain onset, afebrile	O
Bone infarction	Focal bone pain in a patient with a hemoglobinopathy	O
Bursitis	Bursa swelling without joint effusion	O, SA
Cellulitis	Erythematous skin, soft tissue swelling without joint effusion	O, SA
Gout	Intense pain, uncommon in children	O, SA
Hemarthrosis	History of trauma or hemophilia	SA
Juvenile idiopathic arthritis	Morning stiffness, subacute or chronic symptoms, rash, fever	SA
Legg-Calvé-Perthes disease	Hip pain, limp, insidious onset, afebrile	SA
Lyme disease	Large joint effusion, afebrile, knee most commonly involved, no micromotion tenderness	SA
Malignancy	Intermittent symptoms, not responsive to antibiotics, no effusion	O, SA
Nonaccidental trauma	Multiple injuries over time by history or on examination or imaging	O
Rheumatic fever	Small effusion, migratory arthritis	SA
Reactive arthritis	Small effusion, lower WBC count in synovial fluid	SA
Slipped capital femoral epiphysis	Limp because of hip pain in patient with obesity, afebrile	SA
Transient synovitis	Hip pain, afebrile, improvement with nonsteroidal antiinflammatory drugs	SA
Vitamin C deficiency	Food restriction, petechiae, bleeding, coiled hair	O

O, Osteomyelitis; *SA,* septic arthritis; *WBC,* white blood cell.

bear weight, or decreased use of the affected limb along with fever. Neonates and young infants may present with only fever and irritability or decreased activity. Approximately 75% of cases involve joints of the lower extremity with knees and hips being the most common. Hip septic arthritis may manifest as knee or thigh pain complicating localization. The joint symptoms are usually persistent and progressive over time. While typically monoarticular, polyarticular septic arthritis occurs in up to 10% of patients, typically neonates. In older children, polyarticular symptoms may indicate alternative diagnoses (Table 28.1).

On physical examination, the affected joint is often swollen and may have associated erythema and warmth. Movement of the affected joint is often limited by pain and swelling. Pain with small movements of the affected joint, called micromotion tenderness, should raise strong suspicion for septic arthritis. Patients with septic arthritis of the hip rarely have focal swelling, warmth, or erythema, but classically present with ipsilateral hip and knee flexion and hip external rotation. Rashes may provide insight into possible infections such as *N. gonorrhea* or *N. meningitidis* or alternative diagnoses (see Table 28.1).

Diagnosis

Definitive diagnosis requires joint aspiration, which should not be delayed when septic arthritis is suspected (see Fig. 28.4). Initial workup should include WBC, ESR, CRP, blood culture, and synovial fluid studies from the joint aspiration. The synovial fluid is typically cloudy, with a WBC count greater than 50,000 cells/μL with a neutrophil predominance and may have bacteria on Gram stain. However, the synovial fluid WBC count is nonspecific and has been reported as low as 20,000 cells/mcL. Juvenile idiopathic arthritis (JIA) and Lyme arthritis can have similarly elevated synovial fluid WBCs, so serologic testing for JIA and Lyme disease may be useful in patients with the appropriate clinical presentation.

Ultrasound is often useful to assess for joint effusions and guide arthrocentesis. Plain radiographs may show joint capsule swelling and are useful in ruling out fractures or nonaccidental trauma. MRI is useful to assess for deep joint infections or associated osteomyelitis.

Management

Treatment of septic arthritis is focused on drainage of the infected synovial fluid and antibiotic therapy. Large joints may require arthrotomy and washout in the operating room, although repeat needle aspiration may provide similar benefits in some scenarios. Concomitant osteomyelitis usually requires arthrotomy for full evaluation and debridement. Rapid decompression is critical, especially in hip and shoulder septic arthritis, to prevent vascular compromise and subsequent avascular necrosis of the femoral or humeral head.

Empiric parenteral antibiotics should be started in patients with a strong suspicion for septic arthritis and should be started if the diagnostic arthrocentesis is delayed. Antibiotic selection is guided by the patient's age, MRSA history, personal risk factors, and local antibiotic resistance profiles. Vancomycin should be started if gram-positive cocci are observed on Gram stain, and a third-generation cephalosporin can be started if gram-negative rods or no organisms are identified. Otherwise, cefazolin or clindamycin are reasonable empiric options depending on local MRSA rates. Neonates are typically treated with cefotaxime, and vancomycin is added if MRSA is suspected. Sexually active adolescents with concern for *N. gonorrhea* are treated with ceftriaxone or cefotaxime. Transition to oral therapy can occur when there is clinical improvement, which may require up to 7 days. In patients responding to therapy, the duration of antibiotics depends on the implicated organism and joint involved with a typical duration of 3 weeks, although successful shorter courses have been reported.

Long-term complications are more common in septic arthritis than osteomyelitis. Rates have decreased over time, with less than 10% of patients having long-term sequelae, including chronic pain, avascular necrosis, and decreased range of motion (Fig. 28.5). Complications are more common if the hip is involved, treatment is delayed, the patient is younger than 1 year, or the infection is caused by *S. aureus.*

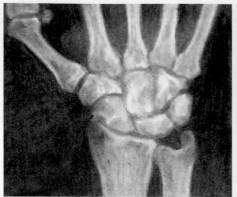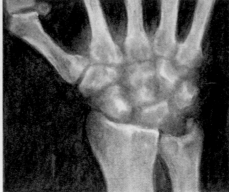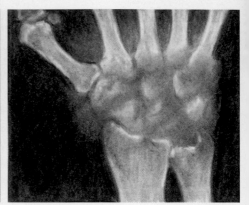

Rapid progression of wrist involvement within 4 weeks, from almost normal (left)
to advanced destruction of articular cartilages and severe osteoporosis (right)

Fig. 28.5 Septic Arthritis: Imaging.

Active areas of research include the shorter treatment courses and strategies to reduce the need for surgical drainage.

DISCITIS

Discitis is caused by inflammation of the intervertebral disk space and is often caused by bacteria. Discitis is much less common than long bone osteomyelitis or septic arthritis, but more common than vertebral osteomyelitis. Discitis tends to affect the lumbar spine and is more common in children younger than 5 years of age.

Patients typically present with subacute symptoms for 2 weeks or longer. Symptoms include irritability, back pain, abdominal pain, limp, or refusal to walk or crawl. Fever is uncommon. On physical examination, patients may have pain with spine or hip flexion, or with percussion of the vertebrae. The WBC may be elevated, and ESR is mildly elevated in more than 90% of patients. Blood cultures are often negative, and tissue cultures are rarely obtained. Given the late presentation of most patients, plain radiographs will often show narrowing of the affected intervertebral space. MRI provides a more definitive diagnosis and rules out other causes of back pain. Empiric antibiotics should provide coverage for *S. aureus* and *K. kingae*, two of the most commonly identified organisms in patients with discitis. Duration of therapy is not well defined. Spine immobilization or bracing, bedrest, and antiinflammatory medications are helpful to control symptoms while assessing response to empiric antibiotics.

SUGGESTED READINGS

Available online.

Cardiology

Matthew Elias

29

Development of the Cardiovascular System

Morgann Loaec and Meghan K. Metcalf

 CLINICAL VIGNETTE

A baby is born by normal spontaneous vaginal delivery at 39 weeks after an uncomplicated pregnancy. The newborn's mother received full prenatal care. At several hours of life, the newborn is noted to be tachypneic. The oxygen saturation in the right upper extremity reveals a saturation of 90%. The remainder of the vital signs are appropriate for age. On examination, the lungs are clear to auscultation and there are no audible murmurs. The abdominal examination is normal without hepatomegaly, and femoral pulses are easily palpable bilaterally. A chest radiograph is performed and demonstrates clear lungs. Further evaluation reveals a blood pressure of 74/38 mm Hg in the right arm and 82/40 mm Hg in the right leg. The pulse oximeter, when placed on the right foot, reveals an oxygen saturation of 81%. An echocardiogram is performed and reveals mild tricuspid regurgitation, a flattened ventricular septum indicative of elevated right heart pressures, and a persistent ductus arteriosus with bidirectional shunting. A diagnosis of persistent pulmonary hypertension of the newborn is made. The patient is placed on 100% FiO_2 by nasal cannula. After a few days, supplemental oxygen is gradually weaned and a repeat echocardiogram demonstrates improved right heart pressures and closure of the ductus arteriosus.

The scope of newborn cardiac disease ranges from the failure to transition appropriately from normal fetal to normal newborn cardiac physiology, to severe malformations of cardiac structures. A full understanding of the embryologic development of the cardiovascular system allows for a better understanding of the physiologic consequences that the newborn and children may face when normal cardiac development or transitions fail.

Knowing the steps involved in the embryologic development of the heart and great vessels can provide a greater understanding of the major congenital anomalies of the cardiovascular system. Furthermore, an understanding of fetal circulation and how this circulation transitions in the perinatal period can allow for a greater anticipation of the needs of a newborn with cardiac disease. This chapter focuses on the embryologic development of the heart and its relationship to fetal and newborn physiology. The formation of the cardiovascular system begins early in embryologic development, and the heart is fully formed and functioning by 8 weeks gestation. Any disruption in this development, whether genetic or environmental, can lead to the development of congenital heart disease. This section describes the process that transforms the primitive heart tube into a four-chambered organ with defined outflow tracts and major vessels and will cover the following major topics:

- Development of the heart tube and derivatives of its major sections
- Folding of the heart tube
- Division of the atrioventricular (AV) junction
- Septation of the atria and ventricles
- Development of the outflow tracts and major vessels
- Development of the conduction system and coronary vessels
- Fetal circulation
- Postnatal transitions of the cardiovascular system

HEART TUBE FORMATION

Cardiac development begins with gastrulation, the formation of the three germ layers, including ectoderm, endoderm, and mesoderm. The splanchnic mesoderm gives rise to the cardiogenic fields, which fuse in the midline to form the cardiac crescent and then further into the primitive heart tube by around 20 days of development. As depicted in Fig. 29.1, the heart tube undergoes a series of segmentations and folds, which give rise to the known structures of the adult heart, a process known as *looping*. The heart tube segments from the cranial to the caudal end include the truncus arteriosus, which gives rise to the ascending aorta and the pulmonary trunk; the bulbus cordis, which primarily gives rise to the right ventricle; the primitive ventricle, which primarily creates the left ventricle; the primitive atrium, which gives rise to both atria; and, finally, the sinus venosus, which contributes to the coronary sinus and the right atrium.

Folding of the Heart Tube

The major step that allows the primitive heart tube to form into a four-chambered heart is the process of cardiac looping occurring between days 23 and 28 of development. The cranial end of the heart tube, including the truncus arteriosus and primitive ventricle, folds caudally, ventrally, and slightly to the right. This folding creates the normal D-loop configuration of the heart, which describes the orientation of the morphologic right ventricle compared with the morphologic left ventricle. Failure of this first stage results in an abnormal L-loop in which the morphologic right ventricle is positioned to the left of the morphologic left ventricle. This defect can be seen commonly in dextrocardia and in a number of complex congenital heart defects in which the position of the ventricles is inverted. This looping brings the common atrium dorsal and cranial to the ventricles, and the bulbus cordis occupies the sulcus between the developing right and left atria, where it will begin to form the outflow tract of both ventricles. Around day 27 of development, this folding creates the first appearance of the recognizable four-chambered heart. Fig. 29.2 depicts the relationship of the heart tube structures at the end of folding and highlights the major divisions giving rise to the AV junction and outflow tracts, which will be discussed further.

Division of the Atrioventricular Junction

Once looping of the cardiac tube positions the atria and ventricles, endocardial cushion tissue begins to form and merge at the AV junction. A superior and inferior cushion meet to divide the right and left sides of the common AV canal. Errors in this fusion give rise to a wide range of common AV canal congenital defects seen commonly in association with trisomy 21.

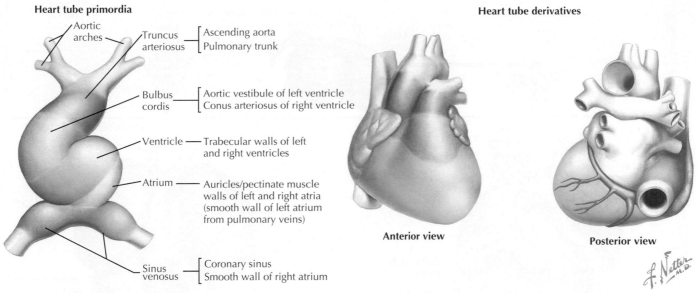

Fig. 29.1 Fate Map of Looped Heart Tube.

Septation of the Atrium and Ventricle

The position of the bulbus cordis in the sulcus of the atrium begins the process of atrial septation. A thin membrane-like structure called the septum primum separates the right and left side of the atrium while growing to meet the endocardial cushion tissue at the AV junction. As septum primum septates the atria and attaches to the endocardial cushions, the connection between the atria created by this diminishing gap (ostium primum) is closed. Perforation in the septum primum though provides a connection between the atria called the ostium secundum. The septum secundum then begins to form from an infolding of the atrial wall, forming a more muscular division. The septum primum decreases in size, with a small remnant remaining near the ostium secundum, creating a flap valve for the foramen ovale.

Septation also occurs between the right and left ventricles starting with the formation of the muscular portion of the septum. The process continues with the formation of the infundibular septum, which separates the right and left ventricular outflow tracts, and finally with closure of the membranous ventricular septum.

Fig. 29.3 highlights the stages of septation occurring among the atria, ventricles, and AV canal, giving rise to the four-chambered heart. Defects can occur in this process leaving septal defects between the atria or the ventricles. The most common form of an atrial septal defect, the secundum atrial septal defect, occurs as a result of a defect in septum primum.

Development of the Ventricular Outflow Tracts

The bulbus cordis must rotate and divide to bring the aortic outflow tract into position with the morphologic left ventricle and the pulmonary artery with the morphologic right ventricle (Fig. 29.4). This process is not completely understood, but migration of neural crest cells is thought to be an integral part of this division. Many major congenital heart defects, including tetralogy of Fallot, common truncus arteriosus, and interrupted aortic arch, can develop from a failure of this process.

Development of the Major Vessels

The truncus arteriosus divides to form the proximal portion of the great arteries and pairs with embryonic aortic arch remnants, which form the distal portions. Abnormalities in this stage may result in coarctation of the aorta, double aortic arch, or right-sided aortic arch. The systemic venous return develops from the sinus venosus, which grows asymmetrically favoring the right-sided portion of the common atria and becomes incorporated within the right atrium. This structure gives rise to the superior and inferior venae cavae and the coronary sinus. A single pulmonary vein then develops from the left atrium and meets with veins growing from the primitive lung. Failure of these veins to grow into the left atrium result in anomalous pulmonary venous return.

Development of the Conduction System and Coronary Vessels

The primitive heart tube already demonstrates peristaltic movements that can be detected as a heartbeat as early as day 22 of development. As the heart loops into its four-chamber system, myocardial cells differentiate into specific conduction myocardial cells. The genes responsible for this differentiation are of great interest in understanding arrhythmia conditions and are not completely characterized. The coronary vessels form late in the development of the heart once the myocardium has become covered by epicardium, which form an ingrowth of cells that give rise to the coronary vessels. After this development of the coronary vessels, the embryonic heart now is recognizable as the four-chambered fetal heart.

FETAL CIRCULATION

In fetal life, the source of oxygenated blood is the placenta, rather than the fetal lungs. Three structures present in the fetus serve to direct this oxygenated blood to vital organs: the ductus venosus, the foramen ovale, and the ductus arteriosus (Fig. 29.5). Oxygenated blood leaves the placenta through the umbilical vein. A large proportion of this blood passes through the liver by the ductus venosus and joins the inferior vena cava before entering the right atrium, and the remainder perfuses the liver and then enters the right atrium by way of the hepatic veins. From the right atrium, oxygenated blood from the ductus venosus is streamed through the foramen ovale to the left atrium, through the mitral valve to the left ventricle, and is then pumped through the aortic valve to the ascending aorta, where it supplies oxygen and nutrients to the coronary circulation and to the developing fetal brain by way of the head and neck vessels.

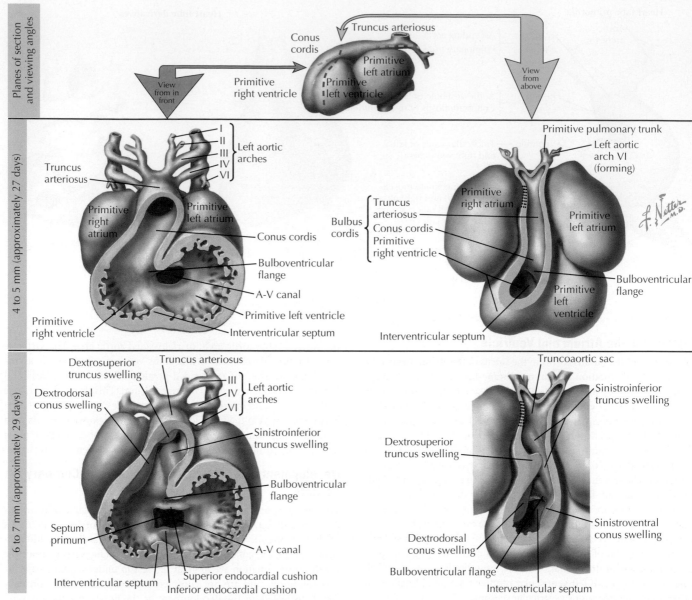

Fig. 29.2 Formation of Cardiac Septa and Structures.

Blood returns from the head and neck through the superior vena cava. Upon entering the right atrium, it combines with blood returning from the liver through the hepatic veins and passes to the right ventricle through the tricuspid valve and then to the pulmonary artery through the pulmonary valve. From the pulmonary artery, approximately 20% of blood flow is directed toward the lungs. The remainder is directed across the ductus arteriosus to the descending aorta, where it supplies the lower half of the body and the two umbilical arteries, which deliver blood back to the placenta.

As a result, the right and left ventricular outputs essentially run in parallel in the fetus. The right ventricular output is slightly larger than the left, which lends to a slightly larger and more hypertrophied right ventricle in the normal fetus.

The formation of fetal heart structures is completed early in gestation; however, the myocardium continues to grow by cell division until birth, after which growth is primarily through cell enlargement. Appropriate myocardial growth is influenced by genetic and molecular signaling as well as by environmental factors, such as blood flow through a structure, which is vital for ongoing normal development

throughout fetal life. For example, aortic stenosis may increase left heart pressures, resulting in decreased blood flow across the foramen ovale and into the left ventricle, resulting in left ventricular hypoplasia.

POSTNATAL TRANSITIONS AND NEONATAL CIRCULATION

After delivery, several transitions must occur for the fetal circulation to evolve and allow for normal neonatal cardiac physiology. These transitions may be disrupted by prematurity, congenital heart disease, perinatal hypoxia, or other stressors.

With the first breath postnatally, a newborn's pulmonary vascular resistance significantly decreases and there is increased blood flow to the lungs. Additionally, with clamping of the umbilical cord and disconnection of the placenta from the fetal circulation, the newborn's systemic vascular resistance rapidly increases. This increase in systemic vascular resistance combined with increased blood return from the lungs results in an increase in pressure in the left atrium, which causes septum primum to press up against septum secundum, effectively

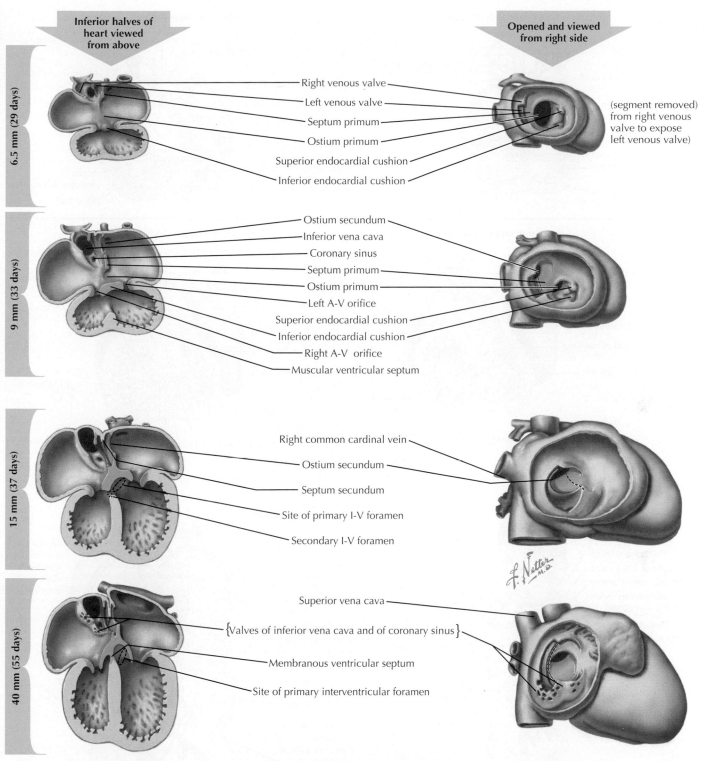

Inferior halves of heart viewed from above

Opened and viewed from right side

6.5 mm (29 days)

Right venous valve
Left venous valve
Septum primum
Ostium primum
Superior endocardial cushion
Inferior endocardial cushion

(segment removed) from right venous valve to expose left venous valve)

9 mm (33 days)

Ostium secundum
Inferior vena cava
Coronary sinus
Septum primum
Ostium primum
Left A-V orifice
Superior endocardial cushion
Inferior endocardial cushion
Right A-V orifice
Muscular ventricular septum

15 mm (37 days)

Right common cardinal vein
Ostium secundum
Septum secundum
Site of primary I-V foramen
Secondary I-V foramen

40 mm (55 days)

Superior vena cava
{Valves of inferior vena cava and of coronary sinus}
Membranous ventricular septum
Site of primary interventricular foramen

Fig. 29.3 Development of Cardiac Septa.

closing the foramen ovale. The foramen ovale will subsequently close anatomically in most; however, it is estimated that it remains open in 25% to 30% of the population. Although a patent foramen ovale is hemodynamically insignificant, it can be a mechanism for a paradoxical embolic stroke if a transient elevation of right atrial pressure leads to right-to-left shunting across it.

The ductus arteriosus is maintained in fetal life by endogenous prostaglandin production, which decreases after birth. In addition, increased oxygen tension leads to ductal constriction, and the ductus arteriosus will close in 90% of full-term infants within 2 to 3 days after birth. Prematurity is often associated with a patent ductus arteriosus, which may require medical or surgical closure because of hemodynamic consequences in the setting of significant left to right shunting and excessive pulmonary blood flow, which increases the risk for pulmonary vascular disease. Some forms of congenital heart disease, such as those with obstruction of pulmonary or systemic outflow, benefit

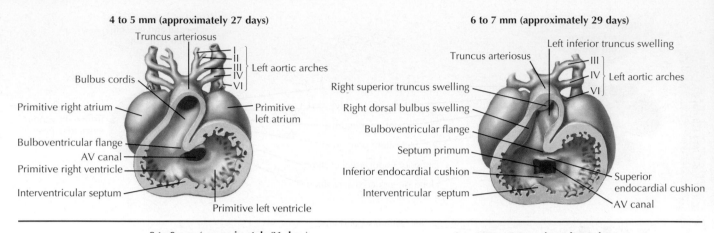

4 to 5 mm (approximately 27 days)

Truncus arteriosus

Left aortic arches (I, II, III, IV, VI)

Bulbus cordis

Primitive right atrium

Primitive left atrium

Bulboventricular flange

AV canal

Primitive right ventricle

Interventricular septum

Primitive left ventricle

6 to 7 mm (approximately 29 days)

Left inferior truncus swelling

Truncus arteriosus

Left aortic arches (III, IV, VI)

Right superior truncus swelling

Right dorsal bulbus swelling

Bulboventricular flange

Septum primum

Inferior endocardial cushion

Interventricular septum

Superior endocardial cushion

AV canal

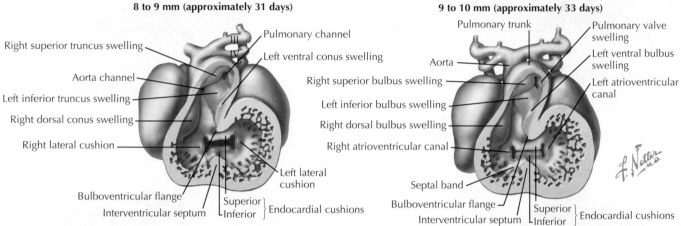

8 to 9 mm (approximately 31 days)

Right superior truncus swelling

Pulmonary channel

Left ventral conus swelling

Aorta channel

Left inferior truncus swelling

Right dorsal conus swelling

Right lateral cushion

Left lateral cushion

Bulboventricular flange

Interventricular septum

Superior / Inferior } Endocardial cushions

9 to 10 mm (approximately 33 days)

Pulmonary trunk

Pulmonary valve swelling

Aorta

Left ventral bulbus swelling

Right superior bulbus swelling

Left atrioventricular canal

Left inferior bulbus swelling

Right dorsal bulbus swelling

Right atrioventricular canal

Septal band

Bulboventricular flange

Interventricular septum

Superior / Inferior } Endocardial cushions

Fig. 29.4 Outflow Tract Septation.

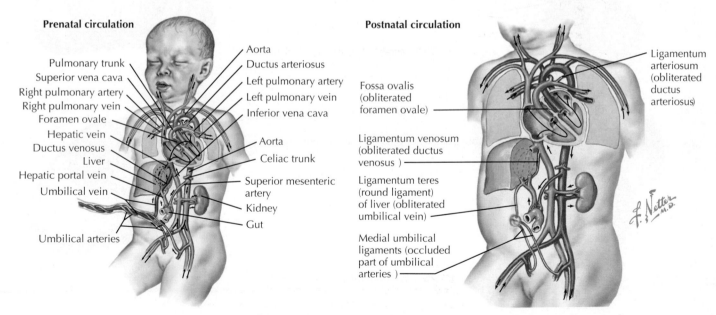

Prenatal circulation

Pulmonary trunk

Superior vena cava

Right pulmonary artery

Right pulmonary vein

Foramen ovale

Hepatic vein

Ductus venosus

Liver

Hepatic portal vein

Umbilical vein

Umbilical arteries

Aorta

Ductus arteriosus

Left pulmonary artery

Left pulmonary vein

Inferior vena cava

Aorta

Celiac trunk

Superior mesenteric artery

Kidney

Gut

Postnatal circulation

Fossa ovalis (obliterated foramen ovale)

Ligamentum venosum (obliterated ductus venosus)

Ligamentum teres (round ligament) of liver (obliterated umbilical vein)

Medial umbilical ligaments (occluded part of umbilical arteries)

Ligamentum arteriosum (obliterated ductus arteriosus)

Fig. 29.5 Prenatal and Postnatal Circulation.

from persistence of the ductus arteriosus, and in these cases ductal patency is maintained with prostaglandin infusion.

Finally, the ductus venosus usually closes 1 to 3 weeks after delivery, but this process may take longer in preterm infants. A specific trigger for closure of this vessel has not been identified.

Although there is a dramatic decrease in pulmonary vascular resistance with a newborn's first breath, it may take weeks to months for pulmonary pressures to decrease to normal. If pulmonary pressures remain significantly elevated after birth, persistent pulmonary hypertension of the newborn may be diagnosed, which is a condition seen in term infants, particularly in those with meconium aspiration syndrome.

FUTURE DIRECTIONS

Despite our current understanding of the development of the cardiovascular system, there are still many unknowns regarding the genetic and environmental factors that drive this normal process. Areas of future research include those focused on achieving a better understanding of the genes responsible for the migration of the neural crest cells needed for proper heart formation and how these are altered in congenital heart disease. By further understanding the development of the heart and the genetic factors involved, the management and outcomes of patients with congenital heart disease should only improve.

SUGGESTED READINGS

Available online.

30

Acyanotic Congenital Heart Disease

Aaron Briggs and Kathryn Restaino

 CLINICAL VIGNETTE

A 6-week-old boy presents to the primary care office for a well-child visit. He has lost 12% of his birth weight. He consumes 1 to 2 ounces every 3 hours over 45 minutes, stopping frequently to catch his breath. He is often diaphoretic with feeds and has no cyanosis. In the office, he is tachycardic and tachypneic with normal oxygen saturation. On examination, he has mild intercostal retractions, mild hepatomegaly, normal femoral pulses, and a harsh holosystolic murmur.

This baby is presenting with heart failure secondary to a large left-to-right shunt and pulmonary overcirculation from a ventricular septal defect. The baby should be referred urgently to a cardiologist for further evaluation, which would include an electrocardiogram, echocardiogram, and likely initiation of diuretics, depending on the final diagnosis.

Acyanotic heart lesions can be separated into two categories: shunt lesions and nonshunt lesions. Shunt lesions, such as ventricular septal defects (VSDs), allow oxygenated blood to bypass the systemic circulation and reenter the pulmonary circulation. Nonshunt lesions consist largely of valvular disease and aortic arch anomalies.

SHUNT LESIONS

Atrial Septal Defect

Atrial septal defects (ASDs) constitute 5% to 10% of all congenital heart defects and occur in approximately 1 in 1500 live births. There are five types of ASDs (Fig. 30.1). The most common type is the *ostium secundum ASD*, which results from a deficiency in septum primum, the thin membrane-like septum that normally closes the foramen ovale. The second most common type is the *ostium primum ASD*, which is a defect in the canal septum. This septum normally divides the common atrioventricular (AV) canal and in so doing creates the tricuspid and mitral valves. Defects in this septum result in AV canal defects, which are discussed later in this chapter. The third type is the *sinus venosus defect*, which is not a defect in the atrial septum but rather a communication between the two atria by way of a "straddling" venous structure, typically either the superior or inferior vena cava. These defects are frequently associated with partial anomalous drainage of the right-sided pulmonary veins. *Coronary sinus ASDs* are the fourth type and again are not true defects in the atrial septum but rather the physiologic consequence of a partially or completely unroofed coronary sinus with left atrial–to–right atrial drainage through the coronary sinus ostium. The fifth type of ASD is seen with *juxtaposition of the atrial appendages*. This defect is extremely rare and results from an absence or misplacement of septum secundum, which normally closes the foramen ovale.

Children with ASDs are usually asymptomatic unless the defect is very large. Cardiac auscultation reveals a systolic ejection murmur at the left upper sternal border from increased blood flow across the pulmonary valve and a fixed, widely split S_2 because of increased venous return to the right heart, leading to the pulmonary valve closing slightly later than the aortic valve. In larger ASDs, there may be a diastolic rumble of an increased amount of blood crossing the tricuspid valve. Electrocardiography (ECG) may show right axis deviation and right ventricular hypertrophy because of volume overload, often with an rSR′ pattern or right ventricular conduction delay. With a significant defect, cardiomegaly may be apparent on chest radiography. Echocardiography is used to confirm the diagnosis.

Management approaches to ASDs vary according to hemodynamic significance and likelihood of spontaneous closure. Small secundum ASDs are likely to close spontaneously during early childhood or remain hemodynamically insignificant. Larger secundum ASDs may become smaller, but if not, may require intervention if/when there is evidence of worsening right-sided volume overload or in the setting of symptoms. Secundum ASDs with well-defined margins are typically amenable to a device closure by cardiac catheterization (Fig. 30.2), but other secundum ASDs and the other forms of ASDs would still need surgical closure. If left untreated into adulthood, hemodynamically significant ASDs can lead to pulmonary hypertension, atrial arrhythmias, risk for stroke, and heart failure.

Ventricular Septal Defect

VSDs account for about 20% of all congenital heart disease and occur in 2 to 10 in 1000 live births. The ventricular septum consists of the inlet (canal septum) along the septal leaflet of the tricuspid valve; the infundibular, conal, or outlet septum superiorly; the muscular or trabecular septum; and the small, membranous septum at the junction of the other three (Fig. 30.3). There are five types of VSDs that result from defects in or between these various components of the ventricular septum.

The most common type of VSD is the *conoventricular VSD*, which is a defect between the conal or infundibular septum and the rest of the ventricular septum. A conoventricular VSD is sometimes referred to as a perimembranous VSD because it may include the membranous septum. These VSDs can be partially closed by tissue from the tricuspid valve leaflets, and many defects become smaller with time. Aortic regurgitation may occur because of prolapse of an aortic valve cusp into the VSD. *Canal-type* or *inlet defects* are usually seen in common AV canal defects (described in more detail later) and occur from absence of the inlet septum; they extend along the full length of the AV valve. *Malalignment* and *conal septal hypoplasia* defects occur as a result of malalignment or absence of the conal or infundibular septum, respectively. Anterior malalignment defects are seen in patients with tetralogy of Fallot (Chapter 31). Posterior malalignment defects are often seen in patients with hypoplastic aortic valves and

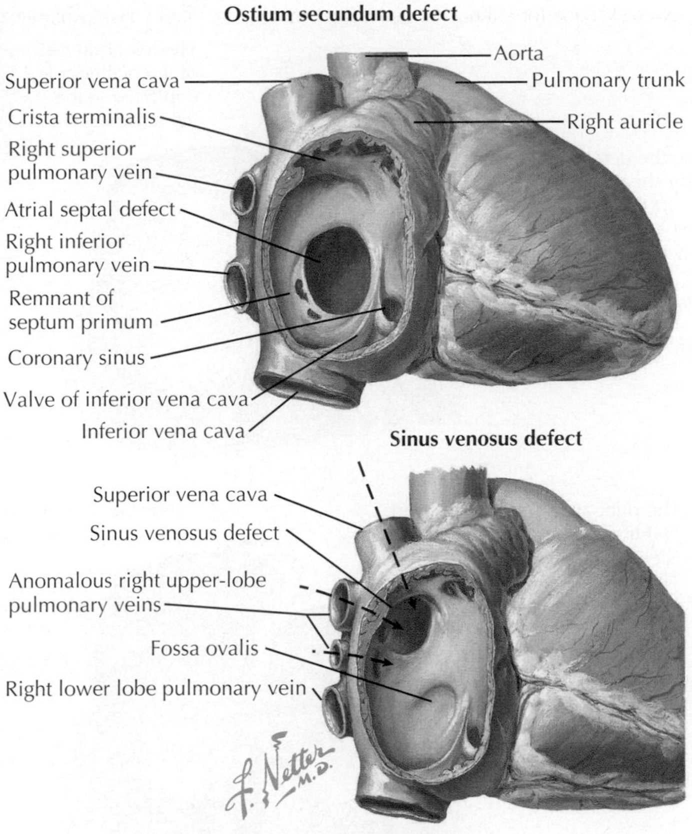

Ostium secundum defect

Aorta
Pulmonary trunk
Superior vena cava
Right auricle
Crista terminalis
Right superior
pulmonary vein
Atrial septal defect
Right inferior
pulmonary vein
Remnant of
septum primum
Coronary sinus
Valve of inferior vena cava
Inferior vena cava

Sinus venosus defect

Superior vena cava
Sinus venosus defect
Anomalous right upper-lobe
pulmonary veins
Fossa ovalis
Right lower lobe pulmonary vein

Fig. 30.1 Arial Septal Defect.

interrupted aortic arch. Conal septal hypoplasia defects also may be associated with prolapse of an aortic cusp, resulting in aortic regurgitation. The second most common type of VSDs are called *muscular VSDs;* these are defects located anywhere other than those described earlier. These defects often spontaneously close if they are small to moderate in size.

In the first 4 to 6 weeks of life, the pulmonary vascular resistance (PVR) decreases, and left-to-right shunting at the ventricular level increases. If the defect is large enough to cause a significant shunt, infants may show signs of pulmonary overcirculation and congestive heart failure such as sweating with feeds, poor weight gain, tachypnea, tachycardia, and hepatomegaly. On cardiac auscultation, moderate-to-large defects may not produce a murmur early in the newborn period. As the PVR decreases, a harsh, holosystolic murmur can be heard at the left sternal border, and large defects can cause a diastolic rumble from an increase in flow across the mitral valve. If left untreated, larger defects can eventually cause irreversible pulmonary hypertension with resulting right-to-left shunting (Eisenmenger physiology).

An ECG can be normal with small defects or show biventricular hypertrophy in larger defects. Chest radiography can show cardiomegaly and increased pulmonary vascular markings in patients with larger VSDs. Echocardiography is used to confirm the diagnosis and characterize the type of VSD.

Both small conoventricular and muscular defects often decrease in size and have a high rate of spontaneous closure within the first several years of life. Canal-type, malalignment, and conal septal hypoplasia defects do not spontaneously close and usually require surgical correction. Among patients with symptomatic VSDs, medical management of symptoms of heart failure is usually pursued initially and often includes diuretics, increased caloric supplementation, and additional

medications, such as an angiotensin-converting enzyme inhibitor or digoxin. In hemodynamically significant VSDs, including those failing medical management and/or demonstrating ongoing significant left-to-right shunting, the VSD is closed surgically, but there are situations in which certain types of VSDs are amenable to catheterization-based device closure.

Common Atrioventricular Canal

Common AV canal (otherwise known as endocardial cushion defect or AV septal defect) accounts for about 4% to 5% of all congenital heart disease and 40% of heart disease in children with trisomy 21. This condition results from the failure of the endocardial cushions to fuse (forming the canal septum), preventing separation of the common AV valve into the tricuspid and mitral valves. The unifying feature of all types of common AV canal defects is a common annulus, but the clinical presentation may be variable and depends on multiple factors, including the type of canal (complete, transitional, or incomplete) and size of the associated defects.

A *complete common AV canal* consists of both an ASD and VSD above and below the level of the AV valve, respectively. The common AV valve is suspended within the septal defect, creating space between the two atria (ostium primum ASD) and space between the two ventricles (inlet-type VSD). Patients with these defects develop symptoms related to the size of the VSD, with symptoms worsening as the PVR decreases during the neonatal period. The degree of common AV valve regurgitation will also affect the clinical presentation. A complete AV canal can be further classified as "balanced" if the common annulus opens equally over both ventricles. If the common annulus opens disproportionately to one ventricle, the patient is at risk of hypoplasia of the neglected ventricle and the defect is termed an "unbalanced" AV canal. Surgical options for an unbalanced AV canal depend on the size of the hypoplastic ventricle.

An *incomplete (or partial) AV canal* has the same septal deficiency but has leaflet tissue adhering to the crest of the ventricular septum such that there is no direct communication between ventricles and thus no VSD component. The morphology of the left side of the common AV valve is described as a cleft because the two components that typically form the anterior leaflet of the mitral valve remain separate. This type of defect has physiology similar to that of an ASD.

A *transitional AV canal* occurs when the AV valve attachments to the ventricular septum result in a small, restrictive VSD component. Transitional AV canal defects can vary in their presentation and symptoms depending on the size and level of restriction at the VSD and the amount of AV valve regurgitation.

The cardiac examination varies with each defect and can reveal a holosystolic murmur at the left sternal border (i.e., VSD), a systolic murmur at the apex (i.e., left AV valve regurgitation), or sometimes no murmur at all. An ECG with a superior or northwest QRS axis is a hallmark of this defect. Chest radiograph may show cardiomegaly with increased pulmonary vascular markings. An echocardiogram will identify and characterize the defect.

Medical and surgical management of complete AV canals are similar to that of large VSDs. Surgical repair is usually performed by 3 to 6 months of life with a concern for developing pulmonary vascular disease with delayed closure, particularly in those with trisomy 21. Medical management and timing of surgical repair of incomplete or transitional AV canals depend on the size of the defects and degree of left-sided AV valve regurgitation. Long-term complications of these defects include AV valve regurgitation or stenosis, heart block, and left ventricular outflow tract obstruction. Even with early surgical repair, a subset of patients, especially those with trisomy 21, may still develop pulmonary vascular disease.

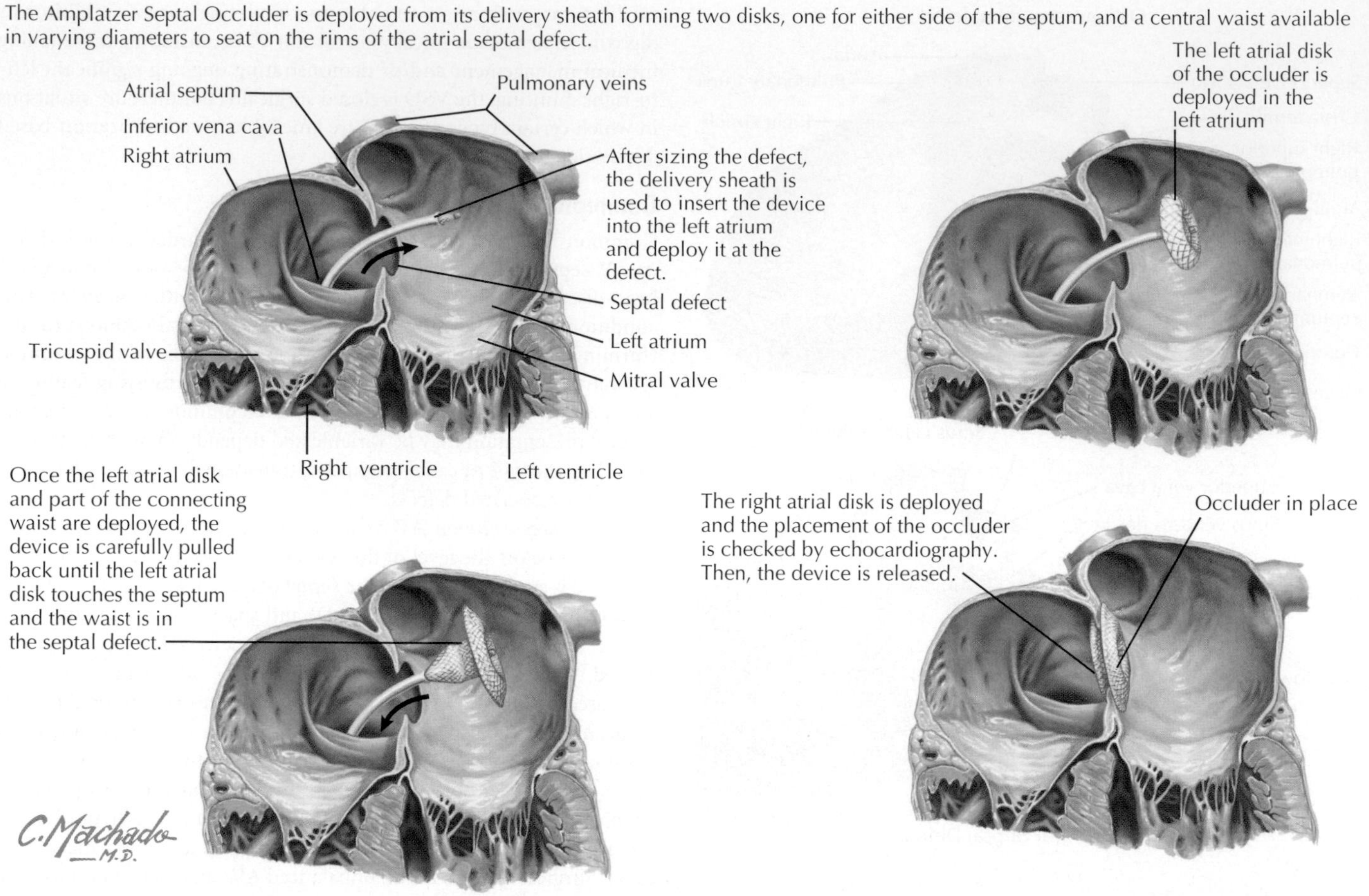

The Amplatzer Septal Occluder is deployed from its delivery sheath forming two disks, one for either side of the septum, and a central waist available in varying diameters to seat on the rims of the atrial septal defect.

Fig. 30.2 Atrial Septal Defect Device Closure.

Patent Ductus Arteriosus

A patent ductus arteriosus (PDA) occurs when the fetal ductus arteriosus fails to achieve functional hemodynamic closure within an appropriate postnatal time frame (Fig. 30.4). In term infants, the PDA often closes within 48 hours after birth. Failure of the PDA to close after birth results in a left-to-right shunt between the aorta and pulmonary artery. The severity and direction of this shunt depends on the pulmonary and systemic vascular resistances and size of the PDA. Typically, patients have left-to-right PDA shunting, but in those with elevated PVR and pulmonary hypertension, there is a right-to-left shunt. Patients with a small PDA are typically asymptomatic, with minimal left-to-right shunting across a restrictive PDA. However, patients with larger PDAs have heart failure symptoms of pulmonary overcirculation. Examination may reveal bounding pulses, widened pulse pressure, and a continuous murmur. ECG and chest radiography findings may appear similar to those of the VSD in larger PDAs. In premature infants, indomethacin is often used to medically close the PDA, if necessary. In children, including premature neonates, the PDA is typically amenable to a device closure by cardiac catheterization, but surgical ligation is still sometimes necessary. In older children, even in smaller, restrictive PDAs with no significant overcirculation, intervention to close the PDA is often considered if the PDA is audible, because of the long-term risk for infectious endarteritis.

Aortopulmonary Window

The aortopulmonary (AP) window is an abnormal shunt located between the proximal or ascending aorta and main pulmonary artery. The AP window is a relatively rare cardiac lesion and may be present in isolation but is commonly found in association with other cardiac defects. Similar to the PDA, the clinical presentation of an AP window is variable and dependent upon the size of the communication and degree of shunting. On examination, a patient with a large, isolated AP window may demonstrate increased work of breathing with a continuous murmur. Chest radiograph may demonstrate pulmonary congestion and cardiomegaly with definitive diagnosis normally achieved by echocardiography, and definitive surgical closure is necessary early in life.

NONSHUNT LESIONS

Aortic Valve Disease

Valvar aortic stenosis (AS) makes up about 3% to 8% of congenital heart defects or 4 in 100,000 live births. There is a strong male predominance (80%). Critical aortic stenosis, most often secondary to a unicuspid aortic valve, presents shortly after birth with symptoms of heart failure or shock. Noncritical AS, often secondary to a bicuspid aortic valve, is often detected via a systolic murmur. *Bicuspid aortic valve* is the most common congenital heart defect and occurs in 0.5% to 2% of the population. Patients with a bicuspid aortic valve are at risk for progressive aortic stenosis, aortic regurgitation, and/or aortic root or ascending aorta dilatation, requiring long-term cardiology monitoring.

Supravalvar AS occurs above the level of the aortic valve and is typically seen in Williams syndrome. It is the least common type of AS and often involves abnormalities in the elastin gene. *Subaortic stenosis* accounts for 10% to 20% of AS in children. It can result from a subaortic membrane (fibrous tissue in the aortic outflow tract), tunnel-like

Conoventricular ventricular septal defect

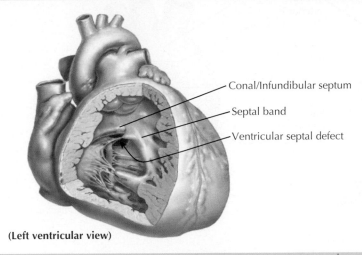

Conal/Infundibular septum

Septal band

Ventricular septal defect

(Left ventricular view)

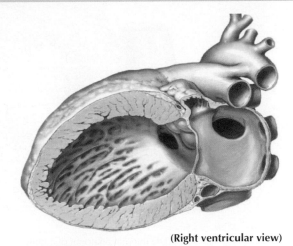

(Right ventricular view)

Muscular interventricular septal defect

Ventricular septal defect

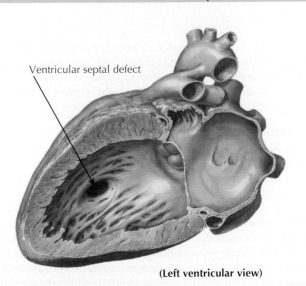

(Left ventricular view)

Conal septal hypoplasia ventricular septal defect

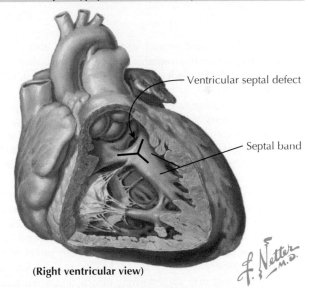

Ventricular septal defect

Septal band

(Right ventricular view)

f. Netter M.D.

Common atrioventricular canal

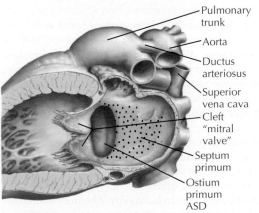

Pulmonary trunk

Aorta

Ductus arteriosus

Superior vena cava

Cleft "mitral valve"

Septum primum

Ostium primum ASD

Incomplete (view from left side)

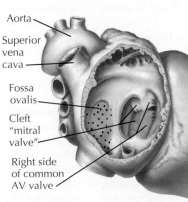

Aorta

Superior vena cava

Fossa ovalis

Cleft "mitral valve"

Right side of common AV valve

Incomplete (view from right atrium)

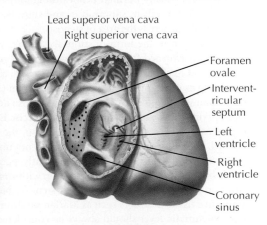

Lead superior vena cava

Right superior vena cava

Foramen ovale

Interventricular septum

Left ventricle

Right ventricle

Coronary sinus

Complete

Fig. 30.3 Ventricular Septal Defect.

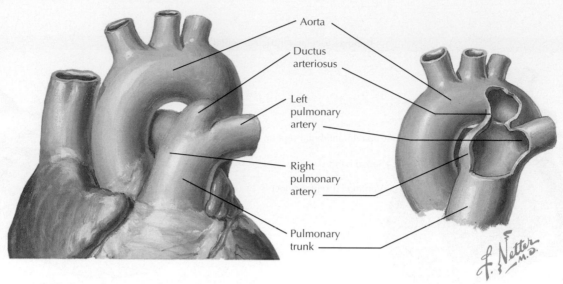

The internal anatomy of a typical "type A" ductus arteriosus, demonstrating the conical aortic ampulla and narrowing near the pulmonary end, making coil placement feasible

Fig. 30.4 Patent Ductus Arteriosus.

narrowing of the outflow tract, or from dynamic obstruction as seen in hypertrophic cardiomyopathy. Subaortic stenosis may be seen with other cardiac defects such as VSDs, common AV canal, and coarctation of the aorta.

AS tends to progress rapidly during periods of rapid growth, such as the first 2 years of life and during puberty. Most children with AS presenting after infancy are asymptomatic. With severe obstruction, children might present with exertional chest pain, syncope, heart failure, or sudden death. Exercise restriction to lower intensity sports is necessary with more significant AS.

On cardiac examination, auscultation reveals a harsh systolic ejection murmur loudest at the right upper sternal border, depending on the severity of the stenosis, and there may be a systolic ejection click with a bicuspid aortic valve. In severe cases, the second heart sound may not be split because of prolongation of left ventricular ejection, although typically still normal. An ECG can show left ventricular hypertrophy and may suggest severe obstruction when accompanied by associated ST changes and left precordial lead T inversion. Chest radiograph is usually normal. Echocardiography is important in the differentiation of valvar, supravalvar, and subvalvar AS and in assessing the gradient across the area of stenosis.

Intervention in the form of surgical valvotomy or balloon valvuloplasty is performed for all infants with critical AS regardless of the gradient and in children with noncritical AS with a gradient of at least 50 mm Hg as measured by cardiac catheterization (Fig. 30.5). The gradient upon which intervention is undertaken also depends on the presence of symptoms, changes on resting or exercise ECG, and the desire to play competitive sports. After intervention, the gradient is usually reduced, but resultant aortic regurgitation is not uncommon.

Aortic insufficiency (AI) very infrequently occurs as an isolated lesion. Instead, it can be seen in association with conoventricular VSDs with a prolapsed aortic leaflet, subaortic stenosis, bicuspid aortic valve, connective tissue disorders such as Marfan syndrome, or endocarditis. Acute rheumatic fever should always be considered in a patient with new-onset AI. The physical examination in patients with AI is typically benign, but with progressive AI, patients will develop an early diastolic murmur typically along the left sternal border, along with a widened pulse pressure. A chest radiograph may reveal a prominent ascending aorta, and an ECG may demonstrate left ventricular hypertrophy, each depending on the severity of the AI and any associated defects. Surgical repair or even replacement of the aortic valve is considered with symptomatic heart failure, decreasing left ventricular systolic function, and/or worsening left ventricular dilatation.

Coarctation of the Aorta

Coarctation of the aorta is a narrowing of the aortic arch, frequently in the form of a discrete narrowing of the distal aorta opposite the entrance of the ductus arteriosus or the ligamentum (after ductal closure) (Fig. 30.6). In rare instances, there may be a narrowing of the abdominal aorta termed abdominal coarctation. Coarctation constitutes about 8% of all congenital heart defects, with males affected about four times more than females. Turner syndrome should be suspected in any female with coarctation. Coarctation is also frequently associated with left-sided lesions such as bicuspid aortic valve, aortic stenosis, mitral valve abnormalities, and VSDs. It can also be associated with noncardiac abnormalities such as intracranial aneurysms.

In neonates with critical or severe coarctation, the presentation is usually shock. Although they sometimes have discrete juxtaductal coarctation, infants often have more long-segment aortic arch hypoplasia proximal to the entrance of the PDA with possible additional intracardiac abnormalities. With slightly less severe coarctation, infants can present with symptoms of heart failure, notably feeding intolerance. Children who have adapted to the gradual development of discrete coarctation are often asymptomatic despite upper extremity hypertension but may experience claudication and rarely chest pain with exercise.

The typical findings in patients with coarctation are elevated systolic pressures in the right arm with lower systolic blood pressures in the lower extremities. Blood pressures should be measured in all four extremities, as the blood pressure differential can vary in location based on the area of coarctation and the arch anatomy. Absent or diminished femoral pulses and a delay between the right upper extremity pulse and the femoral pulse may be noted. Continuous murmurs from collateral vessels can be auscultated in the back in older children. Children with significant collaterals may not have a significant blood pressure differential though, of note. ECGs may show right ventricular hypertrophy

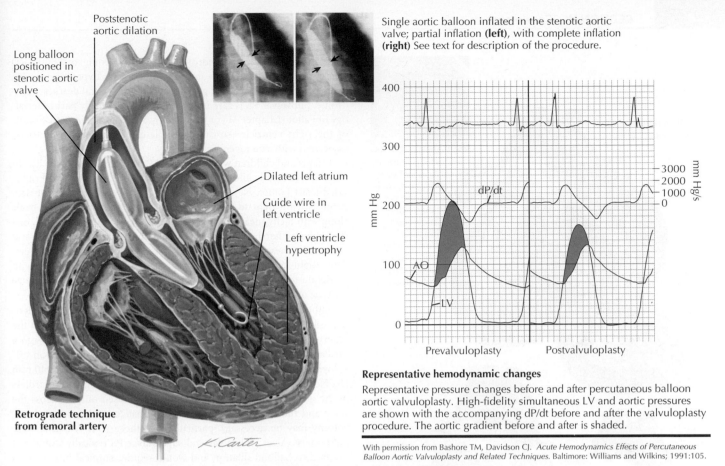

Poststenotic aortic dilation

Long balloon positioned in stenotic aortic valve

Single aortic balloon inflated in the stenotic aortic valve; partial inflation **(left)**, with complete inflation **(right)** See text for description of the procedure.

Dilated left atrium

Guide wire in left ventricle

Left ventricle hypertrophy

Retrograde technique from femoral artery

K. Carter

Representative hemodynamic changes

Representative pressure changes before and after percutaneous balloon aortic valvuloplasty. High-fidelity simultaneous LV and aortic pressures are shown with the accompanying dP/dt before and after the valvuloplasty procedure. The aortic gradient before and after is shaded.

With permission from Bashore TM, Davidson CJ. *Acute Hemodynamics Effects of Percutaneous Balloon Aortic Valvuloplasty and Related Techniques*. Baltimore: Williams and Wilkins; 1991:105.

Fig. 30.5 Balloon Aortic Valve Dilation.

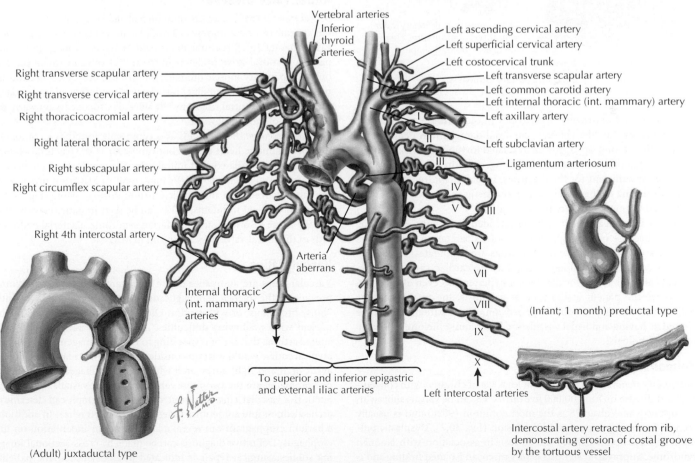

Fig. 30.6 Coarctation of the Aorta.

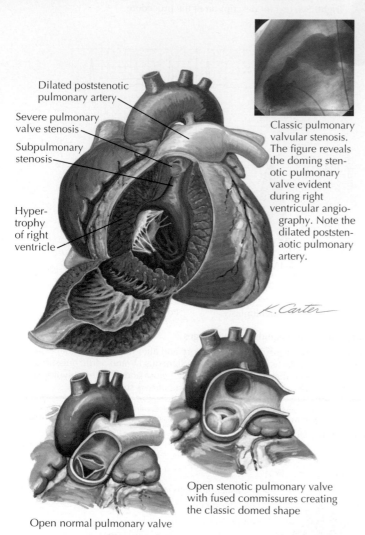

Classic pulmonary valvular stenosis. The figure reveals the doming stenotic pulmonary valve evident during right ventricular angiography. Note the dilated poststenaotic pulmonary artery.

Dilated poststenotic pulmonary artery

Severe pulmonary valve stenosis

Subpulmonary stenosis

Hypertrophy of right ventricle

K. Carter

Open stenotic pulmonary valve with fused commissures creating the classic domed shape

Open normal pulmonary valve

Fig. 30.7 Pulmonary Stenosis.

in infants or left ventricular hypertrophy in older children, depending on the severity. In older children, chest radiography may demonstrate rib notching secondary to erosion by dilated tortuous intercostal arteries that bypass the coarctation. In younger children, echocardiography may be sufficient for the diagnosis. In older children and adults, further imaging of the distal arch by magnetic resonance imaging or computed tomography scan may be required.

Primary surgical repair is recommended in infants and young children because of the high incidence of recoarctation with balloon angioplasty. Older adolescents and adults are candidates for covered stent placement and balloon angioplasty by cardiac catheterization. Patients are still at risk for developing hypertension even after repair. The older the patient at the time of diagnosis, the more likely the patient is to develop chronic hypertension. These patients should be viewed as having abnormal vasculature and require lifelong follow-up with a cardiologist.

Pulmonary Valve Disease

Pulmonary stenosis (PS) occurs in at least 8% of children with congenital heart disease or 7 in 100,000 live births. PS can be valvar, subvalvar, or supravalvar. Valvar PS is the most common (90%) and is usually seen with varying degrees of leaflet fusion (Fig. 30.7). Dysplastic pulmonary valve abnormalities can be seen in association with Noonan syndrome. Supravalvar stenosis is very rarely an isolated finding and is

associated with Williams syndrome, Alagille syndrome, or LEOPARD (lentigines, ECG conduction abnormalities, ocular hypertelorism, PS, abnormal genitalia, retarded growth, and sensorineural deafness) syndrome. Subvalvar PS is rare in isolation and is typically part of tetralogy of Fallot (Chapter 31) or is caused by an additional muscle bundle of the right ventricle (so-called double-chambered right ventricle) associated with a conoventricular VSD.

Infants and children with noncritical PS are rarely symptomatic. In more severe cases, children can have dyspnea with exertion and right-sided heart failure. Newborns with critical or severe PS present with cyanosis from right-to-left shunting through a patent foramen ovale along with tachypnea and poor feeding. On cardiac examination, one should hear a harsh systolic ejection murmur radiating to the back and axillae. On chest radiograph, a dilated pulmonary artery may be evident. Right ventricular hypertrophy is usually present on ECG with moderate-to-severe cases of PS. Echocardiography will characterize the type of severity of stenosis.

Although mild PS often improves over time, patients require ongoing follow-up because of the possibility of worsening disease. On the other end of the spectrum, children with severe PS often undergo a cardiac catheterization for hemodynamic assessment and balloon valvuloplasty, typically if the gradient by catheterization is at least 40 mm Hg. Newborns with critical PS require balloon valvuloplasty regardless of the gradient; severe PS may result in decreased output across the valve and therefore a lower gradient. If unsuccessful, a surgical valvotomy may be necessary, particularly in those with very dysplastic pulmonary valves. Subvalvar and supravalvar PS typically would not respond to balloon dilation and would require surgical intervention if severe.

Mitral Valve Disease

Mitral stenosis (MS) is an uncommon isolated congenital heart defect but appears more commonly as a complication of rheumatic heart disease (Chapter 35). Structural abnormalities that can cause MS include parachute mitral valve (a defect in the mitral valve in which there is only one papillary muscle present), mitral valve arcade (direct attachment of leaflets to the papillary muscles without intervening chordae), or a supravalvar mitral ring. Any left-sided obstructive lesion warrants evaluation of the mitral valve.

Mitral regurgitation (MR) is also commonly found as a complication of rheumatic heart disease but can occur with structural abnormalities as well. Isolated cleft mitral valve is a rare form of congenital MR. *Mitral valve prolapse* (MVP) may result in MR from prolapse of the mitral valve leaflet into the left atrium during systole (Fig. 30.8). Although unusual in infants, MVP can be seen in patients with connective tissue disorders such as Marfan syndrome. Bacterial endocarditis of the mitral valve may also result in MR.

Vascular Ring

Vascular rings are anomalies of the aortic arch that can cause compression of the trachea, esophagus, or both. Infants may present with "noisy breathing" or with stridor. Older children and toddlers might present with swallowing difficulties. Additionally, patients with presumed asthma that is not responding to typical management or has an atypical course would warrant consideration of a vascular ring. Double aortic arch and right aortic arch with a retroesophageal diverticulum of Kommerell are the two most common types of vascular rings (Fig. 30.9). If a vascular ring is suspected, chest radiograph can determine arch sidedness and sometimes indentation of the trachea. In addition, a barium esophagram can reveal a large posterior indentation on the esophagus. Definitive diagnosis can be made by cross-sectional imaging studies. Surgical repair is indicated in any symptomatic patient,

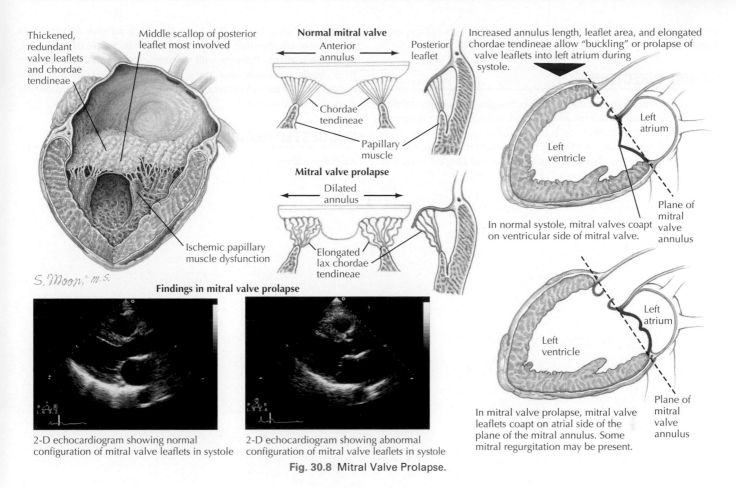

Thickened, redundant valve leaflets and chordae tendineae

Middle scallop of posterior leaflet most involved

Ischemic papillary muscle dysfunction

S. Moon, m.s.

Normal mitral valve

Anterior annulus

Posterior leaflet

Chordae tendineae

Papillary muscle

Mitral valve prolapse

Dilated annulus

Elongated lax chordae tendineae

Findings in mitral valve prolapse

2-D echocardiogram showing normal configuration of mitral valve leaflets in systole

2-D echocardiogram showing abnormal configuration of mitral valve leaflets in systole

Increased annulus length, leaflet area, and elongated chordae tendineae allow "buckling" or prolapse of valve leaflets into left atrium during systole.

Left atrium

Left ventricle

Plane of mitral valve annulus

In normal systole, mitral valves coapt on ventricular side of mitral valve.

Left atrium

Left ventricle

Plane of mitral valve annulus

In mitral valve prolapse, mitral valve leaflets coapt on atrial side of the plane of the mitral annulus. Some mitral regurgitation may be present.

Fig. 30.8 Mitral Valve Prolapse.

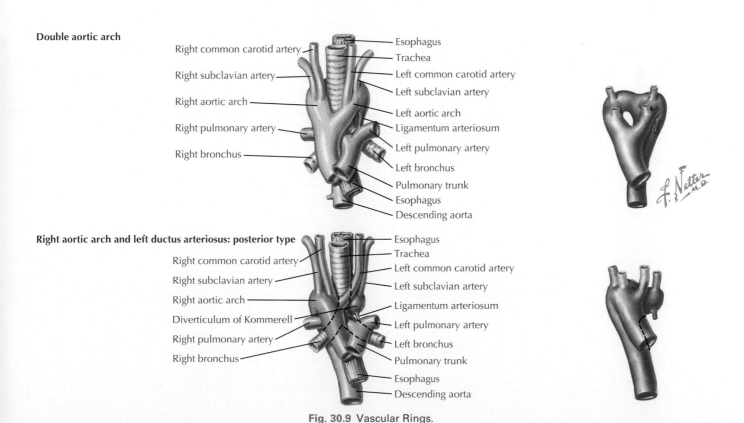

Double aortic arch

Right common carotid artery
Right subclavian artery
Right aortic arch
Right pulmonary artery
Right bronchus

Esophagus
Trachea
Left common carotid artery
Left subclavian artery
Left aortic arch
Ligamentum arteriosum
Left pulmonary artery
Left bronchus
Pulmonary trunk
Esophagus
Descending aorta

Right aortic arch and left ductus arteriosus: posterior type

Right common carotid artery
Right subclavian artery
Right aortic arch
Diverticulum of Kommerell
Right pulmonary artery
Right bronchus

Esophagus
Trachea
Left common carotid artery
Left subclavian artery
Ligamentum arteriosum
Left pulmonary artery
Left bronchus
Pulmonary trunk
Esophagus
Descending aorta

F. Netter M.D.

Fig. 30.9 Vascular Rings.

although symptoms may linger because of prior airway compression in particular.

FUTURE DIRECTIONS

With advancements in prenatal diagnosis, imaging technology, cardiac catheterization interventions, and surgical techniques, the diagnosis and management of patients with congenital heart disease continues to be an evolving field. Certainly, the development of cardiac catheterization techniques has allowed for an alternative to surgical treatment for many of these lesions. Fetal intervention is another exciting new area of investigation that may play a role in the future of congenital cardiac treatment. Patients with acyanotic congenital heart lesions have excellent survival rates, but it is important to realize that most patients with these defects require lifelong follow-up by a cardiologist even after intervention.

SUGGESTED READINGS

Available online.

31

Cyanotic Congenital Heart Disease

Aaron Briggs and David M. Finkelstein

 CLINICAL VIGNETTE

A 37-week-old infant is born to a 24-year-old G1P0 mother with normal pregnancy and regular prenatal care. Delivery and immediate postnatal care are unremarkable. At 24 hours of life, the baby appears slightly "dusky." On examination, the baby is otherwise well-appearing with normal pulses and distal perfusion. The lungs are clear to auscultation with no work of breathing, and there is a normal cardiac examination with no clear murmur. However, the pulse oximeter signals that the oxygen saturation in the right arm and leg are both in the mid-80s. A chest radiograph demonstrates clear lungs. The infant is transferred to the neonatal intensive care unit with initiation of oxygen, and an echocardiogram demonstrates transposition of the great arteries.

CYANOSIS

Cyanotic congenital heart disease (CHD) describes cardiac lesions that manifest with central cyanosis in infancy. Cyanosis describes the blueish discoloration of the tissues observed as a result of an accumulation of deoxygenated, reduced hemoglobin. Skin pigmentation will have an impact on the ease with which this color change is detected. Cyanosis is less readily apparent in infants with darker skin. Mucous membranes and fingernail beds should be carefully assessed during examination of infants with more pigmented skin. Cyanosis in anemic patients may be difficult to appreciate because the absolute content of deoxygenated hemoglobin in the blood may not exceed the threshold to produce a perceptible change in color.

Cyanosis may present peripherally or centrally. Acrocyanosis is a benign, common finding in newborns involving peripheral cyanosis of the hands, feet, and perioral region within the first 24 to 48 hours of life, and intermittent acrocyanosis is often normal in the first 1 to 2 years of life, particularly with colder environmental temperatures. Central cyanosis, discussed in this chapter, results from a decline in systemic arterial oxygen content and presents with blueish discoloration of the trunk and mucous membranes. Cardiac lesions that present with cyanosis are due to deoxygenated blood entering the arterial circulation. This issue can occur in two ways. First, deoxygenated blood from systemic venous drainage may be directed into the arterial circulation, as in transposition of the great arteries (TGA). The degree of cyanosis is related to the amount of mixing between the systemic and pulmonary circulations. Second, there may be mixing of systemic and pulmonary blood with variable pulmonary blood flow, as in tetralogy of Fallot (TOF), single ventricles, and total anomalous pulmonary venous connection (TAPVC). Greater pulmonary blood flow results in less cyanosis.

Critical CHD screening with pulse oximetry increases the likelihood of identifying these conditions soon after birth. These screenings can also detect differential cyanosis, in which the preductal saturation (right upper extremity typically) is higher than the postductal saturation (lower extremity). Differential cyanosis occurs when one ventricle delivers blood to the upper half of the body, and the other ventricle with more desaturated blood provides some of the blood to the lower half via a patent ductus arteriosus (PDA). This issue occurs with coarctation of the aorta, interrupted aortic arch, or pulmonary hypertension. Reverse differential cyanosis (postductal saturation greater than preductal) occurs with TGA in addition to the previously mentioned conditions.

CLINICAL PRESENTATION AND EVALUATION

Severe cyanosis is the most common presenting sign of cyanotic CHD in newborns. In lesions with abundant mixing and excessive pulmonary blood flow, such as truncus arteriosus or unobstructed TAPVC, cyanosis may be less obvious, but tachypnea and respiratory distress are prominent. Other lesions, such as TOF, present variably depending on the severity of obstruction to pulmonary blood flow. Despite the heterogeneity of cyanotic lesions, they are discussed together because they present at the same age and should be considered in the differential diagnosis of a neonate with suspected CHD.

Appropriate evaluation of cyanosis will include a detailed physical examination, preductal and postductal saturations, chest radiography, and electrocardiography. Echocardiography is performed to define the anatomy. CHD is increasingly identified by fetal echocardiography, allowing for delivery of infants with severe forms in tertiary care hospitals. Rates of fetal diagnosis remain subject to significant geographic variability in resources.

Transposition of the Great Arteries

TGA is a cardiac lesion characterized by ventriculoarterial discordance in which the pulmonary artery arises from the left ventricle and the aorta from the right ventricle (Fig. 31.1). TGA accounts for 7% of overall CHD and is the most common cause of cyanotic CHD presenting in a newborn. Incidence is increased among infants of mothers with diabetes. TGA may present with severe cyanosis at birth because of parallel pulmonary and systemic circuits. In *transposition physiologic processes*, oxygenated blood drains from the pulmonary veins to the left atrium and ventricle and reenters pulmonary circulation. Deoxygenated blood returns to the right atrium and ventricle and reenters the systemic circulation. To survive, these parallel circuits require mixing, usually across a patent foramen ovale (PFO).

The clinical presentation of an infant with TGA varies in severity based on the degree of mixing. Physical examination will be remarkable

External appearance of heart

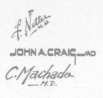
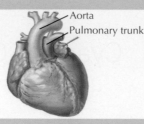

Aorta
Pulmonary trunk

Balloon atrial septostomy (technique)

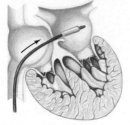
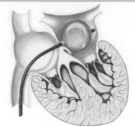
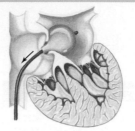
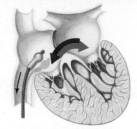

Balloon-tipped catheter introduced into left atrium through
patent foramen ovale

Balloon inflated

Balloon withdrawn
producing large septal defect

Common atrium produced by
septostomy allows mixing of oxygenated and deoxygenated blood

Mustard operation

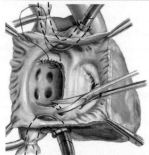
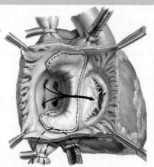
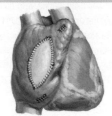

The interatrial septum
has been widely excised,
opening into transverse
sinus at upper end. This
opening is being sutured
and coronary sinus
opened into left atrium.

A patch of pericardium has been
applied so as to channel blood
from pulmonary veins through
tricuspid valve to right ventricle,
then out the aorta. Blood from
venae cavae will now pass to
left ventricle and then to
pulmonary artery.

A patch of pericardium
has been applied to close
incision and enlarge newly
formed right atrium

Arterial repair of transposition of the great arteries

First steps

The aorta and the pulmonary artery are
transected. The cut of the aorta is slanted
and above the Valsalva's sinuses. The
pulmonary artery is divided above its
valve at the same level of the transection
of the aorta. Sinuses of the aorta and
pulmonary artery are excised to
translocate the coronary ostia from the
pulmonary artery to the neo-aorta.
Pericardium is utilized to reconstruct
the neo-pulmonary artery sinuses.

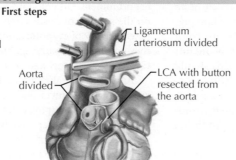

Ligamentum
arteriosum divided

Aorta
divided

LCA with button
resected from
the aorta

Last steps Coronary arteries
anastomosed
to neo-aorta

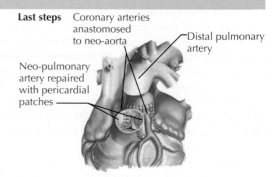

Distal pulmonary
artery

Neo-pulmonary
artery repaired
with pericardial
patches

Fig. 31.1 Transposition of the Great Arteries.

for cyanosis and tachypnea without increased work of breathing. A
murmur is not typically appreciated in TGA, but if one is present, it
may be related to a ventricular septal defect (VSD) or outflow tract
obstruction. Electrocardiography is often normal because findings of
right ventricular hypertrophy and right axis deviation are expected in
the neonatal period. A chest radiograph will typically be normal. There
can be the "egg on a string" appearance because of, among a few reasons, the relationship of the aorta and pulmonary artery that make the
superior mediastinum appear narrow.

Newborns with TGA are initiated on a continuous infusion of prostaglandin E1 to maintain patency of the PDA. Immediate intervention
may be necessary to provide adequate mixing, typically achieved by the
Rashkind balloon atrial septostomy. The contemporary surgical repair

is the arterial switch operation, during which surgical transection and
translocation of the aorta and main pulmonary artery restore ventriculoarterial concordance. Notably, the coronary arteries must also be
translocated in this operation.

Tetralogy of Fallot

TOF is the most common cause of cyanotic CHD and is characterized by anterior displacement of the conal septum (a superior portion of the ventricular septum between the two great vessels). This
malalignment produces the four characteristic findings of TOF: (1)
narrow right ventricular outflow tract (RVOT), which may include
subvalvar, valvar, or supravalvar pulmonary narrowing; (2) VSD
caused by malalignment of the portion of the ventricular septum; (3)

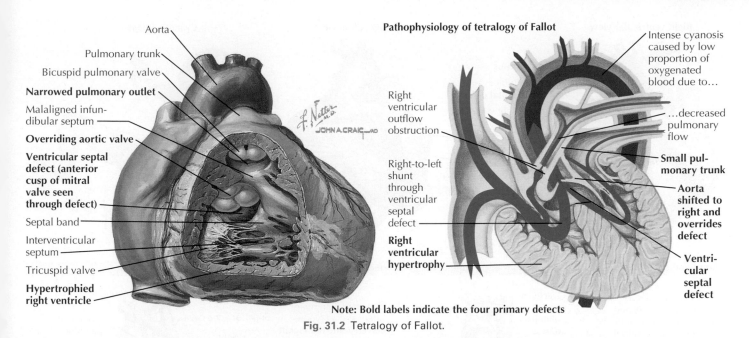

Pathophysiology of tetralogy of Fallot

Aorta

Pulmonary trunk

Bicuspid pulmonary valve

Narrowed pulmonary outlet

Malaligned infundibular septum

Overriding aortic valve

Ventricular septal defect (anterior cusp of mitral valve seen through defect)

Septal band

Interventricular septum

Tricuspid valve

Hypertrophied right ventricle

Right ventricular outflow obstruction

Right-to-left shunt through ventricular septal defect

Right ventricular hypertrophy

Intense cyanosis caused by low proportion of oxygenated blood due to…

…decreased pulmonary flow

Small pulmonary trunk

Aorta shifted to right and overrides defect

Ventricular septal defect

Note: Bold labels indicate the four primary defects

Fig. 31.2 Tetralogy of Fallot.

"overriding aorta" (i.e., the aortic valve sits above both ventricles); and (4) right ventricular hypertrophy caused by pressure overload from the large VSD (Fig. 31.2). TOF accounts for approximately 7% to 10% of all CHD. TOF can be observed in isolation but includes other cardiac anomalies in approximately 40% of cases, most commonly right aortic arch (25%) and atrial septal defects (ASD) (10%). TOF presents as part of a genetic syndrome about 15% of the time, is found in more than 25% of patients with 22q11.2 microdeletion (DiGeorge syndrome), and can be associated with trisomy 21 and Alagille syndrome.

Physical examination in infants with TOF typically includes a systolic murmur loudest at the mid to upper left sternal border, related to restrictive flow across the RVOT. Electrocardiography may show right atrial enlargement, right ventricular hypertrophy, and right axis deviation. Chest radiography may classically demonstrate an abnormal "boot"-shaped cardiac silhouette from right ventricular hypertrophy.

Cyanosis in TOF is variable. There is extensive systemic-pulmonary mixing across the VSD, and cyanosis is dictated by the extent of RVOT obstruction. Neonates with severe RVOT obstruction and inadequate pulmonary blood flow will present with cyanosis in the newborn period, sometimes requiring prostaglandin infusion. Patients with moderate RVOT obstruction permitting an appropriate degree of pulmonary blood flow will be initially asymptomatic but may present later with symptoms as the RVOT obstruction progresses over time. Patients with only mild RVOT obstruction, often called "pink tetralogy" because of lack of cyanosis, are vulnerable to pulmonary overcirculation and have VSD physiologic processes with increasing pulmonary blood flow as pulmonary artery pressures decline. These infants may present with heart failure and must be monitored closely. Patients with TOF may experience episodes of hypercyanosis commonly referred to as "tet spells" during which the RVOT obstruction is transiently increased.

Practice varies with regard to complete surgical repair of TOF in the newborn period. Many institutions proceed with an interim procedure to maintain pulmonary blood flow with either a modified Blalock-Taussig shunt between the aorta and pulmonary arteries or a PDA stent. Historically, the Blalock-Taussig shunt has been the procedure of choice in infants with ductal-dependent pulmonary blood flow requiring operative palliation; however, there is growing evidence for catheter-based PDA stenting. Complete repair involves patch closure of the VSD and relief of the RVOT obstruction. The details of the RVOT surgical intervention depend on the level of obstruction, which may include intervention on the pulmonary valve itself, removal of subvalvar right ventricular muscle bundles, and/or patch augmentation of any supravalvar narrowing. If the pulmonary valve is adequate in size, it can often be dilated surgically, but if not, a transannular patch, an incision and patch enlargement across the pulmonary valve, is often necessary. Patients requiring a transannular patch will have pulmonary insufficiency that is generally well-tolerated during childhood but typically require later pulmonary valve replacement by either surgery or catheterization-based device placement.

Double-Outlet Right Ventricle With Pulmonic Stenosis

Double-outlet right ventricle (DORV) with subaortic VSD and pulmonic stenosis (PS) is often termed "TOF type" DORV. It has similar physiologic processes and presentation to TOF. The surgical approach is similar as well, baffling the left ventricle by way of the VSD to the aorta and either pulmonary outflow augmentation or placement of a right ventricle to pulmonary artery conduit.

Tricuspid Atresia

Tricuspid atresia is characterized by the absence of communication between the right atrium and either ventricle. All blood returning to the right atrium flows across a PFO or ASD to the left atrium, left ventricle, and usually through a VSD to the remnant of the right ventricle. The pathophysiologic processes and presentation of tricuspid atresia vary according to the anatomy of the great arteries and the presence or absence of an associated VSD. In cases with normally aligned great arteries, the size of the VSD affects the amount of pulmonary blood flow and therefore the degree of cyanosis. Many patients have muscular VSDs, which may be large initially with mild cyanosis, but over time a muscular VSD may become smaller, resulting in decreasing pulmonary blood flow and increasing cyanosis. In cases with TGA with tricuspid atresia, the aorta arises from the small remnant of the right ventricle. In these patients, pulmonary overcirculation is common and antegrade systemic blood flow is dependent on the VSD. When the VSD is small, there may be associated coarctation of the aorta. High pulmonary blood flow often results in heart failure and, if not surgically addressed, can eventually cause pulmonary vascular disease.

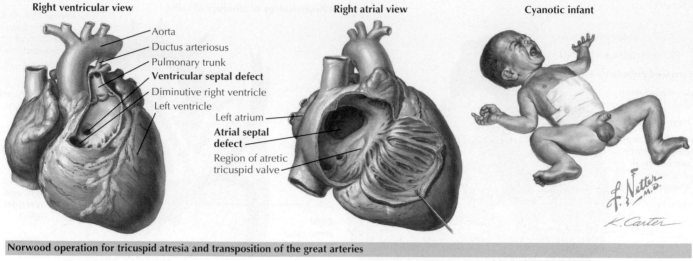

Right ventricular view

- Aorta
- Ductus arteriosus
- Pulmonary trunk
- **Ventricular septal defect**
- Diminutive right ventricle
- Left ventricle

Right atrial view

- Left atrium
- **Atrial septal defect**
- Region of atretic tricuspid valve

Cyanotic infant

Norwood operation for tricuspid atresia and transposition of the great arteries

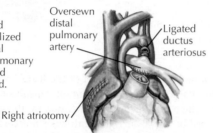

Hypothermic cardio-pulmonary bypass and right atriotomy are utilized to excise the interatrial septum. The main pulmonary artery is transected and a "neoaorta" is created.

- Oversewn distal pulmonary artery
- Ligated ductus arteriosus
- Right atriotomy

The main pulmonary artery and a cryopreserved aortic homograft create a neoaorta. Pulmonary blood flow is established through a systemic-to-pulmonary artery shunt.

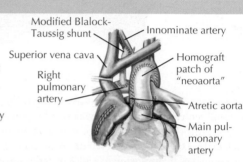

- Modified Blalock-Taussig shunt
- Innominate artery
- Superior vena cava
- Right pulmonary artery
- Homograft patch of "neoaorta"
- Atretic aorta
- Main pulmonary artery

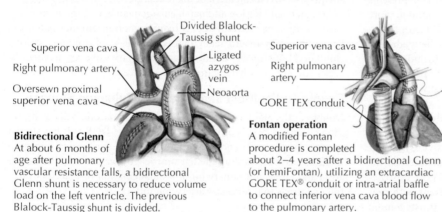

- Superior vena cava
- Divided Blalock-Taussig shunt
- Right pulmonary artery
- Ligated azygos vein
- Oversewn proximal superior vena cava
- Neoaorta

Bidirectional Glenn
At about 6 months of age after pulmonary vascular resistance falls, a bidirectional Glenn shunt is necessary to reduce volume load on the left ventricle. The previous Blalock-Taussig shunt is divided.

- Superior vena cava
- Right pulmonary artery
- GORE TEX conduit

Fontan operation
A modified Fontan procedure is completed about 2–4 years after a bidirectional Glenn (or hemiFontan), utilizing an extracardiac GORE TEX® conduit or intra-atrial baffle to connect inferior vena cava blood flow to the pulmonary artery.

- Neoaorta
- Pulmonary artery
- Extracardiac conduit
- Closure of right atrium
- Closed purse string for bypass cannula in IVC

Systemic venous blood bypasses the right heart directly to the pulmonary arteries and lungs. Oxygenated blood is returned to the left atrium, left ventricle, and is either pumped directly into the aorta in the case of normally aligned great arteries or into the reconstructed aorta after Norwood operation in the case of transpostion of the great arteries.

Fig. 31.3 Tricuspid Atresia.

Physical examination in infants with tricuspid atresia is variable. Cyanosis may be observed and VSD or PDA murmurs may be appreciated. Electrocardiography is classically remarkable for peaked P waves of right atrial enlargement, left ventricular hypertrophy, and left axis deviation. Chest radiograph is typically normal, but infants with pulmonary overcirculation will demonstrate increased pulmonary vascular markings and an enlarged cardiac silhouette.

Patients with tricuspid atresia have a single functional ventricle, and surgical palliation consists of a staged approach. In patients with transposition and a restrictive VSD, a Damus-Kaye-Stansel or a Norwood operation is required to effectively bypass the subaortic obstruction by using the pulmonary valve (arising unobstructed from the left ventricle) as an additional (or only) systemic outlet. These operations involve transection of the pulmonary artery above the valve and combination of the proximal pulmonary stump with the ascending aorta and aortic arch. The distal pulmonary arteries are then supplied by a systemic-to-pulmonary shunt. The ultimate surgery in this pathway is the Fontan operation, in which the systemic venous return passes directly to the pulmonary arteries, without returning to the heart. The Fontan operation depends on low pulmonary resistance to allow systemic venous return without a pump to the pulmonary arteries. As a result, it cannot be carried out until the high pulmonary resistance of the normal newborn has resolved. An intermediary operation, superior cavopulmonary anastomosis (bidirectional Glenn or hemi-Fontan), is typically performed at 4 to 6 months. In this operation, the superior vena cava is connected to the right pulmonary artery so that all venous drainage from the upper body goes to the lungs but inferior vena caval blood mixes with pulmonary venous return and goes to the body. Between 2 and 4 years, typically, the inferior vena cava is connected to the pulmonary arteries by an extracardiac conduit or intraatrial baffle, completing the Fontan (Fig. 31.3).

Pulmonic Stenosis

PS is most commonly localized to the pulmonary valve, but can be found less commonly at the subvalvar and supravalvar levels. PS is typically de novo but has been reported in association with genetic syndromes, including Noonan syndrome. Critical pulmonary stenosis classically describes extreme narrowing of the pulmonic valve orifice.

The pathophysiology by which PS causes cyanosis is limited antegrade pulmonary blood flow with shunting of deoxygenated blood right to left across a PFO. The degree of PS will determine the severity of presenting symptoms. In critical PS, neonates will typically present soon after birth with cyanosis as the PDA begins to close, limiting pulmonary blood flow. Physical examination in an infant with PS is notable for a harsh systolic ejection murmur at the left upper sternal border. An electrocardiogram may suggest right ventricular hypertrophy, and a chest radiograph may demonstrate cardiomegaly.

Critical PS is a ductal-dependent lesion requiring prostaglandin infusion to maintain patency of the PDA in anticipation of a definitive intervention. Most commonly, critical PS can be treated by percutaneous balloon pulmonary valvuloplasty (Fig. 31.4).

Pulmonary Atresia

Pulmonary atresia with intact ventricular septum (PA/IVS) is a more severe form of critical pulmonary stenosis with no antegrade flow across the pulmonary valve. Pulmonary atresia occurs in fetal development, resulting in right ventricular hypertrophy, diminished right ventricular compliance, and halted growth. Patients with PA/IVS have varying degrees of right ventricular hypoplasia, and systemic drainage entering the right ventricle has two means of egress, either tricuspid regurgitation or by the right ventricle to the coronary artery fistulae. Some patients with PA/IVS may have proximal coronary artery obstruction with regions of myocardium exclusively supplied by fistulae. Patients with right ventricular–dependent coronary circulation are at significant risk for mortality.

Infants with PA/IVS present with cyanosis secondary to inadequate pulmonary blood flow and right-to-left shunting of deoxygenated blood across a PFO. Physical examination will typically be remarkable for a cyanotic, tachypneic infant in mild respiratory distress with a continuous PDA murmur and possibly a systolic murmur as a result of tricuspid regurgitation. Chest radiography may demonstrate cardiomegaly but also can be normal. Electrocardiography will typically be notable for increased P wave amplitude because of right atrial enlargement and loss of the normal newborn right axis deviation.

Initial management of PA/IVS involves prompt initiation of prostaglandin to maintain pulmonary blood flow. More stable pulmonary blood flow is achieved with a Blalock-Taussig shunt or PDA stent. While some patients with PA/IVS may undergo percutaneous radiofrequency perforation and balloon dilation of the atretic pulmonary valve or surgical intervention, many never achieve significant right ventricular growth and proceed along the palliative single ventricle pathway toward the Fontan operation.

Ebstein Anomaly of the Tricuspid Valve

Ebstein anomaly is a rare abnormality characterized by displacement of the attachment of the septal and posterior leaflets of the tricuspid valve toward the apex of the right ventricle. The lesion constitutes fewer than 1% of congenital cardiac lesions and is commonly associated with other cardiac lesions. Downward displacement of the tricuspid valve partitions the right ventricle into "atrialized" ventricle above the valve and an apical right ventricle portion below (Fig. 31.5). The tricuspid valve anterior leaflet becomes redundant and "sail-like" with variable tricuspid regurgitation. These patients have a high incidence of ventricular pre-excitation.

Hemodynamically, Ebstein anomaly has a wide range of possible physiologies, depending on the degree of regurgitation or stenosis of the tricuspid valve, the presence of atrial communication, and the degree of right ventricular dysfunction. Patients can present with symptoms of cyanosis, heart failure, or atrial arrhythmias.

Patients with mild symptoms do not require intervention and may have a benign natural history. At the other extreme, patients with severe tricuspid regurgitation have high mortality. Survivors past infancy may develop right heart failure in adolescence or adulthood with cyanosis if an atrial communication exists. Early surgical intervention has had poor results, though tricuspid annuloplasty and valvuloplasty have had improving results in recent years.

Total Anomalous Pulmonary Venous Connection

TAPVC arises from an embryologic failure of all the pulmonary veins to return to the left atrium. Connections to the innominate vein, the portal system of the liver, and the coronary sinus are representative of the main categories noted (Fig. 31.6). Anatomically, patients are divided among those whose pulmonary veins connect above the diaphragm (70%), below the diaphragm (25%), or in mixed fashion (i.e., to more than one connection; 5%). Those connecting above the diaphragm are further divided into those connecting to a vein, most often the innominate vein, and those connecting to the heart, typically the coronary sinus. The majority of these pulmonary veins are unobstructed, but connections below the diaphragm may become obstructed when the ductus venosus closes in the first few days of life.

There are two mechanisms by which TAPVC produces cyanosis: mixing of oxygenated pulmonary venous blood with deoxygenated systemic blood and reduced antegrade pulmonary flow as a result of pulmonary arterial hypertension in cases of severe pulmonary venous obstruction. The presentation of infants with TAPVC is determined by the degree of venous obstruction. Obstructed TAPVC will present during the newborn period with significant cyanosis and tachypnea that may quickly progress to respiratory failure. Patients without obstruction have high pulmonary blood flow and initially have minimal cyanosis, but they may progress to congestive heart failure because of pulmonary overcirculation. Chest radiograph in unobstructed TAPVC may reveal a mildly enlarged cardiac silhouette, but chest radiograph in obstructed TAPVC is notable for marked pulmonary congestion.

Infants with obstructed TAPVC present critically ill and require immediate stabilization before urgent surgical intervention, but all patients with TAPVC require surgical repair to permit pulmonary venous drainage to the left atrium.

Truncus Arteriosus

Truncus arteriosus is a conotruncal defect characterized by the presence of a single arterial trunk that serves as the origin of the aorta, pulmonary artery, and coronary arteries (Fig. 31.7). This condition is almost always associated with a VSD. The truncus is fed by a single truncal valve, most commonly with three cusps, but it may have two to five cusps. The truncal valve typically sits over the VSD. Commonly associated cardiac defects include right aortic arch (33%) and anomalous coronary artery origins. Associated extracardiac anomalies include 22q11.2 microdeletion.

Cyanosis observed in truncus is typically mild related to mixing of systemic and pulmonary venous blood. As pulmonary vascular resistance drops over the newborn period, pulmonary overcirculation will increase resulting in tachypnea and respiratory distress. Signs of heart failure typically develop within the first weeks of life, if not sooner. Patients will often exhibit bounding pulses and a systolic ejection murmur appreciable at the

Pulmonary stenosis

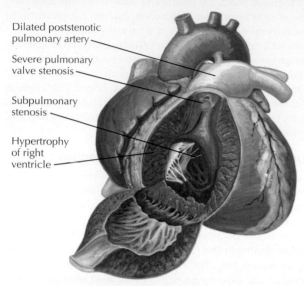

Dilated poststenotic pulmonary artery

Severe pulmonary valve stenosis

Subpulmonary stenosis

Hypertrophy of right ventricle

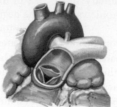

Open normal pulmonary valve

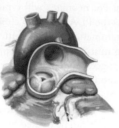

Open stenotic pulmonary valve with fused commissures creating the classic domed shape

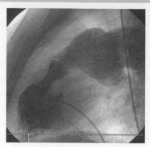

Classic pulmonary valvular stenosis. The figure reveals the doming stenotic pulmonary valve evident during right ventricular angiography. Note the dilated poststenotic pulmonary artery.

Pulmonary balloon valvuloplasty

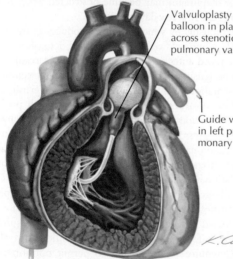

Valvuloplasty balloon in place across stenotic pulmonary valve

Guide wire in left pulmonary artery

Percutaneous catheter from femoral vein

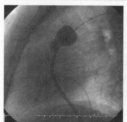

Flouroscopy showing beginning inflation of contrast-filled balloon (**left**) and full inflation with near disappearance of waist from stenotic valve (**right**).

K. Carter

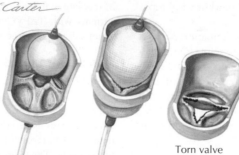

Partially inflated balloon across stenotic pulmonary valve

Fully inflated balloon across stenotic pulmonary valve

Torn valve cusps after balloon inflation

Inoue Balloon Catheter, Toray Industries, Inc., Tokyo, Japan.

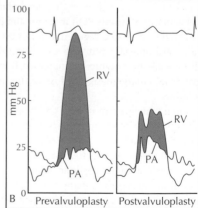

Pressure wave tracings showing difference between right ventricle and pulmonary artery before (**left**) and after (**right**) balloon valvotomy

With permission from Bashore TM, Davidson CJ. Acute hemodynamic effects of percutaneous balloon aortic valvuloplasty. In: Bashore TM, Davidson CJ, eds. *Percutaneous Balloon Valvulopasty and Related Techniques.* Baltimore: Williams & Wilkins; 1991:99–111.

Fig. 31.4 Critical Pulmonic Stenosis.

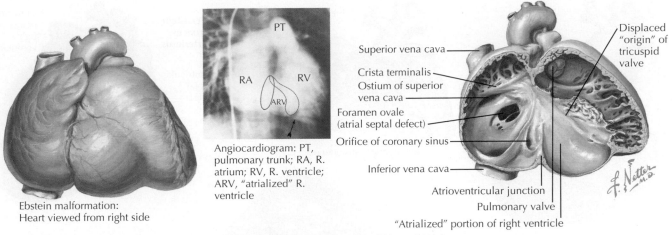

PT

RA RV

ARV

Angiocardiogram: PT, pulmonary trunk; RA, R. atrium; RV, R. ventricle; ARV, "atrialized" R. ventricle

Ebstein malformation: Heart viewed from right side

Superior vena cava
Crista terminalis
Ostium of superior vena cava
Foramen ovale (atrial septal defect)
Orifice of coronary sinus
Inferior vena cava
Atrioventricular junction
Pulmonary valve
"Atrialized" portion of right ventricle
Displaced "origin" of tricuspid valve

Fig. 31.5 Ebstein Anomaly of the Tricuspid Valve.

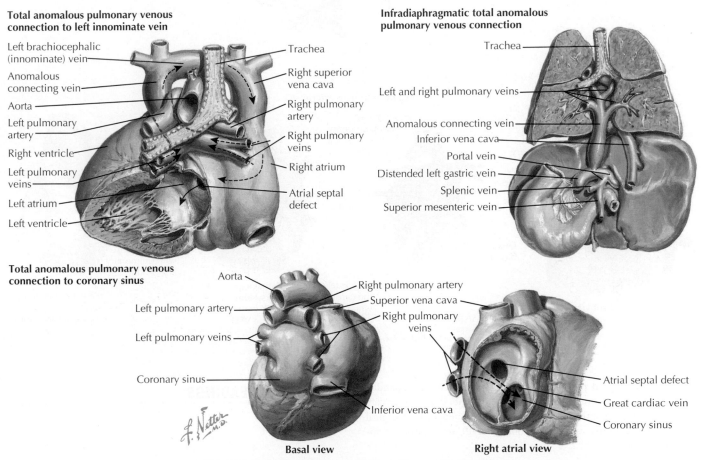

Total anomalous pulmonary venous connection to left innominate vein

Left brachiocephalic (innominate) vein
Anomalous connecting vein
Aorta
Left pulmonary artery
Right ventricle
Left pulmonary veins
Left atrium
Left ventricle

Trachea
Right superior vena cava
Right pulmonary artery
Right pulmonary veins
Right atrium
Atrial septal defect

Infradiaphragmatic total anomalous pulmonary venous connection

Trachea
Left and right pulmonary veins
Anomalous connecting vein
Inferior vena cava
Portal vein
Distended left gastric vein
Splenic vein
Superior mesenteric vein

Total anomalous pulmonary venous connection to coronary sinus

Aorta
Left pulmonary artery
Left pulmonary veins
Coronary sinus

Right pulmonary artery
Superior vena cava
Right pulmonary veins

Inferior vena cava

Basal view

Atrial septal defect
Great cardiac vein
Coronary sinus

Right atrial view

Fig. 31.6 Total Anomalous Pulmonary Venous Connection.

left sternal border. Electrocardiography is nonspecific and chest radiograph may be notable for an enlarged cardiac silhouette. Surgical repair is achieved by surgical separation of aorta and pulmonary artery, placement of a right ventricle–to–pulmonary artery conduit, and VSD closure by baffling the left ventricle to the truncal valve.

FUTURE DIRECTIONS

Progress in the management of patients with cyanotic heart disease is ongoing and reflects the wide range of clinical disciplines involved in the care of these patients. Noninvasive imaging technologies such as cardiac magnetic resonance imaging and computed tomography provide increasingly detailed anatomic and physiologic information, directing care without the risk of more invasive modalities. Treatment continues to improve survival after surgical therapy. These include improvements in surgical technique, intensive care unit management, and long-term medical management. Percutaneous procedures, such as PDA stenting to maintain pulmonary blood flow in ductal-dependent lesions and transcatheter pulmonary valve replacement, are showing promise as alternatives to surgical intervention. Finally, with

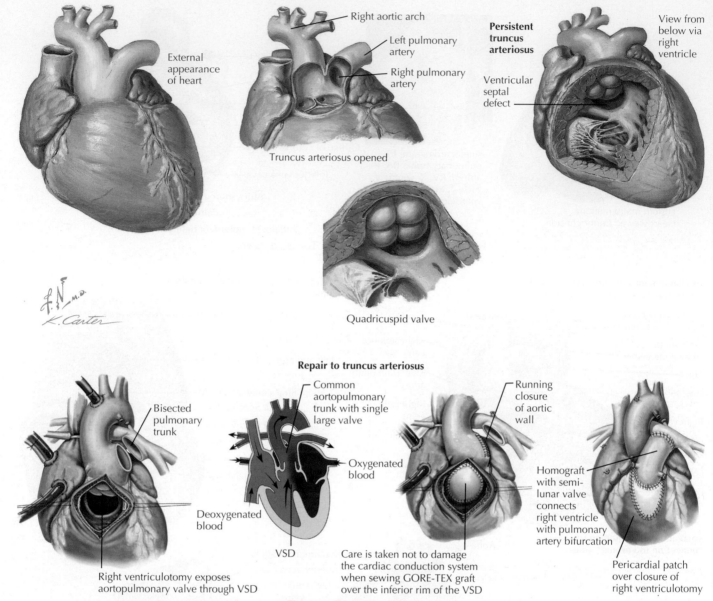

External appearance of heart

Right aortic arch

Left pulmonary artery

Right pulmonary artery

Truncus arteriosus opened

Persistent truncus arteriosus

View from below via right ventricle

Ventricular septal defect

Quadricuspid valve

Repair to truncus arteriosus

Bisected pulmonary trunk

Common aortopulmonary trunk with single large valve

Oxygenated blood

Deoxygenated blood

VSD

Right ventriculotomy exposes aortopulmonary valve through VSD

Care is taken not to damage the cardiac conduction system when sewing GORE-TEX graft over the inferior rim of the VSD

Running closure of aortic wall

Homograft with semi-lunar valve connects right ventricle with pulmonary artery bifurcation

Pericardial patch over closure of right ventriculotomy

Fig. 31.7 Truncus Arteriosus.

dramatically improved postsurgical survival, research has expanded beyond survival to define characteristics of patients that differentiate the success or failure of therapy far beyond the immediate postsurgical period such as objective measures of quality of life and neurodevelopmental outcomes.

SUGGESTED READINGS

Available online.

32

Arrhythmias

Sarah Jaffar and Dustin Nash

✳ CLINICAL VIGNETTE

A 6-week-old boy presents to the emergency department for a chief complaint of fussiness. His parents report that he has felt warm and over the last day has been increasingly fussy and not drinking well. On initial evaluation, his vital signs are notable for temperature of 101.1°F (38.4°C), heart rate of 220 beats/min, blood pressure 93/58 mm Hg, respiratory rate of 20 breaths/min, and SpO₂ 97%. On examination, he is crying and fussy, with mild rhinorrhea but without respiratory distress. He is warm, well perfused with 2+ peripheral pulses, without crackles or hepatomegaly. Acetaminophen is administered, and infectious workup is initiated. His temperature normalizes, but he remains tachycardic with a fixed heart rate of 220 beats/min and now has cold extremities and decreased capillary refill. On continuous heart rate monitor it is difficult to discern P waves. While preparing to administer intravenous antibiotics and fluids for presumed sepsis, a 12-lead electrocardiogram (ECG) is acquired, which confirms absent P waves and narrow-complex tachycardia. Adenosine is administered by rapid intravenous push, and his heart rate acutely drops down to 120 beats/min. Repeat electrocardiography reveals a short PR interval and a delta wave, consistent with Wolff-Parkinson-White syndrome. He is admitted for telemetry monitoring and the cardiology team is consulted.

Although infrequent in the pediatric population, arrhythmias represent significant causes of morbidity and mortality. This chapter describes the cause, clinical significance, and treatment options of common arrhythmias found in pediatric patients.

THE CARDIAC CONDUCTION CYCLE

The diagnosis and management of arrhythmias is aided by understanding of the basic principles of the conduction system (Fig. 32.1). The contraction of the heart relies on spread of depolarizing currents through the myocardium. In a normal cardiac cycle, initial depolarization originates in the sinus node, located in the right atrium. The sinus node is composed of pacemaker cells, which depolarize spontaneously at a rate modulated by the autonomic nervous system. After the sinus node fires, the atria are depolarized resulting in atrial contraction represented by the P wave on electrocardiogram (ECG). The atrial impulse reaches the atrioventricular (AV) node at the base of the intraatrial septum, where the impulse is delayed before conducting to the ventricles via the bundle of His. This conduction tissue splits into the right and left bundle branches, which further divide into Purkinje fibers, allowing for rapid ventricular depolarization and contraction. The AV nodal delay, represented by the PR interval on ECG, allows adequate time for ventricular filling before systole. Ventricular depolarization is represented by the QRS complex.

The ST segment coincides with a relatively isoelectric period before rapid ventricular repolarization, represented by the T wave. The QT interval encompasses the period of ventricular depolarization and repolarization.

Normal sinus rhythm (NSR) is the typical sequential series of events of a heartbeat generated by the sinus node. The characteristics of NSR include a normal P wave morphology and axis (upright P waves in leads I and aVF), a constant PR interval, a P wave before every QRS complex, and a QRS following every P wave.

SINUS ARRHYTHMIAS AND PREMATURE IMPULSES

Sinus Bradycardia

Sinus bradycardia is defined as a heart rate slower than the lower limit of normal for age originating from the sinus node. Sinus bradycardia is often without hemodynamic significance and is commonly seen with increased vagal tone and high level of athletic conditioning. Pathologic conditions associated with sinus bradycardia include increased intracranial pressure, hypothyroidism, hypothermia, hypoxia, hyperkalemia, and drug/toxin exposure.

Sinus Arrhythmia

Sinus arrhythmia refers to physiologic variations of heart rate with respiration resulting from a normal autonomic response. During inspiration, vagal tone decreases with a subsequent increase in heart rate; conversely, during expiration vagal tone increases, with resultant decrease in heart rate.

Premature Atrial Contractions

Premature atrial contractions (PACs) are depolarizations of the atria originating from a separate focus than the sinus node and occur earlier than expected when compared with the prior beats. On ECG, they are represented by a nonsinus P wave. PACs may result in early QRS complexes with normal duration and morphology, wide QRS complexes secondary to aberrant conduction, or absent QRS complexes if the impulse is blocked. PACs are common and often benign in pediatric populations.

Premature Ventricular Contractions

Premature ventricular contractions (PVCs) are depolarizations that originate from a focus within one of the ventricles, resulting in early and wide QRS complexes without preceding P waves. PVCs are classified into two categories: unifocal or multifocal. Unifocal PVCs have the same QRS morphology, whereas multifocal PVCs have different morphologies and are assumed to arise

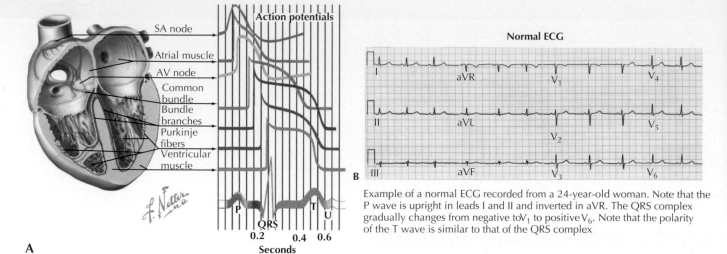

B

Example of a normal ECG recorded from a 24-year-old woman. Note that the P wave is upright in leads I and II and inverted in aVR. The QRS complex gradually changes from negative to V_1 to positive V_6. Note that the polarity of the T wave is similar to that of the QRS complex

Fig. 32.1 Cardiac Conduction System.

from multiple ventricular foci. PVCs may occur in up to 60% of healthy children but can also coincide with pathologic conditions such as myocarditis, cardiomyopathy, long QT syndrome, and congenital heart disease. PVCs may have more significance if they are multifocal, are incessant, occur in couplets or with syncope, or are associated with underlying heart disease or a family history of sudden death. Benign PVCs generally diminish during exercise, but PVCs associated with cardiac disease often persist or increase during exercise.

BRADYARRHYTHMIAS

The most common symptomatic bradyarrhythmias in the pediatric population include sinus node dysfunction and AV block. Infants may present with poor feeding, lethargy, or seizures, and older children can have fatigue, exercise intolerance, or syncope. Severe bradycardia can manifest with signs of poor perfusion and shock.

Sinus Node Dysfunction

Arrhythmias such as severe sinus pause and sinoatrial exit block result from failure of the sinus node to increase the heart rate in response to physiologic stress. Sinus node dysfunction is often due to secondary causes such as cardiac surgery, infection, trauma, ischemia, or medications rather than a primary arrhythmia. Management is based on clinical symptoms and the presence of coexisting heart disease. In symptomatic cases, permanent pacemaker implantation may be needed for definitive therapy.

Atrioventricular Conduction Abnormalities

Abnormal AV conduction occurs when transmission of the sinus node impulse is delayed or blocked because of an abnormality in the AV node or His-Purkinje system (Fig. 32.2).

First-Degree Atrioventricular Block

First-degree AV block results in prolongation of the PR interval due to abnormal delay in conduction through the AV node. This can appear in healthy children as a benign phenomenon, usually related to increased vagal tone. Other causes may include cardiac surgery, rheumatic fever, Lyme disease, digoxin toxicity, and electrolyte imbalance. Isolated first-degree AV block does not require treatment unless there is progression to more advanced AV block.

Second-Degree Atrioventricular Block

Intermittent failure of AV conduction results in two forms of second-degree AV block: Mobitz type I and Mobitz type II, each occurring at different levels within the conduction system. Pathologic causes include myocarditis, cardiomyopathy, myocardial infarction, digitalis toxicity, congenital heart defects, and cardiac surgery.

Mobitz type I (Wenckebach phenomenon) occurs at the level of the AV node, yielding progressive lengthening in the PR interval until one QRS complex or ventricular depolarization fails to occur. This may occur in healthy children with parasympathetic dominance or in trained athletes and is frequently observed during monitoring of heart rates during sleep.

Mobitz type II occurs at the level of the bundle of His and is defined as the intermittent loss of AV conduction without preceding lengthening of the PR interval (i.e., the QRS complex randomly absent). This form is less common and suggests a more serious AV conduction disorder with higher likelihood for progression to complete heart block with hemodynamic compromise.

Third-Degree or Complete Atrioventricular Block

Complete AV block is defined as complete interruption of atrial impulse propagation, resulting in AV dissociation (i.e., atrial and ventricular activity independent of each other). This type of block can be congenital or acquired. ECG will show regular P waves at an appropriate rate for age, with QRS complexes occurring at regular and slower rates than the atrial rate, and no consistent relationship between P waves and QRS complexes.

Congenital Complete Heart Block

Congenital complete heart block occurs in about 1 in 20,000 live births; about 90% of cases occur with associated maternal collagen vascular abnormalities, primarily systemic lupus erythematosus. It can also occur with structural heart disease or as an isolated finding. Fetal bradycardia increases risk for hydrops because of low cardiac output, and congestive heart failure may develop in infancy. However, patients with isolated congenital complete heart block can remain asymptomatic through adolescence. The primary indications for pacemaker implantation in asymptomatic children include an average ventricular rate less than 55 beats/min in infants or less than 70 beats/min in those with congenital heart disease, wide escape rhythms, complex ventricular ectopy, or ventricular dysfunction.

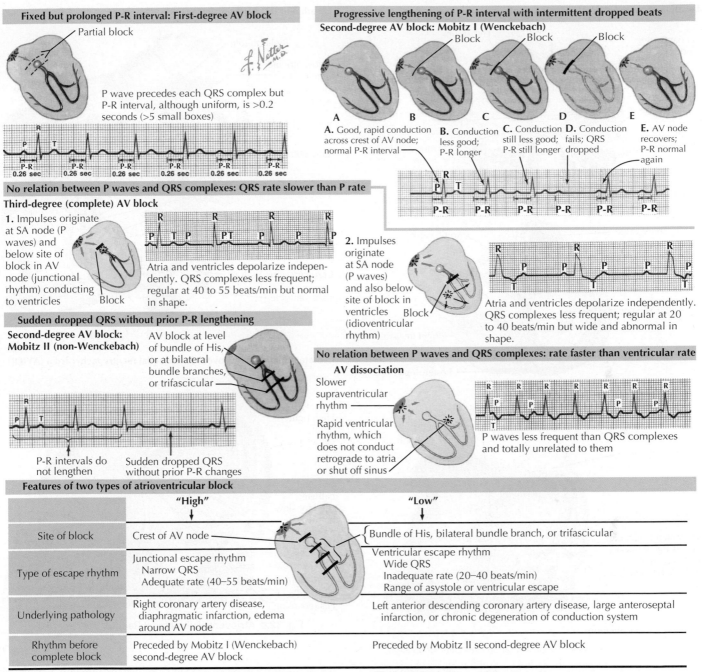

Fig. 32.2 Atrioventricular Conduction Variations.

Acquired Complete Heart Block

Acquired complete heart block occurs most commonly in the postoperative patient population. Other causes include myocarditis, Lyme carditis, acute rheumatic fever, cardiomyopathies, drug overdoses, and myocardial infarction. Symptomatic patients should be treated with atropine or isoproterenol until temporary pacing is available. Permanent pacing is indicated in patients with postoperative complete heart block that persists for at least 7 days after cardiac surgery.

TACHYARRHYTHMIAS

Supraventricular Tachycardia

Supraventricular tachycardia (SVT) involves the conduction system both above and within the AV node and is the most common

tachyarrhythmia seen in the pediatric population, with incidence of 1 in 250 to 1000 live births.

Reentry Tachycardia With an Accessory Pathway: Atrioventricular Reentrant Tachycardia

Atrioventricular reentrant tachycardia (AVRT) is a subset of SVT in which an accessory pathway allows for an electrical circuit to form that involves both the atrial and ventricular myocardium. During SVT, impulses may be carried both in an antegrade (orthodromic conduction) or retrograde fashion (antidromic conduction) through the AV node, with an accessory pathway completing the circuit. AVRT is paroxysmal, occurring with abrupt onset and cessation, and has a rapid, regular heart rate (often over 200 beats/min, especially in neonates and infants). Clinical symptoms in young infants and toddlers are often

Location of atrioventricular accessory pathways and classification

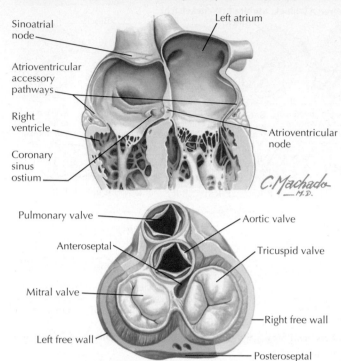

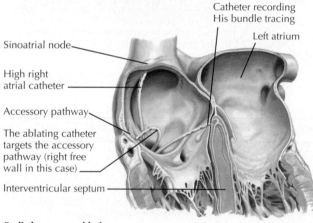

Catheter ablation of accessory pathways

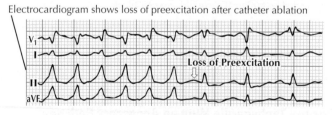

Radiofrequency ablation

Electrocardiogram shows loss of preexcitation after catheter ablation

Fig. 32.3 Accessory Pathways and the Wolff-Parkinson-White Syndrome.

nonspecific, and many children tolerate episodes of SVT very well. If SVT persists or rates are exceptionally elevated, symptoms consistent with heart failure may develop.

The presence of preexcitation (short PR, a widened QRS, and a delta wave) on ECG marks a notable subclass of AVRT called Wolff-Parkinson-White (WPW) syndrome. WPW accounts for 10% to 20% of cases of SVT (Fig. 32.3). This finding may present

Location of the atrioventricular node

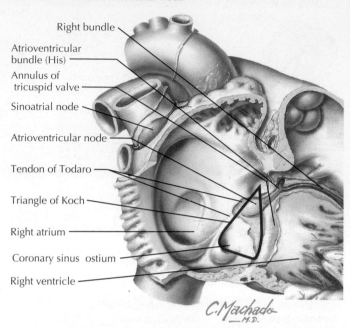

Catheter ablation of atrioventricular nodal reentry tachycardia (AVNRT)

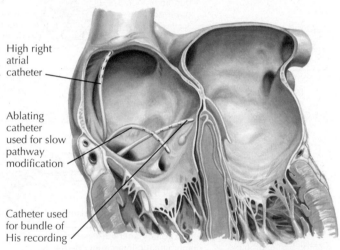

Fig. 32.4 Atrioventricular Nodal Reentry Tachycardia.

at any age and can be associated with Ebstein anomaly, heterotaxy syndrome, and L-transposition of the great arteries. Sudden death may occur because of rapid ventricular responses with 1:1 conduction in the setting of more rapid atrial tachyarrhythmias such as atrial fibrillation.

Reentry Tachycardia Without an Accessory Pathway: Atrioventricular Nodal Reentrant Tachycardia

Atrioventricular nodal reentrant tachycardia (AVNRT) occurs when dual conduction pathways exist within the AV node creating substrate for reentry pathophysiology similar to accessory pathway SVT (Fig. 32.4). Seen more commonly in older children and adolescents, rates can range from 140 to 200 beats/min.

Acute management of hemodynamically unstable patients with reentry tachycardia should seek to restore sinus rhythm either pharmacologically or electrically with synchronized cardioversion. In nonurgent situations, vagal stimulation with the goal of slowing

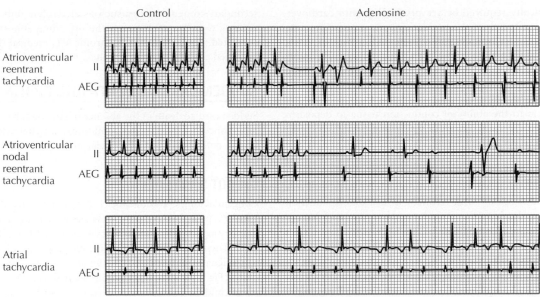

Fig. 32.5 Adenosine Administration.

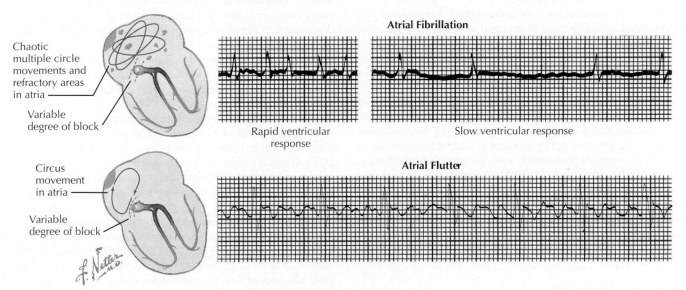

Fig. 32.6 Atrial Flutter and Fibrillation.

conduction through the AV node can be attempted. Commonly used in children, placement of an iced water bag over the face to simulate the diving reflex may abort paroxysmal episodes of SVT. Other vagal maneuvers include the Valsalva maneuver, breath-holding, or blowing against resistance, such as against one's hand or through a straw. Pharmacologic treatment involves rapid infusion of adenosine, which interrupts reentry circuits by blocking AV conduction (Fig. 32.5). Maintenance medications most commonly include digoxin (contraindicated in patients with WPW) or a β blocker such as propranolol. Second-line agents may be necessary but may have negative inotropic effects and should be used with caution.

Definitive treatment for SVT involves radiofrequency ablation of the accessory pathways, bypass tracts, or ectopic foci in the heart. Success rates range from 86% to 96% depending on the location of the accessory pathway and type of SVT.

Intraatrial Tachycardia

Intraatrial reentrant tachycardia (atrial flutter or fibrillation) is caused by reentrant electrical conduction within the atria (Fig. 32.6). Atrial flutter exhibits regular and regularly irregular intervals with atrial rates greater than 250 beats/min. Variable ventricular responses occur as a result of varying degrees of AV block. Risk factors for atrial flutter include structural heart disease with dilated atria, atrial scarring from prior cardiac surgeries, myocarditis, and digitalis toxicity. ECG reveals rapid and regular atrial saw-toothed flutter waves. Atrial fibrillation is much less common in pediatric populations and results from multiple chaotic atrial foci, leading to an irregularly irregular ventricular response. Risk factors for atrial fibrillation are similar to those for atrial flutter. Acute management of atrial fibrillation in hemodynamically stable patients should focus on ventricular rate control.

Synchronized cardioversion can be used in both atrial flutter and fibrillation to restore NSR, but evaluation for intraatrial thrombus is typically required before proceeding with cardioversion, depending on length of the current episode. Long-term anticoagulation should be considered in patients with refractory atrial flutter or fibrillation because of the higher incidence of thromboembolic disease.

Automatic Tachycardias

Automaticity refers to the ability of conduction tissue to depolarize spontaneously. When present outside of the sinus and AV nodes, automaticity can lead to cells firing repetitively, resulting in suppression of pacemaker impulses and tachycardia. Such tachycardias are often susceptible to catecholaminergic stimulation and have characteristic "warm-up" and "cool-down" phases. Automatic tachycardias tend to be chronic and incessant with resultant myocardial dysfunction. Therapies focus on slowing the ventricular response rate and decreasing automaticity of the abnormal foci.

Ectopic atrial tachycardia accounts for approximately 10% to 20% of SVT observed in pediatric patients. Heart rates often range from 140 to 200 beats/min, with ECG revealing P waves with an abnormal axis. Vagal maneuvers and adenosine will yield a gradual slowing in rate with subsequent acceleration after cessation of each maneuver (Fig. 32.5). Spontaneous resolution may occur, but most patients require chronic therapy with multiple agents.

Multifocal or chaotic atrial tachycardia is much less common and is characterized by multiple foci of increased automaticity in the atria, resulting in three or more distinct P wave morphologies on ECG. Often confused with atrial fibrillation, this arrhythmia occurs most often in the newborn period without associated cardiac disease. Spontaneous resolution frequently occurs during the first year of life.

Junctional ectopic tachycardia (JET) occurs when a focus of automaticity is present in the region of the AV node, leading to AV dissociation and a ventricular rate greater than the atrial rate. Congenital JET presents in the neonatal period with symptoms of heart failure, often in association with congenital heart disease. Postoperative JET after cardiac surgery is usually transient and self-limited, lasting from 24 to 72 hours; however, it may cause significant hemodynamic compromise and can be fatal if not controlled. The majority of patients require medical therapy with multiple agents. Radiofrequency ablation is reserved for resistant cases because of the high risk for inducing complete heart block from ablation points near the AV node.

Ventricular Tachycardia

Ventricular tachycardia (VT) is defined as three or more ventricular beats in series at a heart rate above the normal range for age. The spectrum of presentation ranges from the asymptomatic patient with an incidental finding to sudden cardiac death (Fig. 32.7). Acute causes of VT include electrolyte imbalance, infections (myocarditis, pericarditis, rheumatic fever), toxin/drug exposure (cocaine, antiarrhythmics, general anesthetics, sympathomimetics, psychotropics), trauma, and myocardial ischemia (infarction, anomalous coronary arteries, Kawasaki disease). Chronic causes of VT include postoperative congenital heart disease, cardiomyopathies, tumors, infiltrative processes, primary channelopathies, and idiopathic forms. VT should be distinguished from other arrhythmias that present with a wide QRS such as SVT with aberrant conduction; however, any wide QRS complex tachycardia should be considered VT until proven otherwise. Hemodynamically unstable patients must be treated promptly with synchronized cardioversion. For hemodynamically stable patients, intravenous amiodarone and lidocaine are the initial drugs of choice. Ventricular arrhythmias

secondary to acute causes such as electrolyte imbalance, hypoxia, or drug toxicity resolve after the offending abnormality has been corrected. For patients with chronic VT, medical therapies should be aimed at preventing recurrence.

SUDDEN CARDIAC DEATH AND CHANNELOPATHIES

Sudden cardiac death in the absence of structural heart disease should raise concern for inherited conditions and channelopathies predisposing patients toward ventricular arrhythmias and sudden cardiac events.

Long QT Syndromes

Congenital long QT syndrome (LQTS) is a disorder of abnormal ventricular repolarization that results from ion channel genetic mutations, manifesting as prolongation of the corrected QT (QTc) interval on ECG. These alterations in conduction properties predispose patients to malignant ventricular arrhythmias, syncope, and sudden cardiac death (Fig. 32.7). It is commonly defined as a QTc longer than 460 ms in children younger than 15 years old, 450 ms in men and 470 ms in women, but in some forms the QTc can be normal on resting ECG. Other features include abnormal T-wave morphologies (notched T waves, T-wave alternans), bradycardia for age, or history of torsades de pointes. Holter monitor and outpatient exercise testing are both useful diagnostic tests in evaluating patients with syncope and suspected long QT syndrome.

To date, at least 17 genetic mutations have been discovered. Initial familial syndromes were identified as the Jervell and Lange-Nielsen syndrome, a rare autosomal form with sensorineural deafness, along with the autosomal dominant form without deafness, Romano-Ward syndrome. Since that time, multiple genetic mutations have been identified as causes of LQTS with three primary autosomal dominant mutations in potassium and sodium channels: LQT1, LQT2, and LQT3. Whereas patients with LQT1 appear to be at a particularly high risk for sudden death with exercise, patients with LQT2 appear to be at most increased risk in the presence of loud noises and emotional stimuli.

Treatment with β blockers has been shown to markedly reduce the incidence of sudden death, especially in patients with LQT1 and to a lesser extent in LQT2. It is important to avoid QT-prolonging medications when feasible. Patients with syncope despite medical therapy or those who present with aborted sudden cardiac death should be considered for placement of an automatic implantable cardiac defibrillator (ICD).

Brugada Syndrome

Brugada syndrome is a genetic disorder characterized by specific ECG findings in conjunction with increased risk for ventricular tachyarrhythmias and sudden cardiac death. Patients with this condition have a "Brugada pattern" (Fig. 32.7): normal QT intervals, ST-segment elevation with a "coved" appearance, and right ventricular conduction delay, although this pattern can be transient or absent. Initial presentation can include syncope, atrial fibrillation, disordered nocturnal respiration, or sudden death at rest or during sleep, often in the setting of elevated body temperature (e.g., with fever or after vigorous exercise) or in the early morning. Management is focused on prevention of sudden cardiac arrest, with ICD as first-line therapy.

Catecholaminergic Polymorphic Ventricular Tachycardia

Catecholaminergic polymorphic ventricular tachycardia (CPVT) is caused by abnormalities in calsequestrin and ryanodine receptor genes.

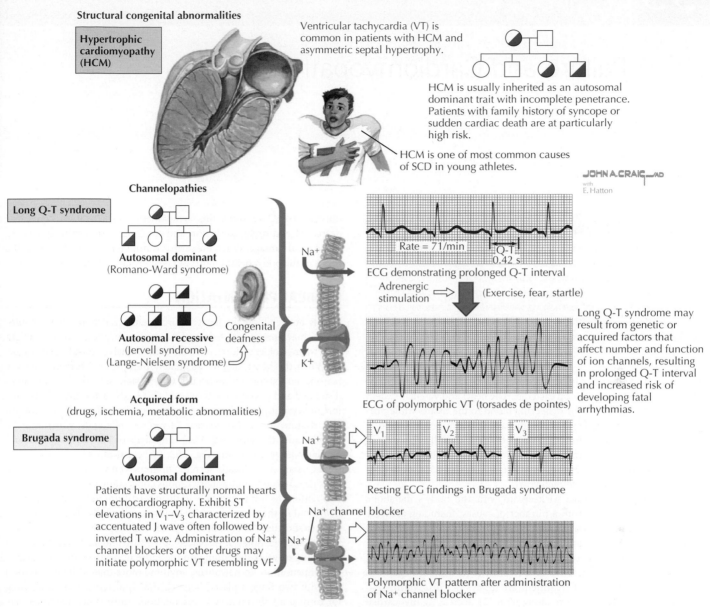

Fig. 32.7 Sudden Cardiac Death.

It predisposes patients to exercise-induced polymorphic VT, syncope, and a high risk for sudden death in the setting of *normal* resting ECGs. CPVT can be diagnosed by stress testing.

FUTURE DIRECTIONS

The diagnosis and management of arrhythmias in the pediatric population have advanced tremendously in recent years, with progress made in electrophysiologic mapping and pacemaker technologies, as well as ablation strategies. The scope of ambulatory monitoring has broadened in recent years with the prevalence of smart watches with ECG capabilities, although the public health implications and impact on clinical practices are still to be determined. Advances in genetic identification of patients with channelopathies will likely improve morbidity and mortality associated with certain arrhythmias.

SUGGESTED READINGS

Available online.

33

Heart Failure and Cardiomyopathy

Gayathri Prabhakar and Travus White

CLINICAL VIGNETTE

A healthy 15-year-old boy presents to the emergency department with chest pain and shortness of breath. Of note, he had a febrile illness approximately 2 weeks ago. He is noted to be tachycardic and tachypneic with a systolic murmur noted over the cardiac apex. He is given an intravenous fluid bolus with no improvement in heart rate. An electrocardiogram shows widened QRS complexes, and a chest radiograph shows cardiomegaly and pulmonary edema. A troponin is elevated. The patient is admitted for management of heart failure secondary to myocarditis.

A healthy child's heart may beat more than 200,000 times and transport more than 3 tons of blood each day. The heart and vascular system are primarily responsible for delivering blood to the tissues while providing oxygen and nutrients and withdrawing waste products. Heart failure is the inability of the heart to meet the metabolic demands of the body because of the inability of the ventricles of the heart to fill with or eject blood. Heart failure affects 12,000 to 35,000 children younger than 19 years of age each year.

The failure of the heart to keep up with the body's metabolic requirements may arise from a number of causes, including arrhythmias, metabolic insufficiencies, and congenital heart defects. Through a careful history and physical examination and with tests such as electrocardiography (ECG), echocardiography, and cardiac catheterization, the cause is often learned and treatment instituted. Regardless of the source, the goals of treatment are always (1) discovering and addressing the cause of failure along with (2) decreasing myocardial workload and oxygen consumption and (3) augmenting and supporting function and systemic oxygenation. With such interventions, the hope is that the heart will remodel, if not recover. Because of the danger of cardiovascular collapse, which may be very rapid, prompt consultation with pediatric cardiologists and intensivists is important, and early recognition requires diagnostic vigilance.

ETIOLOGY AND PATHOGENESIS

The etiology of heart failure can be thought of in two major categories: pump failure (ventricular dysfunction) and overcirculation. Ventricular dysfunction can occur in a structurally normal heart because of a variety of conditions, including cardiomyopathy, myocarditis, arrhythmias, toxins, and metabolic etiologies but also can be due to congenital heart disease. Overload failure can be due to increased pulmonary blood flow, left-to-right shunts, anemia, regurgitant valvular lesions, and increased cardiac output.

Initially the heart is able to compensate by increasing cardiac output. On a molecular level, metabolic pathways are upregulated and downregulated to better use substrates, including oxygen. Sympathetic tone increases, and the renin-aldosterone-angiotensin system is upregulated. Over time, this sympathetic overactivation can cause decreased end-organ perfusion and function and eventually lead to myocardial damage. When the cardiac output is not enough to meet the needs of the body, heart failure can be considered "uncompensated."

CLINICAL PRESENTATION

Infants and children in heart failure present differently from adults. Infants may present with feeding difficulties, tachypnea, and poor weight gain, whereas older children often have abdominal complaints and fatigue.

When the heart fails to adequately pump blood forward for any reason, venous congestion occurs. On the right side, the liver becomes distended and engorged with blood. This leads to abdominal discomfort or vomiting initially, but in certain prolonged cases, may lead to liver dysfunction and distension of venous collaterals, which may be visible under the skin (Fig. 33.1). The signs of peripheral edema and jugular venous distension (Fig. 33.2, *left*) classically seen in adults and teenagers are not typically seen in children. Venous congestion on the left side can lead to pulmonary venous congestion and fluid extravasation within the lungs, typically in the interstitium in infants (Fig. 33.2, *right*) and in the alveoli in older children and adults. This congestion leads to shortness of breath, tachypnea, and dyspnea.

The apex beat may be displaced downward and laterally and may be bounding or weak depending on the cause of heart failure and degree of compensation. In newborns, anything more than a slight pulsation felt with two fingers placed beneath the xiphisternum is concerning for cardiac involvement. On auscultation, muffled heart sounds may signify a pericardial effusion with fluid between the heart and the pericardium. A third or fourth heart sound, or a gallop, is frequently heard in failing hearts. Third heart sounds can be normal in children and are thought to be caused by rapid diastolic filling. A fourth heart sound is indicative of a poorly compliant ventricle.

Murmurs may be heard in the setting of heart failure caused by a primary structural abnormality, and some murmurs represent turbulence across an incompetent valve caused by severe left ventricular dilatation seen in some failing hearts.

As the heart begins to fail in the volume of blood it can pump, the sympathetic nervous system seeks to compensate by increasing the heart rate. Upregulation of the sympathetic nervous system may also cause vasoconstriction and diaphoresis, and the child may present as cold, pale, and diaphoretic. A child in decompensated heart failure may present in cardiogenic shock with poor end-organ perfusion, cool and mottled extremities, delayed capillary refill, and a decreased systolic blood pressure.

DIFFERENTIAL DIAGNOSIS

The heart can fail for multiple reasons (Box 33.1). The most common cause of heart failure in a child with a structurally normal heart

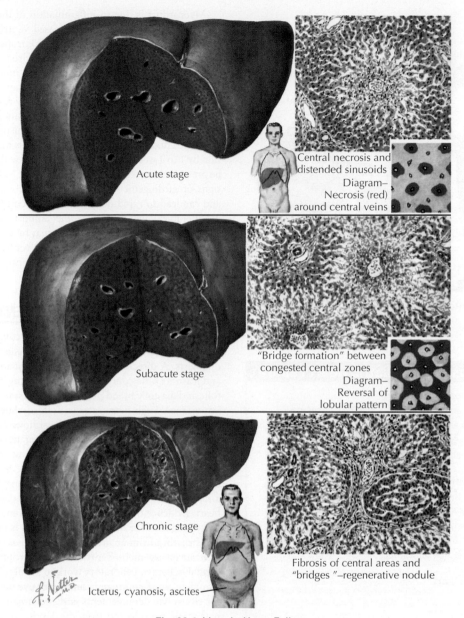

Acute stage

Central necrosis and distended sinusoids
Diagram—Necrosis (red) around central veins

Subacute stage

"Bridge formation" between congested central zones
Diagram—Reversal of lobular pattern

Chronic stage

Fibrosis of central areas and "bridges"—regenerative nodule

Icterus, cyanosis, ascites

Fig. 33.1 Liver in Heart Failure.

is cardiomyopathy. The most common forms of cardiomyopathy are dilated cardiomyopathy, hypertrophic cardiomyopathy, and, less commonly, restrictive.

Dilated cardiomyopathy (DCM) accounts for 50% to 60% of pediatric cardiomyopathy cases. The cause of DCM is typically unknown, but can be due to infection, chemotherapy, or a metabolic disease (including muscular dystrophy). Injury to the myocardium causes ventricular enlargement, leading to impaired ability for the heart to squeeze (systolic dysfunction). Patients can present with palpitations or respiratory symptoms, or in extremis with altered mental status, hypotension, or even sudden death. On auscultation, they can have a gallop rhythm. ECG can show arrhythmias and nonspecific T wave changes. A chest radiograph can show cardiomegaly or pulmonary vascular prominence. Echocardiography demonstrates markedly dilated left and sometimes right ventricles with diminished systolic function.

Hypertrophic cardiomyopathy (HCM) accounts for 25% to 40% of cardiomyopathies. In HCM, there is thickening of the ventricles

without dilation of the chambers. Mutations in sarcomere or components of the cardiomyocyte cytoskeleton genes (typically autosomal dominant inheritance) lead to wall thickening, disproportionately involving the interventricular septum, resulting in impaired filling of the heart and diastolic dysfunction. Systolic function is typically preserved and is often hyperdynamic. Approximately 25% of patients can have obstruction of the flow of the blood out of the left ventricle (left ventricular outflow obstruction) as a result of the septal hypertrophy and abnormal anterior movements of the mitral valve, which is dynamic in nature. Patients are largely asymptomatic, but can present with palpitations, chest pain, fatigability, dizziness, and syncope. Hypertrophic cardiomyopathy is a common cause of sudden cardiac death, particularly in athletes. On auscultation, one may hear a systolic ejection murmur, which is worsened with standing or the Valsalva maneuver because of a decrease in ventricular preload and worsening left ventricular outflow obstruction. Conversely, maneuvers that increase systemic vascular resistance cause the systolic murmur to decrease in intensity. An ECG can demonstrate left ventricular hypertrophy with

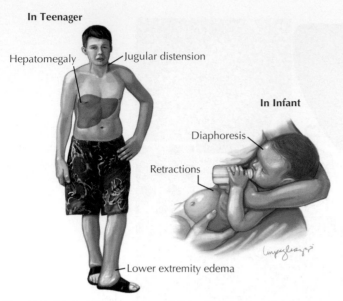

In Teenager

Hepatomegaly — — Jugular distension

In Infant

Diaphoresis

Retractions

— Lower extremity edema

Fig. 33.2 Clinical Presentation of Heart Failure in a Teenager and Infant.

BOX 33.1 Causes of Pediatric Heart Failure

Congenital Heart Disease
- Coarctation of the aorta and obstructive left-sided heart disease
- Anomalous left coronary artery from the pulmonary artery
- Left-to-right shunting defects with pulmonary overcirculation
- Valvular disease with volume overload

Primary Cardiomyopathy
- Dilated cardiomyopathy
- Hypertrophic cardiomyopathy
- Restrictive cardiomyopathy
- Arrhythmogenic right ventricular dysplasia
- Left ventricular noncompaction cardiomyopathy

Structurally Normal Heart
- Myocarditis
- Sepsis
- Inborn errors of metabolism
- Hypertension
- Thyroid disorder
- Tachycardia-induced cardiomyopathy
- Toxin-mediated
- Anthracycline toxicity
- Muscular dystrophy
- Pulmonary hypertension
- Acute rheumatic fever
- Kawasaki disease
- Multisystem inflammatory syndrome in children associated with COVID-19

ST segment and T wave abnormalities. Chest radiography can show cardiomegaly and a prominent left ventricle. Echocardiogram will show hypertrophy of the myocardium. The prognosis is poor for children diagnosed with HCM when younger than 1 year of age or for those with inborn errors of metabolism. First-degree family members of patients with HCM require ongoing, serial screening cardiology evaluations with echocardiograms.

Myocarditis is due to inflammation of the myocardium with cell damage or death leading to decreased ventricular function and cardiac output. In the United States and Europe, most cases are of viral origin, primarily adenovirus and enterovirus. The decrease in myocardial function caused by myocarditis may manifest either suddenly or indolently. Myocarditis may manifest at any age in varying degrees of heart failure, and primary complaints may revolve around chest pain, respiratory distress, or abdominal distress and decreased appetite from venous stasis. There may be a fever or a history thereof from the primary infection; a history of a flulike illness may precede the presentation by 1 to 4 weeks. A resting tachycardia with or without a gallop will be present, along with tachypnea or cough. More severe cases may have signs of cardiogenic shock (hypotension, cool and pale extremities) and can lead to rapid decompensation requiring advanced heart failure therapies, including inotropic support and extracorporeal membrane oxygenation (ECMO). There may be a systolic murmur of mitral regurgitation, typically as a result of left ventricular dilation. Atrial and ventricular fibrillation along with atrioventricular nodal block can be seen and may lead to sudden death.

EVALUATION AND MANAGEMENT

Because of the high risk for cardiovascular collapse, heart failure should be managed in close consultation with pediatric intensivists and cardiologists. A directed history is important to frame the presentation and learn its time course. Resting vital signs, including heart rate, systolic and diastolic blood pressures, and respiratory rate, are of primary importance. High heart rates with borderline or low blood pressures are concerning findings that the cardiovascular system is involved, whether from primary cardiac disease or secondary to another condition such as sepsis. A posteroanterior chest radiograph may be useful in evaluating both the lungs and size of the cardiac silhouette. A child's cardiac shadow should be 50% or less than the diameter of the chest; a larger shadow may indicate an overloaded and potentially failing heart. Evidence of pulmonary infiltration may be secondary to a primary lung cause or heart failure. An ECG is important to differentiate sinus rhythm from an arrhythmia as well as to look for possible signs of heart enlargement, ventricular hypertrophy, heart strain, or myocardial ischemia. Laboratory workup should, at a minimum, include a complete blood count and comprehensive metabolic panel to evaluate for electrolyte derangements and end-organ involvement, and brain-natriuretic peptide and troponin levels. An echocardiogram may be necessary to evaluate heart function and structure. Once the diagnosis of heart failure is made, it is prudent to pursue a more comprehensive workup to confirm the cause and help determine treatment options. Many centers also use cardiac magnetic resonance imaging or catheterization to aid with diagnosis.

If signs of heart failure are present (tachycardia, borderline or low blood pressure, tachypnea, hepatomegaly), judicious use of fluid replacement along with early support with inotropic medications, such as milrinone and dopamine, intubation, sedation, and paralysis may be necessary to reduce metabolic demand in the most serious cases. In cases of complete cardiovascular collapse (shock) when the heart function and blood pressure are unable to maintain adequate perfusion despite maximal support, ECMO may be required to support the child. These large external devices are able to maintain adequate cardiac output and oxygenation to support the patient for days to weeks. If longer periods are necessary, implantable ventricular assist devices are available to support the child until a heart transplant is available.

Volume status is critical in the treatment of heart failure because fluid overload and increased myocardial wall stress exert extra strain on a failing heart. A history of recent weight gain, peripheral or periorbital edema, signs of hepatic distension, and electrolyte abnormalities may indicate a picture consistent with heart failure. Increased central venous pressure along with diminished arterial mean pressure, common in this setting, will diminish renal perfusion and impair fluid excretion. Intravenous diuresis to the patient's estimated dry weight along with the addition of inotropic support may be necessary. Measurement of central venous pressure and mixed venous oxygen saturation through a central catheter is often additionally helpful in estimating cardiac output.

Failing hearts are also more prone to arrhythmias, and inpatient telemetry or 24-hour surveillance Holter monitors should play a routine role in the evaluation of children in heart failure. Finally, hearts that are markedly dilated and hypocontractile are prone to thrombus formation, and such children are at risk for thromboembolism and stroke. Medications to reduce coagulation and platelet function are important in this population.

Because of natural changes in vascular physiology that start at birth, an important clue in the evaluation of a child in heart failure is the patient's age. Infants who present at birth with heart failure most likely have sustained an in-utero insult such as asphyxiation, maternal sepsis, intrauterine myocarditis, prolonged fetal arrhythmia, perinatal hemorrhage, or (rarely) primary valvar regurgitation. An infant who presents at a few days of life typically has structural congenital cardiac anomalies. Finally, children who present from several weeks to a few months of age in heart failure often have shunt defects, coinciding with a decrease in pulmonary vascular resistance. At all of these times or any time thereafter, children may present in heart failure because of underlying genetic, metabolic, or infectious causes.

FUTURE DIRECTIONS

One area of rapid improvement in pediatric heart failure is the continuing development of pediatric ventricular assist devices (VADs). Unlike ECMO, with which a child's heart may be supported for days to weeks in the hope that it will recover from whatever insult it has sustained, VADs allow much longer support and can be used until a child is listed for and receives a heart transplant. VADs also can be used to allow the myocardium to heal in anticipation of eventual device explantation or as a palliative therapy. Devices such as the Berlin Heart EXCOR use extrathoracic pneumatic pumps to help provide pulsatile cardiac output through cannulae that connect to the child's circulation. Newer models include the HeartMate 3 and the HeartWare, which are nonpulsatile devices implanted directly into the heart and are associated with fewer comorbidities. VADs continue to be an exciting area of innovation in the realm of pediatric heart failure, and our use and understanding of these devices will only continue to grow.

SUGGESTED READINGS

Available online.

34

Cardiac Evaluation of Chest Pain, Syncope, and Palpitations

Sarah Jaffar and Catherine E. Tomasulo

 CLINICAL VIGNETTE

A 13-year-old girl presents to her pediatrician after two syncopal episodes with associated palpitations, chest tightness, and nausea occurring during volleyball practice. Family history is unknown because she is adopted. Her vital signs are normal for age, and she is alert and overall well-appearing. Physical examination, including cardiac examination, is normal. She is instructed to avoid strenuous activity and is referred to a pediatric cardiologist for additional evaluation. Echocardiography demonstrates normal biventricular size and function, but the left coronary artery appears to originate from the right sinus of Valsalva. Cardiac magnetic resonance imaging confirms the diagnosis and shows the left coronary artery coursing between the aorta and main pulmonary artery, concerning for compression. She is scheduled for exercise stress testing and referred to a cardiothoracic surgeon for possible intervention.

Chest pain, palpitations, and syncope represent common complaints leading to unscheduled clinic and hospital visits and provoke anxiety in patients and caregivers. However, unlike in adult populations, these complaints in pediatric patients often represent noncardiac issues and are usually not caused by serious disease processes. This chapter will discuss the causes of chest pain, syncope, and palpitations; general approach to management; and indications for pediatric cardiology referral.

CHEST PAIN

Chest pain is one of the most common chief complaints in children and adolescents presenting to the emergency department or outpatient office; however, the majority of pediatric chest pain complaints have benign causes.

Noncardiac Chest Pain
Musculoskeletal

Musculoskeletal or chest wall pain is the most common cause of chest pain in pediatrics and is distinguished by history and reassuring physical examination findings. Trauma and muscle strain are common causes of chest wall pain, especially in adolescents active in sports, often manifesting with localized pain, sometimes with swelling or erythema on examination. History of significant chest trauma with severe chest pain, abnormal cardiac examination, or dyspnea should elicit investigation for myocardial contusion or hemopericardium.

Costochondritis is characterized by sharp pain along the upper costochondral joints that worsens with deep breathing and lasts a few seconds to a few minutes, with chest wall tenderness reproduced by palpation. *Tietze syndrome* is similar, usually developing after an upper respiratory tract infection with excessive coughing, causing nonsuppurative inflammation of the costochondral, costosternal, or sternoclavicular joints. *Slipping rib syndrome* is characterized by pain over the lower chest, attributed to dislocation of the eighth, ninth, or tenth ribs, because these ribs attach to the sternum by a cartilaginous cap and are often hypermobile. Patients may describe a popping sensation or hear clicking. Pain worsens with deep breathing or bending down and can be reproduced with the hooking maneuver, in which the examiner places a finger under the inferior rib margin and pulls the rib edge outward and upward. *Precordial catch*, or "Texidor twinge," can be described as a sudden sharp pain, lasting a few seconds, over the intercostal space at the left lower sternal border or cardiac apex. The cause is unclear but has been associated with poor posture and is thought to be related to nerve impingement.

Pulmonary

Studies have shown approximately 2% to 11% of chest pain in pediatric patients is due to a pathologic respiratory condition. Chest pain is often pleuritic with associated tachypnea or increased work of breathing. Bronchial conditions including exercise-induced asthma are the most common pulmonary causes of chest pain. Chest pain associated with fever, and cough should elicit consideration of infectious conditions. Pulmonary embolism should be considered in cases of chest pain with hypoxemia and shortness of breath and without infectious symptoms. Another noninfectious consideration includes pneumothorax, characterized by unilateral diminished breath sounds and possible hypoxemia and tension physiology. In patients with known sickle cell disease, chest pain should raise concern for acute chest syndrome or pulmonary infarction.

Gastrointestinal

Gastrointestinal causes account for up to 8% of pediatric complaints of chest pain. Common pathologic conditions include gastroesophageal reflux disease, peptic ulcer disease, esophageal spasm, esophagitis, and cholecystitis. Burning chest pain with a temporal relationship to food intake is typical of reflux. Chest pain with swallowing should elicit consideration of esophageal spasm, retained foreign body, or other causes of dysphagia. Chest pain and hematemesis after a prolonged period of forceful vomiting should raise concern for Mallory-Weiss tear.

Psychogenic

Psychogenic chest pain in older children can result from anxiety or panic attacks. There is often an association with other somatic complaints and sleep disturbances. Hyperventilation associated with anxiety can precipitate chest pain as a result of spasm of the diaphragm, gastric distension from aerophagia, or coronary vasoconstriction due to hypocapnic alkalosis.

Miscellaneous

Chest pain resulting from breast-related causes can be seen in pubertal patients. Scoliosis or other deformities that cause spinal cord or nerve

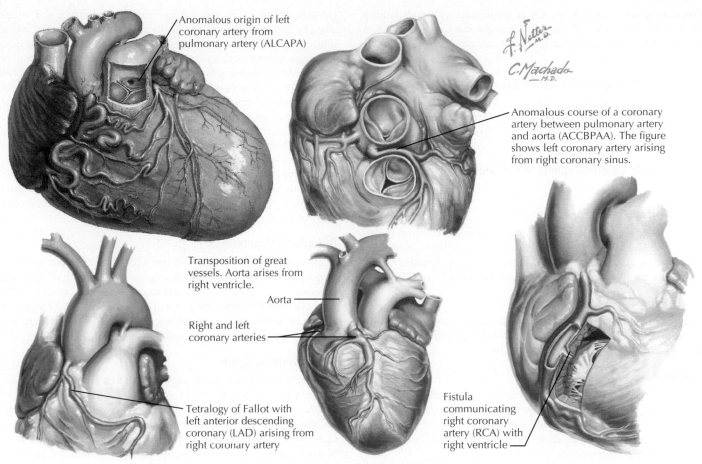

Anomalous origin of left coronary artery from pulmonary artery (ALCAPA)

Anomalous course of a coronary artery between pulmonary artery and aorta (ACCBPAA). The figure shows left coronary artery arising from right coronary sinus.

Transposition of great vessels. Aorta arises from right ventricle.

Aorta

Right and left coronary arteries

Tetralogy of Fallot with left anterior descending coronary (LAD) arising from right coronary artery

Fistula communicating right coronary artery (RCA) with right ventricle

Fig. 34.1 Coronary Artery Abnormalities.

root compression may present with chest pain. Intrathoracic masses can lead to chest pain, typically associated with other systemic signs suggestive of malignancy.

Cardiac Chest Pain

Chest pain due to cardiac conditions is rare in pediatrics, accounting for approximately 5% of patients. However, it is important to consider chest pain as a possible first symptom of potentially life-threatening conditions. Chest pain due to myocardial ischemia can manifest as *angina*, described as substernal squeezing, crushing, tightness, pressure, or burning, with radiation to the left arm, neck, or jaw and is worsened with exertion and associated with diaphoresis, nausea, and/or dyspnea.

Pericarditis

Pericarditis is inflammation of the pericardial membrane and can be accompanied by pericardial effusions. Causes include infectious, immune-mediated, or metabolic conditions; malignancy; trauma; underlying collagen vascular disorder; and postpericardiotomy problems. The chest pain is typically sharp, retrosternal, and pleuritic; worsened when supine; and improved when upright and leaning forward. Examination might reveal a pericardial friction rub. Electrocardiogram (ECG) may show widespread ST-elevation or PR-depression.

Myocarditis

Myocarditis is inflammation of the myocardium, typically secondary to infection or toxin. As inflammatory cells infiltrate the myocardium, interstitial edema and myocyte death with fibrotic replacement occur,

often with left ventricular dysfunction. Children typically present with chest pain resulting from myocardial ischemia or ventricular arrhythmias. Other findings include dyspnea, palpitations, acute heart failure, and ST-changes on ECG.

Coronary Artery Abnormalities

Coronary artery abnormalities are uncommon but important causes of chest pain resulting from myocardial ischemia and can be congenital (Fig. 34.1) or acquired.

Anomalous left coronary artery from the pulmonary artery (ALCAPA) leads to myocardial ischemia and cardiomyopathy because of the relatively low coronary artery perfusion pressure. ALCAPA often presents in infancy as irritability, diaphoresis, feeding intolerance, and eventually circulatory shock.

Anomalous aortic origin of a coronary artery (AAOCA) occurs when the left or right coronary artery arises from the opposite side of the aorta. The most concerning variant occurs when the left coronary artery arises from the right sinus of Valsalva, although the most common variant is the right coronary artery arising from the left sinus of Valsalva. AAOCA may present with either angina due to myocardial ischemia or with sudden death. This presentation is due to limitations in antegrade coronary flow, as the coronary artery arises from a slit-like opening in the aorta and then courses between the two great vessels. Symptoms of chest pain typically occur with exercise, attributed to expansion of the aortic root and pulmonary trunk along with increased myocardial demand, thereby further limiting coronary artery perfusion.

In transplant patients, coronary artery vasculopathy due to rejection can manifest with myocardial ischemia. Patients who have had surgery involving the coronary arteries are at risk for developing coronary artery ostial stenosis. Other considerations include familial hyperlipidemia with associated premature coronary atherosclerosis. A history of Kawasaki disease should raise concern for coronary artery aneurysm or stenosis.

Left Ventricular Outflow Tract Obstruction

Congenital heart disease with associated left ventricular outflow tract obstruction, including hypertrophic cardiomyopathy (HCM) and aortic stenosis can lead to decreased coronary blood flow, with subsequent ischemia and angina.

Hypertrophic Cardiomyopathy and Dilated Cardiomyopathy

See Chapter 33.

Aortic Dissection

Aortic dissection typically presents as severe tearing chest pain radiating to the back. Although this is uncommon in pediatrics, those with predisposing conditions such as Marfan syndrome, vascular Ehlers-Danlos syndrome, and Loeys-Dietz syndrome are at increased risk.

Toxin Exposure

Drug use, including cocaine, methamphetamines, and sympathomimetic agents, may cause chest pain as a result of coronary vasospasm leading to myocardial ischemia or arrhythmias.

Arrhythmias

Prolonged tachyarrhythmias or bradyarrhythmias resulting in ventricular dysfunction and subsequent ischemia can cause chest pain. The sensation of palpitations associated with arrhythmias is often confused with chest pain by patients when describing symptoms. Arrhythmias are discussed in Chapter 32.

SYNCOPE

Syncope is defined as a brief, sudden loss of consciousness and postural/motor tone as a result of decreased cerebral blood flow. This decrease may be attributable to systemic vasodilation, decreased cardiac output, or both. Syncope may be accompanied by brief involuntary movements. Syncope should be distinguished from presyncope (dizziness/lightheadedness without loss of consciousness), vertigo (sensation of spinning), and syncopal-like events (e.g., seizures, migraines, conversion disorder).

Neurally Mediated Syncope

Neurally mediated syncope (NMS) accounts for more than 80% of cases presenting to the emergency department or primary care physician. NMS can be divided into subtypes, although abnormal regulation of the autonomic nervous system is common to all.

Vasovagal Syncope

The most common cause of NMS is *vasovagal syncope*, otherwise known as vasodepressor, neurocardiogenic, or reflex syncope. It is thought to be mediated by an exaggerated response to sudden decreases in ventricular filling pressure. Standing leads to decreased venous return, with reduced left ventricular filling causing decreased signaling from ventricular mechanoreceptors to the brainstem. This pathway stimulates sympathetic activity, eliciting heart rate elevation and systemic vasoconstriction. In patients with vasovagal syncope, there is often a vigorous ventricular contraction in the setting of reduced ventricular filling, resulting in paradoxical central inhibition of peripheral sympathetic tone, vasodilation, relative bradycardia, and then resultant sudden decrease in cardiac output and cerebral blood flow. The prodrome

typically includes dizziness, nausea, pallor, diaphoresis, and visual changes. Loss of consciousness usually lasts less than 1 minute, with a short recovery period accompanied by fatigue, dizziness, and nausea. Vasovagal syncope occurs more often in females and adolescents. It is associated with standing for prolonged periods, particularly in warm temperatures, rising rapidly from supine or sitting positions, taking hot showers, and emotional stressors. *Situational syncope* has a similar mechanism; however, it tends to occur with certain triggers involving an exaggerated vagal stimulus, including micturition, defecation, coughing, hair-combing, or pain.

Patients with NMS should increase water and salt intake to offset decreases in blood pressure that occur with stimulation of the autonomic nervous system. If presyncopal symptoms recur, patients should lie supine with their legs elevated because this maneuver should abort syncope.

Orthostatic Hypotension

Orthostatic hypotension and syncope occur when there is an inappropriate lack of systemic vasoconstriction on sitting up or standing, resulting in a decrease in blood pressure of at least 20 (systolic) or 10 (diastolic) mm Hg within 3 minutes of changing position. This finding may be idiopathic or exacerbated by other conditions or medications, such as diuretics, antihypertensives, and vasodilators.

Breath-Holding Spells

Breath-holding spells typically occur in children ages 6 to 24 months and are outgrown by the age of 5 years, rarely requiring intervention. Classic triggers are emotional insults, such as anger, pain, or fear. Children cry, forcibly exhale, and then seemingly "forget" to inhale. Cyanosis ensues, followed by transient loss of consciousness. Brief posturing or tonic-clonic movements may occur. Children regain consciousness spontaneously.

Cardiac Syncope

A cardiac cause is found in fewer than 2% of previously healthy children with syncope but is important to recognize because it can be associated with an increased risk for sudden death. Cardiac syncope results from an abrupt decline in cardiac output caused by obstructive lesions (aortic stenosis, HCM), myocardial dysfunction (ischemia, cardiomyopathy), and arrhythmias. Many of these conditions can be asymptomatic until syncope or sudden death occurs (Fig. 34.2). Sudden cardiac death (SCD) is fortunately uncommon, with estimated incidence of 1 to 10 per 100,000 population per year. Any concern for cardiac syncope warrants referral to a pediatric cardiologist.

Arrhythmias

Bradyarrhythmias and tachyarrhythmias with inadequate cardiac output and ischemia result in decreased cerebral blood flow and syncope. Arrhythmias can be primary or acquired in the setting of electrolyte disturbances, with myocarditis, or after cardiac surgery. Channelopathies with associated arrhythmia, such as *long QT syndrome, Brugada syndrome,* and *catecholaminergic polymorphic ventricular tachycardia,* often manifest with syncope. Many of these arrhythmias have genetic components, and attention should be paid to family history of sudden death or syncope. Arrhythmias are discussed in Chapter 32.

Cardiomyopathies

HCM is the most common cause of sudden cardiac death in pediatrics and can be associated with syncope secondary to both left ventricular outflow tract obstruction and abnormal myocardium resulting in electrical instability with subsequent risk for tachyarrhythmias. As mentioned previously, *dilated cardiomyopathy* is similarly associated with

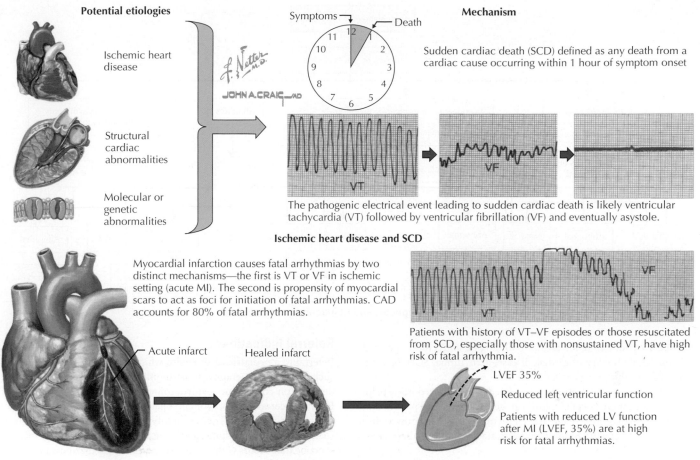

Potential etiologies

Ischemic heart disease

Structural cardiac abnormalities

Molecular or genetic abnormalities

Symptoms — Death

Mechanism

Sudden cardiac death (SCD) defined as any death from a cardiac cause occurring within 1 hour of symptom onset

The pathogenic electrical event leading to sudden cardiac death is likely ventricular tachycardia (VT) followed by ventricular fibrillation (VF) and eventually asystole.

Ischemic heart disease and SCD

Myocardial infarction causes fatal arrhythmias by two distinct mechanisms—the first is VT or VF in ischemic setting (acute MI). The second is propensity of myocardial scars to act as foci for initiation of fatal arrhythmias. CAD accounts for 80% of fatal arrhythmias.

Acute infarct

Healed infarct

Patients with history of VT–VF episodes or those resuscitated from SCD, especially those with nonsustained VT, have high risk of fatal arrhythmia.

LVEF 35%

Reduced left ventricular function

Patients with reduced LV function after MI (LVEF, 35%) are at high risk for fatal arrhythmias.

Fig. 34.2 Sudden Cardiac Death.

myocardial ischemia and tachyarrhythmias, leading to syncope and SCD. Cardiomyopathies are discussed in Chapter 33.

Aortic Stenosis

Valvar stenosis, either congenital or acquired, may lead to syncope from insufficient cardiac output related to fixed narrowing of the valve orifice, secondary arrhythmias from decreased coronary perfusion in the setting of myocardial thickening, or a combination of the two.

Abnormal Coronary Artery Origin

Anomalous coronary artery origin can cause syncope and SCD because of myocardial ischemia with resultant predisposition to ventricular arrhythmias. Up to 40% of patients have symptoms before SCD, and 20% to 30% may have ischemic changes on ECG during exercise.

Pulmonary Hypertension

Children with pulmonary hypertension can experience exercise-induced syncope, which is a late sign associated with decreased cardiac output and hypoxia related to right heart failure.

Myocarditis

Myocarditis can lead to syncope from ventricular dysfunction causing depressed cardiac output, or ventricular arrhythmias due to inflammatory changes, leading to electrical instability of the myocardium.

Congestive Heart Failure

As cardiac output declines, patients with congestive heart failure may experience syncope. This is rarely a presenting sign and is typically accompanied by other signs and symptoms of heart failure, such as exercise intolerance, edema, hepatomegaly, and respiratory distress.

Metabolic Syncope

Metabolic syncope is rare. Typically, metabolic disorders induce a gradual and prolonged impairment of consciousness. They must be considered in the evaluation of syncope, however, because they are often easily identified and treated. Metabolic causes include inborn errors of metabolism, hypoglycemia, and electrolyte abnormalities (e.g., hypocalcemia or hyperkalemia, which can induce arrhythmias). Drug abuse also should be included in the differential diagnoses.

PALPITATIONS

Palpitations refers to the perception of an irregular, rapid, or forceful heartbeat, including an array of sensations such as heart racing, fluttering, or skipping beats. The pathophysiology of palpitations is not well understood, and patient awareness of cardiac activity is highly variable. Palpitations can be perceived in the absence of abnormal cardiac activity, and conversely patients with abnormal cardiac activity may be asymptomatic.

Most commonly, patients reporting palpitations are experiencing sinus tachycardia, which can be a normal physiologic response to fever, anemia, hypovolemia, and pain. Also commonly observed and often benign, premature atrial and ventricular contractions can lead to palpitations, typically lasting a few seconds, in the setting of isolated ectopic beats.

Palpitations can be the initial presenting complaint in tachyarrhythmias such as supraventricular tachycardia. Previously discussed pathologic conditions, including myocarditis, cardiomyopathies, and repaired or unrepaired congenital heart defects, that manifest with chest pain can be accompanied by palpitations secondary to arrhythmia. Palpitations associated with exercise, chest pain, dyspnea, or

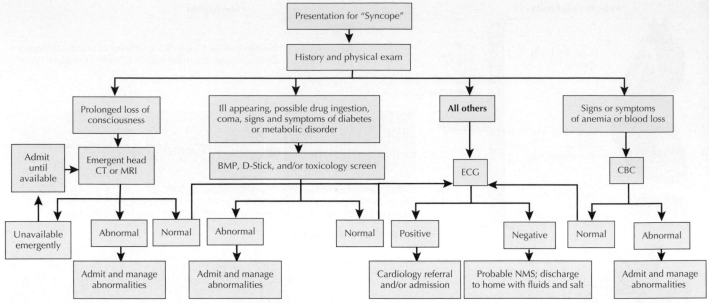

Fig. 34.3 Diagnosis and Management of Syncope.

syncope are concerning for cardiac pathologies, and a thorough medical and family history of cardiac disease, arrhythmia, SCD, or unexplained death should be elicited.

Noncardiac causes should be considered in patients reporting palpitations. For example, hypoglycemia can be associated with palpitations, in addition to diaphoresis and altered mental status. Hyperthyroidism may present with palpitations, with associated weight loss, diaphoresis, and hair loss.

Psychogenic causes of palpitations should be considered, including panic attacks, especially in patients with a history of anxiety or depression. Other important considerations include drug or substance use, such as caffeine, alcohol, or drugs of abuse, and attention-deficit/hyperactivity disorder (ADHD) medications, albuterol, and others.

EVALUATION AND DIAGNOSTIC APPROACH

A thorough history and physical examination alone can suggest the diagnosis in the majority of patients who present with chest pain, syncope, and/or palpitations. History should focus on the description of the symptoms, associated symptoms, and aggravating factors such as exercise. Circumstances leading to palpitations and syncope, including triggers and prodromal symptoms, are important in considering diagnoses (Fig. 34.3). The medical history, such as known congenital heart disease, asthma, sickle cell disease, or neurologic or psychiatric conditions, can guide the differential diagnoses. Family history is key regarding early or sudden cardiac or unexplained death (e.g., motor vehicle accidents, drownings), sudden infant death syndrome, arrhythmias, cardiomyopathies, hypercholesterolemia, and genetic disorders, including connective tissue disorders. Physical examination should include orthostatic vital signs in those with syncope and thorough cardiac, pulmonary, abdominal, and neurologic examinations. Any patient with a suspected cardiac cause should have an ECG. Patients with prolonged loss of consciousness, history of seizure-like movements, or neurologic deficit should undergo neurologic evaluation. Patients with suspected metabolic causes should be evaluated with a basic metabolic panel and toxicology screen, and patients with concern for anemia should be evaluated with a complete blood count. Workup for infectious diseases should be pursued when clinically indicated. Female patients of childbearing age should undergo a urine pregnancy test because hemodynamic shifts in pregnancy predispose to syncope.

Referral Indications

Referral to a pediatric cardiologist, which may include further testing such as echocardiography, heart monitor, and/or exercise stress test, depends on concerning features found on history, examination, and ECG. Concerning history for chest pain includes exertional chest pain, underlying cardiac disorder, angina-type pain, or associated symptoms such as syncope or palpitations. Concerning syncope history includes syncope that occurs without the typical vasovagal dizziness prodrome, exertional syncope, syncope with associated symptoms such as chest pain, or syncope triggered by a sudden stimulus such as a loud noise. Palpitations that occur suddenly or have associated features such as syncope would be concerning for a nonsinus tachycardia and warrant referral. A detailed family history is extremely important to elicit familial cardiac issues that may have an impact on the patient. Examination findings warranting referral include pathologic murmur, gallop, pericardial rub, abnormal second heart sound, hepatomegaly, decreased pulses, and abnormal ECG findings such as pathologic ST-segment or T-wave changes, arrhythmias, or preexcitation. Outpatient versus inpatient cardiology consultation should be based on the severity of presentation and if the child is ill-appearing, requiring hospital admission.

FUTURE DIRECTIONS

With rising health care costs, much attention has been paid to the large number and low yield of ancillary studies ordered in the evaluation of chest pain, syncope, and palpitations, given that primary cardiac pathologic conditions are uncommon in pediatrics. Adding an ECG to a targeted history and physical examination may increase the sensitivity for identifying cardiac disease, although some argue that given the overall low incidence of cardiac abnormalities, there is a low diagnostic yield, risk for false positive test results, and high cost of ECGs per positive result. Ongoing studies targeted at implementing an algorithmic approach to the management of pediatric symptoms is necessary, with the goal of decreasing practice variability and unnecessary resource usage.

SUGGESTED READINGS

Available online.

35

Acquired Heart Disease

Robin Chin and Deborah Whitney

CLINICAL VIGNETTE

A previously healthy 19-year-old female presented to the emergency department with dyspnea and recurrent fevers. Her examination was notable for fever, lung crackles, palpable liver, and grade II/VI blowing systolic murmur. She appeared mildly ill. She had no known cardiac history, but she had recently immigrated to the United States as a refugee and had limited access to medical care as a child. Blood was drawn for culture, and she was started on broad-spectrum antibiotics. Her blood culture was positive for *Streptococcus bovis*. On day 2 of hospitalization, she developed acute dyspnea, chest pain, and desaturation. Chest computed tomography revealed multiple pulmonary emboli. An echocardiogram demonstrated severe mitral regurgitation with an associated vegetation measuring 8 to 10 mm. She was diagnosed with infective endocarditis (IE) and treated with antibiotics accordingly. Future echocardiograms demonstrated resolution of the vegetation, a mildly stenotic mitral valve, and continued mitral regurgitation. She was additionally diagnosed with suspected rheumatic heart disease, a chronic complication of rheumatic fever.

ACUTE RHEUMATIC FEVER AND RHEUMATIC HEART DISEASE

Acute rheumatic fever (ARF) is a nonsuppurative complication after an untreated group A beta-hemolytic streptococcus (GAS) pharyngeal infection. ARF is a self-limited, immune-mediated condition that manifests with a unique constellation of acute symptoms, including pancarditis, migratory arthritis, neurologic findings, and skin findings. A potential chronic sequela of ARF is rheumatic heart disease (RHD), which may arise 10 to 20 years after the initial acute episode of pancarditis. ARF is the leading cause of acquired valvular heart disease globally and remains a significant cause of cardiac morbidity and mortality among poorly resourced populations and developing nations.

Aggressive testing and treatment of GAS pharyngitis has led to near-elimination of ARF in developed countries, with an annual incidence of 2 or fewer cases per 100,000 school-aged children; however, ARF and RHD remain significant public health concerns in countries with poor health infrastructure and limited access to screening or antibiotic treatment. Many patients present to care only after the chronic complications of RHD have developed. ARF is estimated to have an annual incidence of nearly 500,000 cases globally. RHD is estimated to affect 15 to 33 million individuals globally, with 350,000 attributed deaths annually.

ARF is primarily a disease of childhood, peaking between the ages of 5 and 14 years. It is extremely rare to have cases present younger than age 2 or beyond the age of 30. An estimated 40% to 60% of ARF cases will progress to RHD.

Etiology and Pathogenesis

ARF is caused by an antibody-mediated cross-reactivity between GAS bacteria and host cells, likely in the setting of genetic predisposition. During the acute infection, B and T cells eliminate streptococcal colonization of the pharynx by antibody production and T cell activation. The presence of molecular mimicry between the antibody receptors on the surface of GAS cells and host cell antigens triggers an autoinflammatory response approximately 2 to 3 weeks after the initial infection. In ARF, immune complexes bind to specific host tissues, causing localized inflammation affecting the joints, skin, and nervous and cardiac systems. The M protein expressed by GAS in particular has been cited as a structural mimicker of human myosin. Repeated untreated GAS infections may promote recurrent episodes of chronic carditis.

Pharyngeal infection with GAS is most commonly implicated in ARF; other GAS infections, such as cellulitis, are rarely linked to ARF. This finding is thought to be due to particular "rheumatogenic" strains of GAS that colonize the oropharynx and express dense amounts of M protein.

Strong evidence suggests a genetic predisposition for development of ARF, with multiple variants associated with an increased risk.

Clinical Presentation

Patients with ARF most commonly present with fever and arthritis 2 to 3 weeks after a streptococcal pharyngitis. Many pediatric patients will not recall a preceding pharyngitis. The arthritis is often migratory, affecting multiple joints and is likely to improve with nonsteroidal antiinflammatory drugs (NSAIDs). Acute carditis usually manifests by sinus tachycardia, but cardiac inflammation may also lead to exercise intolerance, fatigue, or dyspnea. Physical examination may be notable for a new regurgitant murmur (most commonly mitral but also aortic) and signs of pulmonary congestion. Up to a third of patients will have Sydenham chorea, related to inflammation of the basal ganglia and dopamine dysregulation. This neurologic complication is characterized by intermittent, abrupt, involuntary movements of the limbs, torso, and face, as well as muscle weakness and emotional outbursts of inappropriate behavior. Skin findings of ARF are rare but include an erythematous, annular rash that spreads outward from the torso or proximal extremities (erythema marginatum) and painless subcutaneous nodules overlying bone or tendons (Figs. 35.1 and 35.2).

ARF is a clinical diagnosis aided by use of the Jones Criteria (Table 35.1). A diagnosis of ARF requires the presence of at least two major criteria or one major plus two minor criteria in the setting of a prior GAS infection. An exception is made for chorea, which is considered diagnostic with or without other criteria. Previous GAS infection may be difficult to ascertain through history; in addition, throat cultures are typically negative at time of presentation, although serologic tests

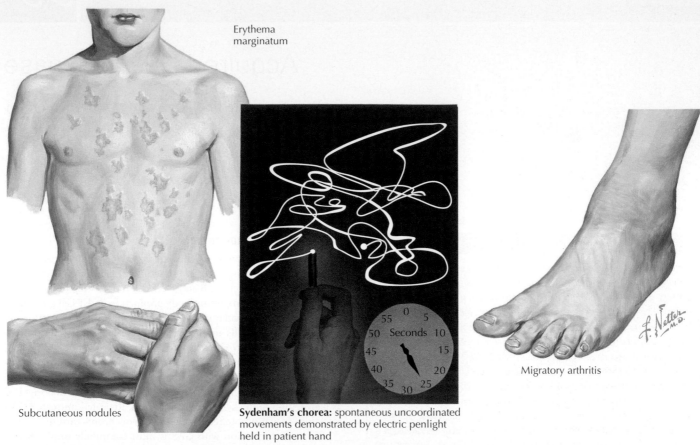

Erythema marginatum

Subcutaneous nodules

Sydenham's chorea: spontaneous uncoordinated movements demonstrated by electric penlight held in patient hand

Migratory arthritis

55 0 5
50 Seconds 10
45 15
40 20
35 30 25

Fig. 35.1 Noncardiac Manifestations of Acute Rheumatic Fever.

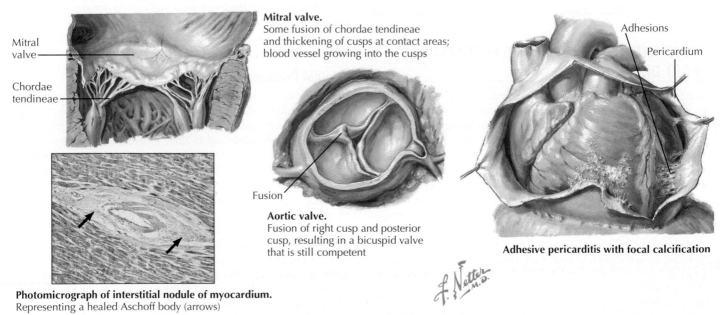

Mitral valve

Chordae tendineae

Mitral valve.
Some fusion of chordae tendineae and thickening of cusps at contact areas; blood vessel growing into the cusps

Fusion

Aortic valve.
Fusion of right cusp and posterior cusp, resulting in a bicuspid valve that is still competent

Adhesions

Pericardium

Adhesive pericarditis with focal calcification

Photomicrograph of interstitial nodule of myocardium.
Representing a healed Aschoff body (arrows)

Fig. 35.2 Manifestations of Acute Rheumatic Carditis.

such as antistreptolysin O (ASO) or antideoxyribonuclease B may be useful (Box 35.1).

Many patients with poor access to medical care will not present during initial or subsequent episodes of ARF. It is common for patients to be diagnosed with advanced RHD with no known history of ARF. Patients with RHD may manifest heart failure symptoms

or other complications of RHD such as infective endocarditis (IE), arrhythmia (most commonly atrial fibrillation), or embolic strokes. Less advanced disease may be asymptomatic but notable for new murmurs. Evaluation consists of an electrocardiogram, sometimes laboratory tests to evaluate for heart failure such as B-natriuretic peptide, and ultimately an echocardiogram (Fig. 35.3).

TABLE 35.1 2015 Revised Jones Criteria for the Diagnosis of Rheumatic Fever

Criteria Type	Low-Risk Populations	Moderate to High-Risk Populations
Major criteria	1. Carditis (clinical and/or subclinical) 2. Polyarthritis, typically migratory 3. Erythema marginatum 4. Subcutaneous nodules 5. Sydenham chorea	1. Carditis (clinical and/or subclinical) 2. Arthritis (mono- or polyarthritis) or polyarthralgia 3. Erythema marginatum 4. Subcutaneous nodules 5. Sydenham chorea
Minor criteria	1. Fever (101.3°F [≥38.5°C]) 2. Polyarthralgia 3. Elevated acute phase reactants: ESR (≥60 mm/hr), CRP (≥3.0 mg/dL) 4. Prolonged PR interval on ECG	1. Fever (101.3°F [≥38.5°C]) 2. Elevated acute phase reactants: ESR (≥60 mm/hr), CRP (≥3.0 mg/dl) 3. Prolonged PR interval on ECG

CRP, C-reactive protein; ECG, electrocardiogram; ESR, erythrocyte sedimentation rate.
From Beaton A, Carapetis J. The 2015 revision of the Jones criteria for the diagnosis of acute rheumatic fever: implications for practice in low-income and middle-income countries. *Heart Asia.* 2015;7(2):7-11. https://doi.org/10.1136/heartasia-2015-010648, Table 1/Page 8.

BOX 35.1 Evidence of Preceding Group A Streptococcal Infection

1. Positive throat culture
2. Rapid antigen test for group A streptococcus
3. Recent scarlet fever
4. Elevated or rising antistreptolysin-O, anti-DNAse B, or other streptococcal antibody titer

Anti-DNAse B, Antideoxyribonuclease B.

Differential Diagnosis

Alternative diagnoses to consider include sepsis, infectious or inflammatory arthritis, myocarditis, pericarditis, IE, and Kawasaki disease (KD) (Box 35.2).

Evaluation and Management

Emphasis is placed on prevention of ARF with appropriate antibiotic treatment of GAS pharyngitis. Timely evaluation and treatment of streptococcal pharyngitis in the primary care setting has nearly eliminated ARF and RHD in developed countries. Screening for GAS can be performed in most offices with rapid streptococcal antigen testing. Given the frequency of sore throat complaints in pediatrics offices, the Centor Score (Box 35.3) was developed to guide testing for streptococcal pharyngitis.

Treatment for known ARF consists of acute management of symptoms followed by daily penicillin prophylaxis to prevent further episodes of ARF and progression to RHD. Episodes of ARF should be treated with antibiotics regardless of culture positivity. Arthritis should be treated with NSAIDs such as naproxen or ibuprofen. The chorea and skin manifestations of ARF are typically self-limiting. Treatment with steroids, NSAIDs, or intravenous immunoglobulin (IVIG) has not been shown to improve carditis or reduce the risk for developing long-term complications. Patients should be evaluated with serial echocardiograms to monitor valve disease and ventricular function. Surgical intervention of affected valves is not typically indicated in the acute setting.

The majority of patients who develop one or more episodes of ARF will develop some degree of RHD, typically involving the mitral and aortic valves. After an initial episode of ARF, treatment with continuous antibiotic prophylaxis is recommended to reduce the risk for recurrent ARF. The optimal duration of prophylaxis is unknown; however, clinical guidelines are based on disease severity. For patients with persistent valvular disease, treatment continues for at least 10 years or until 40 years of age (whichever is longer), and for those without valvular disease, prophylaxis is recommended for at least 10 years or until the patient reaches age 21 (whichever is longer). For patients with ARF but no carditis, the recommended duration is 5 years or until 21 years old (whichever is longer). Adherence to daily oral penicillin is challenging, particularly among populations with limited access to medical care.

Patients with chronic RHD should have routine cardiology follow-up with intermittent echocardiograms. Patients should be monitored carefully for development of ventricular dysfunction or arrhythmia. Patients with severe valvular disease may require repair or replacement. Excellent dental hygiene should be emphasized, given the risk for developing IE.

Future Directions

Although ARF and RHD have been nearly eradicated in developed nations, they remain under-appreciated and neglected globally. Some countries have implemented the use of national registries to track cases of ARF and progression to RHD (Australia and New Zealand). Widespread empiric penicillin treatment among young children has been used to prevent primary infections and ARF, although studies have failed to show significant reduction in cases. Efforts have even been made to perform universal RHD screening among high-risk school-aged children and adults with portable, inexpensive echocardiograms (using devices such as mobile phone attachments) to identify patients who require penicillin prophylaxis.

INFECTIVE ENDOCARDITIS

IE is a bacterial or fungal infection of the endocardium, most commonly affecting the cardiac valves. It is most commonly associated with preexisting congenital heart disease (CHD), prosthetic material, or indwelling devices. IE is characterized by persistent febrile illness and bacteremia, with subsequent risk for mortality or permanent cardiac injury.

IE remains rare in children, with an estimated annual incidence in the United States of 3.3 per 100,000 in infants younger than 1 year to 0.3 to 0.8 per 100,000 in older children and adolescents. The majority of pediatric IE cases arise in the setting of CHD, especially those with cyanotic heart disease. Associated cardiac lesions include aortic valve abnormalities, ventricular septal defects, tetralogy of Fallot, artificial valves, and prosthetic grafts or complex reconstructions. IE also occurs in children with structurally normal hearts but who typically have other risk factors such as an indwelling central venous catheter (CVC), ventriculoatrial shunts, pacemakers, and implantable defibrillators.

Mitral insufficiency

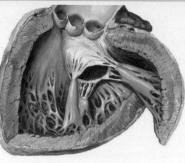

Mitral insufficiency: mitral valve viewed from below; marked shortening of posterior cusp, with only slight commissural fusion and little fusion and shortening of chordae tendineae

Calcific plate at anterolateral commissure of mitral valve, contributing to insufficiency

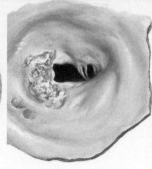

Marked enlargement of left atrium resulting from mitral insufficiency

Thickening and shortening of mitral cusps with "hamstringing" of posterior cusp over the musculature of left ventricle by traction of enlarged left atrium

Aortic insufficiency

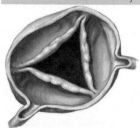

Aortic insufficiency: Valve viewed from above; thickened, short cusps with triangular deficiency

Concentric hypertrophy with some dilatation of left ventricle resulting from aortic insufficiency, causing chordae tendineae to elongate and run in a relatively horizontal direction, thus impeding closure of mitral valve and leading to secondary mitral insufficiency

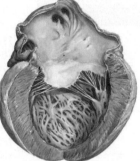

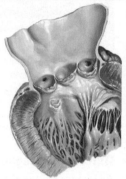

Shortened cusps of aortic valve with exposure of sinuses and dilatation of aorta: "Jet lesion" on septal wall of left ventricle

Fig. 35.3 Clinical Presentation of Rheumatic Heart Disease.

BOX 35.2 Differential Diagnosis of Acute Rheumatic Fever

- Myocarditis
- Pericarditis
- Kawasaki disease
- Other arthritis: traumatic, infectious, inflammatory
- Sickle cell disease
- Infective endocarditis
- Systemic lupus erythematosus
- Lyme disease

BOX 35.3 Centor Criteria for Management of Suspected Streptococcal Pharyngitis

Criteria (Points)
- Absence of cough (1)
- Swollen and tender anterior cervical lymph nodes (1)
- Temperature 100.4°F (>38°C) (1)
- Tonsillar exudates or swelling (1)
- Age
  - 3 to 14 years (1)
  - 15 to 44 years (0)
  - 45 years or older (−1)

Management Options Based on Centor Score
- Score 0 to 1: No testing or antibiotics indicated.
- Score 2 to 3: Throat culture or rapid testing advised.
- Score ≥4: Consider empiric treatment for streptococcal pharyngitis.

From McIsaac WJ, Kellner JD, Aufricht P, Vanjaka A, Low DE. empirical validation of guidelines for the management of pharyngitis in children and adults. *JAMA.* 2004;291(13):1587-1595. https://doi.org/10.1001/jama.291.13.1587-1595.

Etiology and Pathogenesis

IE is thought to arise from transient bacteremia occurring in the setting of disrupted cardiac epithelium or endocardium (Fig. 35.4). Damage may arise from indwelling lines or may occur with turbulent flow from CHD or artificial valves. Once the tissue is injured, fibrin and platelets form a sterile thrombotic deposit on the surface of the valve or endocardium. The resulting platelet-fibrin coagulum is vulnerable to colonization by bloodstream-borne bacteria. Platelets and fibrin envelope bacterial colonies, allowing the vegetation to evade host defenses. The growing vegetation may release infectious emboli into the bloodstream, resulting in multifocal strokes, pulmonary emboli, or distal abscess formation. CVCs also may serve as a nidus for bacterial colonization independent of epithelial injury. Biofilms encasing CVCs or indwelling devices may act as a nidus for bacterial replication, prolonged bacteremia, and eventual thrombus formation.

Gram-positive bacteria are the most commonly implicated organisms in IE. Gram-positive organisms express multiple adhesive surface factors (*adhesins*) that facilitate binding to epithelial surfaces.

Early lesions

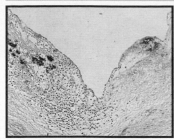

Deposit of platelets and organisms (stained dark), edema, and leukocytic infiltration in very early bacterial endocarditis of aortic valve

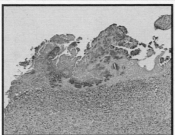

Development of vegetations containing clumps of bacteria on tricuspid valve

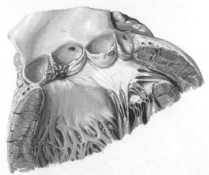

Early vegetations of bacterial endocarditis on bicuspid aortic valve

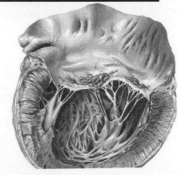

Early vegetations of bacterial endocarditis at contact line of mitral valve

Advanced lesions

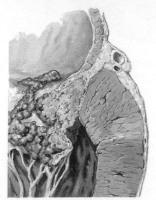

Vegetations of bacterial endocarditis on under-aspect as well as on atrial surface of mitral valve

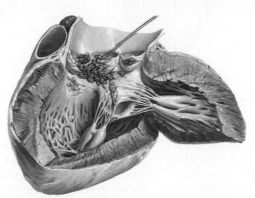

Advanced bacterial endocarditis of aortic valve: perforation of cusp; extension to anterior cusp of mitral valve and chordae tendineae: "jet lesion" on septal wall

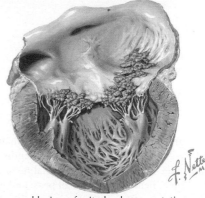

Advanced lesion of mitral valve: vegetations extending onto chordae tendineae with rupture of two chordae; also extension to atrial wall and contact lesion on opposite cusp

Fig. 35.4 Bacterial Endocarditis.

Staphylococcus aureus, Streptococcus pneumoniae, Enterococcus species, and viridans group streptococci are most commonly isolated. *S. aureus* is associated with acute fulminant IE with a high mortality rate. *S. aureus* and coagulase-negative staphylococci are linked to delayed IE of implanted cardiac materials (up to 1 or more years after the procedure). Less commonly, gram-negative bacteria may cause IE. These include the HACEK organisms (a group of oral gram-negative bacilli including *Haemophilus* species, *Actinobacillus actinomycetemcomitans, Cardiobacterium hominis, Eikenella corrodens,* and *Kingella kingae*). These organisms are frequently implicated in culture-negative IE. Fungal pathogens, including *Candida* and *Aspergillus,* are associated with CVC-related infections and parenteral nutrition.

The bacteremia associated with IE is thought to arise most commonly from breakdown of oral mucosa. Although manipulation of gingival tissues from dental procedures is known to cause temporary bacteremia, dental procedures are rarely implicated in the pathogenesis of IE. Rather, the vast majority of IE cases are linked to routine daily activities such as chewing or teeth brushing in the setting of poor oral hygiene. Underlying gingivitis is a risk factor for pathologic bacteremia.

Clinical Presentation

IE can present as an acute or subacute process. Acute IE is rapidly progressive, with high morbidity and mortality. Patients typically have high fevers, appear critically ill, and have rapid destruction of heart valves, abscess formation, embolic phenomenon, and hemodynamic instability. In contrast, subacute IE manifests with indolent, nonspecific symptoms, including prolonged low-grade fever (75% to 100% of patients), fatigue, malaise, and myalgias. Up to half of patients with IE may have some degree of congestive heart failure with symptoms of dyspnea or exertional limitations. Patients may have a normal physical examination, although a new murmur may be appreciated as a result of valvular disruption. Thromboembolic sequelae

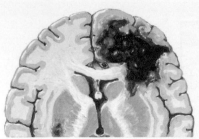

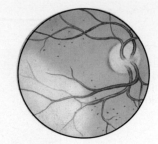

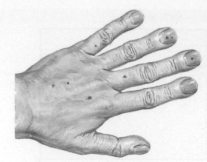

Infarct of brain with secondary hemorrhage from embolism to right anterior cerebral artery; also small infarct in left basal ganglia

Embolus in vessel of ocular fundus with retinal infarction; petechiae

Multiple petechiae of skin and clubbing of fingers

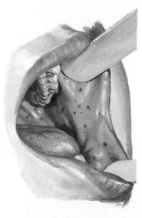

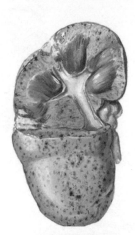

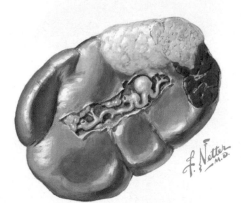

Petechiae of mucous membranes

Petechiae and gross infarcts of kidney

Mycotic aneurysms of splenic arteries and infarct of spleen; splenomegaly

Fig. 35.5 Remote Embolic Effects of Bacterial Endocarditis.

are appreciated less commonly in pediatric patients than in adults. These classically include small, nontender hemorrhages on the palms and soles (Janeway lesions), retinal hemorrhages (Roth spots), linear "splinter" hemorrhages of nail beds, and evidence of septic emboli on head imaging (Fig. 35.5). More severe thromboembolic events include ischemic or hemorrhagic stroke, pulmonary embolism, distal abscess or aneurysms, or renal infarcts. Splenomegaly and petechiae are also frequently noted.

Diagnosis of IE requires a combination of high clinical suspicion with laboratory and echocardiogram findings. The modified Duke Criteria (Box 35.4) has been well studied as a useful tool for diagnosis of IE among adults, with definitive diagnosis in those with two major criteria, one major and three minor criteria, or five minor criteria. Limited studies have demonstrated validation in pediatric populations.

Evaluation includes a detailed fever history and careful cardiac and skin examination. Adolescents should be assessed for intravenous drug use. Initial diagnostic laboratory testing is guided by a high index of suspicion and includes bacterial aerobic and anaerobic blood cultures; fungal blood cultures may be considered among immunosuppressed patients or those with a history of fungal disease. Three separate pretreatment blood cultures from different venipunctures are recommended to avoid misidentifying skin flora contamination as pathologic bacteremia. In patients with suspected IE, an echocardiogram should be pursued to visualize vegetations, abscesses, or valve disease, along with assessment of ventricular function. As opposed to adults, transthoracic echocardiogram often has a sufficiently high sensitivity in pediatric populations. A normal

echocardiogram though does not definitively rule out IE as early vegetations may be too small to visualize. A repeat echocardiogram may be indicated in patients with persistent symptoms but who do not meet full criteria, and a transesophageal echocardiogram is sometimes indicated in those with poor transthoracic echocardiography images. Likewise, serial echocardiograms are necessary in patients with known IE to monitor ventricular function, valve disease, and status of vegetation.

Differential Diagnosis

Clinicians should consider alternative diagnoses for persistent bacteremia (CVC-associated infection, abscess, inappropriate antimicrobial coverage), alternative causes of prolonged fevers (malignancy, inflammatory disease), and other cardiac disease (pericarditis or myocarditis, ARF, noninfective mural thrombus).

Evaluation and Management

The mainstay of treatment for IE is prolonged courses of intravenous antibiotic therapy (minimum 4 weeks). Empiric broad-spectrum antibiotics (vancomycin and gentamicin) should be initiated within 1 hour of presentation of acutely ill patients. Targeted antibiotic selection is guided by the organism, underlying cardiac disease, devices, and resistance patterns. IE affecting artificial valves requires longer duration of therapy with more aggressive regimens. For methicillin-susceptible *S. aureus* (MSSA), nafcillin or oxacillin should be considered; longer courses with vancomycin (>6 weeks) are indicated for MRSA. Streptococcal IE may be treated with shorter courses of intravenous penicillin G; addition of

BOX 35.4 Modified Duke Criteria for the Diagnosis of Infective Endocarditis

Major Criteria

1. Positive Blood Culture
   a. Positive blood cultures (≥2/2) with typical infective endocarditis pathogens (staphylococcus, streptococcus, enterococcus, and HACEK[a] group)
   b. Persistent bacteremia from two blood cultures >12 hours apart; or three positive cultures regardless of timing; or bacteremia from a majority of four or more cultures regardless of timing
   c. Single positive culture for *Coxiella burnetii* or antibody titer against phase I >1:800
2. Endocardial Involvement
   a. Positive echocardiogram result showing oscillating mass, abscess, or dehiscence of prosthetic valve
   b. New regurgitant murmur

Minor Criteria

1. Predisposing heart condition or intravenous drug use
2. Fever 100.4°F (38°C)
3. Vascular factors: Major arterial emboli, septic pulmonary infarct, mycotic aneurysms, intracranial hemorrhage, conjunctival hemorrhage, Janeway lesions
4. Immunologic factors: Glomerulonephritis, Osler nodes, Roth spots, rheumatoid factor
5. Microbiology: Positive blood culture result but not meeting major criteria

[a]HACEK: *Haemophilus* spp., *Actinobacillus actinomycetemcomitans, Cardiobacterium hominis, Eikenella corrodens,* and *Kingella kingae.*
From Li JS, Sexton DJ, Mick N, et al. Proposed modifications to the Duke criteria for the diagnosis of infective endocarditis. *Clin Infect Dis.* 2000;30(4):633-638. https://doi.org/10.1086/313753. Table 4, page 637.

gentamicin or substitution with ampicillin may be considered with artificial valves. *Enterococcal* species should be treated with penicillin G or ampicillin with gentamicin. HACEK organisms may be treated with third-generation cephalosporins; other gram-negative species may require addition of an aminoglycoside because of resistance among *Escherichia coli, Serratia,* and *Pseudomonas aeruginosa.* Removal of inciting devices such as CVCs or nonnative valves should be strongly considered.

IE presents the risk for severe morbidity and mortality, including congestive heart failure, ruptured or regurgitant valves, arrhythmias, and complications of septic emboli. Complications from embolization are managed symptomatically based on the affected organ. Surgery to remove the septic thrombus is sometimes indicated, depending on the size of the vegetation and severity of illness.

Mortality ranges from 5% to 10% of affected patients. Mortality rises with underlying cardiac disease, and *S. aureus* is associated with the poorest outcomes and a nearly 50% mortality rate.

The current guidelines from the American Heart Association recommend antibiotic prophylaxis before dental procedures that involve manipulation of gingival tissue or periapical region of teeth or perforation of oral mucosa. Antibiotics are recommended only in the following subset of patients: prosthetic cardiac valve or involved in valve repair, prior endocarditis, unrepaired cyanotic heart disease, repaired congenital heart disease with prosthetic material or device during first 6 months after repair and then ongoing if residual defects, and cardiac transplantation recipients who develop cardiac valvulopathy.

Future Directions

The current research focus in IE aims to reduce disease incidence through proper oral hygiene and mitigation of high-risk behaviors (intravenous drug use). The cardiology community continues to encourage avoidance of prophylactic antimicrobial treatment for dental or other invasive procedures given poor evidence for outcome improvements. Finally, increased attention has been given to mitigating the role of nosocomial infections in IE with standardized CVC protocols. Antimicrobial biomaterials and targeted therapy aiming to reduce the virulence of adhesins has been an ongoing area of study.

KAWASAKI DISEASE

KD is the leading cause of acquired heart disease in children. It is an acute, inflammatory vasculitis affecting medium-sized arteries throughout the body. A full discussion of KD can be found in Chapter 138, but given the severity of the cardiac complications, it deserves brief mention in this chapter. Although the vasculitis in KD is typically self-limiting, it can lead to acutely life-threatening or severe chronic cardiovascular complications. Acute cardiac manifestations include coronary artery aneurysms and less commonly ventricular dysfunction or cardiovascular shock. Long-term sequelae include coronary artery aneurysms primarily with increased risk for myocardial ischemia and infarction, depending on the aneurysm severity. Timely recognition and treatment of KD is essential in mitigating cardiovascular complications.

The principal cardiac complications associated with KD are coronary artery dilation and development of coronary aneurysms, which occur in approximately 25% of untreated cases. The initial step in the development of coronary artery aneurysms is a necrotizing arteritis with neutrophilic destruction of the arterial wall in the first 2 weeks of illness. Other cardiac tissue may be inflamed, including the endocardium, myocardium, valves, or pericardium. About 5% of KD cases will present with cardiogenic shock requiring volume and pressure resuscitation.

After the acute febrile illness, coronary artery damage may be sustained by a chronic, lymphocyte-mediated vasculitis, followed by luminal myofibroblastic proliferation, a smooth muscle cell–derived myofibroblastic process that can cause progressive coronary artery stenosis over years. Giant aneurysms, in particular, are at risk for rupture acutely, and there is a long-term risk for myocardial ischemia in the setting of progressive stenosis or thrombosis over months to years (Fig. 35.6).

An echocardiogram should be obtained on suspicion or diagnosis of KD, though a normal echocardiogram does not exclude KD (Fig. 35.7). Timely administration of high-dose IVIG is critical to mitigating coronary artery damage. A single infusion of 2 g/kg of IVIG should be administered as soon as a diagnosis of KD is made, ideally within the first 10 days of febrile illness. Timely treatment with IVIG has been shown to reduce the incidence of coronary artery disease from 25% to 4% to 5%. Moderate-to-high doses of aspirin are used initially to combat inflammation but have not been proven to lower the risk for aneurysm development. Low-dose aspirin for antithrombotic effect is a mainstay of treatment initially. Additional anti-inflammatory therapies may be necessary, depending on the response to IVIG. Recent studies suggest that steroids may play a role in decreasing inflammation and cardiovascular sequelae of KD. Thromboprophylaxis with an additional antiplatelet agent and anticoagulation may be necessary, depending on the size of the aneurysms, both in the acute setting and long term.

SUGGESTED READINGS

Available online.

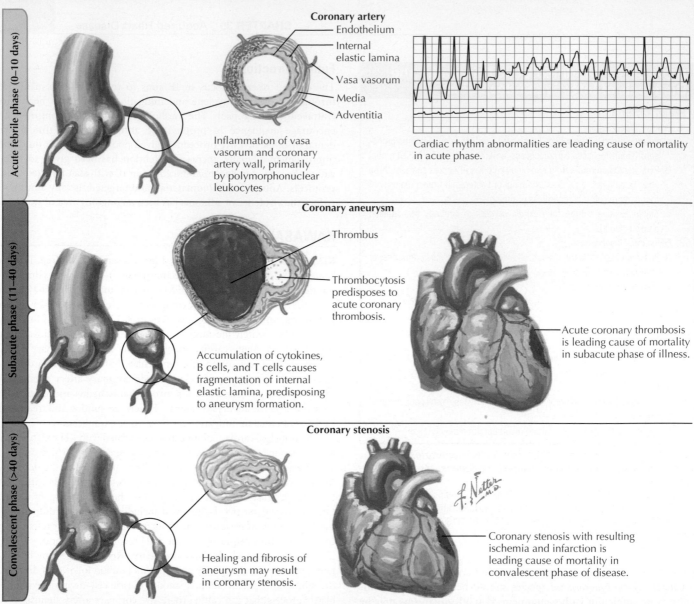

Acute febrile phase (0–10 days)

Coronary artery
- Endothelium
- Internal elastic lamina
- Vasa vasorum
- Media
- Adventitia

Inflammation of vasa vasorum and coronary artery wall, primarily by polymorphonuclear leukocytes

Cardiac rhythm abnormalities are leading cause of mortality in acute phase.

Subacute phase (11–40 days)

Coronary aneurysm

Thrombus

Thrombocytosis predisposes to acute coronary thrombosis.

Accumulation of cytokines, B cells, and T cells causes fragmentation of internal elastic lamina, predisposing to aneurysm formation.

Acute coronary thrombosis is leading cause of mortality in subacute phase of illness.

Convalescent phase (>40 days)

Coronary stenosis

Healing and fibrosis of aneurysm may result in coronary stenosis.

Coronary stenosis with resulting ischemia and infarction is leading cause of mortality in convalescent phase of disease.

Fig. 35.6 Coronary Artery Abnormalities Associated With Kawasaki Disease.

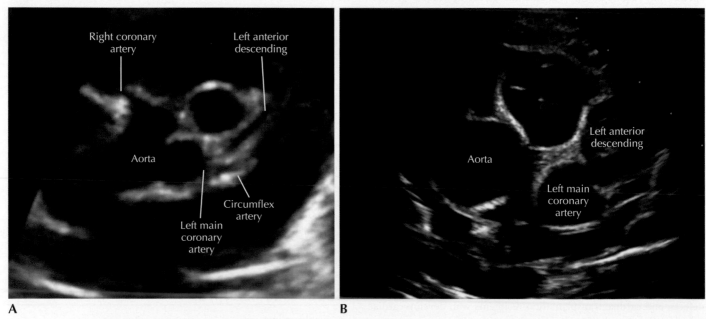

Right coronary artery

Left anterior descending

Aorta

Circumflex artery

Left main coronary artery

Left anterior descending

Aorta

Left main coronary artery

A

B

Fig. 35.7 (A) Normal echocardiographic imaging of coronary arteries and (B) coronary arteries with giant aneurysms secondary to Kawasaki disease, with thrombus visualized in the left anterior descending artery.

SECTION VII

Dermatology

Audrey Jacqueline Chan

36

Dermatologic Morphology

Padmavathi V. Karri and Meena R. Julapalli

 CLINICAL VIGNETTE

A previously healthy 10-year-old girl presents with a 2-day history of pruritus and paresthesias on her neck now with a painful rash in the same distribution. The patient denies fevers, chills, or nausea and is up-to-date on vaccines. Physical examination reveals four clusters of tender vesicles on an erythematous base in a dermatomal distribution on her right anterior neck and jawline (Fig. 36.1). A clinical diagnosis of herpes zoster (shingles) is made and a course of acyclovir is prescribed. As-needed acetaminophen is encouraged to help the patient with discomfort. A week later, the patient's parent calls and says the vesicles ruptured, ulcerated, and left behind a crust. You assure the parent that this is part of the normal healing process.

Although shingles is rare in immunocompetent children, it should remain on the differential for a child with vesicles in a dermatomal distribution and known varicella exposure either through primary infection (particularly before the age of 1 year) or a history of varicella-zoster virus vaccination. Additionally, the pain may continue after the rash is resolved. In this instance, it is important to consult a physician for symptomatic treatment.

BASIC STRUCTURE OF THE SKIN

The skin has three basic layers: the epidermis, dermis, and subcutaneous tissue (Fig. 36.2). Throughout these layers are additional structures and appendages that contribute to the skin's functionality.

Epidermis

The outermost layer of the skin, the epidermis, is composed primarily of keratinocytes, forming a stratified epithelial tissue that functions primarily to protect against the external environment and prevent water loss. The innermost layer of the epidermis consists of the basal cells at the dermal-epidermal junction. Basal cells divide to form keratinocytes, which subsequently flatten to form the stratum granulosum. The keratinocytes eventually die and form the outermost barrier, the stratum corneum, which is continually replenished. The epidermis also has melanocytes, the melanin-producing cells of the skin; Langerhans cells, which are dendritic cells derived from macrophages and perform immune surveillance; and Merkel cells, which are mechanosensory touch receptors.

Dermis

The dermis is composed primarily of a matrix of fibroblasts that synthesize collagen and elastic fibers, which make up the support structure of the skin. The papillary layer of the dermis is closest to the epidermis and is more cellular than the deeper dermis. This layer supports unmyelinated nerve endings that transmit sensations of pain, itch, and temperature. Deep to this is the reticular layer, which is dense in collagen and elastic fibers. Both layers contain blood and lymphatic vessels. In addition, the dermis supports most of the skin's appendages, including the hair follicle, apocrine glands, eccrine sweat glands, and sebaceous glands.

Subcutaneous Tissue

The subcutaneous tissue of the skin serves to conserve body heat and acts as a protective cushion. The subcutaneous tissue is composed primarily of adipocytes, which play important roles in glucose and fat metabolism. In addition, factors released by adipocytes contribute to wound healing, vascular remodeling, and inflammatory and immune responses. A fibrous network anchors the adipocytes to deeper structures, such as muscular fascia and periosteum.

APPROACH TO DERMATOLOGIC MORPHOLOGY AND DISEASE

Recognition of cutaneous lesions begins with basic understanding of dermatologic terminology and morphology. As with any other disease process, diagnosis of cutaneous disease begins with a complete physical examination. A thorough examination includes careful inspection of the body surface, including the mucous membranes, nails, and hair. The differential diagnosis is guided by the distribution and configuration of lesions. More careful examination of individual lesions, including inspection and palpation, helps identify the primary lesion. The primary lesion is defined as the basic, most representative lesion. Lesions often undergo secondary changes as a result of scratching, infection, or treatment. Identification of the primary lesions allows accurate description and aids in generation of a differential diagnosis.

Primary Lesions

Primary lesions (Fig. 36.3) are characterized by their diameter and depth. A *macule* is a flat lesion that can be seen by changes in skin color but cannot be felt. The border may be well circumscribed or may gradually blend into the surrounding skin. It may be of any size, but the term is generally used to describe lesions smaller than 1 cm. Flat lesions larger than 1 cm are termed *patches*. As with macules, *papules* are small (<1 cm) lesions but are palpable, with the greatest mass above the surface of surrounding skin. Elevated skin lesions greater than 1 cm are termed *plaques*. Plaques may be formed by a confluence of papules or can be the primary lesion. Palpable, solitary lesions whose mass is primarily below the surface, in the dermis and subcutaneous tissue, are termed either *nodules* (0.5 to 2 cm) or *tumors*. Tumors may be benign or malignant.

Primary lesions are also characterized by the presence of fluid or debris-filled cavities. Fluid-filled lesions that are less than 1 cm are termed *vesicles;* those larger than 1 cm are termed *bullae*. Discrete, elevated lesions that contain purulent debris are called *pustules;* larger purulent collections that may contain palpable deeper components are referred to as an *abscess*.

Other primary lesions include a *wheal (hive)*, which is a firm, elevated lesion that is secondary to dermal edema. Wheals vary in size and shape and are usually pink to red. Wheals are transient, with individual lesions usually lasting less than 24 hours. A *cyst* is a well-circumscribed, deep lesion that is covered by normal epidermis. It may contain fluid or semisolid debris.

Secondary Lesions

Primary lesions may undergo changes caused by evolution, manipulation, irritation, infection, or application of treatments. Recognition of secondary lesions is important because some changes can aid in diagnosis (e.g., quality of scale can distinguish psoriasis from other papulosquamous entities) whereas others can hinder diagnosis by obscuring the primary lesion (e.g., lichenification). *Scales* are layers of the stratum corneum that have desquamated but remain attached to the skin surface. *Crusts* are thick accumulations of cellular debris, blood, pus, or serum. *Erosions* are superficial loss of tissue, resulting in depression of the surface. They generally heal without scarring because only the epidermis is affected. In contrast, loss that extends into the dermis and even subcutaneous tissue is called an *ulcer*. Ulcers often heal with a scar. Linear ulceration or erosions from scratching are termed *excoriations*. *Fissures* form at sites of chronic inflammation and are characterized by sharply demarcated, linear disruptions in the epidermis and can extend into the dermis. *Lichenification* is a marked thickening of the epidermis that results in exaggeration of skin markings resulting from chronic irritation caused by inflammation, rubbing, or scratching (Fig. 36.4).

Healing of lesions may also result in secondary changes. For example, atrophic changes of the epidermis or dermis result in depressions in the skin surface. Whereas *epidermal atrophy* is demonstrated by very thin, translucent skin with loss of skin markings, *dermal atrophy* manifests as depressions with normal overlying skin.

A *scar* is a permanent change in the skin after an injury that results in fibrosis. An exaggerated response to skin damage may result in hypertrophic scars that remain within the boundaries of the original injury. In contrast, *keloids* continue to grow long after the injury and can grow well outside the boundary of the initial insult.

Color of Lesions

Another important characteristic of lesions is how they compare with the patient's normal skin color. Hyperpigmented lesions are darker than

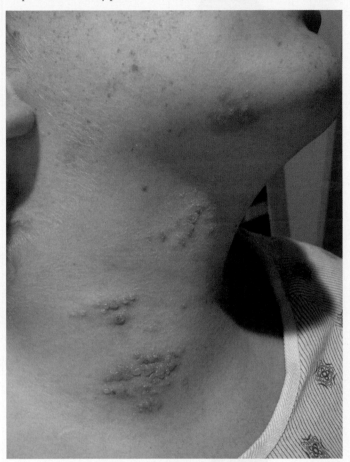

Fig. 36.1 Herpes Zoster (Shingles).

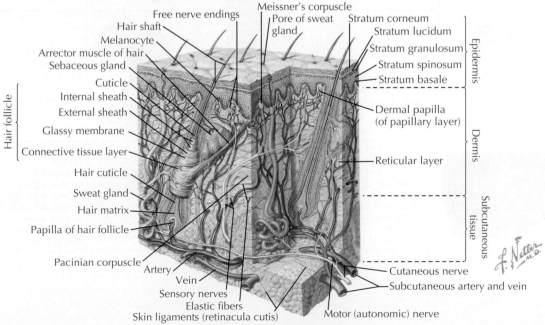

Fig. 36.2 Cross-section of Skin.

Type of primary lesion	Appearance	Description	Example	Type of primary lesion	Appearance	Description	Example
Macules	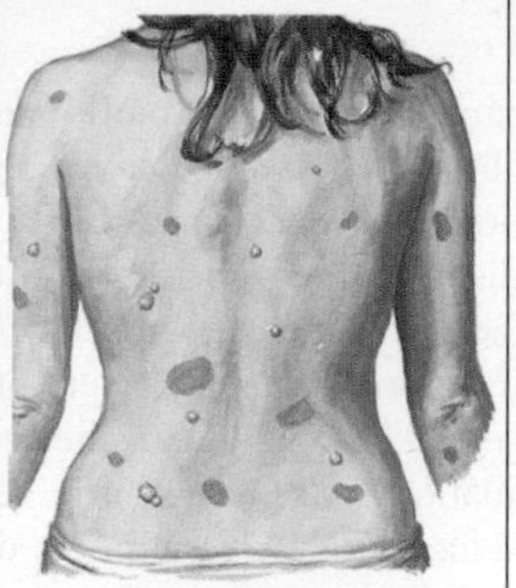	Flat changes in skin color of any size though generally less than 1 cm, may be rounded, irregular or fade into surrounding skin.	Café au lait macules, freckles, capillary malformations	Vesicle	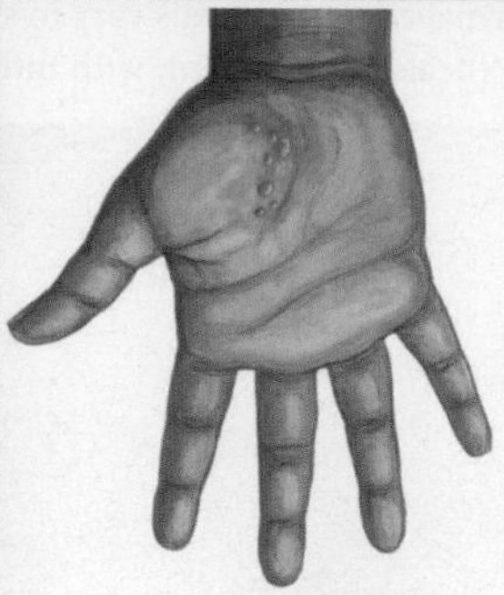	Circumscribed, fluid filled elevation up to 1 cm in diameter	Coxsackie virus, herpes simplex virus, varicella, miliaria crystallina
Patches	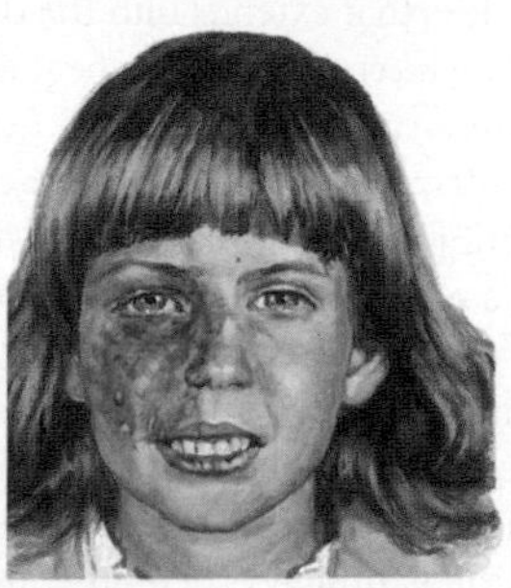	Greater than 1 cm flat lesion with color change, common colors include red (vascular lesion) darker (hyperpigmented) or lighter (hypopigmented or depigmented) than surrounding skin	Capillary malformation (port wine stains) with hypertrophy, dermal melanocytosis, vitiligo	Bullae	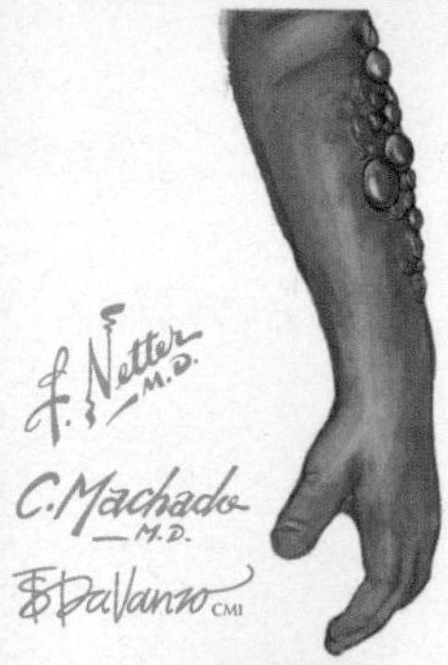	Circumscribed, fluid-filled elevation greater than 1 cm in diameter. Flaccid bullae (superficial, involving the epidermis) rupture easily and intact lesions may not be evident. Tense bullae (subepidermal) remain intact.	Epidermolysis bullosa blistering distal dactylitis, insect bite reaction
Papules	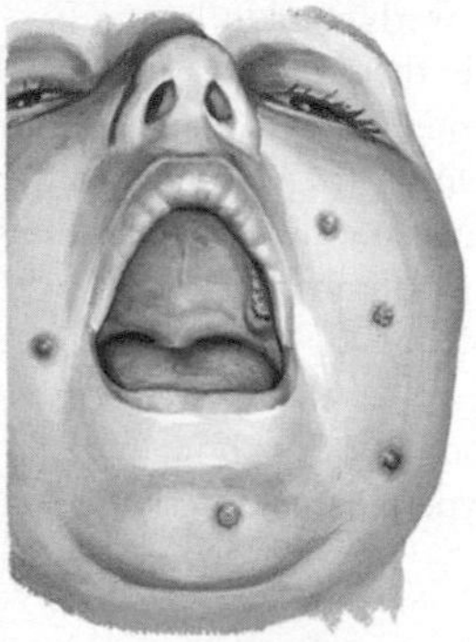	Solid elevations less than 1 cm, may have overlying color change or blend with surrounding skin	Molluscum contagiosum, dermal nevus, verruca/wart, milia	Pustule	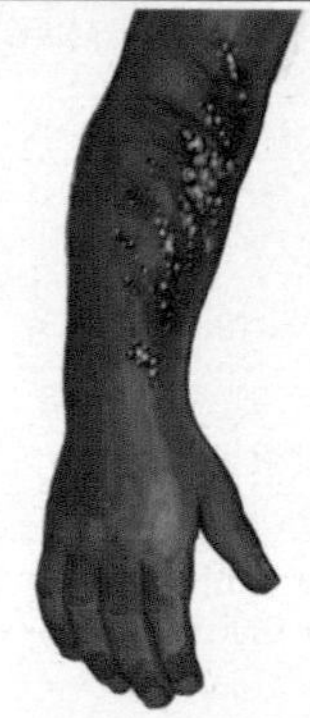	Less than 1 cm, circumscribed elevaton of the skin containing purulent material.	Folliculitis, transient neonatal pustular melanosis, acropustulosis of infancy
Plaques	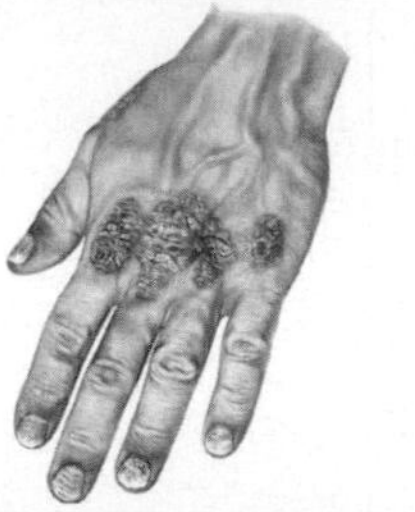	Elevated, flat-topped circumscribed lesion greater than 1 cm in diameter. May be formed by the confluence of papules.	Psoriasis, nevus sebaceus lichen planus	Abscess	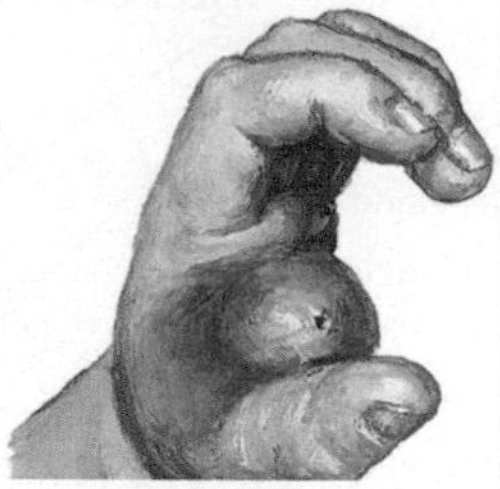	Circumscribed, elevated lesion greater than 1 cm containing purulent fluid.	Staphylococcal abscess, hidradenitis suppurativa, acne conglobata
Nodules or tumors	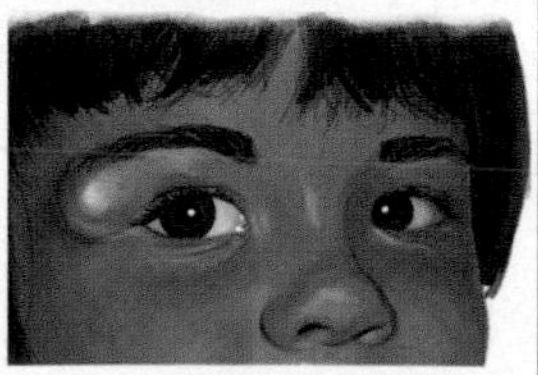	Circumscribed solid lesion less than 2 cm that involves the dermis and may include the subcutaneous tissue. Tumors are greater than 2 cm.	Dermoid cyst, lipoma	Wheal	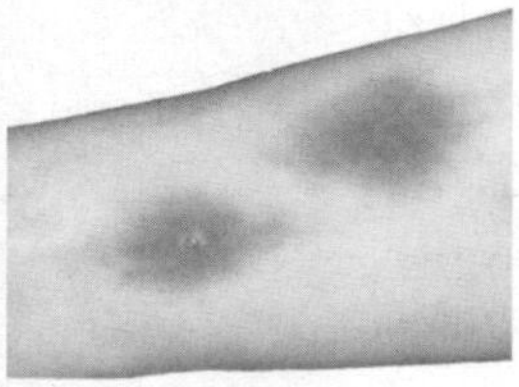	An evanescent, elevated lesion that represents dermal edema. Lesions may vary in size and shape and are often surrounded by macular erythema.	Urticaria (hives), urticarial vasculitis

Fig. 36.3   Primary Lesions.

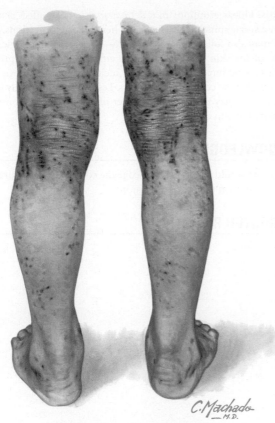

Fig. 36.4 Flexural Lichenification.

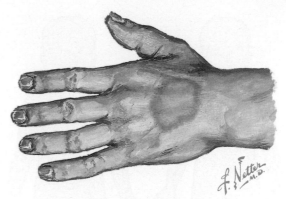

Fig. 36.5 Annular Lesion.

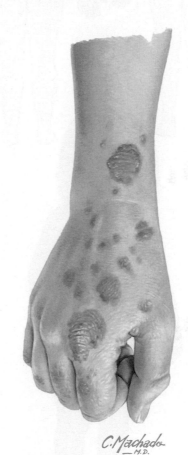

Fig. 36.6 Nummular Eczema.

the surrounding skin. Inflammation can lead to hyperpigmentation. Other examples of hyperpigmentation include nevi and café-au-lait spots (see Chapters 38 and 41). Increased dermal pigmentation often results in a bluish discoloration of lesions, such as in dermal melanocytosis (the former term *Mongolian spot* should be avoided because of racial connotations). Hypopigmented lesions are lighter than the surrounding skin. Examples include postinflammatory hypopigmentation, tinea versicolor, or ash leaf spots of tuberous sclerosis. Depigmented lesions have lost all pigment and can be differentiated from hypopigmented lesions by Wood's lamp examination. An example of a depigmented disorder is vitiligo. Lesions that are pink to red may be inflammatory in origin, whereas more intense red to purple lesions are often vascular.

Configuration of Lesions

Additional diagnostic information can be gained from correct identification of the configuration or shape of individual or grouped lesions. Whereas *discrete* lesions remain distinct and separated from surrounding areas of disease, *confluent* lesions have coalesced or merged. *Clustered* lesions are grouped in one area. In some cases, configuration may suggest an underlying cause. For example, *linear* lesions occurring in a band or line may suggest an exogenous cause, such as poison ivy, or a postzygotic mutation, such as an epidermal nevus.

Specific description of the shape of lesions provides further information. An *annular* lesion (Fig. 36.5) specifies a ring-shaped lesion with a raised or erythematous border and central clearing, providing more information than the adjective "round." Common examples of annular lesions include tinea infections, erythema migrans, and granuloma annulare. *Discoid* lesions are also round but tend to be more confluent. Other "round" lesions include *nummular* (Fig. 36.6), *targetoid* (containing concentric rings), and *guttate* (drop-like) lesions; the latter is commonly used to describe a form of psoriasis in children that occurs after

acute streptococcal infection. *Umbilicated* lesions have a central depression; common examples include molluscum contagiosum and varicella.

Serpiginous describes lesions that have linear and curving elements, as though following the track of a snake. *Reticulated* lesions have a net-like or lacy configuration, such as cutis marmorata or livedo reticularis. *Morbilliform* is a term that refers to a measles-like eruption. It consists of red macules and papules that may be discrete or confluent on large areas of the body surface. Common examples of morbilliform eruptions include Kawasaki disease and drug eruptions. Lesions that have a variety of shapes are described as *multiform*.

Distribution of Lesions

Many cutaneous lesions have predilections for specific areas. Although these are discussed in more detail with specific disease processes, some generalizations about lesion distribution may be helpful in initial diagnosis. Linear eruptions in a *dermatomal* pattern affect skin supplied by a single spinal nerve, such as in herpes zoster infections. Linear lesions may also follow *lines of Blaschko*—lines of embryologic development of the skin (Fig. 36.7). These cutaneous lesions represent a form of genetic mosaicism; examples include epidermal nevi, lichen striatus, and some congenital disorders. Lesions that arise only in sun-exposed areas may represent a disorder of photosensitization or one precipitated by sun exposure.

ACKNOWLEDGMENT

The authors would like to acknowledge the contribution of Lara Wine Lee, MD, PhD, on the previous edition.

SUGGESTED READINGS

Available online.

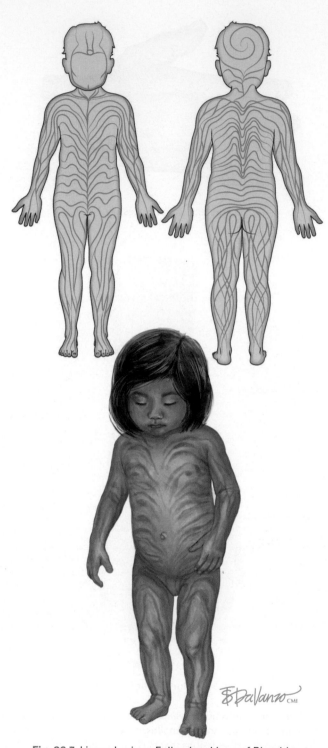

Fig. 36.7 Linear Lesions Following *Lines of Blaschko*.

Acne

Deanna Nardella

✳ CLINICAL VIGNETTE

A 13-year-old girl presents to the clinic for worsening acne. Over the last year, she has noticed increasing skin-colored papules on her forehead and cheeks. She feels that her acne has recently caused her to withdraw from social activities. She has grown along the 65th percentile for height and weight since infancy and is Tanner stage III for breasts and Tanner II for pubic hair. Her first menarche was 6 months ago with regular cycles. Mild acne vulgaris as part of normal adrenarche is suspected. She is initiated on adapalene 0.1% gel nightly with instruction to moisturize and use sunscreen daily. She returns in 2 months with improvement, but not complete resolution. She is advised to continue adapalene nightly, with addition of benzoyl peroxide gel in the morning. She returns 3 months later and is happy with her results, reporting that her mood and social confidence have greatly improved.

Acne vulgaris is a common skin complaint of adolescents. Topical retinoids and benzoyl peroxide products are often effective first-line therapy for mild acne; however, it requires consistent use for 2 to 3 months before improvement may be seen.

Acne vulgaris (AV) affects up to 85% of adolescents, frequently continuing into adulthood. In addition to physical scarring, patients can experience significant psychological morbidity, independent of severity.

ETIOLOGY AND PATHOGENESIS

Acne develops in the pilosebaceous unit (Fig. 37.1) secondary to (1) abnormal keratinization, (2) increased sebum production, and (3) proliferation of *Cutibacterium* (formerly *Propionibacterium*) *acnes* bacteria, which together lead to (4) a proinflammatory cascade. Puberty is associated with increased circulating androgens, resulting in increased sebum secretion. Increased abnormal shedding of keratinocytes is also seen, leading to follicular plugging and formation of the microcomedo. *C. acnes*, a normal skin inhabitant, thrives in this lipid-rich environment, releasing chemotactic factors, leading to inflammatory papules, pustules, and nodules (Fig. 37.2).

Occlusive cosmetics, hair products, and clothing can contribute to AV. A weak association of a high-glycemic index diet and skim dairy products with AV has been observed. However, formal dietary recommendations cannot be made on the current body of evidence.

CLINICAL PRESENTATION

Acne can span from birth to adulthood (Table 37.1).

Neonatal cephalic pustulosis is a common pustular eruption of the head, neck, and chest in neonates, typically seen in the first 6 weeks of life. It is a benign, self-limited, inflammatory reaction to *Malassezia,* a commensal yeast. Although less common, it is

important to consider infectious causes, including bacterial (impetigo, folliculitis, congenital syphilis), viral (herpes, varicella), or fungal/yeast (cutaneous candidiasis) that may require further workup and antimicrobial treatment.

Infantile acne (age 6 weeks to 1 year) is not typically associated with precocious puberty or a hormonal imbalance, yet signs of early adrenarche should be assessed.

Mid-childhood acne (1 to 7 years of age) is almost always abnormal and warrants further workup.

After age 7, AV is likely secondary to normal pubertal adrenarche and typically does not require further studies.

Abnormal age of presentation (ages 1 to 7 years), signs of early adrenarche, expedited growth velocity, or severe acne recalcitrant to treatment should prompt further evaluation (Box 37.1 and Fig. 37.3).

Multiple classification systems exist, though a simple description of the lesion type and spread is most helpful in guiding management (see Fig. 37.2).

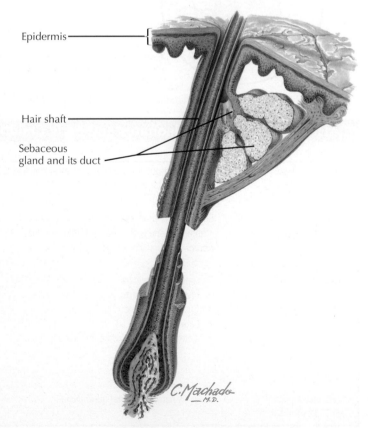

Epidermis

Hair shaft

Sebaceous gland and its duct

Fig. 37.1 Pilosebaceous Unit.

AV can cause postinflammatory dyspigmentation (erythema, hypopigmentation, or hyperpigmentation) that improves weeks to months after resolution of the active AV lesion(s). Moderate to severe AV can leave permanent scarring, with either atrophic (ice-pick, box-car, rolling) or hypertrophic/ keloidal scars. Early, effective treatment can minimize these complications.

DIFFERENTIAL DIAGNOSIS

The differential for AV largely depends on age and cutaneous distribution and includes both local and systemic disease (see Box 37.1).

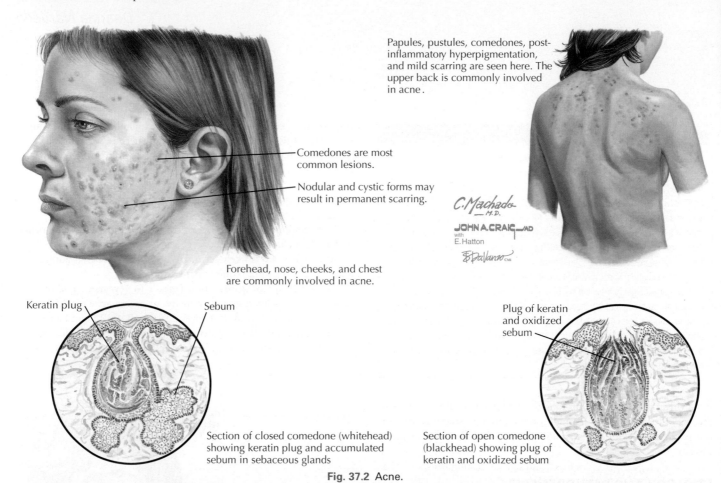

Papules, pustules, comedones, post-inflammatory hyperpigmentation, and mild scarring are seen here. The upper back is commonly involved in acne.

Comedones are most common lesions.

Nodular and cystic forms may result in permanent scarring.

C. Machado M.D.
JOHN A. CRAIG AD
with
E. Hatton
B Dalanzo CMI

Forehead, nose, cheeks, and chest are commonly involved in acne.

Keratin plug   Sebum

Plug of keratin and oxidized sebum

Section of closed comedone (whitehead) showing keratin plug and accumulated sebum in sebaceous glands

Section of open comedone (blackhead) showing plug of keratin and oxidized sebum

Fig. 37.2 Acne.

TABLE 37.1	**Acne in Neonates and Early Childhood**		
	Causes	**Clinical Appearance**	**Expected Course**
Neonatal cephalic pustulosis (<6 weeks)	Commonly a noninfectious inflammatory reaction to commensal *Malassezia* spp.	Pustules on scalp, face, chest	Nonscarring, self-limited Consider 2% ketoconazole cream if numerous lesions
Infantile acne (6 weeks–1 year)	Secondary to prominent fetal zona reticularis of adrenal gland with increased DHEA-S release Adrenals typically normalize by 1 year	Comedones, papules, pustules, nodules Boys > girls	Risk for scarring Treat off label with topical retinoids ± BPO If severe, consider systemic therapies If persistent, rule out underlying cause
Mid-childhood acne (age 1–7 years)	Considered pathologic • Precocious puberty • Cushing syndrome • Late-onset CAH • Adrenal/gonadal androgen-secreting tumor	Comedones, papules, pustules, nodules	Recommend targeted history, linear growth assessment, studies, endocrinology referral Studies: • Free/total testosterone • DHEA-S • 17-Hydroxyprogesterone • Hand x-ray
Preadolescent acne (age 7–12 years)	Typically normal pubertal adrenarche	Comedones, papules, pustules, nodules	Workup usually unnecessary unless rapid virilization is appreciated in females

BPO, Benzoyl peroxide; *CAH,* congenital adrenal hyperplasia; *DHEA-S,* dehydroepiandrosterone sulfate.

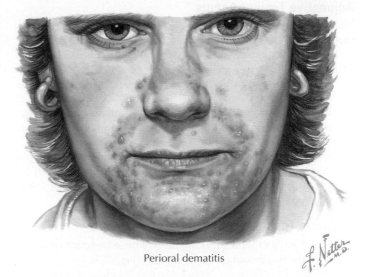

Perioral dematitis

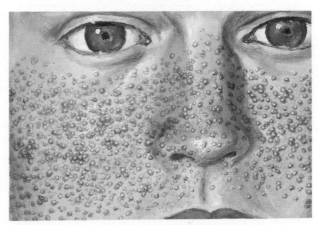

Facial angiofibromas

Fig. 37.3 Perioral Dermatitis and Facial Angiofibromas.

EVALUATION AND MANAGEMENT

Initial evaluation for AV includes a complete history and physical examination. Lesion type (closed or open comedone, papule, pustule, nodule, cyst), distribution, and presence of dyspigmentation and scarring should be noted.

Early adrenarche (before age 8 in girls and age 9 in boys) may manifest with body odor, axillary or pubic hair, advanced bone age, accelerated or stunted vertical growth, and genital virilization. Hyperandrogenism secondary to congenital adrenal hyperplasia (CAH), androgen-releasing adrenal or gonadal tumor, or polycystic ovarian syndrome can together manifest with abnormal weight gain, menstrual irregularities, hirsutism, and signs of insulin resistance (i.e., acanthosis nigricans). Elevated cortisol levels, as seen in Cushing syndrome, may present with stunted growth, hypertension, striae, and a dorsocervical fat pad. Additionally, spondyloarthropathy syndromes associated with acne include PAPA (pyogenic arthritis, pyoderma gangrenosum, and acne), and SAPHO (synovitis, acne, pustulosis, hyperostosis, osteomyelitis).

If there is suspicion for endocrine dysfunction, screening laboratory tests, imaging, and/or referral to endocrinology are recommended (see Table 37.1).

Routine microbial testing is not recommended unless there is concern for gram-negative folliculitis, typically seen after extended treatment with tetracycline antibiotics for acne.

Treatments require 8 to 12 weeks of consistent use to demonstrate maximal effect. Harsh scrubbing and manual extraction should be avoided. Use of noncomedogenic moisturizers may decrease irritation commonly associated with topical therapies. Daily application of sunscreen is recommended to decrease postinflammatory dyschromia and because acne therapies may be photosensitizing.

Fig. 37.4 provides an algorithm of acne classification and treatment.

Benzoyl Peroxide

Benzoyl peroxide (BPO) possesses lipophilic properties that penetrate the subcorneal pilosebaceous unit, working as a bactericidal, comedolytic, and antiinflammatory agent. BPO augments the effect of retinoids and reduces antibiotic resistance. BPO's time in contact with the skin improves its efficacy; cleansers should sit on the skin momentarily before rinsing. Initiate BPO every 2 to 3 days to minimize irritation, titrating to daily use as tolerated. Counsel patients on BPO's bleaching effect on fabrics.

Topical Retinoids

Retinoids are vitamin A derivatives that regulate keratinocyte desquamation, decrease sebum production, and block proinflammatory pathways (i.e., Toll-like receptor 2-like receptor 2). The cornerstone of AV therapy, retinoids demonstrate efficacy after 2 to 3 months of consistent application and are not intended for localized spot treatment. Acne may initially worsen as deeper microcomedones surface. Irritation is commonly associated with retinoids and can be minimized with lower potency creams instead of gels, less frequent application, and use of noncomedogenic moisturizer after application (Table 37.2).

Topical Antibiotics

Topical antibiotics have a bacteriostatic effect on *C. acnes* and reduce proinflammatory cytokines. Clindamycin is frequently used. It is well tolerated, though rapid *C. acne* resistance can develop, mitigated by concomitant BPO use. Combination therapies may improve adherence (see Table 37.2).

Adjunctive Topical Agents

Limited data suggest potential benefit from using adjunctive therapies such as topical dapsone, chemical exfoliants, and niacinamide.

Dapsone is a sulfonamide with antimicrobial and antiinflammatory effects. It is available as a 5% gel twice daily or a 7.5% gel daily.

Alpha and beta hydroxy acids, such as glycolic and salicylic acids, respectively, work as chemical exfoliants to promote desquamation, in turn helping to treat postinflammatory dyspigmentation, prevent follicular plugging, and allow improved penetration of topical AV therapies. They are available over the counter as washes and leave-on therapies.

Nicotinamide, or niacinamide, carries a potential antiinflammatory benefit, protects the skin barrier by minimizing trans-epidermal water loss, and regulates sebum production. It is available in several over-the-counter facial creams and serums.

Systemic Therapies

Systemic therapies (Table 37.3) should be initiated together with topicals when treating moderate-to-severe acne (Fig. 37.5).

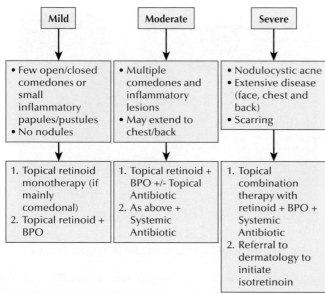

Fig. 37.4 Acne Vulgaris Treatment Algorithm. Use therapies for 2 to 3 months; advance or taper potencies as tolerated. Address poor adherence with combination products. Address dryness with fewer applications, lower concentrations or use of creams over gels. *BPO,* Benzoyl peroxide.

Doxycycline is the preferred oral antibiotic given its favorable side effect profile. In patients who cannot swallow pills, pregnant patients, and those with tetracycline allergies, consider erythromycin or azithromycin. Antibiotics should ideally be tapered by 3 months as topicals take effect.

Isotretinoin is an excellent first-line option for severe, recalcitrant acne or acne complicated by scarring or significant psychosocial stress. Given isotretinoin's well-established teratogenicity, prescribers must be enrolled in the iPledge program, usually requiring referral to a board-certified dermatologist.

Oral hormonal therapies—combined oral contraceptives (COCs) and spironolactone—work by an antiandrogen effect and can be considered as adjunctive therapies for females with moderate-to-severe acne. Before initiating COCs, evaluate for contraindications and counsel that it will take up to three cycles of COCs for efficacy.

Treatment of Scars

Early treatment of AV is crucial to avoid permanent scarring. Variable improvement, but not resolution, of scars may be seen with dermabrasion, subcision, lasers, and dermal fillers.

TABLE 37.2	**Topical Retinoids**		
Retinoid	**Strengths (%)**	**Comments**	**Side Effects of All Retinoids**
Adapalene	0.1	Well tolerated	Irritation
• Gel	0.3	Use day or night and	Exfoliation
• Cream		concomitantly with	Photosensitivity
• Lotion		BPO	Pruritus
Tretinoin	0.025	Destabilized by light,	Teratogenic
• Cream	0.025/0.05/0.1	apply at night	
• Gel	0.025/0.05/0.1		
• Microsphere gel	0.04/0.1		
Tazarotene	0.05	Most irritating	
• Cream	0.05/0.1		
• Gel	0.05/0.1		
• Foam			

BPO, Benzoyl peroxide.

TABLE 37.3	**Systemic Therapies for Acne**		
Medication	**Dose**	**Considerations**	**Side Effects**
Antibiotics			
Doxycycline	40–100 mg daily-BID[a]	Counsel on photoprotection Avoid in children under 8 years of age and pregnant patients Take with food/drink, stay upright for 1 hour after ingestion [a]Subantimicrobial dosing (40 mg daily) yields antiinflammatory effect, minimizes gastrointestinal upset	Gastrointestinal upset Esophagitis Photosensitivity Benign intracranial hypertension
Minocycline	50–100 mg daily-BID	Consider if doxycycline is not tolerated Monitor for new rash, fever, facial swelling	Benign intracranial hypertension Dizziness/vertigo Lupus-like reaction Drug-induced hypersensitivity reaction Blue discoloration of sclera, mucosa, nail beds, scars

TABLE 37.3 Systemic Therapies for Acne—cont'd

Medication	Dose	Considerations	Side Effects
Erythromycin	30–50 mg/kg/day divided TID, 250 mg BID, 500 mg daily	Useful in patients who cannot swallow pills and those with contraindications to tetracyclines High risk for *Cutibacterium acnes* resistance	Gastrointestinal upset Drug interactions Cardiac abnormalities
Hormonal Therapies			
Combined oral contraceptives (COC)	Varies	US Food and Drug Administration (FDA) approved COCs for treatment of acne: • Norgestimate/ethinyl estradiol (Ortho Tri-Cyclen) • Norethindrone/ethinyl estradiol (Estrostep) • Drospirenone/ethinyl estradiol (Yaz)	Headaches Nausea Breast tenderness Thromboembolism
Spironolactone	50–200 mg daily	Generally well tolerated Serial laboratory tests are unnecessary if normal hepatic, renal and adrenal function Avoid in pregnancy	Menstrual irregularity Diuresis Headache Dizziness Hyperkalemia (rare)
Retinoids			
Isotretinoin	~1 mg/kg/day Goal: 120–225 mg/kg total	Avoid use with tetracyclines FDA iPLEDGE requires two forms of contraception for females Screening laboratory tests at baseline and after second month of goal dose	Dry eyes, skin Myalgias Photosensitivity Teratogenicity Hypertriglyceridemia Elevated liver enzymes (Suicidal ideation: may be no greater than background incidence)

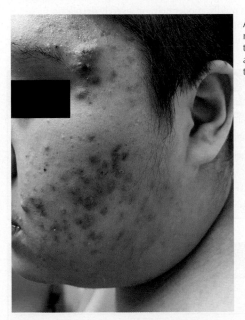

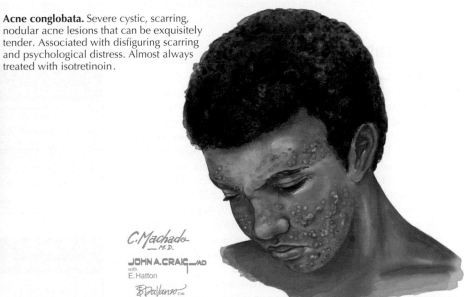

Acne conglobata. Severe cystic, scarring, nodular acne lesions that can be exquisitely tender. Associated with disfiguring scarring and psychological distress. Almost always treated with isotretinoin.

Fig. 37.5 Mixed Moderate Acne Vulgaris.

FUTURE DIRECTIONS

A knowledge gap exists for optimal treatment of AV in nonadolescent children and pregnant patients. Topical antiandrogen therapy is now available, though it requires further pediatric studies. Looking forward, the role of laser and photodynamic therapy, as well as the relationship between skin and gut microbiomes, are areas of great interest.

SUGGESTED READINGS

Available online.

38

Nevi

Deanna Nardella

✳ CLINICAL VIGNETTE

A 9-month-old boy presents with a 2 × 4–cm homogenous brown plaque with well-defined borders on the left lateral thigh. Present since birth, it has grown proportionally to the child. You determine that this is a medium congenital melanocytic nevus (CMN) with benign clinical features. Given its low risk for, melanoma, you, together with the family, decide on routine surveillance, educating the family on high-risk features of which they should be aware.

The risk for melanoma in CMN, at less than 20 cm, is very low. Families should be counseled on routine sun protection and surveillance for concerning intralesional changes (Table 38.1).

Nevi are common in the pediatric population. Up to 6% of neonates have a congenital nevus, and almost 100% of White children develop a nevus by early childhood. Most lesions can be serially followed for features concerning for malignant transformation or possible underlying condition.

ETIOLOGY AND PATHOGENESIS

Nevi in the pediatric population are distinguished by size (small, medium, large, giant), age of presentation (congenital or acquired), cell of origin, and presence of atypia (clinically or histologically dysplastic).

Nevi can be further characterized by depth: junctional (epidermal/dermal junction), compound (epidermis and dermis), or intradermal (dermis only). Lesions may undergo characteristic progression from junctional nevi (macular and brown) to compound nevi (dome-shaped and tan) to dermal nevi (dome-shaped and skin-colored).

Factors affecting nevus development include age, familial tendency, sun exposure, phenotypic skin type, baseline nevi present (high nevus counts or single large congenital melanocytic nevus [CMN]), immunosuppression, medications, and underlying genetic or neuroendocrine diagnoses.

Studies are ongoing, but activating genetic mutations have been associated with certain pediatric nevi (Table 38.2).

Neoplastic change is fortunately rare in children. The 2013 to 2017 Surveillance, Epidemiology and End Results (SEER) database reports a melanoma incidence of approximately 1.5 per 100,000 children ages 0 to 19, and of all new diagnoses, 0.4% are among people under age 20.

CLINICAL PRESENTATION

Nevi typically arise on sun-exposed skin and the scalp but can present on any skin surface, including palms, soles, and genitalia. CMNs are typically present in neonates. Acquired melanocytic nevi appear as early as 6 months of age, increasing in number through the third decade. More unique lesions, such as blue and Spitz nevi can manifest congenitally or later in life. Halo nevi are an immunologic phenomenon to preexisting nevi. Epidermal nevi are congenital; however, they may not be noted until later in life.

Acquired Melanocytic Nevi

Acquired nevi, or common moles, may appear pink, tan, brown, or black (Fig. 38.1). They are typically less than 6 mm, symmetric, homogeneous in color, with well-defined borders.

On the scalp, eclipse nevi are characteristic, with a hyperpigmented, sometimes stellate, rim surrounding a lighter center (Fig. 38.2).

Acral nevi—acquired nevi on the palms, soles, and nail beds—are more common in darker-skinned individuals but can be seen in all ethnicities.

Atypical or Dysplastic Acquired Melanocytic Nevi

Atypical, or dysplastic, nevi are those acquired nevi with clinical or histologic features concerning for dysplasia (see Table 38.1; Fig. 38.3). Histologically, they are categorized as mildly, moderately, or severely dysplastic.

Often arising in puberty, atypical moles favor sun-exposed areas and those with family tendency. Individuals often possess similar

TABLE 38.1 Atypical Features Raising Concern for Pediatric Melanoma

A	Asymmetry, amelanotic
B	Bleeding/ulceration, bump/thickening, irregular borders
C	Color heterogeneity
D	De novo, any diameter for pediatric patients (>6 mm especially concerning)
E	Evolution over time, including pain or itch

TABLE 38.2 Activating Mutations Commonly Associated With Pediatric Nevi

Nevus Subtype	Genetic Mutations (Nonexhaustive)
Congenital melanocytic nevus	NRAS > BRAF
Acquired melanocytic nevus	BRAF > NRAS
Epidermal nevus	FGFR3, PIK3CA, HRAS
Nevus spilus	HRAS
Blue nevus, nevus of Ito, nevus of Ota	G alpha q pathway: GNAQ, GNA11
Spitz	HRAS Receptor tyrosine kinase mutations: ROS1, ALK, MET, NTRK1/3, RET, MERTK

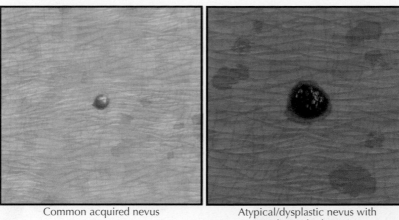

Common acquired nevus

Atypical/dysplastic nevus with surrounding solar lentigines

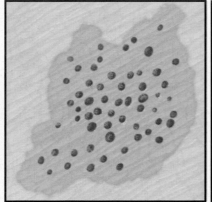

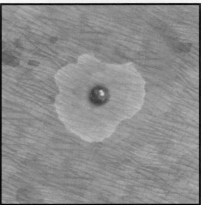

Nevus spilus

Halo nevus

Fig. 38.1 Melanocytic Nevi.

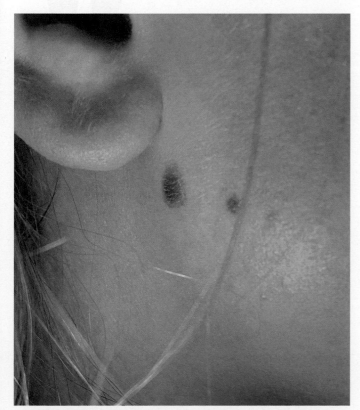

Fig. 38.2 Eclipse Nevus. (Courtesy Nicholas Lowe, MD.)

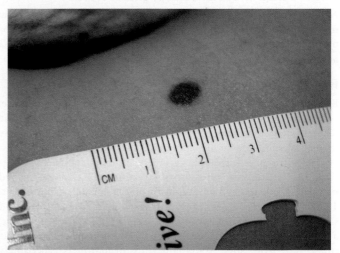

Fig. 38.3 A small melanocytic nevus with benign clinical features of symmetry, well-defined borders, and homogeneous color.

morphology, or "signature" features, among their nevi. Nevi aligned with one's signature are less concerning.

Congenital Melanocytic Nevi

CMNs typically arise in the neonatal period and evolve over time. CMNs extend into subcutaneous tissues, appearing as raised, hyperpigmented lesions with or without hypertrichosis (Figs. 38.4 and 38.5).

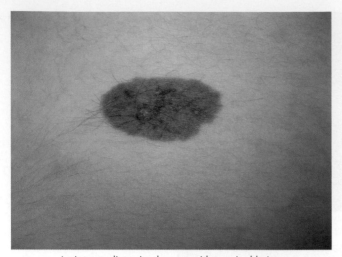

An intermediate sized nevus with terminal hairs.
Fig. 38.4 Medium-Sized Congenital Nevus.

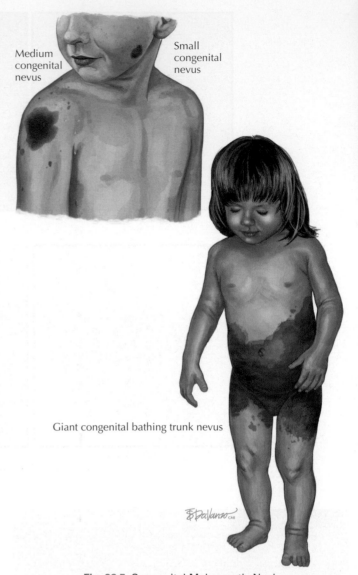

Fig. 38.5 Congenital Melanocytic Nevi.

CMNs are classified by expected size when the patient has achieved full growth: giant (>40 cm), large (>20 cm), medium (1.5 to 20 cm), or small (<1.5 cm). From infancy to adulthood, the estimated size increase of a CMN is twofold on the head and threefold on the trunk and extremities. As a child's rate of growth is most pronounced in the first few years of life, proportional growth of CMNs can alarm families and clinicians but is expected.

Small to medium CMNs have a very low risk for malignancy (~1%). Large and giant CMNs carry a 2% to 5% lifetime risk for melanoma, with half of total cases developing by 5 years of age.

Nevus Spilus or Speckled Lentiginous Nevus

Nevus spilus, a CMN subtype, presents as a tan patch at birth or early infancy, developing superimposed hyperpigmented macules and papules with time (see Fig. 38.1). Development of intralesional melanoma is exceedingly rare.

Blue Nevus

Blue nevi are slow-growing papules or nodules arising in adolescence, commonly on the face, scalp, buttocks, and hands (Fig. 38.6). The depth of dermal melanocytes and melanophages that comprise these lesions is responsible for the blue-gray hue.

There are three histologic variants: common, cellular, and epithelioid. The common type is a solitary blue to black dome-shaped papule, usually under 1 cm, typically on the dorsal hands and feet. The cellular type is more commonly seen on the face, buttock, and sacrum. The epithelioid type can be seen with Carney complex, a disorder of myxomas, lentigines, schwannomas, endocrinopathies, and neoplasms. Malignant transformation is exceedingly rare.

Dermal Melanocytic Nevi (Congenital Dermal Melanocytosis, Nevus of Ota, Nevus of Ito)

Dermal melanocytoses are a family of lesions composed of dermal dendritic melanocytes presenting as blue, green, or gray patches.

Congenital dermal melanocytosis is frequently seen in newborns of Asian, Black, or Native American descent, typically resolving by puberty (Fig. 38.7). They are most commonly located on the lumbosacral area, although they can arise on the extremities, back, and chest.

In contrast, nevus of Ota and nevus of Ito are dermal melanocytoses that do not self-resolve (Fig. 38.8). Both can present congenitally or later in life. Nevus of Ota is distributed along the first or second trigeminal nerve, whereas nevus of Ito is found along the supraclavicular and lateral cutaneous brachial nerves. The development of cutaneous melanoma is exceedingly uncommon. There are rare reports of intraocular or central nervous system melanoma reported with nevus of Ota.

Spitz Nevi

Spitz nevi appear as pink, red, brown, or black, symmetric, well-circumscribed lesions that present rapidly, favoring the face and lower extremities (Fig. 38.9). They are most commonly acquired but can be congenital. Spitz nevi can undergo spontaneous resolution over months to years but should be monitored closely for features that raise concern for atypical Spitz tumors and Spitzoid melanomas (i.e., postpubertal presentation, size >1 cm, asymmetry).

Halo Nevi

Halo nevi describes the phenomenon in which a white rim develops around preexisting nevi, most commonly a melanocytic nevus, but can

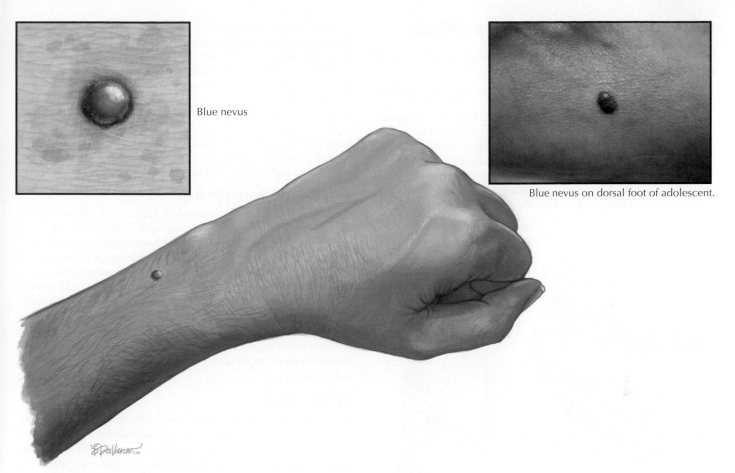

Blue nevus

Blue nevus on dorsal foot of adolescent.

Fig. 38.6 Blue Nevus.

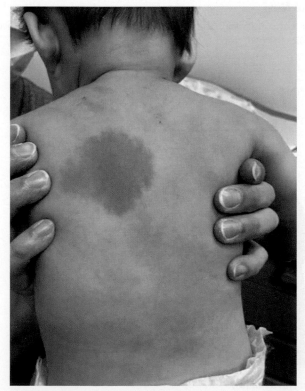

Fig. 38.7 Congenital Dermal Melanocytosis. (Courtesy Danielle N. Brown, MD.)

be rarely seen with blue and spitz nevi. It is thought to be secondary to T cell–mediated destruction of the nevomelanocyte (Fig. 38.10; see Fig. 38.1). These lesions typically occur on the back. The central nevus may lighten and completely regress. Halo nevi in children can be associated with development of vitiligo.

Epidermal Nevi (Keratinocytic Epidermal Nevus, Nevus Sebaceus)

Epidermal nevi are benign hyperplasias of epidermal cells classically manifesting as Blaschko-linear papules coalescing into plaques. Common subtypes include keratinocytic epidermal nevi (Fig. 38.11), which present as skin-colored to brown plaques, whereas nevus sebaceus appear yellow to orange and waxy in texture (Fig. 38.12). Nevus sebaceus are most common on the scalp and associated with alopecia. Both lesions are congenital but may not become apparent until later in life. Both can become increasingly nodular or verrucous with adrenarche.

Becker Nevi

Becker nevi are cutaneous hamartomas presenting as unilateral, hyperpigmented, hypertrichotic patches or plaques classically appreciated with adrenarche. They are outlined in greater detail in Chapter 41.

DIFFERENTIAL DIAGNOSIS

The differential for melanocytic nevi includes both localized and systemic disease, detailed in Box 38.1.

EVALUATION AND MANAGEMENT: BY NEVUS SUBTYPE

All Nevi

Initial evaluation begins with a complete history—prenatal, developmental, medical, and family—and full-body skin examination, including the mucosa, nails, and genitalia. Photographs may help document change, allowing ongoing assessment for high-risk features for pediatric melanoma, as summarized in Table 38.1. Educate families on high-risk features and the importance of sun protection (daily sunscreen, avoid midday sun exposure, protective clothing). If atypia is identified, referral to a dermatology specialist is advised. It is notable that most melanomas develop de novo, not from a preexisting nevus.

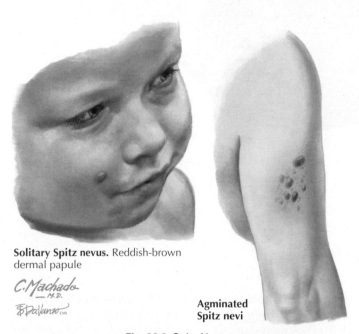

Solitary Spitz nevus. Reddish-brown dermal papule

Agminated Spitz nevi

Fig. 38.9 Spitz Nevus.

For eclipse nevi, despite their two-toned appearance, biopsy is not recommended unless other concerning features are appreciated, such as rapid growth or notable asymmetry.

If extensive involvement, multiple lesions, developmental delay, or focal neurologic deficit is appreciated, concern for genetic or neurocutaneous syndromes should be raised with referral to a dermatologist and possible referral to a genetics specialist.

Surgical removal is a shared decision between provider and family based on clinical and cosmetic concerns, requiring consideration of location, size, and risks of general anesthesia. Excision may decrease, though does not eliminate, the incidence of melanoma.

Congenital Melanocytic Nevi

For singular, small to medium CMNs, referral to a dermatologist is not required unless there are concerning clinical features (e.g., rapid growth out of proportion to patient's overall growth, pain, pruritus, ulceration, new nodules, new-onset asymmetry). However, all large CMNs or those with over 20 satellite lesions warrant referral. Routine surveillance by both a primary provider and family member for change with ABCDEs (see Table 38.1) and palpation for intralesional subcutaneous nodules is crucial to detect neoplastic conversion. If CMNs are cephalic or are postaxially located, magnetic resonance imaging of the brain and spine may be warranted to assess for neurocutaneous melanosis, a rare condition that can carry serious sequelae.

Dysplastic Nevi

Historically, dysplastic nevi were thought to be precursors to melanomas; fortunately, there is increasing evidence that dysplastic nevi and melanoma are distinct entities. If biopsy reveals mild to moderate atypia, close monitoring may be sufficient. Dysplastic nevi with severe atypia may require reexcision; however, pathologic findings should be reviewed by an experienced dermatopathologist.

Blue Nevi

Blue nevi can resemble melanoma; slow versus rapid growth distinguishes the two, respectively.

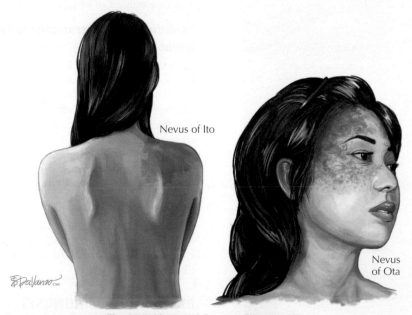

Nevus of Ito

Nevus of Ota

Fig. 38.8 Nevus of Ota and Nevus of Ito.

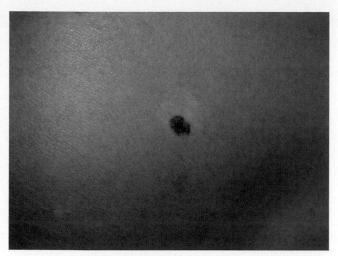

Halo nevus on the trunk of a child.
Fig. 38.10 Halo Nevus.

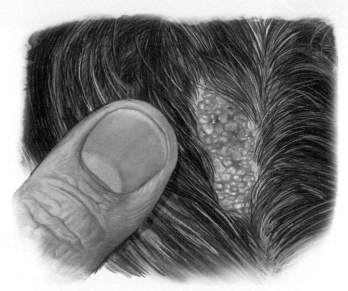

Nevus sebaceus. Flesh- to yellow-colored plaque, typically on the scalp with associated overlying alopecia

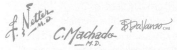

Fig. 38.12 Nevus Sebaceus.

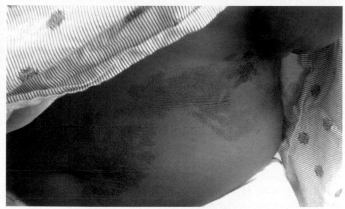

Fig. 38.11 Keratinocytic Epidermal Nevus.

> ## BOX 38.1 Differential Diagnosis of Pediatric Nevi
>
> - Atypical or dysplastic nevus
> - Becker nevus
> - Blue nevus
> - Café-au-lait spot
> - Common acquired melanocytic nevus
> - Congenital melanocytic nevus
> - Dermal melanocytic nevi
> - Halo nevus
> - Keratinocytic epidermal nevus
> - Melanoma
> - Neurocutaneous melanocytosis
> - Nevus sebaceus
> - Spitz nevus

Nevus of Ota

Nevus of Ota can be associated with ipsilateral glaucoma, melanocytosis, and, rarely, melanoma of the choroid. Referral to an ophthalmology specialist should be considered.

Spitz Nevi

Spitz nevi should be closely monitored. If less than 1 cm and stable, clinical monitoring may be sufficient because many Spitz nevi spontaneously involute over years. However, if onset is in adolescence or the lesion possesses atypia (size >1 cm, ulcerated, asymmetric, or heterogenous color), it should be excised for histopathologic evaluation.

Halo Nevus

The appearance of the central nevus dictates management. Biopsy is unnecessary for benign appearing nevi.

Epidermal Nevi

Singular lesions in an otherwise healthy patient can be monitored. Nevus sebaceus, specifically, may develop secondary growths later in life. Although usually benign, less than 1% of secondary growths may be malignant, so, if noted, referral to a dermatologist is recommended. Because of the rarity of malignancy in nevus sebaceus, routine prophylactic excision is no longer recommended.

There exist multiple epidermal nevi syndromes, typically associated with ocular, skeletal, and neurologic abnormalities. If physical examination raises concern for the latter, dermatology referral is recommended.

FUTURE DIRECTIONS

Much research is still needed to best understand the genetics and malignancy potential of various pediatric nevi, because the low incidence of such disease limits the power and generalizability of study findings.

Although surgical excision is the mainstay of therapy, as laser technology advances, there are increasing options for early, cosmetically favorable treatment options.

SUGGESTED READINGS

Available online.

39

Atopic Dermatitis

Sonia A. Havele

CLINICAL VIGNETTE

An 8-year-old girl with a history of asthma and seasonal allergies presents with worsening rash. As a baby, she was noted to have eczematous patches on her cheeks. Over the past 2 years, her mother has noticed involvement of her antecubital fossae, popliteal fossae, and neck, with frequent flares. Recently, her pruritus has become so severe that she is having difficulty sleeping.

For treatment, parents try to apply emollients after showers, though their daughter is often uncooperative. They have also replaced all scented products with fragrance-free alternatives. Although application of mild topical corticosteroids has led to improvement in the past, her parents report that they prefer not to apply steroids because of the risk for skin thinning. Physical examination shows weepy, excoriated plaques with overlying scale and crust present on the antecubital and popliteal fossae bilaterally.

This is a common presentation of atopic dermatitis in childhood. Intense pruritus is a hallmark of this disease, which can significantly impair quality of life for patients and their families. Avoidance of triggers (e.g., contact allergens in soaps) and preservation of the skin barrier with daily moisturization are the cornerstones of management. First-line treatment for flares is topical steroids. Concerns regarding potential side effects of steroid use are common among parents and should be addressed regularly to ensure patients are being treated appropriately.

Atopic dermatitis (AD) is a common, chronic, inflammatory skin disease that affects nearly 11 million children in the United States.

ETIOLOGY AND PATHOGENESIS

Although the cause of AD is unknown, both genetic and environmental factors contribute to an impaired skin barrier and inflammatory cascade that gives rise to this disease.

Loss-of-function mutations in the gene that encodes filaggrin *(FLG)*—a key protein involved in keratinization—are a major risk factor in the development of AD. An intact epidermis provides a barrier to infectious microbes, irritants, and allergens and helps retain moisture. FLG mutations are associated with asthma, allergic rhinitis, and keratosis pilaris—common comorbidities in patients with AD—as well as hyperlinear palms, which also may be noted on examination.

An exaggerated Th2 phenotype has been observed in AD. Elevated Th2 cytokines, especially interleukin-4 (IL-4) and IL-13, lead to increased immunoglobulin E (IgE) synthesis and stimulation of an inflammatory feedback loop. IL-18 impairment, involved in B cell switching between Th1 and Th2, may also favor a Th2 response. IL-31, produced by Th2 cells, binds directly to nerves, leading to itch while also downregulating expression of filaggrin. This imbalance in inflammatory signaling leads to an unremitting cycle of barrier failure and inflammation.

In addition, levels of ceramide, lipid molecules that play a crucial role in maintaining epidermal barrier function, are often decreased. Additionally, external factors such as mechanical injury from scratching and proteases from bacteria and dust mites may also contribute to a weakened skin barrier, facilitating bacterial colonization and penetration of environmental allergens that can further trigger the inflammatory cascade.

CLINICAL PRESENTATION

Most children with AD initially present at a very young age, with more than half presenting in the first year of life and 85% presenting before the age of 5 years. Characteristic lesions involve scaly, erythematous patches, with associated pruritus and xerosis. Distribution varies based on age; thus AD can be divided into three stages: infantile, childhood, and adolescent/adult (Figs. 39.1 and 39.2). Children with AD experience alternating periods of disease flare and symptom resolution, though progression and severity can be difficult to predict.

History

Pruritus is the hallmark symptom of AD. Because pruritus often presents before cutaneous lesions, AD is often referred to as the "itch that rashes."

Patients with AD may have other features of the atopic triad, including asthma and allergic rhinitis. Allergies to nickel and latex, as well as to food products, including egg, cow's milk, and peanut, are also more common in patients with AD; however, elimination of foods rarely results in resolution or notable improvement of underlying AD.

AD can significantly affect quality of life for patients and their families. Nocturnal scratching often leads to poor sleep and chronic fatigue, which can affect school performance and psychological health. Children with AD experience increased levels of stress and anxiety and may struggle with self-image and the ability to socialize with their peers. Providers should always inquire about school performance and mental health when evaluating patients with AD.

Physical Examination

Physical examination findings can be divided into three phases—acute, subacute, and chronic. Acute AD is a vesicular eruption with associated crusting and weeping. Subacute AD is characterized by red papules and plaques with overlying xerosis and scale. Chronic changes involve lichenification, or thickening, of the skin. Xerosis is almost universally present.

The distribution of AD varies by age. In infants, the cheeks, scalp, and extensor surfaces of the arms and legs are most affected (see Fig. 39.1).

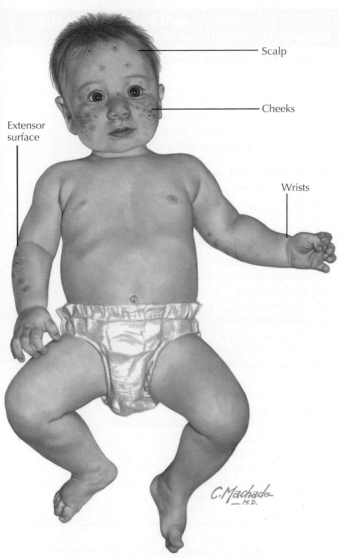

Fig. 39.1 Infant With Atopic Dermatitis.

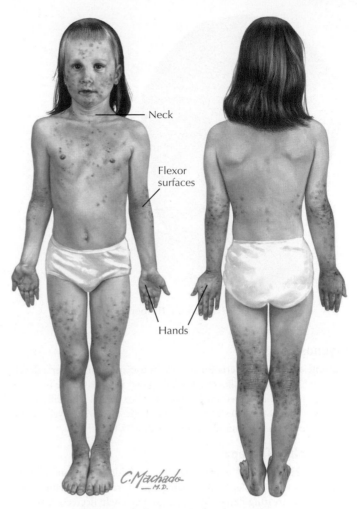

Fig. 39.2 Child With Atopic Dermatitis.

The diaper area is typically spared. The perioral and perinasal areas are rarely involved, leading to the "headlight sign" of pallor. In children and adolescents, the neck, hands, and flexor surfaces of the upper and lower extremities are more commonly affected (see Fig. 39.2). Other findings in AD include thinning of lateral eyebrows (Hertoghe sign) from chronic rubbing of the face and a prominent nasal crease resulting from chronic upward wiping of the nose when allergic rhinitis is present ("nasal salute").

Complications

Defects in the epithelial barrier, decreased expression of antimicrobial peptides, and disruption of the cutaneous microbiome leave the skin susceptible to superinfection by bacteria and viruses, most commonly *Staphylococcus aureus* and herpes simplex virus (HSV).

Staphylococcus aureus

In patients with AD, both normal and affected skin have increased colonization with *S. aureus*. When superinfection occurs, pain, erythema, edema, and warmth may be present. Fever and an elevated white blood cell count can occur if the lesions are extensive or if the bacteria have invaded the bloodstream. Association of *S. aureus* with acute flares in patients with AD has been attributed to IgE antibodies directed against

S. aureus and/or staphylococcal production of superantigens that trigger the inflammatory cascade.

Eczema Herpeticum

Superinfection with HSV can be life-threatening. On history, parents may report the sudden appearance of vesiculopustular, crusted, or "punched out" lesions on areas of inflamed skin (Fig. 39.3). Associated symptoms may include fever, fatigue, and lymphadenopathy. Lesions can spread to involve a larger body surface area. If skin near the eyes becomes affected, urgent ophthalmologic evaluation for herpetic keratoconjunctivitis is required. Superinfections with enterovirus (Coxsackie) or streptococcus may mimic eczema herpeticum. Other viral infections, such as molluscum, may be more widespread in patients with AD.

EVALUATION AND MANAGEMENT

Laboratory Testing

Routine laboratory testing is not typically performed for the diagnosis of AD. If checked for other reasons, a white blood cell count with differential may reveal eosinophilia; a serum IgE also may be elevated. Skin prick testing, patch testing, or IgE assays for specific allergens (also known as radioallergosorbent testing [RAST]) often have high false positive rates, so routine testing is not recommended in the management of AD. If there is suspicion for superinfection, surface cultures with antibiotic sensitivities and/or viral polymerase chain reaction can help guide appropriate therapy.

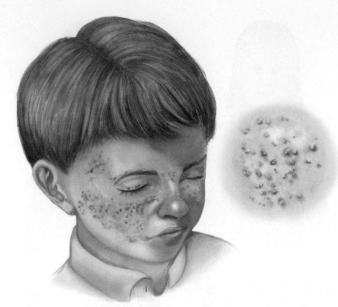

Fig. 39.3 Eczema Herpeticum.

Diagnosis

Multiple diagnostic criteria for AD are in use, including criteria developed by Hanifin and Rajka in 1980. Diagnosis is based on the presence of three major and three minor criteria (Box 39.1). The differential diagnosis of AD includes other dermatologic diseases as well as systemic disease and immunodeficiency (Table 39.1).

Approach to Therapy

The foundation of AD management is twofold: (1) maintaining the skin barrier with frequent moisturizing and (2) reducing inflammation by promptly treating flares. Topical emollients help decrease transepidermal water loss and should be applied at least twice daily. Topical steroids are first-line treatment of acute flares.

Topical Corticosteroids

First-line therapy for AD flares is topical corticosteroids. Ointments are preferred because of decreased burning sensation, fewer ingredients (and thus fewer potential allergens), and better skin penetration. These agents are available in a wide range of potencies. Low-potency corticosteroids, such as hydrocortisone 2.5% ointment, can be used for the face and groin to minimize risk for steroid atrophy. Medium-potency agents such as triamcinolone 0.1% ointment are useful for mildly affected areas or areas such as the trunk, and high-potency agents such as clobetasol 0.05% may be required for areas of severe involvement, lichenification, and/or acral skin.

Cutaneous side effects such as skin atrophy, striae, or telangiectasias can be seen with inappropriate selection (e.g., prolonged use of ultrapotent topical steroid on atrophy-prone areas such as the groin) or inappropriate use of topical steroids (e.g., daily maintenance use of ultrapotent topical steroids, instead of only as needed for flares). Postinflammatory hypopigmentation is often mistaken for steroid atrophy. The former is expected dyschromia after resolution of inflammation, whereas the latter is from inappropriate use of topical steroids, in which white discoloration is accompanied by thinning of the skin with more prominently visible blood vessels and/or striae. Systemic side effects such as Cushingoid syndrome and hypothalamic-pituitary-adrenal axis suppression are extremely rare and typically seen with gross misuse of high-potency topical steroids, such as use of ultrapotent topical steroids to the entire body for months in a young child in

---

BOX 39.1   Hanifin and Rajka Diagnostic Criteria for Atopic Dermatitis

Major Criteria (at Least Three)
1. Pruritus
2. Dermatitis in a distribution characteristic for age
   a. Infants: face and extensor surfaces
   b. Older children and adolescents: flexor surfaces
3. Chronic or relapsing course of dermatitis
4. Personal or family history of asthma, allergic rhinitis, or AD

Minor Criteria (at Least Three)
1. Early age of onset
2. Xerosis
3. Cheilitis
4. Perifollicular accentuation
5. Facial pallor or erythema
6. Ichthyosis, keratosis pilaris, or palmar hyperlinearity
7. Hand and foot dermatitis
8. Nipple dermatitis
9. Pityriasis alba
10. Accentuated infraorbital folds (Dennie-Morgan lines)
11. Infraorbital darkening
12. Cataracts (anterior subcapsular)
13. Recurrent conjunctivitis
14. Keratoconus
15. White dermographism
16. Anterior neck folds
17. Susceptibility to skin Infections (*Staphylococcus aureus*, herpes simplex virus)
18. Sensitivity to emotional factors
19. Intolerance to certain foods
20. Exacerbation of pruritus or dermatitis with sweating
21. Exacerbation of pruritus or dermatitis when wearing wool
22. Immediate (type 1) skin test reactivity
23. Elevated IgE level

AD, Atopic dermatitis; *IgE,* immunoglobulin E.
From Hanifen JM, Rajka G. Diagnostic features of atopic dermatitis. *Acta Derm Venerol (Stockh).* 1980;92(suppl. 92):44-47.

---

lieu of a moisturizer or use in the occluded diaper area of an infant for months.

Referral to a pediatric dermatologist for management of moderate to severe disease should be considered (Box 39.2).

Topical Calcineurin and Phosphodiesterase Inhibitors

The topical calcineurin inhibitors (TCIs) tacrolimus and pimecrolimus and topical phosphodiesterase inhibitor crisaborole are generally considered second-line therapies. They may be useful for eczema on eyelids, because topical steroids should be avoided to minimize risk for cataracts and glaucoma. Burning and stinging sensations are common. Although the US Food and Drug Administration issued a **"black box warning"** for TCIs in 2006 because of concerns about long-term safety, a recent study that followed patients after marketing found no increase in malignancy in over 26,000 patient-years studied.

Systemic Agents

Dupilumab is the first and only targeted systemic therapy for the treatment of moderate to severe AD in children 6 years of age and older. It is a full humanized monoclonal antibody that suppresses Th2-mediated inflammation by inhibition of IL-4 and IL-13, delivered by

TABLE 39.1 Differential Diagnosis of Atopic Dermatitis

Diagnosis	Differentiating Features
Contact dermatitis	History of contact with an allergen Geometric shape or distribution of eruption (exposed extremities for poison ivy, site of contact with button of pants for nickel)
Seborrheic dermatitis	Seborrheic distribution: scalp, glabella, nasolabial folds "Greasy" appearance
Psoriasis	Discrete salmon-colored plaques with well-defined borders Thick scaling
Acrodermatitis enteropathica	U-shaped perioral rash with extremity and perineal involvement Associated with chronic diarrhea, growth delay, hair loss
Wiskott-Aldrich syndrome	T cell immunodeficiency with severe AD, thrombocytopenia, and recurrent infections
Severe combined immunodeficiency	Combined (B and T cell) immunodeficiency with severe AD, diarrhea, failure to thrive, and life-threatening infections
Netherton syndrome	Disorder characterized by ichthyosis in the first 10 days of life, hair shaft abnormalities leading to easy breakage

AD, Atopic dermatitis.

BOX 39.2 Conditions for Referral to a Pediatric Dermatologist

Consider referral in children who:
- Are refractory to topical therapy
- Experience frequent flares
- Experience recurrent infections
- Require hospitalization for atopic dermatitis treatment
- Have associated symptoms that suggest systemic disease

subcutaneous injection. Studies have shown good safety and efficacy profiles in children, with few reported adverse effects.

Immunosuppressants, including cyclosporine and methotrexate, also can be used to treat severe AD and are generally safe in children but require close monitoring for potential side effects.

Additional Pharmacologic Therapies

Sedating antihistamines, such as diphenhydramine and hydroxyzine, can be helpful in improving nighttime pruritus and sleep in children with acute flares. Nonsedating antihistamines have questionable efficacy for AD-related pruritus and are no longer routinely recommended.

Nonpharmacologic Interventions

Patients with AD and their families should be encouraged to avoid known triggers for their AD flares, such as personal hygiene products with fragrance and certain fabrics, such as wool.

Patients and their families should limit bathing to 5 to 10 minutes and avoid very hot water, which can be drying to the skin. After bathing, the skin should be patted dry rather than rubbed. Emollient should be applied at least twice daily, if not more. Keeping fingernails clipped short can help reduce damage to the skin.

Treatment of Complications

Treatment of *S. aureus* superinfection usually involves oral antibiotic therapy with consideration of antibiotics active against methicillin-resistant *S. aureus* (MRSA) as first-line therapy based on local resistance patterns. Small areas may respond to topical mupirocin alone. Hospitalization should be considered in young infants, those with severe disease, and children with signs of systemic illness.

Children with eczema herpeticum should be treated with acyclovir. Hospitalization and intravenous administration of acyclovir may be necessary in severe or disseminated cases.

Treatment of *Staphylococcus aureus* Skin Colonization

Because patients with AD have a high prevalence of *S. aureus* skin colonization compared with the general population, it has been suggested that *S. aureus* eradication may improve AD disease severity independent of secondary infections; however, the evidence for dilute bleach baths (one-half of a cup of bleach in a bathtub filled with water) and intranasal administration of mupirocin ointment is conflicting.

FUTURE DIRECTIONS

Understanding of AD is improving rapidly, with focus shifting toward the altered immune response observed in patients with AD. Targeted systemic therapies such as dupilumab have drastically improved clinical outcomes and quality of life in children with moderate to severe disease, inspiring further investigation into the use of systemic immunomodulators for the management of atopic disease.

SUGGESTED READINGS

Available online.

40

Vascular Disorders

Christopher Teng

 CLINICAL VIGNETTE

A well-appearing 1-month-old male infant presents with a 2-cm bright red, thin vascular plaque with distinct borders over the right scapula without ulceration or bleeding. Parents noted a faint pink marking in that area at birth, but the lesion has become increasingly obvious. A diagnosis of infantile hemangioma is made, and reassurance is given based on the location and lack of complications. It grows until the 3-month visit, after which it stabilizes. In the following months, the plaque thins and becomes fainter. At 5 years, the lesion has flattened and is barely visible.

Infantile hemangiomas (IHs) are common in infants and may be distressing to parents because they are generally subtle at birth and undergo more exuberant growth in the first months of life. For uncomplicated IHs, clinical observation is generally sufficient and most lesions involute completely by early childhood; however, if there is concern for syndromic or visceral involvement or cosmetic and clinical complications, referral to a dermatology specialist before 2 months of age is recommended.

VASCULAR TUMORS

Vascular tumors are grouped by clinical behavior: benign, locally aggressive/borderline, and malignant. Vascular malignancies are extremely rare in children.

Infantile Hemangiomas
Epidemiology and Pathogenesis
Infantile hemangiomas (IHs) are the most common infantile tumors, affecting up to 3% to 10% of infants. These benign proliferations of endothelial cells are thought to develop secondary to tissue hypoxia. Risk factors include prematurity, multiple gestations, assisted reproduction, chorionic villus sampling, increased maternal age, and preeclampsia. Although most hemangiomas are sporadic, both autosomal dominant inheritance and syndromic associations are reported.

Clinical Manifestations
Superficial hemangiomas are bright red protuberant vascular papules/plaques with well-defined borders and often "cobblestoned" texture. Deep lesions may present as vascular swelling with ill-defined margins and normal to blue overlying skin. Most lesions have both superficial and deep components (Fig. 40.1). IHs also may be classified as focal, multifocal, segmental, and indeterminate. IHs are most commonly cervicofacial, but they may be found anywhere on the body.

Although subtle skin changes may be present at birth, most IHs are noted within the first few weeks of life when they begin a period of rapid growth until 2 to 3 months of age, with growth usually complete by 5 months. Regression generally begins at 1 year of age, at which time they flatten, shrink, and fade, with 90% of involution completed

by 4 years of age. Although vascular elements may completely regress, IHs may resolve with residual skin changes, including fibrofatty tissue, scarring, atrophy, telangiectasias, or permanent discoloration.

Management
Most IHs require no therapy. However, rapidly proliferating IHs may bleed or ulcerate, most commonly when perineal, perioral, or intertriginous. Ulcerations are painful and at risk for superinfection. Additionally, IHs may have unique complications. Nasal tip IHs may cause significant bulbous disfigurement. Eyelid IHs may disrupt visual development, requiring early referral to an ophthalmology specialist. IHs along the jawline and neck ("beard distribution") (see Fig. 40.1) have a risk for airway lesions that may cause life-threatening airway obstruction. Spinal dysraphism is associated with midline lumbosacral lesions when greater than 2.5 cm, and magnetic resonance imaging (MRI) is indicated. Currently, abdominal ultrasound in infants with multiple (≥5) IHs is recommended, although the utility of screening in asymptomatic patients is debated. Large visceral hemangiomas may cause high-output heart failure or hypothyroidism as a result of high expression of thyroxine-inactivating enzyme.

Therapy is warranted for significant complications or for lesions with significant cosmetic implications. β-Blockade with oral propranolol or topical timolol is the current standard of medical care. Side effects of propranolol may include hypoglycemia, hypotension, and worsening of underlying cardiac dysfunction, bradyarrhythmia, or reactive airways. Initiation is increasingly done in an outpatient clinical setting, though for infants younger than 5 weeks corrected gestational age or those with medical comorbidities, inpatient initiation may be considered. Should propranolol be contraindicated or ineffective, corticosteroids, pulse-dye laser, and, rarely, surgery may be indicated.

Clinical Associations
Large segmental IHs on the face or lower body warrant referral to a dermatology specialist. Large, segmental IHs on the face, scalp, or neck may be associated with PHACE syndrome (Fig. 40.2) (*P*osterior fossa anomalies, *H*emangiomas, cerebrovascular *A*rterial anomalies, *C*ardiovascular anomalies [particularly coarctation], and *E*ye anomalies). In contrast, LUMBAR syndrome (*L*ower body hemangioma, *U*rogenital anomalies/*U*lceration, *M*yelopathy, *B*ony deformities, *A*norectal malformations, *A*rterial anomalies, and *R*enal anomalies) is associated with lumbosacral or anogenital segmental IHs.

Congenital Hemangiomas
Congenital hemangiomas (CHs) manifest as bright vascular plaques or nodules. However, in contrast with IHs, CHs are fully formed at birth and may be distinguished by histopathologic staining. Noninvoluting CHs (NICHs) do not involute and grow in proportion to the child's

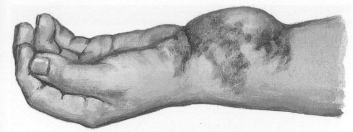

Hemangioma in wrist of young child

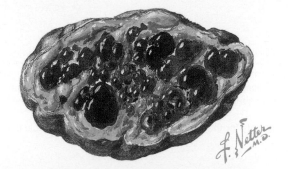

Sectioned hemangioma

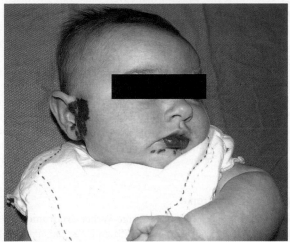

Hemangioma in a beard distribution. *Reprinted with permission for Zaoutis LB, Chiang VW. Comprehensive Pediatric Hospital Medicine. Figure 153-3. Mosby, Elsevier. 2007.*

Fig. 40.1 Infantile Hemangioma.

growth. Rapidly involuting CHs (RICHs) have accelerated regression and may even show signs of involution at birth or within the first year of life. Partially involuting CHs (PICHs) are similar to RICHs but without complete regression.

Tufted Angioma and Kaposiform Hemangioendothelioma

Tufted angiomas (TAs) and Kaposiform hemangioendotheliomas (KHEs) are uncommon, histologically similar tumors thought to represent a spectrum of one underlying entity. Both may exhibit hypertrichosis or hyperhidrosis, which may provide a diagnostic clue. Located most commonly on the thorax, TAs (Fig. 40.3) are slow-growing red to blue subcutaneous nodules and plaques. In contrast, KHEs are locally aggressive vascular tumors that may invade local soft tissue and bone. KHEs may be present at birth and commonly affect children younger than 2 years of age. KHEs may initially mimic infantile hemangiomas, but the lesions become violaceous and sometimes

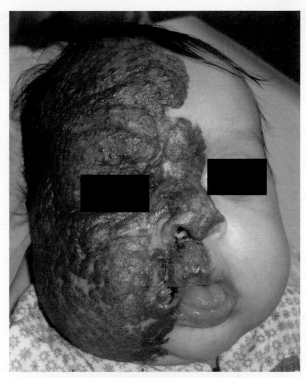

Large segmental facial hemangioma of PHACES syndrome.
Fig. 40.2 PHACES Syndrome.

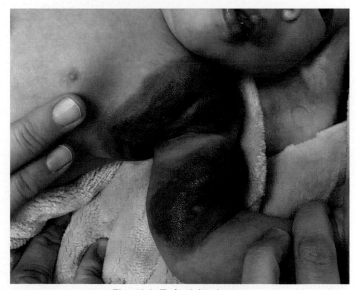

Fig. 40.3 Tufted Angioma.

nodular. Lesions primarily occur on extremities and the trunk, but they may be retroperitoneal.

Although KHEs are benign, diagnosis and appropriate management are critical because of the risk for Kasabach-Merritt phenomenon (KMP), a consumptive coagulopathy with thrombocytopenia and microangiopathic hemolytic anemia that complicates approximately 70% of KHE and 10% to 38% of TA. In KHE, KMP is associated with younger age, retroperitoneal location, and larger lesions. Infants with KMP present with acute, often painful lesion enlargement and bleeding complications, and the mortality rate is as high as 30%. Platelet transfusions should be avoided if possible to avoid exacerbating the underlying pathologic condition, and heparin is contraindicated.

TABLE 40.1   Classification of Vascular Anomalies

| Vascular Tumors | VASCULAR MALFORMATIONS | | | |
	Simple	Combined	Of Major Named Vessels	Associated With Other Anomalies
Benign	CM	CM + VM	Also called "channel type" or "truncal" malformations	Examples
• IH	• NS	CM + LM		• Sturge-Weber syndrome
• CH	• PWS	LM + VM		• Klippel-Trenaunay syndrome
• Pyogenic granuloma	• Telangiectasia	CM + VM + LM		• CLOVES
• TA	VM	CM + AVM		• Proteus syndrome
Locally aggressive or borderline	LM	CM + LM + AVM		
• KHE	• Lymphedema	Others		
Malignant	AVM			
• Angiosarcoma	AV fistula			

AV, Arteriovenous; AVM, Arteriovenous malformation; CH, congenital hemangioma; CLOVES, Congenital Lipomatous Overgrowth, Vascular malformations, Epidermal nevi, Scoliosis/skeletal and spinal; CM, capillary malformation; GVM, glomuvenous malformation; IH, infantile hemangioma; KHE, kaposiform hemangioendothelioma; LM, lymphatic malformation; NS, nevus simplex; PWS, port-wine stain; TA, tufted angioma; VM, venous malformation.
Adapted from ISSVA Classification of Vascular Anomalies ©2018 International Society for the Study of Vascular Anomalies Available at issva.org/classification. Accessed Sept 2020.

For lesions without KMP or symptoms, clinical observation may be an option, but high-risk and symptomatic lesions require treatment, including surgical excision with or without embolization and/or medical management. Previously steroids, vincristine, and antiplatelet agents were used; however, there is growing evidence for sirolimus as the preferred therapy.

Pyogenic Granuloma

Pyogenic granulomas are benign, acquired vascular tumors that manifest as red papules with initially rapid growth. Usually solitary, pyogenic granulomas can occur anywhere on the skin and mucous membranes. Lesions frequently bleed with even slight trauma, and thus treatment is usually required. Shave excision with cauterization at the base is often adequate for resolution of these lesions, though surgical excision is sometimes needed.

VASCULAR MALFORMATIONS

Vascular malformations are grouped into four categories: simple, combined, malformations of major vessels, and malformations associated with other anomalies (Table 40.1). Simple malformations are composed of one type of vessel—capillary, lymphatic, or vein—and also include arteriovenous malformations (AVMs) and fistulae. Combined lesions have more than one type of vascular malformation.

Capillary Malformations
Nevus Simplex

Nevus simplex (NS) is also known as "angel's kiss," "salmon patch," or "stork's bite." NS is benign and found in up to 82% of newborns, typically presenting as pink to red macules or patches with indistinct borders located on the eyelids, glabella, or nape of the neck. Other midline locations include the philtrum, scalp, upper back, and lumbosacral area. Lesions are more noticeable with activity and crying. Lumbosacral NS is not an automatic indication for spinal dysraphism screening unless other cutaneous abnormalities are also present. NS often fades over time, though it may still be evident with crying or straining.

Nevus Flammeus

Nevus flammeus, or port-wine stain (PWS), is the second most common capillary malformation of infancy. It is apparent at birth as a solid flat vascular "stain" that may be pink, red, or purple. PWSs vary in size, from small stains to large segmental lesions. PWS may appear to change color with the Valsalva maneuver, caused by increased flow. Whereas extremity and trunk PWSs are generally stable, facial PWSs may progress in color and induce tissue hypertrophy. The decision to treat is based on the cosmetic impact of the lesion, with the goal to achieve lightening and prevent future hypertrophy or vascular nodules. Vascular-specific laser therapy is the therapy of choice, with earlier initiation of therapy associated with better outcomes.

Although PWS is generally sporadic, familial and syndromic associations are well reported. Sporadic PWS may be associated with other congenital anomalies, including hypoplasia and limb length discrepancy. Underlying spinal dysraphism has been reported with midline lumbosacral lesions, especially with secondary lesions (e.g., dimple, nodule, tuft of hair).

Sturge-Weber Syndrome

PWS is notably associated with Sturge-Weber syndrome (SWS), a neurocutaneous disorder of facial PWSs and vascular malformation of the leptomeninges and eye caused by somatic mutations in GNAQ. Children with facial PWSs involving the forehead, especially if midline or with bilateral/extensive involvement, are at highest risk for SWS and should be referred to neurology and ophthalmology specialists. Children with SWS may have significant neurologic complications, including seizures, progressive hemiplegia, transient focal neurologic defects, and developmental delay. Glaucoma is the most common manifestation in the eye. Cornerstones of SWS treatment include anticonvulsants, glaucoma management, and laser therapy for PWS.

Telangiectasia

Telangiectasias are permanent, blanching dilatations of capillary vessels of the skin with a punctate, red, spidery appearance. They may be primary disorders of vessel development or secondary to sun damage, aging, or systemic disease. Multiple telangiectasias with positive family history may suggest hereditary benign telangiectasia or hereditary hemorrhagic telangiectasia. Other systemic syndromes associated with telangiectasias include ataxia telangiectasia and connective tissue disease.

Venous Malformations

Venous malformations (VMs) most commonly affect cutaneous and mucosal structures but can involve internal structures as well. VMs are often compressible isolated bluish lesions that may enlarge with Valsalva, straining, dependent position, or exercise. Although most VMs are present at birth, they often become more prominent with age, trauma, or pregnancy. A small portion of VMs contain glomus cells and may be more raised and tender, termed glomuvenous malformations. Although VMs are common sporadic lesions, rare familial and syndromic associations are found.

Thrombosis may result from abnormally slow blood flow, and phleboliths may be palpable. Large lesions may be complicated by localized intravascular coagulopathy. Symptoms are secondary to painful thrombi, bleeding, or compression of nearby structures. Significant bony abnormalities may result from deeper involvement.

Ultrasound with Doppler is often first line for diagnosis and anatomic characterization, though MRI is the gold standard. Supportive treatment includes compression garments to reduce thrombosis and anti-inflammatory medications for phlebitis/thrombosis. Coagulopathic lesions may be treated with low-molecular-weight heparin. Sclerotherapy is generally the first choice for definitive treatment or as an adjuvant therapy to surgical excision. Small lesions may be amenable to complete surgical excision, whereas partial excisions may still be indicated for VMs in higher-risk locations. Recently, mammalian target of rapamycin (mTOR) inhibitors have been studied for VMs recalcitrant to other therapies. Other alternatives include cryoablation and laser photocoagulation.

Lymphatic Malformations

Lymphatic malformations (LMs) are aberrantly connected collections of lymphatic channels and/or lymphatic cysts. Localized LMs are characterized as deep "macrocystic," superficial "microcystic," or mixed lesions. Most manifest by 2 years of age as compressible masses with or without overlying cutaneous change. LMs may be bluish because of large cysts or dark red as a result of intralesional bleeding. Continual expansion may be caused by progressive dilatation of the abnormal channels. Depending on location and extent, complications may include extremity overgrowth, airway obstruction, speech impairment, vision impairment, or consumptive sequelae associated with hypoproteinemia, thrombocytopenia, and localized intravascular coagulopathy. Lymphocytic sequestration may lead to lymphopenia. Leakage of lymph fluid may result in chylous effusions or ascites. Ultrasound and MRI are important in the diagnosis and workup of LM. Asymptomatic lesions without aesthetic implications may be observed conservatively. For LM with symptoms or complications, sclerotherapy, laser, or surgical resection may be considered. Radiofrequency ablation and pharmacologic interventions, including sirolimus, are emerging therapies.

Lymphatic malformations resulting in hypoplasia, aplasia, or disruption of lymphatic channels result in *lymphedema*. Primary lymphedema is classified by age of onset: congenital, peripubertal, and late-onset. Management is primarily targeted at compression therapy and infection prevention. The lesions are generally nonprogressive, and resection is reserved for patients with continued significant morbidity.

LMs and lymphedema are associated with a number of genetic syndromes, including Turner, Noonan, and Down syndromes. Prenatally diagnosed cervical macrocystic LMs are associated with unfavorable fetal outcomes, including chromosomal abnormalities in approximately 50% of cases.

Arteriovenous Malformations

AVMs are uncommon vascular malformations that involve a large number of small connections between arterial and venous channels without a capillary bed. Most are present at birth and like other vascular tumors/malformations may feel warm; however, AVMs are uniquely associated with pulsation, a bruit, or a thrill. AVMs may remain quiescent or enter a period of growth. They may be complicated by local tissue hypertrophy or pulsatile, brisk bleeding that is difficult to control, and are rarely associated with congestive heart failure from shunting. Imaging with Doppler ultrasonography, computed tomography, or MRI confirms diagnosis. Treatment with embolization and resection when feasible is most successful when done early.

Capillary Malformation–Arteriovenous Malformation Syndrome

Capillary malformation–arteriovenous malformation syndrome (CM-AVM) is a relatively recently identified autosomal dominant condition resulting from mutations in *RASA1* and *EPHB4*. Patients present with increasing numbers of atypical cutaneous CMs, often geographic red-brown macules, and patches with blanching halo. Importantly, many patients have concurrent AVMs or arteriovenous fistulae, which may occur in the brain or spine. Therefore early diagnosis and further imaging are critical.

Genetic Causes of Vascular Anomalies

In recent years there has been an increasing number of mutations found to be causal in various vascular anomalies. One of the most notable is the *PIK3CA*-related overgrowth spectrum characterized by asymmetric growth and various vascular, visceral, and neurologic anomalies. Examples include CLOVES (Congenital Lipomatous Overgrowth, Vascular malformations, Epidermal nevi, Scoliosis/skeletal and spinal), megalencephaly-capillary malformation (M-CM), and Klippel-Trenaunay syndrome. As genetic underpinnings are better understood, more targeted therapies are becoming available in the treatment of these often-challenging disorders.

SUGGESTED READINGS

Available online.

41

Hyperpigmented Skin Disorders

Raegan D. Hunt and Bernard J. Danna

 CLINICAL VIGNETTE

A 6-year-old uninsured girl is evaluated in clinic for early menses. Her medical history is notable for three prior fractures, including the right humerus at age 4 years, and the left tibia at ages 3 and 5 years.

On examination, she appears older than stated age and is tachycardic. Skin examination shows a large, geographic light-brown patch with jagged, well-demarcated borders on her right chest, neck and back that does not cross the midline torso. Her mother reports that this lesion was present at birth and has grown in proportion to her growth but is otherwise unchanged. Increased lateral spine curvature is noted on examination of the back. Bloodwork shows elevated estrogen; low luteinizing hormone, follicle-stimulating hormone, and thyroid-stimulating hormone; and elevated free thyroxine. A radiograph of the left arm and wrist shows advanced bone age and fibrous dysplasia.

Precocious puberty has a broad differential diagnosis. Although most cases of precocious puberty in girls are idiopathic, a detailed history and physical examination can help identify underlying conditions. In this case, McCune-Albright syndrome is suspected based on a history of multiple fractures and examination findings, including scoliosis, fibrous dysplasia, and a large café-au-lait patch with jagged borders.

Hyperpigmented skin lesions develop for a variety of reasons. Careful assessment of the color, number, shape, demarcation, persistence, and distribution of these lesions offers important diagnostic clues. Skin hyperpigmentation may represent simple cutaneous birthmarks or transient conditions, but it also may be an early physical sign of neurocutaneous disorders, genetic disorders, metabolic conditions, and endocrinopathies. This chapter will review the characteristic clinical features of benign and concerning hyperpigmented skin lesions, associated diagnoses that should be considered, and management of hyperpigmented skin disorders.

ETIOLOGY AND PATHOGENESIS

Hyperpigmented skin disorders result from conditions of increased melanin production. Melanin (eumelanin and pheomelanin) are red-brown pigments produced by melanocytes and transferred to surrounding keratinocytes in the skin. This chapter describes conditions with increased melanin pigment production but not conditions of melanocytic cellular proliferation (e.g., melanocytic nevi). Melanocytic nevi and other disorders of melanocyte overgrowth are discussed separately in Chapter 38.

CIRCUMSCRIBED HYPERPIGMENTED SKIN LESIONS

Ephelides (Freckles)

Ephelides are tiny (<4 mm) tan to medium-brown macules that develop on sun-exposed skin in children. These common, benign acquired lesions develop with ultraviolet (UV) light exposure and fade in the winter months. They are most often seen on the cheeks, nose, and dorsal forearms of individuals with fair skin or red hair. Although benign, freckles occur more often in children with genetically light skin (*MC1R* mutation) and correlate with an increased risk for melanoma; thus parents of children with ephelides should be counseled on sun exposure precautions.

Lentigines

Lentigines are small brown macules that do not fade in the absence of UV light. In contrast to ephelides, lentigines tend to be larger (4 to 10 mm) and darker shades of brown. Lentigines are not restricted to sun-exposed skin and may develop on mucosa.

Although a few lentigines are not worrisome in a child, many lentigines should raise concern for genetic syndromes. Syndromes with multiple lentigines as a recognizable feature include Noonan syndrome with multiple lentigines (NSML), formerly referred to as LEOPARD syndrome (*L*entigines, *E*lectrocardiographic conduction abnormalities, *O*cular hypertelorism, *P*ulmonic stenosis, *A*bnormal genitalia, *R*etardation of growth, and *D*eafness), Peutz-Jeghers syndrome, and Carney complex (Fig. 41.1 and Table 41.1). Lentigines in young children may also indicate xeroderma pigmentosum, a DNA repair disorder that results in extreme UV sensitivity and premature skin cancers. Irregular "ink-spot" lentigines are often seen in type 2 oculocutaneous albinism.

Congenital Dermal Melanocytosis

Congenital dermal melanocytosis (CDM), historically referred to as a "Mongolian spot," is characterized by fairly well-circumscribed gray to blue-green patches, most often over the buttocks or lumbosacral back. The prevalence of CDM varies by ethnicity, occurring in up to 95% of black infants, 85% of Asian infants, 65% of Latino infants, and 10% of white infants. Lesions on the buttocks and lower back generally fade by 5 years of age, but patches of CDM in other anatomic areas may persist longer and sometimes indefinitely. Although CDM is a very common benign skin finding in infants, extensive CDM has been associated with Hurler syndrome, GM1 gangliosidosis, and Hunter syndrome.

Café-au-Lait Spots

Café-au-lait spots (CALS) are very common hyperpigmented lesions. Approximately 25% of school-aged children have one or two CALS. CALS may be noted at birth or develop during childhood. CALS are well demarcated, smooth, and homogeneously tan to light brown macules and patches. They range in size from 2 mm to more than 20 cm in diameter.

As with lentigines, CALS are benign but may be a sign of an underlying condition. The two most common disorders for which CALS offer a major diagnostic clue are neurofibromatosis type 1 (NF1) and McCune-Albright syndrome.

The CALS seen in NF1 are multiple and typically ovoid, with a smooth border which is often compared to the outline of the "coast of California" (Fig. 41.2). To meet one cutaneous diagnostic criterion for NF1, children must have more than five total CALS, each measuring greater than 5 mm prepubertally or greater than 15 mm postpubertally. In NF1, the CALS criterion is frequently met by age 2 years. Other hyperpigmented lesions seen frequently in NF1 include axillary or inguinal freckling (Crowe sign), which typically manifests by age 6 years, and plexiform neurofibromas. Plexiform neurofibromas manifest as large tan or light-brown patches that have an underlying "bag of worms" consistency on palpation; although they are generally present from birth, they may not be recognized until later in childhood. Cutaneous findings of NF1 are reviewed in Table 41.2, and NF1 diagnostic criteria are reviewed in Chapter 111). Legius syndrome, which is due to autosomal dominant mutations in *SPRED-1*, is also characterized by more than five CALS along with axillary and inguinal freckling. However, patients with Legius syndrome lack the other NF1 diagnostic criteria.

In contrast to NF1 and Legius syndrome, the CALS of McCune-Albright syndrome tend to be unilateral and large, often stopping abruptly at the midline (e.g., segmental in appearance). In McCune-Albright syndrome, CALS have a jagged border, likened to the "coast of Maine" (see Fig. 41.2). McCune-Albright syndrome has additional findings of precocious puberty, endocrine abnormalities, and polyostotic fibrous dysplasia, although many children with large segmental unilateral CALS have no associated syndrome.

Becker Nevus

A Becker nevus (also known as Becker melanosis) is an irregular large tan to light-brown patch that tends to break apart into irregular macules at the edges (Fig. 41.3). These lesions typically affect one side of the trunk, most often on the upper chest, and are more common in males. Frequently, overlying hypertrichosis and increased acne are present within the lesion. Because they generally appear around puberty, it is hypothesized that androgens may be involved in the pathophysiologic process of this benign hyperpigmented lesion. Rarely, a Becker nevus on the chest in girls may be associated with ipsilateral breast hypoplasia.

Postinflammatory Hyperpigmentation

Postinflammatory hyperpigmentation is a very common skin finding in children and adolescents. Local skin inflammation, often from atopic dermatitis or acne, stimulates melanin production, resulting in areas of hyperpigmentation in a distribution and pattern consistent with the prior skin eruption (Fig. 41.4). Individuals with darker complexions are most severely affected. These lesions tend to become more pigmented in the presence of UV light. Thus, management includes

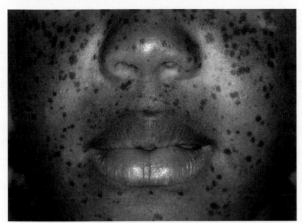

Noonan syndrome with multiple lentigines This patient has multiple lentigines with relative sparing of mucous membranes. (*Reprinted with permission from Cohen BA. Pediatri Dermatology. Mosby, Elsevier. Philadelphia, 2005.*)

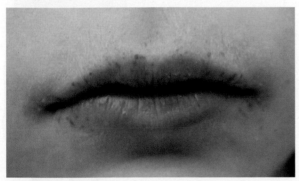

Peutz-Jeghers syndrome Note patient's characteristic mucocutaneous lentigines.

Fig. 41.1 Lentigines.

TABLE 41.1	**Major Lentiginous Syndromes**	
	Distribution of Lentigines	**Associated Features**
Noonan syndrome with multiple lentigines (NSML), formerly known as LEOPARD syndrome	Neck and upper trunk (less often face, arms, palms, soles, and genitalia)	• Lentigines • Electrocardiographic conduction abnormalities • Ocular hypertelorism • Pulmonic stenosis • Abnormal genitalia • Retardation of growth • Deafness (sensorineural)
Peutz-Jeghers syndrome	Mucocutaneous (lips and buccal mucosa; rarely, gums, palate, and tongue); elbows, fingertips, palms, soles, and nasal, periorbital, periumbilical, perianal, and labial regions	• Mucocutaneous lentigines • Gastrointestinal polyps • Increased risk for early-onset adenocarcinomas of the gastrointestinal tract, pancreas, breast, thyroid, and reproductive organs
Carney complex	Face, vermillion border of lips, conjunctiva, vaginal or penile mucosa	• Hyperpigmented cutaneous lesions (lentigines, CALS, and blue nevi) • Myxomas of heart, skin, and breast • Endocrine hyperactivity consistent with multiple endocrine neoplasia syndrome

CALS, Café-au-lait spots.

treatment of any ongoing skin eruption alongside careful sunscreen use and sun avoidance to limit further hyperpigmentation. In the absence of ongoing skin inflammation, the hyperpigmentation will gradually fade over many months to years.

Acanthosis Nigricans

Acanthosis nigricans manifests with velvety thin hyperpigmented plaques, most often found on the posterior and lateral neck, and sometimes involving the axillae, knuckles, elbows, knees, or perioral skin (Fig. 41.5). Acanthosis nigricans is strongly associated with the metabolic syndrome and should raise concern for insulin resistance and type 2 diabetes mellitus.

Mastocytosis

Cutaneous mastocytosis (CM) encompasses a spectrum of conditions resulting from localized mast cell collections within the skin, which are recognizable by overlying tan macules or patches. There are three major subtypes of pediatric CM: solitary mastocytoma(s), maculo-papular CM (formerly termed urticaria pigmentosa), and diffuse CM. Suspected cutaneous mast cell disease can often be confirmed clinically if localized edema, erythema, or blistering develops after the hyperpigmented macule or patch has been stroked firmly several times with the flat edge of a tongue depressor (Darier sign; see Fig. 41.6).

The term mastocytoma(s) is used when cutaneous mast cell infiltration manifests as 1 to 3 solitary large (~1 to 3 cm) tan patches (see Fig. 41.6). Maculopapular CM is characterized by hundreds of widespread small tan macules, often predominantly distributed on the trunk (see Fig. 41.6). Diffuse CM is rare, and the mast cell–infiltrated skin appears slightly yellow and thickened and may have "peau d'orange" texture changes.

Although uncommon, systemic symptoms associated with CM may include skin flushing, itch, wheezing, watery diarrhea, and bone

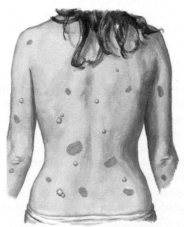

Multiple café-au-lait spots and cutaneous neurofibromas are common manifestations of neurofibromatosis type 1 (NF1).

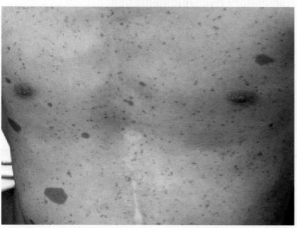

Multiple café-au-lait spots with coast of California contour on the trunk of a teen with NF1.

Café-au-lait spots with coast of Maine contour; sexual precocity in female (McCune-Albright syndrome).

Fig. 41.2 Café-au-Lait Spots.

TABLE 41.2	**Cutaneous Findings in Neurofibromatosis Type 1**	
	Age of Onset	**Clinical Findings**
Café-au-lait spots	Present at birth to early childhood	Prepubertal children must have >5 CALS, each measuring >5 mm; postpubertal children need >5 CALS, each measuring >15 mm
Intertriginous freckling (Crowe sign)	3–5 years old	Small tan macules in the skinfolds of the axilla and inguinal area
Neurofibromas	After puberty	Fleshy subcutaneous skin-toned to pink nodules
Plexiform neurofibromas	Present at birth or shortly thereafter	Soft tissue swelling often underlying a large, irregular tan to light brown patch with overlying hypertrichosis; can grow rapidly; palpation likened to a "bag of worms"

CALS, Café-au-lait spots.

pain. For patients with diffuse CM or extensive maculopapular CM, an abdominal and lymphatic physical examination is recommended, and laboratory screening of complete blood cell count, hepatic function panel, and tryptase levels may be considered. In children with CM, the presence of hepatosplenomegaly is more predictive of systemic mast cell disease than elevated tryptase levels. For those with systemic symptoms or laboratory abnormalities, an evaluation to rule out systemic mastocytosis and mast cell leukemia should be considered, which may include bone marrow biopsy and genetic testing for mutations in the KIT receptor tyrosine kinase.

Management of children with CM involves avoiding potential mast cell degranulation triggers, which include friction, pressure, abrupt temperature changes, and certain medications (aspirin, nonsteroidal anti-inflammatory drugs, opiates, amphotericin B, topical polymyxin B, alcohol, and iodine contrast media). Interestingly, in a small study,

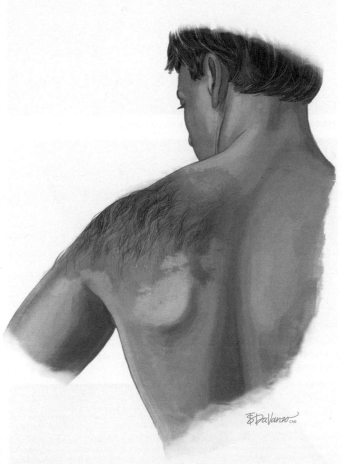

Fig. 41.3 Becker Nevus.

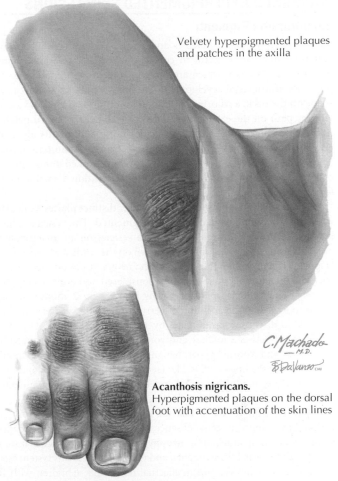

Velvety hyperpigmented plaques and patches in the axilla

Acanthosis nigricans.
Hyperpigmented plaques on the dorsal foot with accentuation of the skin lines

Fig. 41.5 Acanthosis Nigricans.

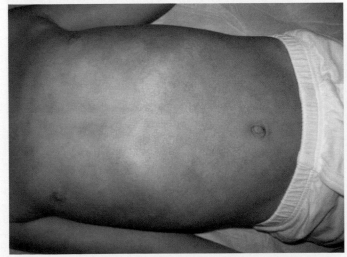

Poorly defined hyperpigmented patches illustrating post-inflammatory changes in a patient with eczema.

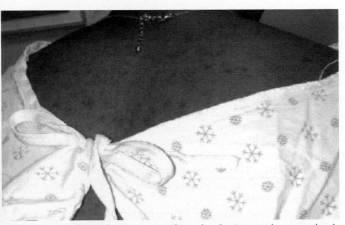

Hyperpigmented macules in an acneiform distribution on the upper back.

Fig. 41.4 Postinflammatory Hyperpigmentation.

all 37 patients with maculopapular CM reported no adverse reaction to past ingestion of ibuprofen. When present, symptoms can generally be controlled with nonsedating type-1 antihistamines such as loratadine or cetirizine, and only rarely is an epinephrine pen indicated in an individual with a history of severe reactions. In addition, topical corticosteroids may offer relief of itch, swelling, or blistering among children with irritated solitary cutaneous mastocytomas.

PATTERNED HYPERPIGMENTED SKIN LESIONS

Incontinentia Pigmenti

When hyperpigmented macules and patches follow curvilinear and patterned lines, it is useful to consider whether the lesions follow the lines of Blaschko, which are thought to represent epidermal cell migration during fetal development. The lines of Blaschko follow a "V" shape on the back, a whorled pattern on the anterior trunk, and a curvilinear path on the extremities (Fig. 36.7). Hyperpigmented patches in this distribution may suggest a diagnosis of incontinentia pigmenti (IP; Bloch-Sulzberger syndrome). IP results from mutations in nuclear factor-κB essential modulator (NEMO). As an X-linked dominant disorder, IP primarily affects girls because the condition is fatal in utero for most males.

The cutaneous component of IP has four distinct phases: vesicular, verrucous, hyperpigmented, and hypopigmented. The vesicular phase is noted in the first 2 weeks of life, with vesicles on an inflammatory base following a whorled or linear pattern on the trunk and extremities (Fig. 41.7). As with any blistering in the neonatal period, herpetic or bacterial infections should always be considered and evaluated appropriately. The vesicular phase typically resolves by 2 months of age and is followed by the eruption of verrucous papules and plaques in a Blaschkoid distribution that fades by 4 to 6 months of age. The third stage, noted between infancy and young adulthood, is recognized by curvilinear and whorled hyperpigmentation on the trunk and extremities following the lines of Blaschko (see Fig. 41.7). The fourth and final stage develops in adulthood and appears as streaks of hypopigmentation most commonly affecting the extremities.

Children with IP are at risk for multiple noncutaneous complications involving the teeth (absence of teeth, conical or peg-shaped teeth), eyes (strabismus, optic atrophy, and retinal neovascularization with possible retinal detachment), and the central nervous system (seizures, spastic paralysis, and intellectual disability). Children with IP should be referred to a genetics specialist for confirmation of the diagnosis and should be monitored closely by a pediatric ophthalmologist and a dentist. If seizures or other neurologic symptoms develop, these children should be referred promptly to a pediatric neurologist.

DIFFUSE HYPERPIGMENTATION

Generalized hyperpigmentation may indicate an underlying endocrinopathy or may result from an adverse effect of a medication. Common disorders leading to hyperpigmentation are Addison's disease, hyperthyroidism, Cushing's disease, acromegaly, hemochromatosis, and chronic renal and hepatic disease. In the case of Addison's disease, Cushing's syndrome and acromegaly, increased production of adrenocorticotropic hormone (ACTH) and its by-product melanocyte-stimulating hormone increases melanin production from melanocytes. This aberrant hyperpigmentation is seen most notably in sun-exposed areas, skin creases on the palms and soles, and mucous membranes.

Medications may also cause hyperpigmentation. Notable examples include antimalarials, amiodarone (blue man syndrome),

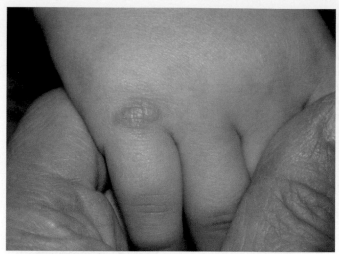

Mastocytoma Tan solitary mastocytoma on dorsum of the hand.

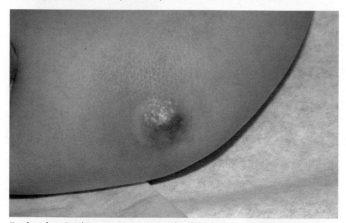

Darier sign Stroking a mastocytoma leads to localized edema and erythema.

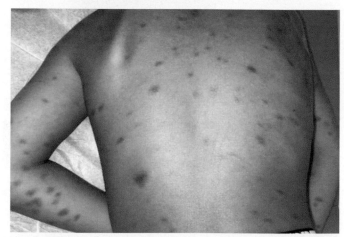

Maculopapular cutaneous mastocytosis Multiple tan macules on the trunk and extremities in child with maculopapular cutaneous mastocytosis.

Fig. 41.6 Mastocytosis.

psychotropic drugs (phenothiazine, imipramine), clofazimine, azidothymidine, chemotherapeutics (5-fluorouracil, bleomycin, cyclophosphamide, daunorubicin, doxorubicin), and heavy metals (gold, bismuth, mercury). The hyperpigmentation associated with medications generally fades over months to years with discontinuation of the medication.

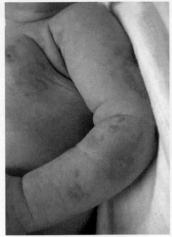

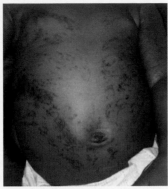

Incontinentia Pigmenti Stage 1
Curvilinear array of vesicles on
an erythematous base.

Incontinentia Pigmenti Stage 3
Hyperpigmentation in whorled
pattern.

Fig. 41.7 Incontinentia Pigmenti.

SUGGESTED READINGS

Available online.

42

Hypopigmented Skin Lesions

Megan Craddock and Jennifer Ruth

✳ CLINICAL VIGNETTE

A 5-year-old girl, accompanied by her mother, presents with complaints of "white spots" to the knee, waistline, and groin. Her mother reports that these began 6 months ago when she fell off her bike and scraped her knee. The area of injury healed but turned white. She has subsequently developed new white spots at the waistline and groin. These have been gradually increasing in size. There has not been any noted pain or pruritus. They deny prior treatment aside from routine use of over-the-counter moisturizers. The patient is bothered by the appearance of her knee and requests to wear pants to school to keep it covered. She is otherwise healthy and meeting developmental milestones. There is no family history of similar skin changes; however, there is a family history of Hashimoto thyroiditis in her maternal grandmother.

Her examination is significant for well-demarcated, depigmented macules and small patches to the waistline, inguinal creases, and right extensor knee.

Therapeutic options are reviewed, and the family and patient elect to treat exposed sites only. Treatment is initiated with a topical corticosteroid, and the importance of sun protection is reviewed. After 3 months, the family and patient are encouraged to note small foci of repigmentation to treated areas.

As in this case, vitiligo classically presents with acquired, asymptomatic, depigmented macules and patches. Friction or trauma may be triggers for disease onset. A family history of autoimmunity is often present, which may be a clue to the diagnosis. Although most pediatric patients are otherwise healthy, it is still advisable to screen those with vitiligo for other autoimmune conditions by performing a thorough review of systems. If therapy is desired, topical corticosteroids are first-line agents for the management of this condition.

Hypopigmentation, a broad term encompassing circumscribed or diffuse lightening of the skin, is the hallmark feature of the cutaneous disorders detailed in this chapter. Disorders of hypopigmentation are common among the general population and can manifest at the time of birth or become acquired over a person's lifetime. Early diagnosis is important, because these skin findings can be associated with an underlying genetic condition with an increased risk for morbidity or cause psychological distress secondary to their cosmetic appearance. This chapter will focus on the recognition and treatment of disorders of hypopigmentation that are most common to the pediatric population.

ETIOLOGY AND PATHOGENESIS

Normal skin depends on healthy melanocytes and melanin production. Melanocytes are neural crest–derived cells found within the skin, eye, inner ear, hair follicles, and leptomeninges. Melanocytes contain special intracytoplasmic organelles called melanosomes in which melanin is produced. These mature melanosomes are then transferred to neighboring keratinocytes. Hypopigmentation may result from either reduced or complete absence of melanin. The underlying cause of melanin deficiency varies widely and may result from errors affecting the melanocyte, melanosome, or melanin itself. This chapter will address disorders of hypopigmentation secondary to an underlying metabolic or genetic cause, followed by disorders associated with loss of preexisting pigmentation.

DISORDERS OF HYPOPIGMENTATION: METABOLIC OR GENETIC CAUSE

Pigmentary Mosaicism

Cutaneous pigmentary mosaicism is secondary to two distinct cell lines that occur from either X-inactivation or postzygotic somatic mutation altering the amount of melanin production within the skin. The cutaneous findings are categorized by linear or segmental patterns, as well as hypopigmentation or hyperpigmentation. The extent of involvement can be limited to a single cutaneous lesion, known as a nevus depigmentosus, or may encompass a larger surface area of the skin. Pigmentary mosaicism can be a cutaneous finding alone, and uncommonly, may be associated with extracutaneous manifestations.

Nevus depigmentosus is a birthmark that occurs in less than 1% of newborns, although it can present as late as 3 years of age. The name is a misnomer, because the affected skin is hypopigmented, not depigmented and may manifest as a solitary patch or in a linear segmental distribution following the lines of Blaschko. These skin findings are most common on the back and buttocks but can occur anywhere on the skin. They grow proportionately with the child and do not require treatment. Differential diagnosis includes hypopigmented macules associated with tuberous sclerosis; three or more hypopigmented macules is a major feature for this neurocutaneous condition.

Belzile et al. (2019) performed a retrospective review of 106 children with pigmentary mosaicism and noted six common patterns (Fig. 42.1). The most common patterns observed were either narrow or broad bands along Blaschko lines (Fig. 42.2). Extracutaneous manifestations such as developmental delay, behavioral disorders, vesicoureteral reflux, and skeletal abnormalities occur in less than one-third of children with pigmentary mosaicism. Because these extracutaneous findings are common among the general pediatric population, it is unclear if pigmentary mosaicism is an independent risk factor. Phylloid hypomelanosis is an uncommon pigmentary pattern characterized by leaf-like and oblong macules and patches (Fig. 42.3). This type of pigmentary mosaicism warrants special mention because it has been associated with abnormalities in chromosome 13. Extracutaneous findings in these children may include conductive hearing loss, skeletal defects, coloboma, and neurologic abnormalities. Most children with pigmentary mosaicism are unlikely to develop serious extracutaneous manifestations when skin findings are limited and they are developing normally for age.

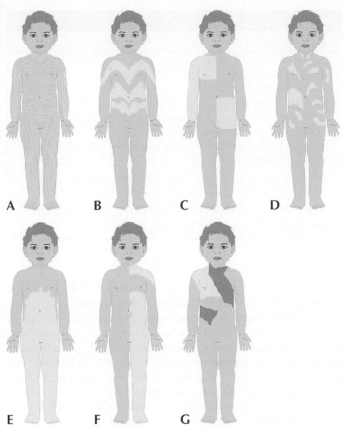

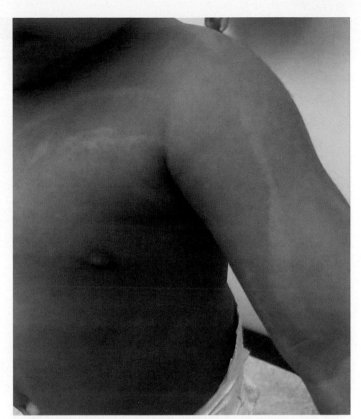

Fig. 42.1 Patterns of Pigmentary Mosaicism. The six archetypal patterns of cutaneous mosaicism. (A) Type 1a, narrow bands along the Blaschko lines. (B) Type 1b, broad bands along the Blaschko lines. (C) Type 2, blocklike pattern (also called checkerboard, flaglike, or segmental pattern). This pattern is characterized by unilateral or bilateral quadrilateral shapes with a sharp midline demarcation. (D) Type 3, phylloid pattern, which is evocative of a floral ornament with oblong, leaflike, or pear-shaped lesions. (E) Type 4, patchy pattern without midline demarcation, with a broad garment-like, bathing trunk or capelike distribution. (F) Type 5, lateralization pattern, with diffuse unilateral involvement and a clear midline separation. (G) Type 6, sashlike pattern, characterized by large oblique patches or round areas reminiscent of a swathed scarf or belt. (Reused with permission from Belzile E, McCuaig C, Le Meur JB, et al. Patterned cutaneous hypopigmentation phenotype characterization: a retrospective study in 106 children. *Pediatr Dermatol.* 2019;36[6]:869-875. https://doi.org/10.1111/pde.13913. Fig. 1.)

Fig. 42.2 Pigmentary Mosaicism. Narrow bands of hypopigmentation along Blaschko lines.

PIEBALDISM

Piebaldism is a rare, autosomal dominant disorder caused by mutations in the *KIT* proto-oncogene. Melanocyte migration from the neural crest is incomplete, with resultant white hair and white patches in midline, ventral locations. Patients present at birth with a white forelock and depigmented macules and patches to the central forehead, mid extremities, and/or midline abdomen. Waardenburg syndrome is the most important entity in the differential diagnosis; however, it can be distinguished by its extracutaneous manifestations. Vitiligo presents with similar appearing depigmented macules and patches, but it is usually not present at birth and is progressive as opposed to stable like piebaldism. If treatment is desired for the white hair and skin, then options include hair dye and cosmetic camouflage or skin-grafting, respectively.

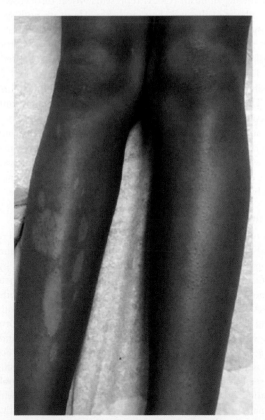

Fig. 42.3 Phylloid Hypomelanosis.

TABLE 42.1   Oculocutaneous Albinism

Type	Percent Affected	Mutation	Description
OCA1 Two forms: A and B	50%	*TYR* (tyrosinase) OCA1A: tyrosinase absent OCA1B: tyrosinase decreased	OCA1A • Most severe form • No melanin production • Severe ocular findings • Highest risk for cutaneous malignancy OCA1B • Variable pigmentation loss; depends on activity of tyrosinase • Most common in Whites
OCA2	30%	*P protein*	Develop more pigment with age, such as lentigines and pigmented nevi Increased risk for cutaneous malignancy, but less than OCA1 Most common in patients of African descent
OCA4	17%	*MATP/SLC45A2*	Most common in Japan, similar to OCA2

Waardenburg Syndrome

Waardenburg syndrome is a rare genetic condition resulting from abnormal neural crest differentiation. There are multiple potential genetic causes, leading to a wide variety of clinical presentations. Four subtypes have been described. Type 1, the most common form, is characterized by well-demarcated white patches of skin and hair, characteristic facial features (e.g., dystopia canthorum), sensorineural deafness, and pigmentary abnormalities of the eyes (e.g., heterochromia irides). Other subtypes are associated with musculoskeletal abnormalities or Hirschsprung disease. Cosmetic camouflage can be used to treat the cutaneous findings.

Albinism

Oculocutaneous albinism (OCA) represents absent or decreased melanin biosynthesis of the eyes, hair, and skin. There are both syndromic and nonsyndromic forms of albinism. The syndromic forms include disorders such as Griscelli syndrome, Chediak-Higashi syndrome, and Hermansky-Pudlak syndrome, which will be discussed later in this chapter. There are seven types of nonsyndromic forms of OCA. These individuals have light skin, hair, and eyes regardless of their ethnic background. The degree of pigmentation and the risk for cutaneous malignancy depend on the specific OCA type. Eye manifestations include photophobia, strabismus, nystagmus, and decreased visual acuity. Table 42.1 describes OCA 1, 2, and 4, which make up greater than 95% of patients who suffer from nonsyndromic OCA. All patients with OCA should be educated on strict sun protection, and multidisciplinary management by an ophthalmologist and dermatologist is advisable.

Syndromic Forms of Albinism

Griscelli syndrome (GS) and Chediak-Higashi are autosomal recessive silver hair syndromes characterized by pigmentary dilution and silver-appearing hair. GS is divided into three types and is caused by mutations affecting melanosomes. GS1 presents with severe neurologic dysfunction without immunodeficiency, GS2 manifests with recurrent infections and hemophagocytosis, and GS3 manifests with silver-appearing hair without neurologic or immunologic abnormalities. Patients with Chediak-Higashi have pigmentary dilution and silver-appearing hair, but may demonstrate hyperpigmentation at acral sites in those with families who have darker skin. Eye abnormalities also may be seen, including photosensitivity, nystagmus, and strabismus. These patients demonstrate recurrent pyogenic infections, with up to 85% of patients developing an accelerated lymphoproliferative phase within the first decade of life. When entering adulthood, these patients

develop neurologic deterioration. Both GS and Chediak-Higashi can be treated with bone marrow transplantation if appropriate.

Hermansky-Pudlak syndrome is an autosomal recessive disorder most prevalent in individuals from Puerto Rico. This condition is divided into nine subtypes. These patients present with pigmentary dilution, bleeding diathesis secondary to platelet dysfunction, and accumulation of ceroid-like material in tissue most commonly leading to a granulomatous colitis and/or pulmonary fibrosis. No curative therapy exists, and thus management is aimed at monitoring for disease complications.

Phenylketonuria

Phenylketonuria (PKU) is secondary to a deficiency in phenylalanine hydroxylase, an enzyme that converts phenylalanine to tyrosinase. As a result of newborn screening, this condition is usually detected early in life and treated with a diet void of phenylalanine. If left untreated, affected children can develop generalized hypopigmentation of the skin, hair, and eyes and progressive neurologic dysfunction.

DISORDERS OF HYPOPIGMENTATION: LOSS OF PREEXISTING PIGMENTATION

Vitiligo

Vitiligo is a common autoimmune condition characterized by depigmentation resulting from immune-mediated destruction of melanocytes. Well-demarcated, depigmented macules or patches often affect the face and extremities, but may affect any area of the skin or hair (Fig. 42.4). A familial genetic tendency toward autoimmune diseases likely predisposes to the development of vitiligo. Other factors such as cutaneous trauma, sunburn, or stress may contribute to disease onset. Clinical subtypes include localized, generalized, universal, and segmental forms. Disease progression is unpredictable in most subtypes. Segmental vitiligo is unique because it manifests as a unilateral depigmented linear patch or block that grows rapidly, but stabilizes quickly and is more resistant to treatment.

Vitiligo is a clinical diagnosis. In patients with light skin, Wood lamp examination can be used to better define the extent of depigmented lesions. Entities in the differential diagnosis include congenital disorders with white patches such as piebaldism or Waardenburg syndrome; however, these entities manifest at birth and are stable. Hypopigmented disorders, such as pityriasis alba or postinflammatory hypopigmentation (PIH), are also in the differential and can be distinguished by poor demarcation, lack of fluorescence on Wood

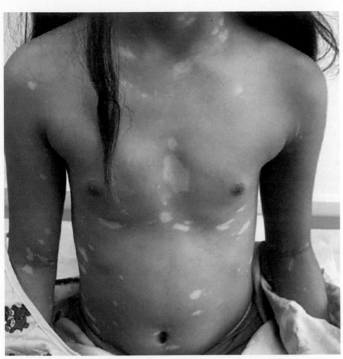

Fig. 42.4 Vitiligo.

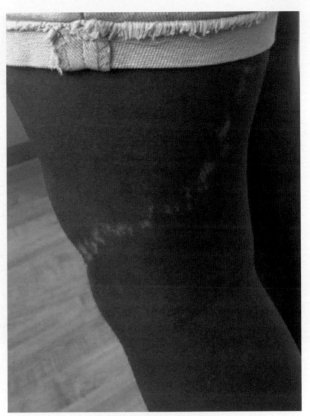

Fig. 42.5 Lichen Striatus.

Lamp examination, and history of atopy or preceding inflammatory dermatosis.

There are many treatments available for vitiligo, but no one curative therapy. Location of involvement, affected body surface area (BSA), and patient preference affect therapeutic selection. First-line therapies in cases of limited involvement (<5% to 10% BSA) are topical corticosteroids applied once or twice daily with steroid holidays or a topical calcineurin inhibitor applied twice daily; the latter is usually favored for delicate sites such as the face or groin. Phototherapy with narrowband ultraviolet B can be helpful for more extensive disease. Screening for other autoimmune conditions, particularly thyroid disease, should be considered given the genetic predisposition to autoimmunity associated with vitiligo.

Pityriasis Alba

Pityriasis alba is a common, low-grade dermatitis. Children classically present with asymptomatic, hypopigmented macules and patches with fine scale to sun-exposed sites, often the cheeks and proximal extremities. A personal or family history of atopy is typically present. Pityriasis alba often presents during the spring and summer months or after sun exposure as the surrounding skin becomes tan, making the color difference between affected and unaffected areas more dramatic. PIH is distinguished by a preceding eruption, and tinea versicolor can be differentiated by a positive KOH test and a distribution that favors seborrheic areas. Treatment for pityriasis alba includes sun protection and moisturization. A low-potency topical corticosteroid can be used for more severe cases.

Postinflammatory Hypopigmentation

PIH refers to a self-limited alteration in pigmentation that follows a preceding inflammatory dermatosis such as eczema, psoriasis, infection, or a burn. Hypopigmented macules or patches appear at sites of prior inflammation. PIH is reversible, and gradual resolution is expected to occur over months to years. Treatment is centered on reassurance, time, and prevention of further irritation and inflammation of the skin. Sun protection should be encouraged to prevent darkening of surrounding skin, which can lead to increased prominence of the hypopigmented areas.

Lichen Striatus

Lichen striatus is an inflammatory dermatosis of unclear cause with a distinct clinical presentation. Pink, flat-topped papules appear in a linear distribution along the lines of Blaschko, typically over a single extremity. These papules often form a single band that appears quickly, over weeks to months. Nail involvement, though infrequent, is possible and manifests as longitudinal onychodystrophy. Over time, the initial papules of lichen striatus flatten and leave behind hypopigmented macules or patches (Fig. 42.5). The eruption is often asymptomatic. The differential diagnosis includes other conditions that manifest in a linear distribution such as inflammatory linear verrucous epidermal nevus (ILVEN). ILVEN is typically more psoriasiform in appearance, persistent, and often symptomatic (pruritic). No treatment is necessary for lichen striatus because self-resolution is expected; however, full clearance of the resultant hypopigmentation can take months to years.

Lichen Sclerosus

Lichen sclerosus (LS) is an inflammatory skin condition that classically affects the anogenital region of prepubertal females or postmenopausal women. Pruritus, pain, and constipation are common presenting complaints. On examination, anogenital involvement is characterized by pink to white, shiny, often atrophic papules or plaques that may involve both the vulvar and perianal skin leading to a figure-of-eight appearance. Purpura and hemorrhagic vesicles may be present. Extragenital involvement is also possible but is typically asymptomatic. The clinical presentation of LS in the genital area can mimic vitiligo, because both may present with loss of pigmentation; however, the symptomatic nature of LS is an important distinguishing feature. Active anogenital LS warrants therapy with high-potency topical corticosteroids to

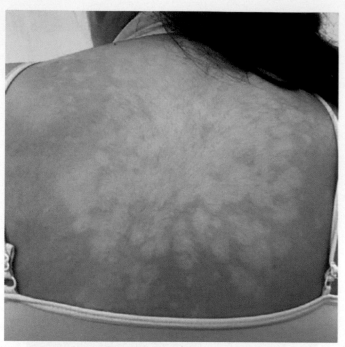

Fig. 42.6 Tinea Versicolor.

prevent distortion of the genital architecture from scarring. Although LS may remit or improve at the time of puberty, the potential for reactivation later in life warrants long-term monitoring.

Tinea Versicolor

Tinea versicolor (TV), despite its name, is not a dermatophyte infection of the skin, but instead is secondary to overgrowth of the yeast form of *Malassezia,* a common dimorphic fungi. TV often manifests during the spring and summer months with pink, hypopigmented or hyperpigmented macules and patches with scant scale often involving seborrheic areas such as the face, chest, and back (Fig. 42.6). The differential diagnosis for the hypopigmented form of TV includes pityriasis alba or PIH. Both often can be ruled out based on history and lesional distribution, or a KOH test can be performed to look for fungal hyphae and clusters of spores. Treatment includes topical agents such as selenium sulfide or ketoconazole, or an oral antifungal agent such as fluconazole can be used for more extensive or recurrent cases.

SUGGESTED READINGS

Available online.

43

Nutritional Dermatoses

Alexander Nguyen and Grace L. Lee

CLINICAL VIGNETTE

A 3-month-old boy presents with a 2-month history of rash. He was born full-term, without complications at birth. He was breastfed until 1 month after delivery. Soon after transitioning to formula, he developed a persistent rash. On physical examination, extensive erythematous, scaly plaques on his groin, anogenital region, dorsal hands, extensor feet, thighs, scalp, and perioral area were noted.

After failing cephalexin for presumptive impetigo and a course of griseofulvin for presumptive tinea corporis, zinc deficiency was suspected. Blood work confirmed a low plasma zinc level (13 μg/dL). He was started on oral zinc supplementation with resolution of rash within a few days.

A well-demarcated rash involving perioral and acral skin is commonly the first sign of zinc deficiency. Diagnosis requires a high degree of suspicion and clinical experience. Most cases respond rapidly to zinc supplementation.

According to the World Health Organization, 45% of deaths among children under 5 years of age are linked to malnutrition. Without sufficient nutrition, infants and children cannot grow or develop normally. Although these nutritional deficiencies are more common in developing countries, they also can be seen in countries with abundant food supplies.

ETIOLOGY AND PATHOGENESIS

In developing countries, inadequate food supply commonly causes protein and caloric deficits. In the developed world, malnutrition is more commonly caused by malabsorptive gastrointestinal (GI) diseases, chronic illnesses, and restrictive diets, including in patients with autism.

CLINICAL PRESENTATION

Protein-Energy Malnutrition

Protein-energy malnutrition is divided into two main categories: protein deficiency and overall caloric deficiency. Protein deficiency with adequate total caloric intake leads to kwashiorkor, whereas inadequate total caloric intake leads to marasmus (Fig. 43.1). These two conditions are more commonly seen in countries without access to sufficient food supplies. Kwashiorkor, however, also can be caused by protein-losing enteropathies or low-protein diets in developed countries.

Protein malnutrition is usually seen in young children because of relatively high protein requirements needed for growth at this stage of life. Children with kwashiorkor typically present with 60% to 80% of expected body weight for their age and edema secondary to hypoproteinemia. Early on, children can appear well-fed and overweight as a result of edema. A distinguishing dermatologic feature is the presence of cutaneous hypopigmentation or hyperpigmentation in areas subject to friction or pressure. In more severe cases, these pigmentation changes can be seen throughout the body. Other findings include superficial desquamation of the skin with an "enamel paint" appearance, which can coalesce into larger areas of cutaneous erosion with a "peeling paint" appearance, typically on the extremities and buttocks. These lesions can be complicated by secondary infection with *Candida* species and skin-dwelling bacteria. These children may also have dry, sparse, and light-colored hair. If periods of protein malnutrition are interspersed with periods of adequate protein intake, the "flag sign" may be apparent, with alternating bands of light and dark hair.

Total caloric deficiency, or marasmus, is defined as less than 60% of expected body weight without edema or hypoproteinemia. This form of malnutrition represents a chronic state of caloric deficiency and is typically seen in young children. These patients enter a catabolic state, using their own body stores of muscle mass and subcutaneous fat to balance their caloric deficit, leading to an emaciated and stunted appearance. The skin in this form of malnutrition is thin, dry, and wrinkled. Other cutaneous findings include lanugo body hair, hyperpigmentation, fine scaling, nail fissuring, and purpura.

Essential Fatty Acid Deficiency

Essential fatty acids (EFAs) are long, polyunsaturated hydrocarbons that can be obtained only through the diet. These EFAs are important in the barrier function of stratum corneum and in the production of prostaglandins, leukotrienes, and thromboxane. Clinically, the two most important EFAs are linoleic acid and linolenic acid. The most common causes of EFA deficiency include inadequate lipid supplementation with total parenteral nutrition and fat malabsorption secondary to GI diseases such as cystic fibrosis or inflammatory bowel disease. Children with pancreatic insufficiency or who have had bowel resection are often treated by supplementation of medium-chain fatty acids, which bypass the intestines and are absorbed directly through the portal vein. Without supplementation of EFAs, these patients are also at risk for EFA deficiency.

Patients with EFA deficiency may present first with cutaneous findings, such as a severely dry, scaly, and generalized dermatitis. Other manifestations include a periorificial rash resembling zinc deficiency, ichthyosis, hypopigmented hair, and alopecia. In addition, patients may exhibit poor wound healing, growth impairment, and increased infection susceptibility.

Vitamin A Deficiency

Vitamin A, or retinol, is a fat-soluble vitamin. Found in animal fats and green leafy vegetables, vitamin A is required for keratinocyte proliferation and differentiation. Typically seen in children in the developing world, vitamin A deficiency can result in phrynoderma, with perifollicular hyperkeratotic papules or "toad skin" distributed symmetrically over the extremities. Patients may also have associated night blindness,

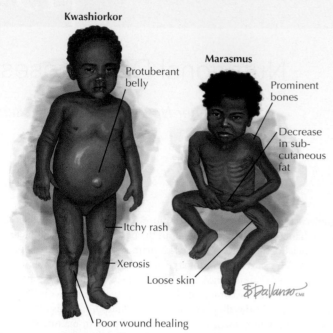

Fig. 43.1 Kwashiorkor and Marasmus.

dry eyes, or Bitot spots (white-gray plaques on the conjunctiva caused by epithelial metaplasia).

Niacin Deficiency

Niacin, or vitamin B_3, is a water-soluble micronutrient. Deficiency in this vitamin leads to a condition commonly known as pellagra. Although niacin is found in most foods, children whose diet consists mainly of corn are at risk because of poor absorption from corn. Children may develop niacin deficiency through other selective eating. Pellagra also can be seen in disorders of tryptophan metabolism because of its essential role in niacin production. The most common genetic disorder of tryptophan metabolism is Hartnup disease, characterized by a mutation in a gene encoding a neutral amino acid transporter *(SLC6A19)*. Carcinoid syndrome can also increase a patient's susceptibility to pellagra by depleting tryptophan reserves to form serotonin. Finally, drug-induced niacin deficiency can be seen with medications such as isoniazid, 5-fluorouracil, or 6-mercaptopurine, which interfere with tryptophan and niacin metabolism.

The classic manifestations of niacin deficiency can be summarized by the "Three Ds": dermatitis, diarrhea, and dementia, although these symptoms are uncommon early on and are rarely seen in conjunction. Characteristically, pellagra presents with well-demarcated, symmetric erythema on sun-exposed portions of the skin with associated pruritus (Fig. 43.2). These lesions resemble severe sunburns and worsen with sun exposure, becoming blistered and forming crusts. Prolonged deficiency leads to hyperpigmented, coarse, and dry skin. Another common cutaneous finding is hyperkeratotic, hyperpigmented plaques on the upper chest, known as Casal necklace. Oral findings include stomatitis and atrophic glossitis; however, this is nonspecific and can be seen in other vitamin B complex deficiencies.

Biotin Deficiency

Biotin, or vitamin B_7, is a water-soluble micronutrient that is an essential cofactor for carboxylation reactions, important in gluconeogenesis and amino and fatty acid metabolism. Biotin deficiency can occur with diets consisting of many raw eggs because avidin, a protein present in raw egg whites, binds to biotin and inactivates it. Children can also acquire this deficiency if they receive total parenteral nutrition without

biotin supplementation. Drugs that alter GI flora and anticonvulsant drugs such as phenytoin and carbamazepine also have been implicated in biotin deficiency. Inherited biotin deficiency, or multiple carboxylase deficiency, can occur with mutations in holocarboxylase synthetase or biotinidase. Holocarboxylase synthetase deficiency typically manifests days after birth, whereas biotinidase deficiency manifests from 3 months to 2 years of life.

Biotin deficiency commonly manifests in infants with neurologic signs such as seizures, hypotonia, ataxia, and developmental delay. Common laboratory findings include metabolic acidosis and organic aciduria. These children are also at risk for fungal infections because of impaired immune function. Dermatologically, biotin deficiency presents with scaly, erythematous dermatitis distributed around body orifices, blepharitis, alopecia, and conjunctivitis. The perioral rash caused by biotin deficiency may resemble that of zinc deficiency. Although biotin supplementation will reverse these cutaneous findings, neurologic impairment is often permanent, and unrecognized genetic biotin deficiency can lead to death. Genetic causes of biotin deficiency are often but not always included in prenatal screening, so clinicians should be aware of signs and symptoms.

Other B Complex Vitamin Deficiencies

Most B complex vitamin deficiencies present with oral findings of stomatitis, glossitis, and cheilitis. Vitamin B_6, or pyridoxine, is an important cofactor in the metabolism of amino acids. Deficiency in this vitamin can be seen with malnutrition, alcoholism, and pyridoxine-inactivating drugs such as isoniazid. Vitamin B_6 deficiency typically manifests with a perioral, scaly rash resembling seborrheic dermatitis. Because of pyridoxine's role in niacin metabolism, children with vitamin B_6 deficiency may also have dermatologic findings resembling pellagra.

Vitamin B_9 (folic acid) and vitamin B_{12} (cyanocobalamin) are important cofactors in the synthesis of nucleotides and amino acids. Although isolated folate deficiency is relatively uncommon because of the fortification of foods, malabsorptive GI diseases, hyperproliferative processes (e.g., pregnancy or sickle cell disease), and medicines inhibiting dihydrofolate reductase may lead to folate deficiency. Isolated cyanocobalamin deficiency can occur secondary to pernicious anemia and strict vegan diets without proper supplementation. Like other B complex vitamin deficiencies, patients with B_{12} deficiency may manifest with painful atrophic glossitis and angular cheilitis; however, characteristic cutaneous findings include hyperpigmentation of the flexural areas, especially in darker-skinned individuals. Laboratory findings include megaloblastic anemia, which may manifest clinically as fatigue. Patients with B_{12} deficiency also may have neurologic findings.

Vitamin C Deficiency

Vitamin C, or ascorbic acid, is an important cofactor for the synthesis of collagen. Although rare in developed countries, vitamin C deficiency, or scurvy, can occur with diets lacking fresh fruit and vegetables and in children with selective diets. Inadequate intake of vitamin C for as little as 3 months can lead to scurvy. Dermatologic findings include follicular hyperkeratosis; hemorrhage; brittle, "corkscrew" hairs classically seen on the extremities and abdomen; and impaired wound healing (Fig. 43.3). Oral findings are also common and include gingival hyperplasia, bleeding gums, and teeth loosening. Patients bruise very easily and may present with widespread ecchymoses. In younger children and infants, scurvy can lead to subperiosteal hemorrhage, resulting in pseudoparalysis.

Zinc Deficiency

Zinc is an essential trace element required for the proper function of metalloenzymes involved in lipid, protein, and nucleic acid

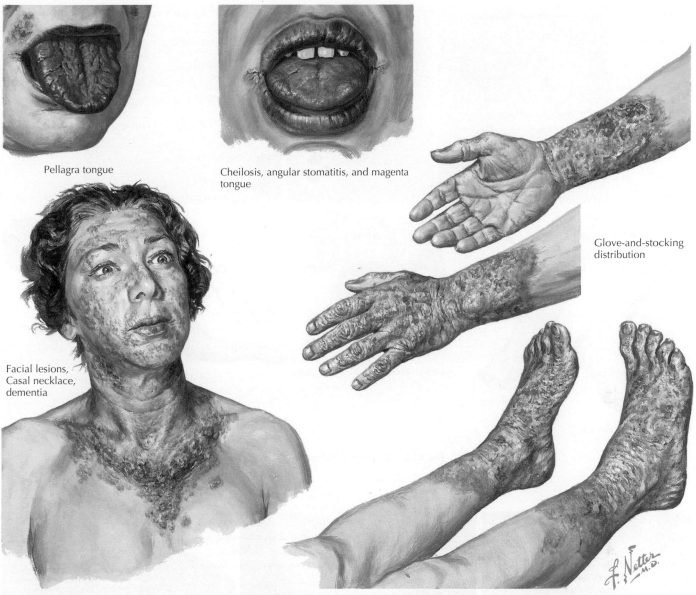

Pellagra tongue

Cheilosis, angular stomatitis, and magenta tongue

Glove-and-stocking distribution

Facial lesions, Casal necklace, dementia

Fig. 43.2 Niacin Deficiency (Pellagra).

synthesis, wound healing, and immune function. The most common cause of zinc deficiency is poor dietary intake but also can be caused by malabsorptive diseases. Acrodermatitis enteropathica is an autosomal recessive disorder resulting from mutation in the gene *SLC39A4,* encoding a zinc carrier protein. Infants typically present after they have been weaned from breast milk, because maternal milk contains compensatory zinc-binding proteins. However, breastfeeding infants with otherwise normal zinc absorption can also become zinc deficient if the mother has a mutation in a zinc transport protein coded by gene *SLC30A2,* leading to inadequate amounts of zinc in the breast milk. Patients with cystic fibrosis are also at risk for zinc deficiency.

Dermatologic findings are often the first indication of zinc deficiency. Classic cutaneous signs of zinc deficiency include well-demarcated, erythematous, and crusted plaques covering the periorificial, anogenital, and acral regions of the body (Figs. 43.4). The characteristic periorificial rash typically spares the upper cheeks and lip, giving a "horseshoe" or "U" appearance (see Fig. 43.4C).

Occasionally, vesicles, bullae, and erosions may develop. Other signs include stomatitis, glossitis, angular cheilitis, onychodystrophy, blepharitis, and alopecia. If zinc deficiency is chronic, these plaques can become lichenified. Superimposed *Candida* species and *Staphylococcus aureus* infections are common. Patients also often present with diarrhea, growth problems, decreased appetite, and irritability. Zinc supplementation will reverse symptoms rapidly, but without prompt diagnosis, zinc deficiency can be fatal. Care must be taken to treat with the lowest effective dose to avoid toxicity.

EVALUATION AND MANAGEMENT

A thorough history, including dietary habits, medications, review of systems, medical history, surgical history, and family history is of paramount importance when investigating nutritional deficiencies. Laboratory testing for nutrient levels is another essential component of diagnosis. Genetic testing also may be considered if treatment does not result in improvement of the symptoms.

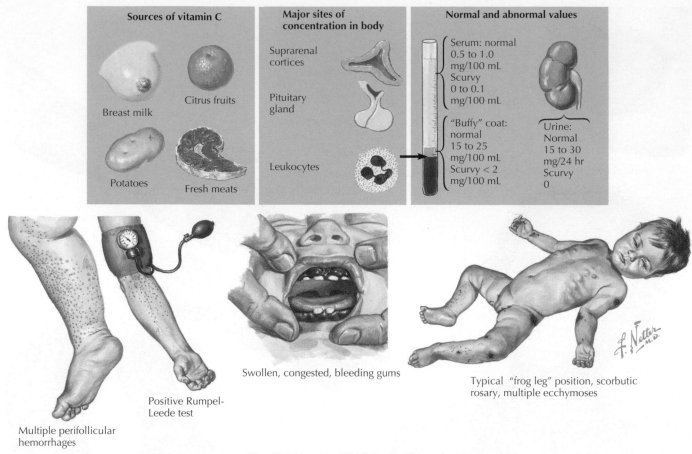

Sources of vitamin C

Breast milk

Citrus fruits

Potatoes

Fresh meats

Major sites of concentration in body

Suprarenal cortices

Pituitary gland

Leukocytes

Normal and abnormal values

Serum: normal 0.5 to 1.0 mg/100 mL Scurvy 0 to 0.1 mg/100 mL

"Buffy" coat: normal 15 to 25 mg/100 mL Scurvy < 2 mg/100 mL

Urine: Normal 15 to 30 mg/24 hr Scurvy 0

Multiple perifollicular hemorrhages

Positive Rumpel-Leede test

Swollen, congested, bleeding gums

Typical "frog leg" position, scorbutic rosary, multiple ecchymoses

Fig. 43.3 Vitamin C Deficiency (Scurvy).

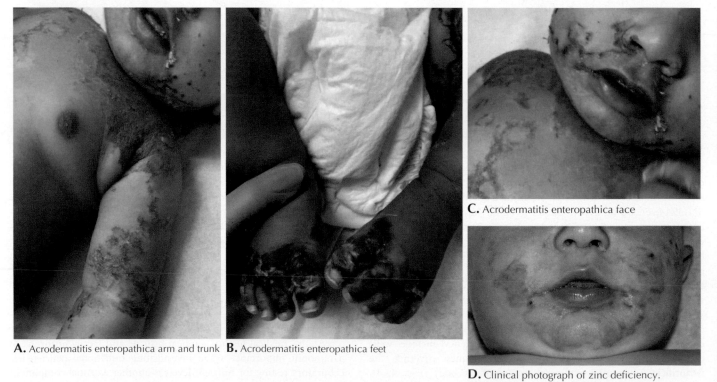

A. Acrodermatitis enteropathica arm and trunk

B. Acrodermatitis enteropathica feet

C. Acrodermatitis enteropathica face

D. Clinical photograph of zinc deficiency. *Photograph courtesy of Albert Yan, MD.*

Fig. 43.4 Acrodermatitis Enteropathica.

FUTURE DIRECTIONS

Several studies are exploring the hypothesis that genetic factors may contribute to a child's risk for developing malnutrition independent of his or her environment using genome-wide association studies. With this knowledge, targeted and more effective interventions can be developed to address the problem of malnutrition.

ACKNOWLEDGMENT

The authors would like to thank Drs. Michael D. Gober and James R. Treat for contributing a chapter on this topic to the prior edition of this work. It has served as the foundation for the current chapter.

SUGGESTED READINGS

Available online.

44

Drug Eruptions

Sonia A. Havele and Lillian Jin

 CLINICAL VIGNETTE

An 8-year-old girl presents to the emergency department (ED) with 2 days of rash. The parents deny fever, and patient is overall well appearing. The patient was started on amoxicillin for an ear infection by her pediatrician 10 days ago. The parents state that the rash began as a few red papules on her trunk that quickly became more generalized.

Vital signs in the ED are stable with no fever. Review of systems is negative for skin pain or pain with swallowing, urinating, or defecating. On physical examination, an erythematous, blanchable maculopapular rash covering her face, neck, arms, back, and abdomen is noted. No facial swelling, lymphadenopathy, mucous membrane involvement, or cutaneous erosions are noted. The patient is diagnosed with a morbilliform drug eruption secondary to amoxicillin. Amoxicillin is discontinued, with resolution of rash over the next 1 to 2 weeks.

Maculopapular or morbilliform drug eruptions (MDEs) are one of the most common cutaneous adverse drug reactions (ADRs) seen in children. Morbilliform eruptions caused by viruses or medications can be indistinguishable; however, history can be helpful because most MDEs occur 7 to 10 days after exposure to the offending agent. Reactions resolve with supportive therapy. The absence of mucosal involvement or skin necrosis helps distinguish from Stevens-Johnson syndrome (SJS)/toxic epidermal necrolysis (TEN). The absence of fever, facial edema, lymphadenopathy, elevated liver enzymes, or eosinophilia helps distinguish uncomplicated MDE from drug-induced hypersensitivity syndrome (DIHS).

Cutaneous adverse drug reactions (ADRs) are common in the pediatric population. Rapid identification and discontinuation of the causative agent is imperative to both treat the ADR and prevent future reactions.

ETIOLOGY AND PATHOGENESIS

Drug eruptions are usually immunologically mediated and encompass a spectrum of hypersensitivity reactions. These reactions are classified according to the Gell and Coombs classification system, which describes the predominant immune mechanisms involved in each reaction (Table 44.1). Most cutaneous ADRs are type I (immediate, immunoglobulin E [IgE]-mediated) or type IV (delayed, cell-mediated—often with activation of T cells).

Several theories explain why certain drugs may trigger an immune reaction. Drug-related risk factors include high-molecular-weight compounds and drugs that haptenate (bind to proteins that trigger an immune response). Larger molecule drugs such as monoclonal antibodies often contain mouse-derived structures, which are recognized as foreign by the immune system and can lead to primarily type I (IgE-mediated) or type III (immune complex–mediated) reactions.

For smaller molecules, such as penicillin, immune reactions may be triggered when the drug or drug metabolite ("hapten") binds to a serum protein such as albumin, forming an immunologically active hapten-carrier complex. In another model, the drug or metabolite binds directly to T cells or Langerhans cells, resulting in the activation of the immune system and production of biologically active molecules.

Patient-related risk factors for developing cutaneous ADRs include previous reaction to the causative agent, age (older children and adolescents > infants), female sex (except in children younger than 3 years of age, when males are more likely to be affected), and genetic predisposition (slow acetylators, certain human leukocyte antigen [HLA] haplotypes). Additionally, patients with immune dysregulation (e.g., systemic lupus erythematosus, human immunodeficiency virus [HIV]) or with Epstein-Barr virus (EBV) have significantly higher rates of eruptions to certain medications.

CLINICAL PRESENTATION

Presentation of drug eruptions depends on the causative agent, morphology of the rash, and presumed immunologic mechanism in play, though morphology seems to be the most helpful framework for characterizing rashes. The most common drug eruption is a generalized maculopapular rash that is raised and erythematous, which often begins on the trunk and spreads to the extremities. In children, viral illnesses should almost always be part of the differential, because they are the most common cause of exanthematous eruptions in this age group. Urticaria may occur as a result of a variety of immune mechanisms. Potentially life-threatening drug eruptions include Stevens–Johnson syndrome (SJS)/toxic epidermal necrolysis (TEN), anaphylaxis, and drug-induced hypersensitivity syndrome (DIHS).

Suspicion for drug eruption can be measured using Naranjo and colleagues' classification system for ADRs, which helps create a framework for evaluation by considering the following questions: (1) Has the patient received a sufficient concentration of the drug in question based on dose and time of administration? (2) Is the morphology a recognized response to the suspected drug? (3) Does the rash improve after the drug is stopped? (4) Does reexposure result in recurrence of the rash?

Morbilliform or Maculopapular Drug Eruptions

An exanthem is a skin eruption that typically occurs in the presence of a viral or bacterial illness. The rash involves small erythematous macules and papules (a few millimeters) that coalesce into larger patches and plaques, which spread from the face or trunk to the extremities bilaterally. When the cause is not infectious, the term maculopapular or "morbilliform" (because of the resemblance of measles) is preferred to exanthem. MDEs are the most common cutaneous ADR in the pediatric population and usually appear within the first 2 weeks

TABLE 44.1 Gell and Coombs Classification of Drug Hypersensitivity Reactions

Immune Reaction	Mechanism	Presentation	Timing	Example Causative Agents
Type I (IgE-mediated)	Drug-IgE complex binds to mast cells, releasing histamine and other inflammatory mediators	Urticaria, pruritus, angioedema, bronchospasm, vomiting, diarrhea, anaphylaxis	Minutes to hours after exposure	β-Lactams, quinolones, neuromuscular blocking agents, platinum-containing chemotherapies, monoclonal antibodies
Type II (cytotoxic)	IgG and IgM antibodies target drug-hapten–coated cells	Hemolytic anemia, neutropenia, thrombocytopenia	Variable	β-Lactams, NSAIDs, quinine, sulfonamides, heparin, propylthiouracil
Type III (immune complex)	Drug-antibody complexes deposit in tissue, leading to complement activation	Serum sickness, rash, fever, arthralgias, lymphadenopathy, glomerulonephritis, vasculitis	1–3 weeks after exposure	β-Lactams, sulfonamides, certain antitoxins (e.g., rabies, botulism), phenytoin, allopurinol
Type IV (delayed, cell-mediated)	Drug molecules are presented to T cells by major histocompatibility complex (MHC), releasing cytokine and other inflammatory mediators	Allergic contact dermatitis, maculopapular drug rash	2–7 days after cutaneous exposure	Local anesthetics (more often benzoic acid ester agents such as lidocaine), antibiotics (neomycin, bacitracin, mupirocin, corticosteroids

Ig, Immunoglobulin; NSAIDs, nonsteroidal antiinflammatory drugs.

of medication administration. Ampicillin is the most common agent associated with exanthematous eruptions, though the frequency of this rash increases significantly during the presence of infection (in particular EBV), and it may be difficult to differentiate the cause. Patients may occasionally experience fever and pruritus. Desquamation may be seen with resolution. Postinflammatory skin changes (e.g., hypopigmentation or hyperpigmentation) may persist for weeks to months, especially in children of darker skin types. Treatment is supportive, with antihistamines and topical corticosteroids as needed for symptomatic relief. If needed, culprit medications can be continued, because maculopapular drug reactions can resolve despite continuation of the offending agent.

Urticaria

Incidence of medication-induced urticaria is difficult to estimate in the pediatric population, given that most acute cases are relatively mild and short-lived, with high frequency in the general population. Urticaria typically occurs within minutes to hours of drug exposure. Most cases are generalized and demonstrate well-circumscribed, pink, or erythematous edematous plaques (e.g., hives, welts). These lesions can range in size (a few millimeters to a few centimeters and can be quite itchy. Angioedema of the subcutaneous or submucosal tissues (e.g., lip, tongue) may also accompany urticarial reactions. The mainstay of treatment is oral antihistamine therapy, including loratadine, cetirizine, or hydroxyzine.

As with exanthematous eruptions, urticaria often occurs in the setting of infection, making it difficult to ascertain whether the infection or treatment is the cause. Penicillins and cephalosporins are most strongly associated with urticarial reactions. In the absence of severe urticaria or anaphylaxis, rechallenge may be considered to confirm causality and avoid unnecessary treatment avoidance in the future.

Fixed Drug Eruptions

A fixed drug eruption (FDE) is a cutaneous ADR that is characterized by well-demarcated, erythematous or edematous plaques that range in color from dusky red to brown/black. Occasionally, FDEs may develop vesiculations, blistering, or bullae. Fixed drug reactions may occur anywhere but are most often found on the lips, genitalia, perianal area, hands, and feet. Lesions may appear acutely 30 minutes to 8

hours after administration but can also occur up to 2 weeks after drug exposure. Lesions typically spontaneously resolve in 7 to 10 days, but often leave postinflammatory hyperpigmentation (PIH) that may last weeks to months. FDEs usually recur in the same location upon reexposure to the same inciting drug or chemically related drug. Diagnosis is made based on lesion morphology and history. Drug classes most commonly associated with FDE are antibiotics (tetracyclines, trimethoprim-sulfamethoxazole) and nonsteroidal antiinflammatory drugs (NSAIDs). Avoidance of inciting drugs is the most important component of managing FDE. Topical corticosteroids and systemic antihistamines may be used as supportive care. No consistently effective therapy exists for PIH.

Photosensitivity Reactions

Photosensitivity reactions may present as phototoxic eruptions or photoallergic eruptions. Phototoxic eruptions present as severe sunburn; common causes include NSAIDs, tetracyclines, amiodarone, and quinolones. It is thought that these drugs can absorb ultraviolet light in the skin, causing cell damage. Photoallergic eruptions present as eczematous dermatitis in photo-exposed areas; common drugs include phenothiazines, sulfa drugs, NSAIDs, and chlorpromazine. The proposed mechanism of photoallergic eruptions is that ultraviolet light converts a drug into an antigen that is presented to lymphocytes, triggering a dermatitis.

Serum Sickness–Like Reactions

Serum sickness–like reactions (SSLRs) are a constellation of symptoms, similar to serum sickness, that usually occur 1 to 3 weeks after administration of certain drugs. Clinically, SSLRs can present with arthralgias, urticarial rash, lymphadenopathy, erythema of hands and feet, and fever. True arthritis, renal disease, and neurologic involvement are uncommon, unlike with true serum sickness. Antibiotics are the leading cause of SSLRs, with cefaclor as the most common inciting agent, in addition to penicillin, amoxicillin, and trimethoprim-sulfamethoxazole. The pathophysiology of SSLRs is not fully understood, but unlike true serum sickness, it is not thought to be immune complex mediated. Diagnosis is usually made clinically, and discontinuation of the inciting drug is the mainstay of therapy, although supportive care with antihistamines, NSAIDs, and, in rare cases, short courses of systemic steroids may be considered.

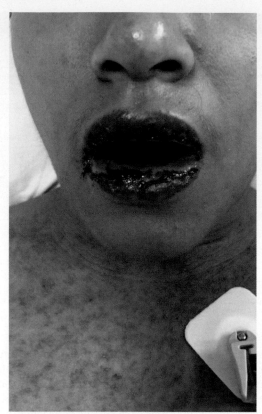

Fig. 44.1 Stevens-Johnson Syndrome/Toxic Epidermal Necrolysis Secondary to Carbamazepine.

Stevens-Johnson Syndrome/Toxic Epidermal Necrolysis

SJS/TEN is a severe, life-threatening, mucocutaneous eruption that is often triggered by medications. SJS and TEN are a disease continuum distinguished by percent of body surface involved. SJS involves less than 10% of skin detachment, and TEN involves more than 30% detachment of body surface area. The estimated incidence of SJS/TEN in the United States is 0.8 per million children. The most common drug triggers of SJS/TEN in children are sulfonamide antibiotics, phenobarbital, carbamazepine, and lamotrigine. The typical onset of SJS/TEN is between 4 days and 4 weeks of first use of a medication. The pathophysiology underlying SJS/TEN is not fully understood, but it is theorized that a cell-mediated cytotoxic reaction against keratinocytes may underlie the presentation of SJS/TEN.

The clinical manifestations of SJS/TEN include high fever, flulike symptoms, photophobia, conjunctival itching, dysphagia, dysuria, and dusky/violaceous exanthematous eruption with subsequent skin tenderness, blistering, and sloughing of the skin. Mucosa are involved in 90% of cases (eyes, mouth, genitalia) (Fig. 44.1). With large areas of skin detachment, patients are at risk for infection and hemodynamic instability secondary to fluid loss. Sepsis and septic shock are the main causes of mortality in SJS/TEN. Treatment consists of prompt withdrawal of inciting drug and supportive care with daily wound care, close fluid and electrolyte management, optimization of nutrition, and appropriate pain control. Admission to a burn care unit is advisable. Gynecologic and ophthalmologic examinations and therapies are necessary to prevent irreversible scarring of urogenital mucosa and eyes. Although studies are lacking, early (preferably within 48 hours) initiation of cyclosporine, etanercept, systemic steroids, or intravenous immunoglobulin (IVIG) may halt skin necrosis, potentially reducing time to reepithelialization and associated morbidities.

Drug-induced hypersensitivity syndrome (DIHS), also known as drug reaction with eosinophilia and systemic symptoms (DRESS), is a rare but severe cutaneous eruption associated with fever, facial edema, eosinophilia, lymphadenopathy, and internal-organ damage. The associated rash is variable but is most commonly morbilliform/maculopapular in appearance. It has been associated with several genetic factors including polymorphisms in CYP450 and N-acetyltransferase that interfere with metabolism, and specific HLA haplotypes. Reaction typically occurs 2 weeks to 2 months after initial drug exposure and can last longer than other cutaneous ADRs. The diagnostic criteria for DIHS are known as the RegiSCAR criteria and include presence of fever, rash, lymph node enlargement, atypical lymphocytes, eosinophilia, internal-organ involvement, and resolution in greater than 2 weeks. DIHS is most commonly reported with anticonvulsant agents (phenytoin, carbamazepine, phenobarbital, and lamotrigine) but has also been seen with antimicrobial drugs, biologic agents, targeted chemotherapies, antiviral agents, and antipyretic agents. Additionally, DIHS may be associated with reactivation of latent human herpes virus (HHV) infections.

The most important step in the treatment of DIHS is discontinuation of the causative drug and consideration of systemic steroids if there is severe internal-organ involvement. The most commonly affected organ is the liver, but nearly every organ can be infected. Long-term sequalae such as autoimmune thyroiditis can develop months after resolution of DIHS. Frequent relapses, even after discontinuation of the offending agent, may occur; thus, if a systemic steroid is initiated, it requires a slow taper over weeks to months.

Vancomycin Flushing Syndrome

Vancomycin flushing syndrome (VFS), previously called "red man syndrome," refers to a bright red macular eruption that can occur in the setting of intravenous vancomycin infusion, possibly as a result of direct toxic effect of vancomycin on mast cells, leading to rapid degranulation and release of histamine in the bloodstream. The eruption usually begins on the back of the neck and will characteristically spread to the face, chest, and upper extremities. Associated features include itching, sensation of heat, angioedema, and hypotension. Therapy involves pretreatment with histamine-1 (H1) and H2 antihistamines and reducing the rate of antibiotic infusion on subsequent administrations. Similar reactions have been reported with antibiotics, including ciprofloxacin, cefepime, amphotericin B, and rifampin, as well as with infliximab, and teicoplanin.

Acute Generalized Exanthematous Pustulosis

Acute generalized exanthematous pustulosis (AGEP) is a very rare, acute drug eruption that leads to the development of multiple, nonfollicular pustules on an erythematous base. AGEP is typically accompanied by fever and leukocytosis. Onset of disease tends to be short (typically within 2 days of drug exposure). More than 90% of cases are triggered by drugs, most commonly β-lactam antibiotics, but also sulfonylureas, tetracycline, antifungals, the calcium channel blocker diltiazem, and antimalarials. Studies have shown an association between AGEP and *IL36RN* gene mutations, which cause susceptibility to pustulosis when exposed to certain medications. Because systemic involvement is extremely rare, most cases of AGEP are limited to the skin and improve with supportive therapy alone. Desquamation occurs within 2 weeks and most patients heal without scarring.

HISTORY

In addition to characterizing cutaneous findings, evaluation of drug eruption should include a detailed history of all the prescription and nonprescription medications (including herbal supplements), timing of administration, onset and duration of clinical symptoms relative to drug exposure, route of administration, drug formulation, dosage, and any previous drug exposures and reactions.

EVALUATION AND MANAGEMENT

Evaluation and management of drug eruptions is usually limited to history and clinical examination with prompt withdrawal of inciting agent.

Laboratory Testing

Laboratory testing is not routinely recommended with most suspected ADRs. DIHS is the exception with recommendations for complete blood count with differential, chemistry tests for liver or kidney involvement, and thyroid-stimulating hormone. Patients with SJS/TEN may require additional monitoring of electrolytes because of insensible losses. Skin biopsy is rarely required because diagnosis is usually made clinically.

Diagnosis

The diagnosis of drug eruptions is based on history of drug exposure with appropriate chronology and clinical features. For any patient with suspected drug eruption, a detailed medication history including current and past medications, an allergy history, and a chronologic relationship between drug exposure and onset of symptoms should be established. If a patient is on multiple medications with a known relation to drug eruptions, it may be difficult to identify which specific drug is the culprit, but all nonessential medications should be discontinued and the patient monitored closely for further symptoms.

Approach to Therapy

The mainstay of therapy for any drug eruption is prompt withdrawal of the inciting agent with supportive care. Few trials have established the efficacy of systemic treatments, but symptomatic treatment may be offered as needed. High-potency topical steroids and oral antihistamines may be used to treat pruritus. For severe drug eruptions (e.g., SJS/TEN, DIHS, recalcitrant AGEP), systemic therapies such as prednisone, IVIG, cyclosporine, or etanercept may be considered.

Prevention

Patients should be counseled to avoid the offending drug and cross-reacting drugs in the future.

Treatment of Complications

For severe drug eruptions that disrupt the skin barrier, such as SJS/TEN, superinfection is a major complication, requiring appropriate antibiotic therapy. Most drug eruptions resolve spontaneously, although usually with PIH. No consistently effective therapy exists for PIH aside from sunscreen and tincture of time. SJS/TEN may heal with scarring, including of the eyes and mucosa requiring management by ophthalmology and gynecology/urology specialists. DIHS may require long-term follow-up by specialty care depending on end-organ involvement.

FUTURE DIRECTIONS

Misattribution of cutaneous eruptions to drugs is extremely common in the pediatric population and warrants closer attention in future years. Tools that can better assist providers in determining whether a cutaneous eruption was truly drug-related, without reexposing a child to a potentially harmful agent, will be useful.

Certain HLA types have been associated with increased risk for drug reactions in specific populations. Personalized pharmacogenomics is an emerging strategy for preventing and treating ADRs, including cutaneous drug eruptions, offering opportunities to reduce morbidity and mortality from these potentially life-threatening reactions.

SUGGESTED READINGS

Available online.

45

Dermatologic Bacterial Infections

Lillian Jin and Yasaman Fatemi

✳ CLINICAL VIGNETTE

An 11-year-old boy presents to the emergency department (ED) with severe pain to his right leg. He was otherwise healthy until the morning of presentation, when he developed a rapidly worsening rash. His leg became increasingly swollen and painful with limited range of motion.

In the ED, his vitals were significant for fever to 103°F (39.4°C), tachycardia, and hypotension. Examination was significant for erythema extending from the mid-thigh to groin with edema. Initial laboratory test results were significant for leukocytosis and elevated inflammatory markers. Blood cultures were obtained before initiation of broad-spectrum antibiotics. On repeat examination, mild crepitus was noted along his right thigh and computed tomography (CT) of his right leg showed gas in the deep soft tissue. A general surgeon was consulted for emergent surgical debridement.

Necrotizing fasciitis, a life-threatening infection of the skin and soft tissue, requires early surgical intervention and antibiotic therapy. Necrotizing fasciitis should be suspected if symptoms progress rapidly and are associated with crepitus on examination or severe pain out of proportion to skin examination findings. Infection can occur in healthy individuals without a clear mechanism of infection, although trauma and immunosuppressive states (e.g., diabetes, cirrhosis, pregnancy) are risk factors.

Skin and soft tissue infections are common problems in the inpatient and outpatient populations. The severity of these infections varies greatly, and management can vary from simple outpatient care to management in the intensive care setting. Early recognition and treatment may prevent progression and complications, including arthritis, nephritis, carditis, and septicemia. It is essential to quickly recognize these infections and begin appropriate therapy (Table 45.1).

ETIOLOGY AND PATHOGENESIS

Most infections occur after there has been breakdown of the skin, allowing normal bacterial colonizers of host flora to invade cutaneous tissues and beyond (Fig. 45.1). Sources of breakdown include direct trauma, excoriation of an insect bite, or underlying conditions such as atopic dermatitis. The seeding point for infection may be caused by microtrauma and not visible to the naked eye. Bacteria can invade to varying depths, determining the severity of the infection. Hair follicles are another source of cutaneous infections, as seen in folliculitis, carbuncles, and furuncles. Host factors also play a role in the severity and progression of illness. Children with underlying illnesses, particularly atopic dermatitis, diabetes mellitus, and renal failure requiring hemodialysis, or those who are immunocompromised, are at higher risk for colonization with pathogenic bacteria and for invasive disease.

Organisms

Most skin infections are caused by gram-positive bacteria that are resident flora on the skin. Gram-negative bacteria also may be implicated; however, this is usually in unique circumstances such as bite wounds, prolonged antibiotic use, patients with extended hospital stays, and immunocompromised hosts. Staphylococci and streptococci cause most gram-positive infections. The predominant staphylococci species in skin and soft tissue infections is *Staphylococcus aureus*, with methicillin-resistant *S. aureus* (MRSA) of particular concern because it is increasingly detected in the community setting. Children with atopic dermatitis are more commonly colonized with *S. aureus*. The predominant streptococcus group for skin infections is group A *(Streptococcus pyogenes)*. Although *S. pyogenes* primarily colonizes the oropharynx, it frequently makes transient appearances on the skin by droplets or the fingers of the host. Other less frequent causes include other *Streptococcus* species, gram-negative bacilli such as *Escherichia coli* and *Pseudomonas* species, and anaerobic bacteria.

CLINICAL PRESENTATION

Nearly all skin and soft tissue infections are characterized by varying degrees of erythema, pain, and warmth.

Impetigo

Impetigo is a superficial bacterial infection, confined to the epidermis, that can present in bullous or nonbullous forms. *S. aureus* is the sole causative agent for bullous impetigo (Fig. 45.2), but it can also cause nonbullous infection. Many species of group A streptococci can lead to nonbullous impetigo. Typically affected are young children, who present with vesicles or pustules, which rupture and form a yellowish-brown crust. The bullous form presents with larger, flaccid lesions that are easily ruptured, leaving a superficial erosion with a collarette of scale. Surrounding erythema is minimal. Lesions are often asymptomatic. Severe cases may have signs of systemic illness. In patients with atopic dermatitis, early infection can be difficult to differentiate from excoriations.

Staphylococcal Scalded Skin Syndrome

Staphylococcal scalded skin syndrome (SSSS) is a bacterial toxin–mediated skin condition. SSSS typically affects children younger than 6 years old; however, it can also affect children older than 6 years. In adults, SSSS occurs only if there is renal dysfunction and inadequate toxin clearance. SSSS is caused by strains of *S. aureus* that produce pathogenic toxins, exfoliative toxin A and exfoliative toxin B, which cleave desmosomal proteins in the skin, resulting in superficial detachment of the epidermis. This contrasts with the full-thickness epidermal necrosis seen in Stevens-Johnson syndrome/toxic epidermal necrolysis. SSSS initially presents with erythema and skin pain, most notably in skinfolds and quickly

TABLE 45.1 **Characteristics and Treatment of Common Pediatric Skin and Soft Tissue Infections**

Infection	Organism(s)	Key Features	Treatment
Folliculitis	*Staphylococcus aureus* *Pseudomonas aeruginosa* and other gram-negative bacteria (rare) *Pityrosporum* (rare)	Follicular distribution Poor hygiene Moist, friction-prone areas Erythema, painless	Improved hygiene with antibacterial soap Topical or oral antimicrobials for severe or refractory cases
Furuncles and carbuncles	*S. aureus*	Nodular or pustular Prone areas similar to folliculitis Erythema, painful	Similar to folliculitis More severe may require drainage, antimicrobials, and hospital admission if systemic signs are present (rare)
Impetigo	*Streptococcus pyogenes* *S. aureus*	Bullous and nonbullous Epidermal vesicles, pustules with yellow or brown crust Minimal pain or erythema	Topical or oral antimicrobials Close follow-up Admission and parenteral medication if systemic signs (rare)
Erysipelas	*S. pyogenes* Other *Streptococcus* species (rare)	Confined to dermis and superficial lymphatics Prodrome Sharply demarcated borders Warmth, tenderness, induration May progress to vesicles or regional lymphatics	Obtain specimen if vesicles or pustules are present Antimicrobials Consider fluid resuscitation, hospital admission, and parenteral medication if systemic signs are present
Cellulitis or abscess	*S. pyogenes* *S. aureus*, attention to MRSA Gram-negative organisms (certain circumstances)	Warmth, tenderness, induration No prodrome Poorly demarcated borders May progress to systemic illness or deeper tissue involvement	Drain collection (may require imaging to define) Antimicrobials Resuscitation, hospital admission, and parenteral medication if systemic signs are present
Necrotizing fasciitis	*S. pyogenes* Other gram-positive organisms, gram-negative organisms, anaerobes	Recent surgery or trauma Pain out of proportion to superficial examination Necrosis, gas formation (crepitus) May appear well or toxic	ABCs Admission with broad antimicrobial coverage Surgery consult Consider intensive care management
Perianal streptococcal dermatitis	Group A beta-hemolytic streptococci	Bright red, sharply demarcated, perianal rash Itching Rectal pain Blood-streaked stools Absence of fever, subcutaneous involvement, and systemic symptoms	Rapid strep or culture of rash site Topical or oral antimicrobials

ABCs, Airway, breathing, circulation; *MRSA,* methicillin-resistant *S. aureus.*

progresses to superficial erosions. There is often crusting, fissuring, and erythema noted prominently in the perioral area. Prodromal and concurrent symptoms of fever, irritability, fatigue, and poor feeding may be present. Diagnosis is made clinically, because bacterial skin cultures will be negative as a result of the toxin-mediated process driving SSSS, but cutaneous or mucosal cultures may be taken from clear sources of infection or to confirm colonization with *S. aureus*. Treatment may involve hospitalization for intravenous antibiotics. Supportive care should be provided to maintain adequate hydration, pain control, and wound care. Patients may continue to have pain, erythema, and desquamation for several days after initiation of antibiotics.

Folliculitis

Folliculitis is a superficial pustule or local inflammation surrounding a hair follicle (Fig. 45.3). It can be solitary, although usually affects multiple follicles. Commonly affected areas include the axillae and inguinal creases, in addition to the scalp, trunk, buttocks, extremities, perioral and paranasal areas. Poor hygiene and a humid environment are risk factors. *S. aureus* is the predominant organism, except for folliculitis that occurs shortly after immersion in a poorly maintained pool or hot tub, in which case *Pseudomonas aeruginosa* is the likely organism. Folliculitis is not usually painful.

Furuncles and Carbuncles

Furuncles (boils) and carbuncles are uncommon in childhood, with the notable exception of children with atopic dermatitis, possibly the result of higher rates of *S. aureus* colonization. Both can be sequelae of poorly managed folliculitis. A furuncle is an acute infection of the hair follicle, that begins as an erythematous papule that progresses to a pustule. Common locations are the neck, face, axillae, groin, and buttocks (Fig. 45.4). Risk factors are the same as for folliculitis, with the addition of hyperhidrosis, anemia, and obesity. A carbuncle is a collection of confluent furuncles, often with multiple drainage points. Both are erythematous and usually painful. Occasionally, carbuncles can progress to the point where the patient develops constitutional symptoms and laboratory evidence of more severe infection.

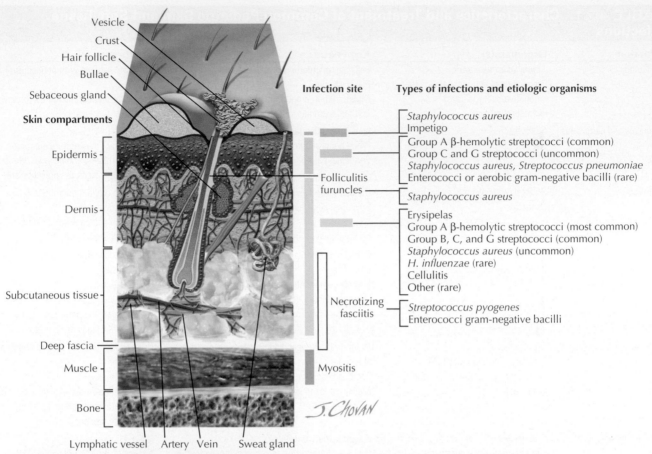

Fig. 45.1 Cross-Section of the Skin Showing Layers and Types of Infections.

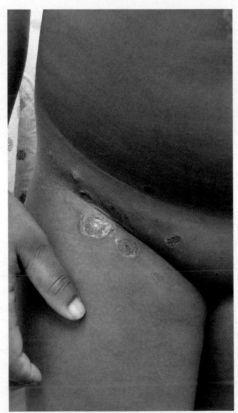

Fig. 45.2 Bullous Impetigo.

Erysipelas

Erysipelas and cellulitis are skin infections that are both characterized by erythema, warmth, and pain (Fig. 45.5). Erysipelas is the more superficial of the two infections, with invasion confined to the dermis. *S. pyogenes* is the most common pathogen. The skin lesions are often preceded by prodromal symptoms of fever, malaise, and chills up to 48 hours before the onset of lesions. Skin lesions begin as brightly erythematous, raised areas with *sharply demarcated*, rapidly advancing borders. Warmth, local edema, and tenderness are nearly universal. Less frequently, there are signs of lymphatic spread such as streaking and regional lymph node inflammation. Severe infection can lead to the formation of vesicles and skin necrosis.

Cellulitis

Cellulitis, unlike erysipelas, extends deeper into the soft tissues below the dermis. It is frequently seeded by relatively minor wounds or skin breakdown. It manifests with erythema, tenderness, warmth, and induration. Erythema may be less clearly demarcated than erysipelas. Lymphatic spread and systemic signs of illness are less common than in erysipelas. Risk factors for infection include recent trauma, local infections, and underlying skin conditions such as atopic dermatitis. Risk factors for more severe or recurrent infections include chronic liver or kidney disease, immune compromise, and poorly controlled diabetes mellitus.

As with erysipelas, *S. pyogenes* is a common pathogen, but other gram-positive cocci such as *S. aureus* play a more prominent role. *S. aureus* may be more likely when significant purulence is identified on examination. Gram-negative and polymicrobial cellulitis can also

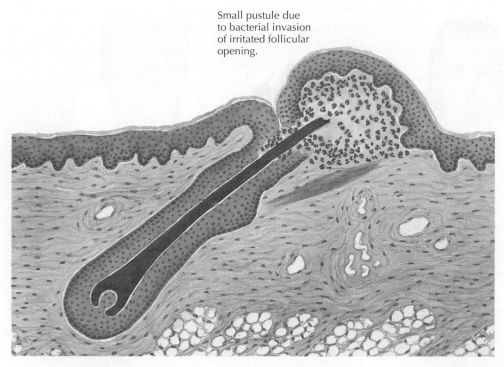

Small pustule due to bacterial invasion of irritated follicular opening.

Fig. 45.3 Follicular Infection.

occur but are usually preceded by a more invasive injury such as bite wounds or other penetrating trauma.

Necrotizing Fasciitis

Necrotizing fasciitis, a severe soft tissue infection that can rapidly progress to severe morbidity or death, is fortunately very rare in the pediatric population. Infection usually begins in the superficial tissues and rapidly spreads along fascial planes into the deeper tissues. Cases are often associated with recent trauma, retained foreign bodies, or recent surgical procedures, although it can be spontaneous. There is initially significant pain; however, anesthesia may develop as infection involves peripheral nerves. Infection can begin with an area of erythema, but induration and warmth may be absent. As the infection rapidly spreads to deeper tissues, there may be evidence of necrosis, gas production (crepitus), bullae formation, and discharge, although none of these findings may be apparent in the superficial tissues. Patients may initially appear well, but more commonly show signs of toxic appearance with fever and cardiovascular instability. Infections can be either monomicrobial or polymicrobial, involving gram-positive, gram-negative, or anaerobic bacteria. Whereas cases with invasive trauma are more likely to involve anaerobes and mixed flora, those caused by minimally apparent trauma are more likely secondary to monomicrobial group A β-hemolytic streptococcal infections.

Blistering Distal Dactylitis

Blistering dactylitis is a localized infection, typically found on the volar aspects of distal phalanges and less commonly on proximal phalanges. It can occur in children and adults. It is characterized by rapid development of single or multiple, tense, ovoid, fluid-filled bullae that may evolve into erosions. Patients may present with pain, fever, or concurrent infections of the eye, upper respiratory tract, gastrointestinal tract, or genitourinary tract. Group A streptococcus and *Staphylococcus aureus* are the most common causative organisms.

Perianal Streptococcal Dermatitis

Perianal streptococcal dermatitis is characterized by a bright red, sharply demarcated rash in the perianal region caused by group A streptococcus. It occurs mainly in children 6 months to 10 years of age. Common concurrent symptoms include perianal dermatitis, perianal itching, rectal pain, and blood-streaked stools. Systemic symptoms are normally absent.

EVALUATION AND MANAGEMENT

After it has been determined that there is a skin or soft tissue infection, management varies based on the severity of the infection, including (1) resuscitation of the patient (if indicated), (2) drainage of purulent material (if indicated) and acquisition of specimens for culture, and (3) appropriate antimicrobial coverage. Except for antimicrobial choice, which will be discussed separately, evaluation and management are best separated by severity of infection.

Mild Infections

Mild infections (e.g., folliculitis, solitary furuncles) require minimal treatment. Bacterial cultures of the affected area may help guide antimicrobial therapy but may also represent the host's colonizing flora, making utility debatable. Decreasing moisture, the use of antibacterial soap, and improved hand hygiene may be beneficial. Mild cases that do not self-resolve within several weeks should be treated with topical or oral antibiotics.

Moderate Infections

Moderate infections include furunculosis, carbuncles, impetigo, erysipelas, and all but the most severe cases of cellulitis. Typically, these infections do not involve hemodynamic compromise.

Obtaining a bacterial culture is important, with implications for both management and treatment. Culture of the material can guide antimicrobial selection, and removal of fluid within a collection or

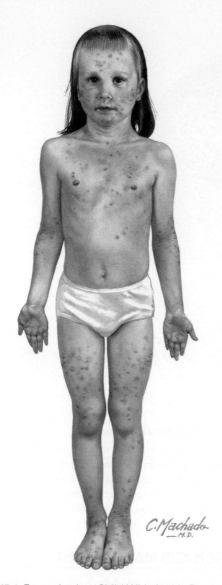

Fig. 45.4 Furuncles in a Child With Atopic Dermatitis.

abscess can be therapeutic as antimicrobials alone may be insufficient. Drainage may be spontaneous or may be achieved with soaks and compresses. In other cases, incision and drainage may be required (Fig. 45.6). If a collection is not apparent but the clinician has a high index of suspicion based on history (abscesses in past, duration, fevers) or there are concerning features on examination (location, size), imaging may be indicated. Optimal imaging modalities may vary by location: ultrasonography may be considered for superficial tissues of an extremity, computerized tomography (CT) scan is preferred when evaluating the head or neck, and magnetic resonance imaging (MRI) may be preferred for evaluation of bony involvement. Blood cultures may be indicated when signs of systemic illness are present.

Severe Infections

Severe infections of the skin and soft tissues include any of the moderate infections that have significant cardiovascular instability and necrotizing fasciitis. Clinicians should consider laboratory testing: blood culture, complete blood count, inflammatory markers (C-reactive protein may be used to monitor response), complete metabolic panel (for possible end-organ damage), and coagulation parameters to evaluate for disseminated intravascular coagulation. Hospital admission

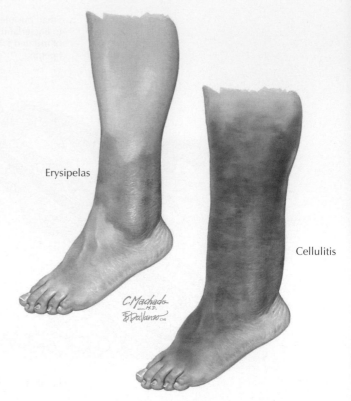

Fig. 45.5 Appearance of Erysipelas and Cellulitis.

is usually required for resuscitation and intravenous antimicrobials. In suspected cases of necrotizing fasciitis, prompt surgical evaluation with possible exploration and subsequent debridement are essential to minimize morbidity and mortality. If cardiovascular compromise is significant, vasopressors and admission to an intensive care unit may be indicated.

Antimicrobials

For most cases, therapy is directed at gram-positive organisms, namely *S. pyogenes* and *S. aureus,* with consideration given to MRSA. For mild and localized infections, mupirocin is the topical agent of choice. If the infection requires systemic antimicrobials, considerations include presence of systemic illness, appearance of the infection on examination, medical history, risk factors for MRSA (prior MRSA infections, hemodialysis, recent antibiotic usage or hospitalization), and the epidemiology of local bacterial flora. For first-time infections, without MRSA risk factors or systemic signs of illness, the clinician may choose to provide coverage for β-hemolytic streptococci and methicillin-susceptible *S. aureus* (MSSA) with oral cephalexin or dicloxacillin. If the patient has any risk factors for *S. aureus,* choices for empiric coverage include clindamycin, trimethoprim–sulfamethoxazole, tetracyclines, or linezolid, depending on the local patterns of resistance. For parenteral coverage, clindamycin and vancomycin are most common, although tetracyclines and linezolid are also options depending on response to therapy and culture results. The parenteral form of trimethoprim–sulfamethoxazole is caustic and should be avoided. For those with severe illness or if there is concern for hospital-acquired strains of MRSA, vancomycin should be considered. For necrotizing fasciitis, surgical debridement is required with empiric regimens of a β-lactam antibiotic (such as a third-generation cephalosporin) plus metronidazole, piperacillin-tazobactam, or a carbapenem, plus vancomycin with the option of clindamycin for antitoxin effects.

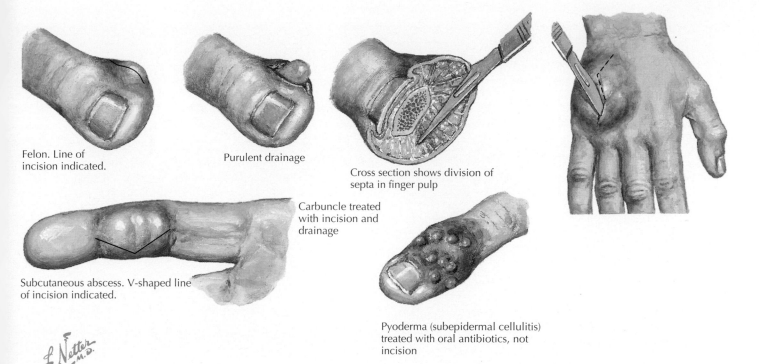

Felon. Line of incision indicated.

Purulent drainage

Cross section shows division of septa in finger pulp

Carbuncle treated with incision and drainage

Subcutaneous abscess. V-shaped line of incision indicated.

Pyoderma (subepidermal cellulitis) treated with oral antibiotics, not incision

Fig. 45.6 Cellulitis and Epidermal Abscess.

SUGGESTED READINGS

Available online.

Endocrinology

Craig A. Alter

Puffpuberty

Talia A. Hitt and Maria G. Vogiatzi

Puberty, a period of physical and psychological transitions from childhood to adulthood, is made up of two distinct processes: gonadarche and adrenarche. Gonadarche is stimulated through the hypothalamic-pituitary-gonadal (HPG) hormonal axis to induce a sex hormone release and the development of secondary sex characteristics and eventual sexual maturity. Adrenarche is an additional process stimulated by the adrenal gland. Puberty also contributes to a growth spurt and subsequent fusion of the growth plates leading to final adult height.

ETIOLOGY AND PATHOGENESIS

Gonadarche

Gonadarche, considered true central puberty or gonadotropin-releasing hormone (GnRH)-dependent puberty, is regulated by the HPG axis: GnRH is secreted in pulses by the hypothalamus, which stimulates the release of the two gonadotropin hormones, follicle-stimulating hormone (FSH) and luteinizing hormone (LH) from the anterior pituitary, which then stimulate the gonads (Fig. 46.1A). The first sign of gonadarche is increased amplitude and frequency of LH pulses during the night. LH induces sex steroidogenesis and secretion of estradiol from ovaries and testosterone from testes. Estradiol in girls induces breast development, pubertal growth spurt, and bone age advancement. Testosterone causes penile enlargement, voice deepening, hair growth, and muscular development and leads to the male growth spurt through conversion of some testosterone to estradiol. FSH promotes gametogenesis and leads to increased size of the gonads.

The HPG axis is active during fetal development and the first couple months of life ("mini-puberty") but then becomes dormant throughout childhood. Reactivation of the HPG axis in puberty is not fully understood, but kisspeptin and makorin ring finger protein (MKRN), encoded by the *KISS1* and *MKRN* genes respectively, appear to be the primary regulators of GnRH release (see Fig. 46.1B). Additional neurotransmitters suspected to regulate GnRH release include neurokinin B, dynorphin, and gamma-aminobutyric acid. Nutritional status may influence GnRH release with stimulation by leptin, reflecting appropriate body energy stores, and inhibition by ghrelin, which is high in physiologic states with low energy stores. Endocrine disruptors such as polychlorinated biphenyls or phthalates may influence pubertal onset by interacting with neuronal networks that regulate GnRH secretion.

Adrenarche

Adrenarche, GnRH-independent puberty, is stimulated by the growth of the zona reticularis in the adrenal gland and release of adrenal androgen hormones: androstenedione, dehydroepiandrosterone, and dehydroepiandrosterone sulfate (DHEA-S). These androgens cause increased body odor, growth of pubic and axillary hair, and acne. The activation of adrenarche is not fully known.

CLINICAL PRESENTATION

Normal Pubertal Development

Pubertal progression is commonly described using the Tanner stage system (Fig. 46.2). Tanner stage 1 is the prepubertal state. Female puberty begins with breast development (thelarche) and with elevation of the subareolar tissue into a breast bud (Tanner stage 2). In girls, the breast and areola continue to enlarge (Tanner stage 3). The areola and papilla then protrude above the breast tissue in a secondary mound (Tanner stage 4) followed by recession of the areola to match the breast contour (Tanner stage 5). Male puberty begins with testicular and scrotal enlargement defined as testicular size 4 mL or greater volume (Tanner stage 2), measured using a Prader orchidometer (Fig. 46.3). In male Tanner stages 3 to 4, penile, testicular, and scrotal growth and maturation continue leading to Tanner stage 5, adult male genitalia. In both sexes, pubic hair development (pubarche) is also measured in Tanner stages (Tanner 2 to 5). Pubertal examination should describe Tanner stages for pubarche separately from breast and testicular development to identify discordances.

The development of secondary sex characteristics and pubertal growth spurts in boys and girls occur at different pubertal stages and at different tempos (Fig. 46.4). Female puberty is shorter, progressing over 3 to 4 years, compared to male puberty, which occurs over approximately 4 years. Female central puberty often starts with thelarche, although 15% start with pubarche. Girls have an earlier growth spurt than boys during Tanner stages 2 and 3, with an average increase in growth velocity to 6 cm/year during the first year of puberty, and

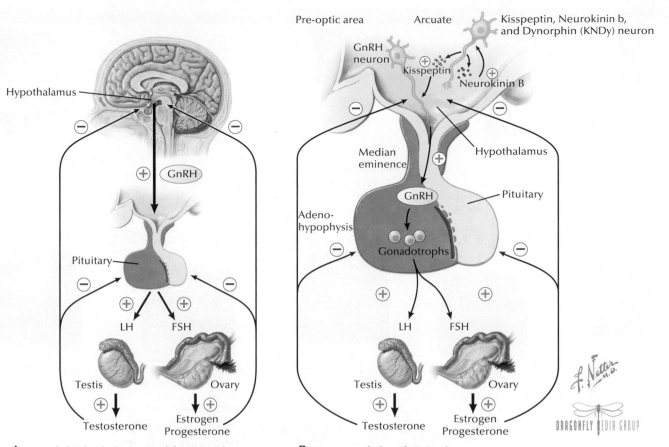

A. Hypothalamic-pituitary-gonadal (HPG) axis   **B. Neuro-regulation of HPG axis**

Fig. 46.1 Hypothalamic-Pituitary-Gonadal (HPG) Axis.

8 cm/year during the second year. Menarche occurs about 2 to 3 years after thelarche during Tanner stage 4 and is followed by a growth deceleration. Male puberty begins with testicular enlargement with pubarche approximately 6 months later. Boys have a pubertal growth spurt during Tanner stages 3 to 4 with growth velocity increase from 5 cm/year on average to 7 cm/year by the second year of puberty, reaching 9.5 cm/year during the subsequent year. Testosterone-induced male secondary sex characteristics include facial hair, voice deepening, increased muscle mass, and nocturnal emissions. The latter signals sperm development (spermarche) and occurs about 3 years after the start of puberty, following the peak growth spurt. In both sexes, bone growth and maturation occur throughout puberty and can be measured using bone age (Chapter 52) radiographs of the wrist, commonly read using the Greulich and Pyle Atlas or the Tanner-Whitehouse method (see Fig. 46.5).

Puberty starts earlier in girls compared to boys: ages 8 to 13 years in girls compared to 9 to 14 years in boys. The mean age of breast development in girls was initially reported at 11.2 years, whereas boys had testicular enlargement at a mean age 11.6 years. More recent epidemiologic studies suggest an earlier onset of breast development in girls, especially among obese girls and certain ethnic groups such as African Americans and Hispanic individuals. Menarche occurs more consistently at a mean age of 12.5 years, suggesting that girls with earlier pubertal onset may have a longer duration before menarche. Pubertal onset timing heritability has been estimated at 50% to 80%, so parental and sibling pubertal history should be assessed for all patients with suspected abnormal puberty.

PRECOCIOUS PUBERTY

Differential Diagnosis

Precocious puberty is defined as secondary sexual characteristic development before age 8 in girls and before age 9 in boys. Precocious puberty includes central precocious puberty (CPP) (gonadotropin-dependent), peripheral precocious puberty (PPP) (gonadotropin-independent), and benign variants, including benign premature thelarche (BPT), benign premature adrenarche (BPA), and benign premature menarche (BPM) (Box 46.1).

CPP is secondary to HPG activation. It can be familial and benign or secondary to a central nervous system (CNS) process such as a brain tumor or anomaly. CPP also can be due to prolonged and severe hypothyroidism, a feature of a genetic disorder such as neurofibromatosis type I, or secondary to genetic mutations of stimulators or inhibitors of the HPG axis, such as *KISS1* activation.

PPP is typically caused by autonomous secretion of sex steroids from gonads or the adrenal gland. The most common cause in girls is a functioning ovarian cyst secreting estradiol. It is characterized by breast development followed by vaginal bleeding once the cyst regresses. Ovarian and testicular tumors can either secrete estradiol or androgens and cause isosexual or contrasexual PPP. Similarly, adrenal tumors can secrete androgens and lead to virilization. In boys, isosexual PPP can be caused by human chorionic gonadotropin (hCG) secreting germ-cell tumors in which hCG activates the LH receptor on Leydig cells, or testotoxicosis secondary to an activating mutation in the LH receptor gene. McCune-Albright syndrome is a rare disorder characterized by the triad of PPP, café-au-lait pigmentation in an irregular distribution,

Breast development

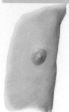

Stage 1
Elevation of
papilla only

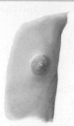

Stage 2
Breast bud: elevation of
breast and papilla as a
small mound and enlarge-
ment of areolar diameter

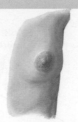

Stage 3
Additional enlargement
of breast and areola with
no separation of their
contours

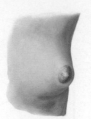

Stage 4
Areola and papilla project
from surface of breast to
form secondary mound

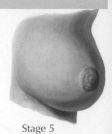

Stage 5
Mature stage with projection
of papilla only with recession
of the areola to the general
contour of the breast

Female pubic hair development

Stage 1
The vellus over the
pubes is the same
as that over the
anterior abdominal
wall

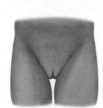

Stage 2
Sparse slightly pigmented,
downy hair along the labia
that is straight or only
slightly curled

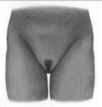

Stage 3
Hair spreads sparsely
over the pubic region
and is darker, coaser
and curlier

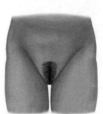

Stage 4
Hair is adult type, but
the area covered is
smaller than in most
adults, and there is no
spread to the medial
surface of the thighs

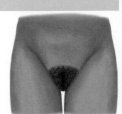

Stage 5
Hair is adult in quantity
and type, distributed as
an inverse triangle and
spreads to the medial
surface of the thighs but
not up the midline
anterior abdominal wall

Male pubic hair and genital development

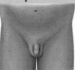

Stage 1
Penis, testes, and scrotum
are the same size and
proportion as in early
childhood

The vellus hair over the
pubic region is the same
as that on the abdominal
wall

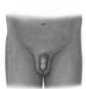

Stage 2
Testes and scrotum
enlarge and scrotal
skin shows a change
in texture and reddening

Sparse growth of straight
or slightly curled pig-
mented hair appearing
at the base of the penis

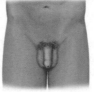

Stage 3
Penile growth in length
more than width; further
growth of the testes and
scrotum

Hair is coarser, curlier,
and darker; spread
sparsely over the
junction of the pubes

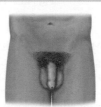

Stage 4
Further penile growth and
development of the
glans; further enlargement
of testes and scrotum

Adult type hair, but area
covered less than in most
adults; no spread to the
medial surface of the thighs

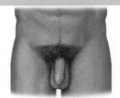

Stage 5
Genitalia are adult in size
and shape

Adult in quantity and type
of hair, distributed as an
inverse triangle; spread is
to the medial surface of
the thighs

Fig. 46.2 Tanner Stages.

and fibrous dysplasia of the bone. PPP can be caused by exogenous sources of sex steroids, such as ingestion of oral contraceptive pills, contact with estrogen or testosterone transdermal products, or contact with lavender or tea tree oil, which may have estrogenic activity.

Benign variants of early puberty occur with incomplete pubertal development such as isolated thelarche, adrenarche, or menarche. The differential diagnosis for isolated adrenarche includes nonclassic congenital adrenal hyperplasia (CAH) and virilizing adrenal or gonadal tumors. Nonclassic CAH or a virilizing adrenal or gonadal tumor, in contrast, is associated with rapid growth and bone age advancement. Nonclassic CAH has been reported in 3% to 5% of cases previously diagnosed as BPA and is diagnosed based on elevated 17-hydroxyprogesterone levels. Virilizing tumors will often have

markedly elevated androgen levels. The differential diagnosis for isolated premature menarche can be secondary to vaginal trauma, foreign body, infection, sexual abuse, or a vaginal or uterine tumor.

Evaluation and Management
Central Precocious Puberty

The initial evaluation for precocious puberty entails a detailed history, including assessment of possible exposures, a focused review of systems (ROS) for CNS pathologic conditions, and a pubertal family history. It should be followed by a complete physical examination, including Tanner staging and skin evaluation to assess for café-au-lait spots, growth monitoring, and bone age evaluation (Table 46.1). Growth acceleration, defined as growth velocity above the 95th percentile, or

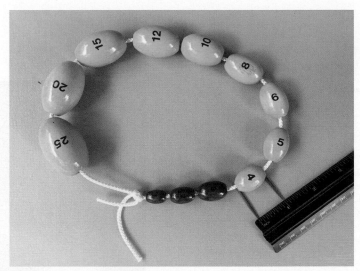

Fig. 46.3 Orchidometer. (Reused with permission from Escobar O, Viswanathan P, Feldman S. Pediatric endocrinology. In: Zitelli BJ, McIntire S, Nowalk, AJ, eds. *Zitelli and Davis' Atlas of Pediatric Physical Diagnosis.* 7th ed. Philadelphia, PA: Elsevier; 2017;341-377, Fig. 9.5.)

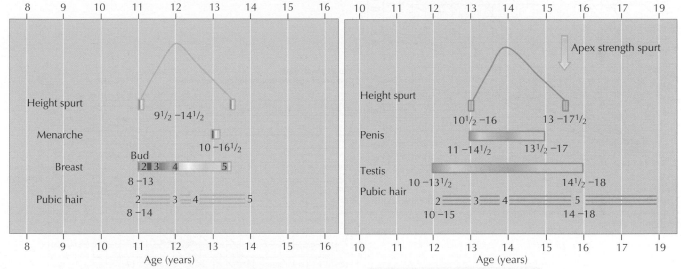

Fig. 46.4 Relationship of Pubertal Milestones. (Adapted from Styne DM, Grumbach MM. Puberty: ontogeny, neuroendocrinology, physiology, and disorders. In: Kronenberg H, Melmed S, Polonsky K, Larsen PR. *Williams Textbook of Endocrinology.* 11th ed. Philadelphia: Saunders; 2007.)

bone age advancement, may indicate precocious puberty over a benign variant (Fig. 46.5A). Laboratory evaluation includes a baseline measurement of LH using an ultrasensitive assay to evaluate for HPG activation and thyroid-stimulating hormone to rule out hypothyroidism. Additional testing, such as a GnRH stimulation test and pelvic ultrasound can be considered.

Because of the possibility of a CNS pathologic condition causing CPP, a pituitary MRI with and without contrast should be considered after its diagnosis. CNS abnormalities causing CPP are more prevalent in boys occurring in as high as 40% to 75% of cases. It is recommended that all boys with CPP undergo a pituitary MRI. In girls, due to the lower prevalence of CNS pathologic conditions and epidemiologic trends in earlier pubertal development, an MRI is recommended for girls with CPP who are younger than 6 years of age. A pituitary MRI can be considered in girls age 7 years when ROS suggests a CNS pathologic condition, such as headaches on

awakening and associated vomiting, vision changes, or abnormal pubertal development, such as fast pubertal tempo. Despite these recommendations, only about 1.6% of girls with CPP have been shown to have an intracranial pathologic condition that requires intervention.

After CPP is diagnosed, treatment can be considered with a long-acting GnRH agonist (GnRHa), which functions through release of GnRH in a constant rather than pulsatile fashion, causing pituitary gonadotrophs to become desensitized and suppressed. The current GnRHa options include injections of leuprolide acetate (various preparations given every 1, 3, or 6 months) or triptorelin pamoate depot, or a histrelin acetate subcutaneous implant that can last at least 12 months. GnRHa treatment benefits may include possible prevention of psychological sequelae of CPP and an increase in the window for growth, which may lead to improved adult height.

A. Growth chart demonstrating rapid linear growth and advanced bone age (approximate bone age demonstrated by arrow) in a child with sexual precocity.

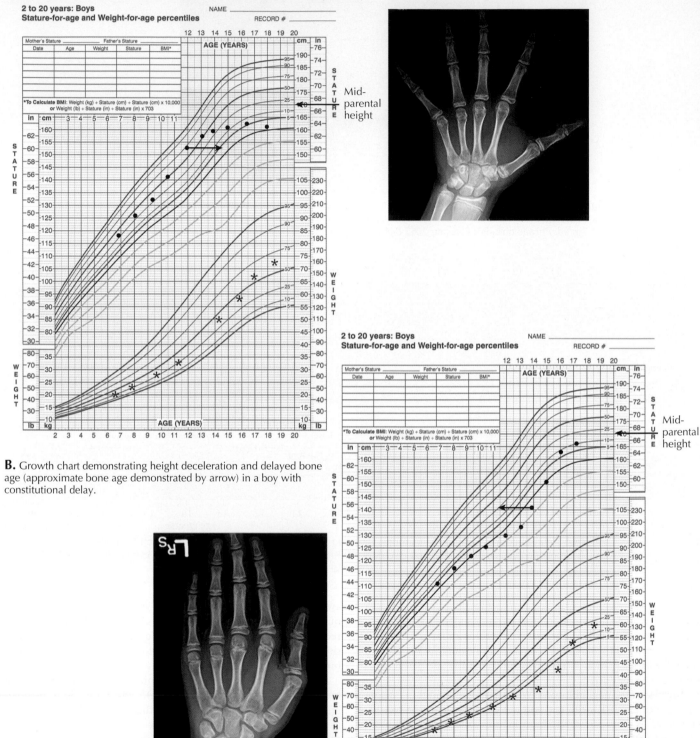

B. Growth chart demonstrating height deceleration and delayed bone age (approximate bone age demonstrated by arrow) in a boy with constitutional delay.

Fig. 46.5 (A) Precocious puberty. (B) Constitutional delay of growth and puberty. (Growth chart from the National Center for Health Statistics in collaboration with the National Center for Chronic Disease Prevention and Health Promotion [2000]. http://www.cdc.gov/growthcharts.)

BOX 46.1 Differential Diagnosis of Precocious Puberty

Central Precocious Puberty

- Idiopathic or familial (most frequent cause)
- Structural CNS process: tumors (optic glioma, astrocytoma, craniopharyngioma, neuroblastoma); congenital anomalies (hypothalamic hamartoma, hydrocephalus)
- CNS inflammation or scarring: trauma, postsurgical, postradiation therapy, postchemotherapy, infection, abscess, infiltrative process
- Mimickers: hypothyroidism
- Syndromes: neurofibromatosis type I, Williams, Prader-Willi, tuberous sclerosis
- Mutations that regulate GnRH secretion
- Adoption from underdeveloped to developed region

Peripheral Precocious Puberty

- Functioning ovarian follicular cysts
- Tumors: gonadal, adrenal, hCG-secreting tumors (liver)
- Testotoxicosis
- McCune-Albright syndrome
- Aromatase excess
- Exogenous sex steroids (estrogen creams, testosterone gels)
- Congenital adrenal hyperplasia

Benign Variants of Premature Puberty

- Benign premature thelarche
- Benign premature adrenarche
- Benign premature menarche

CNS, Central nervous system; GnRH, gonadotropin-releasing hormone; hCG, human chorionic gonadotropin.

TABLE 46.1 Clinical, Laboratory, and Radiologic Features of Precocious Puberty Diagnoses

Features	BPA	BPT	BPM	PPP	CPP
Breast development/ testicular enlargement	—	+	—	±	+
Sexual hair development	+	—	—	±	+
Vaginal bleeding	—	—	+	±	+
Growth acceleration	—	—	—	+	+
Bone age advancement	±	—	—	+	+
Baseline LH elevation (> 0.2 IU/L)	—	—	—	—	+

BPA, Benign premature adrenarche; BPM, benign premature menarche; BPT, benign premature thelarche; CPP, central precocious puberty; LH, luteinizing hormone.

BOX 46.2 Differential Diagnosis of Delayed Puberty

Benign Variants of Delayed Puberty

- Constitutional delay of growth and puberty

Hypergonadotropic Hypogonadism

- Genetic: Turner syndrome (girls), Klinefelter syndrome (boys), DSDs
- Acquired: iatrogenic (radiation, chemotherapy, surgery), trauma, bilateral torsion, infection, autoimmune, cryptorchidism

Hypogonadotropic Hypogonadism

- Functional hypogonadotropic hypogonadism
  - Poorly controlled systemic illness
  - Malnutrition (anorexia nervosa)
  - Excessive exercise
- Permanent hypogonadotropic hypogonadism
  - CNS tumors or infiltrative disease (craniopharyngioma, germinoma, gliomas, prolactinomas, astrocytomas, Langerhans cell histiocytosis), posttrauma, postradiation, post-CNS infection, hypophysitis
  - Anatomic (septo-optic dysplasia, midline defects)
  - Multisystem syndromes (e.g., Prader-Willi, Bardet-Biedl, CHARGE)
  - Isolated gonadotropin deficiency (Kallmann syndrome)
  - Multiple pituitary hormone deficiency (e.g., HESX1, LHX3, PROP1)

CNS, Central nervous system; CHARGE, coloboma of the eye, heart defects, atresia of the nasal choanae, retardation of growth or development, genital or urinary abnormalities, and ear abnormalities and deafness; DSDs, disorders of sexual development.

Peripheral Precocious Puberty

If precocious puberty with growth acceleration and bone age advancement is noted with prepubertal LH, an evaluation for PPP should be initiated. A detailed history should assess for exogenous sources of estrogen and testosterone exposures. A laboratory evaluation should include serum estradiol for feminizing pubertal features and serum testosterone, adrenal androgens, and hCG for virilizing pubertal features. Imaging is guided by the findings on physical examination or laboratory evaluation and may include pelvic or testicular ultrasound or computed tomography of the adrenals. Treatment of PPP depends on the nature of the underlying disorder and can include surgical removal of tumors or other measures to limit sex steroid secretion or block their effects.

Benign Variants of Early Puberty

BPT is isolated unilateral or bilateral breast development that occurs most commonly in girls younger than 2 years of age. Its cause is currently unknown. The breast development can wax and wane and ultimately regress, and growth percentiles do not change. Laboratory evaluation is not needed, and pubertal progression can be monitored. If breast development progresses and is associated with growth acceleration, workup for CPP and PPP can be initiated.

BPM is isolated and self-limited vaginal bleeding, and evaluation should include a detailed history and examination to exclude vaginal trauma, sexual abuse, foreign body, or infection.

BPA occurs in both sexes because of the early onset of production of adrenal androgen hormones and leads to isolated findings of pubarche, axillary hair development, body odor, and acne. Mild elevation of adrenal androgens, most commonly DHEA-S, can be seen. BPA is linked to obesity, insulin resistance, and small-for-gestational-age birth. Benign variants of early puberty do not require therapy beyond monitoring for abnormal progression.

DELAYED PUBERTY

Differential Diagnosis

Delayed puberty is defined in girls as lack of breast development by age 13 or primary amenorrhea by age 16; it is defined by lack of testicular enlargement by age 14 in boys. Puberty delay can occur from a benign constitutional delay of growth and puberty (CDGP; Chapter 52) or hypogonadism (Box 46.2). Hypogonadism can be caused by a primary gonadal defect resulting in failure of gonads to respond to gonadotropin stimulation (hypergonadotropic hypogonadism) or deficient gonadotropin secretion (hypogonadotropic hypogonadism). Lack of pubertal completion within about 4 years of the start of pubertal development should also prompt investigation for hypogonadism.

CDGP is the most common cause of delayed puberty and is characterized by a benign delay of pubertal development and growth associated with a delayed bone age. Family history of delayed puberty is seen in about half of cases.

Hypergonadotropic hypogonadism, also called primary hypogonadism, is secondary to failure of gonads to produce estradiol or testosterone in response to high levels of gonadotropins. Some chromosomal disorders, including Turner syndrome (45,X) and Klinefelter syndrome (47,XXY), are characterized by gonadal failure. In Turner syndrome, because of hypoplastic or "streak" ovaries, the majority of affected girls usually do not experience spontaneous puberty. Boys affected with Klinefelter syndrome develop progressive testicular fibrosis leading to incomplete pubertal development, small testicular size, and infertility. Primary hypogonadism also can be secondary to genetic disorders in sex development. Acquired causes of hypergonadotropic hypogonadism include gonadal injury resulting from chemotherapy, radiotherapy, surgery, trauma, gonadal torsion, infections, or autoimmune attack.

Hypogonadotropic hypogonadism (HH), also called secondary or central hypogonadism, is caused by an ineffective HPG axis leading to low gonadotropin levels. HH can be transient or permanent. Transient HH, also called functional HH, is the result of a poorly controlled systemic illness (e.g., cystic fibrosis, inflammatory bowel disease, hypothyroidism, human immunodeficiency virus [HIV], or renal failure), malnutrition (as seen in anorexia nervosa), or excessive exercise. Individuals with functional HH will have spontaneous pubertal development once their underlying disorder improves. Permanent HH can be secondary to tumors, injury, or malformation of the pituitary or hypothalamus, or various genetic syndromes, such as Prader-Willi syndrome. In these cases, additional pituitary deficiencies can be seen. Congenital isolated GnRH deficiency, or Kallmann syndrome, has variable genetics and presentations. The classic X-linked form is characterized by microphallus in infancy and anosmia. It is due to mutations of the *KAL1* gene that encodes the protein anosmin-1, which is necessary for early fetal migration of GnRH and olfactory neurons.

Evaluation and Management

The evaluation for delayed puberty should begin with a medical history, diet, and exercise history and a complete ROS, including sense of smell (Table 46.2). Family pubertal history and a physical examination with Tanner staging should follow. Assessment of growth records and a bone age radiograph are also important.

In CDGP, family history of delayed puberty is common, growth velocity is prepubertal, and bone age is typically delayed more than 2 years with a predicted adult height appropriate for mid-parental height (Fig. 46.5B). If CDGP is suspected, monitoring for pubertal progression can be implemented without further workup. However, adolescent boys with significant psychosocial distress because of delayed puberty can be treated with a 3- to 6-month course of testosterone for "priming into puberty."

The initial workup for hypogonadism includes a random measurement of serum LH and FSH concentrations along with estradiol for girls and testosterone levels for boys. Elevated gonadotropins with low estradiol or testosterone concentrations is consistent with hypergonadotropic hypogonadism. If hypergonadotropic hypogonadism is found, chromosomal disorders should be considered to rule out Turner syndrome in girls and Klinefelter syndrome in boys.

Low LH, FSH, and gonadal sex steroids are seen in CDGP, functional HH, and other causes of HH. Medical history, including history

TABLE 46.2 Clinical, Laboratory and Radiologic Features of Delayed Puberty Diagnoses

	CDGP	Hypergonadotropic Hypogonadism	HH
Bone age delay	+	±	±
Family history of delayed puberty	+	—	—
Chronic illness, malnutrition, or excessive exercise	—	—	+
Baseline luteinizing hormone elevation (>0.2 IU/L)	—	+	—
Spontaneous progression into puberty after short course of testosterone	+	—	—

CDGP, Constitutional delay of growth and puberty; *HH,* hypogonadotropic hypogonadism.

of weight loss or excessive exercise, or symptoms suggestive of an underlying disease or CNS pathologic condition can tailor the laboratory evaluation. Subsequent workup may include measurement of other pituitary hormones such as prolactin, growth factors, and thyroid function tests, to assess for a prolactinoma or additional pituitary deficiencies consistent with hypopituitarism. Multiple pituitary deficiencies or elevated prolactin should prompt a pituitary MRI to evaluate for an intracranial tumor or malformations. Isolated gonadotropin deficiency and a history of microphallus or anosmia should prompt genetic testing for Kallmann syndrome.

In hypogonadal individuals, sex hormone replacement is initiated at low doses and uptitrated to induce and complete puberty and then maintained at full adult replacement doses. In boys, testosterone can be given intramuscularly or subcutaneously. Testosterone gels or patches for transdermal administration are also available. In girls, estrogen replacement therapy is implemented with transdermal (17β-estradiol) or oral estrogen (equine estrogens or ethinyl estradiol). Once menarche occurs or after 2 to 3 years of estrogen therapy, either cyclic progesterone therapy is added monthly for 10 days to induce endometrial shedding after progesterone withdrawal or estrogen replacement therapy is switched to a low-dosage oral contraceptive pill.

FUTURE DIRECTIONS

Ongoing research is focused on the genetics of CDGP, congenital hypogonadism, and GnRH pulse generation. More research is needed to understand the role of sex hormone replacement on the psychosocial adjustment of treated adolescents and on various health outcomes in children, such as bone accrual and cardiometabolic risk factors. Additional research seeks to develop new biomarkers and testing for diagnosis of CPP, such as urinary LH measurements in a first morning void, or hypogonadism.

SUGGESTED READINGS

Available online.

47

Thyroid Disease

Elizabeth Rosenfeld and Sara E. Pinney

✴ CLINICAL VIGNETTE

A 9-year-old girl was seen by her primary care pediatrician for an annual well visit. Growth parameters were notable for a decline in height-for-age percentiles, from the 85th to 25th percentile over 2 years, despite interval weight gain. On examination, the thyroid gland was slightly enlarged and firm and breast and pubic hair development were prepubertal. Laboratory evaluation revealed a markedly elevated thyroid-stimulating hormone (TSH) level, free thyroxine (fT$_4$) level well below the normal range, and positive thyroid peroxidase and thyroglobulin (TG) antibodies consistent with a diagnosis of autoimmune hypothyroidism (hypothyroidism secondary to Hashimoto thyroiditis). The child and her parents recalled development of decreased energy level and frequency of bowel movements over the past several months. Family history was notable for Hashimoto thyroiditis in her maternal grandmother and aunt. Given the severity and presumed duration of hypothyroidism, treatment was started with levothyroxine (LT4) at half of the conventional age-based dose and gradually increased. Serum TSH and fT$_4$ were obtained after 4 to 6 weeks of full treatment and revealed TSH within goal range (1 to 2 mIU/L). TSH and fT$_4$ were followed every 3 to 6 months until growth was completed and every 6 to 12 months thereafter. Symptoms resolved and linear growth improved markedly with treatment; however, final adult height achieved was slightly below expected.

The most common clinical presentation of hypothyroidism in children is growth failure. Weight gain because of hypothyroidism is typically modest and, in contrast to exogenous obesity, is associated with decreased growth velocity. Although statural growth improves with LT4 treatment and restoration of the euthyroid state, rapid bone age advancement can result in attenuated adult height.

THYROID HORMONE PRODUCTION

Thyroid hormones are produced by the coupling of iodine molecules to the amino acid tyrosine (Fig. 47.1). The principal secreted thyroid hormone is thyroxine (T$_4$). At baseline, the thyroid secretes only small amounts of triiodothyronine (T$_3$), such that most circulating T$_3$ (70% to 90%) is derived from peripheral deiodination of T$_4$. Thyroid hormones circulate bound to carrier proteins, including thyroid-binding globulin (TBG), transthyretin (thyroxine-binding prealbumin), and albumin. Less than 1% of circulating T$_4$ and T$_3$ are unbound or "free."

Hypothalamic thyrotropin-releasing hormone (TRH) stimulates thyrotrope cells in the anterior pituitary to release thyroid-stimulating hormone (TSH), which stimulates production and release of thyroid hormone in the thyroid. When T$_4$ levels are inadequate, a negative feedback loop activates the hypothalamic-pituitary axis and results in increased secretion of TSH, which then acts on the thyroid gland to stimulate increased thyroid hormone synthesis. When circulating levels of T$_4$ and T$_3$ are high, as in Graves disease or overtreatment with exogenous T$_4$, this negative feedback loop acts to reduce TSH secretion.

Circulating levels of T$_4$ are also influenced by peripheral conversion to either T$_3$ or reverse T$_3$ (rT$_3$), an inactive form of thyroid hormone.

Free T$_4$ (fT$_4$) and T$_3$ enter cells by diffusion and carrier-mediated transport processes, and once inside the cell, T$_4$ is converted to T$_3$. T$_3$ binds thyroid hormone receptors with approximately 10 times the affinity of T$_4$ and is the most active form of thyroid hormone. The T$_3$-receptor complex is transported to the nucleus and regulates transcription of a variety of genes, ultimately leading to the synthesis of proteins that manifest thyroid hormone action in peripheral tissues. Thyroid hormone is necessary for normal growth and development and absolutely critical for brain development in utero and during the first 2 years of life.

CONGENITAL HYPOTHYROIDISM

Etiology and Pathogenesis

Congenital hypothyroidism (CH) is one of the most common causes of preventable intellectual disability (Fig. 47.2). Fortunately, early identification and rapid treatment lead to normal neurocognitive development. Although approximately 10% of cases of CH are transient and caused by factors such as iodine exposure, prematurity, or maternal transfer of antithyroid antibodies, in most cases, hypothyroidism is permanent. Worldwide, iodine deficiency is the most common cause of CH. In iodine-sufficient areas of the world, CH most commonly results from thyroid dysgenesis (80% to 85% of cases), thyroid dyshormonogenesis (10%), TSH deficiency (5%), and genetic defects in thyroid hormone signaling pathways are much less common. The incidence of CH is approximately 1 in 1000 to 4000 births, depending on the methods of screening and diagnostic confirmation used. In most cases, CH is sporadic, but mutations in genes encoding proteins required for normal development of the thyroid gland or hormone synthesis are increasingly being identified.

Clinical Presentation

Although there may be few obvious symptoms of CH in the first few weeks of life, a prolonged period of hypothyroidism during infancy can have profound neurocognitive consequences. Therefore newborn screening programs have been established in many countries to identify newborns with CH and facilitate prompt treatment. Infants with untreated CH have an enlarged posterior fontanelle, prolonged jaundice, macroglossia, hoarse cry, distended abdomen, umbilical hernia, hypotonia, poor growth, pericardial edema, and delayed development.

When treatment is initiated before 2 weeks of age, most children with CH achieve normal neurocognitive and physical development. However, subtle deficits in intelligence, attention, memory, and neuromotor performance may exist compared to unaffected control groups and siblings despite prompt treatment with levothyroxine (LT4). In

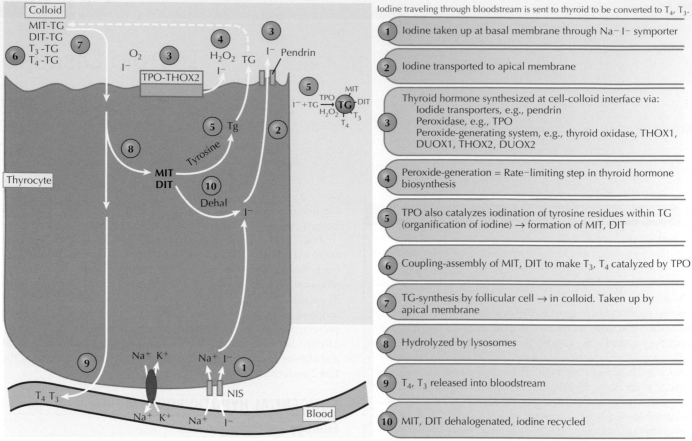

Fig. 47.1 Thyroid Hormone Synthesis.

contrast, long-term untreated CH results in severe intellectual disability and impaired growth.

Evaluation

Newborn screening for CH is based on collection of a blood sample from the newborn between 48 hours and 4 days of life. Measurement before 24 hours of life may lead to erroneous results because of the normal physiologic surge in TSH that occurs soon after birth. Newborn screening programs use blood spots collected on filter paper and use either a primary TSH with or without a backup T_4, or primary T_4 with backup TSH method. An abnormal result should be further evaluated immediately using serum-based assays for TSH and T_4 or fT_4 (Fig. 47.3). Premature or ill infants may have false-negative or false-positive results and should be retested by 2 weeks of age. Any infant with a TSH level above 40 mIU/L with low T_4 is considered to have primary hypothyroidism. In addition to T_4 and TSH measurements, a TG level may be helpful because levels below the lower limit of detection suggest athyreosis.

When there is history of maternal autoimmune thyroid disease, measurement of TSH receptor–binding antibodies in the infant or the mother may identify transient CH. Other diagnostic tests include thyroid ultrasonography and technetium or iodine (I-123) scans to identify functional thyroid tissue, as well as the perchlorate washout test to detect iodine organification defects that might indicate Pendred syndrome (congenital hypothyroidism and deafness). Treatment with LT4 should never be delayed to perform imaging.

Treatment

To avoid neurocognitive deficit, newborns with CH must be treated promptly with LT4 and monitored closely by a pediatric endocrinologist. LT4 is instituted at a dosage of 10 to 15 mcg/kg/day, with a goal to normalize the serum T_4 level within 2 weeks (fT_4 >2 ng/dL) and normalize serum TSH by 1 month of age. There are no suitable liquid preparations of LT4, so tablets must be used. Tablets should be crushed and mixed with a few milliliters of formula or breast milk. Soy-based formula, fiber, calcium, or iron may reduce absorption of LT4 and should be given separately.

Serum levels of T_4, or fT_4, and TSH should be measured every 2 weeks until TSH levels normalize, then every 1 to 3 months during the first 12 months of life, every 2 to 4 months until 3 years of age, and every 3 to 12 months until growth is complete. The half-life of T_4 in the circulation is 1 week, so levels of TSH and T_4 should be repeated 4 to 6 weeks after dose changes to ensure appropriate steady-state levels. An appropriately treated child will have serum T_4 levels that are at or above the upper limit of normal with a serum TSH level of 1 to 2 mIU/L. The serum TSH level is not a reliable indicator of euthyroidism in children with pituitary or hypothalamic disorders, and in these patients, the T_4 level should be maintained within the upper half of the assay's normal range. Infants with suspected transient hypothyroidism should continue LT4 therapy until at least 3 years of age, when thyroid-dependent central nervous system (CNS) myelinization is complete.

CONGENITAL HYPERTHYROIDISM

Neonatal hyperthyroidism is rare (1/25,000), and most cases are caused by transplacental passage of maternal TSH-receptor stimulating immunoglobulins (TSIs). Symptoms of neonatal thyrotoxicosis include goiter, irritability, proptosis, tachycardia, hepatosplenomegaly, jaundice, and cardiac failure, but clinical signs of thyrotoxicosis may be delayed if the mother is taking antithyroid medication. Neonatal Graves

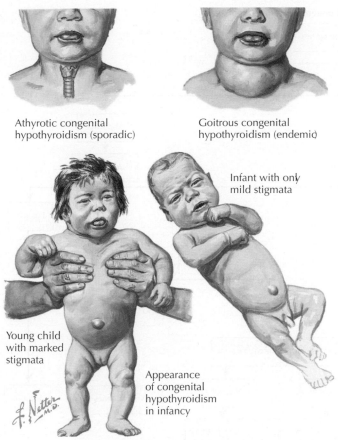

Athyrotic congenital
hypothyroidism (sporadic)

Goitrous congenital
hypothyroidism (endemic)

Infant with only
mild stigmata

Young child
with marked
stigmata

Appearance
of congenital
hypothyroidism
in infancy

f. Netter M.D.

Fig. 47.2 Congenital Hypothyroidism.

disease resolves spontaneously as maternal TSIs are degraded between 3 and 12 weeks of age. Treatment with methimazole is required for symptomatic infants until the maternal immunoglobulins are no longer present, and infants must be closely monitored to ensure normal levels of T_4 and T_3. In some cases, the presence of fetal hyperthyroidism leads to a permanent defect in TSH secretion with a consequent risk for hypothyroidism after maternal TSIs have disappeared.

ACQUIRED HYPOTHYROIDISM

Etiology and Pathogenesis

Hypothyroidism is defined as a deficiency in thyroid hormone and in most cases is associated with an elevated TSH level. Hypothyroidism is more common in females than males and has an increased incidence in adolescents. The most common cause of hypothyroidism is chronic lymphocytic (Hashimoto) thyroiditis, which results in autoimmune destruction of the thyroid gland. Goiter, caused by lymphocytic infiltration or TSH stimulation of thyroid tissue, and circulating antithyroid antibodies (anti-thyroid peroxidase [TPO] and anti-TG) are common but are not universally present. Hashimoto thyroiditis is common in children who have the type 2 autoimmune polyglandular syndrome, which includes Addison disease of the adrenal gland, pernicious anemia, celiac disease, type 1 diabetes mellitus, and juvenile rheumatoid arthritis. Children with chromosomal defects, such as trisomy 21, Turner syndrome, 22q11 deletion syndrome, and Klinefelter syndrome, have an increased incidence of autoimmune diseases, including autoimmune thyroid disease.

Other causes of hypothyroidism include chronic iodine deficiency, excessive iodine exposure, hypothalamic-pituitary dysfunction, acute infection, and medications. Excessive iodine exposure may lead to

acute blockage of thyroid hormone synthesis or release, known as the Wolff-Chaikoff effect. Children with CNS disease are at risk for central hypothyroidism. Medications such as amiodarone, antiepileptics, nitroprusside, and lithium can all affect thyroid hormone production or metabolism; dopamine can reduce TSH secretion.

Clinical Presentation

Symptoms of hypothyroidism include dry skin, constipation, cold intolerance, and a decreased energy level (Fig. 47.4). Severe thyroxine deficiency is associated with linear growth failure and delayed bone age, coarse hair, myxedema, galactorrhea, delayed or, rarely, precocious puberty, bradycardia, pallor, and hyperlipidemia. Although excess weight gain can occur in children with hypothyroidism, height is reduced, which is in contrast to exogenous obesity, in which height is often increased. On examination, the thyroid gland may be enlarged, asymmetric, and/or bosselated. In severe hypothyroidism, the gland may be atrophic. Reflexes are often slowed, the heart rate may be reduced, and the pulse pressure can be decreased. There is a family history of thyroid disease in 50% of patients.

Occasionally, patients with Hashimoto thyroiditis present with elevations in T_4 levels and suppressed TSH, mimicking Graves disease, but without the eye symptoms. This is commonly termed *Hashitoxicosis*, and it may occur as a result of excessive release of thyroid hormone from thyroid destruction. Patients with Hashitoxicosis also can have stimulating TSH-receptor antibodies, although their levels may not reach the high levels that cause hyperthyroidism in patients with Graves disease.

Thyroid uptake scans can differentiate between these two causes of hyperthyroidism with decreased radio-labeled iodine uptake observed in Hashitoxicosis and increased uptake observed in Graves disease.

Evaluation

Typically, patients with hypothyroidism present with elevated TSH, low T_4, and elevated TPO or TG antibodies. In the euthyroid state, TSH, T_4, and T_3 levels are in equilibrium. Decreased thyroid hormone production in hypothyroidism leads to negative feedback on the pituitary, with a concomitant increase in TSH levels. If the gland is unable to respond with an increase in T_4 production, the TSH continues to increase, and there will be very low levels of T_4, fT_4, and T_3.

Children with suspected hypothalamic or pituitary abnormalities should have pituitary function, including thyroid tests (T_4, fT_4, or both), assessed at least once per year. Central hypothyroidism manifests with low fT_4 levels; low-normal T_4 levels; and normal, low, or mildly elevated TSH levels.

Children with slight elevations in TSH (<10 mIU/L) and normal T_4 or fT_4 levels, with or without antibodies, are considered to have subclinical hypothyroidism. In this scenario, treatment may be delayed unless the child has symptoms of hypothyroidism, a goiter, or increasing levels of TSH.

Treatment

Children with confirmed hypothyroidism should be treated with daily LT4 with a therapeutic target of normalizing serum levels of T_4 (or fT_4) and achieving a TSH level of 1 to 2 mIU/L. When there is evidence of long-standing hypothyroidism, LT4 may be started at a low dose and slowly increased to full replacement over several weeks. Serum levels of LT4 and TSH should be measured 4 to 6 weeks after initiation of therapy or change of LT4 dosage to ensure that the expected steady-state levels are achieved. In general, T_4 and TSH levels should be tracked every 3 to 6 months.

When used appropriately, LT4 is a safe medication, and the principal adverse effects are caused by overtreatment or undertreatment. In

Approach to a Newborn with Congenital Hypothyroidism

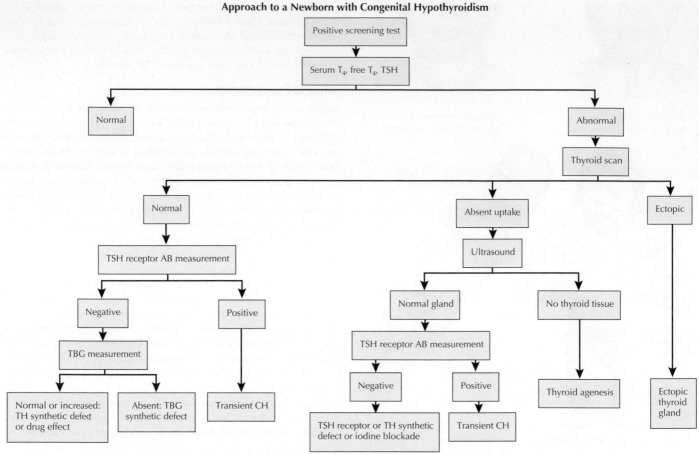

Fig. 47.3 Evaluation of Congenital Hypothyroidism. *AB,* Antibody; *CH,* congenital hypothyroidism; *TBG,* thyroid-binding globulin; *TH,* thyroid hormone; *TSH,* thyroid-stimulating hormone. (From Fisher DA, Gruters A. Disorders of the thyroid in the newborn and infant. In: Sperling MA, ed. *Pediatric Endocrinology.* 3rd ed. Philadelphia, PA: Saunders; 2008:198-226.)

treatment of severe hypothyroidism, bone age may advance rapidly, which can impair ultimate height.

ACQUIRED HYPERTHYROIDISM

Etiology and Pathogenesis

Graves disease accounts for over 90% of hyperthyroidism in children (Box 47.1). Other, less common, causes include a hyperfunctioning toxic ("hot") nodule, transient hyperthyroidism as an early phase of chronic lymphocytic thyroiditis (Hashitoxicosis), and the hyperthyroid phase of subacute thyroiditis. Amiodarone, which contains 37% iodine by weight, causes amiodarone-induced thyrotoxicosis in roughly 2% of pediatric patients on long-term therapy.

Clinical Presentation

Children with hyperthyroidism often have hyperactivity with periods of fatigue and poor sleep (Fig. 47.4). Emotional lability, poor concentration, and a marked decrease in school performance are common. Children often come to medical attention because of cardiovascular complaints such as persistent tachycardia, palpitations, or syncopal episodes. Heat intolerance, weight loss, tremors, and diaphoresis are seen regularly. Although many children with hyperthyroidism indeed lose weight, paradoxical weight gain is common. Hyperthyroidism results in an increased appetite, and in some patients, increased food intake may lead to weight gain despite an increased metabolic rate. Mild polyuria may be seen.

Frequent bowel movements, rather than diarrhea, are occasionally present.

Heart rate and blood pressure may be elevated with a widened pulse pressure. The degree of tachycardia parallels the severity of the hyperthyroidism. There may be normal to accelerated linear growth with concomitant weight loss. The skin is warm to the touch. The eyes may reveal a "lid lag" or prominent eyes, with or without proptosis (exophthalmos) in which the eyes are pushed forward (may be asymmetric). In Graves disease, the more severely hyperthyroid patients have the largest goiters (Fig. 47.5). The thyroid is smooth and diffusely enlarged, and there may be a palpable thrill or audible bruit caused by increased blood flow. Tremors and generalized restlessness are common. A change in mentation associated with hypertension and cardiovascular instability could indicate thyroid storm, which requires urgent hospitalization.

Subacute, or De Quervain, thyroiditis is thought to be viral in origin and lasts weeks to months. In the first few months, hyperthyroidism may be seen because of leakage of thyroid hormone in a damaged gland. In time, transient hypothyroidism can develop as the gland recovers.

Evaluation

Laboratory assessment of patients with hyperthyroidism should include measurement of total or free T_4, T_3, and TSH. In hyperthyroidism, TSH is suppressed (<0.3 mIU/L on most assays). Because of intense stimulation of the gland by TSI, patients with Graves disease

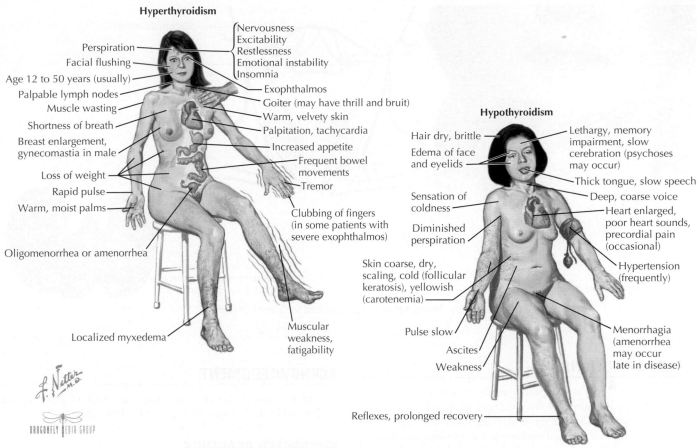

Fig. 47.4 Clinical Features of Hypothyroidism and Hyperthyroidism.

BOX 47.1 Cause of Hyperthyroidism

- Graves disease
- Hashitoxicosis
- Subacute, or De Quervain, thyroiditis
- Toxic adenoma
- Thyroid cancer
- Iodine-induced hyperthyroidism
- Thyroid-stimulating hormone—producing pituitary adenoma
- Thyrotoxicosis factitia (surreptitious levothyroxine)

---

typically have a disproportionately greater increase in T_3 compared with T_4.

Thyroid TPO and TG antibodies can be present in both Graves disease and chronic lymphocytic thyroiditis. Measuring TSI can be helpful when the diagnosis of Graves disease is uncertain in a child with hyperthyroidism. An I-123 scan will show diffusely high uptake of iodine in patients with Graves disease (Fig. 47.5) and patchy areas of uptake in those with chronic lymphocytic thyroiditis. The thyroid gland is hypervascular in Graves disease, and this increased blood flow can be assessed by color-flow Doppler ultrasonography.

Treatment

Treatment of children with hyperthyroidism should be made in collaboration with a pediatric endocrinologist. Families should be informed of three treatment modalities: medication, radioactive iodine (I-131) ablation, and surgery. Most endocrinologists think that initial treatment with antithyroid medication is indicated, especially because

approximately 30% of children may go into a remission within 2 years of starting pharmacologic therapy.

The antithyroid medications available in the United States are propylthiouracil (PTU) and methimazole. Both of these agents block synthesis of thyroid hormone, but only PTU prevents conversion of T_4 to T_3. Since 2008, reports of PTU use and subsequent fulminant hepatic failure in children treated for Graves disease have led to a US Food and Drug Administration (FDA) **"black box warning."** Methimazole has thus emerged as the preferred treatment in the pediatric population. Side effects from both medications occur in up to 20% of children and include skin rash, arthralgia, arthritis, lupus-like reaction, thrombocytopenia, and agranulocytosis. If fever or pharyngitis develop on treatment, methimazole should be immediately discontinued and a complete blood cell count obtained to assess for neutropenia. A β-blocker can be used in patients with more severe cardiovascular signs.

Radioactive iodine ablation of the thyroid is an effective therapy for destroying the thyroid, although it does not ameliorate proptosis of the eyes. The destruction of the thyroid is a gradual process that occurs 2 to 4 months after therapy with I-131. Surgery is another approach to treatment of children with persistent Graves disease. Complications include hypothyroidism, hypoparathyroidism, and damage to the laryngeal nerves so thyroidectomy should be performed by a surgeon with extensive pediatric experience.

Monitoring thyroid function frequently is particularly important in children with hyperthyroidism because of the fluctuating nature of the disease. Monthly laboratory assessments are common. An occasional complete blood count and chemistry panel, including hepatic function tests, may be useful to monitor for medication side effects.

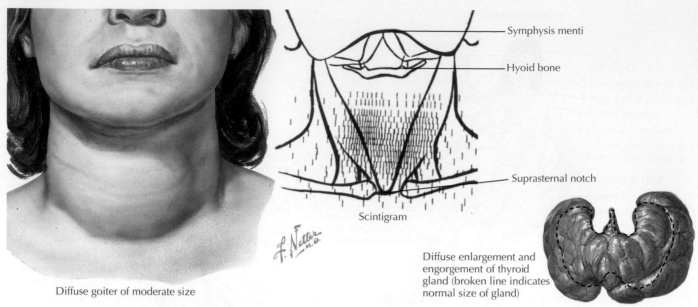

Diffuse goiter of moderate size

Symphysis menti

Hyoid bone

Suprasternal notch

Scintigram

Diffuse enlargement and engorgement of thyroid gland (broken line indicates normal size of gland)

Fig. 47.5 Thyroid Pathologic Features in Graves Disease.

FUTURE DIRECTIONS

In 2020 the FDA approved teprotumumab, an insulin-like growth factor-1 (IGF-1) inhibitor, for the treatment of thyroid eye disease in adults. Use of an IGF-1 inhibitor may negatively affect growth in children who have not attained final height. As the safety and efficacy of teprotumumab has not yet been studied in children, it remains to be seen if this agent will be adopted for use in pediatric or adolescent thyroid eye disease.

ACKNOWLEDGMENT

The authors would like to acknowledge the work of Drs. Vaneeta Bamba and Craig A. Alter on the previous edition chapter.

SUGGESTED READINGS

Available online.

48

Disorders of Calcium and Bone Metabolism

Brittney Newby and Edna E. Mancilla

✳ CLINICAL VIGNETTE

A 19-month-old African American girl, admitted for a respiratory infection, was noted to have bowed legs. She was breastfed until 17 months of age with no vitamin supplementation. Her dairy intake was minimal. Family history was negative for bone disorders. Physical examination revealed a length at the 3rd percentile, body mass index at the 75th percentile, frontal bossing, widened wrists, and bowed legs. She walked with a painful, waddling gait. Laboratory studies revealed calcium of 8.8 mg/dL (8.7 to 9.8 mg/dL), phosphate of 1.9 mg/dL (3.8 to 6.5 mg/dL), alkaline phosphatase of 800 U/L (145 to 320 U/L), and intact parathyroid hormone 400 pg/mL (9 to 56 pg/mL). Wrist and knee radiographs showed physeal widening, metaphyseal flaring, and cupping at the radius, femur, and tibia with obvious bone demineralization. A 25-hydroxyvitamin D level of 5 ng/mL (sufficient >20 ng/mL) confirmed the diagnosis of vitamin D deficiency rickets.

MINERAL AND BONE HOMEOSTASIS

Calcium and phosphate are essential for numerous physiologic processes, including cellular signaling, muscle contractility, neuronal excitation, and skeletal integrity. Approximately 99% of calcium and 85% of phosphate are contained within the skeleton in the form of hydroxyapatite. Plasma calcium is maintained within a narrow range, through regulation by parathyroid hormone (PTH), vitamin D, and fibroblast growth factor 23 (FGF23), acting on the intestines, kidneys, and bone (Fig. 48.1). Approximately half of serum calcium is in ionized form, 35% to 40% is protein bound, mainly to albumin, and 10% is complexed with anions.

PTH is produced by the parathyroid glands, and its secretion is tightly regulated by the calcium sensing receptor (CaSR) expressed on the parathyroid cell membrane. This calcium sensing mechanism maintains calcemia within a narrow physiologic range. PTH directly regulates skeletal remodeling and renal handling of calcium and phosphate. PTH indirectly modulates intestinal absorption of these minerals through formation of 1,25-dihydroxyvitamin D (Fig. 48.1).

PTH induces bone resorption, releasing stores of calcium and phosphate into the circulation. Osteoblasts are responsible for formation and mineralization of new bone and regulate bone remodeling. Activation of the PTH receptor on osteoblasts leads to production and secretion of RANK ligand and macrophage colony-stimulating factor. These molecules stimulate differentiation and proliferation of the osteoclast, the primary cell responsible for resorption of the mineral matrix (Fig. 48.2).

PTH action on the kidney results in a net increase in renal calcium reabsorption and phosphate excretion. Most filtered calcium is passively reabsorbed paracellularly in conjunction with sodium cotransport in the proximal tubule. The CaSR regulates calcium reabsorption in the thick ascending loop of Henle. PTH regulates the active reabsorption of calcium at the distal convoluted tubule and collecting duct through the apical ion channel, TRPV5.

Vitamin D exists as ergocalciferol (vitamin D_2), derived from fungi and plants, and cholecalciferol (vitamin D_3) formed from ultraviolet B irradiation of 7-dehydrocholesterol subcutaneously. Vitamin D undergoes a first hydroxylation step by hepatic CYP2R1 (25-hydroxylase) into 25-hydroxyvitamin D (25[OH]D), its primary storage form. 25-Hydroxyvitamin D is then hydroxylated in the kidney by CYP27B1 (1-α hydroxylase), forming bioactive 1,25-dihydroxyvitamin D. 1,25-Dihydroxyvitamin D binds to its cytosolic receptor within the intestine to stimulate transcellular absorption of calcium and phosphate in the duodenum and proximal jejunum. The principal regulation of vitamin D metabolism is the PTH-mediated α-1-hydroxylation of 25-hydroxyvitamin D. Conversely, elevated serum calcium and fibroblast growth factor 23 (FGF23) inhibit CYP27B1 and stimulate CYP24A1 (24-hydroxylase), which converts 25-hydroxyvitamin D to inactive 24,25-dihydroxyvitamin D. Moreover, 1,25-dihydroxyvitamin D negatively regulates PTH production within the parathyroid gland.

Phosphate homeostasis is largely regulated by the kidney. The majority of phosphate reabsorption occurs at the proximal tubule through the action of renal phosphate (P_i) transporters, NaPi-IIa and NaPi-IIc, which are regulated by FGF23 and PTH. PTH promotes phosphaturia by inducing endocytosis and lysosomal degradation of NaPi-IIa within the proximal tubule. FGF23 is secreted by osteoblasts and osteocytes in response to increasing phosphate levels and 1,25-dihydroxyvitamin D, amongst other factors.

HYPOCALCEMIA

Hypocalcemia is defined as a serum calcium level below the age-specific reference range. Hypocalcemia causes neuromuscular irritability presenting as perioral numbness, paresthesias, and myalgias and can lead to tetany, laryngospasm, cardiac arrhythmias, or seizures. Classic physical examination findings include the Trousseau and Chvostek signs (Fig. 48.3).

Differential Diagnosis

Neonatal hypocalcemia is common and is classified as early or late onset. Early-onset hypocalcemia occurs within the first 72 hours of life as a result of inadequate PTH secretion, PTH resistance, hypercalcitoninemia, and hypomagnesemia amongst other causes. Prematurity, growth restriction, asphyxia, and maternal diabetes are risk factors. Late-onset neonatal hypocalcemia manifests after 72 hours of life, and may be caused by excessive phosphate intake, hypoparathyroidism, hypomagnesemia, maternal hypercalcemia (hyperparathyroidism), or maternal vitamin D deficiency.

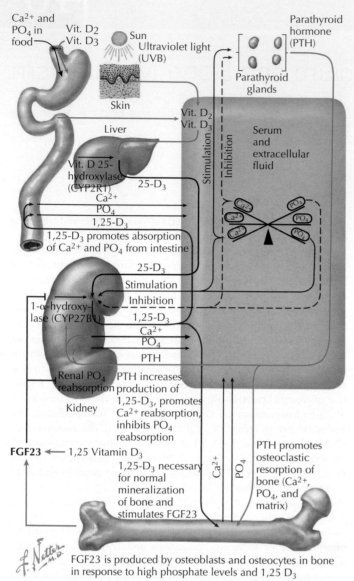

FGF23 is produced by osteoblasts and osteocytes in bone in response to high phosphate levels and 1,25 D₃

Fig. 48.1 Normal Calcium and Phosphate Metabolism.

In children and adolescents, hypocalcemia can be broadly categorized into disorders that are secondary to PTH deficiency or resistance or vitamin D deficiency or resistance.

Hypoparathyroidism, a deficiency in PTH, can be congenital or acquired. Numerous genes have been implicated in PTH gland formation, PTH synthesis, and PTH secretion, including *GCM2*, *GATA3*, and *TBCE*. Congenital 22q11.2 microdeletion syndrome is characterized by hypoparathyroidism resulting from PTH gland hypoplasia. Activating mutations in CaSR or its downstream signaling protein Gα11 cause autosomal dominant hypoparathyroidism, leading to decreased PTH secretion as a result of increased sensitivity to calcium. Immunologic destruction of the parathyroid gland may result from autoimmune polyglandular syndrome type 1 (*AIRE* gene) or in conjunction with other endocrinopathies. Iatrogenic hypoparathyroidism can be acquired from parathyroidectomy or thyroidectomy. Iron or copper deposition from hemochromatosis or Wilson disease can damage the parathyroid gland, and overwhelming infection can stifle PTH release and induce resistance. Pseudohypoparathyroidism results from PTH resistance. Pseudohypoparathyroidism type 1A occurs as a result of maternally inherited mutations in *GNAS*, whereas pseudohypoparathyroidism type 1B results from methylation defects in the maternal allele of *GNAS*.

Severe vitamin D deficiency has reemerged as a cause of hypocalcemia and rickets, resulting from inadequate sunlight exposure, poor dietary intake, or intestinal malabsorption. Vitamin D deficiency is a common problem worldwide and can be easily prevented by supplementation. Acquired disorders of vitamin D metabolism include hepatic dysfunction and renal failure, as well as use of medications that increase cytochrome P-450 activity, including anticonvulsants, rifampin, and theophylline. Hypocalcemia is also observed in hereditary forms of vitamin D resistance. Inactivating mutations of the vitamin D receptor cause hereditary vitamin D–dependent rickets type 2A, and loss-of-function mutations in 1-α hydroxylase (*CYP27B1*) cause vitamin D–dependent rickets type 1A.

Evaluation

Evaluation for hypocalcemia includes measurement of total and ionized calcium, PTH, magnesium, phosphorous, 25-hydroxyvitamin D, and fractional excretion of calcium. Interpretation of total calcium levels should include correction for serum albumin with the formula: Corrected Ca = measured total Ca (mg/dL) + [0.8 × (4 − measured albumin g/dL)]. Vitamin D storage is best reflected in 25-hydroxyvitamin D levels. A recent pediatric consensus defined vitamin D sufficiency as a 25-hydroxyvitamin D level above 20 ng/mL, a level that will prevent rickets all year round. Vitamin D deficiency is diagnosed at a level below 12 ng/mL, and vitamin D insufficiency is defined as 12 to 20 ng/mL. Inappropriately normal or low PTH with hypocalcemia is diagnostic for hypoparathyroidism. Hypomagnesemia represents a reversible cause of hypocalcemia as a result of decreased PTH secretion and action. Vitamin D–related disorders, pseudohypoparathyroidism, and renal insufficiency manifest with elevated PTH levels. Measurement of 1,25-dihydroxyvitamin D is useful when 1-α hydroxylase deficiency or vitamin D receptor defects are suspected.

Management of Neonatal Hypocalcemia

Calcium supplementation is the treatment for neonatal hypocalcemia. Oral calcium supplementation (standard dose range 40 to 100 mg/kg/day) is used in asymptomatic early-onset cases, whereas intravenous calcium gluconate infusion is required for symptomatic cases. In late-onset neonatal hypocalcemia, calcium with a low phosphate formula in a 4:1 ratio helps achieve normocalcemia.

Management of Hypocalcemia in Children and Adolescents

Acute onset or symptomatic hypocalcemia may require hospitalization for intravenous calcium therapy. However, most cases of mild hypocalcemia are treated on an outpatient basis with vitamin D and oral calcium supplementation. The standard regimen starts at 20 to 50 mg/kg of elemental calcium daily. Several calcium salts, which differ in elemental calcium concentration, are available for supplementation. Calcium carbonate (40% calcium) or calcium citrate (21% calcium) can be used for daily replacement, whereas calcium gluconate (9% calcium) is the preferred intravenous preparation. Vitamin D insufficiency/deficiency is best treated with oral vitamin D replacement, either cholecalciferol or ergocalciferol. Typical doses range from 25 to 125 μg daily (1000 to 5000 IU) with close monitoring of 25-hydroxyvitamin D levels. Bolus doses of up to 1250 μg (50,000 IU) vitamin D per week for 6 weeks have been recommended to bring levels toward the normal range. Patients who cannot receive daily doses can continue with a weekly bolus dose adjusted according to 25-hydroxyvitamin D levels. Prevention of vitamin D deficiency by ensuring adequate dietary intake or supplementation is key. In 2010 the Institute of Medicine (now the National Academy of Medicine) suggested a recommended dietary allowance (RDA) of 10 μg (400 IU)

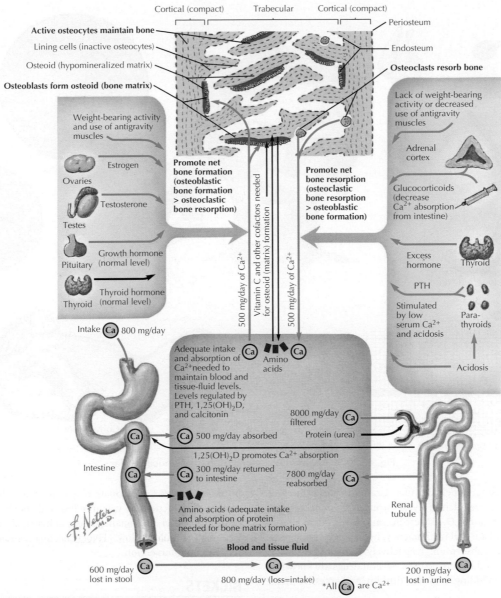

Fig. 48.2 Dynamics of Bone Homeostasis.

per day for infants and 15 µg (600 IU) per day for children older than 1 year of age. Vitamin D supplementation is recommended by an international consensus for all infants younger than 12 months of age, especially in the context of breastfeeding.

Magnesium replacement should be initiated in hypomagnesemia. Calcitriol (1,25-dihydroxyvitamin D), in addition to calcium, is essential for the treatment of hypocalcemia secondary to hypoparathyroidism, pseudohypoparathyroidism, and vitamin D–dependent rickets. Patients with chronic hypocalcemia should undergo regular follow-up with a pediatric endocrinologist to optimize treatment and prevent complications such as hypercalciuria, nephrolithiasis, and nephrocalcinosis.

HYPERCALCEMIA

Hypercalcemia is defined as a serum calcium greater than the age-appropriate normal range. Although often asymptomatic, hypercalcemia can cause a wide variety of symptoms, including hypotonia, weakness, and stupor. Commonly, patients present with nausea, constipation, and

anorexia. Polyuria and nephrolithiasis can develop as a result of impaired urinary concentration and calcium wasting, respectively. Symptoms are often related to the degree and rate of onset of hypercalcemia.

Differential Diagnosis

The differential diagnosis depends on age and includes increased PTH secretion, increased vitamin D levels, increased bone resorption or decreased serum phosphate levels (Fig. 48.4). Neonatal hypercalcemia is often due to maternal disorders of mineral metabolism. Infants may present with hypercalcemia as part of Williams syndrome, subcutaneous fat necrosis, idiopathic infantile hypercalcemia secondary to inactivation of CYP24A1, hypophosphatasia, or familial hypocalciuric hypercalcemia (FHH) as a result of inactivating mutations in the CaSR, Gα11 and AP2σ proteins. FHH is often asymptomatic, but neonatal severe hyperparathyroidism (NSHPT) is a life-threatening, severe form of FHH manifesting in neonates. Primary hyperparathyroidism in children is rare, usually because of a parathyroid-secreting adenoma and may be part of multiple endocrine neoplasia syndromes. Prolonged immobilization and malignancies may lead to enhanced

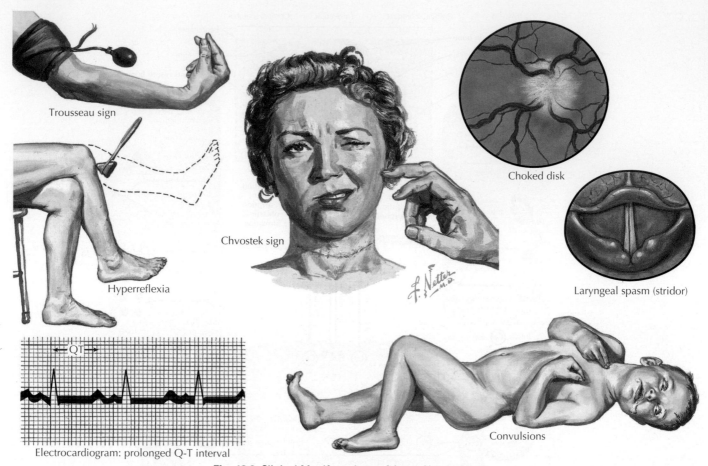

Fig. 48.3 Clinical Manifestations of Acute Hypocalcemia.

bone resorption, causing hypercalcemia. Granulomatous diseases, such as sarcoidosis, increase calcium levels through extrarenal production of 1,25-dihydroxyvitamin D. Hypercalcemia may occur as a result of hyperthyroidism and adrenal insufficiency, by increased bone turnover and renal calcium reabsorption, respectively. Ketogenic diets may lead to hypercalcemia and hypercalciuria. Several drugs are known to cause hypercalcemia, including thiazides, lithium, and excessive intake of vitamins A and D.

Evaluation

Laboratory evaluation of hypercalcemia should include serum calcium corrected for albumin, PTH, 25-hydroxyvitamin D, magnesium, phosphorus, and urine calcium and creatinine. Elevated or inappropriately normal PTH is diagnostic for primary hyperparathyroidism and should prompt further investigation for parathyroid adenomas and/or FHH. In FHH, fractional excretion of calcium is typically less than 1%. PTH suppression should prompt measurement of parathyroid hormone–related peptide (PTHrP) and vitamin D metabolites to evaluate for PTH-independent causes of hypercalcemia.

Management

Mild asymptomatic hypercalcemia is managed on an outpatient basis with adequate oral hydration and avoidance of dietary calcium and vitamin D. Cases of moderate-to-severe hypercalcemia (12 to 14 mg/dL) require inpatient hospitalization, especially those who are symptomatic. Intravenous volume expansion with normal saline is the first step. Loop diuretics should be avoided because they can worsen hypercalcemia. Calcitonin aids in acutely decreasing serum calcium levels; however, tachyphylaxis is a limiting factor. Intravenous

bisphosphonates (zoledronate or pamidronate) help provide a more sustained reduction in calcium levels through inhibition of bone resorption. After acute management of hypercalcemia, disease-specific treatment should follow. Hypercalcemia caused by FHH usually requires no intervention.

RICKETS

Rickets is a disease of the growth plate characterized by decreased apoptosis of hypertrophic chondrocytes secondary to hypophosphatemia. This results in excessive accumulation of cartilage at the growth plate, impaired growth, and skeletal deformities. By contrast, osteomalacia results from impaired bone mineralization and can manifest at any age. Rickets and osteomalacia are classified as calcipenic or phosphopenic.

Calcipenic Rickets

Clinical and radiologic manifestations of rickets are depicted in Fig. 48.5. In calcipenic rickets, insufficient intestinal calcium absorption results in compensatory hyperparathyroidism. PTH stimulation promotes renal phosphate excretion leading to hypophosphatemia, which causes dysregulation of the growth plate. Moreover, PTH increases bone resorption leading to demineralized osteoid. Calcipenic rickets includes nutritional rickets from calcium and vitamin D deficiencies, as well as defects in vitamin D metabolism. Vitamin D deficiency rickets is characterized by low 25-hydroxyvitamin D, hypocalcemia, or eucalcemia, increased levels of alkaline phosphatase and PTH, with low phosphate levels. Treatment consists of vitamin D and calcium as described earlier for vitamin D deficiency.

Condition	Serum Ca^{2+}	Serum P$_i$	Serum PTH	Serum 25(OH)D	Serum 1,25(OH)$_2$D	Associated findings
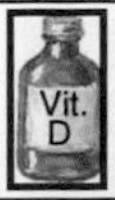 Vitamin D intoxication	↑	N or ↑	↓	↑↑	N or ↑	History of excessive vitamin D intake
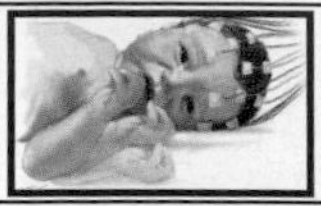 Ketogenic diet–associated hypercalcemia	↑	N or ↑	↓	N	↓↓	Patients with intractable epilepsy. Ketotic hypercalcemia can occur years after initiation. Characterized by impaired bone mineralization, hypercalciuria, and nephrolithiasis.
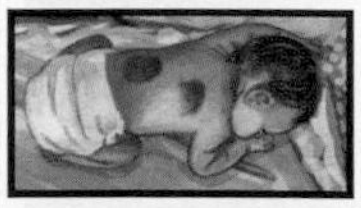 Subcutaneous fat necrosis	↑	N	↓	N	↑	Presents in 1st 6 wk of life, erythematous to purple colored nodules or indurated plaques on the cheeks, back, buttocks, or extremities. Associated with therapeutic hypothermia, sepsis, asphyxia.
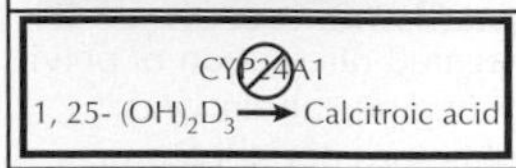 Idiopathic infantile hypercalcemia	↑	N	↓	N or ↑	N or ↑	Inactivating mutation CYP24A1. Severe hypercalcemia with failure to thrive, vomiting, dehydration, and nephrocalcinosis
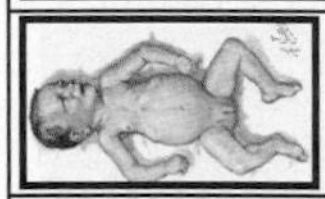 Neonatal severe hyperparathyroidism (NSHPT)	↑↑	N or ↓	↑↑	N	N or ↑	Life-threatening, low urinary calcium excretion, related to familial hypocalciuric hypercalcemia
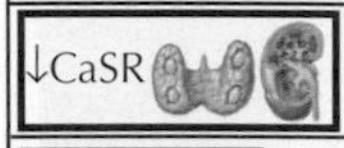 Familial hypocalciuric hypercalcemia	↑	N or ↓	N or ↑	N	N or ↑	Usually asymptomatic
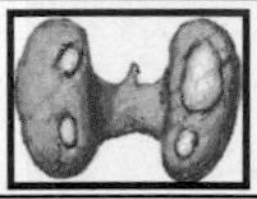 Primary hyperparathyroidism	↑	N or ↓	High N or ↑	N	N or ↑	85% symptomatic. Hypercalcemic symptoms. Nephrolithiasis
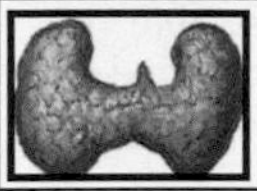 Hyperthyroidism	↑	N	↓	N	N	Symptoms of hyperthyroidism, elevated serum thyroxine
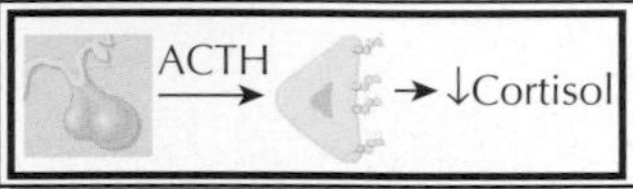 Adrenal insufficiency	↑	N or ↑	N	N	↑	Hypercalcemia occurs due to volume depletion and decreased glomerular filtration of calcium. Absence of cortisol results in increased 1-α hydroxylase and increased intestinal calcium absorption.
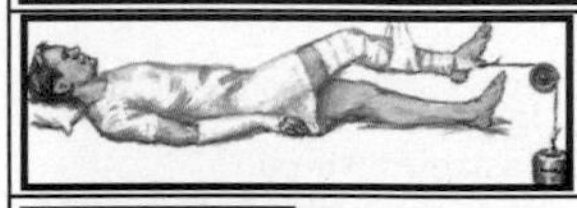 Total body immobilization	↑	N or ↑	↓	N	↓ or N	Multiple fractures, paralysis
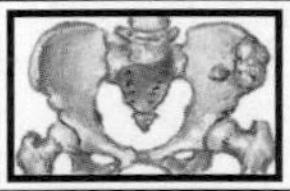 Cancer with extensive bone metastases	↑	N or ↑	↓	N	↓ or N	History of primary tumor, destructive lesions on radiograph, bone scan
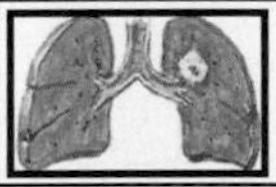 Humoral hypercalcemia of malignancy	↑	N or ↓	↓	N	↓ or N	↑PTHrP. Solid malignancy usually evident
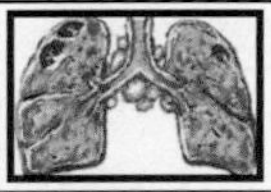 Sarcoidosis and other granulomatous diseases	↑	N or ↑	↓	N	↑	Hilar adenopathy interstitial lung disease, elevated angiotensin-converting enzyme
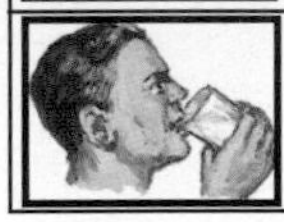 Milk—alkali syndrome	↑	N or ↑	↓	N	N or ↓	History of excessive calcium and alkali ingestion, heavy use of over-the-counter calcium-containing antacids

Fig. 48.4 Differential Diagnosis of Hypercalcemic States.

Phosphopenic Rickets

Phosphopenic rickets presents with hypophosphatemia, which is independent of PTH signaling (Fig. 48.6). It occurs most often as a result of decreased renal reabsorption of phosphate secondary to genetic or acquired disorders and is rarely caused by decreased intestinal absorption of phosphate. Similar to calcipenic rickets, patients often present with bone pain, growth delay, and leg deformities.

Differential Diagnosis

The most common heritable cause of phosphopenic rickets is X-linked hypophosphatemia, an X-linked dominant disorder with an estimated prevalence of 1 in 20,000. Inactivating mutations in *PHEX*, an endopeptidase, are associated with decreased degradation of FGF23, leading to accumulation of FGF23, and renal phosphate wasting.

Other FGF23-related forms of hypophosphatemia include autosomal dominant hypophosphatemia, in which a gain-of-function mutation in FGF23 renders resistance to proteolysis. Mutations in negative regulators of FGF23 action, such as DMP1, ENPP1, and FAM20C have been described in autosomal recessive forms of hypophosphatemia. Other disorders leading to excessive production of FGF23 can result in phosphopenic rickets, including tumor-induced osteomalacia, McCune-Albright, and epidermal nevus syndrome. Hypercalciuric hypophosphatemia is caused by defects in the renal phosphate transporters, NPT2, and is characterized by normal FGF23 levels and

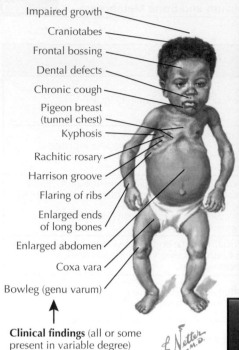

Impaired growth

Craniotabes

Frontal bossing

Dental defects

Chronic cough

Pigeon breast
(tunnel chest)

Kyphosis

Rachitic rosary

Harrison groove

Flaring of ribs

Enlarged ends
of long bones

Enlarged abdomen

Coxa vara

Bowleg (genu varum)

Clinical findings (all or some
present in variable degree)

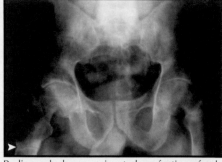

Radiograph of rachitic hand shows decreased bone density, irregular trabeculation, and thin cortices of metacarpal and proximal phalanges. Note increased axial width of epiphyseal line, especially in radius and ulna

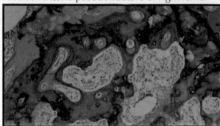

Radiograph shows variegated rarefaction of pelvic bones, coxa vara, deepened acetabula, and subtrochanteric pseudofracture of right femur

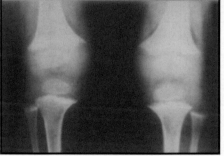

Flaring of metaphyseal ends of tibia and femur. Growth plates thickened, irregular, cupped, and axially widened. Zones of provisional calcification fuzzy and indistinct. Bone cortices thinned and medullae rarefied

Section of rachitic bone shows sparse, thin trabeculae surrounded by much uncalcified osteoid (osteoid seams) and cavities caused by increased resorption

Fig. 48.5 Clinical Manifestations of Rickets.

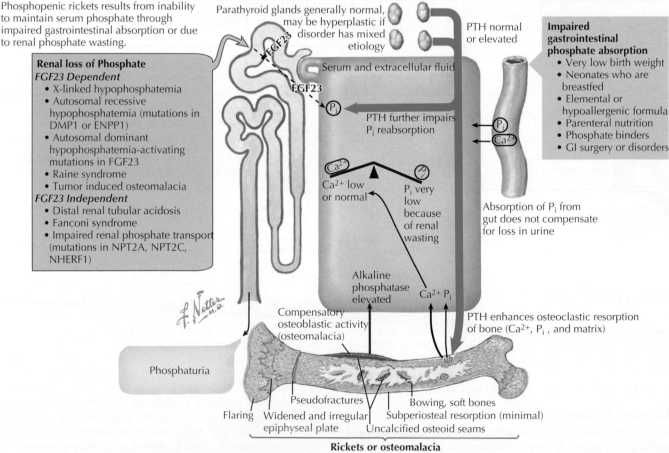

Phosphopenic rickets results from inability to maintain serum phosphate through impaired gastrointestinal absorption or due to renal phosphate wasting.

Parathyroid glands generally normal, may be hyperplastic if disorder has mixed etiology

PTH normal or elevated

Impaired gastrointestinal phosphate absorption
• Very low birth weight
• Neonates who are breastfed
• Elemental or hypoallergenic formula
• Parenteral nutrition
• Phosphate binders
• GI surgery or disorders

Renal loss of Phosphate
FGF23 Dependent
• X-linked hypophosphatemia
• Autosomal recessive hypophosphatemia (mutations in DMP1 or ENPP1)
• Autosomal dominant hypophosphatemia-activating mutations in FGF23
• Raine syndrome
• Tumor induced osteomalacia
FGF23 Independent
• Distal renal tubular acidosis
• Fanconi syndrome
• Impaired renal phosphate transport (mutations in NPT2A, NPT2C, NHERF1)

FGF23

Serum and extracellular fluid

PTH further impairs P_i reabsorption

P_i

Ca^{2+}

Ca^{2+} low or normal

P_i very low because of renal wasting

Absorption of P_i from gut does not compensate for loss in urine

Alkaline phosphatase elevated

$Ca^{2+} P_i$

PTH enhances osteoclastic resorption of bone (Ca^{2+}, P_i, and matrix)

Compensatory osteoblastic activity (osteomalacia)

Phosphaturia

Flaring

Widened and irregular epiphyseal plate

Pseudofractures

Uncalcified osteoid seams

Bowing, soft bones

Subperiosteal resorption (minimal)

Rickets or osteomalacia

Fig. 48.6 Hypophosphatemic Rickets.

appropriately increased 1,25-dihydroxyvitamin D. Genetic or acquired renal tubular defects, such as Fanconi syndrome, result in impaired phosphate reabsorption.

Evaluation

The evaluation of phosphopenic rickets should include PTH, 25-hydroxyvitamin D, 1,25-dihydroxyvitamin D, alkaline phosphatase, and serum and urine calcium, phosphate, and creatinine. Contrary to calcipenic rickets, phosphopenic rickets will manifest with normal PTH levels, and a more modest elevation in alkaline phosphatase. Tubular reabsorption of phosphate (TRP) is calculated by the formula: $1 - [(\text{serum creatinine} \times \text{urine phosphate})/(\text{urine creatinine} \times \text{serum phosphate})]$. A low TRP in the face of hypophosphatemia is diagnostic of renal phosphate wasting. Urinary glucose, amino acids, and bicarbonate are useful when suspecting a generalized tubular dysfunction. Genetic testing may confirm heritable forms of hypophosphatemia.

Treatment

Treatment for heritable forms of phosphopenic rickets resulting from FGF23 excess has consisted of oral phosphate and calcitriol to enhance intestinal phosphate absorption. Unfortunately, this treatment may result in hyperparathyroidism and a predisposition for nephrocalcinosis. In 2018 a human anti-FGF23 antibody, burosumab, was approved for treatment of X-linked hypophosphatemia in patients older than 1 year of age after a trial showed greater improvements than conventional therapy. Tumor-induced osteomalacia is cured with treatment of the underlying cause.

FUTURE DIRECTIONS

New molecular insights regarding the regulation of phosphate and calcium will bring new therapeutic targets. Prevention of vitamin D deficiency rickets is of utmost importance because it has reemerged as an important public health problem.

SUGGESTED READINGS

Available online.

49

Disorders of the Adrenal Gland

Yesenia Sanchez-Kleinberg and Rachana Shah

✳ CLINICAL VIGNETTE

A 13-year-old boy presents to the emergency department with vomiting and abdominal pain for several hours. His mother notes poor appetite and weight loss over the past few months. His pulse is 120 beats/min and blood pressure is 85/40 mm Hg. He appears ill and tired; the remainder of his examination is normal. He is given a bolus of normal saline intravenously. Initial laboratory studies are remarkable for a sodium of 128 mEq/L and potassium of 5.8 mEq/L.

Cortisol and adrenocorticotropic hormone levels are drawn, and he is given 100 mg/m^2 of hydrocortisone intravenously immediately. Vital signs improve and he is admitted to the endocrinology service to continue intravenous steroids. The next day, sodium is 135 mEq/L, potassium is 4.6 mEq/L, and cortisol is less than 1 μg/dL. The patient appears stable. Plasma renin activity, aldosterone level, and anti–adrenal antibody levels are sent. He is switched to oral hydrocortisone and fludrocortisone. Before discharge, the family is instructed on when and how to administer oral and intramuscular stress dose steroids.

A shock-like presentation has a wide differential diagnosis, but the presence of hyponatremia and hyperkalemia strongly suggest primary adrenal insufficiency, with loss of glucocorticoid and mineralocorticoid production. Although demonstrating a low cortisol level is necessary for diagnosis, treatment with steroids should not be delayed awaiting results. Autoimmune destruction is the most common cause of adrenal insufficiency in the Western world. Maintenance treatment with oral steroids and instructions on stress dose steroids for illness or physical stress are crucial.

ADRENAL GLAND PHYSIOLOGY

The adrenal cortex consists of three distinct anatomic zones: the glomerulosa, the fasciculata, and the reticularis. The major adrenal steroid hormones are synthesized in these different areas.

Mineralocorticoid (aldosterone) is produced in the zona glomerulosa under independent control of the renin-angiotensin system. Low blood pressure and intravascular volume contraction lead to renin release from the kidney, activating this system. Aldosterone acts on the distal nephron to increase the reabsorption of sodium, thereby increasing fluid retention and blood pressure, and secretion of potassium and hydrogen (acid).

Glucocorticoid (cortisol) is made in the zona fasciculata, where it is regulated by the hypothalamic-pituitary-adrenal (HPA) axis. Cortisol production is directly stimulated by adrenocorticotropic hormone (ACTH) secreted from corticotropes in the anterior pituitary gland in response to corticotropin-releasing hormone (CRH) released by the hypothalamus (Fig. 49.1). Cortisol plays important roles in cardiovascular stability (maintaining blood pressure by increasing the sensitivity of the vasculature to the vasoconstrictive effects of epinephrine and norepinephrine), metabolism (increasing hepatic gluconeogenesis to prevent hypoglycemia), and fluid and electrolyte balance (sodium retention and potassium excretion). It

also inhibits bone formation and is a potent anti-inflammatory agent (Fig. 49.2). A reduction in circulating cortisol levels activates the HPA axis, leading to increased secretion of ACTH from the anterior pituitary, whereas high levels of cortisol or exogenous steroids downregulate the axis.

Adrenal androgens are produced in the zona reticularis and promote pubarche, or the development of secondary sexual characteristics (i.e., pubic hair) in both males and females during puberty (Chapter 46). Excess production of adrenal androgens can cause early pubic hair production in children. Lack of these hormones may affect pubertal development but is not otherwise known to be detrimental to health.

ADRENAL INSUFFICIENCY

Etiology and Pathogenesis
Primary Adrenal Insufficiency

Primary adrenal insufficiency is caused by congenital or acquired dysfunction of the adrenal cortex or the hormone-producing steroidogenic pathway (Table 49.1). The most common cause in the developed world is autoimmune adrenalitis. In developing countries, tuberculosis remains the most prominent cause. Destruction of the gland ultimately leads to deficiencies in all adrenal cortex hormones, but this process may be asynchronous, and patients may present with deficiency of glucocorticoid only. Enzyme defects can cause cortisol deficiency with an excess of precursor hormones. Loss of negative feedback from low cortisol levels leads to high ACTH in primary adrenal insufficiency.

Secondary and Tertiary Adrenal Insufficiency

Secondary and tertiary adrenal insufficiency reflect a defect in the anterior pituitary and hypothalamic (central) regions that impair secretion of ACTH and CRH, respectively. Central adrenal insufficiency most commonly occurs in patients with congenital or acquired pituitary defects that arise as a consequence of surgery, trauma, radiation, hemorrhage, infiltrative disease, genetic mutation, or structural defect. Patients may have isolated ACTH deficiency (rare) or multihormonal deficiency (panhypopituitarism).

Iatrogenic Adrenal Insufficiency

Long-term use of exogenous steroids is a common cause of tertiary, central adrenal insufficiency. Daily administration of glucocorticoids in doses exceeding normal adrenal production can cause prolonged suppression of the HPA axis and ultimately atrophy of the adrenal cortex. This occurs most commonly from oral administration of potent glucocorticoids but can also occur from inhaled glucocorticoids or even topical steroids. Slow tapering of the daily dosage over weeks to months may be required before adrenal function recovers. Until

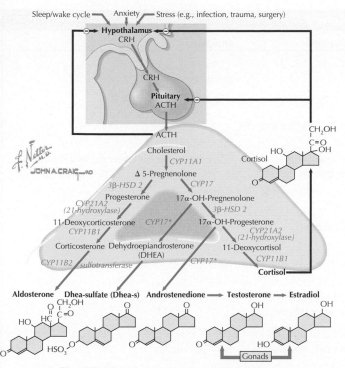

Fig. 49.1 Regulation of Adrenal Hormones.

normal function is proven, the patient remains at risk for adrenal insufficiency during times of stress.

Clinical Presentation

Chronic symptoms of adrenal insufficiency are vague and often unrecognized. Children experience fatigue, malaise, poor growth, and anorexia.

In primary adrenal insufficiency, pituitary secretion of ACTH is markedly increased and is often associated with hyperplasia of corticotropic cells in the pituitary. Generalized hyperpigmentation of the skin and mucosa may occur because of co-secretion of melanocyte-stimulating hormone (α-MSH) with ACTH (Fig. 49.3).

Physical stress can trigger acute adrenal crisis, a shock-like syndrome with tachycardia, hypotension, dehydration, and acute abdominal pain often mistaken for appendicitis. A significant factor precipitating an adrenal crisis is mineralocorticoid deficiency, and the main clinical problem is hypotension. The presence of both hyponatremia and hyperkalemia is indicative of primary adrenal insufficiency. Other laboratory findings include hypoglycemia, hypercalcemia, acidosis, eosinophilia, and elevated blood urea nitrogen and creatinine.

Associated signs and symptoms are often unique to the specific cause of adrenal insufficiency. Patients may exhibit evidence of autoimmune disease (thyroiditis, vitiligo, type 1 diabetes) with autoimmune adrenalitis; hypoparathyroidism and mucocutaneous candidiasis with autoimmune polyendocrinopathy syndromes; neuromuscular dysfunction with adrenoleukodystrophy; and weight loss, fever, and

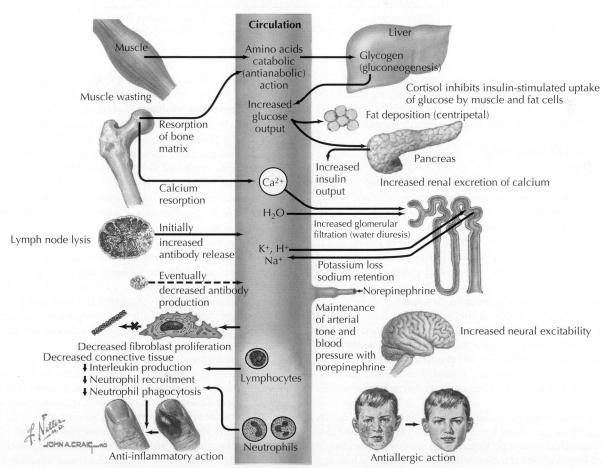

Fig. 49.2 Actions of Cortisol.

TABLE 49.1   Causes of Primary Adrenal Insufficiency

Cause	Associations or Pathogenesis	Diagnosis
Acquired		
Autoimmune adrenalitis	Other autoimmune diseases	Adrenal antibodies
Autoimmune polyglandular syndrome	Type 1: hypoparathyroidism and mucocutaneous candidiasis Type 2: type 1 diabetes, thyroiditis, other autoimmune diseases	*AIRE* gene mutation in type 1
Infiltration or infection	Tuberculosis, fungal, cancer, amyloidosis, sarcoid, hemochromatosis, CMV (HIV patients)	PPD, cultures, imaging, biopsy, ELISA or Western blot
Waterhouse-Friderichsen syndrome	Meningococcemia leading to adrenal hemorrhage	Cultures
Bilateral hemorrhage	Trauma, anticoagulants	Imaging
Medications: mitotane, ketoconazole	Destruction of gland, enzyme blockage	History
Congenital		
Congenital adrenal hyperplasia	Autosomal recessive; mutation of 21-hydroxylase and others	Adrenal steroid profiles, genetic testing
Adrenoleukodystrophy	X-linked; buildup of VLCFA in adrenals and cerebral or spinal cord involvement; neuromuscular disease	Serum VLCFAs; *ALD* gene
X-linked congenital adrenal hypoplasia	X-linked; delayed puberty	*DAX1* or *SF1* gene testing
Triple A syndrome	Autosomal recessive; achalasia, alacrima, *adrenal insufficiency*	AAAS gene testing
Other syndromes: IMAGe, MIRAGE, Smith-Lemli-Opitz	Varies; mutations in *CDKN1C* (IMAGe), *SAMD1* (MIRAGE), DHCR7 (Smith-Lemli-Opitz)	Genetic testing
ACTH resistance	ACTH receptor or melanocortin 2 receptor accessory protein (MRAP) gene mutations	Genetic testing

ACTH, Adrenocorticotropic hormone; *CMV*, cytomegalovirus; *ELISA*, enzyme-linked immunosorbent assay; *HIV*, human immunodeficiency virus; *IMAGe*, intrauterine growth restriction, metaphyseal dysplasia, adrenal hypoplasia congenita, genital abnormalities; *PPD*, purified protein derivative; *VLCFA*, very long chain fatty acid.

cough with tuberculosis. In patients with central adrenal insufficiency, the presence of midline facial defects can suggest structural abnormalities of the pituitary, and poor growth or pubertal progression may reflect a more global disorder of the anterior pituitary gland.

Evaluation and Management
Laboratory Studies
Clinical diagnosis of adrenal insufficiency can be confirmed biochemically by demonstrating inappropriately low cortisol secretion. Testing to determine whether the adrenal insufficiency is primary or central and evaluating for the underlying cause should be completed.

In primary adrenal insufficiency, there is elevated serum ACTH and low cortisol, along with the classic electrolyte abnormalities of hyponatremia and hyperkalemia. An elevated plasma renin activity level and low aldosterone in the presence of hyponatremia or shock indicates concomitant mineralocorticoid deficiency. Conversely, in central adrenal insufficiency, laboratories will demonstrate low ACTH levels. These patients do not have mineralocorticoid deficiency because although lack of appropriate ACTH stimulation leads to atrophy of the zona fasciculata and reticularis, the zona glomerulosa, under independent control of the renin-angiotensin system, is unaffected and aldosterone secretion is preserved. Other pituitary hormone deficiencies also may be seen.

The gold standard test for diagnosis of primary adrenal insufficiency, as determined by the Endocrine Society, is the ACTH stimulation test. The ACTH stimulation test is performed with synthetic corticotropin administered intravenously at a standard dose of 250 µg for adults and children 2 years of age and older or 15 µg/kg for infants. Serum samples

for cortisol are collected at baseline and after stimulation. Peak cortisol levels below 500 nmol/L (18 µg/dL) (collected at either 30 or 60 minutes) indicate adrenal insufficiency. A baseline ACTH level also should be obtained. In patients with confirmed cortisol deficiency, a plasma ACTH greater than twofold the upper limit of the reference range is consistent with primary adrenal insufficiency. Simultaneous measurement of plasma renin and aldosterone to determine the presence of mineralocorticoid deficiency is also recommended. A low-dose (1 µg) corticotropin test with baseline and stimulated cortisol and ACTH levels is preferred for the diagnosis of secondary adrenal insufficiency or recovery from adrenal suppression.

If a corticotropin stimulation test is not feasible, a basal serum cortisol level at 8 AM in combination with ACTH level is recommended (cortisol secretion has diurnal variation and peaks in early morning). For patients in critical condition, a cortisol level should be drawn before administering steroids. A cortisol level less than 140 nmol/L (5 µg/dL) is highly suggestive of adrenal insufficiency; levels greater than 500 nmol/L (18 µg/dL) strongly support sufficient adrenal function. Borderline results necessitate further testing.

Once samples are obtained, suspected adrenal insufficiency should be treated with glucocorticoids while awaiting results. Analyses to determine the underlying cause of adrenal insufficiency should be pursued after the child is stabilized. Common tests include very long chain fatty acids (for adrenoleukodystrophy), adrenal antibodies (for autoimmune adrenalitis), genetic testing, purified protein derivative (PPD) placement (for tuberculosis), and human immunodeficiency virus (HIV) testing (for acquired immunodeficiency syndrome [AIDS]). For patients with suspected central adrenal insufficiency, magnetic

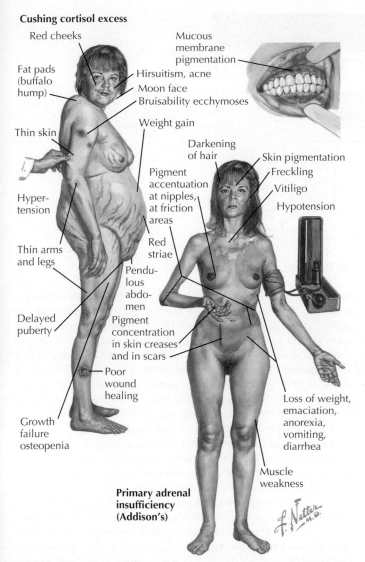

Cushing cortisol excess

Red cheeks

Fat pads (buffalo hump)

Thin skin

Hyper-tension

Thin arms and legs

Delayed puberty

Growth failure osteopenia

Mucous membrane pigmentation

Hirsuitism, acne

Moon face

Bruisability ecchymoses

Weight gain

Darkening of hair

Pigment accentuation at nipples, at friction areas

Red striae

Pendulous abdomen

Pigment concentration in skin creases and in scars

Poor wound healing

Skin pigmentation

Freckling

Vitiligo

Hypotension

Loss of weight, emaciation, anorexia, vomiting, diarrhea

Muscle weakness

Primary adrenal insufficiency (Addison's)

Fig. 49.3 Signs and Symptoms of Primary Adrenal Insufficiency and Cushing Syndrome.

resonance imaging (MRI) of the pituitary gland and hypothalamus, and testing for other pituitary deficiencies (growth hormone, thyroid-stimulating hormone, and gonadotropins) is indicated.

Treatment and Prognosis

Treatment of adrenal insufficiency centers on appropriate replacement of cortisol and aldosterone as necessary. Treatment is divided into maintenance (daily needs) and stress coverage (for illness or other physical stress). Maintenance doses of hydrocortisone are adjusted to provide 8 to 10 mg/m^2 in three to four divided doses. Tablets should be used and can be crushed and mixed with liquids immediately before administration, because commercial suspensions of hydrocortisone are unreliable. In specific cases, liquid prednisolone can replace hydrocortisone.

In secondary and iatrogenic adrenal insufficiency, the adrenal glands continue to produce modest amounts of hormone; maintenance corticosteroids may not be needed, but stress steroids are necessary. Symptoms such as abnormal fatigue and lethargy may suggest underdosing, and increased weight gain and decreased height velocity may suggest overtreatment. Hydrocortisone is the preferred

glucocorticoid because it confers fewer side effects than more potent steroids. Children with confirmed aldosterone deficiency require treatment with fludrocortisone starting at 100 μg/day, and infants often require sodium chloride supplements.

All patients with proven or assumed adrenal insufficiency should be instructed in the use of stress dose steroids for illness, injury, or other physical stress. Instructions for both oral and intramuscular stress dosing should be given and reviewed regularly. During stress, a tripling of the maintenance dosage (i.e., 25 mg/m^2/day) can be given orally in three divided doses. In the event of vomiting, lethargy, or other conditions precluding oral intake, an intramuscular injection of hydrocortisone at a dose of 50 to 100 mg/m^2 should be administered and the child should be brought to the hospital for evaluation. In hospital settings, stress coverage for surgery or critical illness consists of an initial dose of 100 mg/m^2 of hydrocortisone intravenously or intramuscularly and then 100 mg/m^2/day intravenously divided every 4 to 6 hours until recovery, at which time maintenance doses can be resumed. For a child presenting in extremis with suspected adrenal insufficiency, baseline diagnostic laboratory studies and resuscitation with dextrose containing isotonic fluids and glucocorticoid steroids should be initiated immediately.

CUSHING SYNDROME

Etiology and Pathogenesis

Glucocorticoid excess caused by oversecretion of ACTH from a pituitary corticotrope adenoma is called Cushing disease. Cushing syndrome is the general term for glucocorticoid excess of any nonpituitary cause, including ectopic ACTH production, adrenal disease, and exogenous glucocorticoid use. Endogenous Cushing syndrome is rare, with a global incidence of 0.7 to 2.4 per million people per year, of which only 10% occur in children.

Clinical Presentation

Signs and symptoms of glucocorticoid excess include weight gain with decreased growth velocity, fatigue, hypertension, glucose intolerance, and delayed puberty (Fig. 49.3). Osteopenia, acne, facial plethora, hirsutism, a dorsocervical fat pad, and striae can occur. Hyperandrogenism and virilization can indicate an adrenal carcinoma. Exogenous Cushing syndrome may be obvious with a prolonged history of glucocorticoid use.

Evaluation and Management

Documenting loss of diurnal rhythm of cortisol secretion or excessive production of cortisol supports the diagnosis of Cushing syndrome. Options include measurements of free cortisol in a 24-hour urine collection (normal, <40 to 50 μg/day), 11 PM salivary cortisol (normal, <145 ng/dL), or serum cortisol before 9 AM after administration of 1 mg of dexamethasone at 11 PM the evening before (normal, <1.8 μg/dL). Abnormal results should be confirmed by repeating one or more of these tests, because false positive results are common. ACTH measurements should be performed, and a high-dose dexamethasone suppression test can be used to distinguish between ACTH-dependent and ACTH-independent Cushing syndrome (Fig. 49.4).

Pituitary MRI with gadolinium can be used to visualize small adenomas. If the MRI is inconclusive, the best test to confirm the presence or absence of an ACTH-secreting pituitary tumor is petrosal sinus sampling. In this procedure, the inferior petrosal sinuses are catheterized, and blood is sampled for ACTH before and after administration of CRH. Adrenal masses can be identified using ultrasonography or computed tomography (CT).

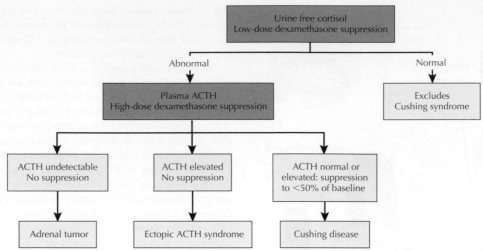

Fig. 49.4 Outline of Tests for the Differential Diagnosis of Cushing Syndrome.

Treatment options include surgery to resect pituitary or adrenal lesions, or chemotherapy to block secretion of adrenal hormones.

CONGENITAL ADRENAL HYPERPLASIA

Etiology and Pathogenesis

Congenital adrenal hyperplasia (CAH) is a group of disorders characterized by defective adrenal steroid synthesis; accumulation of androgenic steroid intermediates; and, variably, cortisol and mineralocorticoid deficiency. The most common form of CAH is caused by homozygous mutation of the *CYP21* gene that encodes 21-hydroxylase, the enzyme that catalyzes the conversion of 17-hydroxyprogesterone to 11-deoxycortisol and the conversion of progesterone to deoxycorticosterone (Fig. 49.1). The absence (or severe deficiency) of 21-hydroxylase results in a deficiency of cortisol and aldosterone.

Clinical Presentation

Deficiency of 21-hydroxylase activity classically manifests as a salt-wasting adrenal crisis during the second week of life; 46 XX females can have varying degrees of virilization with genital ambiguity. Affected children can also present later in childhood with premature development of pubic hair, penile enlargement in boys, or as infertility or a polycystic ovary syndrome (PCOS)-like syndrome in women (Fig. 49.5).

Differential Diagnosis

In infants presenting with shock, the differential includes sepsis, cardiac or metabolic disease, and trauma. Ambiguous genitalia in newborns also can be due to in utero exposure to sex hormones, androgenic enzyme inhibitors, gonadal steroid synthesis defects, or isolated or syndromic malformation of genitals from nonendocrine causes. CAH and late-onset CAH can manifest in childhood or later as virilization and precocious pubarche and must be considered in the context of a differential diagnosis that includes virilizing tumors, particularly adrenal carcinoma, exogenous androgen exposure, or PCOS.

Evaluation and Management

The diagnosis of CAH requires biochemical testing and confirmation through genetic analyses. Newborn screening programs throughout the United States enable early diagnosis of 21-hydroxylase deficiency and timely institution of hormone therapy to prevent life-threatening adrenal crisis. These programs assay 17-hydroxyprogesterone in blood spots and use normal ranges adjusted for gestational age. Patients with abnormal newborn screen results should be referred to a pediatric endocrinologist immediately for confirmatory testing, including measurement of serum levels of adrenal steroid intermediates and cortisol. A high-dose ACTH stimulation test may be required to distinguish between less severe late-onset CAH, and genetic analysis of CYP21 (or CYP11) should be considered to confirm the diagnosis.

Adrenal crisis in patients with CAH requires urgent treatment, as described earlier. Long-term management requires treatment with glucocorticoids to prevent adrenal crisis and suppress overproduction of adrenal steroid intermediates. Suppression of excess adrenal androgens is critical to stop virilization and prevent accelerated skeletal maturation that may compromise adult height. Glucocorticoid doses must be titrated carefully, because overtreatment can suppress growth and cause Cushing syndrome. Hydrocortisone is the preferred oral glucocorticoid because of its shorter half-life and lower growth-suppressing effect. Patients with classic CAH require mineralocorticoid replacement with fludrocortisone to prevent salt wasting and allow reduction in glucocorticoid dose.

In females with CAH who have virilized genitalia, parents should be informed about surgical options, including delaying surgery until the child is older or forgoing surgery altogether. Genital surgery should be performed only in centers with experienced pediatric multidisciplinary teams.

FUTURE DIRECTIONS

Glucocorticoid replacement therapy for adrenal insufficiency has remained unchanged for over 50 years, and this population still experiences high mortality and morbidity. New modified-release hydrocortisone preparations that more closely imitate natural circadian rhythms are being studied and will hopefully improve outcomes.

SUGGESTED READINGS

Available online.

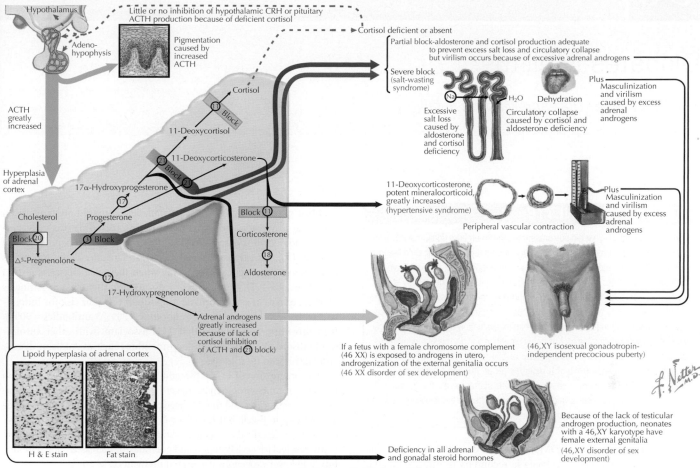

Hypothalamus

Little or no inhibition of hypothalamic CRH or pituitary
ACTH production because of deficient cortisol

Adeno-
hypophysis

Pigmentation
caused by
increased
ACTH

Cortisol deficient or absent

Partial block-aldosterone and cortisol production adequate
to prevent excess salt loss and circulatory collapse
but virilism occurs because of excessive adrenal androgens

Severe block
(salt-wasting
syndrome)

Na

H_2O

Dehydration

Plus
Masculinization
and virilism
caused by excess
adrenal
androgens

ACTH
greatly
increased

Cortisol

Block

11-Deoxycortisol

Excessive
salt loss
caused by
aldosterone
and cortisol
deficiency

Circulatory collapse
caused by cortisol and
aldosterone deficiency

11-Deoxycorticosterone

Hyperplasia
of adrenal
cortex

Block

17α-Hydroxyprogesterone

11-Deoxycorticosterone,
potent mineralocorticoid,
greatly increased
(hypertensive syndrome)

Plus
Masculinization
and virilism
caused by excess
adrenal
androgens

Cholesterol

Progesterone

Block 11

Peripheral vascular contraction

Block 20

Block

Corticosterone

△⁵-Pregnenolone

Aldosterone

17-Hydroxypregnenolone

Adrenal androgens
(greatly increased
because of lack of
cortisol inhibition
of ACTH and 21 block)

Lipoid hyperplasia of adrenal cortex

If a fetus with a female chromosome complement
(46 XX) is exposed to androgens in utero,
androgenization of the external genitalia occurs
(46 XX disorder of sex development)

(46,XY isosexual gonadotropin-
independent precocious puberty)

H & E stain

Fat stain

Because of the lack of testicular
androgen production, neonates
with a 46,XY karyotype have
female external genitalia
(46,XY disorder of sex
development)

Deficiency in all adrenal
and gonadal steroid hormones

Fig. 49.5 Classic Congenital Adrenal Hyperplasia.

50

Diabetes Mellitus

Sandra Vazquez Diaz and Marissa J. Kilberg

 CLINICAL VIGNETTE

A previously healthy 5-year-old boy presents to the emergency department (ED) for evaluation of 1 day of vomiting and tachypnea. Parent reports that the child "seems thirsty all the time" and has been urinating more frequently for the past 2 weeks. The parent also states that he was previously potty-trained, but recently started having "accidents" at night. This morning he complained of nausea and abdominal pain followed by two episodes of emesis. His parent noticed he was tired-appearing and breathing fast and brought him for evaluation. In the ED, his physical examination was remarkable for Kussmaul breathing and dry mucous membranes. Laboratory tests revealed a blood glucose of 554 mg/dL, β-hydroxybutyrate 4.8 mmol/L (reference range 0.1 to 1.0 mmol/L), pH of 7.0, and bicarbonate of 6.7 mmol/L. He received a normal saline bolus, was started on an insulin drip with 1.5× maintenance intravenous fluids, and then admitted to the endocrine service for management of diabetic ketoacidosis.

The term diabetes mellitus (DM) is used to describe a group of disorders characterized by hyperglycemia secondary to impaired insulin action. DM may arise from insulin secretion defects, insulin resistance, or other syndromic causes/combinations (Box 50.1). Type 1 DM (T1D), although accounting for only about 10% of all diabetes, is the most common type seen in pediatrics. However, the SEARCH for Diabetes in Youth study, a multicenter longitudinal study of individuals with youth-onset (diagnosed at younger than 20 years of age) T1D or type 2 DM (T2D) in the United States, has identified an increasing incidence of T2D. This chapter will emphasize T1D but will also provide relevant information regarding T2D.

ETIOLOGY AND PATHOGENESIS

Type 1 Diabetes Mellitus

T1D occurs in a bimodal distribution, with peaks at school age and again in early puberty. Males and females are affected equally. The overall incidence of T1D in the United States is 22 cases per 100,000 and continues to increase, making it the most common chronic disease of childhood.

T1D is thought to involve genetic susceptibility as demonstrated by increased risk for children with affected family members (first degree relative risk of ~8% and monozygotic twin risk of 35% to 65%) and an association with major histocompatibility complex (MHC) class II expressing human leukocyte antigen (HLA) DR3/4-DQ28. However, 85% of new-onset diabetes occurs in individuals with no family history. Other risks include certain viral infections such as enterovirus, coxsackie and congenital rubella, thought to be related to direct β-cell infection or molecular mimicry resulting in autoimmune β-cell damage. The influence of milk/gluten exposure, vitamin D deficiency, perinatal insults, microbiome differences or the protective nature of breast milk have been explored, but there is no conclusive evidence.

Most patients with T1D have circulating autoantibodies against a variety of pancreatic endocrine cell proteins, including islet cells, glutamic acid decarboxylase (GAD65), protein tyrosine phosphatase–like protein (IA2), zinc transporter 8 (ZnT8), and insulin. These antibodies can support the diagnosis, especially when there is a clinical question of T1D versus T2D. Antibodies are also used in the research setting as markers of risk in asymptomatic individuals (10-year risk for individuals with: 1 antibody = 30%, 2 antibodies = 70%, 3 antibodies = 90%). It is also important to note that T1D associates with other autoimmune disorders, including endocrinopathies such as Addison disease and Hashimoto thyroiditis.

The progression of T1D is thought to involve a genetic predisposition followed by an environmental trigger (second "hit") resulting in infiltration by lymphocytes and macrophages and development of autoantibodies resulting in β-cell, but not α- or δ-cell, destruction. This progressive β-cell loss is described in "stages." Patients identified at earlier stages have better residual islet cell function and potential for increased "honeymoon" time and lower exogenous insulin requirements (Fig. 50.1).

DM ultimately results from defective insulin action, making an appreciation of this anabolic polypeptide hormone's normal function essential to understanding this disorder. Insulin works to regulate the body's glucose levels by stimulating the uptake of glucose in the muscle, liver, and fat while inhibiting hepatic gluconeogenesis. Additionally, insulin stimulates lipogenesis, inhibits lipolysis, and stimulates protein synthesis (Fig. 50.2). Thus insulin deficiency results in impaired glucose usage, leading to hyperglycemia and increased lipolysis leading to ketosis. This essentially replicates the starvation state despite presence of food intake and normal to elevated glucose concentration (Fig. 50.3). Hyperglycemia, specifically once blood glucose is about 160 to 180 mg/dL, results in glucosuria because the renal threshold for glucose reabsorption has been exceeded. This osmotic diuresis results in polyuria and subsequent polydipsia. Eventually, dehydration occurs with potential for circulatory compromise and lactic acidosis. Glucosuria is accompanied by renal loss of other electrolytes such as sodium, potassium, phosphorus, magnesium, and calcium. Furthermore, with continued impaired insulin action, ketone body accumulation leads to an anion gap metabolic acidosis known as diabetic ketoacidosis (DKA). Metabolic acidosis and dehydration also stimulate counterregulatory hormones, such as growth hormone, cortisol, and epinephrine, further antagonizing insulin action.

Although DKA can occur in patients with known T1D, specifically in the case of illness or insulin omission/failure, it is most commonly seen in patients with new-onset diabetes.

Type 2 Diabetes Mellitus

The prevalence of T2D continues to increase in pediatrics, owing in part to insulin resistance from obesity and insulin secretion defects of possible epigenetic causes. The incidence is significantly higher in Native Americans, non-Hispanic Blacks, and Hispanic individuals,

BOX 50.1 Diabetes Mellitus Types

Type 1 Diabetes
- Immune mediated
- Idiopathic

Type 2 Diabetes
Other Types
- Genetic forms: β-cell defects
  - Monogenic diabetes of the young
  - Mitochondrial disease
- Genetic forms: insulin action defects
  - Donohue syndrome (formerly leprechaunism)
  - Rabson-Mendenhall syndrome
  - Type A insulin resistance
  - Lipoatrophic diabetes
- Exocrine pancreas defects
  - Pancreatitis
  - Hemochromatosis
  - Pancreatectomy
- Endocrinopathies
  - Cushing syndrome
  - Pheochromocytoma
  - Hyperthyroidism
- Drug or chemical induced
  - Glucocorticoids
  - Diazoxide
  - Tacrolimus
  - β-Adrenergic agonists
  - Pentamidine
  - Nicotinic acid
  - Vacor
  - Phenytoin
  - Thiazides
- Infections
  - Congenital rubella
  - Cytomegalovirus
- Other genetic syndromes associated with diabetes
  - Cystic fibrosis–related diabetes
  - Down syndrome
  - Turner syndrome
  - Klinefelter syndrome
  - Prader-Willi syndrome
  - Friedreich ataxia
  - Wolfram syndrome
  - Myotonic dystrophy
  - Lawrence-Moon-Biedl syndrome
  - Alstrom syndrome
- Uncommon forms of immune-mediated
  - "Stiff man" syndrome
  - Anti-insulin receptor antibodies
- Gestational diabetes

Adapted from American Diabetes Association. 13. Children and adolescents: standards of medical care in diabetes—2020. *Diabetes Care.* 2020;43(suppl 1):S163-S182.

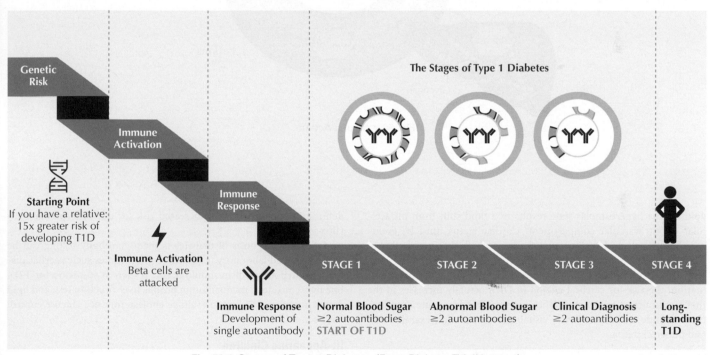

Fig. 50.1 Stages of Type 1 Diabetes. (From DiabetesTrialNet.org.)

and these groups are also disproportionately affected by the trend of increased incidence. Other risk factors include family history, sedentary lifestyles, and female sex.

Insulin resistance can initially be compensated with increased insulin secretion, but ultimately there is an imbalance of supply and demand. Consequently, presentation of T2D is often during puberty, a time of increased insulin resistance.

CLINICAL PRESENTATION

Type 1 Diabetes

Given the progressive nature of β-cell dysfunction (Fig. 50.1), the presentation of T1D can be quite variable from hyperglycemia detected on

laboratory assay in the absence of symptoms to the most feared, life-threatening DKA. The majority of children with diabetes present with symptoms such as polyuria (with nocturia and/or secondary enuresis), polydipsia, polyphagia with weight loss instead of gain, dehydration, abdominal pain, vomiting, blurry vision, or lethargy (Table 50.1).

Physical examination (Table 50.2) begins with evaluation of a patient's airway, breathing, and circulation. In DKA one will notice hyperventilation known as Kussmaul breathing (deep, labored breathing) and circulatory system impairment (tachycardia, hypotension, and delayed capillary refill). Less severe signs of dehydration may include dry mucous membranes and sunken eyes. It is important to note that the physical examination will likely underestimate the degree of dehydration because of an initial preservation of the intravascular

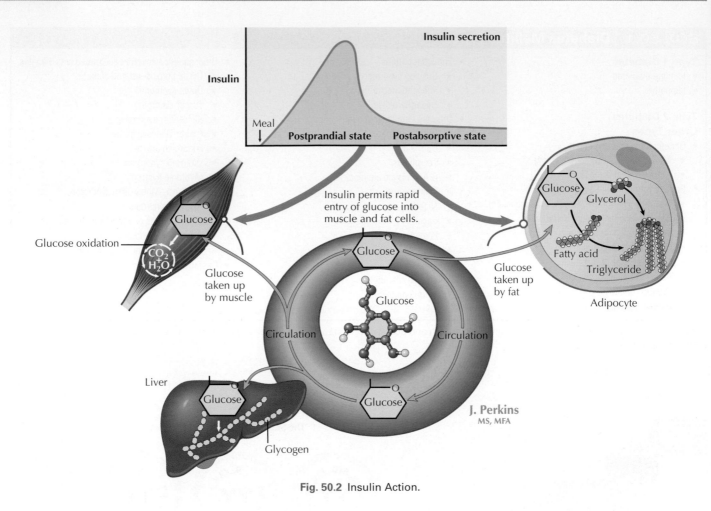

Fig. 50.2 Insulin Action.

volume; the hyperosmolar state results in a fluid shift from intracellular to intravascular compartment. Cardiac status must be evaluated because electrolyte abnormalities confer risk for an arrhythmia. Although patients may present with altered mental status in the early stages of DKA, one should not be reassured by an initial normal examination; the risk for cerebral edema in DKA actually increases in the first few hours of treatment. Other essential but less acute examinations include anthropometrics, visual assessment, skin examination, and pubertal status.

Type 2 Diabetes

Similar to T1D, T2D varies in presentation from asymptomatic hyperglycemia to DKA or hyperglycemic, hyperosmolar syndrome (HHS). In fact, T2D manifests more acutely and with DKA far more frequently in pediatrics than adults. The previously mentioned assessment and examination apply similarly to T2D, but one may also note signs of insulin resistance, including obesity (particularly central adiposity) and acanthosis nigricans.

Initial Evaluation
Well-Appearing Children

Evaluation may consist of a basic metabolic panel, urinalysis, C-peptide and insulin (if not already administered) concentration, and hemoglobin A1c (HbA1c). Oral glucose tolerance testing can be used for T2D diagnosis. The American Diabetes Association (ADA) has established definitions for diabetes and increased risk for diabetes (prediabetes) (Box 50.2).

Once the diagnosis of diabetes is made, antibody testing can be considered and laboratory testing for comorbidities such as celiac disease and hypothyroidism should occur. If there is suspicion for T2D, one may consider a microalbumin profile, liver function test, and lipid panel; however, it is best to evaluate cholesterol once glucose control has been established.

Ill-Appearing Children

In addition to the aforementioned tests, these patients require a comprehensive metabolic panel (including liver function tests, calcium, magnesium, phosphorus), venous blood gas, and complete blood count (CBC) with differential. DKA is present when a patient has marked hyperglycemia (glucose >300 mg/dL), ketonemia or ketonuria, and acidosis (pH <7.3 and bicarbonate <15 mmol/L).

In this insulin deficient state, hypokalemia and hypophosphatemia are common, resulting from the osmotic diuresis and loss through the kidneys. This may be compounded by increased aldosterone secondary to dehydration and enteral losses as a result of emesis. Importantly, the laboratory values may not fully reflect the degree of whole body and intracellular depletion because the intravascular concentration may be normal or even slightly high because of the acidosis and insulin deficiency (promoting efflux of these ions from the cell into the blood). In the case of potassium abnormalities (high or low), electrocardiography

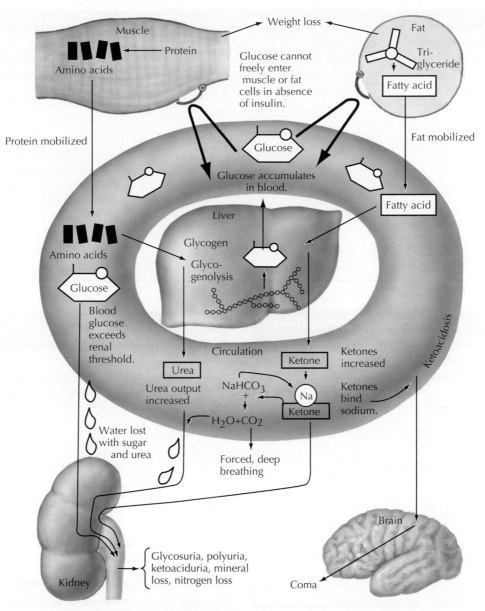

Fig. 50.3 Insulin Deprivation.

TABLE 50.1	Etiology and Differential Diagnosis for the Presenting Signs and Symptoms of Diabetes	
Presenting Sign/Symptom	**Etiology**	**Differential Diagnosis**
Polyuria	Hyperglycemia exceeding renal threshold	Diabetes insipidus, urinary tract infection, psychogenic polydipsia
Glycosuria	Hyperglycemia exceeding renal threshold	Benign renal glycosuria, Fanconi syndrome
Polydipsia	Secondary to polyuria	Diabetes insipidus, psychogenic polydipsia
Polyphagia	Increased metabolic demand	Hyperthyroidism
Weight loss	Proteolysis and lipolysis	Anorexia nervosa, inflammatory bowel disease, celiac disease, infectious etiologies, hyperthyroidism
Abdominal pain/vomiting	Ketonemia, occasionally pancreatitis	Gastroenteritis, inflammatory bowel disease, appendicitis, toxic ingestion, pancreatitis
Blurry vision	Hyperglycemia and fluid compartment shifts	Migraine, near/farsightedness
Respiratory distress	Kussmaul breathing as compensation for metabolic acidosis	Pneumonia, asthma exacerbation
Hyperglycemia	Insulin deficiency	Stress-induced hyperglycemia, medication-induced hyperglycemia

TABLE 50.2   Physical Examination and Interpretation in New-Onset Diabetes Mellitus

Physical Examination	Findings	Interpretation
General	Alert and interactive → obtunded	Obtain a glucose measurement immediately on any patient presenting with altered mental status
Head, Eyes, Ears, Nose, Throat	Dry mucous membranes, blurred vision, fruity odor to breath	Diuresis resulting in dehydration Hyperglycemia resulting in blurred vision Ketosis resulting in fruity odor to breath
Cardiovascular	Tachycardia	Indicative of dehydration
Lungs	Kussmaul respirations	Deep, sighing breaths used as respiratory compensation for metabolic acidosis Lungs are clear to auscultation, indicating the absence of an underlying lung pathology
Abdomen	Diffuse abdominal tenderness	Ileus may result from ketosis and can mislead the diagnosis toward an acute abdominal process
Extremities	Delayed capillary refill, decreased skin turgor	Indicative of dehydration
Skin	Candidal infection	Yeast buildup as a result of hyperglycemia

---

BOX 50.2   American Diabetes Association Criteria for Diagnosis of Diabetes

Criteria for Diagnosis of Diabetes

1. Random blood glucose ≥200 mg/dL *and* symptoms of diabetes
   or
2. Fasting plasma glucose ≥126 mg/dL[a]
   or
3. 2-h glucose ≥200 mg/dL on an OGTT[a]
   or
4. HbA1c ≥6.5% (must be performed using NGSP-certified method, standardized to DCCT assay)[a]

Criteria for Diagnosis of Prediabetes

1. Fasting blood glucose: 100–125 mg/dL (impaired fasting glucose)
   or
2. 2-h plasma glucose 140–199 mg/dL during a standard OGTT (impaired glucose tolerance)
   or
3. HbA1c = 5.7%–6.4%

[a] In absence of obvious hyperglycemia, confirm by repeat testing.
DCCT, Diabetes Control and Complications Trial; *NGSP,* National Glycohemoglobin Standardization Program; *OGTT,* glucose tolerance test.
Adapted from American Diabetes Association. Type 1 diabetes in children and adolescents: a position statement by the American Diabetes Association. *Diabetes Care.* 2018;41(9):2026-2044.

BOX 50.3   Risk Factors Associated With the Development of Cerebral Edema

- Age younger than 3 years
- Severe acidosis (pH <7.1, bicarbonate <5 mmol/L)
- Severe dehydration (elevated blood urea nitrogen)
- Severe hyperosmolarity (corrected sodium >155 mmol/L, glucose >1000 mg/dL)
- Longer duration of symptoms
- New-onset diabetes
- Intravenous insulin bolus, insulin in first hour of treatment
- Bicarbonate bolus
- Too rapid or too slow of changes in electrolyte

---

should be performed immediately. Dilutional hyponatremia may result because of hyperglycemia, although actual sodium concentration may be normal or elevated from dehydration. One can "correct" the sodium value for interpretation by adding 1.6 mEq/L to the measured sodium for every 100 mg/dL of glucose over 100 mg/dL.

Cerebral edema is the most concerning complication of DKA, with a 0.5% to 1% incidence in the United States but a 20% to 25% mortality rate. It is poorly understood with many of the associated risk factors derived from confounded case control studies (Box 50.3). Cerebral edema can be identified on presentation, in the first 12 hours of treatment or even up to 48 hours of treatment. Current understanding suggests injury is related to cerebral hypoperfusion and reperfusion (cytotoxic and vasogenic), and the most recent trials have not demonstrated differences based on rehydration rates.

If cerebral edema is suspected, head CT should be performed and appropriate treatment should ensue.

Diabetes Ketoacidosis Management

The three main components of initial management include treating dehydration with fluids, treating insulin deficiency with insulin, and repleting electrolytes as needed. Treatment begins with a normal saline bolus 20 mL/kg (maximum 1 L), followed by a continuous normal saline–containing infusion at a rate of 1.5 to 2 times the maintenance intravenous fluid rate. Insulin is given by intravenous infusion at a continuous rate of 0.1 unit/kg/h, 1 hour *after* fluid resuscitation, because early insulin initiation may be associated with cerebral edema. As treatment progresses and hyperglycemia resolves, dextrose-containing fluids should be added to allow continued insulin administration. Routine fluid repletion should contain extra potassium (once K is <6 mmol/L) and phosphorous, but additional oral or intravenous potassium phosphate boluses can be given as needed.

Sample DKA monitoring plan is reported in the following section (Table 50.3).

Post–Diabetic Ketoacidosis and Home Management
Type 1 Diabetes

Ideal management of children with T1D requires the expertise of a multidisciplinary team consisting of a pediatric endocrinologist, nurse educator, dietitian, child life specialist, and mental health professional. The treatment plan must be tailored to the child's emotional and cognitive development, social and environmental factors, and pubertal changes.

The goals of therapy are to preserve normal growth and development, promote high quality of life and minimize the risk for acute and long-term complications. HbA1c targets should be individualized, ideally reaching near normal values while avoiding hypoglycemia and excessive burden of care. Previously, the ADA recommended less strict HbA1c guidelines for children because of the risk for hypoglycemia, but with improved diabetes technology for insulin delivery (insulin analogs and pumps) and monitoring (continuous glucose monitor [CGM]), a target of less than 7% can be safely recommended for many children. Less strict targets (<7.5%) are appropriate for children who cannot articulate symptoms of hypoglycemia, have hypoglycemia unawareness, have a history of severe hypoglycemia, or have limited resources.

Insulin replacement therapy is essential in all patients with T1D and is intended to imitate normal physiologic patterns. Normally, plasma insulin levels are low during the fasting and overnight periods and rapidly increase in the postprandial state. A combination of rapid- and long-acting insulin preparations (basal bolus) by multiple daily injections are used to mimic these patterns; furthermore, continuous subcutaneous insulin infusion (insulin pump) can provide the most physiologic insulin replacement therapy (Fig. 50.4). Many insulin formulations are available for pediatric use and are shown in Table 50.4.

Although the previously mentioned basal bolus and pump therapy are currently considered the standard of care, the "mixed-split" regimen was historically used in children to minimize the number of daily injections. This consists of fixed doses of a short-acting insulin mixed in the same syringe with an intermediate-acting analog, given twice daily—one injection with breakfast and one with dinner. Although no longer considered the ideal treatment regimen, it can be used in the setting of unique social or economic circumstances, for example, when a caregiver is not available to provide multiple injections or when a simpler regimen might improve adherence.

Establishment of the initial insulin total daily dose (TDD) must be personalized and depends on many factors such as patient age, clinical presentation, weight, stage of puberty, etc. In general, most prepubertal children require 0.7 to 1 units/kg/day, whereas adolescents, who are experiencing a physiologic phase of insulin resistance, require above 1 and as high as 2 units/kg/day. Consideration should be given to the "honeymoon phase," which refers to the period soon after diagnosis, characterized by endogenous insulin secretion from remaining pancreatic β-cells

TABLE 50.3 Sample Diabetic Ketoacidosis Monitoring Plan

Parameter	Frequency
Point of care glucose (glucometer)	Hourly
BMP, Mg, Phos	Every 2 h
Neurologic checks	Hourly in emergency/intensive care unit
Venous blood gas	Every 2 h until pH >7.0
Urine ketones (serum BOHB if available)	Every 2 h
Intake and output	Hourly

BMP, Basic metabolic panel; *BOHB*, β-hydroxybutyrate; *Mg*, magnesium; *Phos*, phosphorus.

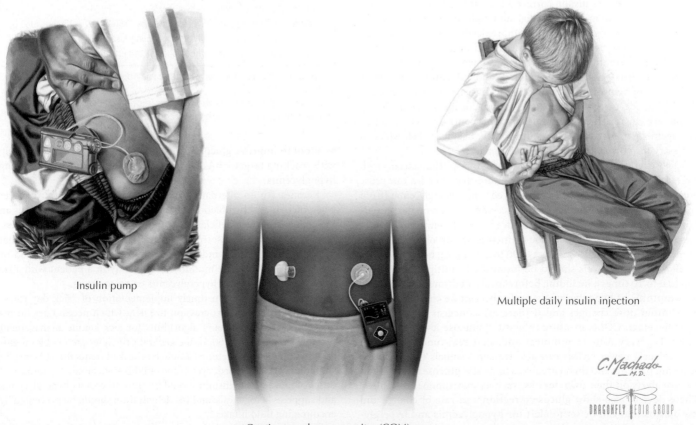

Insulin pump

Continuous glucose monitor (CGM)

Multiple daily insulin injection

Fig. 50.4 Insulin Delivery Methods.

TABLE 50.4   Pharmacokinetic Profiles of Insulin Analogs

Insulin Type (Brand Name)	Onset of Action (h)	Peak of Action (h)	Duration of Action (h)
Ultra-Rapid Acting			
Faster Aspart (Fiasp)	0.1–0.2	1–3	3–5
Rapid-Acting			
Aspart (Novolog)	0.25–0.5	1–3	3–5
Lispro (Humalog)	0.25–0.5	1–3	3–5
Glulisine (Apidra)	0.25–0.5	1–3	3–5
Short-Acting			
Regular	0.5–1	2–4	5–8
Intermediate-Acting			
NPH	2–4	4–8	12–18
Long-Acting			
Detemir (Levemir)	2–4	None	12–24
Glargine (Lantus, Basaglar, Toujeo)	2–4	None	22–24
Degludec (Tresiba)	2–4	None	>24

NPH, Neutral protamine Hagedorn.

and in most cases lower insulin requirements (<0.5 units/kg/day). This stage lasts on average 7 to 9 months and up to 24 months.

In a basal bolus regimen, the basal insulin represents 30% to 50% of the TDD and can be given either by 1 or 2 daily injections of long-acting insulin or by rapid-acting insulin delivered as the basal rate on an insulin pump. The bolus insulin consists of rapid-acting insulin administered by injection or the bolus function on an insulin pump. The insulin bolus doses have two components: (1) a prandial dose or insulin to carbohydrate ratio (ICR), which covers the amount of carbohydrates (in grams) in each meal or snack; and (2) a dose to correct hyperglycemia or insulin correction/sensitivity factor (ISF). Ideal insulin administration is preprandial, although considerations can be made for very young children with unpredictable eating. Regardless, the blood glucose used for correction should be taken before eating commences. An example of a basal bolus regimen is shown in Box 50.4.

Individualized nutrition evaluation and education encompass a vital component of the treatment plan. Initial nutrition education should include carbohydrate counting and pre-meal insulin dosing as they are key in achieving optimal glycemic control. Overall, dietary management must consist of a nutritionally balanced diet, which is necessary for normal growth and development.

Daily exercise is recommended for all children and adolescents with T1D. Patients and families should be aware that exercise can cause both hypoglycemia (immediate or delayed) and hyperglycemia (from an adrenaline effect). Families should receive education on the prevention and management of exercise-induced hypoglycemia with strategies such as reducing insulin dose or increasing carbohydrate intake to maintain a blood glucose target of 90 to 250 mg/dL before exercise.

Blood glucose levels should be monitored multiple times daily (up to 6 to 10 times), including before meals, bedtime, with exercise or symptoms of hypoglycemia. Levels also can be checked at 2 AM with initial dose changes and if there are concerns for overnight hypoglycemia. CGMs measure interstitial glucose levels at regular intervals (every 5 to 15 minutes) and send real-time readings to a "receiver"; newer CGMs can also transmit signals to a "cloud," allowing patients and their caregivers to review glucose tracings and receive alerts on their own devices, such as smartphones or tablets. These devices also show glucose direction and rate of change and use alarms that can be set to alert for hypoglycemia and hyperglycemia. Most CGMs are self-inserted subcutaneously and last 6 to 14 days. A real-time CGM should be considered in youth with T1D

BOX 50.4   Basal Bolus Regimen Example for a 40-kg Child

Total daily dose (TDD) = 40 units (1 unit/kg/day)

Basal insulin = 50% of TDD = 20 units of long-acting insulin (e.g., Glargine) given once per day[a] (usually at bedtime) *or* 0.8 units per hour of rapid-acting insulin (e.g., Aspart) as basal rate on insulin pump.

Bolus insulin

- Insulin-to-carbohydrate ratio (ICR) calculated by the "500 rule" = 500 divided by TDD = 500/40 = Use 1 unit of rapid-acting insulin for every 12 g of carbohydrates in every meal or snack.
- Insulin sensitivity factor (ISF) calculated by "1800 rule" = 1800 divided by TDD = 1800/40 = Use 1 unit of rapid-acting insulin to lower 45 points of blood glucose above the target blood glucose (generally 100 mg/dL[b]).

[a] In younger children long-acting dose may divided in half and administered every 12 hours.
[b] May use higher target blood glucose (e.g., 120 mg/dL) in younger children or if concerns for hypoglycemia.

---

as a tool to improve glucose control, because it can effectively help with reaching target HbA1c, increasing time in range and reducing hypoglycemia.

Ketones are an alternative energy source produced by the liver when there is a lack of blood glucose from insufficient intake, or as an indication of insulin deficiency. Additionally, during an acute illness, there is a physiological secretion of counterregulatory hormones that increase blood glucose and ketogenesis. For these reasons, blood or urine ketones should be monitored frequently in a patient with T1D when there is prolonged hyperglycemia or acute illness.

Educating families on timely implementation of "sick day rules" is essential to prevent progression to DKA, which necessitates hospitalization. There are many algorithms for sick/ketone management (sample shown in Box 50.5); the general principles are (1) blood glucose and blood/urine ketones should be checked frequently; (2) insulin should never be stopped, even if the child is not eating; (3) additional doses of rapid-acting insulin should be given to correct hyperglycemia and suppress ketogenesis; and (4) dehydration should be prevented by encouraging fluid intake.

After the initial intensive education, patients and their families should have routine visits every 3 months for ongoing evaluation of

BOX 50.5   Sample Sick Day Management

1. Check blood glucose level every 3–4 hours while sick.
2. Give a correction factor dose (ISF) with rapid-acting insulin every 3–4 hours, even if not eating.
3. Check urine/blood ketones every 3–4 hours.
4. Encourage oral fluids: drink 1 ounce (30 mL) for every year of age per hour.
   - If glucose level is ≥200 mg/dL, give sugar-free fluids
   - If glucose level is <200 mg/dL, give sugar-containing fluids
5. In the presence of small or greater urine ketones or blood BOHB >1 mmol/L, check blood glucose, ketones and give ISF every 2 hours.

BOHB, β-Hydroxybutyrate; *ISF*, insulin sensitivity factor.

individual goals, home glucose data, glycemic control, insulin regimen, growth, and development. A crucial goal of ongoing diabetes education is independent self-management. With time and practice, families should be able to gain the confidence required to make independent day-to-day decisions about insulin doses, carbohydrate intake, and physical activity.

Type 2 Diabetes Mellitus

As in T1D, a multidisciplinary team is essential in the management of youth-onset T2D. The goals of treatment in T2D, including normoglycemia with minimal hypoglycemia and reduction of comorbidities, can be achieved by a combination of increased physical activity, decreased caloric intake, weight loss, and pharmacologic management. For most children and adolescents with T2D, a target HbA1c should be less than 7%. Compared with T1D, youth with T2D have a lower risk for hypoglycemia and greater risk for complications.

Lifestyle recommendations such as eating a balanced diet, daily exercise, and achieving a healthy weight must be endorsed from diagnosis. A family-centered approach to lifestyle modifications is crucial in pediatric T2D. Individualized dietary adjustments should be provided by a pediatric nutritionist. Common recommendations include reducing portion sizes, avoiding sugar-containing beverages, limiting high-fat foods, and increasing daily fruits and vegetables. Children and adolescents with T2D should be encouraged to participate in at least 60 minutes of daily moderate-to-vigorous physical activity. Non-academic screen time must be limited to less than 2 hours per day.

Pharmacologic therapy in youth with T2D is limited to three approved drugs: metformin, insulin, and liraglutide. Pharmacologic therapy should be started at time of diagnosis. The initial treatment modality is determined by symptoms, degree of hyperglycemia, and presence or absence of ketosis/ketoacidosis.

Metformin is the initial drug of choice in asymptomatic patients with HbA1c less than 8.5% and normal renal function. To decrease the common side effects of metformin (abdominal pain, diarrhea, or nausea), the usual recommendation is to start at a lower dose and gradually increase it to a maximum dose of 1000 mg twice daily given with food. Monitoring of kidney and liver function tests (comprehensive metabolic panel) and complete blood count are recommended while on treatment with metformin because of the rare side effects of lactic acidosis and megaloblastic anemia from vitamin B_{12} deficiency. Additionally, metformin should be withheld 48 hours before and after any procedures requiring intravenous contrast because of increased risk for lactic acidosis.

Patients without acidosis but significant hyperglycemia (blood glucose >250 mg/dL, HbA1c ≥8.5%), and symptoms of polyuria, polydipsia, nocturia and/or weight loss, require initial treatment with basal insulin while metformin is titrated to effect. If ketosis or ketoacidosis are present, metformin initiation should be delayed until resolution of acidosis. Patients who are meeting glycemic targets and were initially treated with insulin and metformin can begin to wean insulin over 2 to 6 weeks. On the other hand, if glycemic control is not achieved with metformin (± basal insulin), liraglutide, a glucagon-like peptide-1 receptor agonist, should be considered in pediatric patients 10 years old and older without a medical or family history of medullary thyroid carcinoma or multiple endocrine neoplasia type 2. The most common side effects of liraglutide are headaches, nausea, diarrhea, and vomiting that frequently manifest upon initiation and decrease over time. Patients and families should be counseled on the risk for hypoglycemia (especially if concomitant use of insulin), and therefore there is a need for frequent blood glucose monitoring and insulin reduction. Although rare, pancreatitis is another side effect of liraglutide that should be considered and evaluated if concerning signs or symptoms.

Complications and Comorbidities

Reducing the risk for acute and chronic complications is a major therapy goal in both pediatric T1D and T2D. Hypoglycemia (blood glucose <70 mg/dL) is the most common acute complication in patients with T1D and T2D if treated with insulin. Patients and their families must receive education on the presentation, prevention, and treatment of hypoglycemia. Mild hypoglycemia should be treated by the 15-15 rule. Patients should ingest 15 g of oral glucose (e.g., glucose tablets, sweetened beverages) and wait 15 minutes before retesting blood glucose. Target blood sugar is >70 mg/dL. The 15-15 rule should be repeated if this is not attained. Severe hypoglycemia requires treatment with glucagon. Families must have an emergency glucagon kit readily available and should be taught to administer intramuscular or subcutaneous glucagon in situations such as loss of consciousness or inability to tolerate oral glucose. Intranasal glucagon is a new alternative for severe hypoglycemia, approved for use in patients ages 4 and older.

Long-term complications of T1D and T2D are related to the noxious effects of chronic hyperglycemia, and present as microvascular disease (retinopathy, nephropathy, neuropathy) and macrovascular disease (coronary artery, cerebrovascular, and peripheral vascular disease). Once the child is 3 to 5 years from diagnosis, and pubertal or age 10 years (whichever is sooner), screening for microvascular and macrovascular diseases in children with T1D should begin. In youth-onset T2D, comorbidities may be found at diagnosis; therefore screening should commence at that time. Recommendations by the ADA for screening methods, initial timing, and frequency are shown in Table 50.5.

Because of the increased incidence of other autoimmune disorders in TID, screening for thyroid dysfunction and celiac disease should be considered soon after diagnosis and every 1 to 2 years.

Additional comorbidities in children with T2D are those associated with pediatric obesity, such as obstructive sleep apnea (OSA), nonalcoholic fatty liver disease (NAFLD), and polycystic ovary syndrome (PCOS). Screening for symptoms of OSA should be done at every visit, and, if present, referral to a pediatric sleep specialist is recommended. Annual measurement of liver function tests to evaluate for NAFLD should start at diagnosis. Evaluation for PCOS should be considered in female adolescents with menstrual irregularities, acne, or hirsutism.

FUTURE DIRECTIONS

Since the discovery of insulin in 1921, there have been countless advances in diabetes care. Automated insulin delivery systems are revolutionizing current diabetes management. These systems have three components: an insulin pump, a continuous glucose sensor, and an algorithm that controls insulin delivery. The majority use a "hybrid" approach, known as hybrid closed-loop, in which basal insulin is

TABLE 50.5   American Diabetes Association Screening Recommendations for Vascular Complications

Complication	Screening Method	Timing of Screening in T1D[a]
Nephropathy	Urinary albumin-to-creatinine ratio	Annually at puberty or ≥10 years (whichever sooner) once 5 years after diagnosis
Retinopathy	Fundal photography or mydriatic ophthalmoscopy	Annually at puberty or ≥11 years (whichever sooner) once 3–5 years after diagnosis
Neuropathy	History and physical examination Clinical tests (e.g., monofilament test, tuning fork test)	Annually at puberty or ≥10 years (whichever sooner) once 5 years after diagnosis
Macrovascular disease	BP, lipid profile	BP at each routine visit Lipid profile—near diagnosis (once glycemia improves) and age ≥2 years; at 9–11 years of age; and then at least every 3 years

[a]In T2D screening must start at diagnosis.
BP, Blood pressure; *T1D*, type 1 diabetes.

determined by the algorithm, but users are required to bolus for meals and snacks. In addition to more advanced closed-loop systems, dual-hormone systems (insulin and glucagon) are under development.

Stem cell–based therapy represents one of the most innovative approaches to cure T1D; nevertheless, results from clinical trials remain unsatisfactory. Another promising area of research in diabetes involves the use of immunomodulatory agents to prevent β-cell loss before or soon after the development of T1D.

Although our understanding of youth-onset T2D has significantly increased over the last decades, evidenced-based data are still limited regarding diagnostic and therapeutic modalities. Newer pediatric study designs have resulted in progress conducting research on drugs that are already approved in adults with T2D, providing hope for expanding the treatment options for T2D in youth.

Parallel to novel technological development, ongoing research is needed to better comprehend the complex epidemiology, pathophysiology, and complications and in addition to improve quality of life and long-term effects of pediatric diabetes.

SUGGESTED READINGS

Available online.

51

Hypoglycemia

Herodes Guzman and Katherine Lord

✳ **CLINICAL VIGNETTE**

A 3-year-old boy with a history of poorly controlled asthma requiring high-dose inhaled corticosteroids and frequent courses of oral steroids presents with altered mental status and hypoglycemia. The family reports that he was well until 2 days before admission, when he developed a fever, rhinorrhea, and anorexia. On the night before admission, he ate a smaller than normal dinner and then went to sleep without his usual bedtime snack. In the morning, his parents found him difficult to arouse and inappropriately answering questions. They took him to the emergency department, where he was found to have a blood glucose of 46 mg/dL. He was given a dextrose bolus and his glucose increased to 90 mg/dL. He was admitted to the hospital and underwent a diagnostic fasting test. A critical sample was obtained when his glucose was less than 50 mg/dL and a glucagon stimulation test was performed. His laboratory evaluation showed elevated β-hydroxybutyrate of 3.1 mmol/L, low cortisol of 2.1 mcg/dL, and no rise in his glucose after administration of glucagon. He underwent a low-dose adrenocorticotropic hormone stimulation test, which demonstrated a low peak cortisol of 9 mcg/dL. He was diagnosed with adrenal insufficiency secondary to steroid exposure. The family was instructed on administering stress dose hydrocortisone with illnesses and procedures. He had no further episodes of hypoglycemia.

Hypoglycemia is rare in children but carries significant consequences such as brain damage and death. The differential for hypoglycemia is large and requires a systematic approach. An accurate diagnosis allows for the timely initiation of disease-specific therapy that can prevent the long-term complications of seizures, developmental delays, and learning disabilities. In children, the most common cause of persistent hypoglycemia is hyperinsulinism (HI), a disorder affecting approximately 1 in 50,000 children.

ETIOLOGY AND PATHOGENESIS

In children, as in adults, blood glucose levels are maintained within a narrow range in both postprandial and fasting states. Thus normal fasting blood glucose levels should be above 70 mg/dL. A lower level of 50 mg/dL is recommended for diagnostic purposes only. Infants and children most commonly present with fasting hypoglycemia.

To recognize the different causes of hypoglycemia, it is helpful to understand the fundamentals of energy homeostasis (Fig. 51.1). In the fed state, as glucose levels increase, so do insulin levels. Insulin stimulates glucose uptake into cells for use as a source of energy or for storage. Insulin has other effects that influence energy metabolism. In the liver, insulin inhibits glycogenolysis, gluconeogenesis, and ketogenesis. In fat, insulin suppresses lipolysis. In the fasted state, insulin secretion is suppressed, allowing glycogenolysis and gluconeogenesis to commence, followed by fatty-acid oxidation, which leads to ketogenesis. In the absence of glucose, the brain uses ketones (e.g., β-hydroxybutyrate and acetoacetate) as energy sources. Additionally, suppression of insulin allows for increased secretion of counterregulatory hormones, glucagon, cortisol, growth hormone, and epinephrine, that maintain

blood glucose levels by stimulating glycogenolysis and gluconeogenesis. Disorders that impair insulin regulation and counterregulatory hormone secretion, as well as storage or production of glucose, can result in hypoglycemia.

CLINICAL PRESENTATION

The classic diagnostic triad of hypoglycemia, also known as Whipple's triad, consists of a documented low blood glucose, symptoms of hypoglycemia, and resolution of symptoms with normalization of the blood glucose level. The symptoms of hypoglycemia result from two different mechanisms. An adrenergic response, manifested by sweating, tremors, and nausea, typically is triggered in response to a rapid decrease in blood glucose. By contrast, the slower decline in blood glucose that occurs with fasting hypoglycemia may not trigger an obvious adrenergic response but can manifest as a loss of consciousness and seizure caused by neuroglycopenia (Fig. 51.2). Hypoglycemia in neonates can present with irritability, shakiness, difficulty feeding, hypothermia, pallor, hypotonia, and seizures. In children, symptoms include sweatiness, unsteadiness, headache, hunger, nausea, weakness, tachycardia, change in mentation, and seizures. It is important to note that infants and toddlers commonly do not manifest symptoms of hypoglycemia.

EVALUATION AND MANAGEMENT

Evaluation for a disorder of hypoglycemia should occur in older children and adolescents if Whipple's triad is documented, or in infants and younger children if blood glucose concentrations less than 60 mg/dL on laboratory quality assays are found. Neonates at high risk for hypoglycemia (those born large or small for gestational age or those with perinatal stress, maternal diabetes, certain congenital syndromes, or family history of genetic hypoglycemia disorders) with glucose values less than 60 mg/dL should also undergo evaluation after the first 48 to 72 hours of life.

Important caveats to blood glucose testing are worth noting. Blood samples that are not processed promptly can have erroneously low glucose levels owing to glycolysis by red and white blood cells (i.e., at room temperature, the decline of blood glucose can be 5 to 7 mg/dL/h). In addition, hospital bedside glucose monitors and similar home glucose monitors are less precise than clinical laboratory methods and can be expected to have an error range of 10% to 15%.

Management of an Unstable Patient With Hypoglycemia

In symptomatic or clinically unstable patients with hypoglycemia, the first step should be administration of a 2 mL/kg bolus of 10% dextrose in water intravenously followed by a continuous infusion of 10% dextrose in an age-appropriate saline concentration at a glucose infusion rate of 5 to 6 mg/kg/min for infants and 2 to 3 mg/kg/min for toddlers

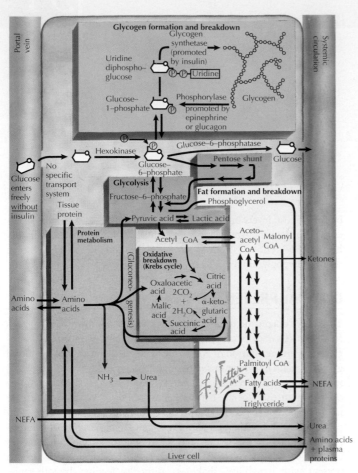

Fig. 51.1 Intermediary
Metabolism in the Liver Cell.

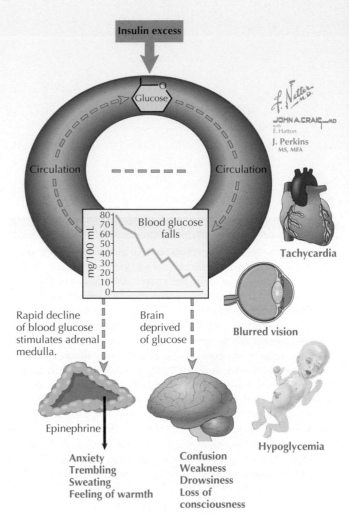

Fig. 51.2 Symptoms of Hypoglycemia.

and older children (Box 51.1). Frequent blood glucose monitoring should follow to ensure correction of hypoglycemia and maintenance of euglycemia.

Management of a Stable Patient With Hypoglycemia

In a stable patient with a glucose value less than 50 mg/dL, a "critical" blood sample can be obtained to establish the underlying cause of hypoglycemia (Box 51.2). The critical sample can be obtained during an episode of spontaneous hypoglycemia or during a supervised diagnostic fasting test. A glucagon stimulation test also should be performed after collection of the critical sample. Children who are conscious and cooperative may be treated with oral carbohydrates. If this treatment fails to correct the hypoglycemia, intravenous dextrose should be administered. Long-term management of children with hypoglycemia depends on the cause of the hypoglycemia (see specific disorders below).

DIFFERENTIAL DIAGNOSIS

The differential diagnosis of hypoglycemia is expansive and includes not only disorders of carbohydrate metabolism but also disorders of fat oxidation, hormone deficiencies, and medication-induced hypoglycemia (Box 51.3). Using the results of the critical sample can help narrow this differential (Fig. 51.3).

Nonacidemia

Patients with hypoglycemia without acidemia (defined as having a bicarbonate level of ≥18 mmol/L) on laboratory workup bring HI,

neonatal panhypopituitarism, infants of mothers with diabetes, and fatty acid oxidation (FAO) defects under consideration.

Low Ketones With Low Free Fatty Acids

A pattern of hypoketotic hypoglycemia and hypofattyacidemia raises the suspicion of HI. Insulinomas, factitious HI, neonatal panhypopituitarism, and infants of mothers with diabetes can also produce these findings.

Hyperinsulinism. The most common cause of persistent hypoglycemia in infants and children is HI. HI can be categorized into three main types: perinatal stress, congenital, and syndromic HI.

Perinatal stress HI occurs in infants exposed to stress in utero or during delivery, such as intrauterine growth restriction, birth asphyxia, or being born with a congenital heart defect. Infants with this form of HI are responsive to diazoxide, and the hypoglycemia commonly resolves within the first 6 months of life.

Congenital HI is due to single-gene defects affecting the insulin secretory pathways of the β cell. The most common and severe form, known as K_{ATP}-HI, is due to inactivating mutations of *ABCC8* and *KCNJ11*, which encode the potassium channel on the β cell membrane. This form occurs in two histologic subtypes, diffuse and focal, and typically does not respond to diazoxide. Children presenting with diazoxide-unresponsive HI require expedited genetic testing of *ABCC8* and *KCNJ11* and potential transfer to a center capable of performing a specialized positron emission tomography (PET) scan to localize focal

BOX 51.1 Treatment of Hypoglycemia

Emergency Treatment
- Dextrose bolus: 2 mL/kg of D10W
- Continuous infusion of D10W with GIR 5–6 mg/kg/min (infants) or 2–3 mg/kg/min (older children)

Specific Treatment
- Hyperinsulinism
  - Diazoxide: 5–15 mg/kg/day divided twice a day
  - Octreotide: 2–20 mcg/kg/day divided every 6–8 hours
  - Glucagon: 1 mg IM or IV or 1 mg/day by continuous infusion
- Disorders of gluconeogenesis or glycogenolysis
  - Limit fasting
  - Cornstarch
- Disorders of fatty acid oxidation
  - Limit fasting
- Adrenal insufficiency
  - Hydrocortisone:
    - IV stress dose: 100 mg/m^2 once then 100 mg/m^2/day divided every 4 hours
    - Oral stress dose: 50 mg/m^2/day divided every 8 hours
    - Maintenance dose: 8–12 mg/m^2/day divided three times daily
- Growth hormone deficiency
  - Growth hormone: 0.3 mg/kg/week divided twice daily
- Postprandial hypoglycemia
  - Prolonged or continuous feeds
  - Dietary modification with fats and complex carbohydrates
  - Acarbose 12.5–50 mg before each meal

GIR (mg/kg/min) =

$$\frac{\text{IV rate (mL/hour)} \times \text{Dextrose conc (g/dL)} \times 1000 \text{ (mg/g)}}{\text{Weight (kg)} \times 60 \text{ (minute/hour)} \times 100 \text{ (mL/dL)}}$$

D10W, Dextrose 10% in water; *GIR,* glucose infusion rate.

BOX 51.2 The Critical Sample and Glucagon Stimulation Test

Blood and Urine Tests at the Time of Hypoglycemia
- Glucose
- Comprehensive metabolic panel
- β-Hydroxybutyrate
- Growth hormone
- Cortisol
- Free fatty acids
- Insulin
- C-peptide
- Lactate
- Ammonia
- Acylcarnitine profile
- Free and total carnitine
- Insulin-like growth factor binding protein-1
- Urine organic acids

Glucagon Stimulation Test
- Check blood glucose (time 0)
- Give 1 mg of glucagon intravascular or intramuscular
- Check blood glucose every 10 minutes for 40 minutes
- If blood glucose does not increase by 20 mg/dL in 20 minutes, rescue patient with dextrose
- Positive response: increase in blood glucose by 30 mg/dL by 40 minutes after glucagon administration

lesions. Infants with focal HI can be cured with surgical resection of the focal lesion.

HI also is associated with certain syndromes, such as Beckwith-Wiedemann, Kabuki, and Turner.

During hypoglycemia, these children have inappropriately normal or elevated serum insulin levels (although insulin may not be detected in all assays), suppressed free fatty acids and β-hydroxybutyrate, and a glycemic response to glucagon (defined as a 30 mg/dL rise in glucose). Additional laboratory tests that help distinguish specific forms of HI include ammonia (glutamate dehydrogenase HI) and 3-hydroxy-butyrylcarnitine (short chain 3-hydroxyacyl Co-A dehydrogenase HI). Genetic testing is used to identify gene mutations responsible for congenital and syndromic forms of HI.

In general, infants with HI present with severe hypoglycemia shortly after birth or in the first few months of life. They require high glucose infusion rates (GIRs) to maintain euglycemia. However, HI is a spectrum and some children may present with normal birth weights and only moderately increased dextrose needs.

The mainstay therapy for HI is diazoxide. Diazoxide suppresses insulin secretion by its action in the K$_{ATP}$ channel. Because a functional K$_{ATP}$ channel is required for diazoxide to exert an effect, most patients with K$_{ATP}$-HI do not respond to diazoxide. The dosage of diazoxide is 5 to 15 mg/kg/day given orally and divided into two equal doses. The side effects of diazoxide include fluid retention and hypertrichosis. Neonates and infants who are treated with diazoxide should also be placed on a diuretic to prevent fluid overload.

The second-line medical therapy for children unresponsive to diazoxide is octreotide, a somatostatin analog. The initial response to octreotide is good in most cases of HI, but tachyphylaxis develops after a few doses, rendering therapy inadequate for long-term use. Additionally, it is associated with cases of fulminant necrotizing enterocolitis so it should not be administered to infants younger than 2 months old. Glucagon can also be given as a continuous intravenous infusion to help maintain euglycemia in the hospital setting.

Insulinoma. An insulinoma should be considered in older children and adolescents presenting with hypoketotic hypoglycemia. Insulinomas are pancreatic islet cell tumors, which are typically benign. Imaging studies that can be useful in the diagnosis of an insulinoma include magnetic resonance imaging (MRI), transesophageal ultrasonography, and somatostatin receptor PET scans. Complete surgical resection of the insulinoma is curative. A diagnosis of multiple endocrine neoplasia syndrome type 1 should be considered in patients with pancreatic islet cell tumors.

Factitious hyperinsulinism. Surreptitious administration of insulin must always be considered in children with hypoglycemia as a result of excess insulin action. These patients may have increased insulin levels, as well as other markers of excessive insulin effects; however, they will have inappropriately low C-peptide levels relative to their insulin level. Administration of sulfonylurea drugs can cause a far more malicious form of factitious HI, because levels of insulin and C-peptide will both be elevated. Sulfonylurea toxicology studies are required to detect this cause of hypoglycemia. Surreptitious insulin and sulfonylurea administration in neonates and children are almost always a result of Munchausen by proxy syndrome.

Neonatal panhypopituitarism. Children with neonatal panhypopituitarism can present with hypoglycemia caused by deficiencies of the counterregulatory hormones cortisol and growth hormone. The presentation in infants can be similar to that in HI,

BOX 51.3 Differential Diagnosis of Hypoglycemia in Infants and Children

- Infant of a mother with diabetes
- Hyperinsulinism (HI)
  - Perinatal stress-induced HI
  - Congenital HI
    - K_{ATP}-HI
    - Hyperinsulinism-hyperammonemia syndrome or GDH-HI
    - Glucokinase-HI
    - HNF4α-HI
    - HNF1α-HI
    - SCHAD-HI
    - UCP2-HI
    - Exercise-induced HI
  - Syndromic HI
    - Beckwith-Wiedemann syndrome
    - Kabuki syndrome
- Turner syndrome
  - Soto syndrome
- Insulinoma
- Postprandial hypoglycemia or dumping syndrome
- Disorders of gluconeogenesis
  - GSD Ia
  - GSD Ib
  - F-1,6-Pase deficiency
  - Pyruvate carboxylase deficiency
- Disorders of glycogen storage
  - GSD 0
  - GSD III
  - GSD VI
  - GSD IX
- Disorders of fatty acid oxidation
  - Medium-chain acyl-CoA dehydrogenase deficiency
- Pituitary hormone deficiency
  - Panhypopituitarism
  - Isolated ACTH deficiency
  - Isolated growth hormone deficiency
- Primary adrenal insufficiency
- Medication-induced hypoglycemia
  - Insulin
  - Sulfonylureas
  - Ethanol
  - β-Blockers
  - Salicylates
- Idiopathic ketotic hypoglycemia

ACTH, Adrenocorticotropic hormone; *F-1,6-Pase,* fructose-1,6-biphosphatase; *GDH,* glutamate dehydrogenase; *GSD 0,* glycogen synthase deficiency; *GSD 1a,* glucose-6-phosphatase deficiency; *GSD 1b,* glucose-6-phosphate translocase deficiency; *GSD III;* debrancher enzyme deficiency; *GSD VI,* glycogen phosphorylase deficiency; *GSD IX,* phosphorylase kinase deficiency; *HNF4α,* hepatic nuclear factor 4 alpha; *HNF1α,* hepatic nuclear factor 1 alpha; *K_{ATP},* adenosine triphosphate–sensitive potassium; *PPH,* postprandial hypoglycemia; *SCHAD,* short-chain 3-hydroxyacyl-CoA dehydrogenase; *UCP2,* uncoupling protein 2.

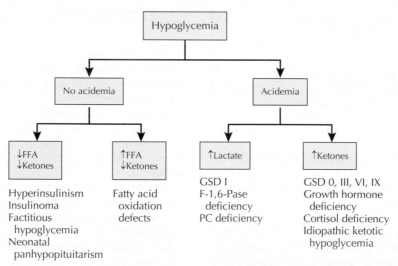

Fig. 51.3 Hypoglycemia Diagnostic Algorithm.

including suppressed ketones and fatty acids and a glycemic response to glucagon. After the first year of life, children with hypopituitarism present with ketotic hypoglycemia. Clues to this diagnosis include midline defects and in boys, a small phallus.

Infant of a mother with diabetes. Infants of mothers with uncontrolled diabetes mellitus (DM) during pregnancy (regardless of type) are at risk for hypoglycemia because of transient HI. These infants are almost always large for gestational age. During gestation, the β cells of the fetal pancreas secrete elevated levels of insulin in response to chronic exposure to elevated glucose. After delivery, there is a sudden removal of the mother's elevated glucose supply, and hypoglycemia quickly occurs in the newborn, who continues to secrete increased levels of insulin. Hypoglycemia typically resolves in the first several days of life as the pancreatic islet cells reduce the insulin secretory rate.

Low Ketones With High Free Fatty Acids

On a critical laboratory sample, FAO disorders present with hyperfattyacidemia and hypoketotic hypoglycemia.

Disorders of fatty acid oxidation. Disorders in the pathway of FAO include defects in β-oxidation, carnitine-based transport of fatty acids into mitochondria, and in the synthesis or usage of ketones. The most common of these disorders is medium-chain acyl-CoA dehydrogenase (MCAD) deficiency. Disorders of FAO can also affect liver, cardiac, and muscle function. Patients become symptomatic in the setting of illness or prolonged fasting. Because hypoglycemia can be a late manifestation of the disease, if an FAO disorder is suspected, treatment with intravenous dextrose should be initiated immediately. The majority of FAO disorders are identified through the newborn screen. The diagnosis also can be made based on metabolites observed in serum acylcarnitine or urine organic acid profiles. The primary treatment for disorders of fat oxidation is to avoid fasting.

Acidemia

The differential diagnosis of a patient found to have acidemia (defined as having a bicarbonate level of <18 mmol/L) in the setting of hypoglycemia, narrows to gluconeogenic disorders, ethanol intoxication, glycogen storage disorders, hormone deficiencies, or idiopathic ketotic hypoglycemia.

Elevated Lactate

An elevated lactate level should point the clinician toward disorders of gluconeogenesis and ethanol intoxication.

Disorders of gluconeogenesis. Glycogen storage disease (GSD) Ia (glucose-6-phosphatase deficiency) and GSD Ib (glucose-6-phosphate translocase deficiency), although typically classified as GSDs, are actually disorders affecting both gluconeogenesis and the release of stored glucose. Patients present with hypoglycemia, lactic acidosis, mild ketosis, hypertriglyceridemia, and hepatomegaly. Hypoglycemia occurs even after brief periods of fasting because patients are unable to access their glucose stores. Gluconeogenic precursors are shunted to alterative pathways in the liver, resulting in elevations of lactate, triglycerides, and uric acid. Life-threatening lactic acidosis develops with any prolonged fasting. A child with suspected or confirmed GSD I who is not tolerating oral feedings should be started immediately on intravenous fluids containing dextrose. Long-term therapy for patients with GSD I includes frequent feedings, avoiding disaccharides containing fructose or galactose, and a regimen of 1 to 2 g/kg of uncooked cornstarch taken orally or by a gastrostomy tube every 4 to 6 hours.

Fructose-1,6-biphosphatase (F-1,6-Pase) deficiency and pyruvate carboxylase deficiency are rare disorders resulting in impaired gluconeogenesis. Both can manifest with hypoglycemia and lactic acidosis. Long-term treatment of F-1,6-Pase deficiency includes limited fasting (8 to 10 hours) and consuming a diet high in carbohydrates (excluding fructose), low in protein, and with a normal fat content. Treatment of pyruvate carboxylase deficiency is primarily symptomatic.

Ethanol. Ethanol intoxication also can result in hypoglycemia and elevated lactate levels. In the liver, ethanol diminishes the supply of nicotinamide adenine dinucleotide (NAD) and results in decreased gluconeogenesis. A drug screen can be used to confirm ethanol ingestion. Hypoglycemia should self-resolve as the ethanol clears the patient's system. Treatment is primarily supportive.

Elevated Ketones

Acidemia with elevated ketones is due to glycogen storage disorders, hormone deficiencies, or idiopathic ketotic hypoglycemia.

Disorders of glycogen storage. Children with glycogen storage disorder (GSD) 0 or glycogen synthase deficiency, GSD III (debrancher enzyme deficiency), GSD VI (glycogen phosphorylase deficiency), and GSD IX (phosphorylase kinase deficiency) present with fasting ketotic hypoglycemia, liver abnormalities, and growth failure. GSD 0 presents as fasting ketotic hypoglycemia and is the only GSD not associated with hepatomegaly. Children with GSD 0 have postprandial hyperglycemia with hyperlactatemia and hyperlipidemia. GSD III is characterized by fasting hypoglycemia with hyperlipidemia, hepatomegaly, and short stature. GSD VI and IX both have hypoglycemia after prolonged fasting and hepatomegaly. Lactate levels are not increased in GSD III, VI, or IX. Treatment of GSDs is regular administration of uncooked cornstarch and limiting fasting time.

Hormone deficiencies. Growth hormone (GH) or adrenocorticotropic hormone (ACTH) deficiency can also present with ketotic hypoglycemia. If central adrenal insufficiency is suspected and the patient is stable, a corticotropin-releasing hormone or low-dose ACTH stimulation test should be performed. If GH deficiency is suspected, the patient should undergo a stimulation test with arginine and clonidine. If a patient has central adrenal insufficiency, GH deficiency, or both, central hypothyroidism should also be considered and a free thyroxine (T_4) level should be measured. Infants with confirmed GH or ACTH deficiency should undergo pituitary imaging by MRI. The hypoglycemia resolves with hormone replacement, although neonates and infants with growth hormone deficiency require twice-daily growth hormone dosing, instead of the standard daily dosing, to prevent ongoing hypoglycemia.

Adrenal insufficiency (Addison disease). Patients with primary adrenal insufficiency resulting in the loss of glucocorticoid production may present with hypoglycemia (Chapter 49). Additionally, these patients can present with hyponatremia, hyperkalemia, and dehydration caused by a loss of mineralocorticoid production. Patients may also appear hyperpigmented secondary to the effects of excess ACTH. The diagnosis can be made by checking 8-AM cortisol and ACTH levels or by performing a high-dose ACTH stimulation test.

These patients should be treated with hydrocortisone (8 to 12 mg/m^2/day divided every 8 hours), plus a mineralocorticoid if they have primary adrenal insufficiency. If the patient is unstable, serum should be obtained and reserved for later measurement of cortisol and ACTH levels, and therapy with stress dose glucocorticoids should be initiated immediately: hydrocortisone (100 mg/m^2) as an intravenous bolus followed by hydrocortisone 100 mg/m^2/day divided every 4 to 6 hours for 24 hours or until the patient is stable.

Idiopathic ketotic hypoglycemia. Children with idiopathic ketotic hypoglycemia (IKH) have a shorter than expected fasting tolerance for their age but become appropriately ketotic at the time of hypoglycemia. Children with IKH typically present during the toddler years in the setting of a precipitating illness. IKH is a diagnosis of exclusion, so other causes of ketotic hypoglycemia must be ruled out. Patients with ketotic hypoglycemia do not typically require medical therapy but instead are instructed to avoid prolonged fasting. During times of illness, their fasting tolerance is even shorter. If a child with ketotic hypoglycemia is not tolerating food or liquid by mouth, he or she should be taken to an emergency department to receive intravenous fluids containing dextrose. Ketotic hypoglycemia usually resolves by age 6 to 8 years.

OTHER DIAGNOSES

In patients with hypoglycemia who do not fit within the hypoglycemia diagnostic algorithm, further history and workup can help elucidate the correct diagnosis.

Postprandial Hypoglycemia (Dumping Syndrome)

Postprandial hypoglycemia (PPH) is extremely uncommon in children except in cases in which PPH (or late dumping syndrome) develops as a consequence of a Nissen or other fundoplication procedures. These children develop hyperglycemia shortly after a meal followed by an acute rise in insulin, and then a reactive hypoglycemia 1 to 3 hours after the feeding. Evaluation of a patient with suspected PPH consists of a mixed meal tolerance test and frequent glucose checks after a meal or feed. The cause of PPH is unclear, but it may involve rapid gastric emptying, overstimulation of enteroendocrine cells, and hypersecretion of glucagon-like peptide-1, an incretin hormone that stimulates insulin secretion. These patients are managed with feeding manipulations, typically through prolonged feeds or adding fats and complex carbohydrates to slow absorption of the food. Acarbose, an α-glucosidase inhibitor that slows the absorption of carbohydrates, may be useful in older patients.

Medication-Induced Hypoglycemia

In addition to exogenous insulin, sulfonylureas, and ethanol (see above), β blockers and salicylates also can cause hypoglycemia. β-blocking medications can lead to hypoglycemia because activation of β-2 adrenergic receptors normally stimulates glycogen breakdown and the release of glucagon from the pancreas. Salicylates may accelerate glucose usage by interfering with gluconeogenesis and by augmenting insulin secretion.

FUTURE DIRECTIONS

In the past few years, significant advances in molecular genetics have contributed to our understanding of the most common causes of hypoglycemia in children. These advances should result in the development of specific, more effective therapies in the next few years that may improve the outcome in these children.

Acknowledgments

The authors would like to acknowledge Andrew Palladino and Diva De León, who contributed the initial version of this chapter.

SUGGESTED READINGS

Available online.

52

Disorders of Growth

Camilia Kamoun and Adda Grimberg

✳ CLINICAL VIGNETTE

A previously well 9-year-old girl presents for a yearly check-up. She weighs 23.5 kg (10th percentile for age) and measures 122 cm (5th percentile for age) with a body mass index at the 28th percentile. Two years ago, she had been tracking at the 35th and 30th percentiles for weight and height, respectively. Her midparental height is 160 cm (30th percentile). She eats a balanced, unrestricted diet. Review of systems is positive only for occasional poor appetite. There is no family history of short stature or abnormal puberty. Physical examination findings are normal, and she has no signs of puberty. Bone age is concordant with chronologic age. Screening laboratory samples submitted for potential causes of short stature include a comprehensive metabolic panel, erythrocyte sedimentation rate, C-reactive protein, complete blood count, celiac panel, thyroid studies, insulin-like growth factor (IGF)-I, and IGF-binding proteins (IGFBP)-3, as well as a karyotype to assess for Turner syndrome. Her celiac antibodies return positive, leading to referral to a gastroenterologist; intestinal biopsy confirms the diagnosis of celiac disease. After 1 year on a gluten-free diet, her weight and height plot at the 30th and 20th percentiles, respectively.

Statural growth is an integral part of childhood development and normally occurs in a predictable pattern. The pediatrician's primary responsibilities are to identify children who may not be growing adequately and then differentiate between physiologic variants of growth and worrisome patterns. Interval growth should be accurately assessed and plotted on a growth chart at each health maintenance visit. The sex-adjusted midparental height (genetic target height) should be calculated by adding together the heights of the biological parents and adding 13 cm for a boy or subtracting 13 cm for a girl and then dividing by 2. This height plus or minus 10 cm represents an estimate of the child's genetic height potential. Deviations from typical growth patterns or the child's genetic height potential should be evaluated; the greater the deviation, the greater are the chances of an underlying abnormality. Early detection is important for diagnosing any underlying conditions and intervening in a timely fashion to maximize health and adult height.

ETIOLOGY AND PATHOGENESIS

Longitudinal Growth and Mediating Factors

Growth is a complex process regulated by multiple factors, including nutrition, hormones, and growth factors, that act either systemically or within the growth plate. The physis (growth plate) is a cartilaginous zone located between the metaphysis (bone shaft) and epiphysis (secondary ossification zone at the end of long bones). Longitudinal growth (bone elongation) occurs by chondrocyte proliferation and subsequent endochondral ossification within the physes.

Growth hormone (GH) is the most important growth-regulating hormone; its pulsatile secretion from the anterior pituitary somatotrophs is mainly regulated by two hypothalamic peptide hormones, GH-releasing hormone (GHRH) and somatostatin, which, respectively, stimulate and inhibit its release (Fig. 52.1). Circulating GH is bound to GH-binding protein (GHBP). Many, though not all, of GH's actions are mediated through insulin-like growth factor (IGF)-I. Serum IGF-I is produced principally in the liver in response to GH and circulates in the bloodstream bound to high affinity IGF-binding proteins (especially IGFBP-3) that control its bioavailability. IGF-I binds cell-surface IGF receptors on target tissues to trigger multiple downstream effects that include cellular hypertrophy and proliferation. IGF-I and free fatty acids also inhibit GH secretion at the level of the pituitary and hypothalamus.

Other systemic hormones that affect growth include insulin (the principal growth-promoting hormone in utero), androgens and estrogens (which induce the pubertal growth spurt and, in the case of estrogens, maturation of growth plates), thyroid hormone (which has a permissive effect on GH secretion and exerts direct action at the growth plates), and glucocorticoids (which inhibit growth both centrally and at the growth plate). These hormones work in concert with signaling cascades local to the growth plate, whose effects are not measurable by routine testing; mutations of genes in these pathways can affect growth (e.g., short stature homeobox-containing [SHOX], Indian hedgehog [IHH], and fibroblast growth factor receptor 3 [FGFR3] genes).

Normal Growth Patterns

Normal growth is depicted in growth charts, which contain sequential percentile curves showing the distribution of selected body measurements in reference children of a select population (see Measurement Techniques and Growth Charts section below). Growth is fastest during the fetal period; fetal size primarily relates to maternal/pregnancy health and nutrition. During infancy, genetic factors come into play. When there is a mismatch between the two, infants cross length percentiles to a percentile more in line with their genetic potential (physiologic rechanneling), with roughly equal numbers rechanneling upward as downward. Growth gradually slows postnatally, with an average increase in length of 25 cm over the first year of life and 10 cm over the second year. After the second birthday, growth proceeds at a slow, relatively constant velocity of 4 to 6 cm/year, and shifting percentile channels is *abnormal*. Childhood growth is slowest just before the onset of puberty and then accelerates during adolescence, resulting in the pubertal "growth spurt" (reaching peak growth velocities of 12 to 13 cm/year). At the end of puberty, growth ceases as the physes fuse.

Poor or Atypical Growth

Poor growth can be caused by systemic illness, psychosocial deprivation, malnutrition, or abnormalities in the secretion or action of any of the

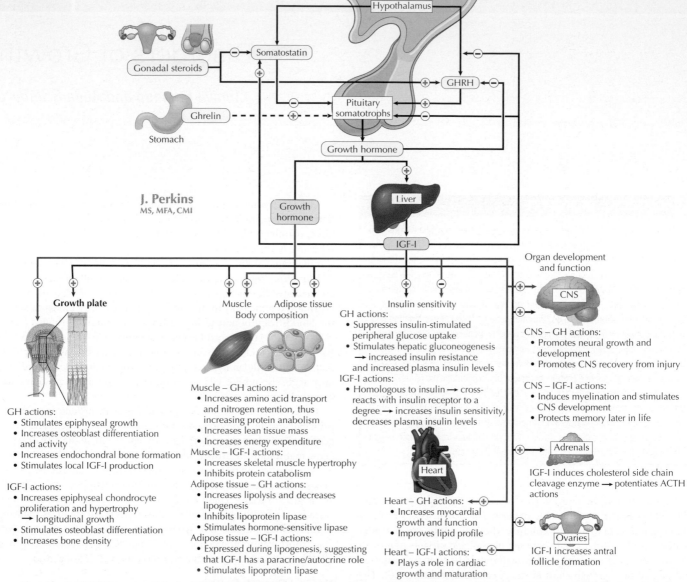

The endocrine GH/IGF-I system is shown, which involves multiple levels of stimulatory and inhibitory signaling. Both GH and IGF-I are made throughout the body. Autocrine and paracrine GH and IGF-I actions contribute to their effects at target tissues. The line for ghrelin is dashed because its physiologic role is unclear.

Fig. 52.1 Growth Hormone and Insulin-Like Growth Factor: Systemic and Metabolic Effects.

previously mentioned hormones and growth factors. Height is a continuum; healthy adult heights differ considerably within the human population. A height more than 2 standard deviations (SDs) below or above the child's genetic potential (i.e., midparental height) or the mean for age and sex in the reference population should prompt evaluation for worrisome growth (Fig. 52.2). *Growth failure* is defined as height velocity that is less than expected for age, sex, and pubertal stage or as the downward crossing of two or more major height percentiles (major percentile curves on standard growth charts) beyond 2 years of age. Growth failure always merits an evaluation. Excessive linear growth, upward crossing of major percentiles, also warrants investigation to assess for underlying pathologic or genetic conditions that can lead to excessive linear growth.

CLINICAL PRESENTATION

Short Stature

The causes of short stature can be divided into categories (Box 52.1). Endocrine diseases are less common causes of short stature and are

usually distinguished from other causes by linear growth failure that is more significant than weight deceleration.

Familial Short Stature

Familial short stature (FSS) is the most common cause of short stature in healthy children living in well-resourced conditions. A child with FSS has a height that falls at the lower end of the population distribution but that is consistent with the child's genetic potential. Usually at least one parent's height is in the lower height percentiles, and the child's growth pattern and predicted adult height are *consistent* with the height of at least one parent (and extended family members). The hallmark is a normal growth velocity, such that the child's growth curve is parallel to the standard population curve. In the absence of a family history of delayed puberty, the timing of puberty is usually average. The medical history, review of systems, physical examination, and laboratory test results are unremarkable. The bone age is within 2 SD of published standards for age (see Bone Age section).

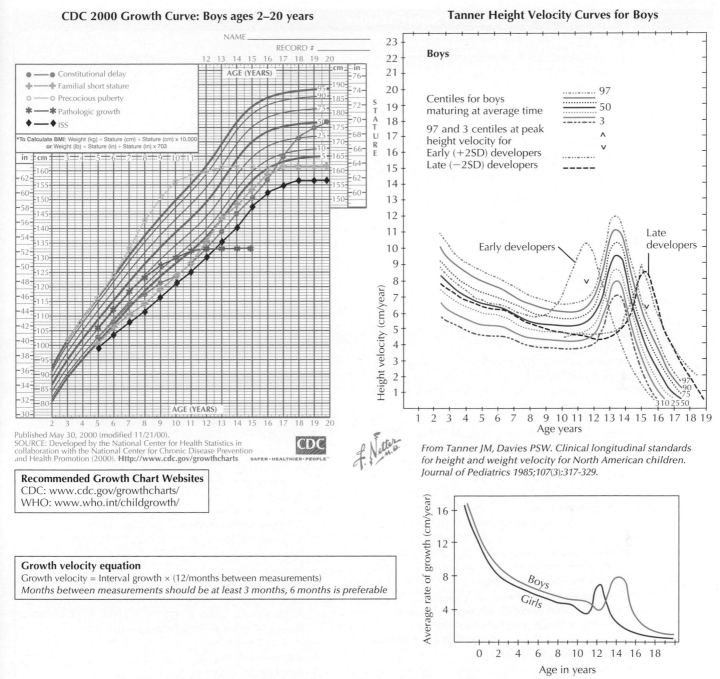

CDC 2000 Growth Curve: Boys ages 2–20 years

- ●——● Constitutional delay
- ✚——✚ Familial short stature
- ○——○ Precocious puberty
- ✱——✱ Pathologic growth
- ◆——◆ ISS

*To Calculate BMI: Weight (kg) ÷ Stature (cm) ÷ Stature (cm) x 10,000
or Weight (lb) ÷ Stature (in) ÷ Stature (in) x 703

Published May 30, 2000 (modified 11/21/00).
SOURCE: Developed by the National Center for Health Statistics in
collaboration with the National Center for Chronic Disease Prevention
and Health Promotion (2000). Http://www.cdc.gov/growthcharts

Recommended Growth Chart Websites
CDC: www.cdc.gov/growthcharts/
WHO: www.who.int/childgrowth/

Growth velocity equation
Growth velocity = Interval growth × (12/months between measurements)
Months between measurements should be at least 3 months, 6 months is preferable

Tanner Height Velocity Curves for Boys

Boys

Centiles for boys
maturing at average time ········· 97
·········· 50
--------- 3
97 and 3 centiles at peak
height velocity for ^
Early (+2SD) developers
Late (−2SD) developers ⌄

Early developers

Late
developers

*From Tanner JM, Davies PSW. Clinical longitudinal standards
for height and weight velocity for North American children.
Journal of Pediatrics 1985;107(3):317-329.*

Fig. 52.2 Growth Curves and Disorders of Growth. (For differential diagnosis of short stature, see Box 52.1.) *ISS,* Idiopathic short stature.

It is important to note that healthy variant short stature (i.e., FSS) is a polygenic trait. Dominantly inherited single gene defects (e.g., *SHOX* gene haploinsufficiency, see later; or hypochondroplasia) can be mislabeled as FSS when the parent is yet undiagnosed, particularly if height is significantly below the third percentile. An extended pedigree of family members' heights can help guide suspicion for such a condition.

Constitutional Delay of Growth and Puberty

Constitutional delay of growth and puberty (CDGP) is the second most common cause of short stature among children living in well-resourced conditions. Children with CDGP usually have a normal birth length, begin crossing height percentiles by age 2 years, and settle in the lower percentiles, where they track until the onset of puberty

BOX 52.1 Differential Diagnosis of Short Stature

I. Normal variants
   A. Healthy variants (excludes dominantly inherited genetic problems)
   B. Constitutional delay of growth and puberty
   C. Idiopathic short stature
II. Abnormal causes
   A. Intrauterine growth restriction
   B. Bone disorders
      1. Osteochondrodysplasias
         a. Achondroplasia and hypochondroplasia
         b. Achondrogenesis
         c. Mesomelic dysplasias
         d. Epiphyseal and metaphyseal dysplasias
      2. Osteogenesis imperfecta
   C. Chromosomal abnormalities
      1. Turner syndrome
      2. Trisomy 21
      3. Trisomies 8, 13, and 18
      4. 18q deletion
   D. Endocrine disorders
      1. Pituitary or hypothalamic dysfunction
         a. Idiopathic GH deficiency
         b. Structural abnormalities:
            • Associated with other midline defects (e.g., holoprosencephaly, septo-optic dysplasia)
            • Isolated hypothalamic or pituitary malformations (e.g., empty sella syndrome, ectopic neurohypophysis)
         c. Genetic causes:
            • Multiple pituitary hormone deficiencies: *HESX1, PROP1, POUF1 LHX3,* and *LHX4* mutations
            • GHRH receptor mutation
            • GH gene (*GH1*) mutations or deletions
            • Growth hormone secretagogue receptor *(GHSR)* mutation
         d. Brain or hypothalamic tumors (e.g., germinomas, gliomas)
         e. Pituitary tumors (e.g., craniopharyngiomas, histiocytosis X)
         f. Surgical resection of the pituitary or pituitary stalk
         g. Brain trauma: generalized or specific to the hypothalamus, pituitary stalk, or anterior pituitary
         h. Pituitary or hypothalamic inflammation
         i. Brain or hypothalamic irradiation
      2. Primary insulin-like growth factor (IGF) deficiency
         a. GH insensitivity (Laron syndrome) or bio-inactivity
         b. Post-GH receptor defects (e.g., *STAT5B, IGFALS,* and *PAPP-A2* mutations, IGF-I deficiency or resistance)
      3. Hypothyroidism
      4. Glucocorticoid excess
      5. Diabetes mellitus (Mauriac syndrome)
      6. Pseudohypoparathyroidism
      7. Rickets
   E. Malnutrition
      1. Protein calorie (kwashiorkor)
      2. Generalized (marasmus)
      3. Anorexia nervosa
      4. Micronutrient deficiencies (especially iron, zinc)
   F. Psychosocial deprivation
   G. Nonendocrine chronic systemic diseases
      1. Malabsorptive disorders
         a. Celiac disease
         b. Inflammatory bowel disease
         c. Short gut syndrome
      2. Renal disease
         a. Fanconi syndrome
         b. Renal tubular acidosis
         c. Uremia or chronic renal failure
      3. Cardiovascular disease
         a. Congenital (especially cyanotic)
         b. Congestive heart failure
      4. Pulmonary disease
         a. Cystic fibrosis
         b. Severe asthma
      5. Hepatic
         a. Chronic liver disease or liver failure
      6. Hematologic
         a. Profound anemia
         b. Thalassemia (especially if transfusion dependent)
         c. Hemosiderosis
      7. Oncologic
         a. Malignancy
         b. Secondary to oncologic treatment (chemotherapy or irradiation)
      8. Infectious
         a. AIDS or HIV infection (untreated)
         b. Tuberculosis
         c. Intestinal parasites
      9. Rheumatologic diseases
   H. Other genetic conditions
      1. *SHOX* gene haploinsufficiency
      2. Russell-Silver syndrome
      3. Prader-Willi syndrome
      4. Noonan syndrome
      5. Others: Cornelia de Lange syndrome, insulin receptor gene mutations (Donohue syndrome), Rubinstein-Taybi syndrome, Aarskog syndrome, Bloom syndrome, Cockayne syndrome, progeria, Seckel syndrome, Dubowitz syndrome, Mulibrey (Perheentupa) syndrome
   I. Inborn errors of metabolism
      1. Glycogen storage diseases
      2. Galactosemia
      3. Mucopolysaccharidoses
      4. Glycoproteinoses
      5. Mucolipidoses
   J. Iatrogenic
      1. Chronic glucocorticoid exposure (e.g., in severe asthma)
      2. Stimulant medications for ADHD

ADHD, Attention-deficit/hyperactivity disorder; *GH,* growth hormone; *GHRH,* growth hormone–releasing hormone; *GHSR,* growth hormone secretagogue receptor; *IGF,* insulin-like growth factor.

in their peers, when they appear to drop further away from the growth curve. This growth pattern is associated with delayed puberty (Chapter 46). CDGP represents the late end of the spectrum of pubertal development. Because children with CDGP enter puberty (and thus accelerate their growth velocity) later than most of their peers, they develop a transient height and sexual maturation gap relative to their age-matched peers. However, children with CDGP continue to grow after their peers stop growing, and thus they eventually attain an adult height within their genetic potential.

Family history often reveals relatives with similarly delayed puberty ("late blooming"). There are no other abnormalities present. While CDGP is not sex-specific, boys with CDGP present more often for short stature evaluation because they are the last of their classmates to have their pubertal growth spurt.

The differential diagnosis of CDGP includes Kallmann syndrome and isolated gonadotropin deficiency; lack of anosmia can exclude the former, but only time or genetic analyses can help distinguish between CDGP and the latter. Bone age is significantly delayed, which provides reassurance that sufficient time for growth remains for the child to reach the predicted adult height. Any physical or biochemical abnormalities should suggest another diagnosis. When CDGP occurs superimposed on FSS, the child's short stature can appear severe; however, the child is still healthy and his or her growth is a normal variant.

Idiopathic Short Stature

Idiopathic short stature (ISS) refers to extreme short stature that does not have a diagnostic explanation after an ordinary growth evaluation. The US Food and Drug Administration (FDA) set the threshold for GH treatment of ISS at a height more than 2.25 SD below the mean, roughly equal to the shortest 1.2% of the population. ISS represents a statistical extreme. In some cases, however, specific genetic mutations may account for poor growth and the idiopathic label is misleading. For example, 3% to 15% of children with ISS have deletions or mutations in the *SHOX* gene (see later).

Intrauterine Growth Restriction and Small for Gestational Age

Intrauterine growth restriction (IUGR) can result in a newborn who is small for gestational age (SGA), commonly defined as a birth weight less than 2.5 kg at a gestational age beyond 37 weeks, or length or weight below the 10th percentile for gestational age. Although most infants with IUGR and SGA experience catch-up growth in the first 2 years of life, approximately 10% to 15% remain below the third height percentile. Note that not all SGA states are due to IUGR. If history or physical examination in a child born SGA suggests an intrinsic abnormality, an appropriate evaluation should be obtained (i.e., genetic evaluation for possible syndromes or radiographs if limbs are disproportionate).

Osteochondrodysplasias

Osteochondrodysplasias (skeletal dysplasias) are a diverse group of genetic disorders (over 450 identified) whose common denominator is abnormality of cartilage, bone, or both. Most children with osteochondrodysplasias grow slowly and disproportionately because these disorders usually affect the limbs and torso differentially. There may be disproportionate rates of growth between limb segments (rhizomelic affecting proximal limbs, mesomelic affecting distal limbs, or acromelic affecting the hands or feet). Osteochondrodysplasias are hereditary. However, many cases represent de novo mutations, so absence of a family history does not exclude the possibility. Careful measurement of body proportions should be taken and combined with radiographic evaluation to determine which bones are primarily involved (long bones, vertebrae, or skull; epiphyses, metaphyses, or diaphyses).

Turner Syndrome

Turner syndrome, a disorder in females associated with the partial or complete absence of one X chromosome, is relatively common (prevalence, 1 in 2500 live-born girls). Girls with Turner syndrome may have a subtle or even normal phenotype (Chapter 65). Short stature is the most common phenotypic manifestation and is caused by loss of the *SHOX* gene.

SHOX encodes a transcription factor expressed in the growth plate that helps regulate chondrocyte differentiation and proliferation. The *SHOX* gene is located in the pseudoautosomal region of the short arm of the sex chromosomes; genes in this region do not undergo X inactivation. Both copies of the *SHOX* gene are required for normal growth. Patients with Turner syndrome who lack the short arm of X (or one entire X chromosome) have only one functional copy of the *SHOX* gene. This condition, termed "*SHOX* haploinsufficiency," accounts for the 20-cm difference in height between women with 45,X Turner syndrome and women of the referent population, as well as for several skeletal defects.

Because of the phenotypic variability, Turner syndrome should be considered and a karyotype determined in all females with unexplained short stature. Multiple organ system abnormalities are associated with Turner syndrome, so, if detected, a comprehensive evaluation and monitoring are needed.

Abnormalities of the Growth Hormone–Insulin-Like Growth Factor Axis

Dysfunction may appear at any level of the GH–IGF axis, including the hypothalamus and higher brain centers (e.g., congenital malformations, trauma, inflammation, central nervous system [CNS] tumors), pituitary (e.g., structural defects, pituitary tumors, hypophysitis, idiopathic GH deficiency), GH receptor (e.g., Laron syndrome or GH insensitivity), or postreceptor signaling defects (e.g., primary IGF-I deficiency and IGF insensitivity).

The prevalence of idiopathic GH deficiency (GHD) is estimated at 1 in 3500 children. Factors that raise suspicion for GHD include a neonatal history of traumatic delivery, prolonged jaundice or hypoglycemia; microphallus; craniofacial midline abnormalities (e.g., septo-optic dysplasia, holoprosencephaly, or a central maxillary incisor); suprasellar tumor, CNS infection, infarction or other insult, cranial irradiation; or family history of similar presentations.

Infants with congenital isolated GHD tend to have average birth size; however, postnatal growth is overtly abnormal. Severe GHD in early childhood results in early growth failure and slower muscular development, resulting in potentially delayed gross motor milestones. Body composition (i.e., the relative amounts of bone, muscle, and fat) is affected in many children with severe deficiency, so that increased adiposity (especially truncal) is common (although GHD alone rarely causes severe obesity). Some children with severe GHD have recognizable, cherubic facial features characterized by mid-face hypoplasia and forehead prominence. Other features of GHD include normal skeletal proportions, poor lean body mass gain, delayed dentition, and delayed age of pubertal onset. A child suspected of having GHD should be referred to a pediatric endocrinologist for diagnostic evaluation.

Poor Nutrition

Malnutrition is the most common cause of poor growth in the global setting. Inadequate food and/or nutrient intake and malabsorption are both important causes of malnutrition that have a multitude of etiologies (Chapter 120). Optimal statural growth requires optimal nutrition.

Total calorie and/or protein-calorie malnutrition suppresses hepatic IGF-I production, decreasing negative feedback to the hypothalamus and pituitary. This results in increased GH production and secretion and thus elevated basal and stimulated serum GH levels.

Poor weight gain generally precedes the decrease, and eventual failure, of linear growth, and drop in body mass index (BMI) percentiles is a major clue. Bone age and puberty are often delayed.

Taking a detailed dietary history is essential to establishing this diagnosis. A 3-day diet log is a useful tool, which can be analyzed for intake of total calories, macronutrients, and micronutrients. Laboratory evaluations should include all those involved in the evaluation for chronic illness.

Psychosocial Deprivation

Psychosocial growth failure (previously termed psychosocial or deprivation dwarfism) is a growth disorder secondary to emotional deprivation, a stressful environment, or both. Malnutrition is commonly, but not always, associated. Failure to thrive is usually seen in infancy, whereas toddlers and older children often manifest bizarre behaviors, as well as emotional disturbances surrounding food and eating. Delayed statural growth and puberty, growth arrest lines in long bones, and temporary widening of cranial sutures have been reported.

Chronic Systemic Illnesses

Many chronic illnesses are associated with poor growth (Box 52.1). General mechanisms include anorexia, nutrient malabsorption, chronic acidosis or hypoxemia, anemia, chronic inflammation, increased energy requirements, and medical therapy (e.g., glucocorticoids). The growth curve typically shows a period of normal growth followed by growth deceleration or cessation consistent with the onset of illness. Bone age is usually delayed and approximates the height age.

Hypothyroidism

Growth deceleration is one of the most significant manifestations of hypothyroidism in children (Chapter 47). Growth failure caused by acquired hypothyroidism can take several years to clearly manifest, but when it is clinically significant, it tends to be severe and progressive. Puberty is often delayed, but in severe cases, precocious puberty with a paradoxically delayed bone age can be seen.

Tall Stature

Although the majority of cases of tall stature are attributable to familial tall stature or constitutional advance of growth (conditions with growth characteristics that mirror FSS and CDGP), pathologic causes of tall stature should not be missed.

Pathologic tall stature can result from endocrine disorders (e.g., precocious puberty, congenital adrenal hyperplasia, GH/IGF-I excess, hyperthyroidism, aromatase deficiency), chromosomal duplication syndromes (e.g., 47,XXY, Klinefelter syndrome; 47,XYY), and genetic syndromes (e.g., Sotos syndrome, Weaver syndrome, Marfan syndrome, homocystinuria, fragile X syndrome). Obesity is associated with increased growth velocity (and hence, taller stature) but also early puberty, which leads to early cessation of growth and an adult height within the individual's genetic range. Other causes should be excluded before attributing increased growth velocity to obesity. Features that raise concern for pathologic tall stature include signs of early puberty, hyperthyroidism, or phenotypic features of genetic conditions associated with tall stature, discordance between child and midparental heights, and continued growth past the typical age of puberty.

BOX 52.2   Growth-Specific Clinical History Questions

- What were birth weight, length and head circumference? Gestational age at birth? Any perinatal complications? Any maternal conditions or medication use during gestation?
- At what age did the child's first infant tooth come in? Fall out?
- Has the child had any head trauma?
- Is the child having symptoms of central nervous system pathologic conditions (e.g., headaches, vision changes, polyuria or polydipsia concerning for central diabetes insipidus)?
- Has the child been on steroid or stimulant medications?
- Has the child had any significant life stressors (e.g., food insecurity, exposure to violence, neglect)?
- In the family, are there any females who are less than 4 feet, 11 inches? males less than 5 feet, 4 inches?
- When did the child's mother start menstruating? father undergo voice deepening in comparison to his peers?
- Is there a family history of puberty onset before age 8 years for a girl or 9 years for a boy?

EVALUATION AND MANAGEMENT

Evaluation and therapy differ greatly depending on the cause of atypical stature. The importance of a detailed history and thorough physical examination cannot be overemphasized because abnormalities of one or both often suggest the diagnosis.

Clinical History

Eliciting the clinical history should focus on learning about the child's growth to date (i.e., birth measurements, growth curves, pubertal status); assessing for a history or symptoms suggestive of chronic illness, malnutrition, or psychosocial stress; determining exposure to medications that may suppress growth; and acquiring a thorough family history of growth and development (Box 52.2). Heights of parents and siblings should be obtained (ideally by measurements in clinic). An extended pedigree if one parent is particularly short or tall assists in guiding the clinical index of suspicion for a genetic disorder.

Measurement Techniques and Growth Charts

Measurement of length or height must be accurate and reproducible to correctly assess the degree of interval growth. Children younger than 2 years should be measured in a supine position. Children older than 3 years should be measured standing. Children in between can be measured either way depending on their ability to stand erect for the duration of measurement. Proper measuring technique with fixed measurement equipment and correct positioning is crucial (Fig. 52.3). Recumbent lengths should be plotted on the length growth charts and standing heights on the height charts, because a person's length usually exceeds his or her height. A child's current height and growth pattern should be interpreted within the context of standards for the local population. In the United States, the Centers for Disease Control and Prevention (CDC) recommends using the World Health Organization (WHO) growth charts for infants and toddlers (ages 0 to 2 years) and the CDC's growth charts for children and adolescents (ages 2 to 20). These percentile curves illustrate age-ased distributions of length or height, weight, head circumference (for ages birth through 3 years), and weight-for-length or BMI (BMI = weight [kg]/height [m]^2) according to data from samples of children from global and US populations, respectively.

A. Supine length

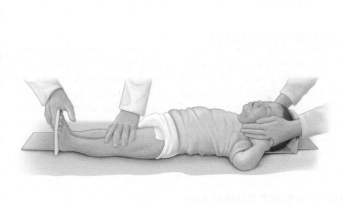

B. Standing height

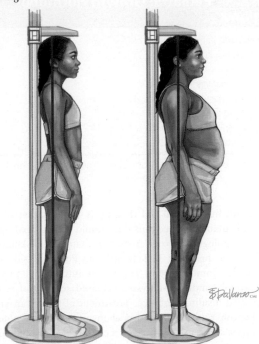

Two adults hold the child firmly in place, with the head against an inflexible board. The head is positioned in the Frankfurt plane (wherein the child's line of vision is straight up, perpendicular to the long axis of the trunk). The legs are held fully extended, and the ankles flexed perpendicularly with the feet flat against a moveable foot board.

Using a wall-mounted stadiometer, the child's feet are placed together in parallel to each other, and heels, buttocks, thoracic spine, and back of head should all be in line and parallel to the stadiometer's vertical axis. The child should be standing fully erect, knees straight, heels touching the ground, and head in the Frankfurt plane, as described above; the child may or may not be fully touching the wall depending on their body habitus.

Fig. 52.3 Proper Measurement Techniques.

Specific Elements of the Physical Examination

During physical examination, the practitioner should look for signs of underlying systemic illness, genetic abnormalities (e.g., dysmorphic features), or midline defects suggesting possible hypothalamic or pituitary malformations (e.g., a central maxillary incisor, or nystagmus, which is often the presenting feature of septo-optic dysplasia). The degree of dental maturation, which correlates with skeletal maturation (delayed dentition can imply delayed bone age), should also be assessed. Determining pubertal status using the Tanner staging criteria is critical (Chapter 46). Disproportionate growth can be ascertained by measurement of the upper-to-lower body segment ratio (upper segment length is the distance from top of the head to the top of the symphysis pubis, and lower segment length is the distance from the top of the pubic symphysis to the floor; normal ratios are 1.7:1 at birth, 1.3:1 at 3 years of age, and 1:1 by age 7 years), arm span (distance between the tips of the middle digits with both arms fully extended; normally arm span is less than standing height before age 8 years, equal to height at ages 8 to 12 years, and greater than height after age 12 years), or sitting height (to determine ratio to standing height).

Bone Age

The child's bone age represents the maturation of the skeleton and is the only quantitative determination of somatic maturation, mirroring the tempo of growth and puberty and indicating the remaining growth potential. After the child is beyond toddlerhood, an anteroposterior radiograph of the left hand and wrist is taken and compared with published standards (Greulich and Pyle or Tanner-Whitehouse); knee radiographs can be used at younger ages when hand and wrist films are

not yet informative. A bone age within 2 SDs of published standards is considered normal but should be interpreted within the context of other clinical findings.

Diagnosis of Growth Hormone Deficiency

The initial laboratory evaluation of potential GHD involves measuring IGF-1 and its carrier protein, IGFBP-3. Because of the circadian rhythm of GH secretion, it is not useful to measure a random serum GH level beyond the newborn period. Further evaluation is best deferred to a pediatric endocrinologist. All children with diagnosed GHD warrant magnetic resonance imaging of the brain with designated pituitary cuts to exclude an intracranial tumor or structural pituitary abnormality as the underlying cause.

MANAGEMENT

Management should be tailored to the cause. Important considerations include the following:
- **FSS** *is a normal variant.* The patient and family should be reassured that the child is healthy and will likely reach an adult height in keeping with family trends.
- **CDGP** *is a benign condition.* One can reassure the patient and family and monitor growth expectantly because spontaneous entry into puberty and attainment of family-appropriate adult height are anticipated.
- **Malnutrition:** refer to Chapter 120.
- **Systemic diseases** should be treated accordingly (e.g., gluten-free diet for celiac disease, levothyroxine replacement for hypothyroidism).

BOX 52.3   Pediatric Growth Hormone Indications

- Growth hormone deficiency
- Chronic renal insufficiency
- Turner syndrome
- Prader-Willi syndrome
- SGA or IUGR without catch-up growth
- Idiopathic short stature
- *SHOX* gene haploinsufficiency
- Noonan syndrome

IUGR, Intrauterine growth restriction; *SGA,* small for gestational age; *SHOX,* short stature, homeobox containing.

- **Recombinant human (rh) GH therapy** is a medication administered by subcutaneous injections that should be managed by pediatric endocrinologists. Box 52.3 provides current FDA-approved indications for pediatric GH treatment. Potential side effects include pseudotumor cerebri (increased intracranial pressure), slipped capital femoral epiphysis, increased severity of scoliosis, and increased insulin resistance. Treatment of GHD can unmask central hypothyroidism and adrenal insufficiency. Of note, evidence supports a permissive but not a causal role, for both GH and IGF-I in cancer development; thus active malignancy is a contraindication to GH treatment. Long-term (into adulthood) effects of pediatric GH treatment are unclear, as rhGH has been commercially available only since 1985.
- **Idiopathic short stature** is an indication for rhGH that warrants careful consideration. In 2003 the FDA approved rhGH therapy for ISS in children with growth rates not expected to lead to attainment of adult height in the "normal range" and in whom other causes of growth failure having been excluded. This indication remains controversial because evidence supporting the treatment's presumed psychosocial benefits is weak and inconsistent. Additionally, rhGH is expensive (estimated at $100,000 for an average gain of 1.9 inches) and often ineffective. In contrast, classic GHD involves health ramifications beyond height, and GH treatment universally increases height as long as adherence to the injections is high.

FUTURE DIRECTIONS

Socioeconomic, sex, and racial disparities in growth evaluations have been identified but no solutions developed to address them. The challenge for the future is to eliminate these disparities that can lead to delayed or missed diagnoses. It also remains necessary to distinguish the various causes of ISS, understand who benefits from pharmacologic height gain, and thereby identify which children warrant pharmacologic treatment versus other interventions (e.g., psychological therapy).

DISCLOSURE SUMMARY

Adda Grimberg served as a Consultant for the Pediatric Endocrine Society Growth Hormone Deficiency Knowledge Center, sponsored by Sandoz.

ACKNOWLEDGMENT

The authors would like to acknowledge the contribution of Dorit Koren, MD, on the previous edition chapter.

SUGGESTED READINGS

Available online.

53

Endocrine Dysnatremias

Stephanie Green and Amanda M. Ackermann

✷ CLINICAL VIGNETTE

A 4-year old boy with no medical history presents to the emergency department with 3 months of polydipsia, polyuria, weight loss, intermittent emesis, decreased appetite, headaches, and behavior changes. His parent reports that he asks for water throughout the day, urinates 10 to 20 times daily, and wakes up overnight to drink and urinate. He was even found drinking from a fish tank. On examination, he is afebrile, crying for water, with sunken eyes, heart rate 118 beats/min, and normal blood pressure. Laboratory test results show serum sodium 144 mEq/L, BUN 12 mg/dL, creatinine 0.5 mg/dL, urine specific gravity less than 1.005, urine osmolality 54 mOsm/kg, and serum osmolality 307 mOsm/kg. Magnetic resonance imaging of the brain and pituitary with and without contrast reveals a 12- × 8- × 9-mm enhancing lesion near the pituitary stalk and hypothalamus, concerning for a germinoma, and absent T1 hyperintensity of the posterior pituitary, consistent with central diabetes insipidus (DI). Anterior pituitary hormone assessments reveal central hypothyroidism and central adrenal insufficiency. He is given desmopressin 0.1 mg orally every 12 hours and stress dose hydrocortisone, and he is allowed to drink to thirst; after receiving hydrocortisone for 24 hours, levothyroxine is started, with plans to perform a biopsy of the lesion.

This is a typical presentation of a child with an intrasellar or suprasellar mass that leads to hypothalamic and/or pituitary dysfunction. Despite having DI, because he has intact thirst, he is able to maintain a relatively euvolemic eunatremic state under normal circumstances.

Serum sodium derangements often represent a physiologic response to physical stress or external stimuli, such as dehydration. However, inappropriate alterations in thirst, vasopressin, aldosterone, natriuretic peptides, or renal function require additional assessment and intervention.

PATHOGENESIS

Water Balance Regulates Extracellular Osmolality and Volume Status

Plasma, serum, or blood osmolality (or tonicity) is defined as the solutes in osmoles in 1 kg of water (mOsm/kg water), as opposed to osmolarity, which is the solutes in osmoles in 1 liter of the solution (mOsm/L). The effective osmolality is the osmotic gradient created by solutes unable to freely cross the cell membrane (e.g., sodium, glucose, urea), equilibrated by water crossing the cell membrane. Serum osmolality is largely determined by sodium (mEq/L), with small contributions from blood urea nitrogen (BUN) (mg/dL) and glucose (mg/dL) normally:

$$\text{Osmolality} = (2 \times Na^+) + (BUN/2.8) + (Glucose/18)$$

Serum osmolality is maintained between 280 and 295 mOsm/kg water by changes in vasopressin release, renal water excretion, and thirst.

Vasopressin

Arginine vasopressin (AVP or antidiuretic hormone [ADH]) is a peptide synthesized by the hypothalamic supraoptic and paraventricular nuclei (SON, PVN), transported by axons in the pituitary stalk to the posterior pituitary gland (neurohypophysis), stored in neurosecretory granules, and released from axon terminals into the systemic circulation. The stored vasopressin granules are responsible for the "posterior pituitary bright spot" seen on T1-weighted magnetic resonance imaging (MRI) (Fig. 53.1) and contain 5 to 30 days' worth of vasopressin.

Osmoreceptors from the anterior hypothalamus continuously monitor serum osmolality through fenestrated capillaries. They can detect as little as a 1% change in serum osmolality. Vasopressin release starts at approximately 283 mOsm/kg and increases linearly up to 320 mOsm/kg. Nausea, hypoglycemia, cortisol, and many medications can also affect vasopressin release (Fig. 53.2).

Vasopressin release is also regulated by baroreceptors in the aortic arch (carotid sinus), cardiac atria, and pulmonary veins, which sense changes in volume status. However, this mechanism is less sensitive for modulating vasopressin release, requiring 8% or greater volume depletion to stimulate exponential vasopressin release. Importantly, vasopressin does not directly regulate blood pressure.

Vasopressin binds and activates the G_s-coupled V2 receptors on principal cells in renal collecting ducts, which stimulate transport of aquaporin-2 water channels to the apical membrane to increase water reabsorption (up to 100-fold). Without vasopressin, urine is dilute (<50 mOsm/kg). Vasopressin-stimulated water retention concentrates the urine to 300 to 600 mOsm/kg and up to 1000 to 1200 mOsm/kg after maximal vasopressin secretion. Vasopressin's half-life is approximately 5 minutes, and aquaporin channels are rapidly shuttled away from the cell membrane after loss of V2 receptor signaling. Thus, changes in vasopressin release lead to precise minute-to-minute variations in urine concentration and serum volume.

Thirst

Thirst is regulated by the hypothalamic ventromedial nucleus and cortical neurons responding to changes in serum osmolality and intravascular volume, similar to the regulation of vasopressin. However, the threshold for thirst activation is higher (~293 mOsm/kg). Immediately after water intake, chemoreceptors in the oropharynx decrease thirst and vasopressin release, in proportion to the volume and coldness of the fluid, before any changes in serum osmolality, which prevents rapid overconsumption of fluids.

Sodium Metabolism Regulates Volume Status

Volume status is largely regulated by sodium intake and excretion, which are modulated primarily by renal filtration, aldosterone, and natriuretic peptides.

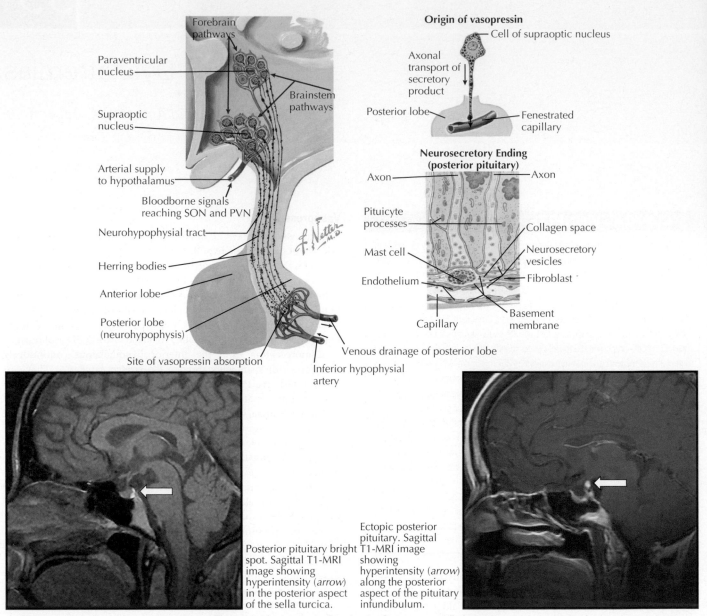

Fig. 53.1 Vasopressin Synthesis, Storage, and Release.

Aldosterone

Aldosterone is a potent mineralocorticoid secreted by the zona glomerulosa of the adrenal cortex. Decreased intravascular volume reduces perfusion of the renal juxtaglomerular apparatus, stimulating the renin-angiotensin-aldosterone system (RAAS). Aldosterone binds the mineralocorticoid receptor in the renal collecting duct principal cells (and to some degree the intercalated cells), increasing sodium reabsorption at the expense of potassium and hydrogen excretion. Aldosterone synthesis and secretion are also stimulated by increased serum potassium, adrenocorticotropic hormone (ACTH), and vasopressin. Aldosterone secretion is inhibited by atrial natriuretic peptide (ANP), somatostatin, and dopamine.

Atrial Natriuretic Peptide

Endothelial and vascular smooth muscle cells secrete ANP in response to volume expansion, increased atrial or ventricular pressure, exercise, tachycardia, and hypoxia. ANP acts on the inner renal medullary collecting ducts and proximal tubules to inhibit sodium reabsorption, and

it decreases and inhibits aldosterone and vasopressin. The net effect of increased ANP is natriuresis and diuresis.

Cerebral Adaptation

Cerebral adaptation to osmolality derangements can occur within 24 to 72 hours. With hypernatremia, brain volume is maintained by water movement from the cerebrospinal fluid into the brain and increased production of intracellular osmoles (e.g., glycine, sorbitol, glutamine) that promote extracellular-to-intracellular water shift. With hyponatremia, electrolytes and osmolytes are extruded, with water following.

HYPERNATREMIA

Clinical Presentation and Differential

Hypernatremia (serum sodium >145 to 150 mEq/L) occurs when free water losses exceed intake, or when sodium intake exceeds excretion. Signs and symptoms of hypernatremia (Box 53.1) may be coupled with symptoms of hypovolemia or hypervolemia depending on the cause.

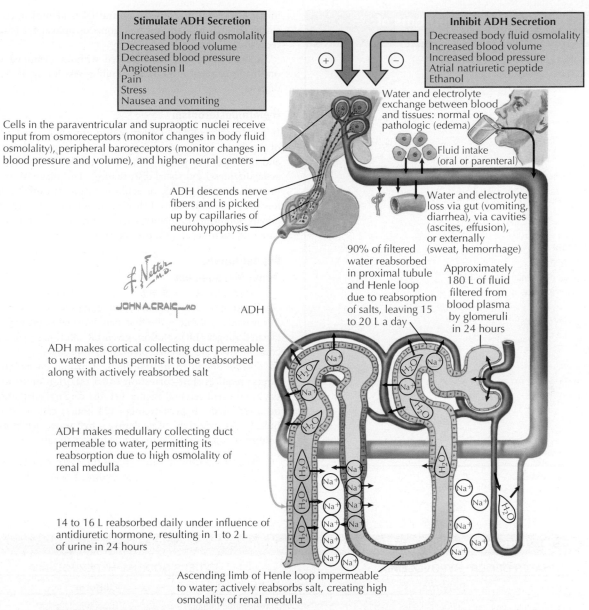

Stimulate ADH Secretion

Increased body fluid osmolality
Decreased blood volume
Decreased blood pressure
Angiotensin II
Pain
Stress
Nausea and vomiting

Inhibit ADH Secretion

Decreased body fluid osmolality
Increased blood volume
Increased blood pressure
Atrial natriuretic peptide
Ethanol

Cells in the paraventricular and supraoptic nuclei receive input from osmoreceptors (monitor changes in body fluid osmolality), peripheral baroreceptors (monitor changes in blood pressure and volume), and higher neural centers

ADH descends nerve fibers and is picked up by capillaries of neurohypophysis

Water and electrolyte exchange between blood and tissues: normal or pathologic (edema)

Fluid intake (oral or parenteral)

Water and electrolyte loss via gut (vomiting, diarrhea), via cavities (ascites, effusion), or externally (sweat, hemorrhage)

90% of filtered water reabsorbed in proximal tubule and Henle loop due to reabsorption of salts, leaving 15 to 20 L a day

Approximately 180 L of fluid filtered from blood plasma by glomeruli in 24 hours

ADH

ADH makes cortical collecting duct permeable to water and thus permits it to be reabsorbed along with actively reabsorbed salt

ADH makes medullary collecting duct permeable to water, permitting its reabsorption due to high osmolality of renal medulla

14 to 16 L reabsorbed daily under influence of antidiuretic hormone, resulting in 1 to 2 L of urine in 24 hours

Ascending limb of Henle loop impermeable to water; actively reabsorbs salt, creating high osmolality of renal medulla

Fig. 53.2 Vasopressin (Antidiuretic Hormone [ADH]) Regulates Urine Volume and Concentration.

Severe hypernatremia (serum sodium >160 mEq/L or a rapid rise in sodium) can cause subarachnoid, subdural, or parenchymal cerebral hemorrhages as a result of brain volume shrinkage and vascular rupture, particularly in infants. Thrombosis may also occur. The differential diagnoses can be categorized based on volume status and urine output (Table 53.1).

Evaluation

If there is concern for an endocrinopathy based on history and examination, initial studies should include serum sodium, potassium, calcium, bicarbonate, glucose, BUN, creatinine, and osmolality; urinalysis; and urine osmolality, sodium, and creatinine (ideally all collected at the same time). Additional studies may include serum renin and aldosterone.

Diabetes Insipidus

Hypernatremia with elevated serum osmolality but inappropriately dilute urine suggests diabetes insipidus (DI). Serum osmolality greater than 300 mOsm/kg with simultaneous urine osmolality less than 300 mOsm/kg is diagnostic. If serum osmolality is less than 270 mOsm/kg or urine osmolality is greater than 600 mOsm/kg, DI is unlikely. If history is suggestive but initial laboratory test results are not definitive, an inpatient water deprivation test should be pursued.

During a water deprivation test, food and fluid intake are prevented and serum and urine sodium and osmolality, urine output, and body weight are serially measured. If urine osmolality is greater than 1000 mOsm/kg at any time, or greater than 600 mOsm/kg for 1 hour or longer, DI is excluded. If serum osmolality is greater than 300 mOsm/kg and urine osmolality remains below 600 mOsm/kg, DI is diagnosed, and administration of vasopressin followed by serial serum and urine measurements can distinguish between central DI (urine output decreases and urine osmolality increases) and nephrogenic DI (no change in urine output or osmolality).

Because central DI can indicate intracranial pathologic conditions, an MRI of the brain and pituitary with and without contrast should be obtained. Of note, germ cell tumors or pinealomas in the area of the hypothalamus-stalk-posterior pituitary are frequently associated with DI. However, germ cell tumors may be too small to detect on

Signs and Symptoms of Hyponatremia and Hypernatremia

Hyponatremia
- Nausea/vomiting
- Anorexia
- Malaise
- Muscle cramps
- Headaches
- Hypothermia[a]
- Apnea[a]
- Altered mental status[a]
- Seizures[a]
- Obtundation[a]
- Coma[a]

Hypernatremia
- Nausea/vomiting
- Increased thirst (if mechanism intact)
- Restlessness/irritability
- Weakness
- High-pitched cry (infants)
- Fever
- Tachypnea
- Hyperglycemia
- Hypocalcemia
- Altered mental status[a]
- Lethargy[a]
- Seizures[a]
- Coma[a]
- Cerebrospinal fluid protein elevation (infants)

[a] Present in severe cases.

initial MRI, so if no cause of central DI is identified, consider measuring serum β-human chorionic gonadotropin and α-fetoprotein and repeating MRIs every 3 months.

If nephrogenic DI is diagnosed without identified cause based on history, a renal ultrasound should assess for cystic or obstructive disease.

Hyperaldosteronism

In primary hyperaldosteronism, aldosterone is secreted independently of the RAAS, leading to aberrant salt and water retention, potassium and hydrogen ion wasting, and hypertension (with associated headache, dizziness, and visual disturbance). This diagnosis is rare in children, but can be genetic or acquired. Patients exhibit hypervolemia, low urine sodium, relatively low urine volume, elevated urine specific gravity and urine osmolality, acidic urine, hypokalemia, alkalosis, elevated aldosterone, and suppressed renin.

Management
Acute Management

Intravascular repletion in hypovolemic hypernatremia. Stabilization of cardiovascular status and organ perfusion by restoring intravascular volume is the first step. Normal saline is preferred over lactated Ringer (LR) solution, given LR solution's hypotonic sodium concentration (154 versus 130 mEq/L, respectively).

Correction of hypernatremia. Chronic hypernatremia (>24 hours) requires slow correction (<0.5 mEq/L/h or 10 to 12 mEq/L/day) to prevent cerebral edema, because cerebral adaptation has likely occurred. Acute hypernatremia (<24 hours) can be corrected more quickly (~1 mEq/L/h). Calculating a free water deficit estimates the volume of water required to correct hypernatremia:

$$\text{Free water deficit (mL)} = (4 \text{ mL/kg}) \times (\text{weight in kg}) \times (\text{current Na}^+ - \text{desired Na}^+)$$

TABLE 53.1 **Differential Diagnosis of Hypernatremia**

WATER DEFICIT: HYPOVOLEMIA		EXCESS SODIUM: HYPERVOLEMIA	
Oliguria	**Polyuria**	**Variable**	**Oliguria**
Gastrointestinal losses (most common cause) • Diarrhea or high ostomy output • Emesis or nasogastric drainage • Osmotic cathartics (lactulose) Inadequate intake • Adipsia or hypodipsia (usually secondary to damage to hypothalamus) • Ineffective breast or formula feeding • Child abuse Increased insensible losses • Premature infants • Radiant warmers • Burns • Excessive sweating • Phototherapy • Mechanical ventilation	Central diabetes insipidus • Genetic • Acquired Nephrogenic diabetes insipidus • Genetic • Acquired Renal losses • Iatrogenic osmotic diuresis (mannitol) • Diabetes mellitus (osmotic diuresis due to glucosuria) • Chronic kidney disease (dysplasia and obstructive uropathy) • Polyuric phase of acute tubular necrosis • Postobstructive diuresis	Improperly mixed formula Ingestion of seawater or sodium chloride Intentional salt poisoning (child abuse) Iatrogenic • Intravenous hypertonic saline • Sodium bicarbonate administration	Hyperaldosteronism Apparent mineralocorticoid excess Cushing syndrome
↑ Urine specific gravity ↓ Urine Na⁺	↓ Urine specific gravity ↓ Urine Na⁺	↑ Urine specific gravity ↑ Urine Na⁺	↑ Urine specific gravity ↓ Urine Na⁺

Maintenance fluid requirements and ongoing fluid losses must be provided in addition to repleting the free water deficit. Oral fluids are generally preferred over intravenous fluids if possible. Sodium should be monitored frequently, and fluid rate and content should be titrated appropriately.

Disease-Specific Management

Central diabetes insipidus. There are many genetic and acquired causes of central DI (Table 53.2). Anterior pituitary hormone abnormalities may be present at the time of diagnosis or may develop later. Importantly, adrenal insufficiency decreases renal free water clearance, which may mask DI until steroids are given. Conditions that also affect the hypothalamus may impair thirst perception and regulation, affecting fluid management.

Trauma to the skull base or neurosurgery near the hypothalamus and pituitary, may result in transient sodium disturbances termed the triphasic (or triple phase) response. Initially, transient DI occurs for 0.5 to 2 days, followed by the syndrome of inappropriate antidiuretic hormone (SIADH) secretion lasting up to 10 days, then a final (likely permanent) phase of DI if greater than 90% of the vasopressin cells are destroyed. Frequent monitoring of sodium and urine output, with management adjustments, is important to avoid critical fluctuations in serum sodium.

The treatment goals for central DI are to maintain euvolemia and quality of life by using medication to reduce urine output and to maintain eunatremia by providing appropriate free water intake.

The vasopressin analog desmopressin (DDAVP) comes in oral, sublingual, intranasal, and subcutaneous formulations. The half-life of oral desmopressin is approximately 2.8 hours, with duration of action of 6 to 18 hours. It is typically given every 8 to 12 hours, allowing for approximately 1 hour of urine output breakthrough (>3 mL/kg/h) at least once daily, to decrease the risk for water intoxication and allow excretion of renal solutes. If thirst is intact, the patient is instructed to drink to thirst, otherwise free water is typically prescribed at approximately two-thirds maintenance volume, which accounts for insensible losses and daily breakthrough urine output.

Aqueous vasopressin has a short half-life (approximately 10 minutes) and rapid onset, so continuous infusion is recommended for patients in the operating room or intensive care.

Infants with central DI are managed differently because their fluid intake cannot be restricted, because it is their only nutrition source, so antidiuresis with desmopressin would put them at high risk for severe hyponatremia. Therefore infants are typically managed with a combination of additional prescribed free water intake, low-solute formula (breast milk or Similac PM 60/40), and/or a thiazide diuretic. Desmopressin may be used in select cases.

Nephrogenic diabetes insipidus. Nephrogenic DI can be genetic or acquired (Table 53.2). Genetic forms typically manifest early in infancy with failure to thrive.

Treatment includes (1) correcting the underlying cause (if able), (2) ensuring adequate fluid intake, and (3) decreasing urine output by limiting solute load and using a thiazide diuretic. Addition of amiloride or an NSAID may be also be required. In infants, solute load is minimized by feeding human milk or Similac PM 60/40. In children, protein and sodium restriction should be targeted to not impair growth.

Primary hyperaldosteronism. Treatment of primary hyperaldosteronism depends on the cause and may include surgical resection or unilateral adrenalectomy, mineralocorticoid receptor antagonists (spironolactone or eplerenone), or glucocorticoids.

HYPONATREMIA

Clinical Presentation and Differential

Hyponatremia (serum sodium <135 mEq/L) results from excess free water reabsorption or sodium excretion, associated with decreased serum osmolality and hypovolemia, euvolemia, or hypervolemia. Mild hyponatremia (serum sodium ~125 to 135 mEq/L) is typically asymptomatic and is often associated with hypovolemia as a result of diarrhea. However, severe (serum sodium <125 mEq/L) or acute (<12 to 24 hours) hyponatremia can cause a wide variety of symptoms with severe symptoms resulting from cerebral edema (Box 53.1).

Pseudohyponatremia (normal serum osmolality with low serum sodium on laboratory test results) is a laboratory artifact resulting from serum dilution in the presence of hyperlipidemia or hyperproteinemia (e.g., intravenous immunoglobulin, myeloma) when sodium is measured indirectly; point of care and blood gas analyzers use direct ion-selective electrodes yielding more accurate measurements in this setting.

Dilutional hyponatremia (normal or high serum osmolality) may result from excess osmolytes (glucose or mannitol) causing intracellular-to-extracellular osmotic shift, without affecting total body sodium or water. Correcting the underlying solute abnormality normalizes serum sodium. The corrected serum sodium concentration must be calculated to account for excess solutes:

$$\text{Sodium correction for hyperglycemia} = Na^+_{measured} \\ + (1.6 \times [\text{glucose (mg/dL)} - 100]/100)$$

The differential for true hypotonic hyponatremia is broad (Fig. 53.3). Ascertaining volume status is imperative. History should assess for emesis, diarrhea, insensible losses, medication and drug use, sodium and fluid intake, urination frequency and volume, trauma, and surgical, neurologic, renal, endocrine, and cardiac histories.

Evaluation and Management

Most causes can be diagnosed by a combination of history, examination, complete metabolic panel (serum sodium, creatinine, BUN, potassium, glucose, calcium, albumin), and urinalysis. When the diagnosis is unclear, simultaneously obtaining serum and urine osmolality, sodium, and creatinine can further guide the differential.

Treatment generally includes saline administration in hypovolemia, fluid restriction in euvolemia, and diuresis and/or fluid restriction in hypervolemia, along with treating any underlying cause. If hyponatremia worsens with initial management, promptly consider alternative diagnoses.

Acute Management

Intravascular repletion in hypovolemic hyponatremia. Stabilization of cardiovascular status with isotonic saline or LR is the first step.

Severe acute hyponatremia. If severe symptoms (e.g., seizures) are present, 3% hypertonic saline boluses should be administered to quickly increase extracellular osmolality, increase serum sodium 4 to 6 mEq/L or less, and resolve symptoms. If hypervolemic, consider adding loop diuretics.

Chronic hyponatremia. Slow correction of hyponatremia (<0.5 mEq/L/h or 10 to 12 mEq/L/day) is warranted in chronic cases (>24 to 72 hours) to avoid brain cell dehydration in the setting of cerebral adaptation. Rapid correction of hyponatremia can lead to osmotic demyelination (previously known as pontine myelinolysis), which occurs within several days of correction and may be irreversible. This syndrome is characterized by agitation, confusion, flaccid or spastic quadriparesis, and death.

Disease-Specific Management

Hypotonic hypovolemic hyponatremia

Appropriate ADH release. Extrarenal sodium and water losses with inadequate volume intake stimulates vasopressin secretion,

TABLE 53.2   Causes of Endocrine Hypernatremias

Condition	Cause	
Central diabetes insipidus	**Genetic** • AD or AR vasopressin mutation (*AVP* gene) • Wolfram (DIDMOAD) syndrome (DI, DM, optic atrophy, deafness) (*WFS1* gene) **Congenital anatomic defects (midline brain anomalies)** • Septo-optic dysplasia with agenesis of corpus callosum • Kabuki syndrome • Holoprosencephaly • Familial pituitary hypoplasia with absent stalk **Trauma** • Skull fracture hemorrhage (e.g., Sheehan syndrome) • Operative **Neoplasms** • Germ cell tumors (e.g., germinoma) • Pinealomas • Craniopharyngioma • Optic glioma • Myelocytic leukemia metastatic disease (infiltration)	**Other** • Empty sella • DI of pregnancy • Hamartoma **Infiltrative, autoimmune, infectious disease** • Langerhans cell histiocytosis • Lymphocytic hypophysitis • Sarcoidosis • Wegener granulomatosis **Drugs/medications** • Ethanol • Phenytoin • Opiate antagonists • Halothane • α-Adrenergic agents

Nephrogenic diabetes insipidus	**Genetic**
	• X-linked V2 receptor mutation (*AVPR2* gene)
	• AD or AR aquaporin-2 mutation (*AQP2* gene)
	Acquired (partial or complete)
	• Intrinsic renal disease
	  • Obstructive uropathies
	  • Acute/chronic renal failure
	  • Renal cystic diseases
	  • Renal dysplasia
	  • Interstitial nephritis
	  • Nephrocalcinosis
	  • Sjögren syndrome
	  • Sickle cell disease
		Acquired (partial or complete)—cont'd
		• Extrinsic
		  • Primary polydipsia
		  • Hypokalemia (chronic)
		  • Hypercalcemia
		  • Medications (lithium, amphotericin B, cisplatin, colchicine, cidofovir, demeclocycline, ifosfamide, foscarnet, methicillin, methoxyflurane, propoxyphene, rifampin, vinblastine)

Increased cortisol activity	**Cushing syndrome** • Pituitary ACTH secreting adenoma (Cushing disease) • Ectopic ACTH production **Apparent mineralocorticoid excess** • AR mutation of 11-β-dehydrogenase type 2 (*HSD11B2* gene) Exogenous glucocorticoid	
Primary hyperaldosteronism	Aldosterone secreting adenoma Bilateral multinodular adrenocortical hyperplasia Unilateral adrenal hyperplasia Adrenocortical carcinomas Glucocorticoid-suppressible hyperaldosteronism (familial hyperaldosteronism type 1)	

ACTH, Adrenocorticotropic hormone; *AD*, autosomal dominant; *AR*, autosomal recessive; *AVP*, arginine vasopressin; *DI*, diabetes insipidus; *DM*, diabetes mellitus.
Note: Renal failure can have variable urine sodium. Syndrome of inappropriate antidiuretic hormone (SIADH) secretion can be mildly hypervolemic.

causing free water reabsorption and decreased serum sodium. This causes increased urine specific gravity and osmolality, decreased urine output and urine sodium (as a result of activation of RAAS), and increased BUN. Treatment includes oral or intravenous fluid resuscitation and assessment of response.

Cerebral salt wasting. Cerebral salt wasting (CSW) is thought to be due to increased ANP secretion after brain injury. Polyuria and hypovolemia with inappropriately increased urine sodium, urine osmolality, and BUN are suggestive of CSW. Treatment includes oral or intravenous fluids to replace losses and sodium supplementation.

Aldosterone deficiency and pseudohypoaldosteronism. Salt craving and failure to thrive with hyperkalemia, metabolic acidosis, and elevated urine sodium and osmolality is suspicious for aldosterone deficiency or resistance (pseudohypoaldosteronism [PHA]). The aldosterone level distinguishes these diagnoses.

Aldosterone deficiency occurs secondary to primary adrenal insufficiency and results in sodium excretion, potassium and

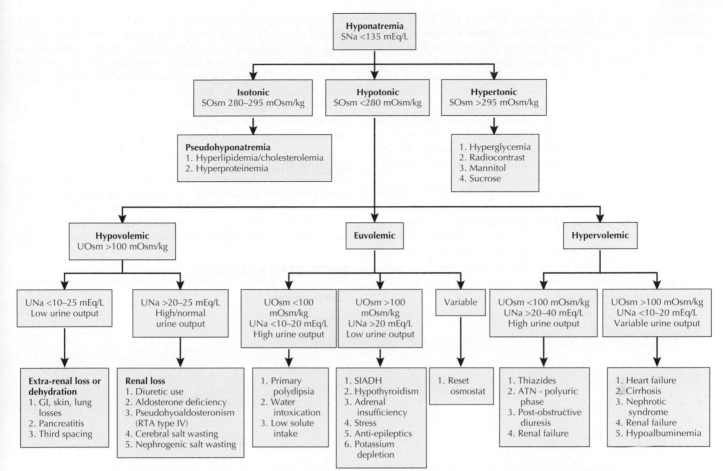

Fig. 53.3 Evaluation Algorithm for Hyponatremia. *ATN,* Acute tubular necrosis; *RTA,* renal tubular acidosis; *SIADH,* syndrome of inappropriate antidiuretic hormone; *SNa,* serum sodium; *SOsm,* serum osmolality; *UNa,* urine sodium; *UOsm,* urine osmolality.

hydrogen ion reabsorption, and hypovolemia. Volume repletion with isotonic fluids is often needed acutely. Fludrocortisone is used to activate the mineralocorticoid receptor. Oral salt supplementation also may be needed.

Pseudohypoaldosteronism (type IV renal tubular acidosis) can be transient in children with urinary tract obstruction or resolving urinary tract infections or the result of a genetic condition (PHA1 or PHA2). PHA1 may be treated with salt supplementation and potassium binders, while PHA2 is treated with sodium restriction and thiazide diuretics.

Euvolemic hyponatremia

Syndrome of inappropriate antidiuretic hormone. SIADH occurs when vasopressin release is not inhibited by low serum osmolality or expanded intravascular volume, leading to excess renal free water retention. This results in euvolemia or very mild hypervolemia. Diagnosis (Fig. 53.3) is based on serum osmolality less than 280 mOsm/kg, urine osmolality of 100 mOsm/kg or greater (usually >300 mOsm/kg and urine greater than serum osmolality), and urine sodium greater than 20 mEq/L. SIADH is suggested by history of brain injury, medication use, lung disease, pain, stress, or vasopressin-producing malignant tumors (Box 53.2), some of which may be transient. Nephrogenic syndrome of inappropriate antidiuresis is a rare X-linked disorder caused by gain of function mutations in the V2 receptor. Findings are identical to those of SIADH, but serum vasopressin is undetectable, and males are typically affected.

BOX 53.2 Causes of Syndrome of Inappropriate Antidiuretic Hormone Secretion

- At-risk hospitalized patients
  - Pain
  - Stress
  - Nausea
- Central nervous system disorders
- Lung disease
- Medications
  - Desmopressin
  - Antiepileptics (carbamazepine, oxcarbazepine, valproate)
  - Barbiturates
  - Opioids
  - Sulfonylureas (chlorpropamide, tolbutamide)
  - Vincristine
  - Selective serotonin reuptake inhibitors
  - Tricyclic antidepressants
  - Diuretics (thiazides)
- Drugs
  - MDMA (Ecstasy)
- Nephrogenic SIADH
- Malignant tumors (ADH producing)

ADH, Antidiuretic hormone; *SIADH,* syndrome of inappropriate antidiuretic hormone.

Treatment requires fluid restriction, typically two-thirds maintenance volume (1000 mL/m²/day). This volume accounts for obligate renal solute excretion and typical insensible fluid losses, but it should be titrated based on subsequent serum sodium, serum osmolality, and volume status. In some cases, enteral sodium supplementation or a loop diuretic may be used. Vasopressin antagonists (vaptans) may be used in rare cases but can result in too rapid/overcorrection of serum sodium as a result of diuresis. Urea is also safe and effective in children but is not used commonly in the United States. If a medication side effect is suspected, the risk and benefit of medication discontinuation versus SIADH treatment should be weighed.

Water intoxication and psychogenic polydipsia. In children, the kidney can dilute urine up to 50 mOsm/kg and can safely excrete up to 10 L/m²/day without developing hyponatremia. Infants and neonates cannot dilute their urine to this degree, so they are at high risk for water intoxication when given excess intravenous hypotonic fluids or free water instead of formula or breast milk. Laboratory results show hyponatremia with dilute urine. Removing excess free water corrects the hyponatremia.

Psychogenic polydipsia and DI often reside in the same clinical differential when a child with intact thirst presents with polyuria, polydipsia, and eunatremia. Laboratory testing of the first morning void before fluid intake may rule out DI, or a water deprivation test may be needed. Once DI is excluded, treatment involves behavioral modifications to limit fluid intake to maintenance volume.

Other endocrine causes. Adrenal insufficiency and hypothyroidism both lead to reduced free water clearance and euvolemic hyponatremia. Hormone replacement is corrective.

FUTURE DIRECTIONS

More specific and sensitive tools for diagnosis and treatment of endocrine dysnatremias are needed. Measurement of hypertonic saline-stimulated serum copeptin (C-terminal segment of vasopressin prohormone) may be useful for diagnosing central diabetes insipidus.

SUGGESTED READINGS

Available online.

Gastroenterology

Melissa Kennedy

54

Diarrhea

Wenjing Zong and Chiara Pandolfi de Rinaldis

 CLINICAL VIGNETTE

A 21-month-old girl with trisomy 21 presents with chronic diarrhea. She has had abdominal distension and two to three loose, foul-smelling stools daily for the past month. Her parents also report that she has had poor appetite and increasing fussiness. They deny any fever, recent illness, rash or bloody stools. She has had no sick contacts or travel history. They deny excessive juice intake. She has not gained weight since her last appointment. Her stool studies are negative for infectious causes, but her bloodwork is positive for immunoglobulin A antibodies against tissue transglutaminase; she therefore undergoes an intestinal biopsy. Biopsy demonstrates increased intraepithelial lymphocytes, crypt hyperplasia, and partial villous atrophy, consistent with a diagnosis of celiac disease. She is started on a gluten-free diet, with resolution of her symptoms within a few weeks.

Acute diarrhea accounts for more than 1.5 million outpatient visits, 200,000 hospitalizations, and approximately 300 deaths annually among children in the United States. It is estimated that diarrhea admissions in the United States cost $1 billion per year. In developing countries, diarrhea is a common cause of mortality among children younger than 5 years of age, with approximately 2 million deaths annually.

PATHOPHYSIOLOGY

A total of 8 to 9 L of fluid enters the healthy intestines on a daily basis. Only 1 to 2 L are derived from food and liquid intake; the rest is from salivary, gastric, pancreatic, biliary, and intestinal secretions. Each day, about 90% of this fluid is absorbed in the small intestine, 1 L enters the colon, and about 100 mL is excreted in stool. Normal stool output is approximately 100 to 200 g/day. Diarrhea is defined as stool output greater than 200 g/day in children older than 2 years of age and greater than 10 mL/kg/day in children younger than 2 years of age. It is also described more practically as an increase in liquidity and frequency of bowel movements, with a common definition being the passage of 3+ loose stools per day. Diarrhea can be categorized by duration, as either *acute* (≤2 weeks) or *chronic* (>2 weeks), or by mechanism, as *osmotic* or *secretory*. It also can be categorized by the presence or absence of malabsorption (Fig. 54.1).

Both secretory and osmotic diarrhea are caused by defective or impaired mucosal absorption. In osmotic diarrhea, excess amounts of nonabsorbed substances, such as lactose, lactulose, fructose, or sorbitol, remain in the intestinal lumen, causing luminal water retention. After these luminal substances enter the colon, they are processed by colonic flora, producing large amounts of organic acids, increased flatulence, and faster transit. The fecal osmolar gap [290 mOsm/L − {2 × (measured stool sodium + measured stool potassium)}] is usually greater than 100 mOsm/L in the setting of osmotic diarrhea. When an abnormal gap is found, reducing substances, stool pH, and fecal fat should be measured. Osmotic diarrhea improves with fasting. Examples of osmotic diarrhea include lactase deficiency, celiac disease, and short bowel syndrome. Secretory diarrhea is the result of abnormal ion transport in epithelial cells, leading to decreased absorption of electrolytes and increased secretion of fluid. The fecal osmolar gap is usually less than 50 mOsm/L, and the diarrhea persists despite fasting. Examples include congenital chloride and sodium diarrhea, cholera, and neuroendocrine tumors.

Another important underlying mechanism of diarrhea is dysmotility. For example, pseudo-obstruction may result in bacterial stasis, overgrowth, and resultant diarrhea, whereas hyperthyroidism may be associated with diarrhea because of rapid intestinal transit.

The character of the stool can help determine the origin of diarrhea. Watery, voluminous, nonbloody stool with few or no white blood cells (WBCs) and low pH (<5.5) is likely to emanate from disease of the small intestine. Low-volume, mucous, often bloody diarrhea with a large number of WBCs and higher pH often originates from the colon.

Bloody diarrhea is a concerning symptom. The most common cause is infection, especially in the setting of fever and acute onset. If bloody diarrhea is progressive and persistent, chronic inflammatory causes should be considered. The age of the patient is also important. In infants, milk protein–induced enterocolitis is a common cause of bloody stools.

ACUTE DIARRHEA

Etiology and Pathogenesis

The most common cause of acute diarrhea is infection (see Chapter 63). In young children, this is most often viral, with the most common agents being rotavirus, adenovirus, astrovirus, sapovirus, and norovirus. Norovirus causes 60% to 90% of nonbacterial gastroenteritis in the United States, affecting 19 to 21 million Americans each year and accounting for up to 1 million pediatric medical visits annually. Rotavirus is a leading cause of death in children younger than 5 years of age worldwide. In immunocompromised hosts, viruses such as cytomegalovirus, Epstein-Barr virus, and BK virus should be considered. It is estimated that 70% of infectious diarrhea is foodborne, and thus a detailed history of exposures is very important (Table 54.1). Exposure to untreated water, for instance, may cause giardiasis. Use of public swimming pools poses a risk for *Shigella, Giardia, Cryptosporidium,* and *Entamoeba* infection, with the last three being chlorine resistant. Home pets can transmit infections. For example, turtles carry *Salmonella* species. History of foreign travel may narrow exposures based on the specific destination. The most common cause of traveler's diarrhea remains enterotoxigenic *Escherichia coli. Cryptosporidium* and *Giardia* species are responsible for most parasitic infections in developed countries. Cyclospora outbreaks have occurred in the United

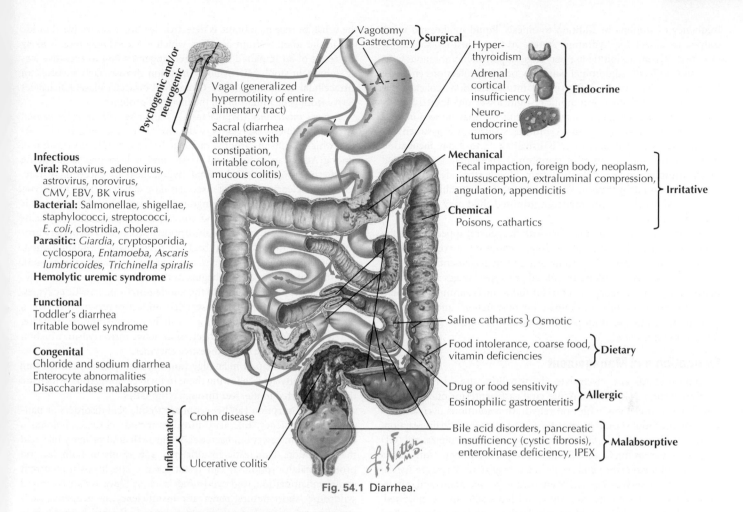

Infectious
Viral: Rotavirus, adenovirus, astrovirus, norovirus, CMV, EBV, BK virus
Bacterial: Salmonellae, shigellae, staphylococci, streptococci, *E. coli*, clostridia, cholera
Parasitic: *Giardia*, cryptosporidia, cyclospora, *Entamoeba*, *Ascaris lumbricoides*, *Trichinella spiralis*
Hemolytic uremic syndrome

Functional
Toddler's diarrhea
Irritable bowel syndrome

Congenital
Chloride and sodium diarrhea
Enterocyte abnormalities
Disaccharidase malabsorption

Psychogenic and/or neurogenic

Vagal (generalized hypermotility of entire alimentary tract)

Sacral (diarrhea alternates with constipation, irritable colon, mucous colitis)

Vagotomy Gastrectomy } **Surgical**

Hyperthyroidism
Adrenal cortical insufficiency
Neuroendocrine tumors
} **Endocrine**

Mechanical
Fecal impaction, foreign body, neoplasm, intussusception, extraluminal compression, angulation, appendicitis

Chemical
Poisons, cathartics
} **Irritative**

Saline cathartics } Osmotic

Food intolerance, coarse food, vitamin deficiencies } **Dietary**

Drug or food sensitivity
Eosinophilic gastroenteritis } **Allergic**

Bile acid disorders, pancreatic insufficiency (cystic fibrosis), enterokinase deficiency, IPEX } **Malabsorptive**

Inflammatory { Crohn disease

Ulcerative colitis

Fig. 54.1 Diarrhea.

TABLE 54.1	**Foodborne Infectious Agents**
Food	**Associated Infectious Agent**
Eggs	*Salmonella* spp.
Dairy	*Campylobacter jejuni*
Vegetables	*Clostridium perfringens*
Pork	*Clostridium perfringens*
	Yersinia enterocolitica
Seafood	*Aeromonas* spp.
	Vibrio spp.
	Plesiomonas spp.
Rice	*Bacillus cereus*
Beef	Enterohemorrhagic *Escherichia coli*

States. *Clostridioides difficile* infection, previously thought to affect only hospitalized patients or those taking antibiotics, is now responsible for 40% of community-acquired diarrhea. A recent increase in *C. difficile* infections has been observed, some attributable to the resistant strain, BI/NAP1. An overgrowth of toxin-producing *Clostridioides* organisms causes pseudomembranous colitis, which may be a potentially life-threatening condition. However, colonization with toxigenic *C. difficile* is also common in children, with colonization detected in up to 50% of neonates and 70% of children younger than 2. *Vibrio cholerae* remains a cause of illness and death in war zones and developing countries. The mechanism of infectious diarrhea is primarily secretory. It can quickly lead to electrolyte abnormalities and acidosis. Infection

may result in villous atrophy, which can add an osmotic component. Mucosal healing after infection may lead to transient postinfectious diarrhea.

Several other causes of acute diarrhea, particularly in afebrile children, may be particularly concerning. Intussusception, a telescoping of two segments of bowel that occurs mostly in children between 6 and 36 months, may manifest with bloody diarrhea (see Chapter 60). The typical manifestation is colicky abdominal pain, vomiting, and an abdominal mass. "Currant jelly" stools occur in a minority of patients with intussusception but are pathognomonic for the condition. Hemolytic-uremic syndrome (HUS) is an uncommon but potentially fatal illness that may manifest with acute bloody diarrhea and is typically caused by Shiga toxin–producing *E. coli*. HUS begins as a mild gastroenteritis that evolves into hematochezia, microangiopathic hemolytic anemia, thrombocytopenia, and acute renal failure (see Chapter 104). Less commonly, appendicitis may manifest with abdominal pain and diarrhea as a result of colonic irritation from the inflamed appendix (see Chapter 4).

Other acute causes of diarrhea include inflammatory bowel disease (IBD; see Chapter 57), overfeeding (caused by increased osmotic loads), antibiotic-associated diarrhea (likely caused by changes in bowel flora), extraintestinal infections (otitis media, urinary tract infection, pneumonia), and toxic ingestions.

Clinical Presentation

In any patient presenting with acute diarrhea, a thorough history and physical examination should guide the immediate and subsequent evaluation and therapy. It is important to quantify the duration and frequency of stooling in addition to emesis, liquid intake, and urine output to assess for hydration status. A travel history should be obtained. Recent antibiotic use may suggest pseudomembranous colitis with *C. difficile.* Abdominal pain may occur in infectious enteritis; however, it also may be indicative of intussusception (colicky, episodic) or appendicitis (periumbilical, right lower quadrant). Bloody diarrhea is more typical in bacterial enteritis but may be seen in viral illness, HUS, or colitis. Associated vomiting suggests viral gastroenteritis. In infectious diarrhea, there is usually a 1- to 8-day incubation period with a sudden onset of symptoms. There may be associated fever, vomiting, crampy abdominal pain, bloody stools, tenesmus, loss of appetite, and dehydration. The immune state of the child should be determined because an immunocompromised child may present with more unusual organisms.

The physical examination begins with the general appearance of the child—does the child look malnourished or appear to have lost weight? Vital signs then help guide evaluation and management. Fever usually indicates infection. Pulse and blood pressure changes may indicate dehydration, shock, or sepsis. A careful abdominal examination should assess for bowel sounds (to evaluate for obstruction) and masses (to evaluate for intussusception). A stool sample should be guaiac tested for microscopic blood.

Evaluation and Management

Hydration status and electrolyte abnormalities should be assessed, with correction as indicated. Acute viral gastroenteritis often requires rehydration, preferably with oral rehydration solutions over intravenous fluids. Stool should be sent for viral polymerase chain reaction, bacterial culture, and *C. difficile* toxin assay. Most gastrointestinal (GI) infections, except for *C. difficile,* do not require treatment. Antibiotics tend to prolong diarrhea and result in a carrier state. There are special circumstances, such as *Salmonella* enteritis in young infants and immunocompromised patients, for which antibiotic therapy is indicated. Most infections resolve in 14 days in healthy children. Antidiarrheal agents are typically not effective and should be avoided in children. Serious complications, such as sepsis, HUS, pancreatitis, urinary tract infection, and perforation, are uncommon.

CHRONIC DIARRHEA

Etiology and Pathogenesis

Chronic diarrhea (Fig. 54.2) manifesting as two to eight large, loose bowel movements per day, typically occurring during the daytime, in an otherwise healthy and normally growing child is usually attributable to functional diarrhea. For instance, chronic nonspecific diarrhea of childhood (toddler's diarrhea) most commonly affects young children 6 months to 5 years of age and is typically due to excessive fluid or carbohydrate intake, low fat intake, or rapid transit. Irritable bowel syndrome (IBS) is another cause of functional diarrhea in older children with a prevalence of 1% to 3% and is two times more common in girls than boys. In some cases, functional diarrhea is caused by osmotic effects of carbohydrates such as sorbitol and fructose or dysmotility with rapid transit.

Congenital diarrheas are rare causes of voluminous, typically watery stools that manifest at birth. These disorders include chloride and sodium diarrhea, structural enterocyte abnormalities (e.g., microvillus inclusion disease and intestinal epithelial dysplasia or tufting enteropathy), and disaccharidase malabsorption (e.g., congenital sucrase-isomaltase deficiency and glucose–galactose transporter deficiency). Sodium and chloride diarrhea are autosomal recessive disorders that present at birth with secretory diarrhea in the presence of normal mucosa. In chloride diarrhea, the Cl^-/HCO_3^- exchanger in

the brush border membrane is defective, leading to excessive chloride loss in the stool. Sodium diarrhea, which is exceedingly rare, is likely the result of an impaired Na^+/H^+ exchanger leading to excessive loss of sodium in stool. Microvillous inclusion disease likely involves an intracellular trafficking defect. Congenital disaccharidase deficiencies derive from gene mutations of the involved proteins.

Lactose intolerance (hypolactasia) is an inherited disorder caused by reduced genetic expression of the enzyme lactase-phlorizin hydrolase, which results in carbohydrate malabsorption. It is most common among American Indians and Asians and is least prevalent among Northern Europeans. Congenital hypolactasia is exceedingly rare. Lactase deficiency (a form of disaccharidase deficiency) in enterocytes results in the rapid passage of ingested lactose to the colon, where it is processed by bacterial flora and converted to short-chain fatty acids and hydrogen gas. Lactose malabsorption also can be a secondary process caused by mucosal injury, bacterial overgrowth, or inflammation.

Malabsorption of fat may also result in chronic diarrhea (Fig. 54.3). Digestion of protein and fat begins in the oral cavity by salivary amylase and lipase and continues in the duodenum by pancreatic enzymes. Pancreatic enzymes are initially secreted as inactive proenzymes, which are activated by enterokinase, a brush border membrane protease. Enterokinase activates trypsinogen to its active form trypsin, which in turn activates the rest of the digestive enzymes.

Bile acids participate in fat digestion and absorption by emulsifying long-chain fatty acids, allowing them to form chylomicrons, which are then transported to the liver through lymphatics.

Fat malabsorption can be secondary to bile acid disorders or pancreatic insufficiency. Bile acid disorders include chronic cholestasis, terminal ileum resection, bacterial overgrowth, and primary bile acid malabsorption. Pancreatic insufficiency can result in both fat and protein malabsorption. It can result from cystic fibrosis, recurrent severe inflammation, and syndromes such as Shwachman-Diamond syndrome (short stature, pancreatic insufficiency, neutropenia, skeletal abnormalities). Enterokinase deficiency in the brush border may result in malabsorption caused by impaired activation of pancreatic proenzymes, which similar to colipase or lipase deficiency, results in failure to thrive and steatorrhea. In cystic fibrosis, the secretion of pancreatic enzymes is diminished by hyperviscosity and mucous plugging of ducts. Abetalipoproteinemia presents shortly after birth with steatorrhea and failure to thrive and if untreated may result in neurologic damage. Diarrhea with protein loss can be caused by a wide spectrum of disorders, including IBD, celiac disease, IPEX (immune dysregulation, polyendocrinopathy, enteropathy, X-linked) syndrome, and lymphangiectasia.

Several conditions causing chronic diarrhea are the result of an abnormal immune response to antigens in food or in the GI tract itself. Celiac disease is caused by gluten sensitivity, causing inflammation of the small intestine (see Fig. 54.3). In celiac disease, exposure to gluten and its active component gliadin results in an abnormal immune activation. This dietary gluten–triggered immune process leads to villous blunting or flattening, crypt elongation, and lymphocytic infiltration of the lamina propria. This disease affects about 1% of the population and can present any time between infancy and adulthood. It is associated with higher prevalence of HLA-DQ2/DQ8; therefore, family history is important. It is also more common in the setting of Down syndrome, type 1 diabetes, immunoglobulin A (IgA) deficiency, Turner syndrome, Williams syndrome, and autoimmune thyroiditis. IBD, including Crohn's disease and ulcerative colitis, usually presents with slow-onset, sometimes bloody, diarrhea with peak incidence in adolescence (see Chapter 57). *Allergic colitis,* which is often the result of milk or soy allergy, may manifest as bloody or non-bloody diarrhea in infants. Similarly, *food protein–induced enterocolitis*

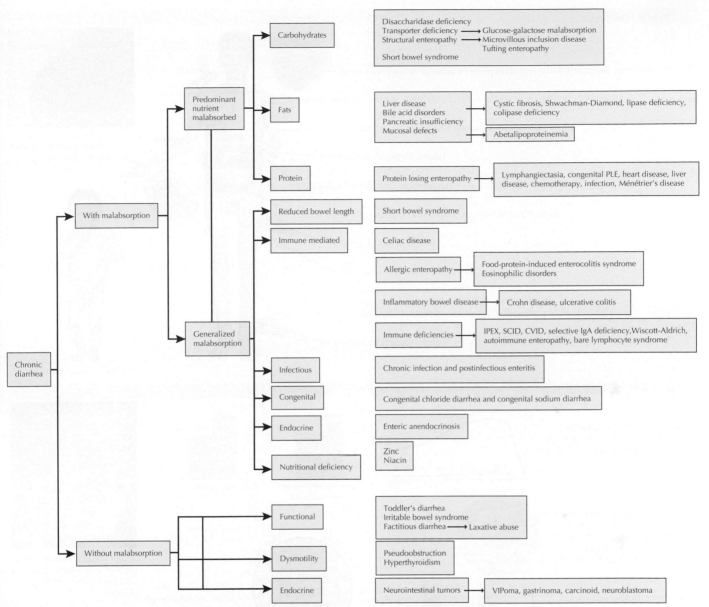

Fig. 54.2 Differential Diagnosis of Chronic Diarrhea.

is a non–IgE-mediated hypersensitivity syndrome that manifests with acute onset, repetitive vomiting with or without diarrhea in infants.

Food allergies resulting in malabsorption may be caused by eosinophilic gastroenteritis (Fig. 54.4). This disorder is often associated with other atopic conditions, such as asthma, eczema, and allergic rhinitis. Mechanisms of eosinophilic disorders that are associated with eosinophilic infiltration of various parts of the GI tract are poorly understood. They seem to involve an interaction among genetic predisposition, environmental exposures to foods and allergens, immunoglobulin E (IgE)-mediated activation of the immune system, and possible interaction with GI microbiota. Rare immune deficiencies that cause diarrhea include IPEX syndrome, severe combined immune deficiency, and autoimmune enteropathy. IPEX syndrome is caused by a mutation in the *FoxP3* gene in T-regulatory cells, resulting in a lack of immune homeostasis. Autoimmune enteropathy, which is associated with antienterocyte antibodies, may occur as part of IPEX but also can be isolated.

Neuroendocrine tumors, such as gastrinoma (Zollinger-Ellison syndrome), carcinoid, and VIPoma (pancreatic cholera), are rare in children and cause secretory diarrhea as a result of overproduction of intestinal hormones. Enteric anendocrinosis is a rare autosomal recessive disorder that causes severe diarrhea and is associated with type 1 diabetes. In this condition, mutation of neurogenin 3 results in deficient enteroendocrine cells perturbing the balance of fluid secretion and absorption, which in turn results in malabsorptive diarrhea.

Motility disorders are both diagnostically and therapeutically complex. They can be primary or secondary processes. Intestinal motility is controlled by the enteric nervous system, which interacts with multiple hormones, neurotransmitters, and extraintestinal stimuli. Hyperthyroidism is a common cause of alterations in intestinal dysmotility leading to mild to moderate diarrhea. Rapid transit time may be the result of increased neuronal stimulation. Lack of proper peristalsis may lead to bacterial overgrowth with associated diarrhea. Hyperthyroidism is associated with rapid transit, hypersecretion, increased adrenergic stimulation, and possibly a small degree of fat malabsorption secondary to rapid transit.

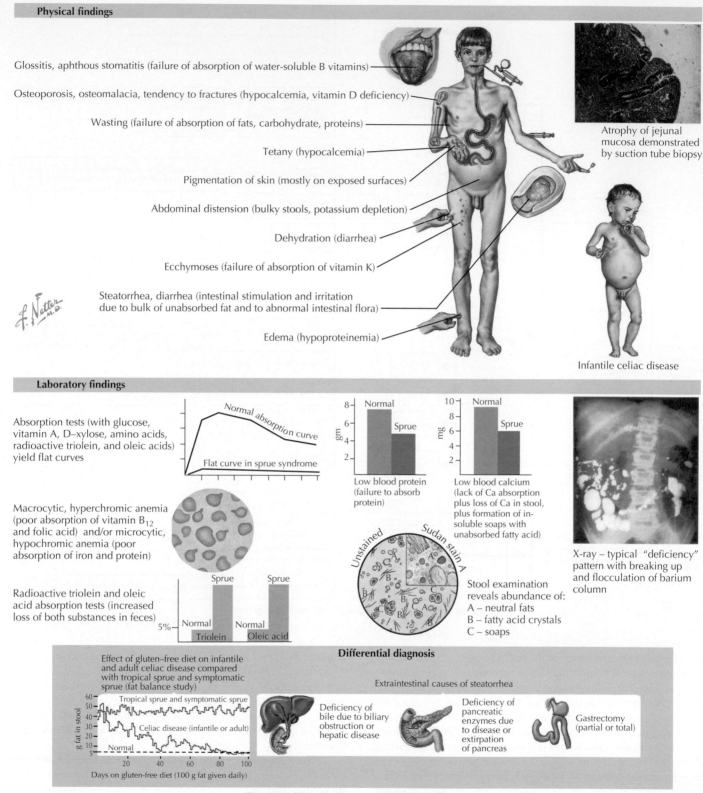

Physical findings

Glossitis, aphthous stomatitis (failure of absorption of water-soluble B vitamins)

Osteoporosis, osteomalacia, tendency to fractures (hypocalcemia, vitamin D deficiency)

Wasting (failure of absorption of fats, carbohydrate, proteins)

Tetany (hypocalcemia)

Pigmentation of skin (mostly on exposed surfaces)

Abdominal distension (bulky stools, potassium depletion)

Dehydration (diarrhea)

Ecchymoses (failure of absorption of vitamin K)

Steatorrhea, diarrhea (intestinal stimulation and irritation due to bulk of unabsorbed fat and to abnormal intestinal flora)

Edema (hypoproteinemia)

Atrophy of jejunal mucosa demonstrated by suction tube biopsy

Infantile celiac disease

Laboratory findings

Absorption tests (with glucose, vitamin A, D–xylose, amino acids, radioactive triolein, and oleic acids) yield flat curves

Normal absorption curve

Flat curve in sprue syndrome

Normal   Sprue

Low blood protein (failure to absorb protein)

Normal   Sprue

Low blood calcium (lack of Ca absorption plus loss of Ca in stool, plus formation of insoluble soaps with unabsorbed fatty acid)

Macrocytic, hyperchromic anemia (poor absorption of vitamin B_{12} and folic acid) and/or microcytic, hypochromic anemia (poor absorption of iron and protein)

Radioactive triolein and oleic acid absorption tests (increased loss of both substances in feces)

Sprue   Sprue

Normal   Normal
Triolein   Oleic acid
5%

Unstained   Sudan stain A

Stool examination reveals abundance of:
A – neutral fats
B – fatty acid crystals
C – soaps

X-ray – typical "deficiency" pattern with breaking up and flocculation of barium column

Differential diagnosis

Effect of gluten–free diet on infantile and adult celiac disease compared with tropical sprue and symptomatic sprue (fat balance study)

Tropical sprue and symptomatic sprue

Celiac disease (infantile or adult)

Normal

Days on gluten-free diet (100 g fat given daily)

g fat in stool

Extraintestinal causes of steatorrhea

Deficiency of bile due to biliary obstruction or hepatic disease

Deficiency of pancreatic enzymes due to disease or extirpation of pancreas

Gastrectomy (partial or total)

Fig. 54.3 Malabsorption and Celiac Disease.

Clinical Presentation and Evaluation
Functional Diarrhea

Functional diarrhea in young children does not result in malabsorption or weight loss. Irritable bowel syndrome (IBS) with diarrhea predominance manifests with a wide range of symptoms, including abdominal pain and diarrhea characterized by frequent loose stools during waking hours, mostly in the morning and postprandially. The Rome IV criteria are currently used for the diagnosis of IBS and are based on symptoms of abdominal pain associated with altered bowel pattern and improvement with defecation in the absence of inflammatory, anatomic, metabolic, or neoplastic processes that would otherwise explain the symptoms.

Symptoms • Dyspepsia
- Malnutrition and malabsorption
- Diarrhea
- Weight loss
- Allergy symptoms (asthma)

Biopsy appearance

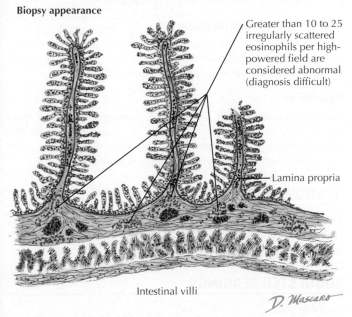

Greater than 10 to 25 irregularly scattered eosinophils per high-powered field are considered abnormal (diagnosis difficult)

Lamina propria

Intestinal villi

D. Mascaro

Fig. 54.4 Eosinophilic Gastroenteritis.

Congenital Diarrhea

Congenital chloride and sodium diarrhea present with voluminous stool output, high in chloride or sodium, respectively, which does not improve with fasting. Polyhydramnios may be noted prenatally. Diarrhea quickly leads to dehydration and acidosis. Structural abnormalities, such as tufting enteropathy and microvillous inclusion disease, manifest at birth with intractable secretory diarrhea and require endoscopic biopsies for diagnosis. Congenital disaccharidase deficiency usually presents with osmotic diarrhea when foods are introduced to the infant's diet and should be suspected if the stool contains reducing substances and the pH is low (<5.5). It is also associated with severe diaper rash. The diagnosis is made by disaccharidase analysis of duodenal tissue.

Carbohydrate Malabsorption

Symptoms after the ingestion of lactose include abdominal pain; bloating; flatulence; diarrhea; and, particularly in adolescents, vomiting. The stools tend to be bulky, frothy, and watery. In older children, the hydrogen produced by intestinal bacteria can be measured by a breath hydrogen test. Enzyme activity can also be determined by small bowel biopsy. Stool-reducing substances are present, and stool pH is low (<5.5).

Fat Malabsorption

Patients with fat malabsorption usually present with steatorrhea and failure to thrive. Fat-soluble vitamins (A, D, E, K) may be deficient. Protein loss may result in hypoalbuminemia, which may present clinically as edema or anasarca. The diagnosis of steatorrhea can be made by assessment of fecal fat in a single specimen, with the Sudan III stain, or by a quantitative assay of fecal fat excretion over 72 hours.

Celiac Disease and Immune-Mediated Diarrhea

Celiac disease may manifest with a wide range of symptoms, including diarrhea, steatorrhea, constipation, abdominal distension, failure to thrive, iron-deficiency anemia, dermatitis herpetiformis, arthritis, and ataxia or may be asymptomatic. Celiac disease is diagnosed by a combination of serologic testing and histopathologic findings. Serologic examination should include antitissue transglutaminase antibodies (anti-tTG) and endomysial antibodies. For children younger than 2 years of age, antigliadin antibodies also should be measured. Most serologic testing is IgA based, but about 10% of patients with celiac disease are IgA deficient, so testing should include a total IgA level to aid in interpretation. In the event of IgA deficiency, the antibodies can be tested using IgG-based assays. Upper endoscopy with duodenal biopsy remains the gold standard for the diagnosis of celiac disease.

Fecal calprotectin levels are increased in intestinal inflammation and therefore can be useful for distinguishing inflammatory from noninflammatory causes of diarrhea. Eosinophilic GI disease may manifest with diarrhea, poor growth, and bloody stools. Peripheral eosinophilia may not be present. The diagnosis is based on histopathologic evaluation of endoscopic biopsies. IPEX syndrome presents with chronic diarrhea, failure to thrive, food allergies, endocrinopathies such as type 1 diabetes and thyroiditis, hematologic disorders, and dermatitis. Suspected immune deficiencies require specialized evaluation with immunoglobulin levels, lymphocyte activities, WBC function tests, and genetic testing.

Endocrine-Mediated Diarrhea

VIPomas present with watery diarrhea, hypokalemia, and hypochlorhydria. Stool volumes are high and may lead to dehydration. Episodic symptoms in VIPoma and carcinoid may be related to sudden intermittent release of large quantities of hormones. Other associated symptoms include skin flushing caused by the vasodilator effects of vasoactive intestinal peptide (VIP) and secretin (commonly produced by carcinoid). The diagnosis is made by clinical symptoms and the presence of high hormone levels in the blood or metabolites in the urine. Gastrinoma (Zollinger-Ellison syndrome) causes large gastric secretion volumes that cannot be reabsorbed by the small intestine, thus leading to diarrhea.

Dysmotility

Diarrhea caused by dysmotility requires a thorough evaluation including motility evaluation, endoscopy and investigation into extraintestinal causes.

Management
Functional Diarrhea

If the child is growing adequately and is otherwise healthy, diagnostic testing and elimination diets are not recommended for functional diarrhea in toddlers and young children as symptoms will likely resolve by age 5. However, reducing fruit juices and dietary sorbitol, and liberalizing fat intake can be helpful for functional diarrhea. Dietary restriction is not typically recommended for children with IBS except on a case-by-case basis if there is a clear correlation between the symptoms and a specific trigger such as lactose or sorbitol. Sorbitol is a dietary ingredient that is often thought to trigger symptoms. Antimotility agents and antidepressants are also not routinely recommended for treatment of IBS in children, unlike in adults. Use of antispasmodics such as peppermint oil has limited evidence in children, but may be considered in the management of associated abdominal pain. Other therapies include behavioral health techniques to manage anxiety and stress.

Congenital Diarrhea

Nutritional support, including parenteral and enteral nutrition, is necessary. Congenital chloride and sodium diarrhea require chronic electrolyte supplementation. Congenital disaccharidase deficiency is managed by eliminating the offending sugar from the diet or in the case of sucrase-isomaltase deficiency, sacrosidase replacement may be used.

Carbohydrate Malabsorption: Disaccharidase Deficiency

Treatment involves an elimination diet, lactase enzyme supplementation, or both. If the disaccharidase deficiency is secondary, treatment of the underlying condition may help restore enzyme activity.

Fat Malabsorption

Fat malabsorption is detected by a 72-hour quantitative fecal fat. Fat-soluble vitamins should be measured in serum. Pancreatic insufficiency can be screened for using a fecal elastase level. Pancreatic enzyme collection and activity measurement can be performed endoscopically by collection of pancreatic secretions after secretin administration. If enzyme activity is low, pancreatic enzyme supplementation is indicated. If abetalipoproteinemia is suspected, serum very low-density lipoprotein and β-lipoprotein levels should be measured. In a patient with diarrhea and peripheral edema, protein loss should be evaluated by concurrent measurement of stool and serum α-1 antitrypsin (AAT). Because AAT is not digested while passing through the GI tract, its amount in stool is a good indicator of protein losses.

Celiac Disease and Immune-Mediated Diarrhea

Treatment of celiac disease is currently limited to a strict gluten-free diet. Dietary adherence is measured by periodic anti-tTG level measurement. Management of eosinophilic disorders involves allergy testing for specific food sensitivities with use of elimination or elemental diets. Sequential endoscopies may be useful to assess treatment success. Antiinflammatory and antiallergy agents have been tried with variable success. Treatment of immune deficiency is determined by the specific disorder and may require a bone marrow or stem cell transplant. Supportive nutritional therapy is indicated.

Endocrine-Mediated Diarrhea

Surgical removal of the offending endocrinologic tumor is optimal. Supportive therapy with somatostatin analogs may be required. Postcancer surveillance is required after treatment.

Dysmotility

Motility disorders remain a therapeutic challenge. If bacterial overgrowth is a cause of diarrhea, it should be treated with antibiotics. Antiadrenergics such as propranolol have been successfully used in hyperthyroidism to slow transit and improve absorption.

ACKNOWLEDGMENTS

The authors would like to acknowledge the contribution of Anna Hunter, MD, and Rose C. Graham, MD, for their work on the previous edition chapter.

SUGGESTED READINGS

Available online.

55

Constipation

Joshua D. Eisenberg and Jennifer Webster

✳ CLINICAL VIGNETTE

A 4-year-old boy presents with a chief concern of infrequent bowel movements. For the past 3 months he has two bowel movements per week. The stools are hard, large in caliber, and occasionally clog the toilet. A few times each week, he has "accidents" of liquid stool passing without him noticing. He has no blood in the stool, is growing well, and is meeting his developmental milestones. As a newborn, he passed meconium on the first day of life. Physical examination is significant for a nontender, firm abdominal mass palpable in the left lower quadrant, and a rectal examination positive for a large, firm stool ball in the rectal vault.

Functional constipation (FC) with encopresis is a common condition, particularly in toddlers and school-aged children. The patient described in the vignette meets the Rome IV criteria for FC with no high-risk historical elements for an underlying condition. He does not require additional evaluation. He will require fecal disimpaction before initiating maintenance therapy for constipation.

Constipation is a common concern in children, accounting for 3% to 5% of all visits to general pediatricians and as many as 30% of visits to pediatric gastroenterologists. When constipation occurs without an underlying medical condition or organic cause, it is considered *functional constipation* (FC) and is defined by clinical symptoms. The Rome IV criteria have provided the most widely accepted consensus definition for FC. This definition requires at least two of the following symptoms occurring weekly for at least 1 month: two or fewer bowel movements per week, at least one weekly episode of incontinence after the acquisition of toileting skills, history of retentive posturing or excessive stool retention, history of painful or hard bowel movements, the presence of a large fecal mass in the rectum, or a history of large-diameter stools that obstruct the toilet. Because FC accounts for the majority of constipation in children, it is the focus of this chapter.

ETIOLOGY AND PATHOGENESIS

FC typically results from a cycle of events involving pain with passing hard stool. Pain causes voluntary withholding of stool, leading to prolonged stasis of feces in the rectum (Fig. 55.1). Stasis promotes fluid reabsorption, hardening of the stool, and increased diameter of the stool. The fear of passing large, hard stools that stretch the anus and cause pain leads to further withholding and avoidance of defecation and can occur at any age. Over time, as it accommodates the enlarging fecal mass, the rectal wall becomes less sensitive to stretch and less efficient at peristalsis. Eventually, the urge to defecate decreases, and this retentive behavior becomes subconscious. In this setting, fecal soiling or encopresis can occur. *Encopresis* is the passage of stool under socially inappropriate conditions, either intentionally or unintentionally, by a child who is developmentally 4 years of age or older. Encopresis

occurs in about 1.5% of all children and is a common complication of constipation.

Clinical Presentation

Children with FC can present with infrequent bowel movements, decreased oral intake, and abdominal pain, distension, or cramping. They may report painful hard bowel movements and demonstrate withholding behaviors. Encopresis may develop if the constipation is severe. FC is often triggered during a dietary transition in infants, toilet training in toddlers, or school entry in older children.

A thorough history is important in discriminating between FC and constipation caused by an underlying illness. It is important to determine how soon after birth the child passed his or her first stool, the onset of constipation, the frequency and consistency of bowel movements, and the presence of blood in the stool, *tenesmus* (ineffectual straining with the urge to defecate), withholding behaviors, and encopresis. The history should probe for red flags (Box 55.1) suggestive of organic disorders resulting in constipation.

The physical examination should include an abdominal examination, external examination of the perianal region, including assessment of the anal wink reflex, and a digital rectal examination (DRE). The DRE evaluates the tone of the anal sphincter, size of the anal canal and rectum, presence or absence of stool, and consistency of the stool.

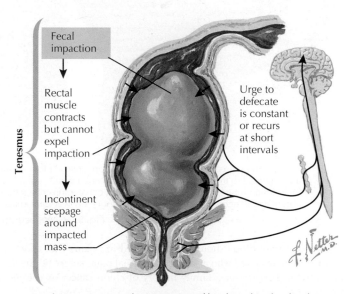

Fecal impaction, or a large amount of hard stool in the distal rectum obstructing the anal outlet. The presence of a fecal impaction can lead to encopresis as more proximal fecal matter seeps around the impacted fecal mass.

Fig. 55.1 Pathophysiology of Defecation.

BOX 55.1   Potential High-Risk Features in Constipation

- Passage of meconium after 48 hours of life
- Family history of Hirschsprung disease
- Ribbon stools
- Blood in stools in the absence of anal fissures
- Failure to thrive
- Bilious emesis
- Severe abdominal distension
- Abnormal thyroid gland
- Abnormal anal position
- Absent anal or cremasteric reflex
- Lower extremity neurologic deficits
- Sacral dimple and/or tuft of hair
- Gluteal cleft deviation
- Anal scars

Adapted from Hyams JS, Di Lorenzo C, Saps M, et al. Childhood functional gastrointestinal disorders: child/adolescent. *Gastroenterology.* 2016;150:1456-1468.

BOX 55.2   Differential Diagnosis of Constipation in Children

- Functional constipation
- Hirschsprung disease
- Hypothyroidism
- Celiac disease
- Cow's milk intolerance
- Tethered spinal cord
- Cystic fibrosis
- Lead poisoning
- Infantile botulism
- Anorectal anomalies:
  - Imperforate anus, anal atresia
  - Anal stenosis
- Anal achalasia

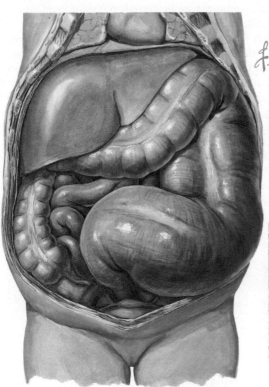

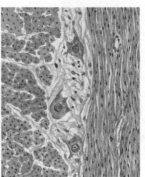

Barium enema; characteristic distal constricted segment

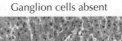

Tremendous distension and hypertrophy of sigmoid and descending colon; moderate involvement of transverse colon; distal constricted segment

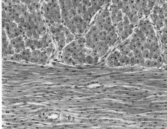

Ganglion cells absent

Ganglion cells present between longitudinal and circular muscle layers

Hirschsprung disease, or congenital aganglionic megacolon, is caused by the congenital absence of ganglion cells in the rectosigmoid region and can lead to the onset of constipaton in early infancy and the development of a bowel obstruction and megacolon. Diagnostic evaluation includes an unprepared barium enema that can demonstrate a transition zone *(top right, above)* and rectal biopsy that demonstrates the absence of ganglion cells *(lower middle above). Lower right* image depicts the presence of ganglion cells.

Fig. 55.2 Megacolon (Hirschsprung Disease).

Testing for occult blood should be performed in infants with constipation and in any child who also has abdominal pain, failure to thrive, intermittent diarrhea, or a family history of colon cancer or colonic polyps.

Differential Diagnosis

Although most constipation in children is functional, it is important to consider the broad differential diagnosis of constipation in children (Box 55.2). Patients with a condition underlying their constipation usually present with a range of high-risk symptoms or physical findings in addition to constipation (see Box 55.1). For example, children with *Hirschsprung disease* (Fig. 55.2) often do not pass meconium during the first 48 hours of life and have problems with constipation beginning in infancy (Table 55.1). On examination, the rectum is generally very small and empty of stool and there is frequently a large amount of eliminated stool after withdrawal of

TABLE 55.1	**Distinguishing Functional Constipation From Hirschsprung Disease**	
	Functional Constipation	**Hirschsprung Disease**
Onset	Rare in infancy	Common in infancy
Delayed passage of meconium	Rare	Common
Encopresis	Common	Unusual
Stool size	Very large	Small, ribbon-like
Failure to thrive	Rare	Common
Abdominal distension	Variable	Common
Painful defecation	Common	Rare
Stool in rectal vault	Common	Rare
Anal tone	Open, distended	Tight

Adapted from Graham-Maar RC, Ludwig S, Markowtiz J. Constipation. In: Fleisher GR, Ludwig S, Henretig FM, eds. *Textbook of Pediatric Emergency Medicine*. 5th ed. Philadelphia, PA: Lippincott Williams & Wilkins, 2006; and Behrman RE, Kliegman RM. *Nelson Essentials of Pediatrics*. 4th ed. St. Louis, MO: Saunders; 2002.

the digit. *Hypothyroidism* can result in constipation in addition to lethargy, hypotonia, short stature, cold intolerance, and/or dry skin. *Celiac disease* can manifest with constipation with poor growth and abdominal pain. *Lead poisoning* can cause constipation with vomiting and intermittent abdominal pain. Patients with a *tethered spinal cord* may have a sacral dimple and lower extremity motor deficits. In general, patients with constipation secondary to an underlying illness have additional findings in the history or physical examination warranting further investigation.

EVALUATION AND MANAGEMENT

The evaluation of constipation depends on the suspected clinical diagnosis. If Hirschsprung disease is suspected, work-up includes an unprepared barium enema to look for a transition zone and a rectal suction biopsy to detect ganglion cells. Other tests to consider include thyroid function tests, celiac antibodies, lead level, calcium level, sweat test, and imaging of the lumbar spine.

If FC is suspected based on the history and physical examination, no laboratory or radiologic investigation is necessary. Routine use of abdominal radiography is not recommended but may be useful if fecal impaction is suspected and the patient will not tolerate a rectal examination. Additionally, colonic motility can be assessed with a radiopaque marker study. For this study, the patient swallows radiopaque markers and completes an abdominal x-ray examination 5 days after ingestion. For refractory cases, anorectal manometry can be performed to assess anorectal sensation and reflex circuits in patients for whom disordered defecation dynamics are suspected.

Initial treatment of FC depends on the presence or absence of a fecal impaction. *Fecal impaction* is defined as a hard mass in the lower abdomen on physical examination, a dilated rectum filled with a large amount of hard stool on rectal examination, or excessive stool on abdominal radiography. Disimpaction must occur before

maintenance therapy can be effective and is best accomplished by the rectal route with phosphate-, saline-, or mineral oil-containing enemas. An oral approach to disimpaction is slower and less effective than rectal disimpaction, but if necessary, can be attempted with high-dose osmotic laxative paired with a stimulant laxative. If enemas and oral laxatives are ineffective, a manual disimpaction is indicated to alleviate colonic obstruction. Treatment after fecal disimpaction includes initiating maintenance therapy and educating the patient and family.

Maintenance therapy should focus on prevention of recurrence. It generally includes a combination of behavioral modification, laxatives, and dietary changes. Osmotic laxatives, when used regularly, help maintain soft stool. These laxatives include polyethylene glycol, magnesium hydroxide, lactulose, and sorbitol. Stimulant laxatives such as senna and bisacodyl can be used for short intervals; the prolonged use of stimulant laxatives in children is not recommended. Dietary interventions consist of increasing dietary fiber and fluid intake. Behavioral modification involves healthy toilet habits, including scheduled toilet sitting, counseling on toilet sitting posture, and a reward system for positive reinforcement. Successful treatment of FC often takes at least 3 to 6 months.

FUTURE DIRECTIONS

Future advances in the diagnosis of constipation include the development of noninvasive measures of colonic motility to focus treatment. Therapeutic advances include novel pharmacologic agents that are already in use for adults with refractory constipation and are being evaluated for effectiveness and safety in children.

SUGGESTED READINGS

Available online.

56

Gastritis and Gastrointestinal Bleeding

Logan Grimes and Steven Fusillo

CLINICAL VIGNETTE

An 11-year-old boy with history of biliary atresia who underwent Kasai portoen-terostomy in infancy presents to the emergency department (ED) with dark stools. He has had progressive epigastric abdominal discomfort and fatigue for the past 3 days, and several episodes of dark "sticky" stools since yesterday. He has had no vomiting, fevers, or other symptoms. In the ED, his vital signs are notable for pulse of 118 beats/min and blood pressure of 95/70 mm Hg. On physical examination, he is tired-appearing and jaundiced, with marked hepatosplenomegaly and ascites. His rectal examination is notable for guaiac-positive tarry black stools without apparent hemorrhoids or fissures. Two peripheral intravenous lines are placed and serum laboratories obtained. His hemoglobin is found to be 6.4 g/dL with a normal platelet count. A type and screen is obtained. His aspartate aminotransferase/alanine aminotransferase are markedly elevated, with an elevated conjugated bilirubin and an international normalized ratio (INR) of 2.2. A right upper quadrant ultrasound with Doppler ultrasound demonstrates an interval increase in hepatomegaly with evidence of worsening fibrosis (as compared to his surveillance imaging). Nasogastric lavage is performed, with copious bright red blood present in the aspirate that clears after 200 mL normal saline flush. He is started on an intravenous proton pump inhibitor, given subcutaneous vitamin K, and transfused 15 mL/kg packed red blood cells. His hemodynamic status stabilizes and he undergoes upper endoscopy which reveals interval worsening of portal gastropathy and two grade 3 esophageal varices. Esophageal banding is performed with complete flattening of the varices. He has no further bleeding, and postprocedure hemoglobin remains stable. He received a total of 3 days of subcutaneous vitamin K, with normalization of his INR. He is discharged home in stable condition and ultimately listed for liver transplant.

Numerous potential causes, combined with the gastrointestinal (GI) tract's extensive surface area, make the assessment and management of GI bleeding exceptionally challenging. Observations of several key clinical features assist clinicians in formulating rational differential diagnoses. Gastritis is an important cause of GI bleeding and abdominal pain that deserves particular attention. Although the inability to arrive at a definitive diagnosis (i.e., obscure GI bleeding) remains a persistent issue, the growing arsenal of diagnostic modalities is making it increasingly possible to localize the source of bleeding, particularly with regard to proximity to the ligament of Treitz, which facilitates a more successful treatment strategy.

ETIOLOGY AND PATHOGENESIS

The causes of GI bleeding are diverse (Fig. 56.1). Grouping the possibilities into pathophysiologic categories aids in constructing a differential diagnosis. Note that comorbid underlying disorders of coagulation (e.g., hemophilias, vitamin K deficiency in neonates) and hepatic dysfunction (because of the liver's role in producing coagulation factors) can exacerbate any of these causes.

Direct Mechanical Injury

Blunt and penetrating trauma can initiate bleeding from any part of the GI tract. Ingestion of certain foreign bodies (e.g., button batteries) may result in mucosal injury and even bowel perforation. Repeated vomiting or retching may create esophageal mucosal defects called Mallory-Weiss tears that bleed. Surgical interventions, such as dental procedures and tonsillectomy, may result in blood loss that is swallowed and subsequently vomited. Anal fissures or rectal trauma may manifest as bleeding from the GI tract.

Mucosal Erosion

The GI tract has a robust and sophisticated mucosal defense mechanism designed to prevent erosion. These protective elements include (1) the superficial "unmixed" layer of mucus, bicarbonate, and other factors that form a neutralizing and buffering barrier against acid, enzymatic, and abrasive injury; (2) the epithelial cells that generate this superficial layer; (3) continuous cell renewal coupled with (4) uninterrupted nutrient blood flow to the mucosa; (5) sensory innervation that optimizes this blood flow; and (6) endothelial production of prostaglandins and nitric oxide, which synergize to promote the aforementioned mechanisms. Disruption of any of these factors may predispose a given region to erosion, local loss of vascular integrity, and resultant bleeding.

Drug-Induced

A number of drugs can precipitate mucosal erosions, the most notorious being those from the nonsteroidal antiinflammatory drug (NSAID) class, which inhibit cyclooxygenase-mediated prostaglandin synthesis. Other culprits include corticosteroids, alcohol, caffeine, and nicotine. Chemotherapeutic agents, such as vincristine, methotrexate, and 5-fluorouracil, may cause GI bleeding via inflammation and mucosal erosion (termed *mucositis*) anywhere along the GI tract by inhibiting epithelial cell turnover, recruiting inflammatory cells, and making the mucosa more susceptible to infectious insults.

Inflammation

Disruption of mucosal integrity may occur in disorders that promote the recruitment of inflammatory cells, such as lymphocytes and neutrophils, which injure the epithelium by direct cell-to-cell contact or by secreted immunologic factors, such as cytokines. Examples include autoimmune enteropathy and eosinophilic gastroenteritis. Another important example is inflammatory bowel disease (IBD), a complex autoimmune disease that encompasses Crohn's disease, which can cause full-thickness inflammation anywhere along the GI tract, and ulcerative colitis, which causes mucosal ulcerations in the colon (see Chapter 57). Children who have undergone bone marrow transplant may experience a form of rejection called graft-versus-host disease (GVHD). When it affects the GI tract, GVHD causes diarrhea,

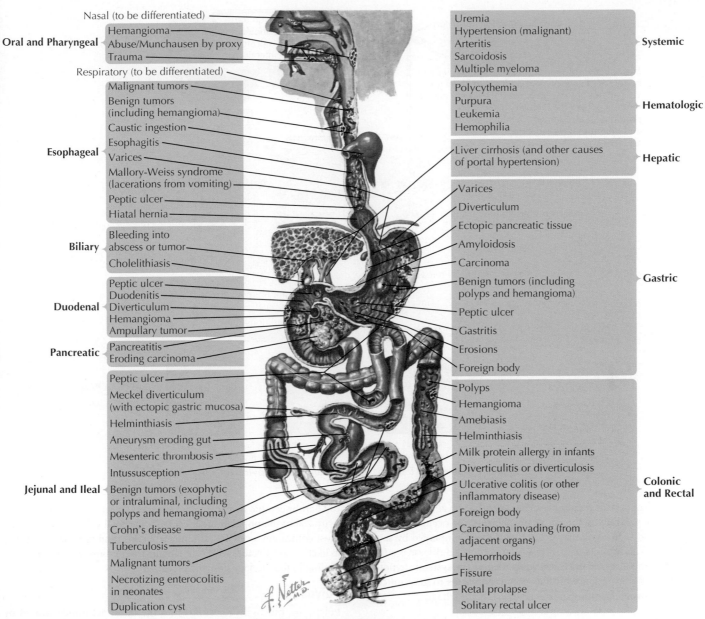

Fig. 56.1 Gastrointestinal Hemorrhage.

vomiting, fever, abdominal pain, and GI bleeding. Certain immunodeficiencies, such as common variable immunodeficiency, precipitate inflammation because of dysregulated immunity that leads to autoimmune responses and GI bleeding may occur.

Infection

Infections disrupt mucosal integrity by direct cytotoxicity and/or by promoting inflammation. For example, herpes simplex virus is known to cause florid esophagitis, particularly in immunocompromised individuals, with nearly one-third of these patients experiencing an acute upper GI bleed. Additionally, infections may elicit specific responses. For example, cytomegalovirus is occasionally associated with massive gastric epithelial proliferation leading to a hypertrophic gastropathy called Ménétrier disease. This causes protein wasting (including coagulation factors) from the leaky mucosa, as well as a higher risk for mucosal erosion and bleeding. *Helicobacter pylori* is perhaps the most infamous of the infectious causes of gastritis and duodenitis because of its chronicity, high prevalence (especially among certain

populations, including immigrants from developing countries, children living in crowded and/or low socioeconomic status households, and those attending daycare centers), its associations with peptic ulcers and adenocarcinoma of the stomach and duodenum, and its resistance to eradication (Fig. 56.2).

Caustic Ingestions

Ingestion of acidic substances causes a coagulation necrosis that results in ulcers and mucosal bleeding. Alkali ingestions can create significantly worse complications through liquefaction necrosis and mucosal sloughing, which can lead to severe ulceration, perforation, and eventual luminal stenosis.

Ischemia

Loss of blood flow to the bowel can lead to ischemic injury and necrosis. Examples of conditions in which this may occur are mesenteric arterial thrombosis; vascular malformations that create regions of suboptimal blood flow; and drug-induced bowel injury, as can occur

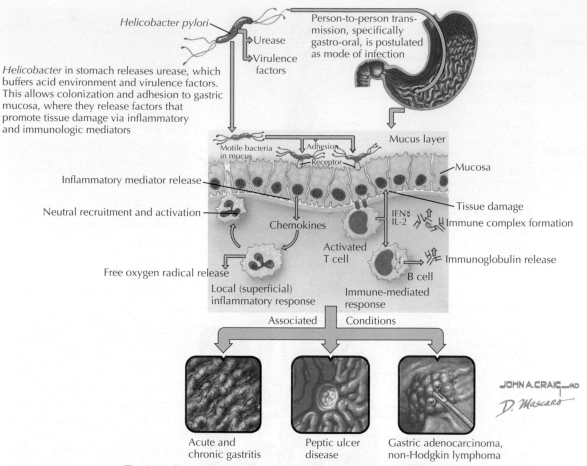

Helicobacter pylori

Urease

Virulence factors

Person-to-person transmission, specifically gastro-oral, is postulated as mode of infection

Helicobacter in stomach releases urease, which buffers acid environment and virulence factors. This allows colonization and adhesion to gastric mucosa, where they release factors that promote tissue damage via inflammatory and immunologic mediators

Mucus layer

Motile bacteria in mucus

Adhesion

Receptor

Mucosa

Inflammatory mediator release

Neutral recruitment and activation

Tissue damage

IFNδ IL-2

Immune complex formation

Chemokines

Activated T cell

Free oxygen radical release

Immunoglobulin release

B cell

Local (superficial) inflammatory response

Immune-mediated response

Associated   Conditions

JOHN A.CRAIG—MD
D. Mascaro

Acute and chronic gastritis

Peptic ulcer disease

Gastric adenocarcinoma, non-Hodgkin lymphoma

Fig. 56.2 Cause and Pathogenesis of *Helicobacter pylori* Infection.

with the use of certain chemotherapeutic agents such as vincristine and cisplatin. Depending on the severity of the vascular occlusion, microscopic or frank bleeding may occur, typically accompanied by severe postprandial abdominal pain. Stress-related mucosal disease is a form of gastritis encountered in critically ill patients. The systemic hypotension frequently experienced in this population leads to local mucosal ischemia, causing erosions and subepithelial hemorrhage.

Infiltration

Although rare in children, tumors involving the GI tract, such as lymphoma, may promote bleeding by direct invasion and by inflammatory cells that may also damage the mucosa.

Hypersecretion

Several rare disorders may result in excessive or ectopic acid secretion. For example, gastrinomas are uncommon tumors arising in the stomach or pancreas that are a major cause of Zollinger-Ellison syndrome, in which pathologically elevated gastrin production promotes excess gastric acid secretion and the formation of refractory peptic ulcers in almost all affected patients. Duplication cysts are developmental disorders in which ectopic gastric tissue within the cyst may cause inappropriate acid secretion in a relatively unprotected portion of the GI tract (potentially anywhere, most commonly the ileum), resulting in erosion and bleeding. They can also cause GI bleeding through other mechanisms, such as by acting as lead points for intussusception, with resultant ischemia, or through the rare development of a malignancy at the cyst site. Meckel's diverticulum is another developmental disorder resulting from incomplete involution of the vitelline duct that

can harbor ectopic gastric mucosa (features summarized by the rule of twos: 2% of the population, 2 feet from ileocecal valve, 2 inches long, most commonly presents around age 2 years, and boys are two times as likely to be affected) with resultant acid secretion within small bowel leading to mucosal erosion and bleeding.

Polyps

Polyps are mucosal projections into the intestinal lumen caused by disordered epithelial growth. Various spontaneous and familial polyposis entities exist. Regardless of the specific underlying process, they are a source of painless bleeding secondary to mechanical irritation or wholesale shearing by passing fecal material. In contrast to adults, the vast majority of polyps in children are juvenile polyps. These nonneoplastic polyps are typically composed of many cystic, dilated glands; copious inflammation; and surface erosions, the last of which is the cause of bleeding. Juvenile polyps have a peak incidence from 2 to 6 years of age, represent more than 90% of all pediatric polyp diagnoses, and are found in about 1% of school-age children.

Vascular Abnormalities

Congenital vascular defects may result in fragile vascular arrangements vulnerable to erosive and mechanical insults. Whereas hemangiomas represent proliferative vessel abnormalities that may regress, true malformations (including disorders such as arteriovenous malformations, blue rubber bleb nevus syndrome, and Osler-Rendu-Weber syndrome) are nonproliferative and do not regress. Processes that compromise the full thickness of bowel, such as Crohn's disease and bowel surgery, may result in vessel-to-bowel fistulas associated with significant bleeding.

Vasculitides, classically Henoch-Schönlein purpura, may result in occlusion of mesenteric vessels and intestinal ischemia.

Portal Hypertension

The final common pathway for many chronic liver diseases is cirrhosis, in which the underlying disease causes excessive production of extracellular matrix; destruction of normal liver architecture; and, ultimately, severe organ dysfunction. Cirrhosis is the most common cause of portal hypertension. Other potential causes include portal venous thrombosis, veno-occlusive disease in patients receiving chemotherapy, and hepatic vein thrombosis (Budd-Chiari syndrome). Backpressure from the high-resistance liver increases the intravascular pressure within the portal venous system, resulting in esophageal varices (abnormally dilated veins within the distal esophagus) and portal hypertensive gastropathy (increased venous pressure throughout the gastric wall). Varices are a known cause of catastrophic GI bleeds. The bleeding from these engorged vessels is often exacerbated by inadequate hepatic synthesis of coagulation factors in the setting of underlying liver dysfunction.

Blood From Extrinsic Sources

In neonates, swallowed maternal blood from delivery or breastfeeding is a potential cause of bloody emesis or stool. Blood swallowed from the airway in patients with frequent, severe coughing (e.g., pneumonia, cystic fibrosis, tuberculosis) may be mistaken for hematemesis. Rarely, hepatic injury from trauma or an abscess may cause hemobilia, with blood draining from the biliary system into the duodenum.

CLINICAL PRESENTATION

The first priority is to establish the patient's clinical stability; the initial impression can provide valuable clues. Pallor, lethargy, and diaphoresis are all immediately concerning signs of significant blood loss. However, the absence of these signs and symptoms in a seemingly well-appearing individual with a history of hematemesis, melena, or hematochezia should not be overly reassuring. Careful evaluation of the vital signs is of the utmost importance; indeed, tachycardia combined with normal blood pressure for age could indicate compensated shock. The most definitive physical examination indicator of significant blood loss is orthostatic hypotension, defined as a decrease in systolic blood pressure of at least 20 mm Hg or diastolic blood pressure of at least 10 mm Hg within 3 minutes of standing from a supine or sitting position.

The clinician should then focus on addressing the following several key questions.

What Are the Route and Appearance of the Bleeding?

Visible GI bleeding manifests differently depending on the location of origin. Traditionally, authors have grouped causes of GI bleeding into upper and lower sources divided by the ligament of Treitz. In 2007 the American Gastroenterological Association promoted the refinement of this classification into upper, middle, and lower GI tract bleeding, with the dividing point between the upper and middle tract being the ampulla of Vater and the dividing point between the middle and lower tract being the ileocecal valve, though the latter classification remains less widely adopted.

Hematemesis, which is vomiting of either fresh blood or coagulated, denatured blood ("coffee ground emesis"), indicates upper GI bleeding. Coffee-ground hematemesis generally represents old blood or bleeding that is occurring at a slow rate, as opposed to red blood, which raises suspicion for active bleeding. *Melena* (black, tarry, foul-smelling stool containing oxidized blood) usually originates from the upper GI tract, but it can emanate from a more distal GI source

if the transit rate is not rapid. *Hematochezia* (red blood per rectum) generally suggests middle or lower GI bleeding, although it may also represent a brisk upper GI bleed. Indeed, hematemesis combined with melena or hematochezia is an ominous combination that must be investigated promptly. Therefore, in any patient with bloody stool, one must always properly screen for possible upper GI bleeding. It is important to remember that many cases of GI bleeding are *occult* (i.e., microscopic), are not visible to the eye, and can occur anywhere along the GI tract. It is also essential to determine whether the blood could be emanating from a non-GI source, epistaxis and menstruation being two common examples.

What Is the Age of the Patient?

Most causes of GI bleeding can manifest in a variety of ages. However, some disorders tend to present more commonly in specific age groups. For example, juvenile polyps have a peak incidence in young school-age children. IBD, although it can manifest at almost any age, is generally rare in very young children, and when it does occur in that group, its presence prompts concerns of a possible underlying immunodeficiency syndrome.

Several disorders appear almost exclusively in neonates and infants. In newborns, particularly premature infants, necrotizing enterocolitis is a life-threatening emergency in which segments of bowel become inflamed and necrotic, leading to hematochezia and/or melena, abdominal distension, and fever. Neonates at delivery or breastfeeding infants may also swallow blood (the latter from cracked maternal nipples), which can then appear in reflux or emesis. The Apt test can help distinguish maternal blood from that of the patient. Milk protein allergy most often manifests in the first few months of life as fussiness and mild hematochezia in an otherwise well-appearing infant who has been exposed to cow's milk proteins, either through formula or indirect transmission via the mother's breast milk.

Is the Bleeding Acute or Chronic?

A history of repeated bleeding episodes over time suggests causes that have the potential for chronicity. For example, IBD does not typically manifest with sudden, catastrophic bleeds but tends to have a more insidious course marked initially by other symptoms such as weight loss or diarrhea. Peptic ulcers are another example in which bleeding may begin as occult but worsen over time if left untreated or exacerbated by other factors such as NSAID use. In such cases, a patient may exhibit pallor and fatigue but can remain functional, at least for a time, because of the body's adaptation to the progressive anemia. On the other hand, rapid onset of significant bleeds and patients with symptomatic anemia should sway the clinician toward other causes. For example, two significant causes of sudden melena or hematochezia are Meckel diverticula and vascular malformations. In patients with known liver disease, esophageal varices are a critical consideration.

Is the Bleeding Associated With Pain?

Abdominal pain associated with GI bleeding may suggest structural compromise. Bleeding coincident with pain in the epigastric region may be caused by peptic disease or necrotizing pancreatitis. If the pain is associated with distension or vomiting, the clinician should consider the causes of intestinal obstruction potentially associated with bleeding, such as intussusception, although blood in the upper GI tract itself can stimulate vomiting. If acute-onset GI bleeding occurs with significant generalized abdominal pain that is disproportionate to a relatively benign abdominal examination, ischemia may be the contributing cause. Bowel inflammation, as occurs with ulcerative colitis, can cause cramping pain. An ill-appearing patient with peritoneal signs may be experiencing bowel perforation and requires urgent medical and surgical evaluation.

What Is the Relationship Between the Blood and Stool?

The answer to this question can help guide the physician toward the region of a pathologic condition as long as one keeps in mind the limitations of these generalizations. Melena indicates bleeding from an upper or middle GI source. If the patient is having frequent, watery stools containing melena, this suggests a small bowel pathologic condition, as in Crohn's disease. Pure melena without watery diarrhea suggests other causes, such as peptic ulcers or esophageal varices. If the patient has profuse diarrhea with cramping and hematochezia (dysentery), this is more suggestive of colitis, as can occur with ulcerative colitis and many infectious causes, such as *Clostridioides difficile* and *Yersinia, Shigella,* and *Campylobacter* species. If the patient has pure hematochezia, infectious and inflammatory causes are still possible, but one also needs to consider other causes, such as Meckel diverticula, polyps, or vascular malformations, particularly if the bleeding is painless. If the patient has formed stool coated with blood (rather than permeating it), this suggests a distal cause such as solitary rectal ulcer (caused by mucosal erosion in the rectum from hard stool) or an anal fissure.

Does the Patient Have Other Prominent Abnormalities by History or Examination?

Any associated findings may provide clues to the cause. Cutaneous hemangiomas raise the possibility of internal hemangiomas affecting the GI tract. A history of failure to thrive or weight loss raises suspicion for small bowel dysfunction, such as occurs with CD, or, less commonly, malignancy. IBD can be associated with a host of other extraintestinal findings, such as erythema nodosum, episcleritis, or joint pathologic conditions. Polyps may often be a part of syndromes with other findings, a classic example being Peutz-Jeghers syndrome, in which hamartomatous polyps occur with mucocutaneous macules. Stigmata of liver disease, including jaundice, icterus, spider angiomas, and hepatosplenomegaly, may raise suspicion for esophageal varices. Assessing for easy bruising or signs of trauma anywhere along the GI tract is of the utmost importance.

EVALUATION AND MANAGEMENT

The first priority is to triage the patient based on the acuity and severity of the bleeding and ensure hemodynamic stability. Each case needs to be assessed individually, but if the amount of blood reported or witnessed is significant, there is repeated bleeding, or particularly if there are any signs/symptoms of hemodynamic instability, the patient should be sent to the emergency department for further evaluation. Extra caution should be paid to infants unless the bleeding source is readily apparent or if the volume of bleeding appears minimal (e.g., stool covered with streaks of blood in a patient with anal fissure). Once the patient has presented for medical attention, management should contain the elements discussed in the following paragraphs.

Determine Hemodynamic Status

Rapid comprehensive assessment of the patient, starting with the ABCs (airway, breathing, circulation) and including general appearance, vital signs, signs of injury, and mental status, should be performed first to determine the patient's stability and the next step in management.

Establish the Presence of Blood

Many ingested products can mimic the appearance of blood: red-colored foods, drinks, candies, and beets can be mistaken for hematemesis, and licorice, spinach, blueberries, bismuth, and iron supplements can mimic melena. It is therefore important at the outset to confirm that the substance is truly blood using an appropriate guaiac test: Hemoccult for stool and Gastroccult for gastric contents. These cards are quick and generally reliable, but occasionally, the presence of significant amounts of vitamin C, myoglobin (from meat), or the peroxidase or catalase activity of certain vegetables when consumed in large quantities may lead to a false positive result. The Apt test, which capitalizes on biochemical differences between fetal and adult hemoglobin, can delineate whether the source is from the mother or baby if swallowed maternal blood is a possibility.

Determine High-Risk Historical Factors

The clinician must determine whether there are exogenous factors that have contributed to the patient's clinical picture, such as a history of trauma, ingestion, drug use, or other illnesses.

Initial Management in the Emergency Department

Any patient with evidence of significant bleeding should receive supplemental oxygen, be placed on continuous hemodynamic monitoring, and have at least two large-bore intravenous catheters placed. If rapid hemodynamic resuscitation is indicated, isotonic fluids may be required, but blood is the preferred product if there is evidence of significant blood loss.

Although it is associated with patient discomfort, nasogastric lavage is a valuable tool in assessing patients with GI bleeding. When bleeding is self-limited in a well-appearing and hemodynamically stable patient and when bleeding is clearly from a discernible source such as epistaxis, lavage may not be necessary. However, if the patient has had frank hematemesis, lavage helps to assess the extent of bleeding and whether bleeding is ongoing, which would increase the urgency for endoscopic evaluation. In melena and hematochezia, lavage can help determine whether there is upper GI bleeding, although a clear aspirate does not definitively exclude this. When performed, a sump-type catheter (not feeding tube) should be used, the patient's head should be at 30 degrees to reduce the risk for aspiration, and the liquid should be room-temperature normal saline. The clinician should infuse 1 to 2 oz for infants, 4 to 6 oz for school-age children, or 1 L for adult-sized patients per infusion and allow the liquid to stand for 2 to 3 minutes before aspirating and repeating until the aspirate is clear. If the lavage does not clear after three attempts, there is limited utility to continuing, and the tube can be left to gravity or low intermittent suction.

Consultation with a gastroenterologist will assist with guiding the evaluation. Intensive care physicians and general surgeons should be consulted in cases of significant blood loss or hemodynamic instability.

Laboratory Evaluations

Initial laboratory studies assess the patient's hematologic status, screen for underlying contributory factors, and prepare for potential procedures. They should include a complete blood count (including platelet count), reticulocyte count, prothrombin and partial thromboplastin times, liver function tests (including aspartate aminotransferase, alanine aminotransferase, total and unconjugated bilirubin, and serum albumin), serum chemistries, and type and screen. The blood urea nitrogen may be elevated relative to the serum creatinine because of the absorption of amino acids produced by the enzymatic degradation of hemoglobin. As discussed earlier, the presence of blood may be confirmed by Hemoccult (stool) or Gastroccult (gastric aspirate), and the Apt test may be indicated in the neonatal setting if there is suspicion of swallowed maternal blood.

Additional Evaluations

Radiologic, endoscopic, and surgical evaluations are summarized in Fig. 56.3. The approach depends on the bleeding acuity and the setting

	Modality	GI Region Assessed	Question Addressed	Notes
Clinical	Nasogastric lavage	Upper GI tract	Is active upper GI bleeding occurring?	Concern for esophageal varices not a contraindication; use of ice-cold fluid not shown to inhibit bleeding
	Apt test	Upper GI tract	Is the origin of hematemesis the mother or the baby?	Pink = fetal Hgb; yellow-brown = adult Hgb
Radiologic	Radiography ("plain film")	All	Is there a foreign body or evidence of perforation?	Use limited to rapid screening early in assessment
	CT with contrast	Abdomen or pelvis	Are there structural lesions that may be responsible? And when performed as CT angiography, is a vascular defect the source?	High level of structural detail; CT angiography provides vascular data; study of choice in trauma and severely ill patients; may be useful in patients with persistent obscure GI bleeding; significant radiation burden
	Bleeding scan (Tc-99m tagged RBC scan)	All	Where is the source of GI bleeding?	Nuclear studies may have limited availability; lower limit of bleeding rate detection = 0.1 mL/min; poor sensitivity and specificity; only helpful in setting of brisk bleeding
	Meckel scan (Tc-99m pertechnetate scan)	All	Is ectopic gastric mucosa present in the ileum?	Nuclear studies may have limited availability; positive scan results justify bypassing endoscopy and proceeding to surgery
	Angiography	Targeted assessment of bowel vasculature	Is a vascular defect the source of bleeding?	Lower limit of bleeding rate detection = 0.5 mL/min; invasive and associated with risk of internal hemorrhage; may be used for therapeutic intervention
	Ultrasound	Liver or pancreas	Is there structural evidence of liver or pancreatic disease?	Helpful if concerned for hepatic disease, hemobilia, or pancreatitis
	Barium enema	Colon	Is a mucosal defect of the colon responsible?	Rarely used in this context given the overall superiority of colonoscopy; exception is evaluation of intussusception, in which it can also be therapeutic
	Upper GI series with small bowel follow-through*	Proximal GI tract to terminal ileum	Is a mucosal defect or anatomic defect of the bowel from the esophagus to the terminal ileum responsible?	Defects can only be inferred by abnormalities in lumen contour but allows noninvasive evaluation of the small bowel; also detects malrotation
	Enteroclysis (fluoroscopic or CT) MRI*	Small bowel Abdomen or pelvis	Are there structural lesions that may be responsible? And when performed as MR angiography, is a vascular defect the source?	High level of structural detail; SBFT may be superior for evaluation of mucosal defects; no radiation burden; not appropriate for acute evaluation; young patients may need sedation
			Is an intestinal mucosal defect responsible?	Permits more complete examination than SBFT; requires introduction of catheter into small intestine; associated radiation burden; most useful for investigation of occult bleeding
Endoscopic	Upper endoscopy (esophagogastroduodenoscopy)	Proximal GI tract to duodenum	Is a mucosal defect of the upper GI tract responsible?	Gold standard evaluation; direct visualization of lesions capable of obtaining biopsies for tissue diagnosis; capable of therapeutic interventions
	Lower endoscopy (colonoscopy)	Colon, terminal ileum	Is a mucosal defect of the colon or terminal ileum responsible?	Gold standard evaluation; direct visualization of lesions capable of obtaining biopsies for tissue diagnosis; capable of therapeutic interventions
	Capsule endoscopy*	Duodenum through terminal ileum	Is a mucosal defect of the small bowel responsible?	Allows direct visualization of the mucosa; no ability to guide the capsule or biopsy tissue
	Balloon enteroscopy*	Proximal GI tract to terminal ileum	Is a mucosal defect of jejunum or proximal ileum responsible?	Limited availability; technically difficult
Surgical	Exploratory laparotomy	Clinician-defined	Where is the source of this major bleed?	Reserved for catastrophic bleeds with goal of surgical intervention
	Push enteroscopy	Jejunum, ileum	Is there a mucosal defect of the jejunum or proximal ileum?	Reserved for evaluation of persistent obscure GI bleeding after endoscopy and radiologic assessments have been repeatedly negative

Fig. 56.3 Diagnostic Modalities for Gastrointestinal Bleeding. *CT,* Computed tomography; *GI,* gastrointestinal; *Hgb,* hemoglobin; *MRI,* magnetic resonance imaging; *RBC,* red blood cell; *SBFT,* small bowel follow-through; *Tc-99m,* technetium-99m. *Studies not suitable for the acute-care setting.

in which the patient is being evaluated. In general, when the source of bleeding is unclear, the goal is to perform endoscopy, in which a fiber-optic camera is inserted into the mouth (upper endoscopy) or anus (lower endoscopy) to directly visualize the lumen of the gastrointestinal tract. Patients with preexisting medical conditions, pulse greater than 20 beats/min relative to mean pulse for age, prolonged capillary refill time, and need for blood product transfusion are more likely to require endoscopic intervention than those without these findings. Endoscopy is the gold standard given its relative safety and its ability to directly visualize the mucosa, obtain tissue for pathologic diagnosis, and potentially administer therapy. However, endoscopy is not without risk, and the presence of active bleeding may create technical challenges by obscuring the intestinal lumen. Other diagnostic methods may be considered before scoping in certain situations. In cases in which a rapid GI bleed is suspected but the source remains unknown, a tagged red blood cell scan, if available, should be considered. A Meckel scan should be obtained if suspicion is high for Meckel's diverticulum, as a positive result would bypass the need for endoscopy.

Therapeutic Interventions

Patients with significant anemia (hemoglobin <8 g/dL), active bleeding, or symptomatic anemia should receive blood replacement with packed red blood cells at a dose of 10 to 15 mL/kg per transfusion. If coagulation abnormalities are found, they should be corrected with vitamin K, fresh-frozen plasma, or both depending on the clinical context. All hospitalized patients with presumptive or confirmed upper GI bleeding should be started on acid-suppression therapy with a proton pump inhibitor administered intravenously, until the patient has stabilized or until an upper GI cause has been excluded. An octreotide drip may be considered in cases of severe upper GI bleeding. Additional interventions depend on the underlying cause. There are multiple therapeutic techniques that may be deployed using endoscopy, including sclerotherapy or banding of varices, electrocautery, argon plasma coagulation, hemoclips, or injection for ulcers or other lesions. Hemospray is a newer technique that may be used to help achieve hemostasis in actively bleeding tissue. In severe bleeding or bleeding not amenable to endoscopic techniques, surgical intervention may be required.

FUTURE DIRECTIONS

Capsule endoscopy and balloon enteroscopy have been exciting additions to the diagnostic arsenal, but the availability of these studies and the expertise required for their interpretation remain limited, particularly in pediatrics. Whereas small bowel follow-through and enteroclysis are no longer routinely used in the evaluation of GI bleeding, radiologic techniques such as computed tomography (CT) angiography and magnetic resonance angiography or venography are becoming more refined, and newer CT protocols are reducing radiation exposure. Several new endoscopic treatment modalities are emerging, including over-the-scope clips, endoscopic suturing, radiofrequency ablation, cryotherapy, and endoscopic ultrasound-guided angiotherapy. Finally, there are multiple studies underway assessing the use of machine-learned artificial intelligence models to aid in the diagnosis and management of GI bleeding, and preliminary results seem promising.

ACKNOWLEDGMENT

The authors would like to acknowledge the contribution of Andrew Chu, MD, for his work in the previous edition's chapter.

SUGGESTED READINGS

Available online.

57

Inflammatory Bowel Disease

Jennifer K. Sun and Trusha Patel

✳ CLINICAL VIGNETTE

A 12-year-old boy with no significant medical history presents with intermittent abdominal pain, diarrhea, nausea, and vomiting. For the last 2 to 3 months, he has had repeated episodes of nonbloody diarrhea accompanied by nonbilious emesis and lower abdominal cramping. He does not awaken overnight to have bowel movements, but often has to have a bowel movement immediately upon awakening. He has not had any fevers, oral ulcers, or joint pain. He has lost approximately 10 lb since his last well-child examination 6 months ago. He has not had any recent sick contacts or recent travel.

The examination is notable for normal vital signs and pallor with mild tenderness to palpation in the right lower quadrant and suprapubic region without rebound or guarding. Laboratory studies are notable for white blood cell count of 9600/μL, hemoglobin of 11.8 g/dL, platelet count of 480,000/μL, C-reactive protein of 8.15 mg/dL (upper limit of normal 0.5 mg/dL), erythrocyte sedimentation rate of 24 mm/h, and albumin of 3.7 g/dL. Stool infection studies are negative. Fecal calprotectin is elevated to 215 μg/mg.

Because of a high suspicion for inflammatory bowel disease, the patient is referred to a gastroenterology specialist, and he undergoes expedited esophagogastroduodenoscopy and colonoscopy. Findings are notable for ulceration throughout the terminal ileum and colon. Pathologic examination shows chronic transmural inflammation with primarily lymphohistiocytic infiltrates and few noncaseating granulomas. He is diagnosed with ileocolonic Crohn's disease.

Inflammatory bowel disease (IBD) is characterized by chronic inflammation of the gastrointestinal (GI) tract. IBD has traditionally been divided into two subtypes: ulcerative colitis (UC) and Crohn's disease (CD) (Fig. 57.1). Ulcerative colitis is characterized by diffuse colonic mucosal inflammation that begins at the anal verge and extends proximally to a variable extent. The disease is limited to the colon, although distal ileal involvement ("backwash ileitis") may occur. Crohn's disease, on the other hand, is characterized by transmural inflammation that may involve any segment of the intestinal tract from the mouth to the anus. In recent years, however, it is increasingly recognized that IBD is a heterogeneous disease with a spectrum of phenotypes. Many patients, especially in the pediatric population, do not clearly fit the characteristics of either subtype, resulting in growing numbers of patients being classified as IBD-unclassified (IBD-U).

The majority of IBD cases are diagnosed in adolescence or early adulthood, with 25% of patients presenting before 20 years of age. In the United States and Canada, the incidence of IBD is approximately 10 per 100,000 children with an overall prevalence of 100 to 200 per 100,000 children. Over the last two decades, the incidence and prevalence of IBD in children has been gradually increasing, especially among those younger than 6 years of age, characterized as very early-onset IBD.

ETIOLOGY AND PATHOGENESIS

The cause of IBD is likely multifactorial because of the interaction of a host of genetic and environmental factors. From a genetic standpoint, there is a high incidence of disease among first-degree relatives, and genome-wide association studies have identified variants in more than 150 genes that confer increased risk for IBD. Monogenic disease, most often caused by a mutation in a primary immunodeficiency gene, may be seen, most commonly in infants and young children. The rising incidence of IBD, especially in developed countries, may be related to multiple factors, including diet, early antibiotic use, and high rates of cesarean delivery. There has also been growing interest in the role of the microbiome in IBD, as individuals with IBD tend to have decreased intestinal biodiversity. Recent studies supporting the efficacy of multi-drug antibiotic regimens in the treatment of steroid-dependent and anti–tumor necrosis factor (TNF)-resistant IBD also lend credibility to the role of intestinal flora dysregulation in IBD.

CLINICAL PRESENTATION

The clinical presentation of IBD is highly variable depending on the location, extent, and severity of disease. Common manifesting symptoms of IBD include abdominal pain, diarrhea (with or without blood in the stools), nocturnal defecation, urgency/tenesmus, low-grade intermittent fever, oral ulcers, joint pain, fatigue, weight loss, decreased appetite, and decelerated growth velocity. Weight loss or stunted growth may be the only initial clinical manifestation in patients presenting with mild or nonspecific symptoms. Clinicians, therefore, must maintain a high index of suspicion for IBD among children who have declining height or weight percentiles. In children with CD, perianal fistulae, intra-abdominal fistulae or signs/symptoms of bowel obstruction secondary to intestinal stricture may be present at the time of diagnosis (Fig. 57.2).

About one-third of patients with IBD also have extraintestinal manifestations (e.g., rheumatologic, cutaneous, hepatobiliary, renal, ocular, vascular, skeletal) (Fig. 57.3). These symptoms may precede or occur in the absence of GI symptoms. Arthralgia and arthritis are the most common extraintestinal symptoms and may involve both axial and peripheral joints. Skin and cutaneous manifestations of IBD can include oral ulcers, erythema nodosum, and pyoderma gangrenosum. The most common hepatobiliary diseases associated with IBD are primary sclerosing cholangitis and autoimmune hepatitis. Ocular findings include episcleritis, uveitis, and iritis and are more common in CD than in UC. There is also an increased risk for thromboembolic disease in IBD patients compared with the general population. IBD-associated osteopenia is multifactorial, with contributions from malabsorption, malnutrition, chronic steroid use, inactivity, and chronic inflammation.

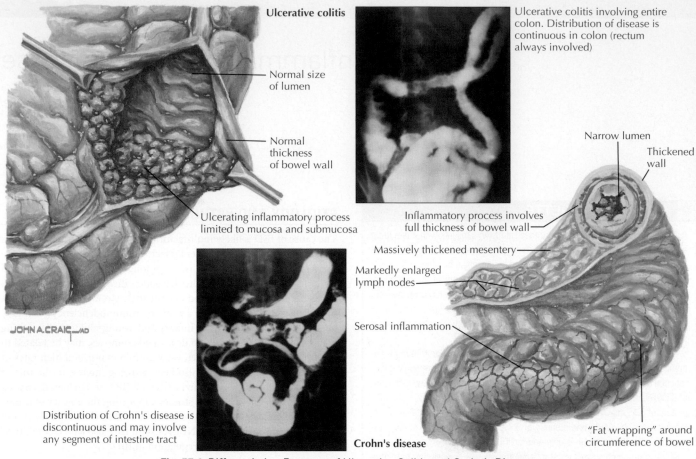

Ulcerative colitis

Normal size of lumen

Normal thickness of bowel wall

Ulcerating inflammatory process limited to mucosa and submucosa

JOHN A. CRAIG—AD

Distribution of Crohn's disease is discontinuous and may involve any segment of intestine tract

Crohn's disease

Ulcerative colitis involving entire colon. Distribution of disease is continuous in colon (rectum always involved)

Narrow lumen

Thickened wall

Inflammatory process involves full thickness of bowel wall

Massively thickened mesentery

Markedly enlarged lymph nodes

Serosal inflammation

"Fat wrapping" around circumference of bowel

Fig. 57.1 Differentiating Features of Ulcerative Colitis and Crohn's Disease.

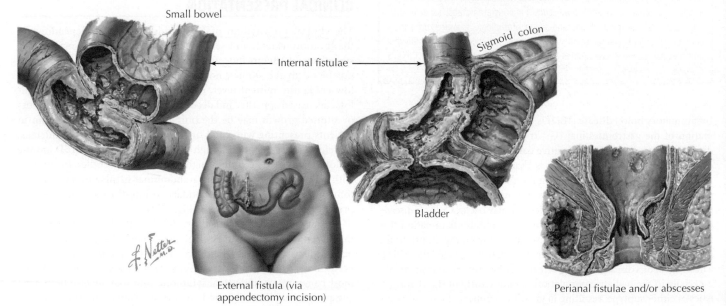

Small bowel

Sigmoid colon

Internal fistulae

Bladder

f. Netter M.D.

External fistula (via appendectomy incision)

Perianal fistulae and/or abscesses

Fig. 57.2 Types of Fistulae in Crohn's Disease.

DIAGNOSIS

The diagnosis of IBD relies on a thorough history and physical examination in conjunction with supporting laboratory findings, imaging, and direct visualization with colonoscopy/esophagogastroduodenoscopy. The differential diagnosis of IBD is broad and largely depends on the presenting symptoms (Table 57.1).

A detailed history and physical examination with comprehensive review of systems should be carefully conducted. Review of the growth chart may reveal growth failure. Abdominal palpation may elicit localized tenderness, but significant rebound, guarding, or signs of peritonitis should prompt urgent evaluation for perforation, toxic megacolon, or other complications. Inspection of the perianal area and perineum

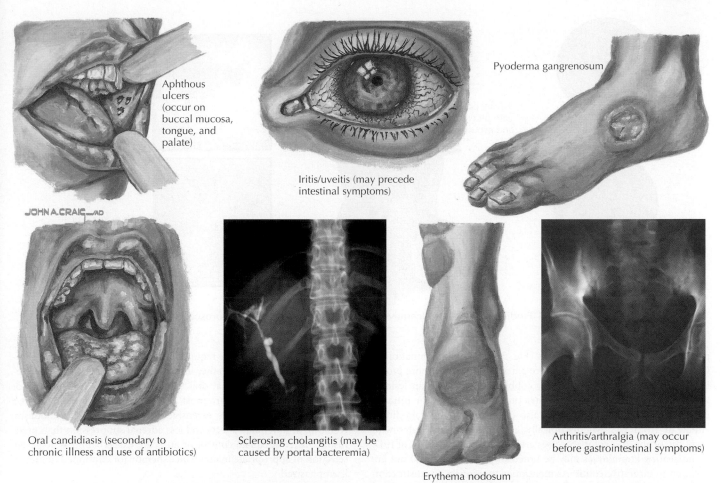

Aphthous ulcers (occur on buccal mucosa, tongue, and palate)

Iritis/uveitis (may precede intestinal symptoms)

Pyoderma gangrenosum

JOHN A. CRAIG—MD

Oral candidiasis (secondary to chronic illness and use of antibiotics)

Sclerosing cholangitis (may be caused by portal bacteremia)

Erythema nodosum

Arthritis/arthralgia (may occur before gastrointestinal symptoms)

Fig. 57.3 Extraintestinal Manifestations of Inflammatory Bowel Disease.

TABLE 57.1 Differential Diagnosis of Inflammatory Bowel Disease

Abdominal Pain	Diarrhea	Hematochezia	Abdominal Obstruction	Growth Failure or Weight Loss
Functional abdominal pain	Infection-bacterial, parasitic, protozoan, *Clostridioides difficile*	Polyp	Lymphoma	Endocrinopathy
Constipation		Meckel diverticulum	Intussusception	Anorexia
IBS	Carbohydrate intolerance	Intestinal AV malformation	Volvulus	Constitutional growth delay
GERD	Celiac disease	Anal fissure	Postsurgical adhesions	Parasitic infection
Appendicitis	Laxative abuse	Hemorrhoids		Neoplasms
Ischemic colitis	Allergic colitis	Infections		
Ovarian cyst	Immune deficiency	Solitary rectal ulcer		
Mesenteric lymphadenitis				
PID				
Vasculitis				

AV, Arteriovenous; *IBS,* irritable bowel syndrome; *GERD,* gastroesophageal reflux disease; *PID* pelvic inflammatory disorder.

may reveal skin tags and fistulae. Skin, joint, and eye examinations are necessary to identify extraintestinal manifestations.

Common laboratory findings in IBD may include anemia, thrombocytosis, hypoalbuminemia, and elevated inflammatory markers (e.g., erythrocyte sedimentation rate and C-reactive protein). Fecal occult blood testing may be positive but is neither sensitive nor specific for the diagnosis of IBD. Fecal calprotectin can serve as a biomarker of intestinal inflammation and is often elevated in IBD. Although they are routinely found on IBD diagnostic panels, antineutrophil cytoplasmic antibody and anti–*Saccharomyces cerevisiae* antibody have low positive and negative predictive values and thus are of limited use in diagnosing

IBD. Stool studies for bacterial pathogens, parasites, *Clostridioides difficile*, *Cryptosporidium* species, and *Giardia* species are indicated to differentiate infectious diarrhea from IBD.

Although the previously mentioned signs and symptoms can indicate IBD, the definitive diagnosis relies on esophagogastroduodenoscopy and colonoscopy for direct visualization and biopsies for histologic evaluation of the intestinal mucosa. In UC, the inflammation is limited to the colon and extends proximally in a continuous and circumferential pattern from the rectum with sharp demarcation between affected and unaffected areas. Common findings in ulcerative colitis include erythema, edema, granularity of the mucosa, friability,

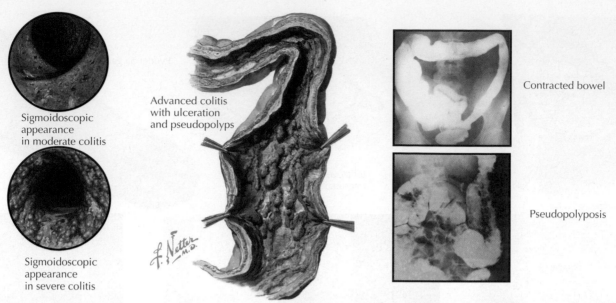

Sigmoidoscopic appearance in moderate colitis

Sigmoidoscopic appearance in severe colitis

Advanced colitis with ulceration and pseudopolyps

Contracted bowel

Pseudopolyposis

Fig. 57.4 Findings Typical of Ulcerative Colitis on Colonoscopy and Fluoroscopy Study.

pseudopolyps, erosions, and ulcers (Fig. 57.4). The inflammation in CD, on the other hand, may be more patchy and include more prominent findings of aphthous ulcers, cobblestoning, and skip lesions. Complications such as intestinal strictures and perianal or intraabdominal fistulae or abscesses may also occur in CD and help differentiate it from UC. Microscopically, inflammatory infiltrates with crypt distortion and crypt abscesses are characteristic findings of IBD. Noncaseating granulomas may be noted in patients with CD but are not seen in ulcerative colitis. As mentioned previously, the distinction between UC and CD is not always clear cut, and some patients may have indeterminate features that make classification difficult, resulting in a diagnosis of IBD-U.

Multiple imaging modalities may be used as adjunctive diagnostic tools to aid in the diagnosis of IBD. The use of cross-sectional imaging in IBD has expanded and has largely replaced fluoroscopic small bowel follow-through as the modality of choice. Magnetic resonance imaging with small bowel enterography, in particular, has gained favor because of its ability to avoid radiation while maintaining high sensitivity for detecting bowel inflammation and potential complications (e.g., stricturing disease, enteric fistula). Other imaging modalities include CT enterography, upper GI series with small bowel follow-through, and contrast-enhanced ultrasound. Video capsule endoscopy also may be used to evaluate the small bowel mucosa.

TREATMENT

Goals of treatment in pediatric IBD include achievement and maintenance of long-term remission, optimization of growth and nutritional status, improvement in quality of life, and prevention of disease- and treatment-related complications. The therapeutic armamentarium for IBD has expanded significantly in recent years, and treatment selection in patients with IBD is individualized based on symptoms and severity and extent of disease.

Medications

Although corticosteroids were previously the mainstay of therapy for moderate to severe disease, steroid-sparing therapies are now preferred, as corticosteroids are ineffective in achieving mucosal healing and simultaneously have a very unfavorable side effect profile. When

steroid-based therapies are required for acute exacerbations, the clinical context will dictate whether intravenous formulations (e.g., methylprednisolone), traditional oral formulations (e.g., prednisone), or newer synthetic steroids are most appropriate. Oral budesonide is a synthetic steroid that has extensive first-pass hepatic metabolism, resulting in fewer side effects and less adrenal suppression than prednisone. After adequate control of an acute exacerbation is achieved, selection of appropriate maintenance therapy for continued remission is emphasized.

Aminosalicylates (5-ASA), such as mesalamine and sulfasalazine, have been used for mild to moderate disease and exert a topical antiinflammatory effect on the GI tract. They function by inhibiting the cyclooxygenase and lipoxygenase pathways of arachidonic acid metabolism, which alters mucosal prostaglandin production. Although 5-ASA therapies are used clinically for the treatment of both CD and UC, systematic reviews have not shown significant efficacy in the treatment of CD. Although aminosalicylates are generally well-tolerated, side effects may include fever, nausea, headache, rash, and, occasionally, worsening of abdominal pain or diarrhea, as well as more severe side effects, including pancreatitis and interstitial nephritis.

Immunomodulators (methotrexate, 6-mercaptopurine [6-MP], azathioprine [AZA]) are used to reduce inflammation by regulating the immune system response. Methotrexate disrupts folate metabolism while 6-MP and AZA inhibit purine nucleotide synthesis and metabolism. Common side effects include nausea, vomiting, diarrhea, hepatotoxicity, cytopenias, and myelosuppression. Although now infrequently used as monotherapy, they are often used as part of dual therapy with biologics for patients with severe disease or to limit antibody formation to biologic therapies.

In the past, monoclonal antibodies directed against TNF-α (e.g., infliximab, adalimumab) were reserved for patients who were refractory to corticosteroid therapy or corticosteroid-dependent despite immunomodulator therapy. More recently, they have been used early in the treatment course for patients presenting with moderate to severe disease. Adverse side effects include injection/infusion site reactions, antibody development, and increased risk for infection, cytopenias, and hepatotoxicity. Before initiation of biologic therapy, patients should be screened for risk for activation of underlying infection such as tuberculosis, hepatitis B, and varicella. Patients should be monitored for rare and other serious side effects such as drug-induced lupus, Guillain-Barré syndrome, and multiple sclerosis.

Although not yet approved by the US Food and Drug Administration for the treatment of IBD in children, additional biologic agents, including anti-integrins (e.g., vedolizumab) and anti–IL-12/ IL-23 agents (e.g., ustekinumab) are currently used in clinical practice with success. Oral small molecule agents which inhibit the Janus kinase (JAK) family of tyrosine kinases (e.g., tofacitinib), have shown success in the management of adult UC.

Surgery

Surgery may be required for patients with disease refractory to medical therapy or with severe complications. With current advanced medical therapies, an estimated 5% to 10% of patients with ulcerative colitis undergo colectomy within 1 year of diagnosis. Colectomy may be performed on an emergent, urgent, or elective basis, depending on the severity of a patient's presentation or the presence of complications (e.g., uncontrolled hemorrhage, toxic megacolon, or bowel perforation) and, in the setting of UC, is considered curative. Surgery for CD, on the other hand, is not curative, given the potential for diffuse involvement of the GI tract. It is typically reserved for patients with CD who develop complications that are not amenable to medical treatment alone (e.g., abscess, fistula, perforation, stricture, obstruction).

Nutritional Therapy

Nutrition optimization is important in both the acute and chronic management of all patients with IBD. In some cases, dietary management may serve as treatment for IBD as well. Exclusive enteral nutrition, typically via nasogastric tube, may serve as first-line therapy for the induction of remission in CD and can be used as an adjunct or alternative to corticosteroids or anti-inflammatory medications. Some pediatric patients, especially those who present with growth failure, may require supplemental enteral nutrition to promote adequate growth and development even in the context of other therapies. There is also great interest in table food diets as therapeutic options for IBD, and numerous studies are ongoing. As a result of chronic inflammation and malabsorption, patients with IBD are at high risk for nutritional deficiencies (e.g., zinc, vitamin B_{12}, iron, vitamin D) and should be screened regularly. Rarely, patients may require total parenteral nutrition (TPN) to allow for bowel rest and provide necessary calories and nutrients in those with intestinal failure. Given significant risks of TPN, including central line–associated blood stream infection, thrombosis, and liver failure, the risks and benefits of longer-term TPN must be considered and enteral feeding should be resumed as soon as it is feasible.

PREVENTION AND SCREENING

Although IBD is a chronic disease that should be managed with the guidance of a pediatric gastroenterologist, pediatricians and other primary care providers play a crucial role in ensuring that patients and families receive all age-appropriate health care maintenance, including vaccinations, screenings, and anticipatory guidance. Furthermore, there are a number of important issues that should be monitored more

closely in patients with IBD, and specific recommendations (from the North American Society for Pediatric Gastroenterology, Hepatology and Nutrition and others) exist to aid primary care providers in caring for this special population.

With regard to vaccinations, children with IBD should receive all inactivated vaccines, including the seasonal influenza vaccine, according to the standard recommended schedule. The pneumococcal vaccine (PPSV-23) should also be administered to children aged 2 years or older because of the increased risk for pneumococcal disease in the setting of chronic inflammation and immunosuppression. Live vaccines are contraindicated in patients receiving active immunosuppressive therapy but can be safely given in children with IBD who are not on immunosuppressive therapies.

Patients and their families should be counseled on the surveillance, treatment, and prevention of infectious complications of IBD. Although frequent antibiotics should be avoided to reduce the risk for *C. difficile* infection and antibiotic resistance, clinicians should have a high index of suspicion for serious infections in patients who develop worsening symptoms of fever, abdominal pain, or diarrhea while on immunosuppressive therapy. Certain immunosuppressive medications may need to be held in the setting of acute infection. Preventive strategies, including routine vaccination, nutritional optimization, and food and travel safety should be emphasized at all well-child visits.

Patients with IBD are at increased risk for certain malignancies, especially intestinal malignancies such as colorectal carcinoma, small bowel adenocarcinoma, and intestinal lymphoma. Starting 7 to 10 years after diagnosis, patients should undergo screening colonoscopies with surveillance biopsies every 1 to 2 years. The risk for dermatologic malignancies, especially melanoma, is also higher in patients with IBD, and any concerning lesions should be serially monitored and referred for biopsy as clinically indicated. Laboratory monitoring with complete blood count and differential can be used to screen for hematologic malignancies.

Finally, IBD can result in significant psychosocial distress, and screening for symptoms of anxiety and depression should be incorporated into a comprehensive model of care.

FUTURE DIRECTIONS

The landscape of pediatric IBD management continues to evolve, with many new approaches and promising treatments on the horizon. Active areas of ongoing research include the use of new cytokine-based biologic treatments (e.g., anti-TL1A, anti-IL6), oral small molecule therapies, stem cell transplantation, and targeted microbiome therapies. As therapeutic options continue to expand, there is great interest in developing personalized management strategies that can be tailored to the clinical phenotype of each patient. Through the identification of novel genetic and serologic markers, it may be possible to predict response and optimize therapy based on individualized risk factors to improve treatment outcomes and quality of life.

SUGGESTED READINGS

Available online.

58

Hernias

Naomi E. Butler Tjaden and Bruce L. Tjaden, Jr.

 CLINICAL VIGNETTE

A 9-month-old boy presents for routine well-child examination. His history is notable for birth at 32 weeks gestational age, requiring care in the neonatal intensive care unit (NICU), including 2 weeks on a ventilator. He is otherwise healthy and up to date on vaccines, and he has been meeting all developmental milestones. He has daily stools and does not have abdominal pain. The only parental concern at this visit is that he has an "outie" belly button that gets more noticeable when he cries or is bearing down to stool. There is no history of trauma or reported pain. On physical examination, an approximately 1-cm reducible mass can be palpated when crying. On auscultation, bowel sounds are heard over the umbilicus. The area is nontender to palpation and is without fluctuance. The child is diagnosed with an umbilical hernia, and the parents are instructed to monitor for signs of strangulation or pain. This defect will likely resolve without surgical intervention by the time he reaches 5 years of age.

Hernias—defined as a protrusion of an organ or part of an organ beyond the anatomic space in which it is normally contained—are encountered frequently in pediatric practice. Hernias in the ventral abdominal wall make up the majority of hernias seen in children. The most common locations are in the umbilical and inguinal regions.

Umbilical hernias involve protrusion of intraabdominal contents, most commonly small bowel, through a dilation at the umbilical fascial opening. These are very common, especially in premature infants, infants of African and African-American descent, and infants with certain diseases or genetic syndromes.

Inguinal hernias involve protrusion of intraabdominal contents, again most commonly small bowel, in the vicinity of the inferior epigastric vessels in the groin. These occur in roughly 1% to 5% of all children, with an increased incidence in those with a family history of inguinal hernia and premature infants. The incidence may be as high as 30% to 42% in those with birth weights less than 1000 g. There is a male predominance, with the right side more commonly affected. Inguinal hernias may cause significant morbidity because of incarceration and strangulation, making it essential that general practitioners and subspecialists alike understand how to approach the condition and recognize when emergent surgery is required.

Rarer pediatric ventral wall hernias may also occur. Epigastric hernias located between the xiphoid process and umbilicus arise as a result of congenitally weakened linea alba through which extraperitoneal fat or omentum may protrude. Spigelian hernias are even more rare in children, located lateral to the rectus muscle. Incisional hernias may occur at sites of prior surgery and can be located anywhere on the abdomen in which the fascia was violated.

Congenital diaphragmatic hernias (CDH) and hiatal hernias are the two most common internal hernias among children. CDH is a neonatal surgical emergency that presents with a scaphoid abdomen, cyanosis, and respiratory distress within minutes of birth as a result of the herniation of abdominal contents into the thoracic cavity (Fig. 58.1).

Hiatal hernias occur when the stomach, intraabdominal esophagus, and/or transverse colon protrude into the thorax. These are less common in children than adults, but remain an important consideration in certain clinical scenarios. Other internal hernias, including paraduodenal and mesenteric hernias, occur within the abdominal cavity. These are largely the result of congenital abnormalities and in rare circumstances become clinically relevant in childhood.

ETIOLOGY AND PATHOGENESIS

Umbilical Hernia

All newborns have a natural fascial defect at the umbilicus, through which the cord vessels pass. In most infants, the umbilical ring closes spontaneously. In some, this closure fails to occur, resulting in an umbilical hernia (Fig. 58.2). Normally, the umbilical vein involutes and becomes the ligamentum teres hepatis, which attaches to the umbilical ring inferiorly. During normal development, the umbilical ring is also supported by the transversalis fascia and peritoneum. Typically, the transversalis fascia thickens at the umbilicus into the umbilical fascia, but a failure or incomplete contribution of this layer to the periumbilical region may leave an area of relative weakness. The closure of the ring is most likely multifactorial as suggested by significant racial differences in incidence of hernia and increased frequency in children with Ehlers-Danlos, Beckwith-Wiedemann, Hurler syndrome, trisomies 13, 18, and 21, and congenital hypothyroidism.

Inguinal Hernia

Indirect inguinal hernias are congenital, arising from incomplete embryogenesis. In boys, the testes initially develop in a retroperitoneal position. A portion of peritoneum called the processus vaginalis attaches to the testes and precedes the testicular descent through the internal inguinal ring into the scrotal sac. The testes are located at the internal inguinal ring by 28 weeks of gestation and reach their final destination by 36 weeks with the left side completing its descent slightly earlier than the right. The processus vaginalis creates a transiently patent conduit between the abdomen and the scrotum via the inguinal canal, and typically obliterates between 36 and 40 weeks of gestation or in the postnatal period. If the processus vaginalis remains patent, abdominal or retroperitoneal contents may escape through the internal inguinal ring and course along with the cord structures via the inguinal canal toward or into the scrotum (Fig. 58.3).

In girls, the ovaries also begin in a retroperitoneal position; however, they do not leave the abdominal cavity. The processus vaginalis descends through the inguinal canal with the round ligament to the labia majoris and usually obliterates between 32 and 36 weeks of gestation. The lack of gonadal descent through the inguinal canal may explain why indirect inguinal hernias occur six times less frequently in females than in males. Boys with cryptorchidism (failure of one or both testicles to descend into the scrotum), infants with urogenital malformations, and those with increased intraabdominal pressure (e.g., by mechanical ventilation) are at increased risk for developing indirect inguinal hernias.

Direct inguinal hernias are rare in children and occur when abdominal or retroperitoneal contents protrude directly into the inguinal canal through a defect in the posterior wall of the canal medial to the inferior epigastric vessels. Femoral hernias, also rare in children, occur when organs herniate through a muscular defect beneath the inguinal ligament medial to the femoral vein. Patients with connective tissue disorders and those who have had previous surgery to correct an inguinal hernia have greater risk for femoral or direct inguinal hernias.

Epigastric hernias occur above the umbilicus through a defect in the linea alba and most commonly contain preperitoneal fat. Such a defect develops when there is failure of complete fusion of the midline fascia during the final stages of abdominal wall formation.

Incisional hernias, resulting from incomplete fascial approximation or healing after a surgical incision, can occur anywhere on the abdomen. They may occur immediately (in which case they represent a technical defect and may be more appropriately termed a fascial dehiscence) or later (as a result of resolution of perioperative tissue edema or suture tearing through fascia which was initially approximated). Obesity, postoperative wound infections, and any process that increases intraabdominal pressure (e.g., mechanical ventilation or ascites) are major risk factors for incisional hernias.

Congenital Diaphragmatic Hernia

CDH refers to an opening in the diaphragm that occurs as a result of a failure of closure of the pleuroperitoneal folds during postconception weeks 4 to 10. This then allows herniation of abdominal viscera into the thoracic cavity. Most defects are located posterolaterally (Bochdalek hernia), though some may be anterior-peristernal (Morgagni hernia), anterior-retrosternal, or central. The presence of additional organs in the thorax may impede normal pulmonary development and lead to pulmonary or cardiac hypoplasia.

Hiatal Hernia

The intraabdominal esophagus and the stomach are secured in place by numerous fascial and ligamentous elements. At its entry into the abdomen, the esophagus is supported by fibroelastic tissue called the phrenoesophageal membrane. This membrane, as well as many other

Sites of herniation
- Foramen of Morgagni
- Esophageal hiatus
- A large part or all of diaphragm may be congenitally absent
- Original pleuroperitoneal canal (foramen of Bochdalek—the most common site)

- Trachea (deviated)
- Right lung (compressed)
- Left lung (atrophic)
- Small bowel
- Colon
- Omentum
- Stomach
- Spleen
- Heart
- Diaphragm
- Foramen of Bochdalek
- Liver
- Cecum (malrotation of bowel often associated)

Fig. 58.1 Congenital Diaphragmatic Hernia.

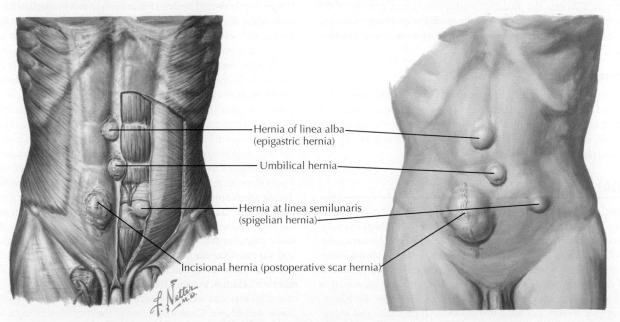

- Hernia of linea alba (epigastric hernia)
- Umbilical hernia
- Hernia at linea semilunaris (spigelian hernia)
- Incisional hernia (postoperative scar hernia)

Fig. 58.2 Abdominal Wall Hernias.

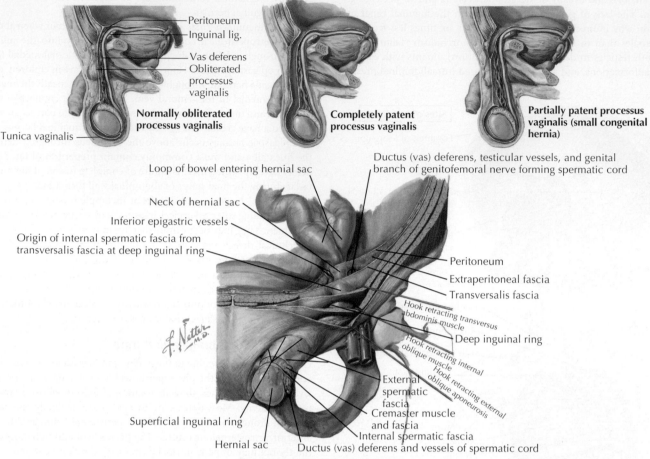

Fig. 58.3 Indirect Inguinal Hernia.

supporting structures, can be structurally deficient at birth or gradually weaken with time and stress, causing laxity of the support and widening of the muscular hiatus. During inspiration, the transdiaphragmatic pressure differential causes the esophagus and stomach to be pulled upward. Depending on the areas of weakness, the gastroesophageal junction may slide into the posterior mediastinum, or a portion of the stomach may pass through the hiatus alongside the esophagus with the lower esophageal sphincter maintained in its correct anatomic position (Fig. 58.4).

Other Internal Hernias

Paraduodenal hernias occur when small bowel protrudes through a fossa created by abnormal mesenteric attachments to the ascending or descending colon. A congenital or acquired defect in the mesentery itself may allow a loop of bowel to pass through the mesentery, leading to a mesenteric hernia.

CLINICAL PRESENTATION

Abdominal wall hernias classically present with the history of an intermittent or persistent swelling without associated pain, which may disappear spontaneously and are most noticeable with crying or straining.

Umbilical hernias are typically detected during the newborn examination, particularly when there is increased intraabdominal pressure, such as during crying or when stooling. The physical examination reveals a soft mass covered by skin protruding from the umbilicus, increasing in size with increased intraabdominal pressure, and reducing easily and completely in all but the rarest of circumstances. The

differential diagnosis for an umbilical mass in a young child also includes umbilical pyogenic granuloma, umbilical polyp, omphalocele, and an omphalomesenteric duct remnant. The umbilical granuloma and polyp are readily differentiated from hernia by the lack of skin covering the mass, reddish color, and serous drainage that may be present. Omphalocele should be detected at birth, if not in utero, with intestine protruding from the umbilicus covered only by a membranous sac. Exceedingly rare umbilical tumors, such as teratomas and sarcomas, have been reported; these are not soft or reducible on examination.

Inguinal hernias can present at birth or at any time during childhood. The history may include a description of the bulge extending to the scrotum or labia majora. The differential diagnosis of an inguinal-scrotal or labial swelling also includes incarcerated inguinal hernia, hydrocele, torsion of an undescended testis, testicular cancer, varicocele, and inguinal lymphadenitis. History and a detailed gastrointestinal (GI) and genitourinary examination should differentiate between these entities (Table 58.1). Observing the mass increasing in size during a period of increased intraabdominal pressure and decreasing in size during relaxation or gentle palpation strongly suggests the diagnosis of inguinal hernia. A smooth mass is often palpable at the external inguinal ring. The smooth sensation of the herniated sac rolling over itself when palpated at the pubic tubercle is known as the "silk glove sign" and supports the diagnosis of hernia, although this sign is not always present. Transillumination is not specific for hydroceles and should be used with caution as a tool to differentiate from hernias, as hernias may transilluminate as well, especially in the incarcerated state with excess bowel wall edema. Close inspection of the contralateral inguinal region is important because 10% to 50% of patients have bilateral inguinal

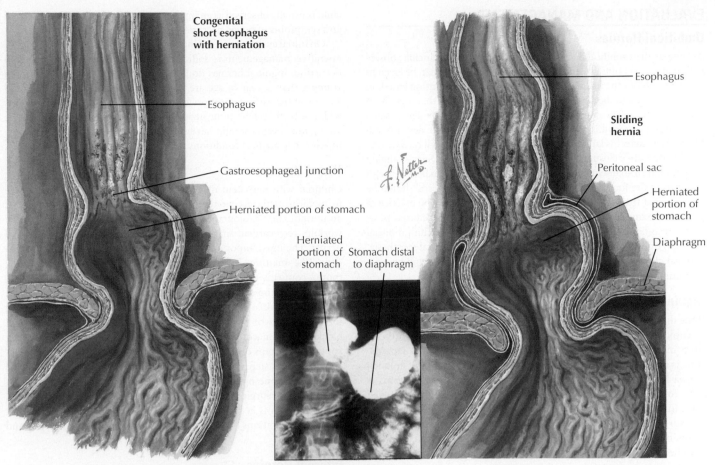

Congenital short esophagus with herniation

Esophagus

Gastroesophageal junction

Herniated portion of stomach

Herniated portion of stomach   Stomach distal to diaphragm

Esophagus

Sliding hernia

Peritoneal sac

Herniated portion of stomach

Diaphragm

Fig. 58.4 Hiatal Hernias.

TABLE 58.1 Differential Diagnosis of Inguinal-Scrotal or Labial Swelling

Clinical Condition	Distinguishing Characteristics
Reducible inguinal hernia	Crying or straining enlarges mass Relaxation or gentle pressure reduces mass Smooth, firm, mobile inguinal mass palpable at external ring
Incarcerated inguinal hernia	Intestinal obstructive symptoms present Mass with significant swelling and lack of mobility
Hydrocele	Gradual onset of swelling, often larger in the evening while the child is ambulating Intestinal obstructive symptoms absent ± Reducible, mobile mass + Transillumination
Torsion of undescended testis	Painful, erythematous groin mass Absence of testicle in scrotum on the ipsilateral side
Inguinal lymphadenitis	Infected or crusted skin lesion possible Multiple discrete palpable nodes in the inguinal region No thickening of spermatic cord or testis
Varicocele	Increase with Valsalva maneuver Decompresses when laying down Soft scrotal mass, "bag of worms"
Testicular cancer	Testicular enlargement or swelling Typically painless Does not change in size or reduce

hernias. Determining if the hernia is indirect or direct is frequently difficult on examination and is often not confirmed until surgery. A femoral hernia is clinically seen as a swelling in the femoral canal (medial to the femoral vessels) and inferior to the inguinal ligament, but also may be confused for an inguinal hernia.

Internal hernias are frequently asymptomatic and may come to the clinician's attention during an unrelated investigation. When symptomatic, the presentation is variable and depends on the site of herniation, but the hernia may manifest as partial or complete small or large bowel obstruction.

The cardinal symptoms of a sliding hiatal hernia are regurgitation and heartburn, which are manifestations of gastroesophageal reflux (GER). When a hiatal hernia is the underlying cause, GER may be associated with complications such as pulmonary infections secondary to aspiration, vomiting, and failure to thrive. Dysphagia also may be described but tends to be a later finding. Paraesophageal hiatal hernias may present in similar fashion to a sliding hernia; however, dysphagia, early satiety, and chest pain tend to be more prominent with paraesophageal hernias. Sliding and paraesophageal hiatal hernias should be considered as part of the differential diagnosis for any of these presenting symptoms. The physical examination may provide insight to the presence of GER but is not helpful in making the diagnosis of either type of hiatal hernia.

Paraduodenal, mesenteric, and other types of visceral hernias contained within the abdominal cavity rarely cause symptoms during childhood. When problematic, these hernias usually manifest with a constellation of symptoms, including abdominal pain, vomiting, decreased stooling, and irritability as manifestations of acute or recurrent intestinal obstruction.

EVALUATION AND MANAGEMENT

Umbilical Hernias

As long as the umbilical hernia is asymptomatic and reducible, observation alone will initially suffice. Anticipatory guidance can be given to the parent about the likelihood of the hernia's self-resolution based on the child's age and the size of the defect. Defects smaller than 1 cm have a greater than 80% chance of closing spontaneously by age 5 years. Referral to a surgeon is recommended at that time if the defect is still open. If the defect is larger than 1.5 cm in diameter, it will rarely close, making operative closure appropriate by 2 years of age. Defects ranging 1 to 1.5 cm in diameter should be observed for a gradual decrease in size during the first 2 to 3 years of life, and surgical referral should be made at that time if the defect fails to become smaller. The practice of strapping material over the hernia to maintain it in a reduced position does not assist in facilitating closure. If a patient with umbilical hernia is undergoing an unrelated procedure under general anesthesia, surgical closure may be discussed at that time with risks and benefits examined on a case-by-case basis.

Inguinal Hernias

If the diagnosis remains uncertain, ultrasonography is the imaging test of choice in differentiating a patent processus vaginalis or hydrocele from inguinal hernia. Infrequently, direct visualization with laparoscopy is needed to confirm the diagnosis. After the diagnosis of inguinal hernia has been made, the first step is to determine if the hernia is reducible or incarcerated. Incarceration of the hernia sac has occurred if it cannot be reduced into the abdominal cavity. An incarcerated sac is a surgical emergency and can proceed rapidly to strangulation, in which blood flow to the contents of the sac is compromised, resulting in ischemia. If the spermatic cord and testis or fallopian tube and ovary are affected, sterility of the involved organ may result. A strangulated bowel viscus is at risk for ischemia and perforation.

If the hernia is incarcerated without strangulation and the patient is in stable condition, manual reduction is often successful and should be attempted. The patient must be relaxed to perform this maneuver; analgesics or sedatives are frequently useful. Placing the patient in slight Trendelenburg position is also beneficial. Mild continuous pressure (taxis) is applied to the hernia to return the hernia sac into the abdominal cavity. If successful reduction cannot be achieved, intravenous fluids and broad-spectrum antibiotics are administered while awaiting emergent surgical correction before strangulation occurs. If manual reduction is successful, however, definitive surgical repair of the hernia may be delayed for 24 to 48 hours. During this period, the child is usually observed as an inpatient to ensure feedings are tolerated and symptoms of bowel necrosis do not develop.

On initial evaluation, if the inguinal hernia is freely reducible, timely operative management is indicated to prevent incarceration from occurring. Inguinal hernias do not resolve without surgery. Children younger than 1 year of age are at highest risk for incarceration, and surgery at the earliest appropriate time is indicated. Premature infants with low birth weight in the neonatal intensive care unit found to have an inguinal hernia should have surgical repair before discharge home unless other medical conditions make the procedure unsafe.

Hiatal Hernia

Children with persistent dysphagia or GER symptoms unresponsive to medical management require evaluation with imaging studies. If an upright chest radiograph has been performed as part of the initial workup, retrocardiac air-fluid levels are highly suggestive of a hiatal hernia. The most important initial test is a contrast upper GI series to define the anatomy. The presence of a portion of the stomach in the thorax confirms the diagnosis. If a sliding hiatal hernia is observed, both medical and surgical management options should be considered. An upper endoscopy may be helpful in guiding therapy by assessing for esophagitis or strictures. If optimal medical management, acid blockade pharmacotherapy and appropriate dietary changes, do not control symptoms or significant esophageal disease is found on endoscopy, the next step is a surgical evaluation for a fundoplication. The presence of paraesophageal hiatal hernia on contrast radiography is an indication for surgical repair. The gastric fundus herniating through the diaphragm is at high risk for incarceration, volvulus, or perforation—complications that carry significant potential for morbidity and mortality.

Internal Hernias

For patients with signs and symptoms of intestinal obstruction, plain radiographs and contrast studies, including computed tomography scans, may give clues to the presence of an internal hernia; however, these often fail to confirm this as the cause for the obstruction. More frequently, an internal hernia is found intraoperatively and the herniated bowel can be reduced and the defect can be repaired. Strangulation and bowel necrosis are possible complications requiring swift treatment.

SUGGESTED READINGS

Available online.

59

Disorders of the Esophagus

Atu Agawu and Amanda B. Muir

✳ CLINICAL VIGNETTE

A 13-year-old boy with a history of asthma and anaphylaxis to peanuts presents to his local emergency department (ED) after eating grilled chicken at a barbecue. He was laughing while he was eating and felt as though the food got stuck. He attempted to dislodge the food by drinking water but vomited twice and the feeling persisted. A neighbor attempted the Heimlich maneuver with no effect. In the ED he was tachycardic with normal oxygen saturations and has been unable to swallow his saliva. There were no visible abnormalities in his oropharynx, and he had no respiratory distress. The remainder of his physical examination was normal. On further history the teen's family notes that he is always the last to finish his meals, and frequently consumes multiple glasses of water or other fluids with his meals. He admits to feeling food get temporarily stuck in his throat multiple times a week, which he typically manages by drinking lots of water.

A chest radiograph was obtained without evidence of a radiopaque foreign body. Upper endoscopy was performed and showed a large mass of white material in the middle third of the esophagus that was removed. There was no stricture present after food was removed, but the mucosa appeared edematous, and there were circumferential rings along the esophagus. Microscopic evaluation of the mucosa revealed esophagitis with many intraepithelial eosinophils (>60/high-power field), basal cell hyperplasia of the esophageal epithelium, and lamina propria fibrosis. He was placed on proton pump inhibitor therapy and had improvement in his symptoms. Repeat endoscopy 8 weeks later showed esophageal edema and furrowing, with normal histologic findings on biopsies.

The esophagus is an epithelium-lined muscular tube connecting the pharynx and the stomach. Its role is to move material from the mouth to the stomach. It does not produce any digestive enzymes and has no active role in digestion. Disorders of the esophagus can manifest with dysphagia, vomiting, poor growth, chest or abdominal pain, or gastrointestinal (GI) bleeding. Disorders involving the esophagus include structural abnormalities (congenital or acquired), mucosal inflammation (allergic, chemical, infectious), and functional disorders (e.g., motility disorders).

CONGENITAL ANOMALIES

Congenital disorders of the esophagus occur in approximately 1 in 3000 to 5000 births. These disorders commonly occur during embryogenesis as the trachea separates from the esophagus, and include atresia with or without tracheoesophageal fistula (TEF), esophageal stenosis, esophageal duplication, esophageal webs and rings, esophageal diverticulum, and esophageal or bronchogenic cysts.

Etiology and Pathogenesis

The esophagus forms from a small ventral diverticulum of the embryonic foregut. This diverticulum separates into the esophagus and trachea around the fourth gestational week of fetal development. One of the most common anomalies is TEF with or without atresia. This occurs when there is a disruption in the elongation and separation of the trachea from the esophagus. There are five types of TEF. The most common is type C, in which there is atresia of the proximal esophagus with a fistula from the trachea to the distal esophagus (Fig. 59.1). Other categories of TEF, in descending frequency, include isolated esophageal atresia without TEF, isolated TEF, esophageal atresia with proximal TEF, and esophageal atresia with proximal and distal TEF. TEF can occur in isolation or with associated genetic syndromes, and as many as 70% of children with esophageal abnormalities may have other congenital anomalies, including imperforate anus, vertebral anomalies, duodenal atresia, and annular pancreas. The VACTERL association is a combination of defects that are commonly found together: *v*ertebral anomalies, *a*norectal atresia, *c*ardiac anomalies, *t*racheoesophageal fistula, *e*sophageal atresia, *r*enal anomalies, and *l*imb anomalies.

Clinical Presentation

Individuals with congenital esophageal disorders typically present in the neonatal period or infancy with a variety of symptoms, including respiratory distress worsened by feeding, regurgitation, recurrent aspiration pneumonia, or failure to thrive. Older children may present with dysphagia, regurgitation, halitosis, or respiratory symptoms. The severity of symptoms depends on the degree of esophageal compression or obstruction. There can be a prenatal history of polyhydramnios as a result of the fetus' inability to swallow amniotic fluid.

Evaluation and Management

Esophageal atresia or complete esophageal obstruction can be diagnosed by an inability to pass an orogastric or nasogastric tube into the stomach. TEF may be suggested on abdominal or chest radiograph; however, an isolated TEF (H-type) is best detected by a water-soluble contrast upper GI performed with the patient in the prone position. Upper GI can also detect stenosis or incomplete obstruction from a web, ring, cyst, or diverticulum. Surgical correction is required to treat most congenital anomalies.

ESOPHAGITIS

Esophagitis is a nonspecific term that refers to inflammation of the esophagus. Esophagitis can result from numerous causes, including chemical irritation (reflux, caustic ingestion), infection, or stasis of esophageal contents (e.g., with motility disorders). Table 59.1 summarizes the endoscopic and histologic findings of common etiologies of esophagitis.

GASTROESOPHAGEAL REFLUX

Gastroesophageal reflux (GER) is the retrograde movement of gastric contents into the esophagus with or without associated emesis.

1. Tracheoesophageal fistula

Most common form (90% to 95%) of tracheoesophageal fistula. Upper segment of esophagus
ending in blind pouch; lower segment originating
from trachea just above bifurcation. The two
segments may be connected by a solid cord

**2. Variations of tracheoesophageal
fistula and rare anomalies of trachea**

Upper segment of esophagus ending in
trachea; lower segment of variable length

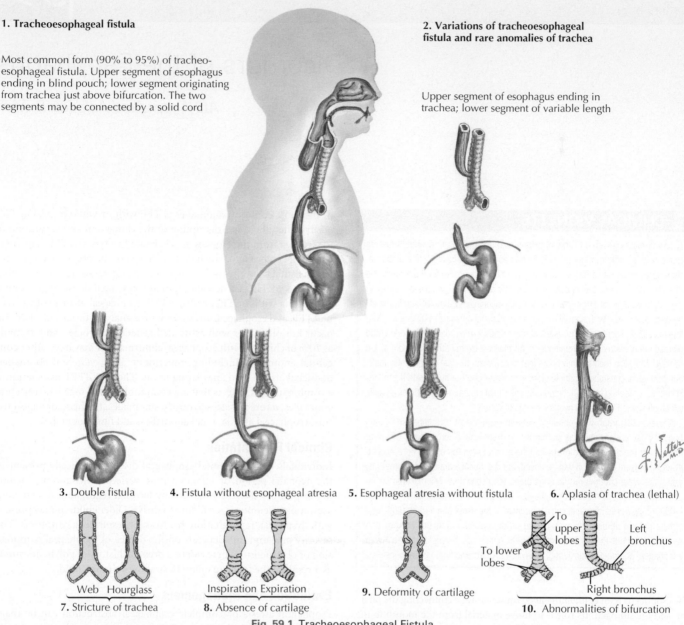

3. Double fistula   **4.** Fistula without esophageal atresia   **5.** Esophageal atresia without fistula   **6.** Aplasia of trachea (lethal)

Web   Hourglass
7. Stricture of trachea

Inspiration   Expiration
8. Absence of cartilage

9. Deformity of cartilage

To upper lobes
To lower lobes
Left bronchus
Right bronchus
10. Abnormalities of bifurcation

Fig. 59.1 Tracheoesophageal Fistula.

Infrequent GER is a normal process in all age groups, particularly in newborns and infants. However, when GER causes bothersome clinical symptoms, it is labeled gastroesophageal reflux disease (GERD). GERD is the most common esophageal disorder in children of all ages. Emesis from GER occurs in 67% of all 4-month-old infants, and heartburn and epigastric pain from GERD occur in 1% to 8% of children. The incidence of GERD is increased in premature infants and in children with neurologic, pulmonary, and developmental disorders.

Etiology and Pathogenesis

GER episodes are typically associated with transient lower esophageal sphincter relaxation (TLESR). The lower esophageal sphincter (LES) is tonically contracted with resting pressures between 10 and 30 mm Hg. This tonic contraction prevents retrograde movement of gastric contents. The primary role of TLESR is venting of gas to prevent gastric distension. TLESR frequency increases after meals and with gastric distension (e.g., food bolus). Infants have a higher frequency of TLESRs

than older children and adults, and the presence of a hiatal hernia can increase the frequency of TLESRs.

Clinical Presentation

GER and GERD manifest differently in infants and children. In infants, the most common symptoms of GER are effortless regurgitation and emesis. GERD typically involves symptoms of GER accompanied by irritability, arching, respiratory distress, refusal of food, or failure to thrive. Infantile GER and GERD usually begin to improve after 6 months of age and typically disappear by 2 years of age. In children over 5 years, GERD most commonly manifests as postprandial abdominal pain or burning chest pain. Children with GERD may also experience cough, dysphagia, odynophagia, or nocturnal worsening of their asthma. GERD may be associated with sore throat, otalgia, oral cavity disease, wheezing, and hoarseness in some children. In infants with vomiting, the differential diagnosis includes food allergies, anatomic abnormality (pyloric stenosis, malrotation, volvulus, rings, webs, and stenosis), infection, metabolic disorder, rumination, toxic ingestion, or increased intracranial pressure.

Evaluation and Management

GERD is a diagnosis made on history and physical examination. Diagnostic testing should be reserved for those with atypical or concerning (red flag) symptoms (Box 59.1), symptoms unresponsive to therapy, or symptoms suggestive of anatomic abnormality or tissue damage (hematemesis, bloody stool, anemia). An upper GI study with barium swallow is used to demonstrate anatomic anomalies. Scintigraphy (also known as milk scan or gastric emptying study) can show delayed gastric emptying. Upper endoscopy assesses for mucosal injury or inflammation (allergic or infectious), and may help distinguish GERD from eosinophilic esophagitis (EoE). Esophageal pH monitoring is helpful to evaluate the frequency of acid reflux events, and multichannel intraluminal impedance studies can demonstrate non–acid reflux events. These measurements are also correlated with clinical symptoms to help establish or refute the relationship between clinical symptoms and GERD.

The goals of treatment of GERD are symptom reduction, healing esophageal mucosal injury, and preventing complications, including esophagitis, Barrett esophagus (metaplasia of the lower esophagus), and stricture formation (Fig. 59.2). In infants with GER who are not

TABLE 59.1 Characteristic Endoscopic and Histologic Findings for Various Causes of Esophagitis

Etiology	Endoscopic Findings	Histology Finding
EoE	Circumferential rings Longitudinal furrows Edema (loss of typical vascular markings) Punctate white plaques Stenosis	>15 eosinophils/high-power field Eosinophilic microabscesses Basal cell hyperplasia Lamina propria proliferation
HSV esophagitis	Ulceration	Mononuclear infiltrate Multinucleate giant cells
CMV esophagitis	Ulceration	Basophilic nuclear inclusions
Candidal esophagitis	Macroscopic white plaques	Pseudohyphae budding yeast

CMV, Cytomegalovirus; *EoE,* eosinophilic esophagitis; *HSV,* herpes simplex virus.

BOX 59.1 Concerning "Red Flag" Symptoms in Vomiting Infants and Children

- Bilious emesis
- Bulging fontanelle, lethargy, morning emesis
- Hematemesis or hematochezia
- Weight loss
- Respiratory distress or history of multiple episodes of pneumonia
- Fever or systemic symptoms
- Skin lesions
- Seizures
- Macrocephaly/microcephaly
- Chronic diarrhea
- Abdominal distension
- Hepatosplenomegaly

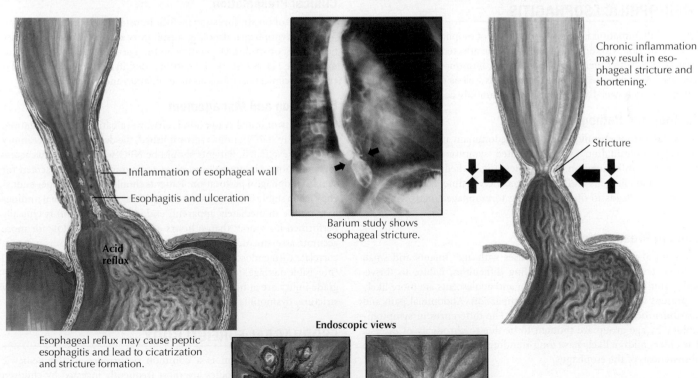

Inflammation of esophageal wall

Esophagitis and ulceration

Acid reflux

Esophageal reflux may cause peptic esophagitis and lead to cicatrization and stricture formation.

Barium study shows esophageal stricture.

Chronic inflammation may result in esophageal stricture and shortening.

Stricture

Endoscopic views

Esophagitis

Esophageal stricture

Fig. 59.2 Complications of Gastroesophageal Reflux Disease.

bothered by emesis and who are growing appropriately, no therapy is necessary. Initial therapy for symptomatic infants without red flag symptoms focuses on reducing gastric distension to decrease TLESR frequency: smaller volume frequent feeds, frequent burping, and maintaining upright position for longer duration after feeds. Recent guidelines have suggested a trial of protein hydrolysate or amino acid–based formula (or cow's milk elimination in maternal diet for breast-fed infants) before pharmacologic therapy if initial interventions are unsuccessful.

Pharmacologic therapy for GERD includes antacids to buffer existing acid and H2 receptor antagonists (e.g., famotidine) or proton pump inhibitors (PPIs; e.g., omeprazole) to decrease secretion of acid from parietal cells. Pharmacotherapy does not decrease the frequency of reflux events but reduces the acidity of the refluxate, which may improve feeding tolerance or pain associated with feeding. Prokinetic use (e.g., metoclopramide, erythromycin) has declined because of unfavorable side effect profiles and is typically not recommended. Surgical fundoplication, a procedure in which the fundus is wrapped around the distal esophagus to reinforce LES tone, is an option for children who are unresponsive to pharmacologic treatment or those who develop respiratory compromise or stricture. The most common fundoplication performed is a Nissen fundoplication, which involves a 360-degree wrap of the fundus around the intraabdominal esophagus. Fundoplication can help prevent refluxate by increasing the strength of the gastroesophageal junction and creating an acute angle at the cardia (angle of His). Side effects of fundoplication include bloating, dysphagia, dumping syndrome, hernia, small bowel obstruction, and recurrence requiring a second fundoplication.

EOSINOPHILIC ESOPHAGITIS

Allergic inflammation is an emerging cause of esophagitis in the pediatric population with up to 1 in 1000 children affected by EoE. EoE can be associated with other atopic disease (e.g., immunoglobulin E [IgE]-mediated food allergies, asthma, eczema) as well as celiac disease and inflammatory bowel disease (IBD) but commonly occurs in isolation.

Etiology and Pathogenesis

EoE results from chronic eosinophil-predominant inflammation (on histologic examination) with associated symptoms of esophageal dysfunction. Inflammation is immune/antigen mediated and caused by both food allergens and aeroallergens. Over time, chronic allergic inflammation leads to fibrosis, leading to esophageal narrowing and stricture.

Clinical Presentation

The clinical presentation of EoE varies with age. Infants and small children tend to present with feeding difficulties, failure to thrive, and vomiting, whereas older children and adolescents are more likely to present with dysphagia and food impaction. Abdominal pain and heartburn occur across all age groups. The differences in symptomatology by age group are thought to be due to chronicity of disease. The older children likely have long-standing inflammation resulting in fibrostenosis of the esophagus.

Evaluation and Management

The diagnosis of EoE is made by endoscopy, with biopsy revealing 15 or more eosinophils per high-power field. Endoscopy may reveal furrowing of the esophagus, rings or trachealization, white plaques representing eosinophilic microabscesses, or a general narrow caliber (Fig. 59.3). Upper GI examinations with barium are standard in the evaluation of dysphagia, recurrent food impactions, and profuse vomiting.

These may reveal narrowing or stricture in the esophagus as a result of fibrosis and are more sensitive at appreciating subtle narrowing than endoscopy.

EoE can be treated with PPI therapy, swallowed corticosteroids (e.g., budesonide, fluticasone), or dietary therapy. Dietary therapy can either focus on empiric elimination of the foods most commonly associated with EoE inflammation (milk, egg, soy, wheat) or initiation of an elemental diet. Remission is defined as improvement in histologic inflammation, specifically less than 15 eosinophils per high-power field. Once remission is achieved, foods are sequentially added back with endoscopic evaluation. Serum immunoglobulins and prick and patch testing are not reliable predictors for food allergens. The goals of EoE therapy are to reduce the eosinophilic inflammation to prevent the development of esophageal stricture. Patients with EoE frequently need serial endoscopic assessment because of the poor correlation between visual findings and histologic findings.

CAUSTIC INGESTION

The ingestion of caustic substances can cause immediate and long-lasting damage to the esophagus, including perforation, stricture formation, stenosis, and squamous cell carcinoma. Common household caustic substances include drain cleaners, dishwasher detergent, bleach, ammonia, and others. The risk for injury to the esophagus is highest with agents with a pH less than 2 or pH greater than 12. Alkaline substances cause liquefactive necrosis with fat and protein digestion, whereas acidic substances cause coagulative necrosis and typically have a lower risk for esophageal injury than alkaline substances.

Clinical Presentation

Symptoms of caustic ingestion include burning of the oropharynx, dysphagia, odynophagia, drooling, respiratory distress, abdominal pain, hoarseness, or stridor. Depending on the age of the child, there may or may not be a clear history of ingestion. Identifying the agent ingested is critical to clinical decisions about evaluation and management.

Evaluation and Management

The priority of initial evaluation is airway evaluation and stabilization. Once airway stabilization is accomplished, the degree of GI tract injury should be evaluated. Patients should be NPO with intravenous access for hydration. Abdominal and chest radiographs can help screen for signs of esophageal perforation. Patients should undergo upper endoscopy when stable to assess the extent of damage. Because visual findings may not be immediately apparent, endoscopic evaluation is typically performed no sooner than 6 hours after ingestion to allow for more accurate assessment. Oropharyngeal findings and symptoms may not correlate with endoscopic findings. Esophageal injury is graded from 0 (no visible damage) to 3 (extensive necrosis), and patients with higher-grade injury are at higher risk for long-term complications, including stricture, dysmotility, and squamous cell carcinoma.

ESOPHAGEAL FOREIGN BODY

Foreign body ingestion is a common occurrence in the pediatric population. Foreign bodies are most frequently ingested by children younger than 3 years, although older children and children with developmental delays or psychiatric disease can also present with foreign body ingestion. The most common locations of esophageal foreign bodies are thoracic inlet (at the level of the upper esophageal sphincter), mid-esophagus at the aortic notch, and just above the LES.

The most common items ingested in the United States are coins, small toys, game pieces, batteries, magnets, and jewelry. In other

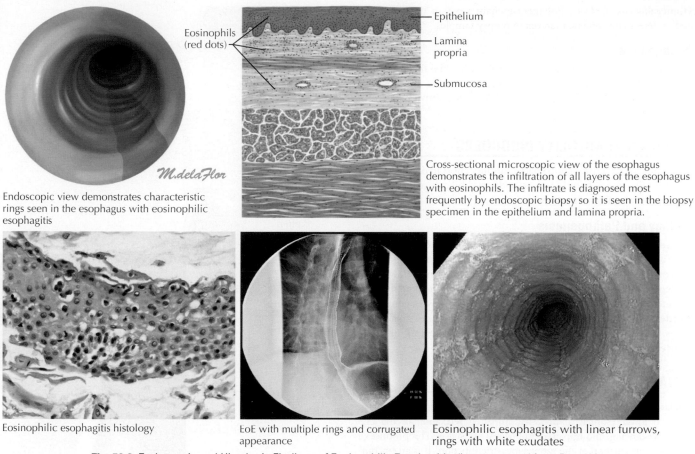

Endoscopic view demonstrates characteristic rings seen in the esophagus with eosinophilic esophagitis

Eosinophils (red dots)

Epithelium

Lamina propria

Submucosa

Cross-sectional microscopic view of the esophagus demonstrates the infiltration of all layers of the esophagus with eosinophils. The infiltrate is diagnosed most frequently by endoscopic biopsy so it is seen in the biopsy specimen in the epithelium and lamina propria.

Eosinophilic esophagitis histology

EoE with multiple rings and corrugated appearance

Eosinophilic esophagitis with linear furrows, rings with white exudates

Fig. 59.3 Endoscopic and Histologic Findings of Eosinophilic Esophagitis. (Images reused from Reynolds JR. *The Netter Collection of Medical Illustrations. Vol. 9: Digestive System, Part I, The Upper Digestive System.* 2nd ed. Philadelphia, PA: Elsevier: Plate 3.28.)

countries, fish, pork, and chicken bones are also frequent causes of esophageal foreign body ingestion.

Clinical Presentation

Patients with esophageal foreign bodies may be asymptomatic depending on the location and nature of the foreign body. Symptomatic patients may have dysphagia, odynophagia, drooling, wheezing or hoarseness, or chest pain. Larger and sharper foreign bodies tend to produce symptoms. Patients with food impaction often require evaluation for anatomic abnormalities (including stricture or vascular ring) or EoE, although not always in the acute phase.

Evaluation and Management

Endoscopy is the primary diagnostic and therapeutic tool for management of esophageal foreign bodies. Chest radiograph may identify radiopaque, but not radiolucent, objects. Contrast studies can be performed in select patients with suspected esophageal foreign bodies; however, they must be performed with caution because of the risk for aspiration if there is an obstructive foreign body and risk for mediastinitis if the foreign body has caused esophageal perforation. Computed tomography (CT) is infrequently used in the diagnosis of esophageal foreign bodies. Endoscopic removal is usually necessary and can be used to evaluate the esophagus after removal of the foreign body. Timing of endoscopic removal is based on the presence or absence of symptoms, the type and location of the suspected object, and the duration since ingestion. In general, all symptomatic patients, or patients with suspected button

battery, sharp object, or magnet ingestion require emergent endoscopic removal. Button batteries have been known to cause erosion through the esophagus to the aorta and cause death, so any suspected button battery in the esophagus represents a true emergency. Nonsharp objects (i.e., coins) typically undergo urgent endoscopic removal (within 24 hours).

INFECTIOUS ESOPHAGITIS

Infectious esophagitis most frequently occurs in immunocompromised children. Infections that commonly cause esophagitis include herpes simplex virus (HSV), cytomegalovirus, *Candida*, and, less frequently, varicella zoster virus, *Helicobacter pylori*, and human immunodeficiency virus (HIV). HSV is the most common cause of esophagitis in immunocompetent patients.

Clinical Presentation

Individuals with HSV esophagitis frequently have odynophagia. The general symptoms of infectious esophagitis are nonspecific, and the diagnosis requires a high degree of clinical suspicion.

Evaluation and Management

Infectious esophagitis is diagnosed on upper endoscopy with compatible visual findings that are confirmed on culture or histologic examination. Fungal esophagitis typically has numerous white plaques that can be brushed for culture. HSV esophagitis is often ulcerative and will show viral inclusions on histologic examination (also seen with cytomegalovirus [CMV]). Polymerase chain reaction (PCR) can be used to detect viral genetic material in biopsy samples.

Management

Management typically involves systemic antimicrobial therapy aimed at the underlying pathogen. Fluconazole is often the antifungal of choice for candidal esophagitis, and acyclovir is the antiviral of choice for HSV esophagitis.

ESOPHAGEAL MOTILITY DISORDERS

The esophagus relies on a coordinated motility effort to drive food forward into the stomach and to clear acidic and bilious secretions that may leak upward from the stomach.

Etiology and Pathogenesis

Striated muscle makes up the upper esophageal sphincter along with the proximal one-third of the esophagus. Smooth muscle composes the remaining two-thirds. The LES is a physiologic sphincter. Motility problems can arise from muscular disorders (achalasia, polymyositis, dermatomyositis, muscular dystrophy, myasthenia gravis), neurologic disorders (stroke, multiple sclerosis, lead poisoning), systemic illness (lupus, scleroderma, sarcoidosis, thyroid disease, diabetes), or infection (tetanus, botulism, *Trypanosoma cruzi*).

ACHALASIA

Achalasia is a progressive motor disorder of the esophagus resulting in increased lower esophageal pressure, impaired relaxation of the LES during swallowing, and impaired esophageal peristalsis. This produces a functional obstruction at the esophagogastric junction. It is an uncommon disorder in children. In the United States, childhood-onset achalasia is most often idiopathic, but systemic disease should be considered in determining the cause. Histologic changes seen with achalasia include loss of ganglion cells, a decrease in the number of myenteric plexus nerve fibers, and degeneration of the vagal nerve. In Latin America, achalasia is associated with chronic infection with *T. cruzi* (the causative agent in Chagas disease), secondary to infectious destruction of the myenteric plexus.

Clinical Presentation

Symptoms of achalasia include food and liquid dysphagia, regurgitation, vomiting, choking, and coughing episodes, a sense of "food getting stuck," a gurgling noise coming from the chest, postprandial and nocturnal chest pain, recurrent episodes of pneumonia, and weight loss. Leiomyoma of the distal esophagus, anorexia nervosa, eosinophilic esophagitis, rumination syndromes, Chagas disease, and candidal esophagitis are other diseases with similar symptoms that need to be considered in the differential diagnosis. Allgrove syndrome is an autosomal recessive disorder that includes achalasia, alacrima, and adrenocorticotropic hormone insensitivity.

Evaluation and Management

Chest radiograph may show widening of the mediastinum, loss of the gastric air bubble, or an esophageal air-fluid level. Barium swallow will show impaired contrast movement, abnormal peristalsis, and tapering of the distal esophagus known as the "bird's beak" sign (Fig. 59.4). Endoscopy should always be performed and often shows esophageal dilatation, erythema, and ulceration from stasis. Esophageal manometry, a measurement of sphincter pressure and esophageal contraction, remains the gold standard for diagnosis. In achalasia, manometry shows increased lower esophageal pressure, abnormal peristalsis, and elevated esophageal pressures.

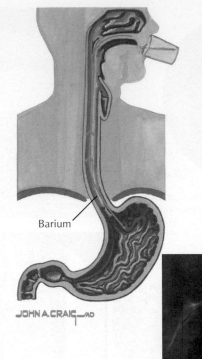

Barium

JOHN A.CRAIG—AD

Barium contrast study shows narrowed esophagogastric junction with more proximal esophageal dilatation

Fig. 59.4 Barium Swallow Findings Seen With Achalasia.

Treatment of patients with achaasia includes pneumatic dilatation, surgical myotomy, botulinum toxin injection to inhibit acetylcholine release at the neuromuscular junction, and more recently per-oral endoscopic myotomy. Pharmacologic therapy with calcium channel blockers and nitrites is largely ineffective and reserved for patients who cannot undergo invasive procedures. Because these therapies permanently open the LES, a long-term complication of achalasia is GER. Chronic inflammation as a result of reflux, as well as stasis and genetic factors, places achalasia patients at higher risk for both esophageal squamous cell carcinoma and adenocarcinoma.

MEDICATION-INDUCED ESOPHAGITIS

Medications, including NSAIDs, potassium, iron, and antibiotics (tetracyclines), can cause esophageal damage, particularly in patients with delayed esophageal motility. Symptoms of odynophagia can occur immediately after ingestion or can be delayed. Endoscopy will reveal inflammation and possibly focal erosion; it provides the opportunity to remove the pill if still retained.

ESOPHAGEAL RUPTURE

Esophageal rupture is a life-threatening event and can result from severe vomiting (Boerhaave syndrome), thoracic or abdominal trauma, instrumentation, or ulcer perforation. Patients with esophageal rupture present with chest, neck, or abdominal pain; dysphagia; hematemesis; subcutaneous emphysema; or signs of shock. Chest and abdominal radiographs may reveal air in the subcutaneous tissue, mediastinum, thorax, or abdomen. In patients with EoE, prolonged food impaction is a risk factor for esophageal perforation. Treatment is typically supportive or surgical.

FUTURE DIRECTIONS

Future directions in esophageal disorders are focused on developing new therapies and on decreasing the need for recurrent general anesthesia exposure. In EoE, trials are underway to investigate alternative medication options, particularly for patients for whom dietary therapy is not tolerable and who cannot tolerate swallowed corticosteroids. Transnasal endoscopy is not standard of care but is being investigated for older children to reduce the burden of frequent exposure to general anesthesia. Studies are underway to investigate potential biomarkers for esophageal inflammation that could replace the need for recurrent endoscopic evaluation.

SUGGESTED READINGS

Available online.

60

Intestinal Obstruction and Malrotation

Kanak Verma and Atu Agawu

✳ CLINICAL VIGNETTE

A 1-month-old previously healthy male infant presents to the emergency department after several episodes of vomiting. He has had 8 to 10 episodes of dark green emesis over the last 24 hours. He is now not tolerating any oral intake and his urine output has decreased. He has had no recent fevers, diarrhea, or recent sick contacts at home. On examination, he is moderately ill-appearing, with delayed capillary refill and diminished skin turgor. His abdomen is mildly distended and tender, with hypoactive bowel sounds. An abdominal radiograph shows a dilated, air-filled duodenum with a paucity of gas distally. An upper gastrointestinal series is obtained and demonstrates a misplaced duodenum with the ligament of Treitz on the right side of the abdomen, consistent with malrotation with volvulus. The patient is referred for emergent laparotomy with the Ladd procedure.

Patients with intestinal malrotation are at risk for acute bowel obstruction as a result of midgut volvulus. Early detection and prompt surgical intervention are imperative to restore perfusion and prevent catastrophic bowel injury.

The gastrointestinal (GI) tract is designed for active, unidirectional flow (Fig. 60.1). Any barrier to forward propulsion can lead to accumulation of intestinal contents and luminal distension proximal to the obstruction. Prompt identification, triage, and management of intestinal obstruction is imperative to prevent postobstructive complications, including bowel infarction and perforation, peritonitis, and septic shock.

ETIOLOGY AND PATHOGENESIS

Intestinal obstruction leads to progressive proximal bowel dilation, often leading to vomiting, and decreased blood flow to the abdominal wall, resulting in ischemia. Stagnant bowel contents can allow rapid bacterial proliferation. This common pathway can facilitate bacterial translocation into the bowel wall, leading to bacteremia, endotoxemia, and sepsis.

A variety of congenital and acquired defects may cause throughput failure (Fig. 60.2). Intestinal obstruction can be characterized as partial or complete based on the degree of blockage and as simple or strangulating based on impairment of intestinal blood flow. Causes of intestinal obstruction can be further classified based on the origin of the obstruction: extrinsic, intrinsic, and functional obstruction.

Extrinsic Obstruction

Extrinsic obstruction involves compression of the bowel lumen by surrounding tissue, masses, organs, or vessels. Adhesions are fibrous bands of tissue within the peritoneum that arise spontaneously in response to injury, such as peritonitis or abdominal surgery, and can encircle and constrict loops of bowel. The risk for postoperative obstruction due to adhesions varies greatly based on the type of surgery

performed, with 5-year readmission rate for obstruction secondary to adhesions ranging from 0.3% for appendectomy to 25% for ileostomy formation or closure.

Enlarged mediastinal lymph nodes, caused by infection or neoplasm, can compress the esophagus. Similarly, intraabdominal masses, such as Wilms tumor or mesenteric lymphatic cysts, can obstruct the small bowel. Annular pancreas is an anatomic variant in which a ring of pancreatic tissue encircles the duodenum and can cause obstruction. In superior mesenteric artery (SMA) syndrome, the SMA compresses the third segment of the duodenum against the aorta; it can be seen in patients after precipitous weight loss, resulting in loss of the mesenteric fat pad that protects the duodenum from compression; external body cast application; or recent intestinal or spinal surgery causing downward traction on the SMA over the duodenum. A closed loop obstruction occurs when a loop of bowel passes through a mesenteric defect or similar orifice (e.g., inguinal hernia) and becomes trapped, resulting in occlusion of both the proximal and distal ends of the bowel loop.

Malrotation is an important entity to consider when evaluating intestinal obstruction at any age. Intestinal development is a complex, continuous process that transforms the primitive gut into a long, highly specialized organ. During fetal development, the rapidly growing midgut protrudes through the umbilical ring out of the abdominal cavity, then subsequently returns to the peritoneum and rotates 270 degrees counterclockwise. This process is completed by the 8th week of gestation and positions the intestine such that the duodenum, ending at the ligament of Treitz, is in the left upper quadrant, and the cecum is fixed in the right lower quadrant.

Malrotation refers to any abnormality in fetal intestinal rotation, resulting in an atypical spatial arrangement within the abdomen and inadequate mesenteric attachment of the intestine to the abdominal wall. As a result, the bowel is at risk for volvulus, or twisting upon its mesenteric stalk, causing auto-obstruction and ischemia (Fig. 60.3). Malrotation is frequently associated with the presence of Ladd's bands, congenital intraperitoneal fibrous adhesions that can encircle and obstruct the duodenum.

Intrinsic Obstruction
Congenital Defects

Congenital abnormalities in lumen structure and function can present as bowel obstruction in infancy. Intestinal atresia is total or near-total discontinuity of a bowel segment, whereas stenosis refers to narrowing of the intestinal lumen. Intestinal webs are mucosal membranes within the intestinal lumen that can precipitate obstruction. Intestinal atresia has an estimated incidence of 1.3 to 3.5 per 10,000 live births. There is a strong association between intestinal atresia and chromosomal abnormalities (e.g., trisomy 21). The most common intestinal atresia is duodenal atresia, followed by jejunal/ileal atresia, with colonic atresia being the least common type. Duodenal atresia occurs as a result of

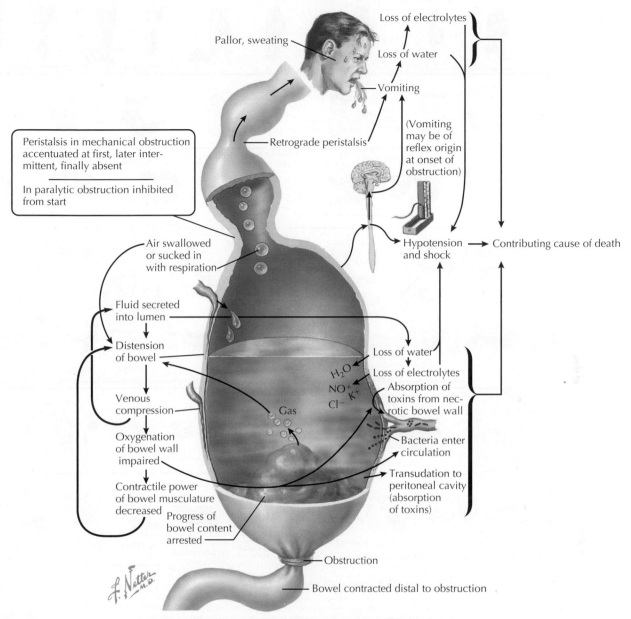

Peristalsis in mechanical obstruction accentuated at first, later intermittent, finally absent

In paralytic obstruction inhibited from start

Pallor, sweating

Loss of electrolytes

Loss of water

Vomiting

Retrograde peristalsis

(Vomiting may be of reflex origin at onset of obstruction)

Air swallowed or sucked in with respiration

Hypotension and shock → Contributing cause of death

Fluid secreted into lumen

Distension of bowel

Loss of water

Loss of electrolytes

H_2O
NO^+
Cl^- K^+

Absorption of toxins from necrotic bowel wall

Venous compression

Gas

Oxygenation of bowel wall impaired

Bacteria enter circulation

Transudation to peritoneal cavity (absorption of toxins)

Contractile power of bowel musculature decreased

Progress of bowel content arrested

Obstruction

Bowel contracted distal to obstruction

Fig. 60.1 Intestinal Obstruction, Adynamic Ileus.

recanalization failure and is on the same spectrum as a duodenal web. Jejunal and ileal atresia are thought to result from a prenatal vascular insult with subsequent ischemic necrosis.

Hirschsprung disease is caused by an interruption in neural crest cell migration during fetal development, resulting in absent enteric innervation of the rectum and colon. Patients typically present with severe constipation and lower intestinal obstruction in infancy. Meconium ileus can cause small bowel obstruction in neonates. Meconium, an intestinal conglomeration of sloughed mucosa, bile salts, and other debris, accumulates during fetal development and typically passes within the first day of life. When the meconium is exceedingly inspissated, frequently as a result of pancreatic dysfunction from cystic fibrosis, patients may present with failure to pass meconium, abdominal distension, and vomiting.

Acquired Defects

Areas in the gastrointestinal tract that are inherently narrow (upper esophageal sphincter, esophagus adjacent to the carina, lower esophageal sphincter, pylorus, ileocecal valve) are particularly vulnerable to intrinsic obstruction. Gastric outlet obstruction as a result of pyloric stenosis, a disorder of smooth muscle hypertrophy, is typically seen in infants during the first 3 to 6 weeks of life (Fig. 60.4). Gastric outlet obstruction can also occur in the setting of an impacted bezoar, a foreign body composed of accumulated indigestible material (e.g., hair, fiber from vegetables). Blunt abdominal trauma, including seatbelt or bicycle handlebar injuries in children, can instigate a small bowel hematoma and obstruction because of the small luminal caliber. Duodenal hematomas are a rare complication of diagnostic upper endoscopy that occur exclusively in children. Intussusception, the invagination of one portion of bowel into another, can also cause intestinal obstruction and is most common in the first 3 years of life.

Bowel inflammation and injury can lead to luminal narrowing. Inflammatory strictures due to caustic ingestion can cause upper esophageal narrowing, and peptic strictures can occur in the lower esophagus. Over time, persistent inflammation due to eosinophilic esophagitis can cause esophageal strictures and dysphagia. In Crohn's

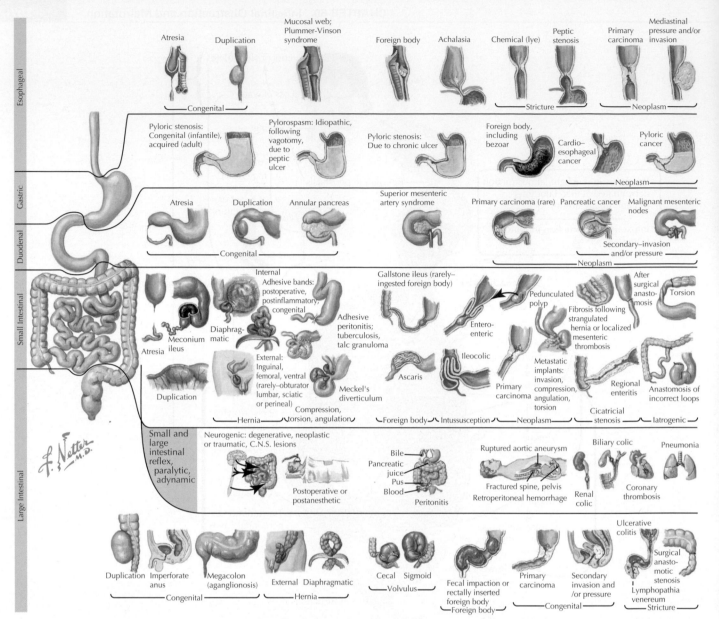

Fig. 60.2 Causes of Intestinal Obstruction.

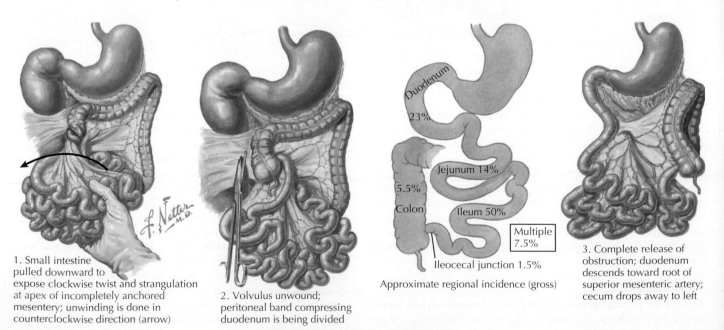

1. Small intestine pulled downward to expose clockwise twist and strangulation at apex of incompletely anchored mesentery; unwinding is done in counterclockwise direction (arrow)

2. Volvulus unwound; peritoneal band compressing duodenum is being divided

Approximate regional incidence (gross)

Duodenum 23%
Jejunum 14%
Colon 5.5%
Ileum 50%
Ileocecal junction 1.5%
Multiple 7.5%

3. Complete release of obstruction; duodenum descends toward root of superior mesenteric artery; cecum drops away to left

Fig. 60.3 Malrotation and Volvulus.

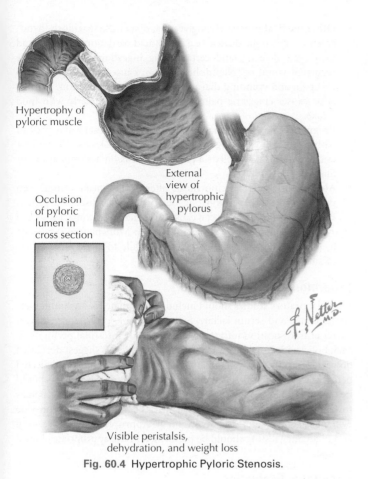

Hypertrophy of pyloric muscle

External view of hypertrophic pylorus

Occlusion of pyloric lumen in cross section

Visible peristalsis, dehydration, and weight loss

Fig. 60.4 Hypertrophic Pyloric Stenosis.

disease, chronic transmural inflammation can lead to stricture formation (see Chapter 57). Malignancy, although relatively uncommon in children, can lead to tumor infiltration of the bowel wall and decreased luminal diameter.

Functional Obstruction

In the absence of a mechanical obstruction, failure of coordinated peristalsis can also result in obstructive symptoms. Achalasia causes functional esophageal obstruction as a result of aperistalsis and inadequate lower esophageal sphincter relaxation. Chronic intestinal pseudo-obstruction refers to a spectrum of rare primary and secondary disorders caused by failure of the enteric nervous system or intestinal smooth muscle to coordinate peristalsis. The most common cause of acute colonic pseudo-obstruction is Ogilvie syndrome.

Postinfectious ileus, commonly seen after gastroenteritis, pneumonia, or peritonitis, is usually mild and self-limited; in rare instances, it can result in severe and prolonged gastroparesis, feeding intolerance, and the need for postpyloric nasogastric feeding. Abdominal surgery can cause a postoperative ileus; symptoms typically resolve within 72 hours of surgery, but may be prolonged with concurrent use of opioid medications due to their intrinsic antimotility effect.

CLINICAL PRESENTATION

Clinical presentation can vary widely based on the nature and severity of the obstruction. The presence or absence of specific signs and symptoms can provide helpful clues to the underlying cause. Classic obstructive symptoms include vomiting, abdominal distension, and

change in bowel habits. Abdominal pain may be present and is typically relieved by vomiting.

It is important to elicit the character of the emesis, which can reflect the location of the obstruction. Gastric outlet obstruction as a result of pyloric stenosis causes nonbilious vomiting, because bile is secreted by the liver into the duodenum at the ampulla of Vater, beyond the point of obstruction. Small bowel obstruction typically leads to rapid abdominal distension, crampy discomfort in the middle or upper abdomen, and recurrent bilious vomiting. Large bowel obstruction tends to produce milder symptoms with slower onset in comparison to small bowel obstruction. Patients develop bowel distension and cramping abdominal pain and may develop vomiting with severe or prolonged obstruction.

Patients with esophageal obstruction frequently report dysphagia. Low-grade esophageal obstruction can cause difficulty swallowing solid foods without vomiting, whereas high-grade obstruction can interfere with swallowing liquids, resulting in sialorrhea and regurgitation of undigested food.

Abdominal pain is frequently described as crampy and intermittent. The pattern of abdominal pain can also reflect the degree of obstruction. Patients with partial bowel obstruction may experience waxing and waning symptoms. Older children with a history of recurrent partial small bowel obstruction, as seen in Crohn's disease–associated strictures, may even self-limit oral intake with onset of characteristic symptoms. Patients with intussusception report recurrent bouts of intense pain and vomiting that resolve between episodes. With complete obstruction, symptoms typically persist until the obstruction is relieved and the bowel is mechanically decompressed.

Stool character and frequency can also inform the differential diagnosis. Complete bowel obstruction, including extrinsic compression or intrinsic obstruction due to strictures, may cause severe constipation or obstipation. Alternating constipation and diarrhea can signal either a partial mechanical obstruction or a functional obstruction. Hematochezia in association with obstructive symptoms is concerning for intestinal vascular compromise and can be seen with intussusception or volvulus.

A patient's medical history may reveal severe prior reflux symptoms or recurrent abdominal pain episodes, raising suspicion for malrotation or mild congenital anomalies such as webs. Children with trisomy 21 are at increased risk for duodenal atresia and stenosis, as well as esophageal atresia with tracheoesophageal fistula. Heterotaxy, or abnormal lateralization of the thoracoabdominal organs, is associated with intestinal malrotation and an increased risk for volvulus. Intussusception is a rare complication of Henoch-Schönlein purpura. Additional important historical information includes prior abdominal or spinal surgery and any history of blunt or penetrating trauma.

EVALUATION AND MANAGEMENT

All patients should undergo a thorough physical examination. Patients with severe or prolonged obstruction may be ill-appearing (e.g., pallor, lethargy, diaphoresis, restlessness), raising concern for postobstructive complications such as bowel ischemia or perforation. Level of consciousness, distal perfusion, and mucous membranes can be used to assess hydration status.

Abdominal inspection may reveal distension. Gastric obstruction can produce mild to moderate epigastric distension, whereas obstruction distal to the duodenum typically results in more prominent abdominal distension. Auscultation may reveal normal bowel sounds, hyperactive, tinkling, high-pitched bowel sounds suggesting complete bowel obstruction, or diminished to absent bowel sounds late in obstruction. Palpation may elicit focal tenderness as a result of pressure applied to gas- or fluid-filled bowel loops or more diffuse tenderness concerning for peritoneal inflammation. Additional peritoneal signs, including involuntary guarding, rebound tenderness to palpation, and exquisite sensitivity to movement raise concern for peritonitis (potentially associated with perforation). A sausage-like mass in the right upper quadrant may be palpated with intussusception, whereas a nontender, "olive"-shaped mass in the epigastrium is consistent with pyloric stenosis. An inguinal hernia may present as a discrete, tender, smooth mass originating from the external ring lateral to the pubic tubercle with surrounding edema.

The rectal examination may be notable for a hard-palpable stool "ball" with obstruction resulting from fecal impaction or may be devoid of stool with a more proximal colon obstruction. Explosive stooling may be precipitated by rectal examination in a patient with obstipation due to Hirschsprung disease.

Initial Care in the Emergency Department

The goal of the initial evaluation is to determine the severity of the child's illness. Vital signs should be evaluated for fever, tachycardia, low-normal blood pressure with widened pulse pressure (concerning for compensated shock), and hypotension (consistent with decompensated shock). Physical examination should include assessment of mental status, level of dehydration, evidence of trauma, and systemic stigmata of disease, as well as a thorough abdominal and rectal examination.

Initial interventions should be directed at stabilization, fluid resuscitation, and gastric decompression to prevent further bowel distension and possible aspiration. Intravenous fluid therapy with isotonic fluids should be initiated to correct electrolyte and fluid imbalances. Patients with severe dehydration may require isotonic fluid boluses to achieve hemodynamic stability. A nasogastric Salem sump catheter can facilitate decompression and help relieve pain and vomiting. If the sump catheter aspirates large volumes of gastric contents, losses should be replaced by intravenous fluid administration. For febrile or ill-appearing patients, broad-spectrum intravenous antibiotic therapy with adequate coverage for common gut flora (including gram-negative and anaerobic organisms) should be initiated after appropriate cultures are obtained. Early surgical evaluation is imperative to determine whether the patient will require operative intervention.

Vomiting is a ubiquitous symptom, often caused by nonobstructive processes. This can make the assessment of a vomiting child challenging. For example, viral gastroenteritis can present with acute recurrent vomiting. Key clinical features that can distinguish viral gastroenteritis include a history of recently ill contacts, nonbilious emesis (or perhaps "highlighter" green after repeated vomiting episodes, as opposed to the "spinach green" color of true bilious emesis in obstructed patients), associated diarrheal symptoms, and a benign, nondistended abdominal examination. *Several red-flag symptoms raise concern for alternative, more serious causes of vomiting:*

- **Intracranial lesions:** Although rare, intracranial tumors can manifest with recurrent emesis. Distinguishing characteristics include a concurrent history of neurologic symptoms, including headaches, vision changes, loss of motor coordination, regression of developmental milestones, or changes in speech. The vomiting typically occurs without associated nausea, abdominal pain, or distension. Physical examination should include a fundoscopic examination and thorough neurologic assessment. If there is clinical concern, the team should obtain intracranial imaging (typically computed tomography [CT] in the emergency setting, although higher resolution imaging with magnetic resonance imaging [MRI] may eventually be required to detect small lesions or lesions localized to the posterior fossa).

- **Other medical illness:** Hypoglycemia, diabetic ketoacidosis, hypokalemia, metabolic disease (e.g., fatty acid oxidation disorders and urea cycle defects), and certain drug ingestions can also cause recurrent vomiting. Nephrolithiasis can cause significant abdominal pain and vomiting that mimic intestinal obstruction. Pancreatitis causes epigastric pain and vomiting, particularly with food intake.

- **Pregnancy:** Postmenarchal women who are pregnant may present with significant vomiting because of morning sickness or hyperemesis gravidarum, as well as a palpable uterus on abdominal examination.

- **Abuse:** Intracranial hemorrhage after severe head trauma can produce symptoms mimicking obstruction, as discussed earlier. Blunt abdominal trauma can cause duodenal hematoma, leading to symptoms of small bowel obstruction. In Munchausen syndrome by proxy, a caretaker may force a young child to ingest medications or substances to induce illness symptoms.

Laboratory Evaluation

Initial laboratory studies should include a complete blood count, metabolic panel, and serum lactate. Significant leukocytosis may suggest bacterial translocation into the bloodstream or intestinal perforation. Metabolic acidosis with elevated serum lactate levels suggest decreased bowel perfusion and ischemia. Blood cultures should be collected before initiating broad-spectrum antibiotic therapy. Urinalysis should be obtained to assess for evidence of urinary tract infection or hematuria due to nephrolithiasis. Normal amylase and lipase levels provide evidence against pancreatic involvement. Appropriate drug screening and pregnancy testing should be performed in the appropriate clinical context.

Radiologic Evaluation

Upright and supine abdominal radiographs should be obtained for all patients with suspected obstruction to assess bowel gas pattern and identify intraabdominal free air, foreign bodies, volvulus, and masses. Obstruction is generally associated with significant proximal intestinal distension, either with fluid or air. Gaseous distension of the stomach alone suggests gastric outlet obstruction or, rarely, gastric volvulus. The "double-bubble" sign, in which air localizes to the stomach and proximal duodenum, is suggestive of duodenal atresia. Air-fluid levels denote stasis of intraluminal contents, resulting from either obstruction or ileus. Pneumatosis (or gas in the bowel wall) is frequently a sign of intestinal ischemia, which can result from prolonged obstruction.

Bedside ultrasonography is a useful tool for assessment of pyloric stenosis and intussusception, without radiation exposure. Significant bowel gas and large body habitus can limit yield of abdominal ultrasound.

Fluoroscopic contrast studies can provide an enhanced assessment of bowel anatomy and function in clinically stable patients. Water-soluble contrast (e.g., Gastrografin) is the recommended contrast media in the setting of obstruction because of the risk for severe chemical peritonitis from barium if a perforation is present.

There are several types of contrast fluoroscopy. An upper GI series follows contrast medium to the ligament of Treitz and can visualize malposition in malrotation with volvulus. In an upper GI series with small bowel follow-through, contrast media is followed to the terminal ileum. This can be a valuable tool for assessment of distal small bowel obstruction beyond the ligament of Treitz; however, it is inappropriate in the acute setting because of the length of time required to perform imaging and the need for barium contrast to effectively assess the distal small bowel.

Contrast enemas may be useful in delineating colonic obstruction, such as Hirschsprung disease or meconium ileus. Air enema can be both diagnostic and therapeutic for patients with suspected intussusception; air is used to insufflate the rectum and colon, with the generated hydrostatic pressure serving to reduce the intussuscepted bowel.

In patients who are clinically unstable, CT imaging should serve as the initial imaging modality. The risk for radiation exposure is typically outweighed by the benefits in the acute setting. Abdominal CT can define the cause and level of obstruction, identify emergent postobstructive complications, and assist with surgical planning. Thickened bowel wall suggests ischemic injury, and pneumoperitoneum or pneumatosis intestinalis suggests necrosis and perforation. When available, MRI can provide an alternative imaging modality in more stable patients.

Endoscopy can serve as a useful diagnostic and therapeutic tool in the nonacute setting, allowing direct visualization of the mucosa, tissue sampling for histologic evaluation, and stricture dilation. Rectal suction biopsy is the gold standard for diagnosis of Hirschsprung disease.

Surgical Management

Surgical exploration is indicated for severe intestinal obstruction or acute clinical deterioration. Signs of peritonitis, ischemia, or perforation mandate immediate surgical exploration. Incarcerated hernias are also an indication for immediate surgical correction. The Ladd procedure for malrotation with volvulus involves detorsion and reorientation of the small bowel and cecum, lysis of Ladd's bands, and appendectomy (see Fig. 60.3). Although laparotomy may be indicated in some patients, advances in minimally invasive surgical techniques have made laparoscopy an acceptable approach for correction of some causes of pediatric bowel obstruction.

FUTURE DIRECTIONS

The increasing availability and use of laparoscopy for correction of pediatric obstruction promises improved morbidity, reduced lengths of stay, and decreased cost of care when compared with laparotomy. Refined protocols for pediatric chest and abdominal CT imaging have demonstrated substantial reductions in radiation dose. Advances in fetal surgery also offer an alternative treatment for a growing number of congenital anomalies.

SUGGESTED READINGS

Available online.

61

Disorders of the Pancreas

Logan Grimes and Jefferson N. Brownell

✳ CLINICAL VIGNETTE

A 14-year-old girl with no chronic medical problems presented to the emergency department (ED) with acute-onset epigastric abdominal discomfort. She describes the pain as burning and states that it radiates to her back. She has no appetite, is nauseated, and vomited nonbloody, nonbilious contents once en route to the ED. Her vital signs are stable, and her examination is notable for generalized abdominal discomfort that is worse in her epigastric and right upper quadrant regions. Her laboratory data are notable for mild leukocytosis with left shift and lipase level that is 10 times the upper limit of normal along with mild increase of her aspartate aminotransferase (AST) and alanine aminotransferase (ALT). Abdominal ultrasound is read as "normal ultrasound of the abdomen, normal appearance of pancreatic head and body, pancreatic tail is obscured by bowel gas." The patient is admitted to the hospital and is made nil per os (NPO), aggressively fluid resuscitated and provided isotonic fluids at two times her maintenance rate, analgesia, and antiemetics. Within 18 hours, her abdominal discomfort is much improved and her appetite returns. The team diagnoses acute pancreatitis, and the patient reports that this is her third episode of pancreatitis. Evaluation is expanded to assess for causes of acute recurrent pancreatitis. Magnetic resonance cholangiopancreatography (MRCP) shows pancreatic divisum. Her markers of exocrine pancreatic function are reassuring, and her genetic/autoimmune pancreatitis panel is negative. She is referred to general surgery for consideration of surgical amelioration of her pancreatic divisum in attempts to prevent subsequent bouts of acute pancreatitis.

Disorders of the pancreas (Fig. 61.1) are rare in childhood but can be associated with significant morbidity and mortality. Pancreatitis, or inflammation of the pancreas, occurs less frequently in children than in adults and can be acute, recurrent, or chronic (Table 61.1). Complications are rare, although they include shock, hypocalcemia, pseudocyst formation, or necrosis. Exocrine pancreatic insufficiency (EPI), defined as insufficient pancreatic enzyme and bicarbonate secretion resulting in nutrient malabsorption and malnutrition, occurs in patients with significant pancreatic parenchymal volume loss due to disorders such as chronic pancreatitis or cystic fibrosis (CF); it affects about 80% to 90% of patients with CF. Congenital anomalies of the pancreas are found in approximately 10% of the healthy population and are generally asymptomatic but can be associated with pancreatitis (pancreas divisum) or duodenal obstruction (annular pancreas).

ETIOLOGY AND PATHOGENESIS

Pancreatitis

Pancreatitis occurs when intracellular trypsinogen and other digestive enzymes are prematurely activated, leading to autodigestion of the pancreatic acinar cells. This damage leads to a localized inflammatory response and edema (Fig. 61.2). Acute pancreatitis may occur as a single episode or may be recurrent. Chronic pancreatitis is often due to recurrent episodes of pancreatitis and is characterized by permanent structural damage such as fibrosis and parenchymal volumes loss. Most cases of chronic pancreatitis in children are due to genetic variants, including *CFTR* (in patients with or without pulmonary manifestations of CF), *SPINK1*, *PRSS1*, and *CTRC*. A large percentage of cases remain idiopathic.

The incidence of acute pancreatitis in children and adolescents has been increasing worldwide over the past 20 years. Causes of pancreatitis broadly include mechanical (trauma, anatomic abnormalities, and obstruction), toxic (including medications and metabolic byproducts), infectious, autoimmune, or genetic. Contrary to adults, alcohol and tobacco use are rarely implicated in pediatric pancreatitis. More narrowly, obstructive causes include choledocholithiasis, tumors, and choledochal cysts. Toxic causes include scorpion envenomations and most viral infections, such as enterovirus, Epstein-Barr virus, hepatitis A, rubella, coxsackievirus B, cytomegalovirus, human immunodeficiency virus (HIV), and influenza. Medications can cause pancreatitis as well, particularly chemotherapeutic agents, such as thiopurines and L-asparaginase, glucocorticoids, valproate, and tetracycline antibiotics. Acute pancreatitis also can be the result of systemic diseases and metabolic abnormalities, including CF, diabetic ketoacidosis, hypercalcemia, hypertriglyceridemia, and hemolytic-uremic syndrome.

Exocrine Pancreatic Insufficiency

Exocrine pancreatic insufficiency (EPI) occurs in patients with CF, chronic pancreatitis, and sometimes as part of a genetic syndrome. In patients with CF, EPI is caused by dysfunction of the *CFTR* gene (Fig. 61.3), leading to impaired secretion of sodium, chloride, and bicarbonate in the pancreatic ducts and increased viscosity of pancreatic fluid. This pancreatic duct obstruction results in destruction of pancreatic acini. In patients with chronic pancreatitis and CF, acinar destruction leads to diminished enzyme secretion and impaired enzymatic activity in the duodenum as a result of a more acidic pH. Children with Schwachman-Diamond syndrome, caused by variants in the *SDS* gene, present with short stature, variable neutropenia, and EPI that improves as they grow older. The cause of poor growth in patients with Johanson-Blizzard syndrome, otherwise characterized by facial abnormalities and hearing loss, is progressive EPI.

Congenital and Inherited Anomalies

Congenital anomalies of the pancreas arise in utero, as the pancreas forms from fusion of dorsal and ventral buds from the embryonic foregut. The ventral process rotates at about the eighth week of gestation and settles posteroinferiorly to the dorsal portion of the pancreas. Failure of the portions to fuse results in pancreas divisum, the most common pancreatic anomaly. Annular pancreas occurs when the ventral bud fails to rotate with the duodenum and instead surrounds it (Fig. 61.4).

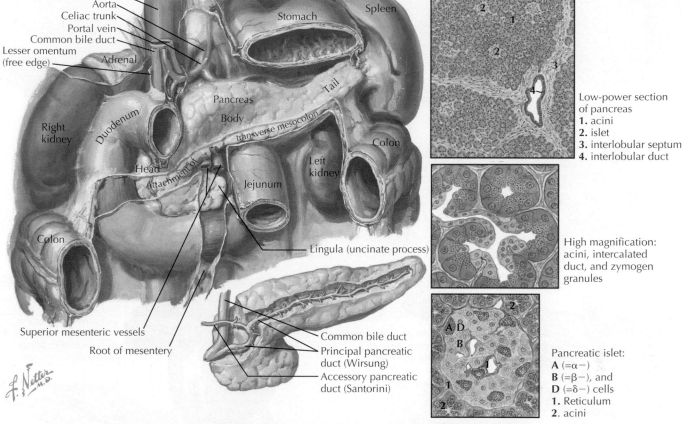

Fig. 61.1 Anatomy and Histology of the Pancreas.

TABLE 61.1 Pediatric Pancreatitis Definitions

Clinical Entity	Diagnostic Criteria
Acute pancreatitis	Requires ≥2 of the following criteria: 1. Abdominal pain consistent with acute pancreatitis 2. Elevation of serum lipase and/or amylase ≥3 times the reference limit of normal 3. Imaging findings commonly seen in acute pancreatitis
Acute recurrent pancreatitis	Requires ≥2 distinct episodes of acute pancreatitis with intervening return to baseline by symptoms or laboratory data
Chronic pancreatitis	Requires ≥1 of the following criteria: 1. Persistent abdominal pain typical of pancreatitis *with* imaging findings suggestive of chronic pancreatic damage 2. Evidence of exocrine pancreatic insufficiency and suggestive imaging 3. Evidence of endocrine pancreatic insufficiency and suggestive imaging

CLINICAL PRESENTATION

Pancreatitis

Acute pancreatitis in children most commonly presents with nausea, vomiting, and epigastric abdominal pain that may radiate to the back. Additional symptoms may include anorexia, fever, tachycardia, and hypotension, as well as symptoms related to the underlying cause, such as jaundice in the case of biliary obstruction. Physical examination findings include abdominal tenderness, rebound, or guarding, as well as hypoactive bowel sounds. Patients with a pseudocyst may present with abdominal distension and a tender, palpable epigastric mass. Acute hemorrhagic pancreatitis is a rare entity in children and is life-threatening. These patients may present in shock and have physical examination findings that include a bluish discoloration of the flank (Grey-Turner sign) or periumbilical area (Cullen sign). The differential diagnosis of pancreatitis includes disorders of the stomach, intestines, gallbladder, kidneys, lungs, and liver (Box 61.1).

Exocrine Pancreatic Insufficiency

The most striking symptoms of EPI are related to fat malabsorption as a result of decreased lipase activity and include steatorrhea, diarrhea, and abdominal pain. Over time, chronic malabsorption leads to malnutrition with poor growth, as well as symptoms of fat-soluble vitamin deficiencies.

In children with CF, the prevalence of EPI increases with age, with only about 60% of neonates affected as compared with 80% to 90% of older children as the pancreas is progressively destroyed.

Congenital and Inherited Anomalies

Congenital anomalies of the pancreas are often asymptomatic and are typically found incidentally on imaging or at autopsy. Pancreas divisum is the most common pancreatic congenital anomaly, present in up to 10% of the population. There is an association between divisum and pancreatitis, although the mechanism is unclear. It should be on the differential diagnosis list for patients with recurrent pancreatitis. Annular pancreas is the second most common congenital anomaly of the pancreas and can cause duodenal obstruction in some patients.

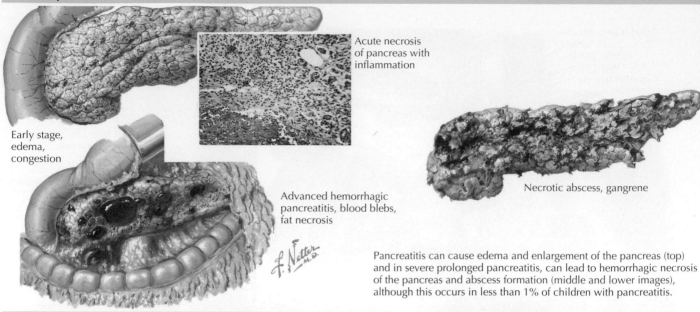

Acute necrosis
of pancreas with
inflammation

Early stage,
edema,
congestion

Advanced hemorrhagic
pancreatitis, blood blebs,
fat necrosis

Necrotic abscess, gangrene

Pancreatitis can cause edema and enlargement of the pancreas (top)
and in severe prolonged pancreatitis, can lead to hemorrhagic necrosis
of the pancreas and abscess formation (middle and lower images),
although this occurs in less than 1% of children with pancreatitis.

Chronic pancreatitis

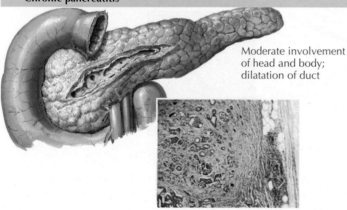

Moderate involvement
of head and body;
dilatation of duct

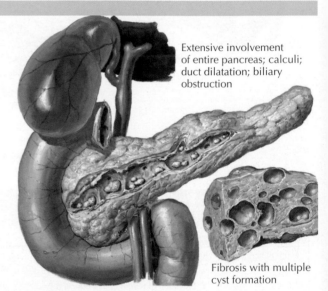

Extensive involvement
of entire pancreas; calculi;
duct dilatation; biliary
obstruction

Chronic pancreatitis can lead to calculi formation and fibrosis.

Fibrosis with multiple
cyst formation

Fig. 61.2 Pancreatitis.

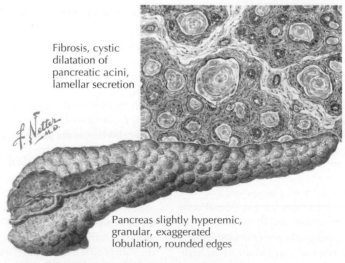

Fibrosis, cystic
dilatation of
pancreatic acini,
lamellar secretion

Pancreas slightly hyperemic,
granular, exaggerated
lobulation, rounded edges

In cystic fibrosis, sodium and chloride transport is impeded, leading to obstruction of the pancreatic
ducts with viscous exocrine fluid. This results in cystic dilatation and pancreatic fibrosis.

Fig. 61.3 Pancreatic Disease in Cystic Fibrosis.

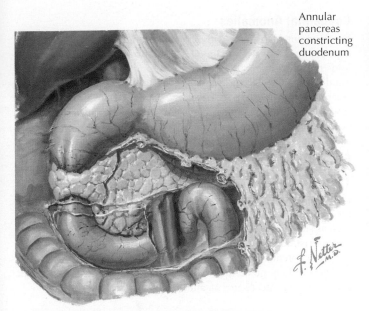

Annular pancreas constricting duodenum

Annular pancreas occurs when the ventral bud fails to rotate with the duodenum and instead surrounds it. This may result in duodenal obstruction.

Fig. 61.4 Annular Pancreas.

BOX 61.1 Differential Diagnosis of Pancreatitis

- Peptic ulcer disease
- Gastroenteritis
- Acute cholecystitis
- Biliary colic
- Small bowel obstruction
- Early appendicitis
- Renal colic
- Basilar pneumonia

TABLE 61.2 Causes of Elevated Amylase and Lipase Levels

Amylase	Pancreatitis and resulting complications
	Pancreatic ductal obstruction
	Intestinal disease (perforation, obstruction)
	Peritonitis
	Celiac disease
	Severe gastroenteritis
	Biliary tract disease (choledocholithiasis and cholecystitis)
	Macroamylasemia
	Decreased amylase clearance (renal, liver disease or failure)
	Pancreatic trauma (blunt trauma, abdominal surgery, ERCP)
	Malignancies
	AIDS
	Drugs
	Female reproductive tract disease and pregnancy
	Acidosis
	Parotitis
	Cystic fibrosis
	Pneumonia
	Burns
	Anorexia nervosa and bulimia
	Abdominal aortic aneurysm
Lipase	Pancreatitis
	Pancreatic duct obstruction or calculus
	Intestinal disease (perforation, obstruction)
	Duodenal ulcer or perforated peptic ulcer
	Celiac disease
	Gastroenteritis
	Acute cholecystitis
	Macrolipasemia
	Renal disease
	Pancreatic trauma (blunt trauma, abdominal surgery, ERCP)
	Pancreatic malignancies
	AIDS
	Drugs
	Diabetic ketoacidosis

AIDS, Acquired immunodeficiency syndrome; *ERCP,* endoscopic retrograde cholangiopancreatography.

This obstruction can present with a range of symptoms depending on the degree of obstruction; the range includes feeding difficulty, vomiting, and abdominal distension in a newborn with severe obstruction to postprandial fullness, nausea, and weight loss in an older child with a lower grade obstruction.

EVALUATION AND MANAGEMENT

Pancreatitis

A thorough history is important to distinguish pancreatitis from other causes of acute abdominal pain. It is important to determine the onset and the character of the pain, as well as any other associated symptoms. A complete list of current medications should be obtained because many medications may cause pancreatitis. The primary laboratory evaluation should include serum amylase and lipase, as well as a complete metabolic panel to evaluate for renal injury, hepatitis, and other metabolic consequences. Other causes of elevated lipase and amylase should be considered (Table 61.2). Recurrent episodes of pancreatitis should prompt further laboratory evaluation, such as serum triglyceride levels, immunoglobulin G subtypes (for autoimmune causes), and genetic testing for hereditary causes including *SPINK1, CFTR, PRSS1,*

and *CTRC.* An ultrasound may reveal an enlarged pancreas with altered echogenicity because of edema. Sonography can also provide clues to the cause, such as gallstones, dilated bile ducts, biliary sludge, choledochal cysts, abnormal pancreatic ducts, or long-term complications of pancreatitis like pseudocysts or fibrosis. Magnetic resonance cholangiopancreatography (MRCP) can be helpful in further identifying ductal abnormalities.

Treatment of children with pancreatitis is generally supportive and includes aggressive hydration, pain control, and appropriate nutrition. Current consensus suggests against use of antibiotic therapy in the absence of documented infection or pancreatic necrosis. Physicians should remain vigilant for signs of severe complications such as shock, peritonitis, or hypocalcemia. Trending serial amylase and lipase values is of no prognostic value, and treatment decisions should be based primarily on the patient's clinical status and symptoms. Relative to the prior standard of care, early introduction of oral or enteral feeds (within 48 hours of admission) is not only tolerated well, but associated with better outcomes. In patients who cannot tolerate oral intake for more than 48 hours, nasogastric or nasojejunal feeding should be used to safely provide nutrition as an alternative to parenteral nutrition. There is no role for dietary fat restriction to prevent future attacks of pancreatitis. Patients who develop a pseudocyst may require drainage if it is associated with clinical symptoms and does not resolve spontaneously. Cholecystectomy is indicated in patients with gallstone pancreatitis or biliary sludge. Endoscopic retrograde cholangiopancreatography (ERCP) may be required if there is evidence of acute biliary or pancreatic duct obstruction or in cases of recurrent pancreatitis in which there is concern for a ductal or structural abnormality. Pancreatic necrosis occurs in fewer than 1% of children with pancreatitis and may require debridement or necrosectomy in patients with persistent fevers or other associated symptoms. For patients with chronic pancreatitis, surgical interventions may reduce pain and cancer risk.

Exocrine Pancreatic Insufficiency

The gold standard for diagnosis of EPI is the coefficient of fat absorption, in which dietary fat intake is compared to fecal fat over a 72-hour period. A simpler test, the fecal elastase test, measures a protease resistant to degradation in the gastrointestinal tract from a single formed stool sample; values lower than 200 µg/g stool suggest EPI. The treatment of EPI is pancreatic enzyme replacement therapy. Additional fat-soluble vitamin provision is often necessary, particularly in patients with CF. Response to therapy is monitored by anthropometrics and serum vitamin concentrations.

Congenital Anomalies

Management of patients with congenital anomalies of the pancreas depends on the degree of clinical significance. If an annular pancreas leads to a duodenal obstruction, it can be surgically repaired with a duodeno-duodenostomy bypassing the annulus. In patients with pancreas divisum who have recurrent episodes of pancreatitis and a narrowing of the minor papilla, surgical or endoscopic intervention may be an option.

FUTURE DIRECTIONS

There are no current therapies to arrest the cascade of pancreatic autodigestion seen in pancreatitis, and surgeries present radical therapies for patients with recurrent or chronic pancreatitis. Genetic studies such as genome-wide association studies may continue to reveal causative or risk-modifying alleles for congenital and other pancreatic diseases and potential therapeutic targets. There is a need for higher-level evidence to help guide the evaluation and management of pediatric patients with acute, recurrent, and chronic pancreatitis.

SUGGESTED READINGS

Available online.

62

Hepatobiliary Disease

Kanak Verma and Amit A. Shah

 CLINICAL VIGNETTE

A 1-month-old female infant presents to her primary care physician with persistent jaundice. She was born at full term with no complications after birth. Her parents first noticed "eye yellowing" 2 weeks ago, which progressed to yellowing of her skin. She was initially diagnosed with physiologic jaundice but was brought back by parents after she developed pale stools and dark urine. On examination, she is awake and alert, with scleral icterus, facial and truncal jaundice, and an enlarged, nontender liver. Laboratory evaluation demonstrates total bilirubin 14.3 mg/dL, direct bilirubin 13.0 mg/dL, and mildly elevated serum aminotransferase levels. Liver biopsy reveals portal tract fibrosis, bile duct proliferation, and bile plugs consistent with obstructive cholestasis. She is immediately referred for laparotomy with intraoperative cholangiogram to evaluate for biliary atresia (BA) and subsequent hepatoportoenterostomy as treatment if diagnosed with BA.

Cholestatic jaundice in infancy indicates hepatobiliary dysfunction and requires early identification and timely referral for evaluation and management.

An estimated 15,000 children are hospitalized for liver disease in the United States annually, with important age-related differences in cause and frequency. Compared to adult liver disease, pediatric hepatobiliary disease is relatively rare, but accounts for significant morbidity and mortality as a result of progression to end-stage liver disease. Successful identification, treatment, and prevention of pediatric liver disease has significant implications for the health and quality of life of children.

NORMAL ANATOMY AND PHYSIOLOGY

The liver arises from endoderm between the third and fourth weeks of gestation and plays an important role in bile production and excretion, synthesis of coagulation factors, glucose and protein metabolism, and biotransformation of food, drugs, and toxins. It consists of four lobes: right, left, caudate, and quadrate (Fig. 62.1). The liver receives a dual blood supply from the portal vein and the hepatic artery. The portal vein, supplied by the splenic vein and mesenteric veins, delivers approximately 75% of the liver's blood supply, and the hepatic artery originates from the celiac axis and delivers oxygenated blood to supply the remaining 25%. Blood exits the liver through the hepatic veins, which empty into the inferior vena cava (Fig. 62.2). Bile exits the liver by way of the intrahepatic bile ducts that lead to the right and left hepatic ducts, which merge to form the common hepatic duct. The common hepatic duct courses caudally to merge with the cystic duct from the gallbladder and form the common bile duct, which allows bile drainage into the duodenum.

ETIOLOGY AND PATHOGENESIS

The most common pediatric liver diseases reflect metabolic, anatomic, infectious, autoimmune, toxic, and oncologic causes. Metabolic liver diseases include Crigler-Najjar syndrome, galactosemia, tyrosinemia, hereditary fructose intolerance, urea cycle defects, bile acid synthetic disorders, and α-1-antitrypsin (AAT) deficiency. Anatomic liver diseases may be congenital (e.g., biliary atresia [BA], choledochal cysts, Alagille syndrome) or acquired (e.g., cholelithiasis, Budd-Chiari syndrome). Common infections include viral hepatitides, Epstein-Barr virus (EBV), and cytomegalovirus (CMV). Common autoimmune diseases are autoimmune hepatitis and primary sclerosing cholangitis. Toxins or medications that frequently cause liver injury include acetaminophen, ethanol, chemotherapeutic agents, and total parenteral nutrition (TPN). Pediatric hepatic tumors include hepatoblastoma and hepatocellular carcinoma. Systemic processes, such as hypothyroidism, panhypopituitarism, congestive heart failure, celiac disease, and obesity can also affect the liver.

Each disease process causes alterations in liver structure or function, manifesting as unique patterns of cell injury. Elevations of aspartate aminotransferase (AST) and alanine aminotransferase (ALT) arise from hepatocyte inflammation and injury. Elevations of γ-glutamyl transpeptidase (GGT) and alkaline phosphatase (ALP) result from impaired bile flow. Elevated unconjugated or conjugated bilirubin results in jaundice. Unconjugated hyperbilirubinemia occurs in about 60% of full-term infants and is most commonly physiologic jaundice secondary to immature hepatic bilirubin conjugation. Unconjugated hyperbilirubinemia may also arise from increased bilirubin production (as seen in hemolysis) or defects in bilirubin conjugation. Conjugated hyperbilirubinemia arises from decreased bilirubin excretion by damaged hepatocytes or from biliary tract disease and is always considered pathologic (see later).

CLINICAL PRESENTATION

Hepatobiliary diseases can present as acute fulminant liver failure or with an insidious onset. A thorough history, with close attention to the timing of symptom onset, can be helpful in narrowing the differential diagnosis. For example, both breastfeeding jaundice and breast milk jaundice present with unconjugated hyperbilirubinemia; however, breastfeeding jaundice occurs in the first week of life, whereas breast milk jaundice develops after the seventh day of life.

Dark urine, acholic (light-colored) stools, easy bruising, epistaxis, pruritus, fractures, and palmar erythema can occur in patients with liver disease. Portal hypertension may manifest with hematemesis from esophageal or gastric variceal hemorrhage. Hepatic encephalopathy may manifest as deteriorating school performance, depression, or sleep disturbances. The medical provider should ask about medications or possible ingestions by the mother (for a breastfed infant) or child. Additional important historical information includes travel and infectious exposures. Family history of hepatitis B, C, or other liver diseases may raise concern for familial transmission.

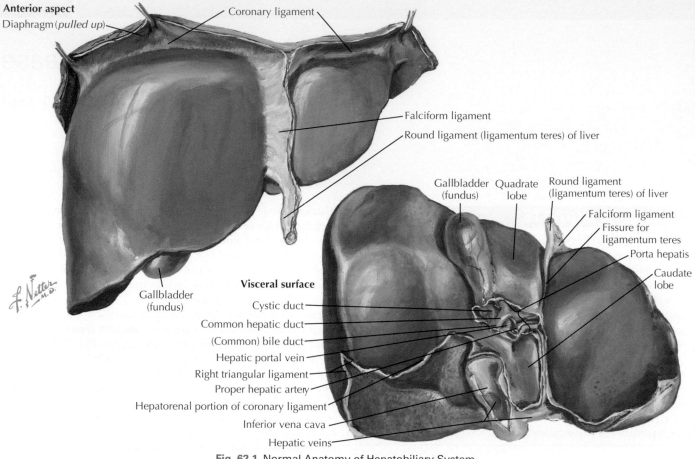

Fig. 62.1 Normal Anatomy of Hepatobiliary System.

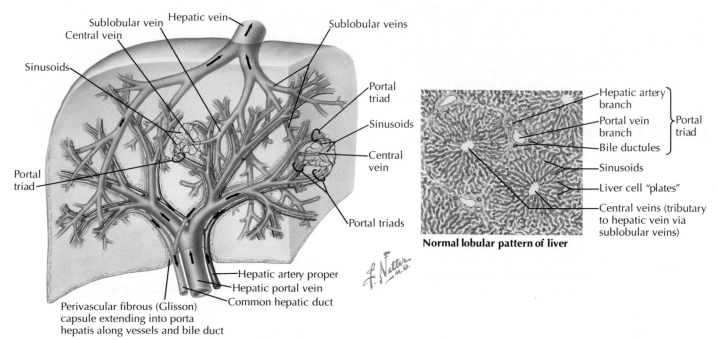

Fig. 62.2 Intrahepatic Structure and Blood Supply.

All patients should undergo a comprehensive physical examination. Scleral icterus is a sign of hyperbilirubinemia (conjugated or unconjugated). Yellow discoloration of skin and mucous membranes may also be present but can be difficult to ascertain particularly in dark-skinned patients. Evaluation of the skin may also reveal bruises secondary to coagulopathy or petechiae secondary to thrombocytopenia from portal hypertension and hypersplenism. Heart murmurs may be present secondary to persistent pulmonic stenosis, which is seen in Alagille disease. The lung examination may reveal signs of pleural effusions in patients with significant ascites.

Abdominal inspection may reveal distension secondary to ascites, hepatosplenomegaly, or prominent superficial abdominal veins (caput medusae) in a patient with portal hypertension. Hepatomegaly can be present; however, liver volume may decrease with progression to cirrhosis. Right upper quadrant tenderness can be seen with cholecystitis, choledocholithiasis, or acute hepatitis.

Differential Diagnosis

The differential diagnosis is vast and can be divided by age (Table 62.1).

Neonates and Infants

Inborn errors of metabolism generally present in the neonatal period, as do congenital TORCH (*Toxoplasma gondii*, **o**ther infections, **r**ubella, **C**MV, and **h**erpes simplex virus) infections. Gestational alloimmune liver disease (GALD), a complement-mediated process in which maternal immunoglobulin G (IgG) antibodies target fetal liver tissue, typically presents in the first days of life with acute liver failure. Patients with Alagille syndrome, characterized by paucity of interlobular bile ducts, can present with neonatal cholestasis, as well as additional ocular, cardiovascular, renal, and vertebral abnormalities. Cystic fibrosis (CF), tyrosinemia, and galactosemia, which are all part of the newborn screen, may cause neonatal jaundice. Urinary tract infections (UTIs) can cause cholestasis with conjugated hyperbilirubinemia. Hereditary fructose intolerance can present in infants after introduction of fruit juices, sucrose, or sorbitol.

Biliary atresia (BA) should be considered in infants with new or persistent jaundice beyond 2 weeks of life. BA is a progressive, fibroinflammatory process involving the biliary tree, which leads to obstruction of bile flow (Fig. 62.3). At presentation, most infants are well-appearing despite being jaundiced. Early diagnosis and treatment of BA is imperative to a good outcome. BA is treated surgically with hepatoportoenterostomy (see Fig. 62.3), a procedure whose success rate is greater in high-volume centers with experienced surgeons. Despite intervention, BA remains the most common indication for pediatric liver transplantation. To facilitate early detection, the evaluation of jaundiced infants beyond the first few days of life should always include a fractionated bilirubin level. Any infant with a conjugated bilirubin greater than 1.0 mg/dL requires further evaluation (Fig. 62.4).

Older Children and Adolescents

Infectious causes are the most common reason for liver disease beyond infancy, including hepatotropic viruses (hepatitis A through E), systemic viral infections (e.g., adenovirus, CMV, EBV), and nonviral infections (e.g., abscesses, bacterial sepsis, and Fitz-Hugh-Curtis syndrome). Autoimmune hepatitis can manifest with only laboratory changes suggesting liver dysfunction, signs of chronic hepatitis, or acute fulminant hepatic failure. Cholecystitis and choledocholithiasis should be considered in a child with acute right upper quadrant pain. Patients with chronic hemolytic diseases (including sickle cell disease, hereditary spherocytosis, thalassemia) are at increased risk for cholelithiasis. With rising childhood obesity rates, the prevalence of pediatric nonalcoholic fatty liver disease (NAFLD) has increased over the last two decades. These patients are typically asymptomatic at presentation with mildly elevated serum transaminase levels, but disease can progress over time to cirrhosis.

Use of various prescription medications (isoniazid, valproate, other antiepileptics) and recreational drugs can lead to acute liver failure. Intentional or unintentional overdose of acetaminophen is a common cause of liver failure in older children and adolescents.

AAT deficiency and Wilson disease should be included in the differential diagnosis of acute or chronic hepatitis in children and

TABLE 62.1 Differential Diagnosis of Hepatobiliary Disease in Children[a]

All Ages	Patients (%)
Viral infection: EBV; CMV; hepatitis A–E; herpes simplex virus, echovirus, enterovirus, rubella, parvovirus, adenovirus, toxoplasmosis, syphilis, HIV, varicella	12.0
Bacterial infection: sepsis, UTI, tuberculosis, *Listeria*, *Treponema pallidum*	
Extrahepatic obstruction (choledochal cyst, bile duct stricture or tumor, cholelithiasis)	
Drugs (valproate, isoniazid, acetaminophen)	
Parenteral nutrition	
CF	
Congestive heart failure	
Ischemia secondary to congenital heart disease, asphyxia, cardiac surgery, ECMO	
Metabolic: AAT deficiency, fatty acid oxidation defect, urea cycle disorders	16.3
Intrahepatic cholestasis: PFIC; Alagille syndrome	12.4
Idiopathic	
Neonates and Infants	
Biliary atresia	33.1
Endocrine (hypothyroidism, panhypopituitarism)	
Metabolic (galactosemia, glycogen storage disease, hereditary fructose intolerance, tyrosinemia, urea cycle defects)	
Disorders of lipid metabolism (Wolman disease, Niemann-Pick disease, Gaucher disease)	
Bile acid synthesis defects	
Idiopathic neonatal hepatitis	
Mitochondrial disorders	
Neonatal lupus erythematosus	
GALD	
Congenital hepatic fibrosis and autosomal recessive polycystic kidney disease	
Peroxisomal disorders (Zellweger syndrome)	
Children and Adolescents	
Malignancy	7.3
Acetaminophen overdose	
NAFLD	
Autoimmune hepatitis	
Primary sclerosing cholangitis (≈68% have IBD)	
Wilson disease	
Fatty liver disease of pregnancy/HELLP syndrome/intrahepatic cholestasis of pregnancy	

[a]Percentages of total cases of liver transplant recipients (UNOS 2016–2018) identified as having the listed diagnosis are shown.

AAT, α-1 Antitrypsin; *CF*, cystic fibrosis; *CMV*, cytomegalovirus; *EBV*, Epstein-Barr virus; *ECMO*, extracorporeal membrane oxygenation; *GALD*, gestational alloimmune liver disease; *HELLP*, hemolysis, elevated liver enzymes, and low platelet count; *IBD*, inflammatory bowel disease; *NAFLD*, nonalcoholic fatty liver disease; *PFIC*, progressive familial intrahepatic cholestasis; *UTI*, urinary tract infection.

Biliary atresia   Hepatoportoenterostomy

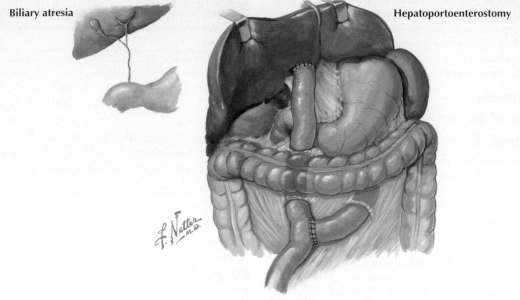

Fig. 62.3 Biliary Atresia.

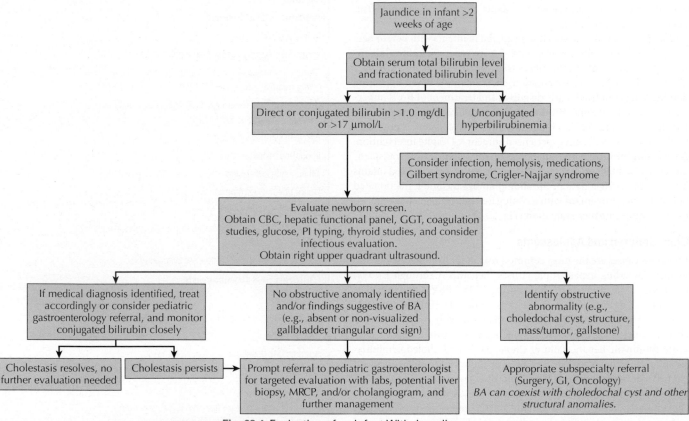

Fig. 62.4 Evaluation of an Infant With Jaundice.

adolescents. AAT deficiency can present at any age with variable presentation, including neonatal cholestasis, asymptomatic hepatomegaly, or advanced liver disease. Wilson disease results in impaired biliary copper excretion, with progressive accumulation of copper in the liver. As hepatocytes becomes overloaded, copper is redistributed to other tissues, causing toxicity to the brain, kidneys, corneas, and other organs. The presentation of Wilson disease is also variable; patients may first seek medical attention for neuropsychiatric symptoms,

including fatigue, worsening school performance, behavioral symptoms, or declining motor coordination.

EVALUATION

Laboratory evaluation can be used to screen for liver abnormalities, determine the nature of these abnormalities (hepatocellular versus cholestatic injury), and assess their impact on liver synthetic function

TABLE 62.2 Laboratory Evaluation of Hepatobiliary Disease

Test	Significance
AST, ALT, LDH	Elevated from hepatocyte injury
GGT, ALP	Elevated from impaired bile flow
Fractionated bilirubin	Conjugated bilirubin elevated in cholestasis
Complete metabolic panel	Albumin low with compromised liver synthetic function
PT time	PT prolonged with abnormal synthetic function, vitamin K deficiency
CBC	Thrombocytopenia, leukopenia with hypersplenism
Ammonia	Elevated in advanced liver disease and some metabolic disorders
Sweat test	Most state newborn screens include most common CF mutations only; therefore, sweat test should be obtained if CF suspected
Serum AAT level, PI type	PI type is needed to make the definitive diagnosis
Serum ceruloplasmin	Serum level is low in Wilson's disease

AAT, α-1 Antitrypsin; *ALP,* aspartate aminotransferase; *ALT,* alanine aminotransferase; *AST,* aspartate aminotransferase; *CBC,* complete cell count; *CF,* cystic fibrosis; *GGT,* γ-glutamyl transpeptidase; *LDH,* lactate dehydrogenase; *PI,* protease inhibitor; *PT,* prothrombin time.

TABLE 62.3 Examples of Specific Therapies for Liver Diseases

Disease	Therapy
Chronic hepatitis B	Nucleoside analogues (entecavir, tenofovir); IFN-α
Chronic hepatitis C	Dependent on age and HCV genotype; ledipasvir/sofosbuvir, glecaprevir/pibrentasvir, or sofosbuvir with ribavirin
Galactosemia	Elimination of dietary galactose
Acetaminophen overdose	*N*-Acetylcysteine
Wilson disease	Copper chelating agents, zinc salts, low-copper diet
Autoimmune hepatitis	Corticosteroids, azathioprine
Nonalcoholic fatty liver disease	Weight loss, physical activity
Bile acid synthesis disorders, peroxisomal disorders	Cholic acid
GALD	IVIG and double-volume exchange transfusion

GALD, Gestational alloimmune liver disease; *HCV,* hepatitis C; *IFN,* interferon.

(Table 62.2). AST and ALT levels are typically elevated in liver disease, although they may decrease in hepatic failure because of significant hepatocyte loss. High alkaline phosphatase and GGT levels suggest biliary tract inflammation or obstruction, with the rare exception of some types of bile acid synthetic disorders or progressive familial intrahepatic cholestasis. The total serum bilirubin level can quantify degree of jaundice. Prolonged international normalized ratio or prothrombin time reflect compromised liver synthetic function.

Abdominal ultrasonography can provide information regarding liver size, structure, and hepatic blood flow. Ultrasound can also identify anatomic abnormalities, such as choledochal cysts, choledocholithiasis, tumors, or vascular anomalies. Small or absent gallbladder may be noted in diseases involving the biliary system, such as BA and Alagille syndrome.

Neonates and Infants

The evaluation of neonates with conjugated hyperbilirubinemia should focus on exclusion of disorders requiring immediate treatment (see Fig. 62.4). The newborn screen should be reviewed to exclude thyroid abnormalities, galactosemia, CF, and rare metabolic disorders. A catheterized urine culture should be obtained to assess for UTI. Additional urine tests should also be obtained, including urine succinylacetone (present in tyrosinemia), urine organic acids (abnormal in organic acidemias, peroxisomal diseases), and urine bile acids (assess for bile acid synthetic defects). Plasma amino acids, acylcarnitine profile, and lactate/pyruvate ratio can be sent as a screen for metabolic or mitochondrial disorders. A sweat test should also be obtained if CF was not part of the patient's newborn screen.

If BA is suspected, the infant should be promptly referred to a pediatric gastroenterologist. The diagnostic approach varies by institution and may include ultrasound and liver biopsy. If the evaluation supports a diagnosis of BA, the patient should undergo an intraoperative or percutaneous cholangiogram, the gold standard for the diagnosis of BA.

Children and Adolescents

All patients in this age group should be tested for viral hepatitis (EBV, CMV, enterovirus, adenovirus, and hepatitides A, B, and C). Testing should also include an autoimmune hepatitis panel to assess for autoantibodies to constituents of the nucleus, liver-kidney-microsome antigens, and smooth muscle. Acetaminophen level should be sent in acute liver failure. Low serum AAT level is suggestive of AAT deficiency, but protease inhibitor (PI) typing is necessary to make a definitive diagnosis. Low ceruloplasmin is suggestive of Wilson disease and should be followed with a 24-hour urine collection to measure copper excretion. Ultrasound is the best initial imaging for cholelithiasis. Magnetic resonance cholangiopancreatography can be used to assess for primary sclerosing cholangitis. Children with persistent cholestasis or hepatitis and an otherwise nondiagnostic evaluation should undergo liver biopsy, which can identify the cause and assess disease severity based on the degree of fibrosis present.

MANAGEMENT

Many liver diseases are managed supportively. Patients with acute liver failure should be admitted to an intensive care unit for monitoring of fluids, glucose, electrolytes, coagulopathy, and encephalopathy (Table 62.3). *N*-Acetylcysteine improves survival in acetaminophen-induced liver injury. Endoscopic retrograde cholangiopancreatography can be therapeutic in choledocholithiasis; these patients should undergo eventual cholecystectomy.

Complications of chronic liver disease include coagulopathy, ascites, and portal hypertension. Significant GI bleeding due to hemorrhage from esophageal, gastric, duodenal, or rectal varices can occur. Once hemodynamically stable, these patients typically require endoscopic intervention, such as sclerotherapy or banding. Diuretics can be used for the management of ascites. Abdominal paracentesis may be both diagnostic (for suspected spontaneous bacterial peritonitis) and therapeutic. β-Blockers and portosystemic shunts are sometimes used in children with portal hypertension.

For cholestasis, the most common choleretic agent is ursodeoxycholic acid. Some patients develop pruritus secondary to the accumulation of bile salts and may benefit from rifampin, naltrexone, sertraline, or surgical biliary diversion. Increased metabolic demands and fat malabsorption secondary to cholestasis can lead to fat-soluble vitamin deficiencies, hepatic osteodystrophy, and generalized malnutrition in patients with liver disease. Growth and nutritional status should be monitored and fat-soluble vitamins should be supplemented as needed.

Liver transplantation can provide definitive therapy for children with end-stage liver disease. The liver is the most commonly transplanted solid organ in children, with more than half of children listed for transplant age 5 years or younger. See Table 62.1 for data from the United Network for Organ Sharing to see the most common diagnoses among pediatric liver transplant recipients.

FUTURE DIRECTIONS

Ongoing research offers promising advances for the management of pediatric liver disease. The growing incidence of NAFLD has led to an increased focus on delineating its natural history, developing non-invasive methods to assess steatosis, and identifying pharmacologic interventions. With the success of direct-acting antiviral HCV therapy, continued evaluation of pediatric pharmacokinetics, safety, and efficacy is needed to facilitate HCV eradication. With advances in genetic testing and precision medicine, gene therapy for Wilson disease and AAT deficiency also provides a promising frontier. For patients requiring liver transplantation, efforts to optimize and eventually minimize immunosuppression, develop biomarkers for rejection, and explore alternatives such as human hepatocyte transplantation may improve long-term outcomes.

SUGGESTED READINGS

Available online.

63

Infections in the Gastrointestinal Tract

Alexandra R. Linn and Arthur J. Kastl, Jr.

 CLINICAL VIGNETTE

A 10-year-old boy presented to an emergency department (ED) with 3 days of nausea, vomiting, and watery diarrhea. He complained of generalized abdominal pain and poor oral intake. He denied recent health care exposures or antibiotic use. He had no sick contacts, but his mother received a phone call earlier that day from his school that a diarrheal illness was affecting several classmates. His vital signs were notable for a fever to 100.76° F (38.2° C) without other abnormalities. On physical examination he appeared tired and had dry mucous membranes. His abdomen was mildly tender to palpation. He had another episode of large volume watery diarrhea, and his stool was sent for testing, including bacterial stool culture, viral stool polymerase chain reaction (PCR), ova and parasite (O&P) analysis, and *Clostridioides difficile* toxin testing. Stool viral PCR returned positive for norovirus, and the patient was diagnosed with acute enterocolitis. He received intravenous fluids and ondansetron in the ED and passed an oral challenge of liquids before being discharged home. He recovered without complications.

Dehydration secondary to acute enterocolitis is a common cause of hospitalizations in the United States. Acute infectious enterocolitis can be caused by bacteria, viruses, or parasites and is typically classified as invasive (bloody) or noninvasive (nonbloody). Norovirus is the most common cause of viral diarrheal outbreaks and can be readily spread by surface fomites. Outbreaks are common in childcare centers, cruise ships, and nursing homes. The differential diagnosis for vomiting and diarrhea is broad and includes enterocolitis from other microbes, acute appendicitis, irritable bowel syndrome, inflammatory bowel disease, celiac disease, and many others. Treatment for norovirus is supportive with antiemetics and oral rehydration therapy and rarely results in complications.

Gastrointestinal (GI) infections cause significant morbidity and mortality in pediatric populations worldwide. This chapter discusses common infections of the digestive system, organized anatomically.

ESOPHAGUS

Infectious esophagitis is most frequently caused by fungi and viruses. The most common pathogen causing esophagitis in children is the fungal genus *Candida*. *Candida albicans* is the most common species, although *Candida glabrata* is an increasingly prevalent cause of fungal esophagitis. Herpes simplex virus (HSV) is the second most common cause of infectious esophagitis and should be considered in immunocompromised patients. Cytomegalovirus (CMV) is less common, but has been described in solid organ transplant recipients and patients with rheumatologic diseases. General risk factors for infectious esophagitis include recent antimicrobial use; chemotherapy/radiation; medical immunosuppression, including steroids; history of transplantation; and human immunodeficiency virus (HIV) or other immunodeficient states.

The clinical presentation of infectious esophagitis is variable but often involves odynophagia and/or dysphagia. Patients may also have substernal chest or epigastric pain resembling Gastroesophageal reflux disease (GERD), as well as cough, fever, vomiting, and diarrhea. *Candida* esophagitis can be asymptomatic and may be discovered incidentally during endoscopy. Whereas thrush (oropharyngeal candidiasis) can signal the possibility of esophageal involvement, a lack of oral involvement does not rule out *Candida* esophagitis. In HSV esophagitis, half of patients present with retrosternal pain and fever. Concomitant oral and genital lesions are reported in about 20% of cases. CMV esophagitis may be associated with hematemesis.

Definitive diagnosis is made by an upper endoscopy with tissue sampling, and the highest yield area for tissue sampling depends on the organism (Fig. 63.1). Typical endoscopic findings for *Candida* esophagitis include white exudate on plaque-like lesions. Biopsy samples taken from plaques in the mid-esophagus will show yeast and pseudohyphae on culture. Brushings for cytologic examinations are often performed in conjunction with biopsies, because it has higher sensitivity. HSV esophagitis shows characteristic well-circumscribed ulcers in the distal esophagus, where the virus infects the squamous epithelium. Biopsies are taken from the ulcer margin, where viral load is highest. In CMV esophagitis, endoscopy shows large distinct solitary ulcers in the distal esophagus, often linear with overlying white plaque. Biopsy samples are taken from the ulcer base and sent for anti-CMV antibody testing.

Treatment in the pediatric population is organism specific. *C. albicans* esophagitis is often treated with fluconazole, and treatment duration is typically at least 2 weeks. Herpes simplex virus (HSV) and cytomegalovirus (CMV) may be self-limiting in immunocompetent patients, but treated with antiviral therapy (acyclovir and ganciclovir, respectively) in immunocompromised populations. Dosing and duration of the antimicrobial depends on the patient's age, clinical status, and response time. All infectious presentations benefit from decreasing the amount of immunosuppressive therapy, if applicable and possible.

STOMACH

Inflammation of the stomach is termed gastritis, which can be due to several infectious causes. Although the acidic environment of the stomach is hostile to many types of organisms, *H. pylori* is a notable exception, which is specifically highlighted because of its community prevalence.

H. pylori is the most common cause of infectious gastritis, accounting for 80% of gastric ulcers and nearly all duodenal ulcers (Fig. 63.2). *H. pylori* is a urease-producing spirochete that survives the acidic environment of the stomach by producing an ammonia coat. The organism can cause infection in some, but acts commensal in others, and

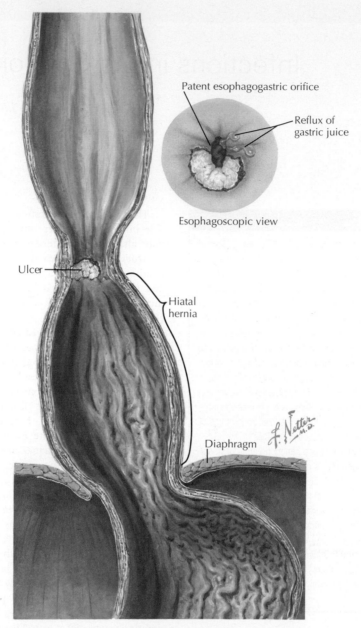

Patent esophagogastric orifice

Reflux of gastric juice

Esophagoscopic view

Ulcer

Hiatal hernia

Diaphragm

Fig. 63.1 Esophagitis.

the reasons for this variation remain unclear. The organism can be acquired at any point in life and may be challenging to eradicate. Other pathogens that can cause gastritis include CMV, *Histoplasma capsulatum, Mycobacteria, Giardia, Mucor,* and *Strongyloides,* but these are all far rarer than *H. pylori.*

The gold standard test for *H. pylori* is endoscopy with tissue sampling, where surface organisms can be seen microscopically. Additional biopsy specimens for rapid urease testing and culture/sensitivities are only recommended if gastritis is confirmed and treatment likely to be offered. It is important to wait at least 2 weeks after stopping a proton pump inhibitor (PPI), or 4 weeks after stopping an antibiotic, before testing for *H. pylori.* A stool antigen test is also available, but its use is limited to select scenarios after endoscopically proven infection is established.

Treatment is recommended for symptomatic patients who have positive test results. It is not indicated for asymptomatic patients who test positive incidentally and who do not have gastritis. Treatment options include triple therapy with a combination of PPI and antibiotics, and quadruple therapy with the addition of bismuth subcitrate. See Table 63.1 for treatment details.

INTESTINE

Enterocolitis is inflammation of the small and/or large intestine causing symptoms of diarrhea, abdominal pain, and nausea. Diarrheal illnesses are responsible for one in nine pediatric deaths worldwide and are the second leading cause of death in children under 5 years. In the United States, it is estimated that diarrheal illnesses lead to approximately 200,000 hospitalizations annually and 300 to 400 deaths per year. Pathogens can be acquired by fecal-oral spread, from contact with fomites on surfaces, and from undercooked food. Additional risk factors for acquiring infectious enterocolitis include acid suppressive medications, recent travel or antibiotic use, and underlying immunosuppression.

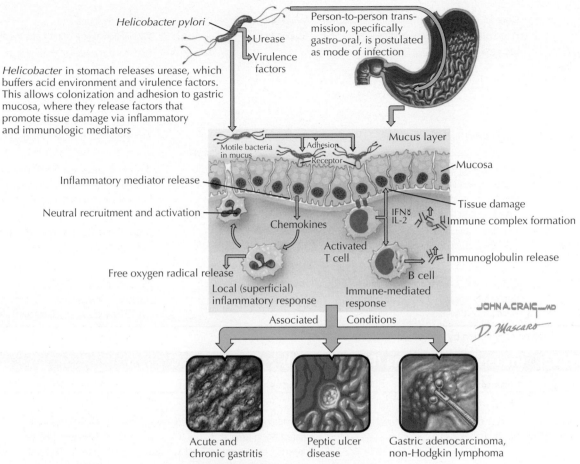

Helicobacter pylori

Person-to-person transmission, specifically gastro-oral, is postulated as mode of infection

Helicobacter in stomach releases urease, which buffers acid environment and virulence factors. This allows colonization and adhesion to gastric mucosa, where they release factors that promote tissue damage via inflammatory and immunologic mediators

Urease

Virulence factors

Motile bacteria in mucus

Adhesion

Receptor

Mucus layer

Mucosa

Inflammatory mediator release

Neutral recruitment and activation

Chemokines

Activated T cell

IFNδ
IL-2

Tissue damage

Immune complex formation

Free oxygen radical release

B cell

Immunoglobulin release

Local (superficial) inflammatory response

Immune-mediated response

JOHN A. CRAIG—MD

D. Mascaro

Associated   Conditions

Acute and chronic gastritis

Peptic ulcer disease

Gastric adenocarcinoma, non-Hodgkin lymphoma

Fig. 63.2 *Helicobacter pylori* Gastritis.

TABLE 63.1 Treatment for *Helicobacter pylori*

Triple Therapy			Quadruple Therapy
PPI[a]	PPI	PPI	PPI
Amoxicillin	Amoxicillin	Clarithromycin	Bismuth subcitrate[b]
Clarithromycin	Metronidazole	Metronidazole	Tetracycline
14 days	14 days	14 days	Metronidazole 10–14 days

[a]For specific dosing information, see Chey WD, Leontiadis GI, Howden CW, Moss SF. ACG clinical guideline: treatment of *Helicobacter pylori* infection. *Am J Gastroenterol.* 112(2):212-239, Table 3.
[b]Bismuth quadruple therapy should be considered for patients with previous macrolide exposure or who are allergic to penicillin.
PPI, Proton pump inhibitor.
Adapted from Chey WD, Leontiadis GI, Howden CW, Moss SF. ACG clinical guideline: treatment of *Helicobacter pylori* infection. *Am J Gastroenterol.* 112(2):212-239, Table 2; and Koletzko S, Jones NL, Goodman KJ, et al. *H. pylori* Working Groups of ESPGHAN and NASPGHAN. Evidence-based guidelines from ESPGHAN and NASPGHAN for *Helicobacter pylori* infection in children. *J Pediatr Gastroenterol Nutr.* 2011;53(2):230-243. doi: 10.1097/MPG.0b013e3182227e90. PMID: 21558964.

Enterocolitis can be caused by both invasive and noninvasive pathogens. Invasive pathogens cause direct and extensive mucosal damage, leading to bloody diarrhea. In contrast, noninvasive pathogens cause a secretory and nonbloody diarrhea. Of the various causes, viruses are the most common cause in children globally. The clinical presentation of these infections typically involves either watery or bloody diarrhea, vomiting, abdominal discomfort, and occasionally constitutional symptoms. The vast majority of infections are self-limited and require only supportive care. See Tables 63.2 and 63.3 for descriptions of various organisms.

Most cases of enterocolitis are self-limited and do not require diagnostic testing; however, it is appropriate to test for severe, bloody, or persistent diarrhea, if patients have constitutional symptoms and/or are immunocompromised. Although it is impossible and impractical to test for all organisms, there are numerous culture, PCR, enzyme-linked immunosorbent assay (ELISA), and other tests targeting common pathogens. For example, many stool culture panels capture frequently seen invasive bacterial species, and PCR panels can screen for a variety of viruses. Bacterial toxin testing is used to identify toxins A and B from *C. difficile*, as well as Shiga-type toxins. For *C. difficile* specifically, there is a high prevalence of asymptomatic carriage in infants and thus testing should not be pursued in children under 1 year of age. In children older than 2 years, testing for *C. difficile* is recommended in those with persistent diarrhea, known antibiotic exposures, or immunocompromising conditions. Stool testing is sufficient in these populations, but if pursued, colonoscopy may reveal characteristic yellow plaques diagnostic of pseudomembranous colitis (Fig. 63.3).

The mainstay of management for enterocolitis, regardless of cause, is supportive care with oral rehydration therapy (ORT) because electrolyte losses and dehydration are so prominent. ORT involves a rehydration phase followed by a maintenance phase. The World Health

TABLE 63.2 Noninvasive Organisms (Nonbloody Stool)

Pathogen	Clinical Presentation	Diagnosis and Treatment	Clinical Pearls
Viruses			
Rotavirus	Fever Potentially severe disease in infancy	Stool PCR Supportive care[a]	Fall to early spring Vaccination at age 2 and 4 months of age
Norovirus Human calicivirus	Most common viral cause		Outbreaks at childcare centers and cruise ships
Adenovirus			Concomitant upper respiratory infections, pharyngitis, conjunctivitis
Bacteria			
Enterotoxigenic *Escherichia coli* (ETEC)	Recent travel, undercooked meals	Stool culture Azithromycin, fluoroquinolone	Also known as "traveler's diarrhea"
Vibrio cholera	Spread via feces contaminated water and undercooked shellfish Often cause mild watery diarrhea but 1/10 can have profuse diarrhea, vomiting and cramping	Stool culture Supportive care[a]	If severe disease, death can occur within hours due to dehydration and electrolyte losses Vaccine exists but not routinely recommended
Staphylococcus aureus/ Bacillus cereus	Vomiting, cramping and diarrhea 4–6 hours after ingestion of contaminated food		Acute illness occurs as a result of ingestion of preformed bacterial enterotoxins
Parasite			
Giardia	Greasy stools, cramping and gas/flatulence Symptoms appear 1–3 weeks after exposure and last 2–6 weeks	Stool antigen Metronidazole	Can lead to chronic diarrhea Acquired in daycare centers; by backpackers/hikers; drinking fresh water; international travelers

[a]Supportive care involves rehydration by oral rehydration therapy.

TABLE 63.3 Invasive Organisms (Bloody Stool)

Pathogen	Clinical Presentation	Diagnosis and Treatment	Clinical Pearl
Bacteria			
Enterohemorrhagic *Escherichia coli* (EHEC) or (STEC)	Stomach cramping, vomiting, fever starting 3–4 days after exposure	Stool culture; may require MacConkey agar to detect Shiga toxin Supportive care; avoid antibiotics to avoid progression to HUS	Makes Shiga toxin Can lead to HUS (5%–10% of infections), TTP, Screen for diabetes mellitus
Shigella spp.	Causes shigellosis with fever, abdominal pain; starts 1–2 days after exposure and lasts 5–7 days	Stool culture Supportive care Severe disease, dysentery, or immunosuppressed: ceftriaxone, fluoroquinolone, or azithromycin	Acquired in child care settings May have seizures or encephalopathy
Salmonella typhi	Severe infection may manifest with constipation Typhoid fever Rose spots: rash on neck or torso, leukopenia, anemia, bacteremia, hepatosplenomegaly, altered mentation	Stool culture Supportive care Infants younger than 3 months, HIV, hemoglobinopathies, immunocompromised: ampicillin/amoxicillin, Bactrim (if not resistant); if resistant: ceftriaxone	Contaminated food, water pets, amphibians Reported MDR strains in Pakistan in 2019
Campylobacter jejuni	Cramping, fever; starts 2–5 days after exposure Abdominal pain can mimic appendicitis or intussusception	Stool culture Supportive care Severe disease: azithromycin, erythromycin, or fluoroquinolones	Undercooked food, especially poultry Complications include immunoreactive postinfectious acute idiopathic polyneuritis; Guillain-Barré syndrome
Clostridioides difficile	Profuse diarrhea, cramping and pain Shed in feces and spread via contact with contaminated surfaces	Stool toxin PCR assay; bacteria antigen, PCR or culture See suggested readings for treatment	Spore forming and toxin-mediated (A and B toxins) Recent antibiotic use (especially clindamycin, cephalosporins, fluoroquinolones), recent hospitalizations Complications include toxic megacolon and bowel perforation
Yersinia enterocolitica	Fever, abdominal pain, develops 4–7 days after exposure and can last 1–3 weeks	Stool culture Supportive care Sepsis, immunodeficiency: cefotaxime, Bactrim, fluoroquinolones, or aminoglycosides	Raw or undercooked pork Pseudoappendicitis syndrome
Parasite			
Entamoeba histolytica	Luminal amebiasis often asymptomatic; amebic colitis causes bloody diarrhea	Stool ova and parasite testing Asymptomatic—paromomycin or iodoquinol; symptomatic—metronidazole or tinidazole	Amebic liver abscess most common extraintestinal manifestation See Chapter 90 for more information

EHEC, Enterohemorrhagic *Escherichia coli; HIV,* human immunodeficiency virus; *HUS,* hemolytic-uremic syndrome; *MDR,* multidrug resistant; *PCR,* polymerase chain reaction; *STEC,* Shiga toxin–producing *Escherichia coli; TTP,* thrombotic thrombocytopenic purpura.

Organization's components for rehydration solution consist of a complex carbohydrate or 2% glucose and 50 to 90 mEq/L of sodium, which couple together for direct transport of electrolytes across the gut epithelium. Diet reintroduction is recommended once previous losses are corrected. A more detailed discussion about ORT can be found in the Suggested Readings section.

Certain pathogens also require specific treatment with antibiotics, as outlined in Table 63.4. *C. difficile* warrants extra attention, because treatment for *C. difficile* colitis is more complicated due to antibiotic resistance and reinfection rates. Metronidazole and vancomycin are considered first-line antibiotic treatments for *C. difficile*. Fidaxomicin has recently been approved in children and has shown effectiveness in treating *C. difficile* infection (CDI) in children. Fecal microbiota transplant (FMT) is reserved for recurrent or refractory cases.

APPENDIX

Inflammation of the vestigial appendix is known as appendicitis, which often is a localized bacterial infection. Appendicitis remains the most common indication for abdominal surgery in childhood and should be in the differential diagnosis for patients presenting with symptoms suggestive of infectious enterocolitis (Fig. 63.4). (See Chapter 4 for further information on appendicitis.)

PERITONITIS AND OCCULT ABSCESSES

Peritonitis and intraabdominal abscesses can manifest after acute appendicitis or enterocolitis and in patients with hepatic dysfunction. Peritonitis is the inflammation of the peritoneum, either from infectious or noninfectious causes. Primary peritonitis, also known as spontaneous bacterial peritonitis (SBP), denotes bacteria in the peritoneal fluid without a clear intraabdominal source. Hematogenous or lymphoid seeding of bacteria into ascites is often how SBP is initiated. Secondary peritonitis is more common and represents inflammation from a source such as a perforated viscera. Foreign materials in the abdomen, particularly chronic peritoneal dialysis catheters and ventriculoperitoneal (VP) shunts, are associated with secondary peritonitis. Microbial causes frequently include staphylococcal and streptococcal species, as well as gram-negative enteric bacilli.

Clinical presentation of peritonitis is variable. Fever, abdominal pain, distension, and lethargy are symptoms commonly associated with peritonitis. Patients with abscesses often present with fever and poorly localized abdominal pain. Patients may also be asymptomatic.

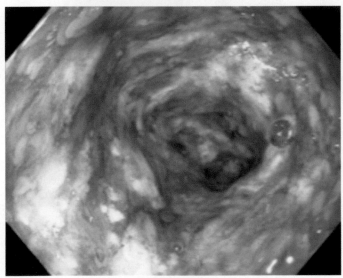

Pseudomembranous colitis

C. difficile colitis

Fig. 63.3 *Clostridioides difficile* **Pseudomembranous Colitis.** (Photograph reused with permission from Reynolds JR. *The Netter Collection of Medical Illustrations.* 2nd ed. Vol. 9, *Digestive System, Part II: Lower Digestive Tract.* Philadelphia, PA: Elsevier, 2016; Plate 3.69.)

TABLE 63.4 *Clostridioides difficile* Treatment in Children

Clinical Definition	Recommended Treatment	Pediatric Dose
Initial episode, nonsevere	Metronidazole[a] × 10 days (PO) or Vancomycin[b] × 10 days (PO)	7.5 mg/kg/dose TID 10 mg/kg/dose QID
Initial episode, severe	Vancomycin[b] × 10 days (PO)	10 mg/kg/dose QID
First recurrence, nonsevere	Metronidazole[a] × 10 days (PO) or Vancomycin[b] × 10 days (PO)	7.5 mg/kg/dose TID 10 mg/kg/dose QID
Second or subsequent recurrence	Tapered and pulsed regimen Vancomycin[b]; or vancomycin for 10 days followed by rifaximin for 20 days, or fecal microbiota transplantation	10 mg/kg/dose QID followed by prolonged taper over weeks; rifaximin—no pediatric dosing

[a]Metronidazole dosing is 7.5 mg/kg/dose (max 500 mg/dose).
[b]Vancomycin dosing is 10 mg/kg/dose (max 125 mg/dose).
Of note, the only regimen with strong/moderate evidence is for vancomycin in initial severe/fulminant infections; all others have weak/low evidence.
Adapted from McDonald LC, Gerding DN, Johnson S, et al. Clinical practice guidelines for *Clostridium difficile* infection in adults and children: 2017 update by the Infectious Diseases Society of America (IDSA) and Society for Healthcare Epidemiology of America (SHEA). *Clin Infect Dis.* 2018;66(7):e1-e481, Table 2. https://doi.org/10.1093/cid/cix1085.

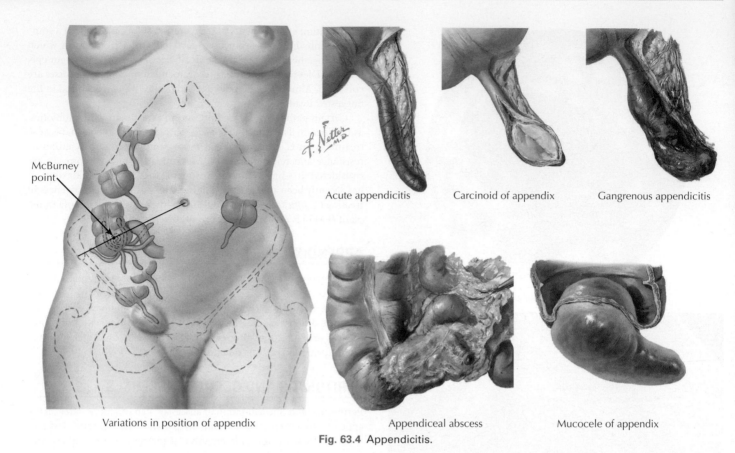

McBurney point

Variations in position of appendix

Acute appendicitis

Carcinoid of appendix

Gangrenous appendicitis

Appendiceal abscess

Mucocele of appendix

Fig. 63.4 Appendicitis.

Blood cultures and paracentesis studies can be helpful for both diagnostic and antimicrobial selection. Plain X-ray testing can reveal free peritoneal air from a ruptured viscus, and ultrasound can aid in visualizing free fluid and also guide paracentesis if applicable for diagnosis. Treatment typically consists of antibiotic therapy tailored to the organisms' sensitivities, and, if refractory, interventional radiology/surgical drainage may be needed for source control.

SUGGESTED READINGS

Available online.

SECTION X

Genetics and Metabolism

Sanmati Rao Cuddapah

64

Overview of Genetic Testing and Newborn Screening

Jessica R.C. Priestley and Rebecca C. Ahrens-Nicklas

 CLINICAL VIGNETTE

A 36-month-old boy with a history of a repaired ventricular septal defect presents for his well-child appointment. The parents report speech delays, but have no other concerns. On physical examination, a bulbous nose and slightly low-set ears are noted. Given concern for a genetic syndrome, a chromosomal microarray is ordered. Results show a 3-megabase (Mb) deletion involving 22q11.2, and the family is referred to a geneticist for parental testing and counseling.

The clinical features of 22q11.2 deletion syndrome are heterogeneous and can include facial dysmorphism, hypoparathyroidism, immunodeficiency, intellectual disability or psychiatric diagnoses, palate abnormalities, and congenital differences of the renal, cardiac, or gastrointestinal systems. Chromosomal microarray is the diagnostic test of choice for this syndrome because its resolution permits finer mapping of the boundaries of the deletion to elucidate which genes are deleted.

PRINCIPLES OF HUMAN GENETICS

Deoxyribonucleic acid (DNA) is the core of the genetic code for living organisms. It comprises complementary pairs of purines (adenine, guanine) and pyrimidines (thymine, cytosine) condensed with proteins into chromosomes. A human diploid cell contains 22 pairs of autosomes (numbered by descending size, 1 to 22) and 1 pair of allosomes (sex chromosomes, X and Y). Additionally, there is a small circular mitochondrial chromosome. Chromosome pairs connect at the centromere, resulting in two arms—a shorter *p* arm and the longer *q* arm (Fig. 64.1). Each chromosome contains 50 to 150 million base pairs and hundreds to thousands of genes.

Inheritance

A gene is a unit of heredity, providing instructions on synthesis of a protein or ribonucleic acid (RNA) product. An allele is a copy of a gene, with an individual inheriting a maternal and paternal allele. This genotype yields a characteristic, called a phenotype. There are different modes of inheritance for various genetic disorders, depending on the nature of the gene. These are summarized in Table 64.1. Heterozygous implies that the two copies of an allele are not identical (e.g., one copy is normal, and the other carries a mutation), and homozygous means that both copies of the gene are identical (i.e., both carry the same mutation). A patient with a disorder can be compound heterozygous if the patient inherits two different mutations, one on each allele.

GENETIC TESTING

Genetic differences underlying human disease result from large or small alterations in chromosomal structure, deletions, duplications, repeat expansions, imprinting anomalies, or point mutations.

Testing modalities differ in ability to detect different types of variation. Choosing an appropriate testing strategy depends on the differential diagnosis for a given patient's phenotype.

Cytogenetic Testing

Cytogenetic testing, including karyotype, fluorescent in-situ hybridization, and microarray, detects abnormalities in chromosomal structure resulting in imbalances in genetic material on the scale of whole chromosomes, arms of chromosomes, or chromosomal regions. Microdeletion or microduplication syndromes occur when subsections of a chromosome are either missing or duplicated and are variable in size. They can also arise from the loss or gain of genetic material when chromosomes adopt abnormal structures (e.g., ring chromosome, translocations, and inversions).

The foundation of cytogenetic testing is the karyotype. A patient's karyotype describes cellular chromosomal content; the laboratory procedure by the same name allows for visualization of chromosomes. Condensed chromosomes are fixed to a microscope slide and visualized by Giemsa staining, in which dark bands of heterochromatin contrast with light bands of euchromatin (Fig. 64.1). Karyotype abnormalities are reported according to the International System for Human Cytogenetic Nomenclature (ISHCN). By convention, the report will state the total number of chromosomes, sex chromosomes, and any observed abnormalities.

Resolution of a karyotype is limited to changes visible under a light microscope. A standard karyotype contains 400 to 500 bands, each representing millions of base pairs and dozens of genes. It is well-suited for detection of aneuploidies or monosomies, for which it is the diagnostic test of choice. Although experienced technologists and advanced staining techniques can impart additional resolution, the karyotype is not well-suited for detection of abnormalities smaller than 1 to 2 Mb. Because karyotypes are repeated on multiple cells, the technique can sometimes detect mosaicism, in which only a proportion of cells are affected by an abnormality. Karyotypes also can be useful in cancer genetics, in which tumors often demonstrate polyploidy, or abnormal numbers of chromosomes.

When detection of smaller microdeletions or translocations is desired, fluorescent in-situ hybridization (FISH) can be used. FISH uses DNA fluorescent probes designed to be complementary to a specific DNA sequence of interest. The probe then hybridizes with the patient's single-stranded DNA and results in a signal visible using fluorescent microscopy (Fig. 64.2). This technology allows for identification of smaller chromosomal subregions than can be visualized by karyotyping. However, FISH requires identification of a target for which a specific probe can be selected before testing—a diagnostic hypothesis, rather than scanning across the genome.

Chromosomal microarray provides a high-resolution, pan-genome approach. It relies on polymorphisms to map the genome.

Karotypes

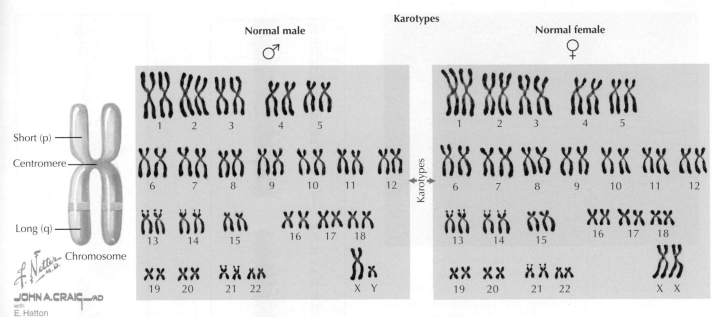

Fig. 64.1 Chromosome Structure and Karyotype.

TABLE 64.1 Genetic Inheritance

Mode of Inheritance	Definition	Example(s)
Autosomal dominant	A trait arising from a mutation on a single allele of a gene on a nonsex chromosome; heterozygous mutation	Marfan syndrome Neurofibromatosis type I
Autsomal recessive	A trait arising from a mutation on both alleles of a gene; homozygous or compound heterozygous mutations	Cystic fibrosis Most inborn errors of metabolism
Sex-linked	A trait arising from a gene on a sex chromosome, typically the X chromosome	Duchenne muscular dystrophy Rett syndrome
Mitochondrial	A trait arising from a gene encoded by the mitochondrial genome (mtDNA), inherited maternally	MERRF MELAS
Mosaicism	Two distinct genotypes in a single individual occurring from postzygotic mutation	Mosaic Turner syndrome Pallister-Killian syndrome (tetrasomy 12p)
Imprinting	Traits arising from genes expressed in a parent-specific manner as a result of epigenetic modifications	Beckwith-Wiedemann syndrome Angelman syndrome
Polygenic or multifactorial	Traits arising from the combined contributions of multiple genes	Obesity Hypertension

MERRF, Myoclonic epilepsy with ragged red fibers; *MELAS,* mitochondrial encephalopathy, lactic acidosis, stroke-like episodes.

By using thousands of evenly spaced markers, gains or losses in material as small as 1 to 2 kilobases (kb) can be detected. Patient DNA is isolated, amplified, and fragmented. Fluorescent probes are used to detect specific alleles at polymorphic sites. Deleted or duplicated regions are identified through differences in probe binding patterns and visualized as a plot of allele frequencies (Fig. 64.3). Results are communicated according to the ISHCN nomenclature; the report will also contain a prediction regarding the pathogenicity of detected anomalies and a list of the involved genes. There are many deletions/duplications for which only a portion overlaps with that of a known syndrome or no phenotype is yet described. The clinical consequences of such a variant may be unclear ("variant of unknown significance" or VUS). In these cases, a clinical geneticist can help interpret results. Some deletions and duplications are seen in unaffected individuals and are thus benign. Microarray can also identify areas of homozygosity resulting from either consanguinity or uniparental disomy.

Microarray is the first-line genetic test for individuals with multiple congenital anomalies or autism/intellectual disability, with a diagnostic yield approaching 20%. It can be particularly useful for neurodevelopmental phenotypes that can be caused by dozens of microdeletion or microduplication syndromes.

Gene Sequencing

A host of genetic conditions are the result of single-gene mutations from alteration of a single base. Sequencing technologies seek to identify these disease-causing differences by "reading" the genetic code to reveal "misspellings" in the adenine, thymine, cytosine, and guanine base language. Selection between single-gene, panel-based, or whole exome/genome sequencing strategies depends on the clinical scenario at hand. Single-gene sequencing can be employed for monogenic conditions with a defined phenotype (e.g., cystic fibrosis). Gene panels can be useful or phenotypes that exhibit locus heterogeneity (e.g., epilepsy). However, in cases of complex phenotypes or critical illness, a

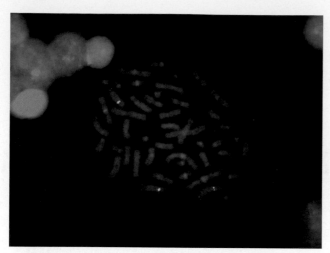

The photograph demonstrates fluorescence in situ hybridization (FISH) carried out on a metaphase spread demonstrating trisomy 8 in this cell. The chromosome 8 centromere is labeled in green, and a chromosome 8q subtelomeric probe is labeled in red. Note the presence of three copies of chromosome 8 in this cell.

Fig. 64.2 Fluorescent In Situ Hybridization (FISH) Detection of Aneuploidy. (Courtesy Nancy B. Spinner, CytoGenomic Laboratory, The Children's Hospital of Philadelphia.)

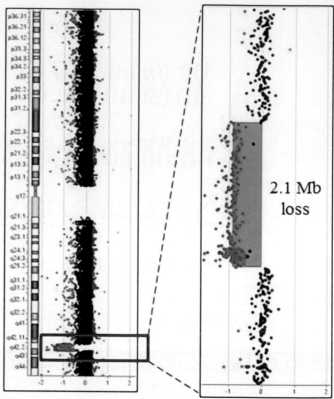

2.1 Mb loss

Fig. 64.3 Microarray Analysis of Chromosome 1. A microarray scatter plot from the long arm of chromosome 1 *(left)* with a 2.1-Mb deletion *(right)*. For each data point representing a marker, the patient sample is compared to a control sample. The x-axis is the normalized log ratio between the two, where negative values suggest deleted patient material, and positive values suggest duplicated patient material.

broader approach may be desired. This can be achieved through whole exome or genome sequencing.

There are two strategies for genetic sequencing: Sanger sequencing, the original sequencing methodology, and "next-generation" sequencing. In Sanger sequencing, patient DNA is cleaved into fragments, denatured into a single strand, and amplified in a solution containing di-deoxynucleotide triphosphates (ddNTPs). As a fragment is amplified, the ddNTP is randomly incorporated and terminates chain elongation at that base. Originally, termination products were separated by size by gel electrophoresis and the sequence was determined by starting at the bottom of the gel (smallest fragments) and working upward. Today, Sanger sequencing utilizes fluorophore-labeled ddNTPs for increased efficiency. Fragments are separated by size on a much smaller capillary gel and the fluorophore is detected using a laser, resulting in a chromatograph (Fig. 64.4). Sanger sequencing is limited to pieces of DNA less than 1 kb in size. It is highly accurate and relatively fast, but would be prohibitively expensive for analysis of the whole genome. These factors have made it the method of choice for single-gene sequencing and for analysis for known variants of which only a very small portion of the entire genome is interrogated.

Next-generation sequencing encompasses a variety of technologies that build on the Sanger strategy to allow high-throughput analysis with improved cost/time efficiency. This makes it ideal for both whole exome (30 million bases, limited to only coding portions of DNA) and whole genome (3 billion bases) sequencing. The cost-effectiveness of next-generation sequencing methods has improved dramatically, permitting commercial availability of whole exome sequencing. Some larger gene panels employ next-generation sequencing to sequence the exome and limit mutation analysis to the genes of interest.

The clinical utility of sequencing depends on reliable and accurate interpretation of sequencing results. First, the patient sequence is compared to a reference sequence that is an amalgam of genomes from unaffected individuals. Genetic changes existing in the patient but not the reference are identified and classified as benign, pathogenic, or VUS. Pathogenic variants are straightforward when they have been

previously identified in someone bearing phenotypic similarity to the patient. For variants not previously reported as disease-causing, analytic software can help to identify "likely pathogenic" variants. These differences may occur in a highly conserved part of the gene, result in a nonsynonymous amino acid substitution at a highly conserved amino acid, introduce a predicted splice site or stop codon, and/or be absent in large populations of unaffected individuals. When these analyses are inconclusive, a variant is a VUS. This can be challenging for both clinicians and families because it means that a definitive link between patient phenotype and genetic difference was not elucidated. However, a VUS can be reclassified as pathogenic or benign as additional information and research are available. For this reason, sequencing results may be reanalyzed periodically.

Given that exome and genome sequencing are not targeted to specific genes of interest, it is possible to find clinically actionable pathogenic variants that are not related to the patient's phenotype but have medical implications. These findings are termed secondary findings.

Methylation Analysis

Imprinting disorders (e.g., Prader-Willi or Angelman syndromes) are the result of abnormal epigenetic methylation patterns that can activate (hypomethylation) or silence (hypermethylation) genes without changes to the DNA code. Detection of imprinting disorders requires methylation analysis, based on methylation sequencing technology. This relies on bisulfite deamination of unmethylated cytosine bases to uracil. Methyl groups protect cytosine residues from bisulfite deamination and are left unaltered. Uracil bases are then "read" as thymine bases during polymerase chain reaction (PCR) amplification of the

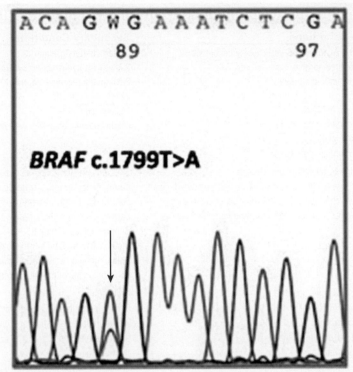

Fig. 64.4 Sample Result of Sanger Sequencing of a Lung Nodule. A Sanger sequencing result demonstrating a T > A transversion at the 1799 position of the *BRAF* gene. At the *arrow,* note the presence of signal for adenine (green) and thymine (orange), representing heterozygosity at this position.

region of interest. Methylation patterns are revealed by comparing that of bisulfite-treated and untreated samples. Because of inherent methylation differences between some maternally and paternally inherited alleles, this analysis can reveal uniparental allele inheritance for imprinting disorders.

Prenatal Genetic Testing

Prenatal genetic testing includes noninvasive and invasive modalities and can provide information regarding a fetus's sex, aneuploidies, or even specific genetic conditions. Preimplantation genetic testing permits identification of genetic disease at the zygotic stage. After in vitro fertilization, the embryo is biopsied to collect a small amount of genetic material without affecting the growth potential of the zygote. From that sample, karyotype, microarray, or gene sequencing can be performed. This allows for subsequent intrauterine implantation of only embryos without a specific genetic syndrome.

Noninvasive prenatal testing (NIPT) or "cell-free DNA testing" analyzes small fragments of fetal DNA that exist in maternal blood because of the placental interface. Such fragments occur randomly and should be evenly represented across the genome; therefore, when a particular region is overrepresented or underrepresented, the pregnancy is at increased risk for aneuploidy. If the analysis reveals an amount of chromosome 21 material 50% higher than what would be expected, the pregnancy is predicted to be at higher risk for Down syndrome (trisomy 21). Sex of a fetus can be determined by applying the same principles to sex chromosomes, where the presence of Y-chromosome material indicates a male fetus. Some laboratories also offer NIPT of smaller chromosomal regions. Importantly, while NIPT is highly sensitive, it is not a diagnostic test. Results depend on normalization to the total fetal DNA in maternal circulation, which is influenced by multiple variables, and results are sometimes uninterpretable.

When abnormalities are identified by NIPT or on ultrasonography, or there is increased risk for genetic abnormalities such as in

advanced maternal age, or there has been an affected sibling, parents may be offered amniocentesis or chorionic villus sampling with follow-up diagnostic genetic testing. These techniques allow for direct sampling of fetal cells and thus provide a complete genetic sample for any of the genetic testing modalities previously described. In utero diagnosis of chromosomal, subchromosomal, and single-gene disorders can then aid in pregnancy management and delivery decisions, allow families to learn and prepare, or inform termination of the pregnancy.

NEWBORN SCREENING

Newborn screening (NBS) is not a single test but a collection of tests that screen for dozens of conditions present at birth for which early interventions can improve health outcomes. The US Department of Health and Human Services maintains the Recommended Uniform Screening Panel, a list of conditions that are recommended, but not required, for states' NBS programs. Table 64.2 provides the most recent iteration of core conditions as well as secondary conditions that may be identified in the process of screening but are not primary testing targets. Final decisions regarding which conditions to screen for and which procedural, genetic, or biochemical testing modalities to employ for that screening, are made by individual states. Although the majority of screened conditions are genetic, NBS uses genetic testing modalities only in some states for some conditions. NBS is universal, although in most states there are mechanisms in place by which parents can opt out.

NBS occurs in the neonatal period: babies are screened for hearing loss with a hearing test, critical congenital heart disease with preductal and postductal pulse oximetry, and a blood sample is collected on a designated filter paper as per individual state protocol. The blood sample must be collected within the appropriate time frame because normal values are time- and age-dependent. Babies born outside of a

TABLE 64.2	**Conditions on the Recommended Uniform Screening Panel as of July 2018**	
	Core Conditions	**Secondary Conditions**
Organic acid conditions	3-Methylcrotonyl-CoA carboxylase deficiency Cobalamin disorders Glutaric acidemia type I Holocarboxylase synthase deficiency Isovaleric acidemia Methylmalonic acidemia Propionic acidemia β-Ketothiolase deficiency	2-Methylbutyrylglycinuria 2-Methyl-3-hydroxybutyric aciduria 3-Methylglutaconic aciduria Isobutyrylglycinuria Malonic acidemia Methylmalonic acidemia with homocystinuria
Fatty acid oxidation disorders	Carnitine uptake/transport defects Long chain L-3 hydroxyacyl-CoA dehydrogenase deficiency Medium-chain acyl-CoA dehydrogenase deficiency Very-long-chain acyl-CoA dehydrogenase deficiency	2,4 Dienoyl-CoA reductase deficiency Carnitine acylcarnitine translocase deficiency Carnitine palmitoyltransferase type I deficiency Carnitine palmitoyltransferase type II deficiency Glutaric acidemia type II Medium/short-chain L-3-hydroxyacyl-CoA dehydrogenase deficiency Medium-chain ketoacyl-CoA thiolase deficiency Short-chain acyl-CoA dehydrogenase deficiency
Amino acid disorders	Argininosuccinic aciduria Citrullinemia type I Homocystinuria Maple syrup urine disease Phenylketonuria Tyrosinemia type I	Argininemia Benign hyperphenylalaninemia Biopterin defect in cofactor biosynthesis or regeneration Citrullinemia type II Hypermethioninemia Tyrosinemia type II Tyrosinemia type III
Endocrine disorders	Congenital adrenal hypoplasia Congenital hypothyroidism	
Hemoglobinopathies	S-β-thalassemia SC disease SS disease	Other hemoglobinopathies
Other disorders	Biotinidase deficiency Critical congenital heart disease Cystic fibrosis Galactosemia Hearing loss Hurler syndrome Pompe disease Severe combined immunodeficiencies Spinal muscular atrophy X-linked adrenoleukodystrophy	Galactose epimerase deficiency Galactokinase deficiency T cell–related lymphocyte deficiencies

hospital setting should have their screen sent by a medical provider. The filter paper is dried and sent to the state laboratory for analysis. Results are generally available in 4 to 7 business days, often by an online portal, and are also sent to the infant's pediatrician for review and communication to the family.

Because this process is designed to screen rather than diagnose, an abnormal result warrants confirmatory testing. In some cases, this entails sending a second dried blood spot for repeat analysis. In other cases, the result is reported directly to a specialist, such as one with expertise in metabolic conditions, to recommend appropriate secondary testing. The pediatrician plays a critical role in communication with the family and coordination of confirmatory testing. States identify NBS centers to facilitate this process and ensure follow-up for babies with positive results. The American College of Medical Genetics and Genomics produces action sheets and algorithms. Available online, these provide a differential diagnosis, condition description, next steps with a timeline for completion, components of the diagnostic evaluation, clinical considerations, and resources for additional information and referral centers.

ETHICAL CONSIDERATIONS

Because genetic testing reveals something fundamental, intrinsic, and permanent to a patient as well as his or her family, with implications for future family members, a discussion of genetic testing cannot and should not be separated from ethical considerations.

Although families can be eager for a diagnosis, they may not be aware of additional information that can come from testing, including nonpaternity and consanguinity. State requirements for informed consent vary. Although the 2008 Genetic Information Nondiscrimination Act protects patients from use of genetic information by employers and health insurance companies, it does not protect use of that information by disability or life insurance companies. In exome sequencing, there are important consent decisions regarding "secondary findings." These are genetic variants unrelated to the reason for sequencing that may be medically actionable, such as cancer predisposition variants. Parents can often opt-in to secondary findings for their children, who may not be affected by the variant until adulthood. Patients and their families should be made aware of these issues and limitations as part of the consent process. Genetic counselors are useful resources in obtaining informed consent and counseling families.

SUGGESTED READINGS

Available online.

65

Chromosomal Disorders

Steven D. Klein and Jennifer M. Kalish

> ## ✳ CLINICAL VIGNETTE
>
> A 6-month-old boy presents to the pediatrician for an initial visit after the family has relocated. His medical records indicate that was born at term and had a complicated neonatal course. Postnatally, he was observed in the neonatal intensive care unit for respiratory distress, feeding difficulties, and hypoglycemia. He was discharged after 1 month and has been bottle feeding on fortified formula. He continues to gain weight and is growing along the 3rd percentile in all domains. On physical examination, he is a small, alert boy in no acute distress. His head is microcephalic, symmetric, and atraumatic. His face displays a flattened nasal bridge, bulbous nasal tip, large protuberant ears and a visible tongue when the mouth is closed. On examination of the mouth, he has one tooth and a high-arched but not clefted palate. Cardiovascular examination reveals a loud harsh holosystolic murmur at the left lower sternal border. Abdominal examination is significant for hepatomegaly, with the liver edge palpable 1 cm below the costal margin. Examination of the digits shows fifth finger clinodactyly bilaterally. On neurologic examination, the child has slightly low tone with head lag and cannot sit unassisted.
>
> The child has a constellation of findings spanning multiple organ systems that include functional and developmental abnormalities. His presentation raises concern for an underlying genetic syndrome. Many of these are chromosomal disorders. We present a systematic approach and organization to these disorders focusing on the stepwise clinical workup and comorbidities that merit medical surveillance. This approach will help guide the management of the undifferentiated dysmorphic child.

Chromosomes are the macro-organizational unit of deoxyribonucleic acid (DNA). They allow for large amounts of DNA to be wrapped and tightly packaged into the nucleus. Furthermore, their dynamic state allows for genes to be accessed and silenced based on a number of stimuli and regulators. Their role in DNA replication and separation during the cell cycle is paramount. Disruptions in chromosome number, structure, and composition can result in human disease. The implementation and widespread application of genome-wide single nucleotide polymorphism (SNP) arrays have allowed for better understanding of the pathogenic nature of even small disruptions in these essential cellular components.

CLINICAL PRESENTATION

The clinical presentations of chromosomal disorders are as varied as the genes they disrupt.

Dysmorphology Examination

Dysmorphic features are defined as atypically formed facial or physical features. A pattern of congenital anomalies and/or dysmorphic features arising from a common cause is called a *syndrome*. In evaluating a patient with dysmorphic features, it is essential to obtain a thorough medical history detailing the prenatal and birth history, developmental milestones, and medical issues, as well as a detailed family history. Then, a detailed physical examination is essential and should include anthropomorphic measurements and detailed observation of dysmorphic features (Table 65.1). It is important to consider how features may differ based on the racial and ethnic background of a patient.

Etiology and Pathogenesis

There are three major groupings of chromosomal disorders: disorders of chromosome number, disorders of chromosome structure, and disorders of chromosome accessibility (Fig. 65.1). Chromosome number is dictated largely by consistent meiotic division during gametogenesis. Aneuploidy in gametes is directly correlated to parental age and is thought to be due to numerous molecular mechanisms, including mitochondrial dysfunction and cohesin deterioration. Disorders of chromosome number (Table 65.2, Figs. 65.2 and 65.3) are the target of prenatal screening, including serum screening and noninvasive prenatal testing (Chapter 64).

Conversely, disorders of chromosome structure (Table 65.3 and Fig. 65.4) are thought to be largely premitotic and result from disruption of key cellular machinery involved in chromosome maintenance such as DNA repair and replication. Numerous intrinsic and extrinsic factors can culminate to cause stress to the DNA replication pathway, which in turn interrupts the replication fork and results in double-stranded breaks. Breaks preferentially happen at sites of genomic instability, which can include telomeres, centromeres, and ribosomal DNA. It is the recombining of double-stranded breaks that result in the deletions, duplications, and rearrangements of the genome.

Disorders of chromosome accessibility (Table 65.4) arise from altered methylation and/or other epigenetic modifiers at key imprinted regions in the genome that normally require allelic contribution from both the maternal and paternal alleles. One such example includes disorders arising from uniparental disomy (UPD) or when both copies of a chromosome carry the methylation pattern from one parent. The mechanism underlying this is a cell compensatory "rescue" from an aneuploidy state. In the event of a trisomy, the cell can expel one of the chromosomes leading to two retained copies from one parent. In the event of monosomies, the cell can replicate the one chromosome to the same end result. Methylation changes can furthermore be present in small regions of a chromosome, not globally, a phenomenon referred to as partial uniparental disomy. These partial UPD cases are thought to arise from mitotic recombination events. The process of imprinting or silencing of a parent-specific copy is essential for balancing the expression of dosage-sensitive genes in the human transcriptome. These imprinting disorders caused by the disruption of methylated and imprinted regions leads to overexpression or underexpression of affected genes, which results in human phenotypes.

TABLE 65.1 The Dysmorphology Examination

System	Features	Examples	System	Features	Examples
Growth parameters	Weight	Overgrowth, failure to thrive	Chest	Cardiac	Murmurs
	Length	Small or large for gestational age		Lung	Absent breath sounds, stridor, wheeze, bowel sounds
	Head circumference	Microcephaly, macrocephaly		Sternum	Pectus deformity
Head	Size	Microcephaly, microcephaly		Shape	Narrow, barrel shaped
	Shape	Dolichocephaly, brachycephaly, premature fusion of sutures		Nipple placement	Wide or narrow, supernumerary
	Fontanelles	Size, number, premature or delayed closure	Abdomen	Umbilicus	Hernia, omphalocele, two-vessel cord
	Hair	Sparse, hirsute, unusual hairline, whorls		Organs	Hepatomegaly, splenomegaly
	Forehead	Bossed, temporal narrowing	Back	Shape	Scoliosis
	Jaw	Micrognathia, retrognathia		Sacrum	Dimple, tuft, myelomeningocele
Eyes	Shape	Almond	Genitourinary	Phallus or clitoris	Hypospadias, chordee, clitoromegaly, ambiguous genitalia
	Spacing	Hypoteloric (narrow), hyperteloric (wide)		Labia, scrotum, or testes	Bifid scrotum, undescended testes
	Structure	Sclera color, cataract, coloboma	Extremities	Limb form	Brachymelia (short), rhizomelia (shortening of proximal limbs), mesomelia (shortening of intermediate segments of long bones), acromelia (shortening of distal limbs)
	Palpebral fissures	Small, lengthened, upslanted, downslanted, epicanthus			
	Setting	Deep set, proptotic			
	Eyebrows	Synophrys			
Ears	Placement	Low set, posteriorly rotated		Digit form	Clinodactyly, camptodactyly
	Form	Short, long, square, overfolded or crumpled helix		Digit number	Polydactyly, preaxial, postaxial, oligodactyly
	Auricles	Preauricular pits or tags, postauricular pits		Digit fusion	Syndactyly
Nose	Tip	Small, bulbous	Dermatoglyphics	Digits	Predominance of arches or whorls
	Alae nasi	Hypoplastic		Palm	Single crease, distal triradius
	Bridge	Depressed, broad	Skin	Pigmentation	Café-au-lait macules, hypopigmented macules, pigmentary variation
	Choanae	Atretic, stenotic			
	Philtrum	Long, short, smooth		Vasculature	Hemangioma, telangiectasia, port-wine stain
Mouth	Size and shape	Small, bow shaped			
	Lips	Thin, thick, downturned, cleft		Sweat glands	Absent
	Frenulum	Absent, tight	Neurologic	Mental status	Alertness, lethargy, unresponsiveness
	Teeth	Natal, absent, single central incisor, enamel defects		Tone	Hypertonic, hypotonic
	Tongue	Macroglossia, protuberant		Movements	Seizures, chorea, fasciculations, symmetry
	Palate	Hard or soft cleft, high, narrow		Vision and hearing	Response to vision and auditory stimuli
	Uvula	Wide, bifid			
Neck	Length	Short			
	Skin	Webbed, excess nuchal			

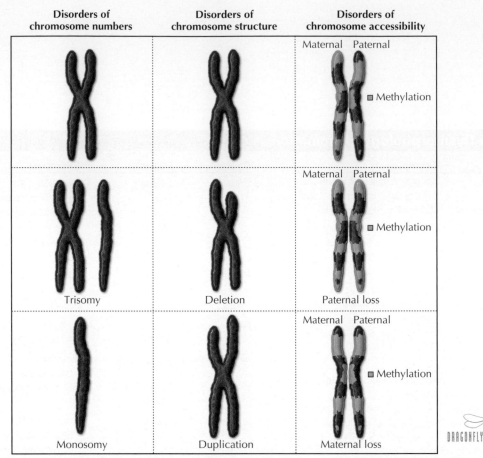

Disorders of chromosome numbers · Disorders of chromosome structure · Disorders of chromosome accessibility

Trisomy · Deletion · Paternal loss

Monosomy · Duplication · Maternal loss

Fig. 65.1 **Organization of Chromosomal Abnormalities.** Three main categories exist: disorders of chromosome number, structure, and accessibility. Chromosome number abnormalities result in aneuploidies, including monosomy and trisomy. Disorders of chromosome structure include deletions and duplications of regions of chromosomes. Disorders of chromosome accessibility alter the epigenetic patterning on chromosomes.

TABLE 65.2	**Disorders of Chromosome Number**		
Name	**Chromosome Alteration**	**Dysmorphic Features**	**Other Features**
Edwards syndrome	Trisomy 18	Microcephaly, short palpebral fissures, micrognathia, rocker-bottom feet	VSD, PDA, pulmonary hypertension, cryptorchidism
Patau syndrome	Trisomy 13	Microcephaly, holoprosencephaly, anophthalmia or microphthalmia	Large cystic kidneys
Down syndrome	Trisomy 21	Flattened face, upslanting palpebral fissures, microtia, short neck, protuberant tongue, single palmar crease	Congenital heart disease, duodenal atresia, hypothyroidism
Klinefelter syndrome	47,XXY or 46,XY/47,XXY	Increased height, narrower than average shoulders, broader than average hips, scoliosis or kyphosis (Fig. 65.2)	Cryptorchidism, hypospadias, or a small phallus
Turner syndrome	45,X	Webbed neck, short stature, shield chest (Fig. 65.3)	Lymphedema, coarctation of the aorta, premature ovarian failure

PDA, Patent ductus arteriosus; *VSD,* ventricular septal defect.

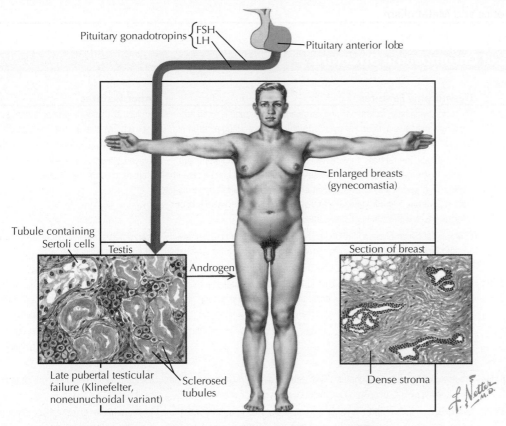

Pituitary gonadotropins { FSH LH

Pituitary anterior lobe

Enlarged breasts (gynecomastia)

Tubule containing Sertoli cells

Testis

Androgen

Section of breast

Late pubertal testicular failure (Klinefelter, noneunuchoidal variant)

Sclerosed tubules

Dense stroma

Nuclear chromatin often positive (female); usually XXY chromosomal pattern but XXX Y , XXXX Y , XXY Y , and mosaic patterns have been described

XXY

Fig. 65.2 Klinefelter Syndrome. Testicular growth is arrested, leading to oligospermia or azoospermia and low testosterone levels. This condition also manifests with gynecomastia, eunuchoid habitus, and decreased hair. Testosterone replacement therapy aims at increasing muscle mass, libido, energy, and improving mood through support of androgen-dependent processes.

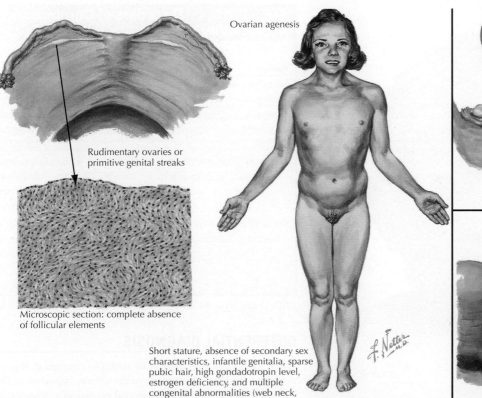
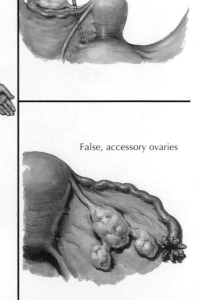

Ovarian agenesis

Rudimentary ovaries or primitive genital streaks

Microscopic section: complete absence of follicular elements

Homolateral absence of ovary, tube, and kidney, and broad and round ligaments

False, accessory ovaries

Short stature, absence of secondary sex characteristics, infantile genitalia, sparse pubic hair, high gonadotropin level, estrogen deficiency, and multiple congenital abnormalities (web neck, shield-like chest, cubitus valgus)

Fig. 65.3 Turner Syndrome. Gonadal dysgenesis is a hallmark of Turner syndrome and typically leads to ovarian failure. Puberty occurs spontaneously in 10% of patients, and hormonal replacement therapy is necessary to achieve development of secondary sexual characteristics as well as to avoid osteoporosis and other postmenopausal complications. Physical features are a consequence of lymphatic abnormalities that include webbed neck, puffy hands and feet, dysplastic fingernails and toenails, protuberant ears, and a broad chest.

TABLE 65.3	**Disorders of Chromosome Structure**		
Name	**Chromosome Alteration**	**Dysmorphic Features**	**Other features**
1p36 deletion syndrome	Deletion of 1p36	Microbrachycephaly, frontal bossing, large anterior fontanelle, marked midface hypoplasia, deep-set eyes, straight eyebrows, long philtrum, abnormally shaped ears	Intellectual disability with poor or absent speech, hypotonia, short feet, brachyc-amptodactyly, brain abnormalities
Wolf-Hirschhorn syndrome	Monosomy 4p	Microcephaly, frontal bossing with a high frontal hairline and prominent glabella, a broad nasal bridge and beaked nose, hypertelorism, epicanthal folds, highly arched eyebrows, downturned mouth with short upper lip and short philtrum, micrognathia, and low-set, large ears often with pits or tags; "Greek warrior helmet" appearance	Delayed growth and development, failure to thrive, hypotonia
Cri-du-chat syndrome	Deletion of 5p	Characteristic high-pitched (cat-like) cry, low birth weight, microcephaly, round face, large nasal bridge, hypertelorism, epicanthal folds, downslanting palpebral fissures	Heart defects, intellectual disability and delayed development
Williams syndrome	Deletion of 7q11.23	Broad brow, bitemporal narrowing, periorbital fullness, a stellate iris pattern, strabismus, short nose, full nasal tip, malar hypoplasia, long philtrum, full lips, wide mouth, malocclusion, small jaw, prominent earlobe	Difficulty with visual-spatial tasks, supra-valvular aortic stenosis, joint problems and soft, loose skin, hypercalcemia
Miller-Dieker syndrome	Deletion of 17p13.3	Front bossing, midface hypoplasia, a small, upturned nose, micrognathia, microtia	Intellectual disability, hypotonia, developmental delay, seizures, spasticity, feeding difficulties
Smith-Magenis syndrome	Deletions of 17p11.2	Brachycephaly, midface hypoplasia with a broad nasal bridge, prognathism, a tented upper lip, deep-set, close-spaced eyes, dental anomalies	Disrupted sleep, personality disorders, self-injury
22q11.2 deletion syndrome	Deletion of 22q11.2	Overfolded or squared-off ear helices, small and protuberant ears with pre-auricular pits or tags, prominent nasal root and bulbous nasal tip, hooded eyelids, ocular hypertelorism, cleft lip and palate, asymmetric crying facies, and craniosynostosis (Fig. 65.4)	Congenital heart disease, hypocalcemia, immune deficiency

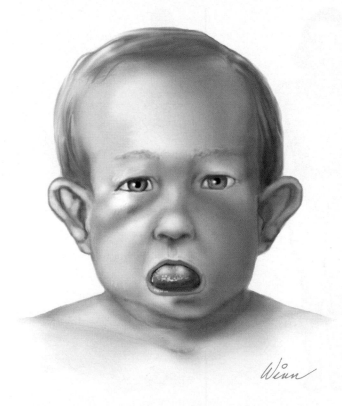

Fig. 65.4 22q11.2 Deletion Syndrome. Common dysmorphic features include overfolded or squared-off ear helices, small and protuberant ears with preauricular pits or tags, a prominent nasal root, and bulbous nasal tip, hooded eyelids, ocular hypertelorism, cleft lip and palate, asymmetric crying facies, and craniosynostosis.

TABLE 65.4	**Disorders of Chromosome Accessibility**		
Name	**Change**	**Dysmorphic Features**	**Other Features**
Beckwith-Wiedemann syndrome (BWS)	Alterations of methylation on 11p15.5	Omphalocele, lateralized overgrowth/hemihypertrophy, macroglossia	Macrosomia, visceromegaly, hypoglycemia, Wilms tumor, hepatoblastoma
Angelman syndrome	Paternal UPD of chromosome 15	Microcephaly, prominent chin, deep-set eyes, flat occiput, wide mouth	Developmental delay, speech impairment, hyperactivity
Prader-Willi syndrome	Maternal UPD of chromosome 15	Narrow forehead, almond-shaped eyes, triangular mouth, short stature, small hands and feet	Hypotonia, poor growth, polyphagia, obesity

UPD, Uniparental disomy.

DIFFERENTIAL DIAGNOSIS

When evaluating the child with multiple congenital abnormalities, pregnancy and birth history are of the utmost importance. The differential diagnoses list includes maternal exposures to teratogens, maternal diabetes, and congenital infections. In the neonatal period, ruling out congenital TORCH (**T**oxoplasmosis, **O**ther [syphilis, varicella-zoster, parvovirus B19], **R**ubella, **C**ytomegalovirus [CMV], and **H**erpes) infections are an important consideration in an infant with congenital anomalies.

FUTURE DIRECTIONS

There is an emerging role for the use of whole genome sequencing in the detection of small duplications and deletions. This in combination with its ability to detect noncoding variants presents a comprehensive approach to the undiagnosed child. These technologies are not yet first line; however, with the speed and rapid implementation of large-scaling, this sequencing may be available in the near future. Additionally, the role of cell-free DNA for screening of aneuploidies is a noninvasive first-line test.

SUGGESTED READINGS

Available online.

66

Syndromes With Congenital Anomalies

Linh Thi Tran and Rose Guo

 CLINICAL VIGNETTE

A 27-year-old woman was referred for prenatal screening and diagnostic testing at 27 weeks gestation for sonographic abnormalities, including a mass in the left upper quadrant, an enlarged right kidney, and a cystic mass in the pelvic cavity. Serial ultrasonography showed increased fetal abdominal circumference above the 97th percentile. A 4.5-kg infant was delivered by cesarean delivery. The infant had an umbilical hernia, macroglossia, and a crease in the left ear lobe. Neonatal ultrasonography and magnetic resonance imaging revealed diastasis recti and visceromegaly of the pancreas, liver, bilateral kidneys, and adrenal glands. Postnatal molecular analysis identified uniparental disomy at chromosome 11p15, consistent with a diagnosis of Beckwith-Wiedemann syndrome.

Infants with multiple congenital anomalies and/or dysmorphic features should undergo evaluation for underlying genetic syndromes. A diagnosis is essential to appropriate screening, management, and recurrence risk assessment.

A congenital anomaly is defined as a structural defect that is present at birth. These defects can be caused by genetic abnormalities and/or environmental exposures. Anomalies can be classified based on the developmental process involved in their formation, including malformations, deformations, disruptions, and dysplasias (Box 66.1).

Major congenital malformations occur in approximately 2% to 4% of live births. Deformations are more common in the limbs and head and are seen in approximately 3% of newborns. The prevalence of disruptions depends on the type of anomaly but ranges from 0.5 to 4 per 10,000 births.

DIAGNOSIS OF A CONGENITAL ANOMALY

The basis for diagnosis of a congenital anomaly syndrome in a neonate involves a combination of a comprehensive history, physical examination, and diagnostic genetic testing. Making a diagnosis is important to evaluate for additional anomalies that may not be overtly obvious or to anticipate future associated medical complications. Various methods of genetic testing (Chapter 64) are available and are constantly evolving; however, a thorough history and physical examination are critical in the diagnosis of genetic disorders (Box 66.2).

CHROMOSOMAL SYNDROMES

The most common congenital anomaly syndromes diagnosed in the neonatal period are chromosomal disorders, discussed in Chapter 65, Chromosomal Disorders.

SYNDROMES WITH CRANIOFACIAL MALFORMATIONS

As with most congenital anomaly syndromes, the disorders classified here cause craniofacial malformations, but not exclusively; most disorders presented are multisystemic and may cause malformations in numerous tissues.

Craniosynostosis

Craniosynostosis is defined as the premature fusion of the cranial bones and occurs in 1 in 2000 live births. Causes can be isolated or syndromic. Evaluation for syndromic causes should include characterizing which cranial sutures are affected (sagittal, coronal, metopic, lambdoid, or multiple) and performing a thorough physical examination with particular attention for additional musculoskeletal differences, such as syndactyly, broad digits, or caudal appendages. Genetic syndromes to consider include Crouzon, Apert, Pfeiffer, Muenke, Jackson-Weiss, and Saethre-Chotzen. Because of the variety of genetic causes (e.g., FGFR-related genes), there are gene panels to aid diagnosis.

Treacher Collins Syndrome

Treacher Collins syndrome (TCS) is a disorder manifesting with midface hypoplasia, downslanting palpebral fissures, micrognathia and retrognathia, external ear anomalies, and abnormalities of the lower eyelids (Fig. 66.1). TCS can be inherited in an autosomal dominant manner (pathogenic variants in *TCOF1*, *POLR1D*, or *POLR1B*) or in an autosomal recessive manner (biallelic pathogenic variants in *POLR1C* or *POLR1D*). Respiratory and feeding difficulties result from hypoplasia of the zygomatic bones and mandible, and up to half of patients have conductive hearing loss. Intellect is typically normal.

Branchiootorenal Spectrum Disorder

Branchiootorenal spectrum disorder (BORSD, previously known as Melnick-Fraser syndrome) encompasses a group of disorders characterized by branchial defects with lateral cervical fistulas or cysts, ear pits, hearing loss, and renal anomalies, including renal aplasia and hypoplasia. This spectrum includes the clinical entities of branchiootorenal (BOR) syndrome and branchiootic syndrome (BOS). An autosomal dominant disorder with incomplete penetrance and variable expressivity, mutations in the *EYA1* gene have been identified in approximately 40% of patients with BORSD. Mutations in *SIX1* and *SIX5* genes have also been reported, though a significant percentage of cases do not yet have an identifiable molecular cause. The incidence is 1 in 40,000 infants, and BORSD is found in approximately 2% of profoundly deaf children. Hearing loss of varying degrees is seen in more than 90% of patients with this disorder.

CHARGE Syndrome

CHARGE syndrome is characterized by a nonrandom association of anomalies (**c**oloboma, **h**eart defect, **a**tresia choanae, **r**etarded growth and development, **g**enital hypoplasia, and **e**ar anomalies) caused by mutations in the *CHD7* gene. Individuals with all four major characteristics (choanal atresia/stenosis, coloboma, cranial nerve anomalies, and characteristic ears [Fig. 66.2]), or three major and three minor characteristics (cardiovascular malformations, genital hypoplasia, cleft lip/palate, tracheoesophageal fistula, distinctive CHARGE facies, growth deficiency, developmental delay) are likely to have CHARGE syndrome. Children with CHARGE syndrome require extensive medical management and surgical interventions. The most common neonatal emergencies involve cyanosis due to bilateral posterior choanal atresia and/or congenital heart defects. The primary focus of management should be airway stabilization and circulatory support.

SYNDROMES CHARACTERIZED BY ABNORMAL GROWTH

Beckwith-Wiedemann Syndrome

Beckwith-Wiedemann syndrome (BWS) is a pediatric overgrowth disorder involving a predisposition to tumor development. Dysregulation of imprinted gene expression in the chromosome 11p15.5 region can result in BWS phenotype, as well as mutations in the *CDKN1C* gene. BWS usually occurs sporadically (85%), but familial transmission can occur. The characteristic features of BWS include omphalocele, macroglossia, and macrosomia. Other findings associated with BWS include hemihyperplasia, visceromegaly, embryonal tumors (Wilms tumor, hepatoblastoma, neuroblastoma, rhabdomyosarcoma), renal abnormalities, neonatal hypoglycemia resulting from hyperinsulinism, and cardiac anomalies. Management includes prompt treatment of hypoglycemia to reduce the risk for

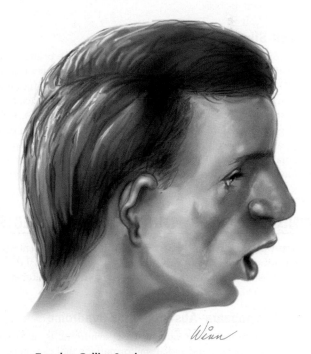

Treacher Collins Syndrome

Fig. 66.1 Facial Features in Treacher Collins Syndrome. Features of Treacher Collins syndrome include midface hypoplasia, microretrognthia, and external ear anomalies.

central nervous system (CNS) complications. Surgical correction (abdominal wall repair) is performed soon after birth for an omphalocele. Management of problems arising from macroglossia include anticipation of difficulties with endotracheal intubation, pulmonary assessment to address concerns regarding potential sleep apnea, and management of feeding difficulties. Abdominal ultrasonography and serum alpha-fetoprotein levels are monitored routinely in childhood to screen for tumors.

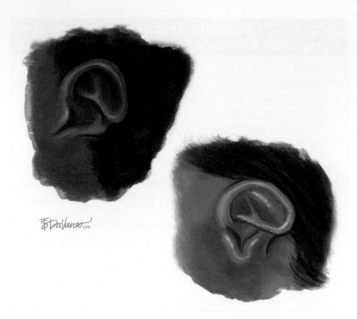

Fig. 66.2 Ear Abnormalities in a Patient With CHARGE Syndrome. Ear abnormalities in CHARGE syndrome include auricular manifestations: a short, wide ear with a small/absent lobe and an abnormal helix with prominent antihelix.

Russell-Silver Syndrome

Russell-Silver or (Silver-Russell) syndrome (RSS) primarily presents with growth delay, typically with intrauterine growth restriction (IUGR) or postnatal failure to thrive that is head-sparing (i.e., normal head circumference). Facial features include triangular facies with a broad forehead, blue sclerae, and micrognathia (Fig. 66.3). Delayed bone age, limb-length discrepancy, and café-au-lait spots can be seen. RSS is associated with imprinting defects at chromosome 11p15.5 or maternal uniparental disomy for chromosome 7. However, up to 40% of individuals who meet clinical diagnostic criteria for RSS have negative genetic testing.

SYNDROMES PRESENTING WITH LIMB DEFECTS

The representative diagnoses presented in this section present primarily but not exclusively with limb defects. Several additional disorders can manifest similarly, including Holt-Oram syndrome, Roberts syndrome, and Duane–radial ray syndrome.

Thrombocytopenia–Absent Radius Syndrome

Thrombocytopenia–absent radius (TAR) syndrome is characterized by thrombocytopenia and radial malformations that can range from complete absence to mild hypoplasia, but are always bilateral (Fig. 66.4). Additional musculoskeletal features can include abnormalities of the ulna, humerus, hips, knees, tibia, and fibula; however, the thumbs are always unaffected. Cardiac and renal anomalies also may be present. TAR syndrome is inherited in an autosomal recessive manner as a result of complex changes involving the *RBM8A* gene.

Townes-Brocks Syndrome

Townes-Brocks syndrome (TBS) should be suspected when the triad of thumb, ear, and anal anomalies are present. Thumb differences include broad, bifid, hypoplastic, or triphalangeal thumbs. Ear differences include small/cupped or overfolded ears or preauricular skin tags. Anal anomalies range from imperforate anus to anterior placement. Additional considerations include renal anomalies and progressive

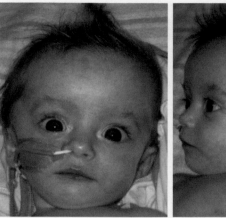
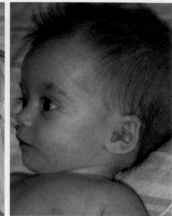

Fig. 66.3 Infant With Russell-Silver Syndrome. Facial features in Russell-Silver syndrome include a broad forehead, triangular facies, blue sclerae, and micrognathia. (Reused with permission from Chopra M, Amor DJ, Sutton L, Algar E, Mowat D. Russell–Silver syndrome due to paternal H19/IGF2 hypomethylation in a patient conceived using intracytoplasmic sperm injection. *Reprod BioMed Online.* 2010;20(6):843–847, Figs. 1 and 2. Copyright © 2010 Reproductive Healthcare Ltd.)

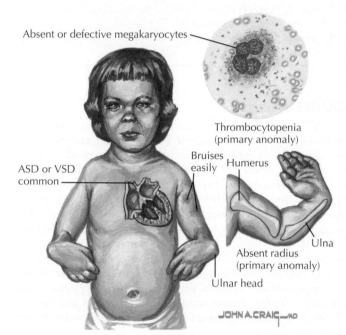

Fig. 66.4 Features of Thrombocytopenia–Absent Radius (TAR) Syndrome.

hearing loss. TBS is inherited in an autosomal dominant manner, most commonly as a result of pathogenic variants in the *SALL1* gene.

ECTODERMAL DYSPLASIAS

Ectodermal dysplasias encompass a broad category of genetic disorders that affect tissues with full or partial ectodermal origin (hair, teeth, nails, epidermis, hair follicles, and sweat glands). These disorders may have additional associated congenital anomalies. One example is ectrodactyly–ectodermal dysplasia–clefting (EEC) syndrome, also known as ankyloblepharon–ectodermal dysplasia–clefting (AEC) or Hay-Wells syndrome. EEC is characterized by cleft lip and/or palate; in addition to dry skin with variable hypohidrosis; sparse, fair, and dry hair; absent eyebrows and eyelashes, hypodontia; and thin brittle nails. It is inherited in an autosomal dominant manner because of variants in the *TP63* gene. In the absence of defining anomalies, the best diagnostic approach is to perform a gene panel given the heterogeneity of ectodermal dysplasias.

DISORDERS OF THE GENITOURINARY AND REPRODUCTIVE SYSTEMS

Disorders of the genitourinary and reproductive systems include causes stemming from sex chromosome aneuploidy (Chapter 65), embryologic development of the kidneys and urologic system (Chapter 106), cholesterol metabolism, endocrinologic abnormalities, and disorders of sexual development.

Sex Chromosome Abnormalities

Aneuploidies of the sex chromosomes (Chapter 65) are associated with abnormalities of the reproductive system. In Turner syndrome (45,X), gonadal dysgenesis is a common feature, often resulting in ovarian failure. Klinefelter syndrome (47,XXY) can result in decreased testicular growth and atypical development of secondary sex characteristics. In both conditions, mosaicism is possible, with some patients with Turner syndrome exhibiting a 45,X/46,XY karyotype and some individuals with Klinefelter syndrome exhibiting 46,XY/47,XXY karyotype. These conditions can have varied implications in the development of internal gonads. Multidisciplinary evaluation is critical for appropriate medical and psychosocial management.

Congenital Adrenal Hyperplasia

Congenital adrenal hyperplasia (CAH) is a group of disorders caused by defective synthesis of adrenal steroids and accumulation of androgenic steroids. Certain types of CAH can cause overproduction of androgens and virilization in 46,XX infants. Most cases of CAH are due to deficiency of 21-hydroxylase, caused by autosomal recessive mutations in the *CYP21A2* gene. Infants can have a salt-wasting adrenal crisis in the neonatal period, making prompt diagnosis essential. Measurement of serum 17-hydroxyprogesterone is part of the Recommended Uniform Screening Panel (Chapter 64) for newborn screening for infants with 21-hydroxylase and less commonly, 11-hydroxylase deficiencies. The phenotypic spectrum of CAH is further discussed in Chapter 49.

WAGR Syndrome

Wilms tumor-aniridia-genital anomalies-retardation (WAGR) syndrome is caused by deletions of the *PAX6* gene and the adjacent *WT1* gene, often associated with recurrent 11p13 microdeletion. Clinical features include significant risk for Wilms tumor during childhood, aniridia (affecting the cornea, iris, lens, fovea, and optic nerve), genitourinary abnormalities (including cryptorchidism, hypospadias, uterine and ovarian abnormalities, and gonadoblastoma), intellectual disability, and/or neuropsychiatric disorders. An isolated ocular anomaly (*PAX6*-related aniridia) is caused by heterozygous pathogenic variants or deletions in *PAX6* alone. Conversely, heterozygous pathogenic variants in *WT1* alone cause a distinct disorder of steroid-resistant progressive glomerulopathy in association with disorders of testicular development and Wilms tumor. This includes the continuum of disorders previously defined as Frasier syndrome and Denys-Drash syndrome.

Smith-Lemli-Opitz Syndrome

Smith-Lemli-Opitz syndrome (SLOS) is a disorder of cholesterol biosynthesis caused by deficiency of the 7-dehydrocholesterol reductase enzyme resulting from pathogenic variants in the *DHCR7* gene. Abnormal cholesterol metabolism leads to decreased androgen production that can manifest as underdeveloped external genitals in males. This syndrome is also characterized by congenital anomalies and intellectual disability (Fig. 66.5) and is discussed further in Chapter 67.

Androgen Insensitivity Syndrome

Androgen insensitivity syndrome (AIS) is caused by hemizygous pathogenic variants in the *AR* (androgen receptor) gene on the X chromosome. There is a spectrum of phenotypes seen in individuals with a 46,XY karyotype, typically characterized by varying degrees of undermasculinization of the external genitalia, abnormal development of secondary sexual characteristics in puberty, and infertility.

Disorders of Sexual Development

The definition of disorders of sexual development (DSD) has evolved with improved understanding of the embryologic and genetic

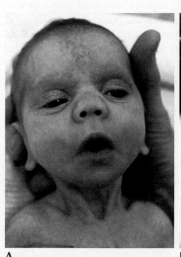
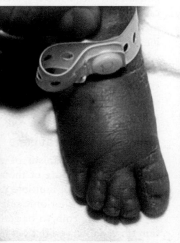
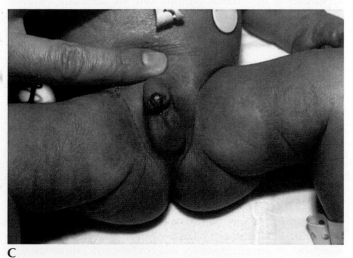

Fig. 66.5 Smith-Lemli-Opitz Syndrome. Note the narrow frontal area, somewhat prominent glabella, ptosis, broad nasal tip with anteverted nares, and micrognathia (A), two-three syndactyly of the toes (B), and hypospadias (C). (Reused with permission from Jones KL, Jones MC, Del Campo MD. In: Jones KL, Jones MC, Del Campo MD. *Smith's recognizable patterns of human malformation.* 8th ed. Philadelphia, PA: Elsevier; 2022: 134-173, Smith-Lemli-Opitz Syndrome, Figs 1C, 2C, 2D.)

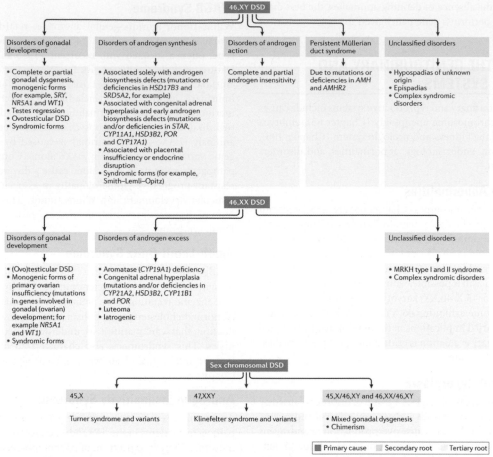

Fig. 66.6 Classification of Disorders of Sexual Development. (Reused with permission from Cools M, Nordenström A, Robeva R, et al; COST Action BM1303 working group 1. Caring for individuals with a difference of sex development (DSD): a consensus statement. *Nat Rev Endocrinol.* 2018;14[7]:415-429. doi: 10.1038/s41574-018-0010-8. PMID: 29769693; PMCID: PMC7136158, Figure 1.)

mechanisms of these conditions. Historically, the term DSD has been used to define conditions in which the chromosomal sex and the appearance of the external genitalia were not congruent. However, more recent discussions have emphasized a broader approach to classification and definition of these DSDs (Fig. 66.6), encompassing some of the disorders discussed previously.

SEQUENCES AND ASSOCIATIONS

Pierre Robin Sequence

Pierre Robin sequence (PRS) is a triad of micrognathia, glossoptosis, and a U-shaped cleft palate (Fig. 66.7). The incidence is approximately 1 per 10,000 births. Most cases result from hypoplasia of the mandible that occurs before the ninth week of development, leading to posterior displacement of the tongue, preventing palatal closure and producing a cleft palate. PRS can occur as an isolated abnormality; however, it can also occur as part of a genetic syndrome. The most common syndromes associated with PRS are Stickler syndrome, 22q11.2 deletion syndrome, and Treacher Collins syndrome. Detailed evaluation for associated congenital anomalies and confirmatory genetic testing is essential for an infant with PRS.

Oligohydramnios Sequence (Potter Sequence)

Potter sequence is caused by oligohydramnios secondary to renal agenesis or other renal anomalies that reduce fetal urine output production.

In some cases, the underlying cause of Potter sequence may be a genetic disorder, such as a chromosomal disorder or polycystic kidney disease. Often, Potter sequence is sporadic and not associated with a genetic cause. The decreased volume of amniotic fluid results in external compression of the fetus, restricts fetal movements, alters the dynamics of lung liquid movement, and results in the associated anomalies. This condition is characterized by pulmonary hypoplasia, limb deformities, growth restriction, and distinctive facial features such as depression of the nasal tip, abnormal ear folding, and wrinkled skin. Potter sequence is often lethal secondary to severe pulmonary hypoplasia and pneumothorax.

Amniotic Band Sequence

The primary mechanism of amniotic band sequence (ABS) is thought to be rupture of the amnion in early pregnancy causing the development of multiple loose mesodermic strands (amniotic bands) from the chorionic side of the amnion that adhere to and/or entangle the embryo or germ disc. This can result in constriction rings, and in severe cases lead to vascular disruption and autoamputation of the involved structure. Constriction rings and limb or digital amputation are the most common findings, present in at least 80% of cases. The cause of amnion rupture is unknown in most cases, though evaluation for underlying genetic causes of limb abnormalities should be considered before attributing symptoms to ABS.

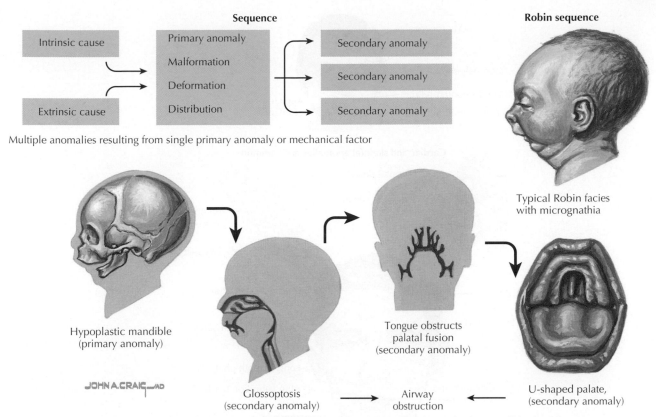

Fig. 66.7 Pierre Robin Sequence. Sequence of anomalies initiated by hypoplastic mandible that causes glossptosis. Resulting palatal defect with glossoptosis may obstruct airway.

VACTERL Association

VACTERL is a spectrum of various combinations of **v**ertebral defects, **a**nal atresia, **c**ardiac defects, **t**racheoesophageal fistula with **e**sophageal atresia (TE), **r**adial or **r**enal dysplasia, and **l**imb anomalies. In addition to the features described in the acronym, other features include a single umbilical artery and prenatal growth deficiency. VACTERL is typically a sporadic disorder; there is currently no known genetic cause. Genetic disorders with features in common with VACTERL syndrome include Feingold syndrome, CHARGE syndrome, Fanconi anemia, Townes-Brocks syndrome, and Pallister-Hall syndrome. Clinical evaluation for these conditions should be considered before a diagnosis of VACTERL is made.

TERATOGENIC MALFORMATIONS

A teratogen is an agent that can cause abnormalities in the form or function of a developing fetus. It acts by producing cell death, altering normal growth of tissues, or interfering with normal cellular differentiation or other morphologic processes. Approximately 4% to 6% of birth defects are caused by exposure to teratogens in the environment. Teratogenic exposure in a fetus may mimic any number of genetic syndromes. A thorough history and evaluation is necessary to determine whether congenital anomalies are due to a genetic or teratogenic cause.

Infectious Agents

Fetal defects secondary to infection are usually due to direct invasion of fetal tissues, leading to damage from inflammation and cell death. Agents known to be toxic to the fetus include toxoplasmosis, rubella, cytomegalovirus, herpes, syphilis, varicella, parvovirus B19, Zika virus, and lymphocytic choriomeningitis virus. Anomalies such as microcephaly, cerebral or hepatic calcifications, intrauterine growth restriction, hepatosplenomegaly, cardiac malformations, limb hypoplasia, and hydrocephalus are suggestive of fetal infection.

Maternal Conditions

Insulin-dependent diabetes mellitus is associated with a twofold to threefold increase in risk for congenital anomalies, including congenital heart disease, cleft palate, colobomas, and spina bifida. Maternal phenylketonuria, if phenylalanine levels are not adequately controlled in the pregnant mother, can cause with microcephaly, intellectual disability, and congenital heart disease in the fetus (Chapter 69).

Intrauterine Drug Exposure

Folic acid antagonists increase the risk for neural tube defects and possibly cardiovascular defects, oral clefts, and urinary tract defects. Oral isotretinoin is associated with ear anomalies, CNS malformations, hydrocephalus, neuronal brain migration defects, cerebellum abnormalities, severe intellectual disability, seizures, optic nerve/retinal abnormalities, conotruncal heart defects, thymic defects, and dysmorphic features. Cholesterol-lowering agents disrupt cholesterol biosynthesis, which is important in cell membrane morphogenesis, leading to limb malformations, congenital heart disease, and CNS abnormalities. Alcohol has the potential to cause deleterious effects at all stages of gestation. Significant alcohol exposure during the first trimester is associated with facial anomalies and major structural anomalies, including

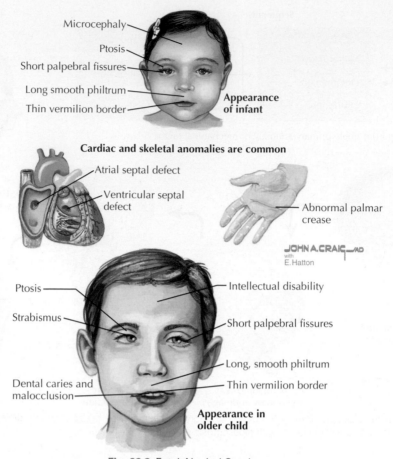

Cardiac and skeletal anomalies are common

Fig. 66.8 Fetal Alcohol Syndrome.

microcephaly, short palpebral fissures, smooth philtrum with thin and smooth upper lip, joint anomalies, and congenital cardiac effects (Fig. 66.8). The neurodevelopmental features of fetal alcohol syndrome are discussed in Chapter 67.

FUTURE DIRECTIONS

Congenital anomalies are a physical manifestation of a spectrum of causes, from genetic syndromes to teratogenic exposures to embryologic defects. A thorough history and physical examination are essential to understanding whether an underlying cause is present. As genetic testing continues to improve and clinical exome and genome sequencing become more common, novel genes and mechanisms contributing to patterns of congenital anomalies will surely be elucidated.

SUGGESTED READINGS

Available online.

67

Syndromic Intellectual Disability

Katherine M. Szigety and Sarah E. Sheppard

✳ CLINICAL VIGNETTE

A 5-year-old boy presents for a well-child check as a new patient. His medical history is significant for macrocephaly, asthma, history of speech therapy through early intervention, and concerns for autism spectrum disorder.

His examination shows weight 70th percentile, length 75th percentile, and head circumference greater than 95th percentile (50th percentile for an adult). He has a pectus excavatum and joint hyperextensibility. There is a soft, mobile mass measuring about 2 × 2 inches on the abdomen. There are multiple hyperpigmented macules on the penis.

This presentation is highly suspicious for PTEN hamartoma syndrome. PTEN hamartoma syndrome should be considered in an individual with developmental delay or autism spectrum disorder and macrocephaly.

Intellectual disability (ID) is defined as limitation in cognitive and adaptive behaviors, including conceptual, social, and practical skills, that occurs before the age of 18. The etiology of ID is multifactorial, including genetic, metabolic, mitochondrial, environmental, and perinatal contributions. In the pediatric population, the prevalence of ID in children from ages 3 to 17 years old is 1.1%. The prevalence of milder ID tends to be more labile due to variability in environmental and perinatal factors, whereas the prevalence of severe ID is generally stable, as genetics play a more substantial role.

This chapter provides an overview of the evaluation and differential diagnosis of the most common syndromic causes of ID, including the etiology, pathogenesis, epidemiology, and clinical presentation. In addition to the diseases presented here, ID can be found in a subset of chromosomal disorders, such as Williams, Cri-du-Chat, and 22q11.2 deletion syndromes (Chapter 65) as well as metabolic disorders (Chapters 69 through 71). At the time of publication, almost 1300 syndromes with ID have been described. The following differential diagnosis is by no means exhaustive but should serve as a framework for the initial evaluation of the patient with suspected syndromic ID.

EVALUATION AND MANAGEMENT

Evaluation of an individual with ID includes a thorough history, including pregnancy history (maternal age, medication or substance use, infection), birth history (prematurity, delivery complications), perinatal history, developmental history, and family history (Fig. 67.1). It is important to distinguish ID from developmental delay, which is a delay in the acquisition of language, motor, and/or cognitive milestones typically occurring before 5 years of age. Not all children with developmental delay will be diagnosed with ID.

Workup of ID can include laboratory testing for lead and ferritin. A comprehensive physical evaluation is critical to assess somatometric measurements and dysmorphic features. Subspecialty evaluations to be considered include:

- Audiology for hearing loss
- Developmental pediatrics for concomitant behavioral concerns
- Neurology for structural brain abnormality as a cause for ID
- Pediatric genetics and/or metabolism for genetic causes and metabolic evaluation

A genetic evaluation for ID is essential. Identification of the underlying cause is crucial for anticipatory guidance, recurrence counseling and, in some cases, targeted treatment. The initial genetic evaluation includes screening for fragile X and chromosomal disorders by *FMR1* CGG repeat testing and chromosomal microarray (Chapter 64). This testing strategy is estimated to yield a molecular cause in about 10% to 20% of individuals with ID, with higher diagnosis rate in those with coexisting neurodevelopmental disorders or congenital anomalies. Additional syndrome-specific single-gene or multigene panel testing may be warranted depending on the patient's presentation. If not done previously, negative preliminary genetic testing should prompt referral to a clinical geneticist for further evaluation and genetic testing. A clinical geneticist may choose whole exome sequencing as a first- or second-line test, depending on the patient phenotype. If a specific syndrome is identified, specific management guidelines based on the manifestations of the disorder should be recommended by a pediatric geneticist.

FRAGILE X SYNDROME

Fragile X syndrome (FXS) is an X-linked disorder caused by a CGG repeat expansion greater than 200 in the promoter of the *FMR1* gene, leading to abnormal gene methylation and silencing (Fig. 67.2). ID in FXS is typically mild to moderate. Additional clinical features include autism spectrum disorder (ASD), hyperactivity, hypersensitivity to stimuli, mood lability, and disordered sleep. Typical physical features include a long face with large ears, a prominent jaw and forehead, and macroorchidism (in males). In infancy and early childhood, individuals with FXS may present with hypotonia, gastroesophageal reflux, seizures, strabismus, joint laxity, pes planus, scoliosis, and recurrent otitis media. Females who are heterozygous for an *FMR1* full mutation can have milder features and can have premature ovarian failure. Anticipation, a phenomenon in which the trinucleotide repeat expands and causes a more severe phenotype in subsequent generations, can occur in FXS.

NEUROFIBROMATOSIS TYPE 1

Neurofibromatosis type 1 (NF1) is an autosomal dominant disorder caused by monoallelic loss-of-function pathogenic variants in *NF1*,

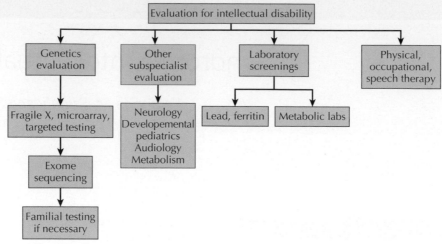

Fig. 67.1 Suggested Evaluation for an Individual With Intellectual Disability.

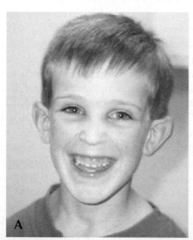

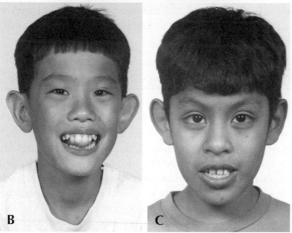

Fig. 67.2 Facial Features of Children With Fragile X Syndrome. Boys with fragile X syndrome. Note the long faces, prominent jaws, large ears, and similar characteristics of children from different ethnic groups: Caucasian (A), Asian (B), and Hispanic (C). (Reused with permission from Jorde LB, Carey JC, Bamshad MJ, White RL. *Medical genetics*. 3rd ed. Philadelphia, PA: Elsevier; 2003:99, Figure 5-13.)

which encodes the tumor suppressor neurofibromin (Fig. 67.3). Approximately half of cases of NF1 are caused by de novo pathogenic variants and the other half of cases are inherited. Diagnostic criteria are described in Chapter 111. Up to 80% of patients have learning or

behavioral difficulties, with 6% to 7% of NF1 patients diagnosed with ID. Examination is notable for macrocephaly; short stature; café-au-lait macules with smooth, regular borders; axillary and/or inguinal freckling; neurofibromas; and juvenile xanthogranulomas. Ocular findings can include Lisch nodules and optic gliomas. Any young child with typical café-au-lait macules should be evaluated for NF1, and radiographs of the lower legs should be performed to identify tibial pseudoarthrosis. NF1 patients should be monitored for scoliosis and hypertension secondary to NF1-associated vasculopathy.

TUBEROUS SCLEROSIS COMPLEX

Tuberous sclerosis complex (TSC) is an autosomal dominant disease caused by monoallelic pathogenic variants in *TSC1* or *TSC2*, arising de novo in about two-thirds of patients (see Fig. 111.1). Over 60% of TSC patients have ID. Patients are at risk for developing TSC-associated neuropsychiatric disorder, which includes ID, autism spectrum disorder (ASD), attention-deficit/hyperactivity disorder (ADHD) and psychiatric issues, such as self-injurious behavior, anxiety, and depression. Physical changes manifest in multiple organ systems because of loss of TSC1 or TSC2 tumor suppressor activity. Skin findings include hypomelanotic macules, facial angiofibromas, shagreen patches, fibrous cephalic plaques, confetti lesions, and ungual fibromas. TSC patients also may have retinal hamartomas and achromic patches. Central nervous system lesions include subependymal nodules, cortical tubers, and giant cell astrocytomas. Seizures and infantile spasms may develop. Renal imaging may identify renal angiomyolipomas and epithelial cysts. Cardiac anomalies include rhabdomyomas, which are largest during the neonatal period and can cause outflow obstruction. Rhabdomyomas typically regress spontaneously; in some patients arrythmias may develop secondary to residual tumor cells in the myocardium.

RETT SYNDROME

Rett syndrome is an X-linked dominant disorder caused by pathogenic variants in *MECP2*. It primarily affects females and is most often caused by de novo pathogenic variants. Children typically present with developmental regression at 6 to 18 months of age. Regression is most pronounced in language and motor skills, and children classically display stereotypical hand movements and bruxism (Fig. 67.4). ID is moderate to severe. Individuals with Rett syndrome can have additional behavioral concerns, such as ASD, disrupted sleep patterns, paroxysmal laughing, and episodes

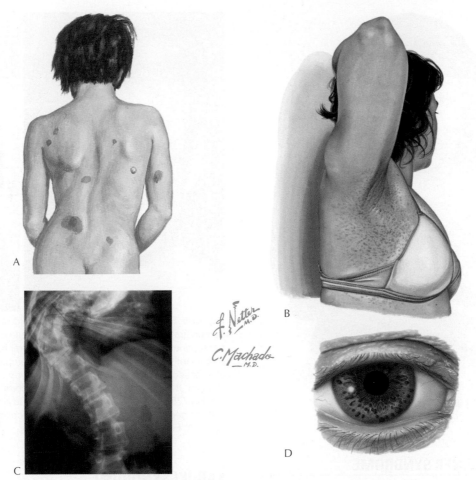

Fig. 67.3 Characteristic Features of Neurofibromatosis. (A) Girl with typical café-au-lait spots but only a few skin nodules. Relatively mild neurobromatous scoliosis is present. Café-au-lait spots are uniformly hyperpigmented flat macules—6 or more café-au-lait spots are highly suggestive of NF1. Cutaneous neurofibromas are soft and fleshy tumors that arise from the peripheral nerve sheath, the trunk being the most common location. (B) Dense axillary and inguinal freckling is rarely found in the absence of NF1. (C) Severe scoliosis. X-ray lm showing typical sharp angulation unresponsive to corrective measures, often seen in neurobromatosis. (D) Lisch nodules are hamartomas on the iris. They are raised and frequently pigmented.

of inconsolable crying. Physical anomalies include growth retardation, acquired microcephaly, and scoliosis. Patients should be monitored for seizures, episodic apnea, hyperpnea, and QTc prolongation.

SMITH-LEMLI-OPITZ SYNDROME

Smith-Lemli-Opitz syndrome (SLOS) is an autosomal recessive disorder caused by pathogenic variants in *DHCR7*, encoding 7-dehydrocholesterol reductase. ID is typically moderate to severe, although patients with milder disease can have mild ID. Behavioral concerns include ASD, sensory hyperreactivity, irritability, sleep cycle disturbances and self-injury. SLOS should be considered when ID is seen in combination with genital differences and two-three syndactyly of the toes. Physical examination is additionally notable for small size, microcephaly, cleft palate, dental anomalies, and characteristic facies, including narrow forehead, epicanthus, ptosis, short nose with anteverted nares, low-set ears, and micrognathia (Chapter 66, Fig. 66.5). Additional features include postaxial polydactyly, underdeveloped external genitalia, hypospadias, and congenital heart defects, including atrioventricular canal defects, anomalous pulmonary venous return, and pulmonary stenosis. Hypotonia, gastrointestinal

and feeding problems, and photosensitivity are common. The diagnosis is supported by elevated serum 7-dehydrocholesterol. Serum cholesterol is typically low but can be normal in some patients and is therefore not clinically reliable for diagnosis. Cholesterol supplementation may be beneficial.

SOTOS SYNDROME

Sotos syndrome is an autosomal dominant disorder caused by monoallelic loss-of-function pathogenic variants in *NSD1*, with more than 95% of cases arising de novo (Fig. 67.5). ID is found in up to 85% of patients and ranges from mild to severe, with particular difficulty with quantitative reasoning. Common behavioral concerns include ASD, ADHD, phobias, aggression, and impulsivity. A hallmark of Sotos syndrome is overgrowth, manifesting as macrocephaly and tall stature. Characteristic facial features include a prominent forehead, long and narrow face, downslanting palpebral fissures, and malar flushing. Additional concerns include seizures, hypotonia in infancy, scoliosis, joint hyperlaxity, and hyperinsulinism. Cardiac and renal anomalies can occur and should be screened for during evaluation.

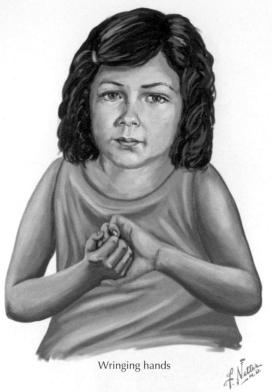

Wringing hands

Fig. 67.4 Rett Syndrome.

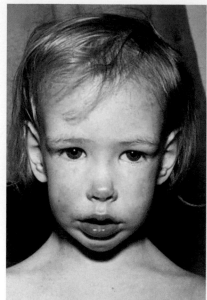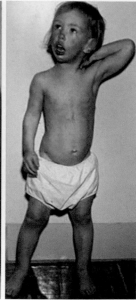

Fig. 67.5 Sotos Syndrome. This 3-year-old girl with Sotos syndrome demonstrates typical facial features: macrocephaly, dolichocephaly, frontoparietal balding, downslanted palpebral fissures, flushed cheeks, prominently pointed chin, with premature eruption of teeth and accelerated osseous maturation. (Reused with permission from Burkardt DD, Graham JM. Abnormal body size and proportion. In: Pyeritz R, Korf B, Grody W. *Emery and Rimoin's principles and practice of medical genetics and genomics: clinical principles and applications.* 7th ed. Philadelphia, PA: Elsevier; 2018:81-143, Fig. 4.15.)

WIEDEMANN-STEINER SYNDROME

Wiedemann-Steiner syndrome is a clinically recognizable syndrome caused by monoallelic pathogenic variants in *KMT2A*, most often arising in a de novo fashion. ID is mild to moderate, and children also may have speech and language delay. Behavioral issues include anxiety and aggression. Patients typically have short stature, hypertrichosis of the elbows and back, and characteristic facial features, including long eyelashes, thick or arched eyebrows, downslanting palpebral fissures and wide nasal bridge (Fig. 67.6). Other issues include failure to thrive, constipation, vertebral and other skeletal anomalies, structural brain anomalies, congenital heart disease, renal anomalies, immune differences, and dental anomalies.

KABUKI SYNDROME

Kabuki syndrome is caused by pathogenic variants in *KMT2D* (autosomal dominant) or *KDM6A* (X-linked); both genes encode members of the ASCOM complex, which plays a role in gene activation (Fig. 67.7). As an X-linked disease, *KDM6A*-related Kabuki syndrome primarily affects males, but heterozygous females typically have a mild disease manifestation. ID is mild to moderate, with patients demonstrating particular difficulty with adaptive skills and delayed speech. Additional behavioral features include ADHD, disrupted sleep, anxiety, and ASD. Physical examination is notable for characteristic facies of long palpebral fissures with

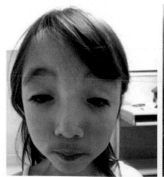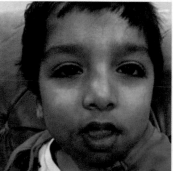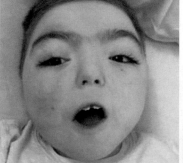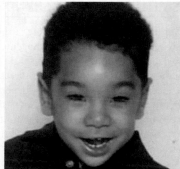

Fig. 67.6 Wiedemann-Steiner Syndrome—Facial Features. Typical facial features of WSS include thick or arched eyebrows, hypertelorism, long eyelashes, downslanting palpebral fissures, and a wide nasal bridge. (Reused with permission from Sheppard SE, Campbell IM, Harr MH, et al. Expanding the genotypic and phenotypic spectrum in a diverse cohort of 104 individuals with Wiedemann-Steiner syndrome. *Am J Med Genet* Part A. 2021;1-17, Fig. 2a, 2c. https://doi.org/10.1002/ajmg.a.62124.)

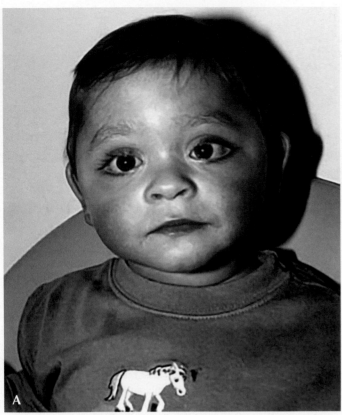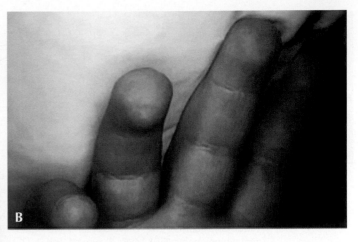

Fig. 67.7 Kabuki Syndrome. An 18-month-old boy with Kabuki syndrome with long palpebral fissures and eversion of the lateral portion of the lower eyelid (A) and protruding prominent finger pads (B). (Reused with permission from Jones KL, Jones MC, Del Campo MD. In: Jones KL, Jones MC, Del Campo MD. *Smith's recognizable patterns of human malformation.* 8th ed. Philadelphia PA: Elsevier; 2022:152-187, Kabuki syndrome, Figs. 1A and 2D.)

everted lower eyelids, arched eyebrows, long eyelashes, short columella with flattened nasal tip, and large, cupped ears. Additional findings include a high arched palate, cleft lip and/or palate, hypotonia, short stature, scoliosis, joint laxity, and persistence of fetal finger pads. Patients may have gastrointestinal anomalies, such as congenital diaphragmatic hernia, left-sided heart lesions, such as aortic coarctation, urogenital anomalies including renal dysplasia, cryptorchidism and hypospadias, hyperinsulinism, hearing loss, and immunodeficiency. Patients may have gastrointestinal anomalies, such as congenital diaphragmatic hernia; left-sided heart lesions, such as aortic coarctation; urogenital anomalies including renal dysplasia, cryptorchidism and hypospadias; hyperinsulinism; hearing loss; and immunodeficiency.

RUBINSTEIN-TAYBI SYNDROME

Rubinstein-Taybi syndrome (RSTS) is an autosomal dominant disorder resulting from monoallelic pathogenic variants in *CREBBP* or *EP300*. Most cases arise from de novo pathogenic variants, although parental germline mosaicism has been reported. ID is generally moderate, and children also can have developmental delay, with a subset remaining nonverbal. Patients also may have behavioral challenges, including impulsivity, distractibility, aggression, and self-injury. Classic findings on physical examination are broad and angulated thumbs and halluces, brachydactyly, and characteristic facies of downslanted palpebral fissures, convex nasal bridge with low-hanging columella, grimacing smile and high arched palate.

Children with RSTS have normal prenatal growth, but postnatal growth deficiency results in short stature. Additional medical concerns include ophthalmologic anomalies, such as coloboma, ptosis, and strabismus; dental anomalies; urogenital anomalies, such as vesicoureteral reflux, cryptorchidism, and hypospadias; and congenital heart disease. Patients also can have frequent infections, obstructive sleep apnea, gastroesophageal reflux, and constipation. There is an increased incidence of meningiomas and pilomatricomas.

PTEN HAMARTOMA SYNDROME

PTEN hamartoma syndrome is caused by monoallelic pathogenic variants in *PTEN*, encoding the PTEN tumor suppressor (Fig. 67.8). An autosomal dominant disorder, it may arise de novo or can be inherited from a parent with a *PTEN*-related disorder. This group of disorders includes clinical entities such as Cowden syndrome and Bannayan-Riley-Ruvalcaba syndrome. Patients present with ID, developmental delay, and/or ASD. Physical examination is notable for macrocephaly, macrosomia, hamartomas, penile freckling, pectus excavatum, joint hyperextensibility, and lipomas. The penile freckling is pathognomonic and seen in about 60% of individuals with *PTEN*-related disorders. About 50% of individuals will have vascular malformations. *PTEN*-related disorders have a cancer predisposition, and patients should be monitored for thyroid, endometrial, and breast cancer. Children should have yearly thyroid ultrasounds and skin examinations.

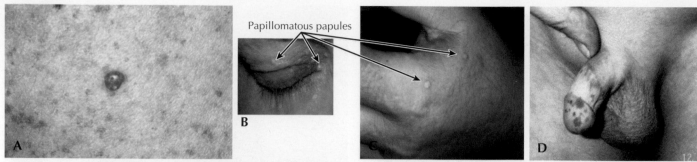

Fig. 67.8 Dermatologic Findings in PTEN-Related Disorders. (A) Trichilemmoma. (B) Papillomatous papules in the periocular region. (C) Papillomatous papules on the dorsum of the hand. (D) Lentigines on glans and shaft of penis. ([A–C] (Reused with permission from Yehia L, Eng C. PTEN Hamartoma Tumor Syndrome. 2001 Nov 29 [Updated February 11, 2021]. In: Adam MP, Ardinger HH, Pagon RA, et al., eds. *GeneReviews* [Internet]. Seattle, WA: University of Washington, Seattle; 1993-2021. Available from: https://www.ncbi. nlm.nih.gov/books/NBK1488/, Figures 1 and 2. D, reused with permission from Erkek E, Hizel S, Sanlý C, et al. Clinical and histopathological findings in Bannayan-Riley-Ruvalcaba syndrome. *J Am Acad Dermatol.* 2005;53(4):639-643. doi: 10.1016/j.jaad.2005.06.022. PMID: 16198785, Figure 2.)

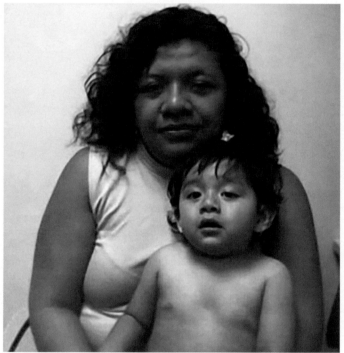

Fig. 67.9 Noonan Syndrome. Parent and child with Noonan syndrome with hypertelorism and downslanting palpebral fissures. Note low-set and posteriorly rotated ears in the child. (Reused with permission from Jones KL, Jones MC, Del Campo MD. In *Smith's recognizable patterns of human malformation.* 8th ed. Philadelphia, PA: Elsevier; 2022:152-187, Noonan syndrome, Fig. 2C.)

NOONAN SYNDROME

Autosomal dominant Noonan syndrome (NS) is caused by pathogenic variants in genes associated with the RAS pathway, most commonly *PTPN11* (50% of cases), *SOS1, RAF1, RIT1, KRAS, NRAS, BRAF,* or *MAP2K1,* with up to 75% of patients inheriting the disorder from an affected parent (Fig. 67.9). Pathogenic variants in *LZTR1* can cause both dominant genetics and recessive forms of Noonan syndrome. Children can present with ID, learning difficulties, and

developmental delay. Behavioral concerns include inattention, poor social skills, anxiety, and depression. Physical examination is notable for short stature, widely spaced nipples, hyperconvex nails, relative macrocephaly, and classic facial features, including hypertelorism, downslanting palpebral fissures, low-set and posteriorly rotated ears, a low posterior hairline, and excess nuchal skin. With age, the face appears more triangular in shape and the webbing of the neck is more prominent. Medical complications of NS include cardiovascular anomalies such as pulmonic stenosis and hypertrophic cardiomyopathy and urogenital anomalies such as renal hypoplasia and cryptorchidism. Lymphatic dysfunction bleeding disorders and myeloproliferative disorders are additional features of this syndrome.

CORNELIA DE LANGE SYNDROME

Autosomal dominant Cornelia de Lange syndrome (CdLS) is caused by pathogenic variants in *NIPBL* (60% of cases), *RAD21,* or *SMC3,* whereas X-linked CdLS is due to pathogenic variants in *HDAC8* or *SMC1A.* The large majority of cases arise de novo, although X-linked CdLS can be inherited from a carrier female. ID is severe, and children may also present with ASD and self-injurious behavior. Characteristic facial features include microbrachycephaly, low anterior hairline, synophrys (fusion of eyebrows) with arched brows, long and thick eyelashes, ptosis, low-set and posteriorly rotated ears with thick helices, depressed nasal bridge with upturned nasal tip and anteverted nares, long and smooth philtrum, thin upper vermilion border with downturned corners of the mouth, small and widely spaced teeth, high-arched palate, and micrognathia (Fig. 67.10). Additional features include growth failure, upper limb anomalies such as micromelia and oligodactyly, cardiovascular anomalies such as ventricular septal defect and pulmonic stenosis, gastrointestinal anomalies such as congenital diaphragmatic hernia and malrotation, and urogenital anomalies such as vesicoureteral reflux and cryptorchidism. Patients may also develop recurrent infections and thrombocytopenia.

ANGELMAN SYNDROME

Angelman syndrome is caused by loss of *UBE3A* expression, most commonly caused by lack of maternal imprinting of chromosome

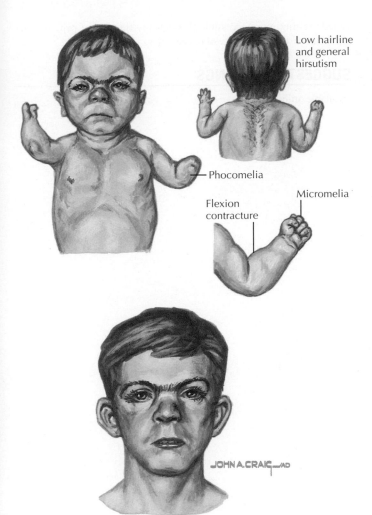

Fig. 67.10 Facial Features and Limb Differences in Cornelia De Lange Syndrome. (A) Infant facies with thick, conjoined eyebrows (synophrys) and thin lips. (B) Adult facies with synophrys and long eyelashes.

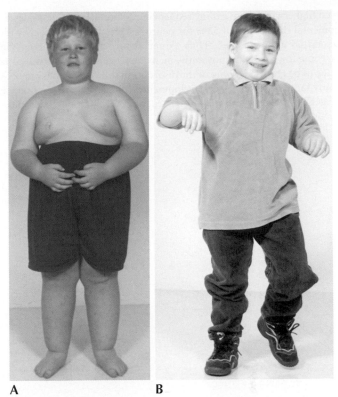

Fig. 67.11 Prader-Willi and Angelman Syndromes. Illustration of the effect of imprinting on chromosome 15 deletions. (A) Inheritance of the deletion from the father produces Prader-Willi syndrome (note the inverted V-shaped upper lip, small hands, and truncal obesity). (B) Inheritance of the deletion from the mother produces Angelman syndrome (note the characteristic posture). (Reused with permission from Jorde LB, Carey JC, Bamshad MJ, White RL. *Medical genetics*. 3rd ed. St. Louis, MO: Mosby; 2003:78, Figure 4.20.)

15q11.2-q13, or in approximately 10% of cases, a pathogenic variant of *UBE3A* (Fig. 67.11). ID is typically severe to profound, with particularly pronounced language deficits. Developmental delay is first apparent around 6 months of age. Characteristic behavioral features include a happy disposition with frequent laughing and excitability, often manifested as repetitive hand flapping. Physical examination findings include acquired microcephaly, tongue protrusion, and widely spaced teeth. Neurological features include hypotonia, ataxia, a characteristic wide-based gait with arms held in flexion, hyperreflexia, and seizures.

PRADER-WILLI SYNDROME

Prader-Willi syndrome (PWS) is due to absence of paternally inherited chromosome 15q11.2-q13 (see Fig. 67.11). Most often it results from maternal uniparental disomy, but it can also arise secondary to an imprinting defect. ID is generally mild, with average IQ scores in the 60s to 70s. Infants have severe hypotonia, which can present as decreased fetal movement before birth, and often

results in poor feeding and failure to thrive. Children present with global developmental delay. Characteristic behaviors include food-seeking, temper tantrums, compulsions such as skin picking, and disordered sleep. Individuals with PWS are short in stature and may develop obesity because of hyperphagia. Physical features include a narrow bifrontal diameter, almond-shaped palpebral fissures, a thin upper vermilion border, down-turned corners of the mouth, micrognathia, and small hands and feet. Genital hypoplasia and cryptorchidism are typical. Additional findings include scoliosis and albinism (hypopigmentation of the skin, eyes, and hair) because of pathogenic changes in the *P* gene which is in the same locus.

FUTURE DIRECTIONS

Genetic evaluation is an essential part of the workup for intellectual disability to provide information about prognosis, management, and recurrence risk. It is important to recognize the indications for genetics referral. Current guidelines recommend fragile X testing and chromosomal microarray as first-line genetic testing for individuals with ID.

Recent work has evaluated the diagnostic yield of different types of genetic testing in individuals with neurodevelopmental disorders. In one study, fragile X testing showed 1.2% yield compared to previous yield of 10% to 20% from microarray. A meta-analysis showed an even higher yield from exome sequencing: about 36% for neurodevelopmental disorders and 53% for neurodevelopmental disorders with associated abnormalities. Thus exome sequencing is becoming the first-line test for ID. Importantly, many novel genetic causes will continue to be reported. Some of the disorders in this chapter have molecularly targeted therapies in development, highlighting the importance of genetic diagnosis. Future infrastructure development may make genetic testing more accessible through the training of primary care clinicians or the availability of telegenetics.

SUGGESTED READINGS

Available online.

68

Musculoskeletal and Connective Tissue Disorders

Michaela B. Reinhart and Staci Kallish

 CLINICAL VIGNETTE

A 10-year-old girl presents to her pediatrician for back pain. She has had back pain for the past year that has progressively gotten worse despite using a brace, though she does not report any physical limitations. She has a family history of scoliosis. On physical examination, her spine has thoracic curvature and pectus excavatum is noted. Her fingers appear long and her growth chart shows she has been growing in height rapidly. Radiograph confirms she has scoliosis.

The presentation of increased growth velocity, scoliosis, and physical features raise concern for an inherited connective tissue disorder, specifically Marfan syndrome. Given the risk for cardiovascular disease and other comorbidities, expedited diagnosis and management are important.

Inherited connective tissue disorders comprise a group of multisystem disorders, some most notable for their cardiac morbidity and mortality. More than 200 inherited connective tissue disorders exist; this chapter will focus on the most common. Many patients with these syndromes have relatively normal lifespans with regular preventive care, though some disorders may have initial manifestations with life-threatening sequelae.

ETIOLOGY AND PATHOGENESIS

Inherited connective tissue disorders result from genetic mutations that compromise the supportive function of connective tissues for the body (Table 68.1). Fibrillin, collagen, and elastin build the extracellular matrix, a principal component of connective tissue that offers support and structure. Mutations of the genes coding for these three proteins, or those with which they interact, lead to connective tissue disorders. The mutations themselves can alter not only the structure of the proteins but also their ability to perform standard molecular interactions that maintain the integrity of the connective tissue.

CLINICAL PRESENTATION

Clinical findings for inherited connective tissue disorders vary both among and within the disorders depending on the specific pathogenic variant involved, as well as penetrance. Ocular, cardiovascular, and musculoskeletal findings are often the primary signs. The marfanoid habitus (Fig. 68.1), characterized by disproportionately long limbs (dolichostenomelia), arachnodactyly, joint hyperlaxity, and arched palate with tooth crowding, may manifest with some or all of these characteristics in disorders outside of Marfan syndrome. Ocular findings include myopia and ectopia lentis, and patients may present with decreased visual acuity or vision loss. Cardiovascular abnormalities tend to lead to the most serious complications. Those with an inherited connective tissue disorder may present emergently with aortic dissection. This chapter will also discuss inherited disorders of the skeletal system, including osteogenesis imperfecta and skeletal dysplasias.

EVALUATION AND MANAGEMENT

The clinical examination is key to evaluation in inherited connective tissue disorders. Physical examination findings should guide the provider's clinical suspicion to prompt further workup, given the potential for devastating morbidity and mortality if clinical signs go unrecognized. Laboratory results are helpful for diagnostic confirmation, and imaging plays an important role in diagnosis and monitoring of disease progression.

Laboratory Tests

Inherited connective tissue disorders are primarily diagnosed by clinical evaluation. Molecular genetic testing can be useful for confirming diagnosis and for testing at-risk family members before clinical features develop. Single-gene testing, genetic panels, or

TABLE 68.1 Inheritance Patterns of Inherited Connective Tissue Disorders

Disorder	Inheritance	Gene
Marfan syndrome	Autosomal dominant	FBN1
Classic Ehlers-Danlos syndrome	Autosomal dominant	COL5A1/2
Hypermobile Ehlers-Danlos syndrome	Unknown	Unknown
Vascular Ehlers-Danlos syndrome	Autosomal dominant	COL3A1
Loeys-Dietz syndrome	Autosomal dominant	SMAD2/3, TGFB2, TGFBR1/2
Congenital contractural arachnodactyly	Autosomal dominant	FBN2
Stickler syndrome	Autosomal dominant or autosomal recessive	COL2A1, COL9A1/2/3, COL11A12
COL1A1/2 osteogenesis imperfecta	Autosomal dominant	COL1A1/2

Marfan syndrome

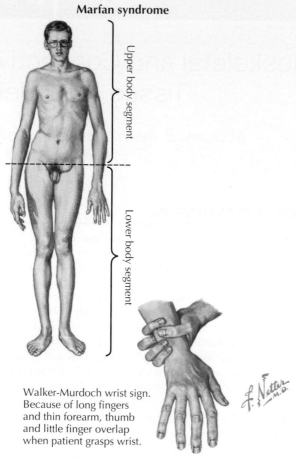

Walker-Murdoch wrist sign.
Because of long fingers
and thin forearm, thumb
and little finger overlap
when patient grasps wrist.

Fig. 68.1 Marfanoid Habitus.

whole exome sequencing are appropriate options depending on the presence of pathognomonic clinical signs and symptoms. Biochemical screening may be indicated if homocystinuria is suspected.

Imaging

Many inherited connective tissue disorders are associated with cardiovascular effects, such as aortic root dilatation. Echocardiogram or magnetic resonance angiography (MRA)/computed tomography angiography (CTA) can be used to evaluate cardiac function and aortic root dilatation. Radiography is useful for characterizing skeletal deformities and guiding orthopedic intervention as necessary, and dual-energy x-ray absorptiometry (DEXA) scan is useful in disorders associated with diminished bone density or demineralization.

MARFAN SYNDROME

Marfan syndrome is marked primarily by ocular, skeletal, and cardiovascular findings and is caused by pathogenic variants in the *FBN1* gene. History may be notable for myopia or ectopia lentis (lens dislocation). Physical features include disproportionately long extremities, pectus excavatum or carinatum from rib overgrowth, and joint laxity. Scoliosis is common and can be progressive. Facial features are notable for malar hypoplasia, micrognathia, arched palate and dental crowding.

Diagnosis is made based on criteria involving genetic testing for an *FBN1* pathogenic variant, imaging for aortic root dilatation, ophthalmologic evaluation, and systemic scoring. The revised Ghent criteria (Box 68.1) and the systemic scoring system (Box 68.2) are used to accomplish this evaluation.

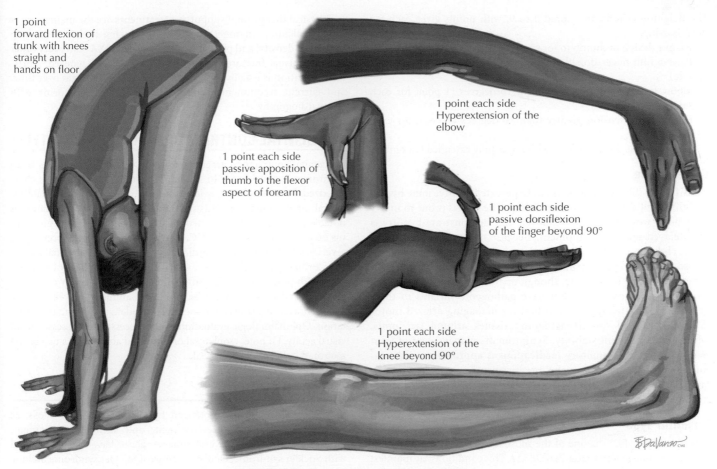

1 point
forward flexion of
trunk with knees
straight and
hands on floor

1 point each side
passive apposition of
thumb to the flexor
aspect of forearm

1 point each side
Hyperextension of the
elbow

1 point each side
passive dorsiflexion
of the finger beyond 90°

1 point each side
Hyperextension of the
knee beyond 90°

Fig. 68.2 Beighton Criteria for Hypermobility.

Cardiovascular abnormalities create the greatest source of morbidity and mortality in Marfan syndrome, which may manifest as aortic dilatation, mitral valve and tricuspid valve prolapse, and proximal pulmonary artery enlargement. Individuals with Marfan syndrome need monitoring for heart failure and worsening aortic dilatation, that may require aortic repair depending on the rate of dilation and level of aortic regurgitation. Annual ophthalmologic evaluation is necessary and can show myopia, ectopia lentis, and possibly retinal detachment or cataracts. Orthopedic evaluation is necessary for progressive scoliosis. Individuals with Marfan syndrome should avoid medications that cause vasoconstriction such as caffeine, and they should avoid heavy weight lifting and contact and competitive sports. Because of a predisposition for pneumothorax, positive pressure ventilation and breathing against resistance, such as playing brass instruments or scuba diving, should be avoided.

LOEYS-DIETZ SYNDROME

Loeys-Dietz syndrome (LDS) has skeletal, cutaneous, and vascular manifestations and is caused by pathogenic variants in *TGFBR1, TGFBR2, TGFB2, TGFB3, SMAD2,* or *SMAD3.* Physical examination may be notable for wide-spaced eyes, bifid uvula, and cleft palate. Pectus excavatum or carinatum, joint laxity, scoliosis, and arachnodactyly also may be observed. The skin can be translucent with easy bruising.

LDS can cause aneurysms and dissections of cerebral, thoracic, and abdominal arteries, along with arterial tortuosity. Aortic dissection can occur at a young age; beta-blockers and angiotensin receptor blockers are prescribed to reduce vascular resistance. MRA and CT of head, chest, abdomen, and pelvis are necessary to identify aneurysms and arterial tortuosity. Patent ductus arteriosus, atrial septal defect, and bicuspid aortic valve are relatively common, and heart function must be monitored over time.

Orthopedic evaluation can be necessary to manage scoliosis. LDS is associated with cervical spine instability, which may require surgery to protect the spinal cord. Radiography of the cervical spine should be performed for any procedure that will manipulate the neck given this predisposition. Individuals with LDS, similar to Marfan syndrome, have increased incidence of pneumothoraces and should therefore avoid breathing against resistance or positive pressure ventilation. They may require pleurodesis or removal of pulmonary blebs depending on the severity of recurrence.

EHLERS-DANLOS SYNDROME

Ehlers-Danlos syndrome (EDS) describes a group of disorders characterized by hyperextensibility and hypermobility. The types listed below (classic, hypermobile, and vascular) are the three most common forms of EDS, yet they also have a wide variety of clinical signs and severity. Other rare forms of EDS include arthrochalasia, dermatosparaxis, and kyphoscoliotic types, among others. The Beighton criteria (Fig. 68.2) are useful in characterizing joint hypermobility.

The Beighton criteria are scored 0 to 9, with points given each for the following:

- Passive flexion of thumb to forearm (1 point for each side)
- Passive fifth finger dorsiflexion greater than 90 (1 point for each side)
- Elbow hyperextension greater than 10 degrees (1 point for each side)
- Knee hyperextension greater than 10 degrees (1 point for each side)
- Ability to rest palms on floor with knees fully extended (1 point)

Classic Type

Classic EDS (cEDS) causes tissue hyperextensibility, joint hypermobility, and abnormal wound healing. The skin is prone to injury with poor wound healing. Children can demonstrate hypotonia and delayed motor development. Because of tissue hyperextensibility, children may have multiple hernias or rectal prolapse. cEDS is associated with pathogenic variants in the *COL5A1* and *COL5A2* genes, and rarely in *COL1A1*, though up to 10% of individuals who have clinical features may not have pathogenic variants in these genes. Physical therapy is important for managing delayed motor development and for strengthening tissues around lax joints, which improves joint stability. Symptomatic management of joint pain with antiinflammatory medications is appropriate, and vitamin C supplementation may help reduce bruising. Stitches for skin lacerations should be left in twice as long as normal for adequate healing.

Vascular Type

Vascular EDS (vEDS) is one of the most severe forms of EDS and is caused by pathogenic variants in *COL3A1*. This condition may manifest with decreased subcutaneous adipose tissue, a thin vermilion border, micrognathia, translucent skin, and aged appearance of extremities. Children often have distal joint hypermobility, club feet, and easy bruising. vEDS is characterized by arterial fragility and can cause arterial rupture without preceding dilation or aneurysm. Individuals with vEDS are also at increased risk for bowel or uterine rupture and this can be the manifesting symptom. A diagnosis of vEDS necessitates periodic arterial screening and blood pressure monitoring, and hypertension must be treated if it develops. Patients are instructed to seek medical care immediately for unexplained pain, and they should also avoid contact sports.

Hypermobile Type

Hypermobility spectrum disorders are classified by type of joint involvement and presence (or lack thereof) of syndromic features, and hypermobile EDS (hEDS) comprises the most extensive of these disorders. hEDS has primarily musculoskeletal findings with joint dislocations being common, which can lead to chronic pain. There is no known genetic cause for hEDS at the present time, and it is thought to be multifactorial in etiology. The diagnostic criteria include joint hypermobility, systemic features and family history, and exclusion of other diseases. Beighton scoring is helpful to elucidate hypermobility history. Systemic features encapsulate a broad range of involvement such as skin findings, hernias and pelvic floor prolapse, dental crowding, arachnodactyly, mitral valve prolapse, and aortic root dilatation. Physical examination may show bruising of the skin and piezogenic papules, but characteristic features found in other connective tissue disorders are less prominent. Patients may experience functional gastrointestinal disorders, autonomic cardiovascular dysfunction, and psychological disorders.

Physical therapy and supportive treatments are the mainstays for hEDS. Calcium, vitamin D, and weight-bearing exercise may help with bone density, and patients should have a DEXA scan every other year if unusual fractures occur and bone loss is diagnosed. Aortic root dilatation is usually mild when present and stabilizes over time, and current recommendations do not endorse monitoring with echocardiography.

CONGENITAL CONTRACTURAL ARACHNODACTYLY

Congenital contractural arachnodactyly (CCA), also known as Beals syndrome, is associated with mutations in the *FBN2* gene. It is characterized by multiple large joint contractures, marfanoid habitus, helical ear abnormalities, and arachnodactyly. Physical examination is notable for micrognathia, arched palate, muscle hypoplasia, and pectus excavatum or carinatum. CCA has a wide phenotypic spectrum of severity, which can include cardiovascular and gastrointestinal anomalies. Primary management of CCA includes management of contractures with physical and occupational therapy or surgery, if necessary. Kyphosis and scoliosis should be monitored annually, as well as aortic root diameter, because of the increased incidence of aortic root dilatation. Ophthalmologic evaluation is also necessary for assessment of visual acuity. Of note, esophageal or duodenal atresia and small bowel malrotation have been observed.

STICKLER SYNDROME

Stickler syndrome is characterized by vision and hearing loss, as well as midfacial underdevelopment, and skeletal involvement. Pathogenic variants in several collagen genes have been associated with Stickler syndrome. Ocular findings of Stickler syndrome include myopia, cataracts, and retinal detachment, and hearing loss can be both conductive and sensorineural. Physical examination often shows cleft palate, malar hypoplasia, micrognathia, and scoliosis (Fig. 68.3). Cleft palate can be isolated or part of Pierre-Robin sequence, and Stickler syndrome is one of the conditions that should be considered in an infant with Pierre-Robin sequence (Chapter 66, Fig. 66.7). Early-onset osteoarthritis occurs, as well as slipped capital femoral epiphysis and kyphoscoliosis. Referral to pediatric otolaryngology and/or plastic surgery is often required for correction of midface anomalies, and individuals with Stickler syndrome should have close surveillance by ophthalmology and audiology specialists.

OSTEOGENESIS IMPERFECTA

Osteogenesis imperfecta (OI) encompasses a group of disorders with a wide spectrum of phenotypic severity. There are four main types of OI caused by *COLA1/2* pathogenic variants.

- Type I (classic nondeforming OI with blue sclerae) manifests with normal stature, though often less than mid-parental height, and frequent fractures, occurring as early as birth. Fractures briefly become less frequent during puberty and early adulthood.
- Type II (perinatally lethal OI) typically causes demise in the postnatal period, with 80% of infants dying from pulmonary insufficiency within the first week of life.
- Type III (progressively deforming OI) is characterized by many fractures in the neonatal period that may lead to pulmonary insufficiency and death. Individuals who survive have short stature and progressive skeletal deformation with or without the occurrence of fractures.

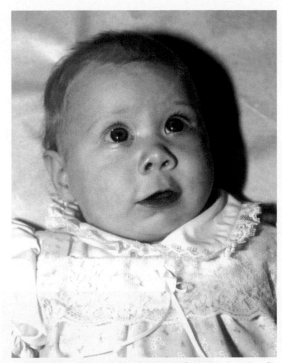
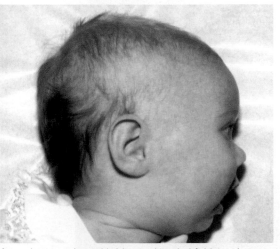

Fig. 68.3 Stickler Syndrome. Infant girl showing flat face, depressed nasal bridge, epicanthal folds, a short nose with anteverted nares, maxillary hypoplasia, and micrognathia. (Reused with permission from Jones KL, Jones MC, del Campo M. Facial-limb defects as major feature. Jones KJ, ed. In: *Smith's Recognizable Patterns of Human Malformation.* 8th ed. Philadelphia: Elsevier; 2022:370-427, Stickler syndrome, Fig. 1.)

- Type IV (common variable OI with normal sclerae) typically leads to short stature and hearing loss as an adult. It has a range of severity and variable presentations.

There are other forms of OI caused by mutations in genes other than *COL1A1/2* that can show autosomal dominant or recessive patterns of inheritance. On physical examination OI is characterized by a triangular face, blue sclerae, short stature, abnormal dentition, and ligamentous laxity (Fig. 68.4). Patients have a predisposition for fractures with minimal trauma and often develop hearing loss over time. Individuals with OI are usually followed by clinical genetics, orthopedics, rehabilitation medicine, and otolaryngology specialists. They often require bracing of limbs and orthotics to aid in joint stabilization. Physical and occupational therapy are necessary to maximize functionality. Those with severe OI may need surgery for progressive scoliosis. Some patients will also have low bone mass or osteoporosis, which can be identified by DEXA scan.

SKELETAL DYSPLASIAS

Skeletal dysplasias have marked effects on bone and cartilage and can manifest prenatally or in the neonatal period. There are over 400 skeletal dysplasias that may affect multiple parts of the bone, including short-rib dysplasias, metaphyseal dysplasias, diaphyseal dysplasias, rhizomelic and mesomelic dysplasias, craniosynostoses, and overgrowth syndromes. Diagnosis is guided by the physical examination and skeletal survey, though molecular genetic testing plays a considerable role because many genetic causes have been identified for this group of disorders. Affected newborns may have a narrow chest relative to the abdomen, short extremities, brachydactyly, and facial findings such as a flattened nasal bridge and midface hypoplasia. Prenatal imaging is important in recognizing these dysplasias early, including those that may be lethal in the perinatal period, allowing for appropriate counseling of parents. Lethality in the perinatal period is often attributed to respiratory insufficiency as a result of physical restriction of lung development in the setting of abnormal thorax development. Dysplasias with milder characteristics tend to be recognized late in pregnancy or shortly after birth, though the mildest forms may not be recognized until later in life.

Achondroplasia

Achondroplasia is one of the most common skeletal dysplasias and one of several dysplasias resulting from pathogenic variants in the *FGFR3* gene. Affected infants will have uniformly shortened extremities (especially proximal extremities), brachydactyly, relative macrocephaly with frontal bossing, limitation of elbow extension, and redundant skinfolds (Fig. 68.5). Complications tend to manifest early in life and may include hydrocephalus or sleep apnea from a tight foramen magnum, kyphosis, and lordosis. Motor milestones are usually delayed, but intelligence is normal as long as secondary neurologic complications such as hydrocephalus are prevented. These children should be evaluated for potential complications by a neurosurgeon or orthopedic surgeon and routinely monitored. For the pediatrician, there are standardized growth curves for achondroplasia to aid in monitoring head circumferences and weight-for-height ratio. Affected individuals may have recurrent otitis media and dental crowding and are at risk for early-onset obesity. New targeted therapeutic options are becoming available to increase linear growth in children with achondroplasia.

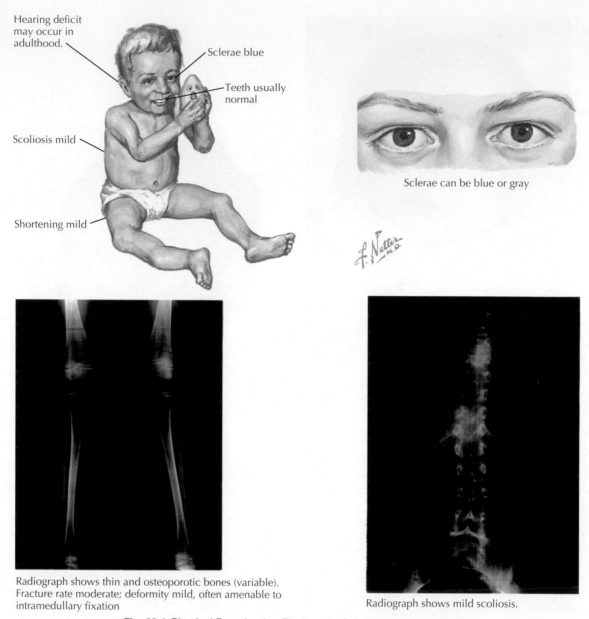

Hearing deficit may occur in adulthood.

Sclerae blue

Teeth usually normal

Scoliosis mild

Shortening mild

Sclerae can be blue or gray

Radiograph shows thin and osteoporotic bones (variable). Fracture rate moderate; deformity mild, often amenable to intramedullary fixation

Radiograph shows mild scoliosis.

Fig. 68.4 Physical Examination Findings in Osteogenesis Imperfecta.

CONNECTIVE TISSUE MIMICS

There are several disorders whose underlying cause is not in genes involved in the structure or function of connective tissue, but whose phenotype involves features of connective tissue diseases. A primary example is homocystinuria, a metabolic disorder of amino acid metabolism, which can manifest with marfanoid habitus and ectopia lentis. In contrast to Marfan syndrome, most individuals with homocystinuria have intellectual disability and are at risk for thromboembolism rather than aortopathy. Another disorder that can manifest with marfanoid habitus is Klinefelter syndrome, a chromosomal disorder resulting from a 47,XXY karyotype (Chapter 65, Fig. 65.2). Other chromosomal and single-gene disorders, including Williams syndrome and Sotos syndrome, are notable for having features of connective tissue disorders, such as joint laxity and scoliosis. Therefore it is important to consider a broad differential diagnosis in a patient presenting with features of connective tissue disease.

FUTURE DIRECTIONS

Genotype-phenotype correlations for inherited connective tissue disorders are still being established to determine which individuals are at risk for specific manifestations or complications. The full spectrum of these disorders requires further study because some individuals may have milder forms of the disorder identified by molecular testing despite lacking obvious signs and symptoms. However, understanding the complexity of polygenic disorders and their possible environmental contributors, such as in hEDS, also must be further elucidated because molecular testing is limited. Finally, research in adjunctive therapies, such as specific antihypertensives in connective tissue disorders with aortic dilatation, the use of bisphosphonates in those with decreased bone density, and targeted therapies for skeletal dysplasias, show promise in improving the management of comorbidities in inherited connective tissue disorders.

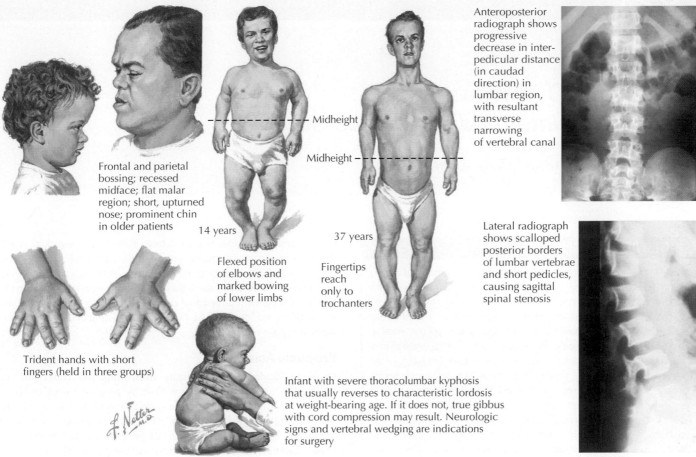

Frontal and parietal bossing; recessed midface; flat malar region; short, upturned nose; prominent chin in older patients

Midheight

Midheight

14 years

Flexed position of elbows and marked bowing of lower limbs

37 years

Fingertips reach only to trochanters

Trident hands with short fingers (held in three groups)

Anteroposterior radiograph shows progressive decrease in interpedicular distance (in caudad direction) in lumbar region, with resultant transverse narrowing of vertebral canal

Lateral radiograph shows scalloped posterior borders of lumbar vertebrae and short pedicles, causing sagittal spinal stenosis

Infant with severe thoracolumbar kyphosis that usually reverses to characteristic lordosis at weight-bearing age. If it does not, true gibbus with cord compression may result. Neurologic signs and vertebral wedging are indications for surgery

Fig. 68.5 Features of Achondroplasia.

SUGGESTED READINGS

Available online.

69

Metabolic Disorders I
Disorders of Intermediary Metabolism

Jessica R.C. Priestley and Hana Alharbi

 CLINICAL VIGNETTE

A full-term male infant is born by uncomplicated spontaneous vaginal delivery after an uneventful pregnancy. Growth parameters are normal. He is his parent's first child, and their family history is unremarkable. He receives routine care in the newborn nursery and is breastfed. Two days later, he develops difficulty feeding and frequent emesis. On transfer to the neonatal intensive care unit, examination reveals tachypnea, hypotonia, dry mucus membranes, and a sunken anterior fontanelle. Laboratory evaluation shows metabolic acidosis and hypoglycemia. Because of concern for sepsis, blood cultures are collected, empiric antibiotics are initiated, and intravenous dextrose is introduced. Additional laboratory evaluation reveals hyperammonemia and ketonuria. His glucose infusion rate is increased, and breastfeeding is discontinued. Newborn screening (NBS) results show elevated propionylcarnitine (C3), concerning for propionic acidemia, methylmalonic acidemia, or a disorder of cobalamin metabolism. Confirmatory biochemical testing is consistent with propionic academia. The infant receives metabolic formula and carnitine supplementation. His hyperammonemia and ketonuria resolve. He is discharged with metabolic specialist follow-up.

The goal of NBS is to identify infants with treatable disorders before onset of symptoms when possible; however, several metabolic disorders can manifest in the first days of life. Early diagnosis and prompt management allow for improved long-term outcomes, though there are chronic long-term complications despite adequate treatment.

Intermediary metabolism acts on nutritional molecules (monosaccharides, amino acids, and fatty acids) to yield the fundamental components of bioenergetics and biosynthesis (Fig. 69.1). Disorders therein yield phenotypes that are the consequence of accumulation of by-products, paucity of end-products, or both. Pathogenic variants in enzyme- or cofactor-coding genes cause most of these conditions. Although individually rare, the collective incidence of inborn errors of metabolism is about 1 in 5000 live births. This chapter focuses on the most common and relevant disorders and highlights their features, summarized in Table 69.1. Disorders of intermediary metabolism relate to many common complaints, including feeding intolerance, growth restriction, developmental delay/intellectual disability (DD/ID), and hypoglycemia. Thus they are an important consideration on any pediatric differential diagnosis.

ORGANIC ACIDEMIAS AND AMINOACIDOPATHIES

Organic acidemias (or organic acidurias) result from amino acid metabolism defects and accumulation of organic acid(s). They share similar, nonspecific neonatal presentations, including feeding intolerance, hypotonia, and lethargy. Aminoacidopathies are also caused by specific amino acid metabolism defects. Pathologic conditions result from accumulation of specific compounds, and there is more phenotypic variability among these conditions. Although classic, severe phenotypes are best described, these conditions exist on a phenotypic spectrum dependent on residual enzyme activity. As more asymptomatic patients are identified by expanded NBS, milder disease phenotypes are better recognized.

Propionic Acidemia

Propionic acidemia (PA) results from impaired conversion of propionyl-CoA to methylmalonyl-CoA by propionyl-CoA carboxylase and resulting accumulation of propionic acid. Newborns present with feeding intolerance, lethargy, irritability, vomiting, seizures, or hypotonia. Untreated, symptoms can progress to cardiorespiratory failure. Laboratory evaluation can reveal anion-gap metabolic acidosis, lactic acidosis, ketosis, hypoglycemia, hyperammonemia, and pancytopenia. Milder PA manifests in childhood with growth restriction, hypotonia, DD/ID, psychiatric problems, and/or movement disorders. Complications include cardiomyopathy, arrhythmias, vision and hearing changes, osteopenia/osteoporosis, seizures, and basal ganglia lesions ("metabolic strokes").

Acute management is emergent, limiting catabolism by providing alternative energy sources (glucose and lipids) and avoiding protein intake. Accumulation of ammonia may require treatment with nitrogen-scavenging medications or hemodialysis. Patients with frequent and severe metabolic crises may require liver transplantation. Long-term PA management includes avoidance of physiologic stressors and limiting dietary protein. Levocarnitine supplementation can enhance propionic acid excretion, and biotin cofactor supplementation is also used.

Methylmalonic Acidemia

Methylmalonic acidemia (MMA) results from impaired conversion of methylmalonyl-CoA to succinyl-CoA by methylmalonyl-CoA mutase. Because adenosylcobalamin is a cofactor for this enzyme, MMA can also result from cofactor synthesis defects (i.e., disorders of cobalamin metabolism). Neonatal presentation of MMA shares phenotypic similarity to PA. Laboratory studies can show anion-gap metabolic acidosis, ketosis, hyperammonemia, pancytopenia, and/or evidence of renal tubular acidosis or renal failure. Imaging can reveal basal ganglia injuries. Milder forms of MMA may manifest with a later initial crisis or may present with growth restriction, DD/ID, and/or hypotonia. Long-term complications include renal insufficiency, movement disorders, pancreatitis, and bone marrow failure.

Acute management of MMA also involves limitation of dietary protein and avoidance of catabolism. Cobalamin supplementation can be

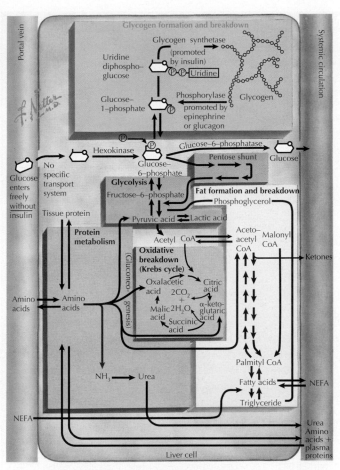

Fig. 69.1 Intermediary Metabolism of the Liver Cell. A schematic of integrated hepatic intermediary metabolism. Note the intersections between carbohydrate, protein, and fat metabolism.

helpful. Liver and kidney transplantation can prevent exacerbations and address renal failure but cannot avoid neurologic sequelae.

Isovaleric Acidemia

Isovaleric acidemia results from impaired conversion of isovaleryl-CoA to 3-methylcrotonyl-CoA by isovaleryl-CoA dehydrogenase in the process of leucine metabolism. Neonatal metabolic crisis can occur in patients with isovaleric acidemia but is less common than in patients with PA or MMA. A characteristic "sweaty sock" odor may be appreciated during acute decompensation. Laboratory studies can show anion-gap metabolic acidosis, hyperammonemia, hyperglycemia or hypoglycemia, ketosis, hypocalcemia, and pancytopenia. Complications include pancreatitis, myeloproliferative syndromes, Fanconi syndrome, and arrhythmias. Management seeks to avoid decompensation and restrict dietary protein. Supplements can be helpful: levocarnitine for secondary carnitine deficiency and glycine to increase isovaleric acid excretion.

Glutaric Acidemia Type 1

Glutaric acidemia type 1 (GA1) results from impaired conversion of glutaryl-CoA to glutaconyl-CoA by glutaryl-CoA dehydrogenase in lysine and tryptophan metabolism. Physiologic stress, particularly fever, can precipitate encephalopathic crises. There can be motor regression and/or progressive macrocephaly. Imaging can reveal a variety of brain abnormalities, notably frontotemporal hypoplasia. Decreased cerebral volume with macrocephaly increases risk for bridging vein disruption

and subdural hematomas. Movement disorders are common. Dietary lysine restriction and carnitine supplementation can improve outcomes, particularly when initiated presymptomatically. Patients often require hospital admission to avoid fever-induced catabolism and metabolic stroke; prompt treatment with intravenous dextrose fluids and carnitine decreases the risk for basal ganglia injury during febrile illness.

Maple Syrup Urine Disease

Maple syrup urine disease (MSUD), named for the sweet odor noticed in urine and cerumen in affected patients, results from impaired branched-chain amino acid (leucine, isoleucine, and valine) metabolism by branched-chain α-ketoacid dehydrogenase (BCKDH). Ketoacid accumulation results in acidosis and neurotoxicity. Leucine encephalopathy can manifest in infants with bradycardia, apnea, seizures, opisthotonos, and "fencing" or "bicycling" posturing. Older patients can present with ataxia and encephalopathy. Laboratory evaluation can show anion-gap metabolic acidosis, ketosis, and ketonuria. Left untreated, cerebral edema, coma, and cardiorespiratory failure can ensue. Although most neurologic sequelae of acute decompensations are reversible, prolonged leucine encephalopathy results in permanent damage manifesting as cognitive impairment, psychiatric problems, and movement disorders. Prompt management with branched-chain amino acid restriction is critical. Thiamine, a BCKDH cofactor, is often supplemented. Liver transplantation can avoid frequent exacerbations in severe cases.

Tyrosinemia Type 1

Tyrosinemia type 1 (TT1) results from impaired cleavage of fumarylacetoacetate to fumarate and acetoacetate by fumarylacetoacetase (FAH) in tyrosine metabolism (Fig. 69.2). Infants present in liver failure. Succinylacetone in blood or urine is pathognomonic for TT1. A more insidious onset in children includes liver and renal dysfunction, poor growth, and rickets. Untreated, patients experience porphyric crises presenting with pain, altered mental status, and/or respiratory failure. Untreated patients are at risk for hepatocellular carcinoma in late childhood or adolescence, necessitating liver transplantation.

TT1 management is dietary with tyrosine restriction and pharmacologic with 2-(2-nitro-4-trifluoro-methylbenzyol)-1,3 cyclohexanedione (NTBC), which prevents toxic intermediate accumulation (Fig. 69.2). These interventions have reduced the incidence of hepatocellular carcinoma and need for liver transplantation over recent decades.

Phenylketonuria

Phenylketonuria (PKU) results from impaired conversion of phenylalanine to tyrosine by phenylalanine hydroxylase (PAH). PAH requires a tetrahydrobiopterin cofactor, and tetrahydrobiopterin deficiency or disorders of biopterin synthesis can lead to elevated phenylalanine.

The pathologic condition in PKU is chronic from prolonged hyperphenylalaninemia and reduced tyrosine and its metabolites, including neurotransmitters. Phenylalanine impairs neurodevelopment, and untreated PKU results in DD/ID, behavioral and psychiatric disorders, seizures, parkinsonism, eczema, musty body odor, and decreased pigmentation. Management limits dietary protein and phenylalanine-rich foods, including artificial sweeteners such as aspartame. When appropriately managed from birth, neurodevelopmental outcomes can be normal.

Phenylalanine is teratogenic. Hyperphenylalaninemia in utero increases risk for intrauterine growth restriction, congenital heart differences, tracheoesophageal fistula, microcephaly, DD/ID, and behavioral problems. Plasma phenylalanine should be closely monitored in PKU patients of reproductive age to prevent toxic exposure of phenylalanine to a fetus.

TABLE 69.1   Important Defects of Intermediary Metabolism

Disorder	Enzyme(s)	Gene(s)	Inheritance	Prevalence	Suggestive Newborn Screening Result	Clinical Features
Organic Acidemias						
Propionic acidemia	Propionyl-CoA carboxylase	PCCA, PCCB	AR	1 in 35,000–75,000	Elevated C3	Severe metabolic acidosis, hyperammonemia, pancytopenia, basal ganglia injuries, growth restriction, hypotonia, developmental delay, psychosis, cardiomyopathy, seizures
Methylmalonic acidemia	Methylmalonyl-CoA mutase Enzymes related to cobalamin metabolism	MMUT MMAA MMAB MCEE MMADHC	AR	1 in 50,000–100,000	Elevated C3	Severe metabolic acidosis, hyperammonemia, pancytopenia, renal failure, basal ganglia injuries, pancreatitis, hypotonia, growth restriction, developmental delay
Isovaleric acidemia	Isovaleryl-CoA dehydrogenase	IVD	AR	1 in 230,000	Elevated C5	"Sweaty sock" odor, metabolic acidosis, hyperammonemia, pancreatitis, myeloproliferative syndromes, renal dysfunction, arrhythmias
Glutaric acidemia type 1	Glutaryl-CoA dehydrogenase	GCDH	AR	1 in 40,000	Elevated C5-DC	Encephalopathic crises, basal ganglia injuries, frontotemporal hypoplasia, bilateral subdural hematomas, progressive macrocephaly
Amino Acidopathies						
Maple syrup urine disease	Branch-chain α-ketoacid dehydrogenase complex	BCKDHA, BCKDHB, DTB, DLD	AR	1 in 185,000	Elevated leucine, isoleucine and allo-isoleucine	Leucine encephalopathy: bradycardia, hiccups, apneas, seizures, opisthotonos, and "fencing" or "bicycling" posturing; metabolic acidosis
Tyrosinemia, type 1	Fumarylacetoacetase	FAH	AR	1 in 100,000	Elevated tyrosine Presence of succinylacetone	Liver and renal dysfunction, hepatocellular carcinoma, growth restriction, rickets, porphyric crises
Phenylketonuria	Phenylalanine hydroxylase	PAH	AR	1 in 10,000–15,000	Elevated phenylalanine Low tryosine	DD/ID, behavioral and psychiatric disorders, seizures, parkinsonism, eczema, musty body odor, decreased pigmentation
Urea Cycle Defects						
Ornithine transcarbamylase deficiency	Ornithine transcarbamylase	OTC	X-linked	1 in 14,000	Low citrulline Elevated glutamate or glutamine-to-citrulline ratio	Hyperammonemia: feeding intolerance, vomiting, altered mental status, seizures, tachypnea, respiratory alkalosis, cerebral edema; growth restriction, hepatic dysfunction, psychiatric disorders
Citrullinemia, type 1	Argininosuccinate synthetase	ASS1	AR	1 in 57,000	Elevated citrulline	Hyperammonemia, hepatic dysfunction, growth restriction, psychiatric disorders
Argininosuccinate lyase deficiency	Argininosuccinate lyase	ASL	AR	1 in 70,000	Elevated citrulline Presence of argininosuccinate	Hyperammonemia, hypertension, trichorrhexis nodosa, neurocognitive delays
Arginase deficiency	Arginase	ARG1	AR	1 in 300,000	Elevated arginine	Growth restriction, DD/ID, seizures, spastic diplegia

TABLE 69.1 Important Defects of Intermediary Metabolism—cont'd

Disorder	Enzyme(s)	Gene(s)	Inheritance	Prevalence	Suggestive Newborn Screening Result	Clinical Features
Disorders of Fatty Acid Metabolism						
Primary carnitine deficiency	Carnitine transporter	*SLC22A5*	AR	1 in 100,000	Low C0	Poor fasting tolerance, hypoketotic hypoglycemia, cardiomyopathy, weakness
SCAD deficiency	Short-chain acyl-CoA dehydrogenase	*ACADS*	AR	1 in 40,000	Elevated C4	Asymptomatic
MCAD deficiency	Medium-chain acyl-CoA dehydrogenase	*ACADM*	AR	1 in 15,000	Elevated C8, C8/C2 and C8/C10	Poor fasting tolerance, hypoketotic hypoglycemia, liver dysfunction
VLCAD deficiency	Very long-chain acyl-CoA dehydrogenase	*ACADVL*	AR	1 in 30,000	Elevated C14, C14:1	Poor fasting tolerance, hypoketotic hypoglycemia, cardiac failure, liver dysfunction, myopathy
LCHAD deficiency	Long-chain 3-hydroxyacyl-CoA dehydrogenase	*HADHA*	AR	Unknown	Elevated C16-OH and C18:1-OH	Poor fasting tolerance, hypoketotic hypoglycemia, liver dysfunction, tachyarrhythmias, cardiomyopathy, rhabdomyolysis, sudden death,
Trifunctional protein deficiency	Hydroxyacyl-CoA dehydrogenase trifunctional multienzyme complex α or β subunits	*HADHA, HADHB*	AR	Unknown	Elevated C16-OH and C18:1-OH	Poor fasting tolerance, hypoketotic hypoglycemia, liver dysfunction, cardiomyopathy, arrhythmias, myopathy
Carbohydrate Metabolism Defects						
Classic galactosemia (GALT deficiency)	Galactose 1-phosphate uridyltransferase	*GALT*	AR	1 in 30,000–60,000	Increased galactose or galatose-1-phosphate Low/no GALT activity	Hypoglycemia, liver dysfunction, *Escherichia coli* sepsis, speech and motor delays, premature ovarian failure, osteopenia, cataracts
GALK deficiency	Galactokinase	*GALK*	AR	<1 in 100,000	Increased total galactose Normal GALT activity	Cataracts
GALE deficiency	UDP-galactose 4'-epimerase	*GALE*	AR	1 in 6700–70,000 depending on ethnicity	Increased total galactose Normal GALT activity	Feeding intolerance, growth restriction, liver dysfunction, most often asymptomatic
Hereditary fructose intolerance	Fructose-1-phosphate aldolase	*ALDOB*	AR	1 in 20,000–30,000	Not included	Hypoglycemia, emesis, abdominal pain/distension, liver dysfunction, hyperuricemia
Glycogen storage disorders	Multiple enzymes	*Multiple*	AR	1 in 20,000–25,000	Not included	Ketotic fasting hypoglycemia, hepatomegaly, lactic acidosis, myopathic forms with exercise intolerance and rhabdomyolysis

AR, Autosomal recessive; *C0*, free carnitine; *CoA*, coenzyme A; *DD/ID*, developmental delay/intellectual disability; *UDP*, uridine diphosphate.

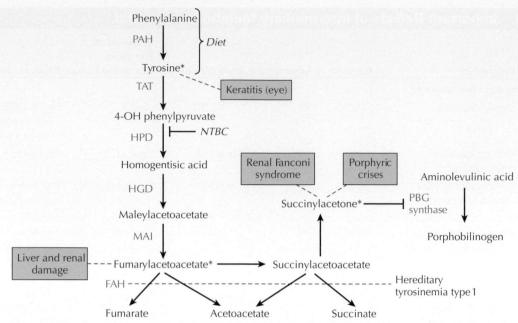

Fig. 69.2 Tyrosine Metabolism. Illustration of the relationship between key intermediates (fumarylaceto-acetate and succinylacetone) in tyrosine metabolism and pathology in tyrosinemia type 1. Note inhibition of 4-hydroxyphenylpyruvate dioxygenase (HPD) by the pharmacologic agent NTBC and its effect on intermediate accumulation.

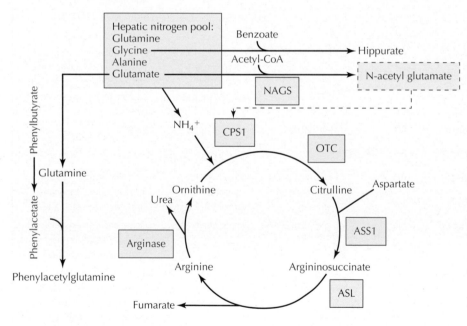

Fig. 69.3 The Urea Cycle. Carbamylphosphate synthetase 1 (CPS1), which requires the activator N-acetylglutamate, catalyzes the first step, the synthesis of carbamylphosphate from ammonia. The enzyme N-acetylglutamate synthetase (NAGS) is necessary for synthesis of the activator from acetyl-CoA and glutamate. Ornithine transcarbamoylase (OTC) catalyzes the condensation of carbamylphosphate (containing a nitrogen atom) and ornithine to make citrulline. Citrulline then reacts with aspartate (which introduces another waste nitrogen atom into the cycle) to make argininosuccinate, a reaction catalyzed by argininosuccinate synthetase (ASS1). Argininosuccinate lyase (ASL) catalyzes the formation of arginine and fumarate from argininosuccinate, after which arginase converts arginine to urea and reforms ornithine to replenish the cycle. Urea is cleared by the kidneys. Nitrogen scavenger medications, including sodium benzoate, sodium phenylbutyrate, and sodium phenylacetate, can convert nitrogen sources into renally excretable metabolites (hippurate and phenylacetylglutamine) via the reactions shown in the diagram.

UREA CYCLE DISORDERS

The proximal hepatic urea cycle begins in the mitochondria with the combination of carbon dioxide and ammonia by carbamoyl phosphate synthetase, forming carbamoyl phosphate (Fig. 69.3). Ornithine transcarbamylase (OTC) converts this to citrulline, which is shuttled into the cytosolic space where the reactions of argininosuccinate synthetase, argininosuccinate lyase, and arginase ultimately yield urea. Deficiencies in any of these enzymes result in urea cycle disorders (UCDs). These cause accumulation of ammonia, which is neurotoxic and results in symptoms of feeding intolerance, vomiting, altered mental status, seizures, and tachypnea. Cerebral edema can occur and result in fatal cardiorespiratory compromise. Blood gas analysis can show respiratory alkalosis secondary to ammonia-mediated stimulation of brainstem breathing centers. Partial enzyme deficiency could result in a delayed and atypical manifestation with hepatic dysfunction, poor growth, protein aversion, or psychiatric disorders.

Management of UCDs includes dietary protein restriction, dextrose delivery for prevention of catabolism, and use of nitrogen scavengers (sodium benzoate, sodium phenylacetate) to address hyperammonemia. Severe hyperammonemia may require hemodialysis. Supplementation of intermediates, citrulline or arginine, can support the cycle, except in arginase deficiency. Liver transplantation can avoid frequent crises but cannot reverse existing neurologic complications. In addition to the specific disorders described below, deficiencies in the NAGS and CPS1 enzymes are rare causes of proximal urea cycle disorders. Defects in orthinine translocase (ORNT1) and citrin, two amino acid transporters, can also cause hyperammonemia.

Ornithine Transcarbamylase Deficiency

The most common UCD is OTC deficiency, unique for its X-linked inheritance pattern. It classically manifests with severe hyperammonemia in male neonates. Laboratory evaluation can reveal low plasma citrulline and arginine with elevated urinary orotic acid. Manifestations in heterozygote females are variable owing to skewed X-inactivation. In these patients, OTC deficiency can be unmasked by childbirth or other physiologic stressors.

Citrullinemia and Argininosuccinate Lyase Deficiency

Argininosuccinate synthetase deficiency (citrullinemia type 1) and argininosuccinate lyase (ASL) deficiency bear considerable phenotypic similarity to OTC deficiency. ASL deficiency is differentiated from other UCDs by hypertension and trichorrhexis nodosa (coarse, brittle hair), the latter of which is pathognomonic. Neurocognitive delay is reported at higher rates in ASL deficiency than in other UCDs and is independent of severity of hyperammonemia. Elevated plasma citrulline and low plasma arginine are common to both conditions. Plasma argininosuccinate helps distinguish citrullinemia from ASL deficiency: levels are low in the former and elevated in the latter.

Arginase Deficiency

Arginase deficiency results in impaired cleavage of arginine to urea and ornithine. The pathologic condition is the result of arginine neurotoxicity. Unlike other UCDs, hyperammonemia is rare. Instead, untreated patients present with poor growth, DD/ID, seizures, and spastic diplegia. Optimal control is difficult, despite appropriate protein restriction and nitrogen scavenging.

FATTY ACID OXIDATION DISORDERS

Fatty acid metabolism occurs by β-oxidation. This requires carnitine, obtained nutritionally and synthesized endogenously. Carnitine palmitoyltransferase localizes intracellular carnitine to the mitochondrial intermembrane space, where it complexes with acyl-CoA to form acylcarnitine. As acylcarnitine, the carnitine/acylcarnitine translocase shuttles acyl-CoA across the inner mitochondrial membrane. Different sets of mitochondrial matrix enzymes catalyze the steps of β-oxidation depending on fatty acid carbon chain length. Among these, the steps of β-oxidation remain the same: conversion of acyl-CoA to its 2,3 enoyl-CoA counterpart, hydration of the resultant double bond to 3-hydroxyacyl-CoA, reduction to 3-ketacyl-CoA, and finally cleavage into an acetyl-CoA and 2-carbon shorter acyl-CoA. The reducing equivalents and acetyl-CoA in turn fuel the Krebs cycle or drive gluconeogenesis. Fatty acid oxidation disorders (FAODs) can involve any of these steps, resulting in acylcarnitine and/or fatty acid accumulation, leading to lipotoxicity and mitochondrial dysfunction.

Primary Carnitine Deficiency/Carnitine Uptake Disorder

Primary carnitine deficiency results from impaired carnitine uptake by the carnitine transporter, and secondary carnitine deficiency is caused by intake. The latter is more common and should be ruled out when low carnitine is detected on NBS. Confirmed cases of primary deficiency should receive carnitine supplementation to prevent cardiomyopathy, skeletal muscle weakness, and metabolic decompensation.

Short-Chain Acyl-CoA Dehydrogenase Deficiency

Short-chain acyl-CoA dehydrogenase (SCAD) deficiency is the mildest FAOD and considered by many a benign biochemical phenotype rather than a true inborn error of metabolism. It is discussed here because it can be identified by NBS. Patients do not present with metabolic acidosis or hypoketotic hypoglycemia, likely because SCAD catalyzes the final steps of β-oxidation and the products of preceding steps meet cellular energy requirements. There also may be some substrate usage by medium-chain acyl-CoA dehydrogenase that can partially compensate for the deficiency. SCAD deficiency was historically associated with ketotic hypoglycemia, feeding intolerance, poor growth, hypotonia, and seizures. However, NBS identification of predominantly asymptomatic individuals calls this into question, and metabolic specialists agree that SCAD deficiency is unlikely to be of clinical significance.

Medium-Chain Acyl-CoA Dehydrogenase Deficiency

Medium-chain acyl-CoA dehydrogenase (MCAD) deficiency is the most common FAOD and impairs the first step of β-oxidation for 6 to 10 carbon fatty acid moieties. Manifestation can include feeding intolerance, vomiting, lethargy, and seizures. Laboratory studies can show hypoglycemia without ketosis or ketonuria, and evidence of liver dysfunction, including hyperammonemia. Imaging may show cerebral edema and/or fatty infiltrates of the liver, heart, and kidneys. Fasting tolerance typically improves with age, although some patients may present at older ages when their fasting tolerance is challenged. Adult presentations have been reported and are sometimes precipitated by ethanol intoxication.

Acute decompensation in patients with MCAD deficiency is managed by providing sufficient levels of glucose to avoid catabolism and sustain energy demand. Long-term management entails avoidance of fasting, with frequent feeding for infants and bedtime cornstarch supplementation for toddlers/children. These interventions may place patients at higher risk for obesity.

Very-Long-Chain Acyl-CoA Dehydrogenase Deficiency

Very-long-chain acyl-CoA dehydrogenase (VLCAD) deficiency impairs the first step of β-oxidation for 14 to 20 carbon moieties, which are common in dietary fats. It includes three phenotypes: early-onset cardiac failure, hepatic, and late-onset myopathic. Patients are generally placed on a low-fat diet with medium-chain triglyceride supplementation.

Early-onset VLCAD deficiency is the most severe phenotype, characterized by cardiomyopathy and arrhythmias, hepatomegaly, hypoglycemia, and hypotonia. Sudden cardiac death can occur, and cardiac dysfunction can be, but is not always, mitigated through dietary modifications. When cardiac dysfunction is avoided, cognitive outcomes are usually normal. Hepatic VLCAD deficiency is phenotypically similar to MCAD deficiency, characterized by hypoketotic hypoglycemia with hepatomegaly in early childhood. Hypotonia and cardiomyopathy are sometimes features. With age, patients can better tolerate fasting and muscle symptoms may predominate. The mildest phenotype in VLCAD deficiency is the late-onset myopathic form, characterized by muscle pain, exercise intolerance, and episodes of rhabdomyolysis, often precipitated by exercise or fasting. Supportive care with hyperhydration and glucose is critical to avoiding renal failure.

Long-Chain 3-Hydroxyacyl-CoA Dehydrogenase Deficiency

Long-chain 3-hydroxyacyl-CoA dehydrogenase (LCHAD) deficiency impairs the third step in β-oxidation for 12 to 16 carbon moieties. LCHAD is part of the mitochondrial trifunctional protein, but isolated deficiency of the LCHAD enzyme does occur. Infants present with nonspecific symptoms progressing to seizures, coma, and death without intervention. Hepatomegaly and jaundice may be appreciable on examination. Laboratory evaluation can show hypoketotic hypoglycemia, evidence of liver dysfunction, and hypocalcemia. Cardiac manifestations are common: tachyarrhythmias precipitating sudden cardiopulmonary arrest and death and/or cardiomyopathy. The sudden death phenotype is sometimes confused for sudden infant death syndrome (SIDS), and LCHAD deficiency should be ruled out when babies die unexpectedly.

Acute management is symptomatic: mechanical ventilation for respiratory failure, inotropes for cardiac dysfunction, and adequate hydration. Like management of VLCAD deficiency, LCHAD deficiency management aims to supply sufficient glucose to avoid metabolism of long-chain fatty acids by avoiding fasting or supplying complex carbohydrates (e.g., bedtime cornstarch) to prolong fasting tolerance.

The neurodevelopmental consequences of LCHAD deficiency are variable and depend on the frequency and severity of metabolic decompensation(s) early in life. Peripheral neuropathy can develop later in childhood or adolescence. Retinopathy develops despite early treatment, and patients should receive regular ophthalmologic follow-up. Myopathy and episodes of rhabdomyolysis can develop, with concurrent weakness, pain, and exercise intolerance.

Mitochondrial Trifunctional Protein Deficiency

Mitochondrial trifunctional protein (TFP) is a complex of four α-subunits and four β-subunits. Deficiency impairs three steps in long-chain β-oxidation—LCHAD, enoyl-CoA hydratase, and thiolase—and results in variable phenotypes. Severe TFP deficiency manifests as a neonate with hypoglycemia, liver dysfunction, cardiorespiratory distress, and myopathy. Early mortality in these patients is common. There is also a milder myopathic phenotype. Management is similar to that of LCHAD deficiency.

Importantly, fetal LCHAD deficiency and TFP deficiency are associated with maternal pathologic liver conditions, including acute fatty liver of pregnancy and HELLP syndrome (**h**emolysis, **e**levated **l**iver **e**nzymes, and **l**ow **p**latelets). Although the precise mechanism is unknown, 3-hydroxy fatty acids from the fetus can cross the placenta and accumulate in maternal tissues, including hepatocytes, resulting in lipotoxicity and subsequent pathology.

DISORDERS OF CARBOHYDRATE METABOLISM

Galactosemia

Galactose is a glucose epimer liberated by lactose cleavage. Three enzymes participate in its conversion to uridine diphosphate (UDP) glucose: galactokinase (GALK), galactose-1-phosphate uridyltransferase (GALT), and UDP-galactose 4'-epimerase (GALE). Deficiencies in these enzymes cause the galactosemias.

GALT deficiency causes classic galactosemia and pathologic accumulation of galactose-1-phosphate, galactose, and galactitol. Metabolic crisis is precipitated by initiation of breastmilk or lactose-based formula feeds. Presentation includes feeding intolerance and poor growth, lethargy, seizures, and/or liver dysfunction, including jaundice, bleeding diatheses, or ascites. Sepsis may occur, with *Escherichia coli* being a common offending organism. Laboratory testing may show hypoglycemia, abnormal coagulation tests, transaminitis, elevated erythrocyte galactose-1-phosphate, and urinary excretion of galactitol. Initiation of a galactose-restricted diet can prevent severe manifestations, but patients remain at risk for DD/ID, speech problems, and motor dysfunction. Premature ovarian failure, osteopenia, and cataracts are also complications.

GALK deficiency is milder, presenting with cataracts. It features galactosemia and elevated urinary galactitol without the galactose intolerance or neurologic manifestations seen in classic galactosemia. GALE, or epimerase deficiency can manifest with feeding difficulties, poor growth, and liver dysfunction, though the more common milder form, peripheral epimerase deficiency, is asymptomatic and does not require treatment. In these patients, erythrocyte galactose-1-phosphate is elevated but GALT activity is normal.

Hereditary Fructose Intolerance

Hereditary fructose intolerance results from impaired cleavage of fructose-1-phosphate to dihydroxyacetone phosphate and glyceraldehyde by fructose 1-phosphate aldolase (aldolase B). Manifestation generally coincides with the introduction of dietary sucrose and fructose and includes poor growth, feeding difficulties, vomiting, and abdominal pain or distension. Symptom severity depends on the magnitude of fructose exposure, and a sizeable fructose ingestion can precipitate profound hypoglycemia. Glucagon cannot rectify this hypoglycemia because of inhibition of gluconeogenesis and glycogenolysis by fructose-1-phosphate. Hepatomegaly and jaundice may be present. Laboratory investigation may show lactic acidosis, hyperuricemia, liver dysfunction, and electrolyte derangements, including hypophosphatemia and hypermagnesemia. Reducing substances can be detected in urine samples. Diagnosis is molecular. Fructose tolerance testing, once a diagnostic mainstay, is no longer recommended.

In the acute setting, hypoglycemia should be promptly addressed. Dietary restriction of fructose, including sucrose and sorbitol, yields normal neurodevelopmental outcomes. Fructose should also be avoided in medications. Poor adherence to these restrictions can cause hepatic and renal dysfunction. Limitation of fruits and many vegetables can precipitate vitamin deficiencies requiring supplementation.

Glycogen Storage Disorders

Glycogen is a branched polysaccharide polymer made of glucose molecules and serves as the storage form of glucose in the liver and muscle. Defects in the breakdown of stored glycogen can primarily affect the liver, the muscles, or both. Glycogen storage disorders (GSDs) encompass a group of disorders caused by specific enzyme deficiencies important in the metabolism of glycogen. In general, GSDs can manifest with ketotic hypoglycemia with fasting, lactic acidosis, and elevated levels of lipids, creatine kinase, and uric acid. The most common GSD is type Ia (von Gierke disease), which typically manifests in infancy with poor growth, hepatomegaly, fasting hypoglycemia, and "doll-like" facies. Type II GSD is Pompe disease (acid maltase deficiency), which is also a lysosomal storage disorder that in the infantile form can manifest with hypertrophic cardiomyopathy. This condition can be treated with enzyme replacement therapy, and early diagnosis is crucial, making it a target for NBS in several states. Other forms of GSD, such as type V (McArdle disease), manifest primarily with exercise intolerance and skeletal myopathy. The clinical phenotypes of GSD are varied but are important to diagnose, because early management can have a significant long-term impact on morbidity and mortality.

FUTURE DIRECTIONS

Disorders of intermediary metabolism are a broad and varied group of conditions, characterized by deficiencies of specific enzymes involved in the metabolism of proteins, fatty acids, and carbohydrates. NBS (Chapter 64) has vastly improved diagnosis and proactive management, as well as prognosis, for many of these disorders. Various therapeutic options already exist, including dietary therapy, substrate reduction, cofactor supplementation, and preventive measures such as avoidance of fasting. The promise of novel therapies such as gene therapy brings a new frontier to the treatment of metabolic disorders, along with improved testing strategies for early diagnosis.

SUGGESTED READINGS

Available online.

70

Metabolic Disorders II
Disorders of Complex Molecules

Michaela B. Reinhart and Jessica I. Gold

 CLINICAL VIGNETTE

A 12-year-old boy presents to his pediatrician for leg pain. His pain has progressively worsened over the past few weeks, and he describes it as an aching pain that is not worsened with activity. He plays soccer at school and has been able to participate as usual. Family history is significant for an aunt who has a history of intermittent pains in her extremities. His vital signs are all within normal limits. On physical examination, he has hepatosplenomegaly and multiple ecchymoses on his extremities. His laboratory test results are notable for a white blood cell count of 5000/μL, hemoglobin of 10 g/dL, and platelets of 40,000/μL. Radiographs of his extremities show multiple lytic lesions of his bones.

This presentation raises concern for Gaucher disease, a lysosomal storage disorder that causes accumulation of sphingolipids in the bone marrow, liver, and spleen. Patients with type 1 Gaucher disease may present with symptoms of anemia, thrombocytopenia, hepatosplenomegaly, or symptoms of bone disease. Prompt treatment is essential because enzyme replacement therapy is available and can halt disease progression and improve symptoms.

Disorders of complex molecules encompass many inherited disorders involving defects in biogenesis or processing within cellular organelles, as well as molecular modifications to proteins required for cellular metabolism and signaling. Lysosomal storage disorders (LSDs), peroxisomal disorders, and congenital disorders of glycosylation (CDG) are broad classifications of these disorders and have a wide spectrum of presentation and disease severity. Many of the disorders discussed tend to have a progressive and degenerative course, though outcomes have improved with the promise of novel therapeutic options in recent years.

ETIOLOGY AND PATHOGENESIS

Cell function depends on precise communication between organelles, and disruption in trafficking or function of this complex network can lead to multisystem disorders. Lysosomes play a large role in intracellular molecule degradation as home to more than 50 hydrolytic enzymes (Fig. 70.1). Genetic mutations causing specific lysosomal hydrolase deficiencies or lysosomal export defects lead to metabolite accumulation, manifesting as a multitude of LSDs. The specific storage material, for example, mucopolysaccharides, sphingolipids, or mucolipids, defines the type of LSD. Lysosomal protein transport out of the lysosome may also be defective. Most LSDs are inherited in an autosomal recessive pattern, with the exception of Hunter syndrome (mucopolysaccharidosis type II) and Fabry syndrome, which are X-linked disorders.

Peroxisomes are organelles responsible for catabolism of very-long-chain fatty acids and synthesis of bile acids and plasmalogen. Genetic mutations, affecting peroxisomal formation or specific enzyme activity, interrupt these metabolic pathways and lead to accumulation of metabolites. Peroxisomal disorders are less common than LSDs.

CDGs are caused by defects in glycosylation, the process of adding sugar molecules to polypeptide chains. These glycoproteins populate the cell membrane and account for most extracellular proteins, including transferrin and clotting factors. Nearly 150 genes that cause deficiency in glycan synthesis or conjugation have been identified, leading to multisystemic disorders. CDGs, also referred to as carbohydrate-deficient glycoprotein syndromes, may have defects in either N- or O-linked glycosylation or both. Defects of lipid glycosylation and biosynthesis of the glycosylphosphatidylinositol (GPI) anchor (glycolipids that reside on plasma membranes for cell surface binding) are also types of CDG.

CLINICAL PRESENTATION

Peroxisomal disorders and LSDs commonly manifest with signs of metabolite accumulation. Symptoms depend on where deposition occurs and frequently include the nervous system, liver, spleen, and bone. Common findings across peroxisomal disorders and LSDs include seizures, intellectual disability, developmental regression, skeletal abnormalities, hepatomegaly, and hypotonia. Infants frequently present with failure to thrive or a loss of developmental milestones. The clinical presentation and age of onset vary from the neonatal period to adulthood. Characteristic physical examination findings include corneal clouding, coarse facies, organomegaly with liver disease, and skeletal abnormalities.

CDGs often manifest with multisystem involvement, many with developmental delay, failure to thrive, hypotonia, and hypoglycemia. These diseases often cause hepatopathy, coagulopathy, and neurologic abnormalities. Symptoms may present throughout the lifespan. Infants often present with neurologic abnormalities, hepatic disease, and nephrotic syndrome. Children often have failure to thrive and developmental delay but may develop stroke-like episodes and seizures. Adults can have endocrine abnormalities on presentation and may exhibit cognitive delay and neurologic symptoms.

DIFFERENTIAL DIAGNOSIS

The differential diagnosis for the disorders of complex molecules is broad. Hepatosplenomegaly also occurs in cirrhosis, steatohepatitis, congenital infections, biliary tract obstruction, venous congestion from cardiac pathologic conditions, neoplasms, and Wilson disease, among other pathologic conditions. Skeletal dysplasia may have an isolated inherited cause such as achondroplasia and osteogenesis imperfecta, along with LSDs and peroxisomal disorders. More generalized

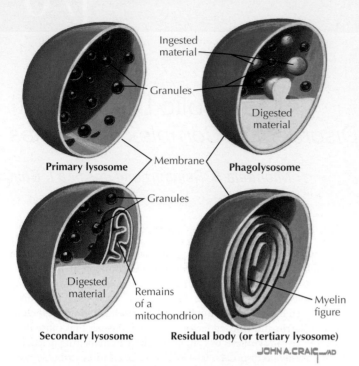

Ingested material

Granules

Primary lysosome

Membrane

Digested material

Phagolysosome

Granules

Digested material

Remains of a mitochondrion

Secondary lysosome

Myelin figure

Residual body (or tertiary lysosome)

JOHN A. CRAIG—AD

Fig. 70.1 Lysosomal Activity.

symptoms such as failure to thrive, developmental delay and intellectual disability, and hypotonia have a wide range of pathologic conditions such as trisomy 21, muscular dystrophy, disorders of amino acid metabolism, fetal alcohol syndrome, hyperthyroidism, protein-losing enteropathy, celiac disease, inherited neurologic disorders, and lead poisoning. The constellation of findings involving multiple systems and progressive deterioration should aid in narrowing the differential diagnosis and help direct the clinician toward disorders of complex molecules.

EVALUATION AND MANAGEMENT

Laboratory Studies

Laboratory analysis and genetic testing are key to diagnosing disorders of complex molecules. Clinical evaluation and suspicion in conjunction with consultation with a clinical geneticist should guide decision-making on specific laboratory testing. In some states, specific LSDs and peroxisomal disorders are included in newborn screening (Chapter 64).

Urine and blood screening tests to detect accumulated metabolites alongside measuring enzyme activity aids in diagnosis of LSDs. Diagnosis of peroxisomal disorders may include analyzing very-long-chain fatty acid levels, α-oxidation of phytanic acid, biosynthesis of plasmalogens, bile acid synthesis, or specific peroxisomal enzymatic assays. For CDGs, serum carbohydrate-deficient transferrin analysis is first-line screening, followed by N-glycan and O-glycan analysis. Flow cytometry can detect GPI anchors, or their deficiencies, on the cellular surface. For each of these classes of disorders, genetic testing can confirm a diagnosis by identifying causative pathogenic variants. Genetic testing is quickly becoming a first-line test in diagnosing these disorders.

Imaging

For disorders of complex molecules, imaging is a helpful modality for diagnosis, establishing disease severity, and monitoring comorbidities. Skeletal radiographs play a key role in identifying skeletal dysplasia, a key finding in rhizomelic chondrodysplasia punctata (Fig. 70.2), and

dysostosis multiplex, common in the mucopolysaccharidoses. Many of these disorders are complicated by poor bone health, and bone density (DEXA) scans are useful for monitoring bone mineral density. Abdominal ultrasound is commonly used to evaluate the hepatosplenomegaly found in many storage disorders or define any renal differences. Finally, cardiac disease, specifically valvar abnormalities, can be seen in many disorders of complex molecules, and serial echocardiograms are often needed.

LYSOSOMAL STORAGE DISORDERS

Gaucher Disease

Gaucher disease (Fig. 70.3) is the most common LSD and is due to accumulation of sphingolipids in the bone marrow, liver, and spleen. There are three types of Gaucher disease, defined by the age at onset, the presence of neuronopathic symptoms, and rapidity of progression. Patients with type 1, nonneuronopathic Gaucher disease tend to have hepatosplenomegaly, thrombocytopenia, and anemia. They are at risk for bone pain crises and osteonecrosis. These individuals have a normal life expectancy but may be at a higher risk for parkinsonism and malignancy. Gaucher disease types 2 and 3 are characterized by primary neurologic disease with a phenotypic spectrum. Neuronopathic Gaucher disease can manifest with strabismus, dysphagia, and limb rigidity with increased deep tendon reflexes. There is a perinatal lethal form at the severe end of this spectrum that is associated with hydrops fetalis or congenital ichthyosis. Gaucher disease type 2 is defined as onset before 2 years of age with a rapidly progressive course that often results in death by age 2 to 4 years. Type 3 Gaucher disease can have early onset but a slower progressive course with longer survival into adolescence or early adulthood. Enzyme replacement therapy (ERT) and substrate reduction therapy have helped with systemic symptoms, including cytopenias, splenomegaly, and bone pain but does not improve neurologic symptoms. Therefore ERT is more effective in patients with type 1 Gaucher disease.

Niemann-Pick Disease

Niemann-Pick disease (NPD), another disorder of sphingolipid storage, manifests as progressive neurologic deterioration leading to childhood death. NPD may manifest with hepatosplenomegaly, lymphadenopathy, and yellow-brown skin pigmentation on examination. Ophthalmologic evaluation may show a macular cherry red spot (Fig. 70.3) or a vertical gaze palsy. NPD types A and B are part of the spectrum of acid sphingomyelinase deficiency, caused by mutations in the *ASMD* gene. Patients with neonatal-onset (NPD type A) typically do not live beyond 4 years of age. NPD type B typically spares the nervous system and allows survival into adulthood. Individuals with NPD type B often have hypercholesterolemia and hypertriglyceridemia and can develop restrictive lung disease with age. Bone marrow transplant has been effective in correcting metabolic defects but will not correct neurologic involvement. Recent therapeutic advances could make enzyme replacement therapy a viable option for some patients with ASMD. NPD type C is caused by pathogenic variants in the *NPC1* or *NPC2* gene, and has variable age of onset. Early infantile, late infantile, juvenile, and adolescent/adult-onset forms are all seen. Symptoms range from isolated splenomegaly to ascites and liver disease in the infantile form to ataxia, developmental delay and regression, and progressive dystonia in the juvenile- and adult-onset forms.

Krabbe Disease

Krabbe disease, a disorder of lysosomal leukodystrophy, is marked by progressive neurologic dysfunction. Infants present with hypertonicity and hyperreflexia followed by hypotonia. They also often

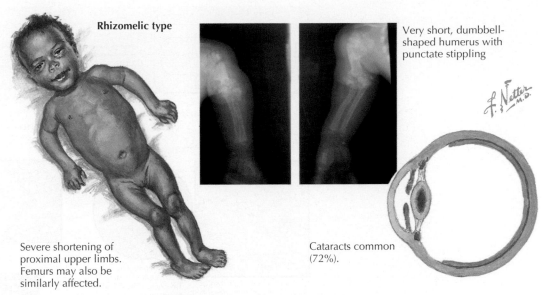

Rhizomelic type

Very short, dumbbell-shaped humerus with punctate stippling

Severe shortening of proximal upper limbs. Femurs may also be similarly affected.

Cataracts common (72%).

Fig. 70.2 Findings of Chondrodysplasia Punctata.

have blindness and deafness. However, there are some progressive, late-onset types of Krabbe disease that may be mistaken for multiple sclerosis or motor neuron disease. Stem cell transplant within the first month of life has been attempted to ameliorate symptoms. As a result, Krabbe disease is now part of NBS in some states.

Fabry Disease

Fabry disease (Fig. 70.4) is an X-linked disorder of sphingolipid storage, and therefore more predominant in males. The nervous, cardiovascular, and renal systems are affected. Common findings on examination include distal extremity paresthesias, hypohidrosis or anhidrosis, and angiokeratomas of the skin. Chronic kidney disease is common as the disease progresses and can lead to end-stage renal disease. Management of cardiac and cerebrovascular disease is imperative, because Fabry disease can cause mitral valve insufficiency, left ventricular hypertrophy, and electrocardiogram changes. Symptoms vary in hemizygous females; females often have acroparesthesias and can have cardiac disease, but few progress to renal failure. ERT is available for Fabry disease, and supportive measures remain important for pain and stroke prevention.

GM₂ Gangliosidoses

Tay-Sachs disease and Sandhoff disease comprise the GM$_2$ gangliosidoses. Tay-Sachs disease develops in infancy, and affected infants will have hypotonia and blindness with a macular cherry red spot on examination (Fig. 70.3). Sandhoff similarly manifests in infancy, though there are some late-onset cases. Patients may have doll-like facies in addition to hypotonia and motor delays. Individuals with Sandhoff disease often have a history of seizures and show neurologic deterioration leading to dementia and death by 5 years. Supportive treatment for epilepsy and nutrition are necessary, because there are currently no effective therapies for GM$_2$ gangliosidoses.

Metachromatic Leukodystrophy

Metachromatic leukodystrophy (MLD), caused by deficiency of the enzyme arylsulfatase A, has three subtypes defined by the general age of onset: infantile, juvenile, and adult (Fig. 70.3). Later onset correlates with slower progression and subsequently longer lifespan. The disease is marked by progressive demyelination and psychiatric disorders. The classic finding on T2-weighted brain magnetic resonance imaging (MRI) is periventricular deep white matter abnormalities with sparing of the subcortical U-fibers. Patients may have proximal renal tubular acidosis that worsens with illness. In children, early signs include a loss of milestones, ataxia, and incontinence. Stem cell and bone marrow transplantation have been shown to slow progression of symptoms if used early in the course of disease.

Mucopolysaccharidoses and Mucolipidoses

Mucopolysaccharidoses (MPSs) are marked by hepatosplenomegaly, facial dysmorphism, hirsutism, and skeletal dysplasia (dysostosis multiplex). Medical history often includes recurrent upper respiratory tract infections, obstructive sleep apnea, and learning disabilities. Hunter (MPS I) and Hurler (MPS II) syndromes are notable for their coarse facial features, hepatomegaly, and valvular heart disease (Fig. 70.5). MPS II is X-linked and thus predominantly affects males. Patients with MPS I respond to hematopoietic stem cell transplant, which may significantly affect disease progression if it is performed before 2 years of age. ERT is also established for MPS I, II, IVA, VI, and VII, but cannot penetrate the blood-brain barrier and therefore does not improve the neurologic features of disease. ERT is still under development for other MPS disorders, and clinical trials are underway for gene therapy and other treatment modalities.

The mucolipidosis (ML) disorders include four clinical phenotypes with a spectrum of severity. I-cell disease (ML II), a disorder of intracellular targeting of lysosomal proteins, manifests in infancy with coarse facial features and dysostosis multiplex. Morbidity and mortality are largely derived from feeding and respiratory difficulty. The other ML disorders have a broad range of severity regarding clinical findings on examination as well as complications. They are all marked by progressive neurodegeneration, learning disabilities, cardiac involvement, and skeletal dysplasia. There are no therapies for mucolipidoses at this time, and supportive treatment is indicated.

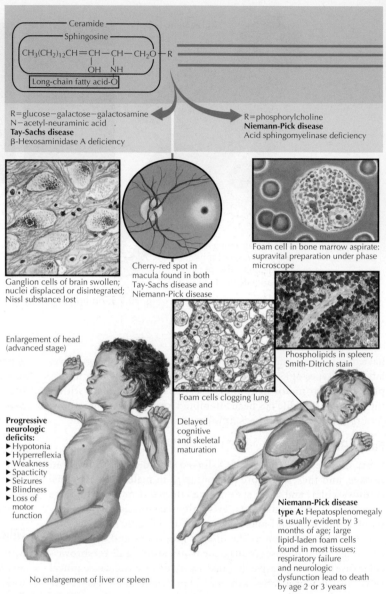

Ceramide
Sphingosine

$CH_3(CH_2)_{12}CH=CH-CH-CH_2O-R$
  $\underset{OH}{|}$ $\underset{NH}{|}$
Long-chain fatty acid-O

R=glucose–galactose–galactosamine
N–acetyl-neuraminic acid
Tay-Sachs disease
β-Hexosaminidase A deficiency

R=phosphorylcholine
Niemann-Pick disease
Acid sphingomyelinase deficiency

Ganglion cells of brain swollen;
nuclei displaced or disintegrated;
Nissl substance lost

Cherry-red spot in
macula found in both
Tay-Sachs disease and
Niemann-Pick disease

Foam cell in bone marrow aspirate:
supravital preparation under phase
microscope

Phospholipids in spleen;
Smith-Ditrich stain

Foam cells clogging lung

Enlargement of head
(advanced stage)

**Progressive
neurologic
deficits:**
► Hypotonia
► Hyperreflexia
► Weakness
► Spasticity
► Seizures
► Blindness
► Loss of
   motor
   function

Delayed
cognitive
and skeletal
maturation

**Niemann-Pick disease
type A:** Hepatosplenomegaly
is usually evident by 3
months of age; large
lipid-laden foam cells
found in most tissues;
respiratory failure
and neurologic
dysfunction lead to death
by age 2 or 3 years

No enlargement of liver or spleen

Fig. 70.3 Signs and Symptoms of Sphingolipidoses, a Subset of Lysosomal Storage Disorders.

PEROXISOMAL DISORDERS

Peroxisomal disorders can be classified into two primary categories: peroxisomal biogenesis disorders and disorders of single peroxisomal enzymes. Examples of each are described here.

Zellweger Spectrum Disorders

Zellweger spectrum disorders are defects of peroxisomal biogenesis, typically due to biallelic pathogenic variants in one of the *PEX* genes. Zellweger syndrome is the most common and most severe, manifesting in infancy with seizures, hepatomegaly, and dysmorphic features. On examination, affected individuals will have a large anterior fontanelle, epicanthal folds, an arched palate, and anteverted nares. Cataracts are commonly seen on ophthalmologic evaluation. Other findings include hepatorenal abnormalities and renal cysts. Death usually occurs within the first year of life. Neonatal adrenoleukodystrophy has milder findings than Zellweger syndrome, but is slowly progressive. Signs and symptoms of liver dysfunction may be present, and many patients have vision impairment and hearing loss. Infantile Refsum disease (IRD) is the mildest of the Zellweger spectrum disorders, usually having some dysmorphic features along with hearing loss and retinopathy. Those with neonatal adrenoleukodystrophy and IRD have intellectual disability but may live for decades. There are no curative therapies, and supportive management is indicated.

Rhizomelic Chondrodysplasia Punctata

Rhizomelic chondrodysplasia punctata (RCDP) is a disorder of peroxisomal biogenesis characterized by shortened limbs, high arched palate, dysplastic pinna, and cataracts on examination (Fig. 70.2), in addition to severe developmental delay and spasticity. RCDP is typically caused by pathogenic variants in the *PEX7* gene. This disease is often complicated by recurrent respiratory infections and breathing problems, which generally limits lifespan to childhood. Treatment is predominantly supportive, though dietary phytanic acid restriction may be helpful in some cases.

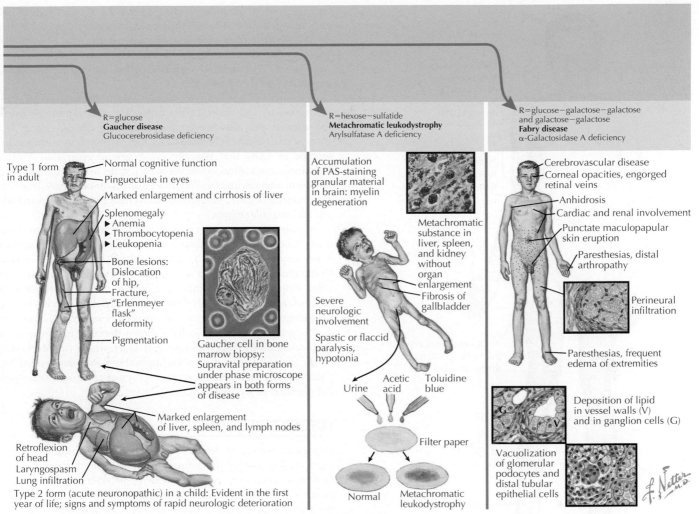

R=glucose
Gaucher disease
Glucocerebrosidase deficiency

R=hexose—sulfatide
Metachromatic leukodystrophy
Arylsulfatase A deficiency

R=glucose—galactose—galactose
and galactose—galactose
Fabry disease
α-Galactosidase A deficiency

Type 1 form in adult
— Normal cognitive function
— Pingueculae in eyes
— Marked enlargement and cirrhosis of liver
— Splenomegaly
  ▶ Anemia
  ▶ Thrombocytopenia
  ▶ Leukopenia
— Bone lesions: Dislocation of hip, Fracture, "Erlenmeyer flask" deformity
— Pigmentation

Gaucher cell in bone marrow biopsy: Supravital preparation under phase microscope appears in both forms of disease

Retroflexion of head
Laryngospasm
Lung infiltration
— Marked enlargement of liver, spleen, and lymph nodes

Type 2 form (acute neuronopathic) in a child: Evident in the first year of life; signs and symptoms of rapid neurologic deterioration

Accumulation of PAS-staining granular material in brain: myelin degeneration

Metachromatic substance in liver, spleen, and kidney without organ enlargement
Fibrosis of gallbladder

Severe neurologic involvement

Spastic or flaccid paralysis, hypotonia

Urine   Acetic acid   Toluidine blue

Filter paper

Normal   Metachromatic leukodystrophy

Cerebrovascular disease
Corneal opacities, engorged retinal veins
Anhidrosis
Cardiac and renal involvement
Punctate maculopapular skin eruption
Paresthesias, distal arthropathy

Perineural infiltration

Paresthesias, frequent edema of extremities

Deposition of lipid in vessel walls (V) and in ganglion cells (G)

Vacuolization of glomerular podocytes and distal tubular epithelial cells

Fig. 70.3, cont'd

X-Linked Adrenoleukodystrophy

X-linked adrenoleukodystrophy (X-ALD) is a peroxisomal enzyme defect caused by variants in *ABCD1* and typically manifests in childhood with progressive neurologic deterioration, regression, and changes in behavior. Adrenal insufficiency is commonly seen and should be monitored and managed appropriately. Hematopoietic stem cell transplantation may help with symptoms if done early in the disease course and before significant leukodystrophy on brain magnetic resonance imaging (MRI). Given the possibility for therapeutic intervention, X-ALD was added to the Recommended Uniform Screening Panel (RUSP) for NBS (Chapter 64, Table 62.4). Late-onset and adult forms of X-ALD exist and have a delayed course with milder neuropathy and ataxia, as well as spared cognitive deterioration.

Refsum Disease

Refsum disease results from accumulation of phytanic acid in plasma as a result of defective catabolism within peroxisomes. Children with Refsum disease present with anosmia, deafness, and ichthyosis. Retinitis pigmentosa and polyneuropathy with ataxia also may be found on evaluation. Age of onset typically occurs in childhood but may vary because of the differing degrees of enzyme activity in individuals. Dietary restriction of phytanic acid is the mainstay of treatment, and plasmapheresis can be useful if phytanic acid levels become too high.

Congenital Disorders of Glycosylation

CDGs tend to affect multiple organ systems. Phosphomannomutase 2 CDG (PMM2-CDG), previously known as CDG-1a, is the most common N-linked disorder and classically manifests in infancy with failure to thrive, developmental delay, abnormal subcutaneous fat distribution, cerebellar hypoplasia, liver disease, and facial dysmorphism. Patients may have nephrotic syndrome, hypertrophic cardiomyopathy, and hepatic disease. Treatment options are limited to supportive care, and up to 20% of those with the disorder will have multiorgan failure within the first year of life. Individuals with milder forms of disease may have a normal lifespan with intellectual disability and endocrine abnormalities such as hyperprolactinemia, insulin resistance, and hypogonadotropic hypogonadism. Some patients may have decreased coagulation factors, such as protein C and S, leading to increased thrombosis risk.

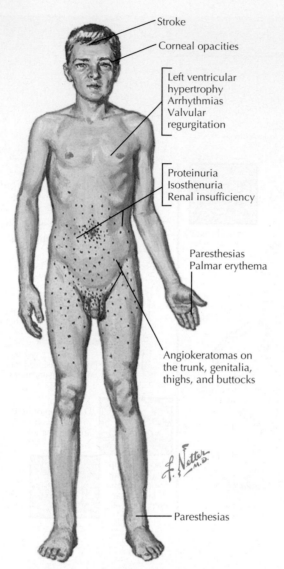

Stroke

Corneal opacities

Left ventricular
hypertrophy
Arrhythmias
Valvular
regurgitation

Proteinuria
Isosthenuria
Renal insufficiency

Paresthesias
Palmar erythema

Angiokeratomas on
the trunk, genitalia,
thighs, and buttocks

Paresthesias

Fig. 70.4 Clinical Findings of Fabry Disease.

Glucosyltransferase 1 deficiency (ALG6-CDG) is the second most common N-glycosylation defect that has a milder presentation than PMM2-CDG. Along with the similar neurologic findings, facial dysmorphism, and failure to thrive, many patients have protein-losing enteropathy and skeletal abnormalities.

Mannosephosphate isomerase deficiency (MPI-CDG) is an N-linked disorder characterized by hepatic and gastrointestinal findings without neurologic involvement. As a result, MPI-CDG often manifests with failure to thrive, recurrent emesis, hypoglycemia, chronic diarrhea from protein-losing enteropathy, and liver disease. These patients are also at increased risk for thrombosis. Symptoms are responsive to oral mannose supplementation, making early diagnosis important for this treatable CDG.

Disorders of O-linked glycosylation lead to neuromuscular, connective tissue, and skeletal phenotypes. Hereditary multiple osteochondromas and muscle-eye-brain disease are clinical entities that are now recognized as O-linked CDG. GPI-anchor defects are another subtype of CDG that typically cause neurodegenerative diseases. Examination can reveal spastic paraplegia, skeletal dysplasia, abnormal skin pigmentation, and facial dysmorphism. X-linked PIGA deficiency is an example of a GPI-anchor defect and manifests with hypsarrhythmia and infantile spasms.

Management of CDG relies largely on symptomatic management. Understanding baseline liver, renal, and endocrine function is key to monitoring and managing a large extent of the disease. Ophthalmologic evaluation is recommended to detect and treat retinitis. Patients with CDG may have poor immunologic response to vaccines, and antibody levels should be checked after immunizations. Coagulation factors may need repletion before surgeries if coagulopathy is present. Other CDGs have shown response to simple sugar supplementations (e.g., mannose, galactose), which vary depending on the specific disease. Given the implications for management and possible treatment, it is important to recognize and diagnose congenital disorders of glycosylation.

FUTURE DIRECTIONS

Important targets of research encompass discovering efficacious therapies for many of these disorders. Substrate reduction therapies to reduce accumulation of metabolic by-products are also a target of investigation for disorders of complex molecules. ERT, which has been used with success in many disorders, is expanding into more LSDs, including the possibility of direct CNS therapies for some disorders. The utility of stem cell transplant for many of these diseases continues to be of question given variable responses in clinical trials. Some of the clinical research limitations arise from the rarity of these diseases, which slows the advancement of potential therapies. However, recent advances in gene therapy offer hope for future therapeutic opportunities for these rare disorders.

SUGGESTED READINGS

Available online.

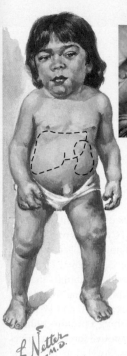

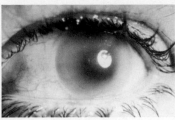

Hurler syndrome (MPS I-H)
Marked dwarfism with protruding
abdomen, hepatosplenomegaly,
coarse facies, and umbilical
hernia. Joint contractures (hips,
knees, elbows), developmental delay,
corneal clouding (above), and
cardiac anomalies. Usually fatal by
ages 6 to 12. Autosomal recessive.

Hunter syndrome (MPS II)
Dwarfism less severe than in
Hurler syndrome; hepatosplenomegaly and umbilical hernia.
Corneal clouding can occur late
in childhood; intelligence may
be normal. Life expectancy,
adulthood. X-linked.

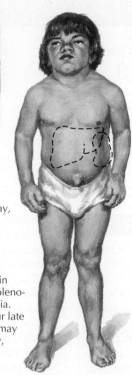

Morquio syndrome (MPS IV)
Marked dwarfism with short trunk,
severe flexion deformities,
knock-knee, corneal clouding
(may occur), and normal
intelligence. Life expectancy,
adulthood. Autosomal recessive.

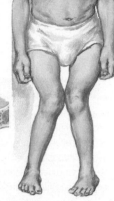

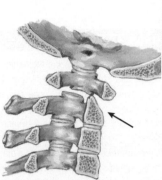

Odontoid hypoplasia, common in Morquio
syndrome, may lead to atlantoaxial subluxation with spinal cord compression injury

Fig. 70.5 Common Findings of Mucopolysaccharidoses.

71

Mitochondrial Disorders

Margaret Means and Edward C. Shadiack III

✳ CLINICAL VIGNETTE

At a 9-month check-up, parents are concerned about their child's development. Since a febrile illness 2 months ago, she can no longer sit on her own and has stopped babbling. She is not growing as well as she once was, and her parents mention that she has not been feeding well. Examination is significant for hypotonia. Brain magnetic resonance imaging reveals bilateral T2-hyperintense lesions in the basal ganglia and brainstem.

This clinicoradiographic presentation is consistent with a diagnosis of Leigh syndrome, a genetically heterogenous neurodegenerative disorder caused by impaired mitochondrial energy production. It is the most common pediatric mitochondrial disease, usually manifesting between 3 months and 2 years of age. Presentations include failure to thrive, developmental delay or regression, hypotonia, and neurologic features such as nystagmus or seizures. Lactic acidosis is common, as is renal tubular acidosis, which may require bicarbonate supplementation.

Primary mitochondrial diseases (PMDs) represent the most common category of metabolic disorders of genetic cause and the most common neurometabolic disorder of childhood, with a prevalence of approximately 1 in 5000 individuals. PMDs may be inherited in any fashion (e.g., autosomal recessive, autosomal dominant, X-linked) and are caused by defects in either nuclear deoxyribonucleic acid (nDNA) or the mitochondria's own distinct DNA (mtDNA) (e.g., maternal inheritance). Approximately 1 in 200 healthy females harbor a pathogenic mtDNA variant capable of causing disease in offspring. Pathogenic variants in more than 350 genes have been implicated in PMDs. Substantial phenotypic overlap exists despite different genetic causes (locus heterogeneity), and each genotype may produce a different phenotypic expression, even within families (pleiotropy). For example, Leigh syndrome is caused by more than 90 individual genetic changes involving both nDNA and mtDNA. Given the ubiquity of mitochondria, multi–organ system dysfunction is the norm in PMD, and organs with higher energy demand (e.g., brain, heart, retina/optic nerve, kidney, and muscle) are more typically affected. This chapter will provide an overview of PMD, an approach to evaluation, and suggested management.

MITOCHONDRIAL ANATOMY AND FUNCTION

Mitochondria are subcellular cytoplasmic organelles present in almost all cells of the body (a classic exception is the erythrocyte). Mitochondria are the chief source of energy production in the form of adenosine triphosphate (ATP) and are also integral in other cellular processes including fatty acid oxidation, the tricarboxylic acid (TCA) cycle, calcium homeostasis, free radical handling, and cellular apoptosis. Each cell has hundreds to thousands of mitochondria, and each mitochondrion has multiple copies of its own distinct mtDNA. The five-complex electron transport chain (ETC) resides on the inner membrane of the mitochondrial double membrane and is responsible for oxidative phosphorylation, which produces ATP (Fig. 71.1). Each ETC complex is a multimeric enzyme composed of subunits that are encoded by both nDNA and mtDNA (the exception being complex II, which is entirely encoded by nDNA). Complexes I, III, and IV pump protons into the intermembrane space, establishing a proton gradient, which is then discharged to provide a proton motive force that drives a spinning mechanism in complex V, phosphorylating adenosine diphosphate to energy-rich ATP.

ETIOLOGY AND PATHOGENESIS

Nuclear DNA

The nuclear genome encodes for over 1500 proteins imported into the mitochondria and provides the majority of ETC proteins and machinery responsible for other essential functions. About 80% of childhood-onset disease is attributable to nDNA defects, and most are inherited in an autosomal recessive manner. The most common nDNA gene causing PMD is *POLG*, which encodes for mtDNA polymerase gamma. nDNA causes often affect the replisome, impairing mtDNA replication and repair, resulting in multiple mtDNA deletions or mtDNA depletion.

Mitochondrial DNA

The mitochondrial genome contains 37 genes, coding for 13 ETC polypeptides, 22 transfer ribonucleic acids (tRNAs), and 2 ribosomal RNAs (rRNAs). mtDNA is circular, lacks introns, and has a high mutation rate without good mechanisms for repair (*POLG* is its only polymerase). A pathogenic variant in mtDNA or a single large-scale mtDNA deletion may cause disease. The ratio of mutant to wild-type mtDNA is known as heteroplasmy (also known as mutation load). As heteroplasmy increases, disease is more likely to become clinically evident because of a threshold effect. mtDNA pathogenic variants are responsible for most adult-onset PMD.

CLINICAL PRESENTATION

PMD can present at any age and with symptoms in any organ system. Although the most commonly reported symptoms are nonspecific, there are some findings that should raise suspicion for PMD.

History

Although classic phenotypic syndromes exist, most patients do not fit neatly under one of these labels. Nonspecific complaints that may present in infancy or childhood include hypotonia, generalized weakness, failure to thrive, dysautonomia, fatigue, exercise intolerance, vomiting, seizures,

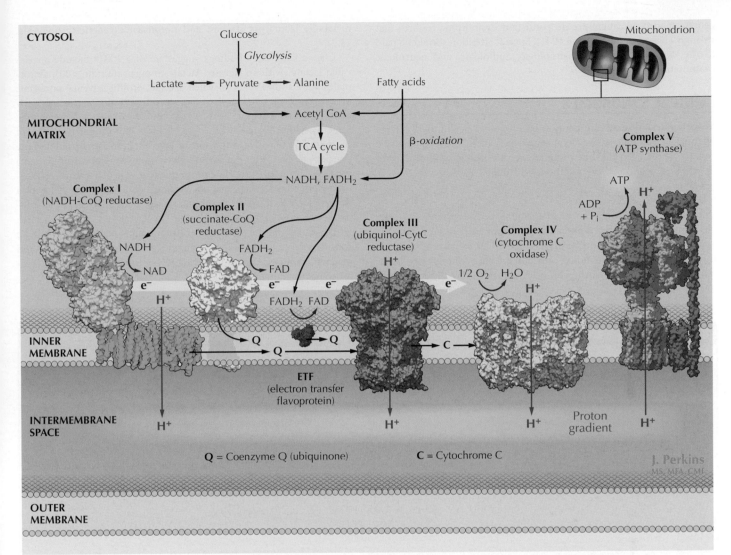

Fig. 71.1 Functions of Mitochondria. Mitochondria are essential in many processes, including the electron transport chain located in the inner membrane, which creates a proton gradient to produce adenosine triphosphate (ATP) for cellular energy.

and encephalopathy. In general, if symptoms or pathologic findings exist in three or more organ systems, especially those with high metabolic demand, PMD should be considered. Table 71.1 lists symptoms that may be more specific for PMD, especially when seen in combination with each other.

Family History

Depending on method of inheritance, there may or may not be a family history of similar clinical features. Symptoms that segregate in the maternal lineage suggest an mtDNA inheritance pattern but can be mild and vary with each family member. There may be no family history of disease in cases of sporadic mutations, single large-scale mtDNA deletions, or autosomal recessive nDNA defects. Symptoms and conditions that should be inquired about in the family include seizures, stroke, migraine, diabetes, deafness, nyctalopia, choking, arrhythmias, cardiomyopathy, muscle pain/weakness/cramps, fatigue and exercise intolerance, ataxia/dyscoordination, neuropathy, or gastrointestinal concerns such as constipation and impaired transit.

Physical Examination

Because any organ system can be affected in PMDs, a wide range of abnormalities can exist on physical examination. Unlike other

TABLE 71.1 Signs and Symptoms of Mitochondrial Disease

System	Symptom/Condition
Neurologic	Hypotonia, epilepsia partialis continua, occipital/metabolic stroke in nonvascular pattern, seizures, myoclonus, ataxia, developmental regression, encephalopathy
Ophthalmologic	Ophthalmoplegia, ptosis, retinal dystrophy, optic atrophy
Otolaryngology	Sensorineural hearing loss
Cardiac	Cardiomyopathy, Wolf-Parkinson-White, conduction defects
Gastrointestinal	Pseudo-obstruction, liver failure, cyclic vomiting
Endocrine	Diabetes mellitus, growth failure, sexual maturation issues
Renal	Fanconi syndrome, steroid-resistant nephrotic syndrome
Musculoskeletal	Exercise intolerance, increased fatigability

genetic syndromes, there are no consistent dysmorphic features that strongly suggest an underlying PMD. Special attention should be paid to the cardiovascular, ophthalmologic, audiologic, and neurologic examinations.

CLINICAL SYNDROMES

Mitochondrial disease can manifest in myriad ways, and there is large phenotypic heterogeneity even among family members with the same genetic defect. Despite this, there are certain classic syndromes that should be recognizable to practitioners (Table 71.2).

Evaluation

The diagnosis of PMDs can be challenging because there is no single biomarker that can define the condition. An initial diagnostic approach explores multiorgan involvement. This consists of ophthalmology examination, including optical coherence tomography; audiology evaluation for sensorineural hearing loss; cardiology evaluation;

metabolic laboratory studies; and noninvasive genetic testing (Fig. 71.2).

Classic laboratory findings suggestive of a PMD include an elevated lactate (with an elevated lactate to pyruvate ratio >20), abnormal plasma amino acids (elevated alanine, proline, glycine, sarcosine, or tyrosine), elevated acyl-to-free carnitine ratio, abnormal acylcarnitines and organic acids (TCA intermediates, ethylmalonate, 3-methyl-glutaconate, dicarboxylic acids). Unfortunately, none of these are very sensitive or specific for PMD. It is also important to note that lactate elevations (in an otherwise nontoxic-appearing patient) can result from inappropriate technique (e.g., use of a tourniquet, failure to place on ice) and are not evidence enough to proceed with a workup for a PMD. Note that lactate is not a sensitive or specific biomarker of mitochondrial disease.

Depending on the phenotype, certain organ-specific studies can be considered, including brain magnetic resonance imaging (MRI) and magnetic resonance spectroscopy (MRS) or lumbar puncture for cerebrospinal fluid metabolic studies.

TABLE 71.2   Clinical Syndromes

Syndrome	Genetics	Onset	Clinical Features	Brain MRI	Special Considerations	Specific Treatment
Primary lactic acidosis	>100 different nDNA and mtDNA mutations	Neonatal	Overwhelming lactic acidosis (classically with lactate/pyruvate ratio >20) Hyperammonemia, congenital malformations (e.g., arthrogryposis, brain malformations), intrauterine growth restriction, premature delivery, hypotonia, central respiratory failure, and congenital cardiomyopathy	Agenesis of the corpus callosum Periventricular and intraventricular cysts, atrophy, delayed myelination	Rule out sepsis, necrotizing enterocolitis, seizures, hypoxic-ischemic encephalopathy and other treatable causes of lactic acidosis	Sodium bicarbonate for acidosis Dialysis may temporize life-threatening lactic acidosis
Leigh syndrome	>90 nuclear genes (most commonly *SURF1*) and 14 mtDNA genes (most commonly *MT-ATP6*, *MT-ND3*, *MT-ND5*, and *MT-ND6*)	Infancy-childhood	Neurodevelopmental regression, encephalopathy, epilepsy, hypotonia, dystonia, and failure to thrive Onset commonly follows a viral infection	Bilateral, typically symmetric, hyperintensities on T2-weighted MRI in the basal ganglia and/or brainstem		Trial of biotin and thiamine with basal ganglia disease of unknown cause Trial of riboflavin for complex I deficiencies
Neuropathy, ataxia, and retinitis pigmentosa (NARP)	*MT-ATP6*	Childhood-early adulthood	Sensorimotor neuropathy, ataxia, pigmentary retinopathy/optic atrophy Clinical continuum with Leigh syndrome	Cerebral or cerebellar atrophy may be noted on brain MRI	Plasma amino acids may reveal citrulline deficiency	Citrulline supplementation
Alpers-Huttenlocher	*POLG*	Childhood	Progressive encephalopathy, intractable epilepsy, movement disorder, myopathy, ataxia, psychomotor regression, endocrinopathy, liver failure	Possible nonspecific gliosis and global atrophy Peri-Rolandic sign, occipital and pulvinar lesions	Avoid valproic acid because of potential for fulminant liver failure	High-dose N-acetylcysteine Folinic acid for secondary cerebral folate deficiency Liver transplant is contraindicated
Chronic progressive external ophthalmoplegia (CPEO)	mtDNA deletion syndromes (typically associated with *POLG*, *SLC25A4*, *TWNK*, *RRM2B*, and *DNA2*) or single large-scale mtDNA deletion	Childhood-adulthood	Ophthalmoparesis, ptosis Possible hearing loss, myopathy, and parkinsonism	Possible leukoencephalopathy, cerebral/cerebellar atrophy, basal ganglia and brain stem lesions		Sling or surgical correction of ptosis; prisms for ophthalmoplegia Lutein for retinal involvement

TABLE 71.2 Clinical Syndromes—cont'd

Syndrome	Genetics	Onset	Clinical Features	Brain MRI	Special Considerations	Specific Treatment
Pearson syndrome	Single large-scale mtDNA deletion	Infancy-childhood	Sideroblastic anemia, exocrine pancreatic dysfunction, endocrinopathy, renal tubulopathy (Fanconi syndrome)	White matter disease	Often go on to develop Kearns-Sayre syndrome in childhood	Folinic acid for secondary cerebral folate deficiency Pancreatic enzymes for abnormal fecal elastase
Kearns-Sayre syndrome (KSS)		Childhood (younger than 20 years)	Progressive external ophthalmoplegia, pigmentary retinopathy, and cardiac conduction abnormalities Can also have cerebellar ataxia, myopathy, endocrinopathies, sensorineural hearing loss, cognitive decline, short stature, failure to thrive, and feeding intolerance	Possible leukoencephalopathy, cerebral/cerebellar atrophy, basal ganglia and brain stem lesions	Transition to complete heart block may be rapid; have a low threshold to place pacemaker at first sign of arrhythmia or bundle branch block Hypocalcemia may develop as a result of hypoparathyroidism	
Mitochondrial myopathy, encephalopathy, lactic acidosis, and stroke-like episodes (MELAS)	mtDNA mutations (most commonly *MT-TL*, m.3243A>G)	Typically, 2-20 years	Stroke-like episodes, deafness, diabetes mellitus, pigmented retinopathy, cardiomyopathy, cerebellar ataxia, seizures, encephalopathy, lactic acidosis, myopathy, short stature, failure to thrive	Metabolic Stroke: slowly spreading T2-hyperintense lesion with diffusion restriction, not in a vascular distribution, typically involving the posterior cerebrum. MRS may show decreased N-acetyl aspartate and increased lactate	Maternal family members with maternally inherited deafness and diabetes (MIDD), renal failure	Intravenous arginine during stroke-like episodes Oral arginine, citrulline, and/or taurine as prophylaxis
Myoclonic epilepsy with ragged red fibers (MERRF)	mtDNA mutations (most commonly *MT-TK*, m.8344A>G)	Childhood	Initial symptom is usually myoclonus Epilepsy, ataxia, myopathy, peripheral neuropathy, neuropsychiatric features, optic atrophy/pigmentary retinopathy, ophthalmoparesis, cardiomyopathy, and elevated lactic acid levels Multiple lipomas in the cervicothoracic region	Possible atrophy and basal ganglia calcification		
Leber's hereditary optic neuropathy (LHON)	mtDNA mutations (most commonly *MT-ND4*, *MT-ND6*, and *MT-ND1*)	Young adults, typically males	Subacute, painless, bilateral, central vision loss ± Dystonia, cardiac preexcitation syndromes, or multiple sclerosis–like symptoms	Variable white matter lesions and/or increased signal intensity in the optic nerves		Multiple clinical trials involving gene therapy or medications Idebenone approved by EMA

EMA, European Medicines Agency; *MRI*, magnetic resonance imaging; *MRS*, magnetic resonance spectroscopy.

The definitive diagnosis of PMD requires that a molecular genetic cause be identified. Noninvasive methods of genetic testing are initially preferred, most often including whole exome sequencing in blood or saliva, with analysis of proband and parent samples if possible; mtDNA sequencing in blood, urine, or buccal cells may be performed in the patient, mother, and other maternal relatives. If noninvasive genetic testing does not identify a cause, genetic testing in an affected organ (muscle, liver) may be necessary.

Functional testing (ETC enzyme analysis) of muscle, liver, or skin can help validate a novel variant identified on genetic testing. Other advanced testing includes mtDNA content determination to rule out depletion syndromes and evaluation of the structure of ETC complexes. Testing of this kind should be performed in coordination with a medical center specializing in the diagnosis of PMDs.

The following are two key points regarding the diagnosis of PMDs: (1) It is counterproductive to provide a label of PMD (or even "possible mitochondrial disease") without a definitive molecular diagnosis, and (2) it is inappropriate to attribute symptoms or conditions to an established diagnosis of a PMD without first ruling out other, potentially treatable, causes.

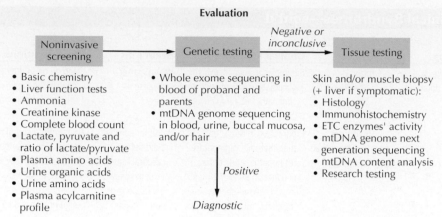

Fig. 71.2 Evaluation for Primary Mitochondrial Diseases. A suggested schema for initial diagnostic investigation.

MANAGEMENT

Acute

Patients with a PMD may have acute worsening of symptoms during times of increased metabolic demand, such as fever, illness, anesthesia, fasting, or other stressors. During these times, it is important to provide adequate hydration and nutritional support, which may necessitate hospital admission for intravenous dextrose to prevent catabolism. Further treatment will depend on specific symptoms and extent of organ dysfunction. Treatment may include arginine for metabolic strokes (± high-dose intravenous steroids for vasogenic edema) or treatment of lactic acidosis with sodium bicarbonate.

Chronic

Most important in the management of PMDs is attention to organ-specific clinical manifestations of the disorder. Referral to appropriate specialists for monitoring and management is critical. Standard advice includes at least annual follow-up with cardiology, ophthalmology, and audiology specialists. A screening assessment with an endocrinologist is recommended, especially in those with single large-scale mtDNA deletion disorders, because of the high prevalence of endocrinopathies. Annual laboratory assessments should be performed to investigate for the development or progression of other organ-specific conditions. Annual developmental, cognitive, neuropsychiatric, and growth assessments are recommended at each visit. Other screening assessments may be performed based on the particular condition.

Supportive care and health maintenance are essential, including avoiding fasting, ensuring proper nutrition, minimizing febrile illness, and achieving restful sleep. Vaccination is recommended given the elevated risk for decompensation with illness.

Exercise (aerobic and isotonic) has been shown to increase the number of healthy mitochondria, improve ETC enzyme activities, increase oxygen uptake, and lower mutant heteroplasmy levels. Supervised exercise programs after cardiac clearance are encouraged.

There are currently no US Food and Drug Administration (FDA)-approved medications for the treatment of PMDs. Supplements and vitamins are a low-risk treatment, often used for patients with PMDs despite lack of decisive evidence of benefit. Antioxidants, such as coenzyme Q10 (CoQ10), alpha-lipoic acid, N-acetylcysteine, and vitamin E, are often used with the aim of reducing oxidative stress and allowing for improved mitochondrial functioning. Vitamins and nonvitamin cofactors are used to support the enzymatic reactions and serve as a building block for complexes in the ETC. Other nutrients are used for specific indications. L-arginine is used for the prophylaxis and acute treatment of metabolic stroke.

MEDICATION SAFETY

Historically, many medications have been considered relatively contraindicated because of theoretical concerns of mitochondrial toxicity. Most of this has been dispelled, though there are some that require specific caution. Certain mtDNA mutations (m.1555A > G and m.1494C > T) do increase the risk for aminoglycoside-induced ototoxicity; however, if these medications would be lifesaving, it would be inappropriate to withhold them. It is suggested that mtDNA mutations be screened for before initiation of long-term aminoglycoside treatment. Valproic acid should be avoided in patients with *POLG* mutations, because this can precipitate fulminant liver failure. Neuromuscular blocking agents should be used with caution in patients with myopathic phenotypes. Anesthetics are generally considered safe; however, it is suggested that prolonged courses of propofol be avoided if possible, and care should be taken during surgery to ensure adequate energy source and hydration with glucose-containing intravenous fluids. Recent consensus guidelines suggest that it is acceptable to use statins as long as symptoms are monitored and creatine kinase levels followed, though this remains controversial.

FUTURE DIRECTIONS

Current therapies for PMDs are mostly symptomatic and preemptive. There are promising studies investigating disease-modifying therapies, including small-molecule therapies, manipulating the amount of cellular mitochondria, metabolic reprogramming, modulating production of reactive oxygen species, and manipulation of the mitochondrial genome. Studies are also being performed to attempt to prevent transmission of mitochondrial diseases to offspring.

SUGGESTED READINGS

Available online.

Head and Neck Disorders

Michelle Dunn

72

Disorders of the Eye

Eden Kahle and Papa Kwadwo Morgan-Asiedu

 CLINICAL VIGNETTE

A 3-year-old boy with a recent upper respiratory tract infection presents with 2 days of a red, swollen eye and 1 day of fever. On examination the patient is fussy and febrile, his right eye is swollen, and the conjunctiva is injected. He has pain with eye movements and limitation of lateral gaze in the right eye. Contrast-enhanced computed tomography of the orbits reveals inflammation in the orbit, an abscess along the periosteum of the right medial orbital wall, and an opacified ethmoid sinus. The patient underwent surgical drainage and was given intravenous antibiotics. Culture of the abscess revealed methicillin-sensitive *Staphylococcus aureus*.

ABNORMAL RED REFLEX

All children should have an examination of the red reflex within the first 2 months of life. Children with dark spots in the red reflex, a blunted or absent red reflex, a white reflex (leukocoria), or asymmetry of the reflexes (Bruckner reflex) should be referred to an ophthalmologist. An abnormal red reflex can result from corneal opacities, aqueous opacities, vitreous opacities, retinal lesions, or the presence of foreign bodies such as mucus in the tear film. Leukocoria may indicate a pathologic condition, including metabolic, inflammatory, infectious, toxic, oncologic, and traumatic causes; the most common are congenital cataracts and retinoblastoma.

Cataracts

Congenital cataracts occur in 2 in 10,000 births (Fig. 72.1). Of these, 20% to 25% of cases occur secondary to a congenital infection (rubella, cytomegalovirus, or toxoplasmosis) or as a component of a genetic or metabolic condition, such as Turner syndrome, Down syndrome, trisomies 13 and 18, galactosemia, and peroxisomal disorders.

Retinoblastoma

Retinoblastoma occurs in 1 in 15,000 to 20,000 live births. Of these, 95% present before the age of 5 years and 75% have unilateral disease. In the hereditary form, caused by a mutation in the retinoblastoma tumor suppressor gene, *Rb1*, approximately 60% of cases are bilateral and are associated with other cancers, notably osteosarcoma. Retinoblastoma can manifest with leukocoria and strabismus, and in more advanced cases, proptosis, eye pain, or hyphema. The extent of the disease should be evaluated by computed tomography (CT) or magnetic resonance imaging and orbital ultrasonography. Urgent referral to an ophthalmologist for potentially vision-sparing and life-saving treatment is imperative.

DISORDERS OF EYE MOVEMENT

Strabismus

Misalignment of the eyes affects approximately 4% of children younger than 6 years of age (Fig. 72.2). Heterophoria is the intermittent tendency for eyes to deviate and can be seen with stress, fatigue, or illness; heterotropia is a constant misalignment. The prefixes eso- (inward), exo- (outward), hyper- (upward), and hypo- (downward) indicate the direction of the misaligned eye. Tropias can be tested using the Hirschberg method, which assesses the corneal light reflex. The examiner shines a light onto both corneas and notes the symmetry of the light reflex; asymmetry indicates strabismus. For the cover test, the child looks at an object in the distance. The examiner covers one eye and watches for movement in the uncovered eye. If movement occurs in the uncovered eye, a misalignment exists in that eye. Phorias can be detected by covering the affected eye; when the eye is uncovered, the practitioner will note the eye moving back into alignment.

Early detection of strabismus is essential because amblyopia can develop if misalignment persists, resulting in permanent visual impairment. Strabismus that is constant or intermittent strabismus that does not correct by age 3 months should prompt ophthalmology referral to begin treatment. The unaffected eye is patched or blurred with atropine eye drops, thereby forcing the strabismic eye to provide a retinal image to the brain and stimulate the proper visual development. In some cases, surgery is necessary to achieve proper alignment.

New-onset eye deviation can be a sign of cranial nerve palsy, which can be caused by increased intracranial pressure, intracranial mass, or infection and should prompt immediate evaluation.

Amblyopia

Amblyopia is one of the most common causes of vision loss in pediatric populations. Amblyopia is vision impairment caused by an interference with a clear retinal image in one or both eyes during the development of visual acuity in infancy and early childhood. Amblyopia occurs during the critical period of development before the cortex has become visually mature, mainly within the first decade of life. It can be caused by a deviated eye (strabismus), difference in refractive error (anisometropia), or opacity within the visual axis (deprivation). Treatment is specific to the cause such as strabismus correction, corrective glasses, or removal of the opacity.

RED EYE

Red eye is one of the most common pediatric complaints in primary care, emergency care, and outpatient encounters. The differential diagnosis is broad, including infectious, allergic, and inflammatory causes such as Kawasaki disease and Stevens-Johnson syndrome, as well as trauma and

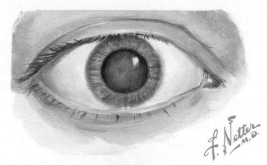

Fig. 72.1 Cataract.

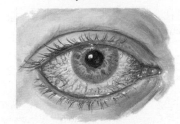

Conjunctivitis   Cobblestoning of tarsal conjunctiva

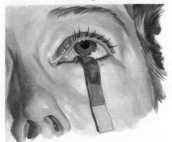

Fluorescein staining and HSV keratitis

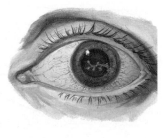

Technique of applying fluorescein strip in previously anesthetized eye

Dendritic keratitis (herpes simplex) demonstrated by fluorescein

Fig. 72.3 Red Eye.

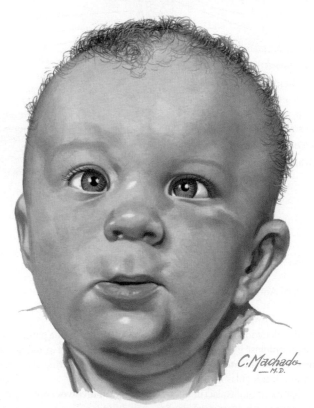

Fig. 72.2 Strabismus.

topical antivirals and, depending on the extent of infection, oral or intravenous acyclovir. Topical steroids are contraindicated. HSV conjunctivitis in neonates should prompt a full workup and intravenous acyclovir because they are at risk for invasive HSV infection.

Bacterial Conjunctivitis

Bacterial conjunctivitis presents with hyperemia, edema, mucopurulent discharge, ocular pain, and early morning crusting. Common organisms involved are nontypeable *Haemophilus influenzae* (often associated with ipsilateral otitis media), *Staphylococcus* and *Streptococcus* species, and *Moraxella catarrhalis*. Treatment involves topical antibiotic drops or ointment such as polymyxin-trimethoprim, and patients who wear contact lens should be treated for *Pseudomonas aeruginosa* with fluoroquinolone drops.

Practitioners should suspect *Neisseria gonorrhoeae* or *Chlamydia trachomatis* infection when symptoms of conjunctivitis are present in the first 4 weeks of life, termed *ophthalmia neonatorum*. After the neonatal stage, *N. gonorrhoeae* should raise concern for sexual abuse. Referral to an ophthalmologist for *Neisseria* conjunctivitis is recommended.

Allergic Conjunctivitis

The hallmark of allergic conjunctivitis is itching along with clear tearing, injected conjunctivae, and conjunctival edema (chemosis) in both eyes. In more severe cases, cobblestoning of the tarsal conjunctivae is present (Fig. 72.3). Acute allergic conjunctivitis includes seasonal allergic conjunctivitis (caused by pollen, weeds, molds, grasses) and perennial allergic conjunctivitis (caused by indoor allergens). Elimination of the offending agent and symptomatic treatment with cold compresses is recommended. Topical therapy with mast cell stabilizers or antihistamines can be used, as can oral antihistamines.

Chemical Conjunctivitis

Various substances can cause chemical conjunctivitis. Alkali exposure lingers in the conjunctival tissues and continues to cause damage for hours or

glaucoma. The most common cause is conjunctivitis, or inflammation of the conjunctivae, which is the mucous membrane that covers the surface of the eye up to the limbus (the junction of the sclera and the cornea) and continues on to the inside surface of the eyelids. Emergency referral to an ophthalmologist is recommended if there is vision loss, significant purulent discharge, involvement of the cornea, traumatic eye injury, history of recurrent ocular infections, or recent ocular surgery.

Viral Conjunctivitis

Viral conjunctivitis manifests with watery or mucopurulent discharge, eye irritation, scleral injection (Fig. 72.3), and foreign body sensation. Both eyes are usually affected simultaneously or in sequence.

Adenovirus, the most common pathogen causing viral conjunctivitis, is highly contagious. Treatment is symptomatic care, including cool compresses. Topical antibiotics should be used if large epithelial defects are present. Other agents such as influenza, enterovirus, measles, and herpes simplex virus (HSV) can also cause conjunctivitis. Primary or recurrent HSV can cause keratitis (corneal inflammation) with a dendrite pattern seen on fluorescein staining (Fig. 72.3). Treatment of ocular HSV should be undertaken in consultation with an ophthalmologist. Options include

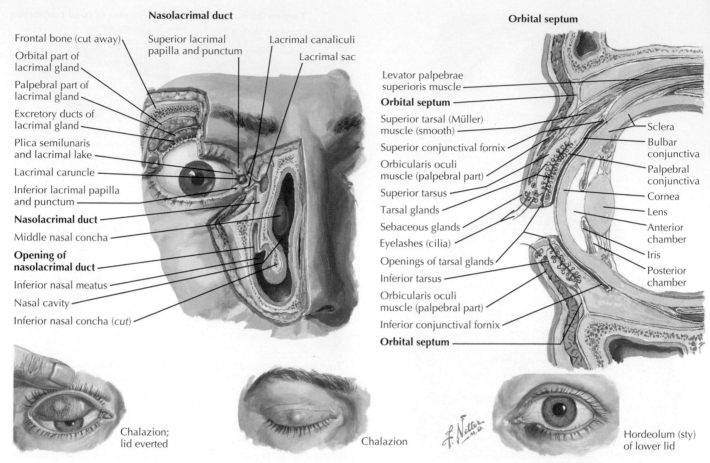

Fig. 72.4 Anatomy of the Eye; Disorders of Adnexal Structures.

days. Acids precipitate proteins and produce their effect immediately. In every patient with a chemical exposure, the eyes should be irrigated thoroughly with normal saline to remove the noxious substance. Irrigation should continue until a neutral pH ($\approx$7.4) of the eye is achieved.

Uveitis

Uveitis is inflammation of the inner vascular coat of the eye (iris, ciliary body, and choroids). Posterior uveitis involves the choroid and manifests with visual changes such as floaters and decreased vision. Anterior uveitis is synonymous with iritis and involves inflammation of the iris and ciliary body. Patients may have circumlimbal redness, eye pain, headache, photophobia, decreased vision, miosis, hypopyon (layering of white blood cells in the anterior chamber), and keratic precipitates. Uveitis can be seen in systemic immune-mediated diseases such as juvenile idiopathic arthritis, inflammatory bowel disease, and sarcoid, as well as infections such as toxoplasmosis, tuberculosis, cytomegalovirus, and syphilis. Patients should be referred to an ophthalmologist for management.

DISORDERS OF ADNEXAL STRUCTURES

Nasolacrimal Duct Obstruction

Nasolacrimal duct obstruction occurs in 2% to 4% of full-term babies and is even more common in premature babies. Congenital obstruction is usually caused by an imperforate membrane at the distal end of the nasolacrimal duct (Fig. 72.4). Patients present with tears overflowing the eyelid (epiphora) and mucoid matter crusting the eyelashes.

If the patient has excessive tearing associated with photophobia, blepharospasm, or corneal and ocular enlargement, the physician should consider glaucoma as a cause of the symptoms and refer the patient to an ophthalmologist immediately. Glaucoma is a rare entity in infancy but can be vision-threatening. Other causes of excessive tearing are corneal abrasion, intraocular inflammation, and foreign body.

Treatment of nasolacrimal duct obstruction involves applying digital pressure with downward strokes several times a day. Approximately 90% of cases resolve before 1 year of age. Patients can be referred to an ophthalmologist if symptoms do not resolve, in which case probing of the duct may be necessary. If mucopurulent discharge is expressible with palpation of the lacrimal sac, and the sac is swollen, red, and tender, the patient may have an associated dacryocystitis, or inflammation of the lacrimal sac. Dacryocystitis requires treatment with topical and often oral or intravenous antibiotics and sometimes surgical drainage.

Hordeolum and Chalazion

A hordeolum is inflammation or impaction of a sebaceous gland of the eyelid. Whereas an internal hordeolum involves the meibomian glands and occurs on the conjunctival surface, infection of the glands of Zeiss or Moll causes an abscess on the eyelid margin known as an external hordeolum (stye). A chalazion is a chronic granulomatous inflammation resulting from obstruction of a meibomian gland, which is noted as a small, rubbery nodule located more centrally on the eyelid (Fig. 72.4).

Treatment of an external hordeolum involves warm compresses to encourage drainage and rarely incision and drainage. Topical antibiotics can be used for lesions that appear infected or are accompanied by discharge. Resolution may take several weeks. A chalazion, if persistent, may be removed by an ophthalmologist by incision and curettage or steroid injection.

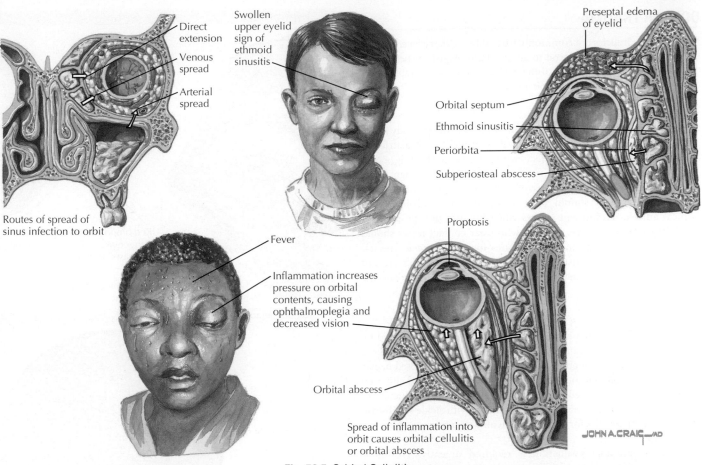

Fig. 72.5 Orbital Cellulitis.

PERIORBITAL AND ORBITAL CELLULITIS

Periorbital (Preseptal) Cellulitis

Periorbital cellulitis is inflammation of the eyelids and periorbital tissues anterior to the orbital septum, usually caused by contiguous infection of the periorbital soft tissues of the face. The most common pathogens are *Staphylococcus aureus, Staphylococcus epidermidis,* group A β-hemolytic streptococci, and *Streptococcus pneumoniae.* Differential diagnosis includes allergic reactions and edema. Patients present with erythema and swelling of the eyelids and conjunctival injection.

Mild cases can be managed on an outpatient basis with antibiotics such as amoxicillin-clavulanate or clindamycin; more severe cases require intravenous antibiotics. If there is any suspicion for orbital cellulitis, the patient should have a CT scan of the sinuses and orbits.

Orbital Cellulitis and Abscess

Orbital cellulitis (Fig. 72.5) presents with the previously described symptoms of periorbital cellulitis, but also with limitation of eye movement, diplopia, and in severe cases proptosis and decreased visual acuity, which distinguish it from a preseptal infection. Paranasal (ethmoid) sinusitis is the most common cause, but it can also result from seeding from bacteremia as well as direct extension or venous spread of infection from contiguous sites such as the eyelids, conjunctiva, globe, lacrimal gland, and nasolacrimal sac. *S. aureus,* group A streptococcus, *Streptococcus pneumoniae, Haemophilus influenzae,* and anaerobes are commonly implicated as pathogens. More serious cases may involve the optic nerve and cause loss of vision or extend intracranially and result in complications such as cavernous sinus thrombosis, meningitis, epidural and subdural empyema, or brain abscesses.

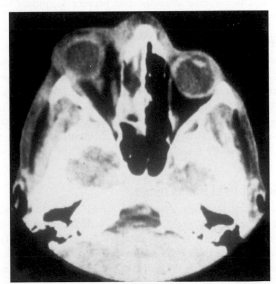

Fig. 72.6 Computed tomography scan showing orbital cellulitis with ethmoid sinus opacification and right eye proptosis.

A CT of the sinuses and orbits with contrast (Fig. 72.6) should be performed to confirm infection within the orbit and to detect subperiosteal abscess or intracranial extension. Treatment with broad-spectrum parenteral antibiotics such as high-dose ampicillin–sulbactam is indicated. Clindamycin or vancomycin may be used for coverage of methicillin-resistant *S. aureus* (MRSA) where it is prevalent. Surgical intervention is likely necessary in cases with abscess or empyema formation.

OCULAR TRAUMA

Minor ocular injuries are commonly treated by pediatricians. Injuries that require immediate referral to an ophthalmologist are penetrated or ruptured globe, laceration of the eyelid margin, or entrapment of the extraocular muscles after orbital fracture.

Corneal Abrasion

Corneal abrasion presents with the sensation of a foreign body in the eye, pain, scleral injection, tearing, and photophobia. Pediatricians can detect corneal epithelial defects with fluorescein dye (Fig. 72.3). The eyelid should be everted to check for retained foreign body. Vision testing also should be performed, and if vision changes are present, the patient should be referred to an ophthalmologist. Topical antibiotic ointment is prescribed for infection prophylaxis and lubrication of the eye. Patients who wear contact lenses should be treated with topical fluoroquinolones for *Pseudomonas* species. Oral analgesics can be used for pain. Topical anesthetics are not recommended because they slow epithelial healing and decrease the protective blinking reflex.

Hyphema

Hyphema is blood in the anterior chamber that is usually caused by blunt trauma or, less commonly, lacerating injury. Layering of blood cells can be seen by penlight or slit lamp (Fig. 72.7). Increased ocular pressure may develop if the trabecular meshwork is affected either by the original injury or by red blood cells causing a blockage. Patients are at risk for rebleeding 3 to 5 days later. Patients with sickle cell disease or trait are at higher risk for complications and require more aggressive intervention.

An ophthalmology evaluation is required urgently. Treatment involves wearing an eye shield and maintaining a 30-degree angle of the head to promote drainage and prevent secondary bleeding. Nonsteroidal antiinflammatory drugs should be avoided.

Retinal Hemorrhage

Retinal hemorrhages can be caused by increased intrathoracic pressure or by acceleration–deceleration injuries. They are common in newborns delivered vaginally and resolve within 2 to 6 weeks without sequelae. They can also occur during trauma and are present in 85% of cases of shaken babies. The hemorrhages seen in nonaccidental trauma have a distinctive pattern and are often bilateral, are flame-shaped, and include preretinal structures and the macula (see Fig. 72.7).

Subconjunctival Hemorrhage

Subconjunctival hemorrhage is the presence of blood between the conjunctiva and sclera (Fig. 72.7), is extremely common in newborns after vaginal birth, and resolves spontaneously within 2 weeks. In older children and adults, these hemorrhages are usually caused by increased intraocular pressure from coughing or sneezing or result from infection such as adenoviral conjunctivitis.

FUTURE DIRECTIONS

Advances continue to be made in diagnostic techniques and treatments of pediatric ophthalmologic conditions. Ocular ultrasonography is an emerging technique for evaluating patients in the emergency department. For traumatic eye injuries, ultrasound can identify penetrating globe injury and intraocular foreign body. Ultrasound also can be used to measure the optic nerve sheath diameter, which correlates with increased intracranial pressure.

SUGGESTED READINGS

Available online.

Hyphema

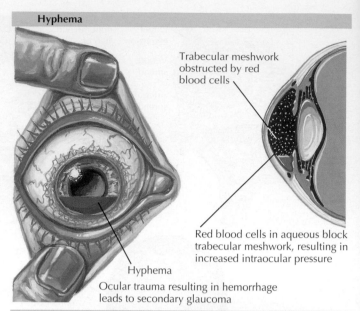

Trabecular meshwork obstructed by red blood cells

Red blood cells in aqueous block trabecular meshwork, resulting in increased intraocular pressure

Hyphema

Ocular trauma resulting in hemorrhage leads to secondary glaucoma

Retinal hemorrhage

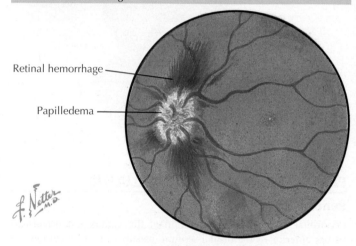

Retinal hemorrhage

Papilledema

In older children, frank papilledema may accompany increased intracranial pressure caused by subdural bleeding

Subconjunctival hemorrhage

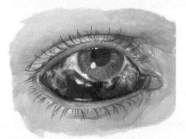

Fig. 72.7 Ocular Trauma.

73

Disorders of the Ear and Audition

Hannah Connor and Holly Benz

✳ CLINICAL VIGNETTE

A 5-year-old previously healthy boy presents to the emergency department (ED) with ear pain and fever. Symptoms started 5 days earlier, with left ear pain. Four days ago, he visited his pediatrician, who diagnosed a viral illness and recommended symptomatic care. Since that time, the pain in his left ear has worsened and he developed a high fever. Parents are also concerned that his left ear seems to be "bulging out" from his head today. In the ED, vital signs are significant for a fever to 104°F (40°C) and tachycardia to the 140s. Physical examination is notable for a dull, bulging left tympanic membrane with surrounding erythema, protrusion of the left ear from the skull base with tenderness, swelling, and erythema over the mastoid bone. Diagnostic workup shows a white blood count of 22,000/μL, with 87% neutrophils, C-reactive protein of 25 mg/dL (normal 0 to 1), and computed tomography scan concerning for opacification of the mastoid air cells and middle ear and loss of definition of the septae that define the mastoid air cells, consistent with mastoiditis. Otolaryngology performs myringotomy, and he is admitted for intravenous antibiotics. Fluid cultures from the ear grow *Streptococcus pneumoniae*, and after improvement on intravenous therapy, he is transitioned to oral antibiotics and discharged home in good condition.

The ear is divided into three parts: the outer, middle, and inner ear. The outer ear consists of the auricle and ear canal up to the tympanic membrane (TM). The middle ear is bound by the TM and the round window. The middle ear contains three bones that conduct sound—the malleus, the incus, and the stapes—and the eustachian (pharyngotympanic) tube that connects the middle ear cavity to the pharynx. The inner ear contains the cochlea and semicircular canals (Fig. 73.1). This chapter will organize ear pathologic conditions by the outer, middle, and inner ear.

THE OUTER EAR

Outer Ear Malformations

Microtia, a small or deformed pinna, and anotia, an absent pinna, can occur in isolation or can be related to a genetic syndrome. Preauricular pits anterior to the helix and superior to the tragus are common, occurring in 8 in 1000 children. Identification of ear malformations, such as ear skin tags or pits are very important on a newborn examination, because they can be clues to underlying genetic or structural pathologic conditions, in particular hearing loss and kidney abnormalities. Infants with microtia, anotia, or preauricular pits should receive audiologic testing. Beyond audiologic testing, if a newborn has an ear malformation in concert with other malformations or dysmorphic features, family history of deafness, or is born to a mother with a history of gestational diabetes, it is recommended that they undergo renal bladder ultrasonography.

Ear malformations should alert the examiner to search for other dysmorphic features that could suggest an underlying genetic disorder, which, if present, should be referred to a pediatric genetic specialist. Skin tags, composed of skin, subcutaneous fat, and/or cartilage, can be removed for cosmetic purposes. Major malformations may require surgery.

Foreign Body

Foreign bodies in the ear are most often found in children younger than 6 years of age. Foreign bodies are often asymptomatic and present if the caregiver has concern that an object was placed in the ear or are found incidentally on examination. Children might also present with hearing loss or otorrhea. If there is evidence of injury or penetration, or the foreign object is a button battery, urgent referral to an otolaryngologist is needed. The foreign body should be removed, and irrigation is often necessary.

Otitis Externa
Etiology and Pathogenesis

Otitis externa (OE), commonly called "swimmer's ear" is inflammation of the external auditory canal. Of cases of OE in the United States, 90% are due to bacterial causes, with *Pseudomonas aeruginosa* and *Staphylococcus aureus* being the most common. OE is characterized by a breakdown in the cerumen-skin barrier, which can be caused by prolonged exposure to water, trauma to the ear canal, dermatologic conditions, or hearing aids.

Clinical Presentation

The symptoms of OE include rapid-onset otalgia, pruritus, otorrhea, and a sensation of "fullness" in the ear canal. The hallmark sign of acute OE (AOE) is tenderness of the tragus or the pinna when manipulated. Otoscopic examination may be painful and shows a swollen ear canal, possibly with visible debris (Fig. 73.2). Other conditions on the differential diagnoses list include otitis media with perforation, malignant OE (necrotizing osteomyelitis), furunculosis, contact dermatitis of the ear canal, and other generalized dermatologic conditions occurring in or around the ear canal (Fig. 73.2).

Evaluation and Management

Uncomplicated OE should be treated with pain management and topical antibiotics. Oral antibiotics should be used only for complicated OE or for immunocompromised patients. Wicks can be used if the ear canal is obstructed. Treatment duration should be 7 to 10 days, with improvement typically seen within 3 days.

Future Directions

Future research should focus on preventive strategies for OE, which is currently not evaluated in any randomized trial.

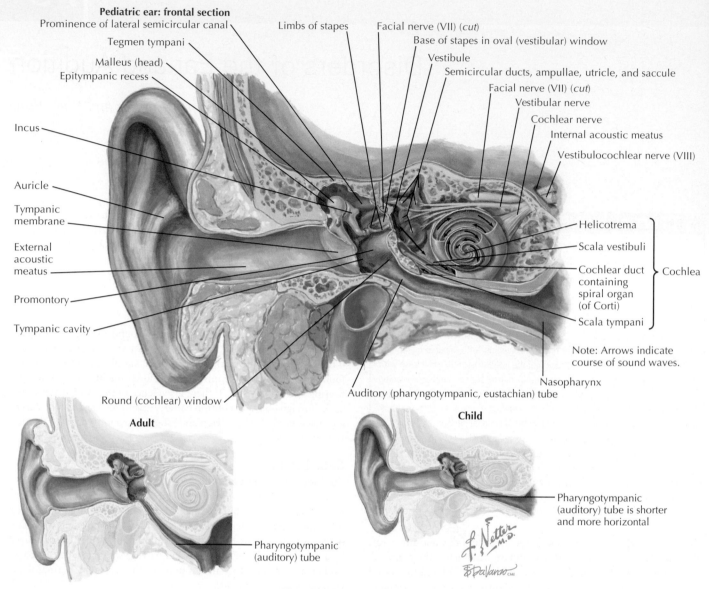

Pediatric ear: frontal section

Prominence of lateral semicircular canal
Tegmen tympani
Malleus (head)
Epitympanic recess
Incus
Auricle
Tympanic membrane
External acoustic meatus
Promontory
Tympanic cavity
Limbs of stapes
Facial nerve (VII) (*cut*)
Base of stapes in oval (vestibular) window
Vestibule
Semicircular ducts, ampullae, utricle, and saccule
Facial nerve (VII) (*cut*)
Vestibular nerve
Cochlear nerve
Internal acoustic meatus
Vestibulocochlear nerve (VIII)
Helicotrema
Scala vestibuli
Cochlear duct containing spiral organ (of Corti)
Cochlea
Scala tympani
Note: Arrows indicate course of sound waves.
Round (cochlear) window
Auditory (pharyngotympanic, eustachian) tube
Nasopharynx

Adult
Pharyngotympanic (auditory) tube

Child
Pharyngotympanic (auditory) tube is shorter and more horizontal

Fig. 73.1 Anatomy of the Ear.

THE MIDDLE EAR

Otitis Media

Etiology and Pathogenesis

Otitis media (OM) is subdivided into acute otitis media (AOM) and otitis media with effusion (OME). AOM is defined by rapid onset of symptoms, evidence of middle ear effusion, and signs and symptoms of middle ear inflammation. OME is characterized by the presence of middle ear fluid without signs of an acute infection. AOM is the most common illness pediatricians encounter and the most common reason for antibiotic prescriptions in children.

OM is usually preceded by a viral upper respiratory tract infection, which leads to the accumulation of inflammatory edema in the nasopharynx. This edema can obstruct the eustachian tube, leading to negative middle ear pressure that allows aspiration of contents and bacteria from the pharynx into the middle ear. In young children, the eustachian tube has a more horizontal orientation, further complicating the flow of middle ear fluid.

In patients with AOM, cultures of middle ear fluid have shown various organism types, with 15% of cultures growing a mixture of bacteria and viruses, and 55% growing only bacteria. The most common bacterial pathogens isolated in AOM are *Streptococcus pneumoniae*, nontypeable *Haemophilus influenzae*, and *Moraxella catarrhalis*.

Clinical Presentation

Children with AOM often present with ear pain, ear tugging, fever, and/or ear drainage. OME is often seen on a routine well-child examination or on examination for follow-up of AOM. OME is generally asymptomatic but can lead to hearing loss.

A normal TM, visible with otoscopy, should be translucent; the umbo, handle of the malleus, shadow of the incus, and cone of the light reflex should be visible (Fig. 73.3). On pneumatic otoscopy, the TM should be freely mobile. An immobile TM suggests the presence of a middle ear effusion (MEE), which occurs in AOM and OME. A bulging TM helps differentiate AOM from OME. Tympanometry or acoustic reflectometry can be used to confirm the presence of MEE.

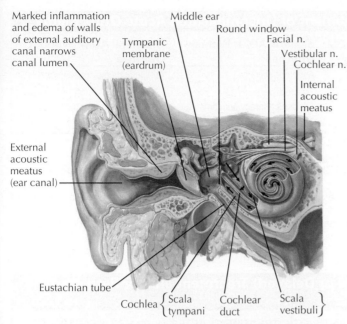

Marked inflammation and edema of walls of external auditory canal narrows canal lumen

Middle ear

Round window

Facial n.

Tympanic membrane (eardrum)

Vestibular n.

Cochlear n.

Internal acoustic meatus

External acoustic meatus (ear canal)

Eustachian tube

Cochlea { Scala tympani

Cochlear duct

Scala vestibuli }

In otitis externa, inflammation, edema, and discharge are limited to external auditory canal and its walls

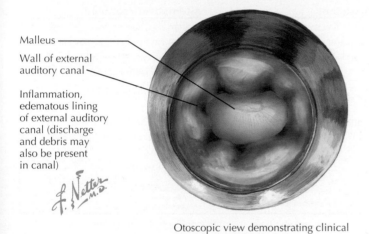

Malleus

Wall of external auditory canal

Inflammation, edematous lining of external auditory canal (discharge and debris may also be present in canal)

Otoscopic view demonstrating clinical appearance of otitis externa

Fig. 73.2 Acute Otitis Externa.

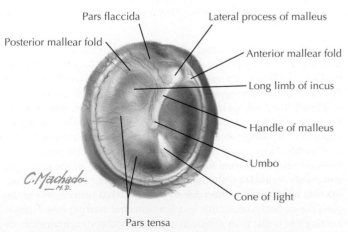

Pars flaccida

Lateral process of malleus

Posterior mallear fold

Anterior mallear fold

Long limb of incus

Handle of malleus

Umbo

Cone of light

Pars tensa

Fig. 73.3 Otoscopic View of Right Tympanic Membrane.

Evaluation and Management

OM can manifest with various signs and symptoms of inflammation, complicating the ability of a physician to diagnose OM and to differentiate between AOM and OME. According to the American Academy of Pediatricians (AAP), AOM should be diagnosed in a child with acute onset of symptoms, MEE, and signs of middle-ear inflammation (otalgia or distinct erythema) (Fig. 73.4). AOM should not be diagnosed if the child does not have MEE.

The management of AOM is continuously evolving as more studies show resolution of AOM independent of antibiotic use. Children 6 months of age or younger with AOM and children 6 to 24 months of age with bilateral AOM should be treated immediately with antibiotics. Children of any age with AOM and severe symptoms (fever ≥102.2°F [≥39°C], otalgia for >48 hours) should be treated with antibiotics. Children 6 to 24 months with nonsevere unilateral AOM and children older than 24 months with unilateral or bilateral nonsevere AOM should either be prescribed antibiotics or offered observation with close follow-up. If observation is chosen, there must be a mechanism in place to ensure follow-up with the patient. Antibiotic therapy should be initiated if symptoms do not improve within 48 to 72 hours of onset (Table 73.1). The first-line antibiotic for AOM is high-dose amoxicillin; see Table 73.2 for comprehensive antibiotic recommendations. Additionally, children with AOM should be prescribed analgesics for pain. AOM in a patient with draining tympanostomy tubes only requires treatment with a topical antibiotic (usually a fluoroquinolone).

More than 75% of cases of OME resolve spontaneously within 3 months. Therefore the AAP recommends watchful waiting of patients with OME for 3 months.

Complications

Mastoiditis is a rare, but serious complication of AOM. The middle ear space is connected to mastoid air cells through the aditus ad antrum. Blockage of the aditus ad antrum leads to inflammation of the mastoid. Physical examination reveals tenderness and swelling of the mastoid area, and sometimes protrusion of the auricle. Imaging of the temporal bone through computed tomography (CT) is not necessary but may assist in the diagnosis. Patients with mastoiditis require treatment with intravenous antibiotics. Intracranial complications such as meningitis, epidural abscess, and cavernous sinus thrombosis are rare. Recurrent AOM can lead to hearing loss and cholesteatoma.

Future Directions

For AOM, an important research question is whether amoxicillin will remain a first-line antibiotic as the pneumococcal vaccine continues to change the prevalence of *S. pneumoniae*. Continual monitoring of outcomes in the United States is a necessity to ensure that serious bacterial infectious complications do not increase as more physicians adopt the observation option before treatment.

Cholesteatoma

Cholesteatomas are spherical, cyst-like lesions in the middle ear or mastoid formed by squamous epithelium and keratin debris. Acquired cholesteatomas most commonly arise from chronic otitis media. Congenital cholesteatomas are less common and are most likely due to the development of squamous inclusion cysts in utero. Warning signs for a cholesteatoma include a white lesion behind an intact TM, a deep retraction pocket, focal granulation on the TM, ear drainage for more than 2 weeks despite treatment, and new-onset hearing loss. Cholesteatomas require surgical resection.

TABLE 73.1   Recommendations for Initial Management of Uncomplicated Acute Otitis Media

Age	Otorrhea With AOM[a]	Unilateral or Bilateral AOM[a] With Severe Symptoms[b]	Bilateral AOM[a] Without Otorrhea	Unilateral AOM[a] Without Otorrhea
6 months to 2 years	Antibiotic therapy	Antibiotic therapy	Antibiotic therapy	Antibiotic therapy or additional observation[c]
≥2 years	Antibiotic therapy	Antibiotic therapy	Antibiotic therapy or additional observation[c]	Antibiotic therapy or additional observation[c]

AOM, Acute otitis media.

[a]Applies only to children with well-documented AOM with high certainty of diagnosis.

[b]A toxic-appearing child, persistent otalgia more than 48 hours, temperature ≥102.2°F (≥39°C) in the past 48 hours, or if there is uncertain access to follow-up after the visit.

[c]This plan of initial management provides an opportunity for shared decision-making with the child's family. If observation is offered, a mechanism must be in place to ensure follow-up and begin antibiotics if the child worsens or fails to improve within 48 to 72 hours of AOM onset.

Reused with permission from Lieberthal AS, Carroll AE, Chonmaitree T, et al. The diagnosis and management of acute otitis media. *Pediatrics.* 2013;131(3):e964-e999; DOI: 10.1542/peds.2012-3488, Table 4, https://pediatrics.aappublications.org/content/131/3/e964.

TABLE 73.2   Recommended Antibiotics for (Initial or Delayed) Treatment and for Patients Who Have Failed Initial Antibiotic Treatment

INITIAL IMMEDIATE OR DELAYED ANTIBIOTIC TREATMENT		ANTIBIOTIC TREATMENT AFTER 48–72 HR OF FAILURE OF INITIAL ANTIBIOTIC TREATMENT	
Recommended First-Line Treatment	Alternative Treatment (If Penicillin Allergy)	Recommended First-Line Treatment	Alternative Treatment
Amoxicillin (80–90 mg/kg/day in two divided doses)	Cefdinir (14 mg/kg/day in one or two doses)	Amoxicillin-clavulanate[a] (90 mg/kg/day of amoxicillin, with 6.4 mg/kg/day of clavulanate in two divided doses)	Ceftriaxone, 3 days Clindamycin (30–40 mg/kg/day in three divided doses), with or without third-generation cephalosporin
OR	Cefuroxime (30 mg/kg/day in two divided doses)	*OR*	Failure of second antibiotic
Amoxicillin-clavulanate[a] (90 mg/kg/day of amoxicillin, with 6.4 mg/kg/day of clavulanate [amoxicillin-to-clavulanate ratio, 14:1] in two divided doses)	Cefpodoxime (10 mg/kg/day in two divided doses)	Ceftriaxone (50 mg/kg/day [max 1 g] IM or IV for 3 days)	Clindamycin (30–40 mg/kg/day in three divided doses) plus third-generation cephalosporin
			Tympanocentesis[b]
	Ceftriaxone (50 mg/kg/day [max 1 g] IM or IV for 1 or 3 days)		Consult specialist[b]

[a]May be considered in patients who have received amoxicillin in the previous 30 days or who have the otitis-conjunctivitis syndrome.

[b]Perform tympanocentesis/drainage if skilled in the procedure, or seek a consultation from an otolaryngologist for tympanocentesis/drainage. If the tympanocentesis reveals multidrug-resistant bacteria, seek an infectious disease specialist consultation.

[c]Cefdinir, cefuroxime, cefpodoxime, and ceftriaxone are highly unlikely to be associated with cross-reactivity with penicillin allergy on the basis of their distinct chemical structures.

IM, Intramuscular; *IV,* intravenous.

Reused with permission from Lieberthal AS, Carroll AE, Chonmaitree T, et al. The diagnosis and management of acute otitis media. *Pediatrics.* 2013;131(3):e964-e999; DOI: 10.1542/peds.2012-3488, Table 5, https://pediatrics.aappublications.org/content/131/3/e964.

INNER EAR

Labyrinthitis

Labyrinthitis, also known as vestibular neuritis, is an acute inflammatory process that affects the vestibular nerve (Fig. 73.5). Clinical presentation is characterized by the rapid onset of vertigo with nausea, vomiting, imbalance, and nystagmus. Symptoms are normally self-resolving within a few days, but glucocorticoids and symptomatic treatment may be given (Fig. 73.5).

Hearing Loss
Etiology and Pathogenesis

Hearing loss is one of the most common congenital anomalies, occurring in 1 to 3 in 1000 healthy newborns and 2 to 4 in 1000 newborns with other risk factors. Causes of pediatric hearing loss can be genetic, infectious, traumatic, or the result of a physical blockage, such as otitis media with effusion or presence of a foreign object. Cytomegalovirus is the most common nongenetic cause of congenital hearing loss.

Conductive hearing loss (CHL), the most common type of hearing loss in children, is due to a disruption of sound in the external or middle ear. A foreign object in the ear canal, impacted cerumen, otitis media with effusion, and ossicular malformations can all cause CHL.

Sensorineural hearing loss is due to malfunction of the inner ear, commonly caused by destruction of stereocilia, cochlear malformation, or damage to the auditory nerve. Mixed hearing loss is the presence of both conductive and sensorineural hearing loss. Central hearing loss is due to dysfunction in the cerebral cortex, brainstem, or the eighth cranial nerve.

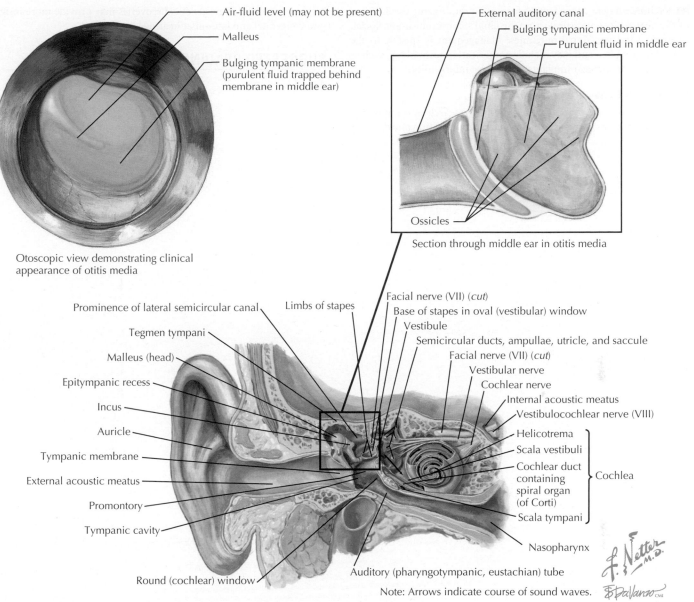

Air-fluid level (may not be present)

Malleus

Bulging tympanic membrane (purulent fluid trapped behind membrane in middle ear)

Otoscopic view demonstrating clinical appearance of otitis media

External auditory canal

Bulging tympanic membrane

Purulent fluid in middle ear

Ossicles

Section through middle ear in otitis media

Prominence of lateral semicircular canal

Limbs of stapes

Facial nerve (VII) (*cut*)

Base of stapes in oval (vestibular) window

Vestibule

Tegmen tympani

Semicircular ducts, ampullae, utricle, and saccule

Malleus (head)

Facial nerve (VII) (*cut*)

Epitympanic recess

Vestibular nerve

Cochlear nerve

Incus

Internal acoustic meatus

Auricle

Vestibulocochlear nerve (VIII)

Tympanic membrane

Helicotrema

External acoustic meatus

Scala vestibuli

Promontory

Cochlear duct containing spiral organ (of Corti)

Cochlea

Tympanic cavity

Scala tympani

Nasopharynx

Round (cochlear) window

Auditory (pharyngotympanic, eustachian) tube

Note: Arrows indicate course of sound waves.

Fig. 73.4 Acute Otitis Media.

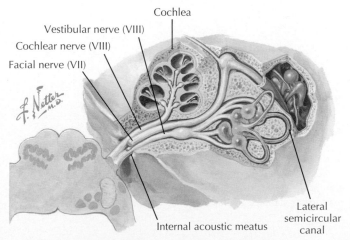

Cochlea

Vestibular nerve (VIII)

Cochlear nerve (VIII)

Facial nerve (VII)

Internal acoustic meatus

Lateral semicircular canal

Fig. 73.5 Vestibulocochlear Nerve (CN VIII).

Clinical Presentation

Speech delay is a hallmark of congenital deafness. Hearing-impaired infants generally develop early language milestones, such as babbling and gesturing, at a normal pace until 6 to 9 months of age. Around this time, those with severe hearing loss may present with loss of language milestones or overt language delay. Hearing loss can develop at any time, so it is important for providers to be aware of its warning signs and pursue further evaluation when indicated.

Evaluation and Management

The Joint Committee on Infant Hearing recommends that all infants receive screening for hearing loss by age 1 month, follow-up testing by age 3 months, and intervention by 6 months. Universal newborn hearing screenings use otoacoustic emission testing and auditory brainstem response testing.

Once hearing loss has been identified, early intervention with speech-language pathologists, audiologists, and educators should be started immediately. Management focuses on minimizing the duration of the hearing loss and supporting the child's communication, social, academic, and vocational outcomes. Management is specific to the type of hearing loss and may include amplification technology, such as hearing aids or cochlear implants, or surgical intervention.

Future Directions

For hearing loss, it is important to continue research into improving screenings, diagnosis, and treatment such as amplification and cochlear implant protocols. New genetic discoveries may provide more insight into congenital and late-onset hearing loss.

SUGGESTED READINGS

Available online.

74

Disorders of the Nose and Sinuses

Kristine A. DellaBadia and Rahael Borchers

 CLINICAL VIGNETTE

A 2-year-old girl presents with unilateral nasal drainage. Four days ago, she developed clear rhinorrhea on the right side. The drainage has become thicker and yellow and now has a foul odor. She has a normal appetite and no fever or cough, but has been sneezing frequently. On examination, purulent nasal discharge with scant blood is noted from the right nare. Anterior rhinoscopy reveals a gray foreign body on the right nasal floor.

Nasal complaints are common in the pediatric population. The differential is broad and variable based on the age of the patient. Evaluation should include an examination of both the exterior and interior of the nose. Interior examination can be accomplished using an otoscope with a wide speculum or a nasal speculum and flashlight. For a more thorough examination, nasal endoscopy is required, which typically requires referral to an otorhinolaryngologist (ear, nose, and throat [ENT] specialist).

CONGENITAL DISORDERS OF THE NOSE

Choanal Atresia

Choanal atresia is the complete or partial obstruction of the posterior nasal aperture by either soft tissue (membranous) or bone. Choanal atresia occurs in 1 in 7000 live births. Up to 50% of children with choanal atresia have other congenital anomalies, often as part of a genetic syndrome, most notably CHARGE (*c*oloboma, *h*eart defect, *a*tresia choanae, *r*etarded growth and development, *g*enital hypoplasia, *e*ar anomalies/deafness) syndrome.

Because infants are obligate nasal breathers, bilateral choanal atresia presents at birth with acute respiratory distress that improves with crying. Less commonly, these infants present with choking and feeding difficulties because of an inability to breathe during feeding. Unilateral choanal atresia is more common and usually manifests within the first 2 years of life with unilateral nasal obstruction and chronic mucoid drainage. Older children may present with chronic sinusitis.

Presumptive diagnosis of choanal atresia is made by failure to pass a 6-French catheter though the nares. Definitive diagnosis is made with computed tomography (CT) evaluation.

For bilateral choanal atresia, initial management involves establishing a stable airway, often requiring intubation. Definitive therapy is surgical recanalization.

Congenital Nasal Masses

Congenital nasal masses such as dermoid cysts, gliomas, and encephaloceles are another important consideration when evaluating a young child with nasal obstruction. Less commonly, these children may present with recurrent nasal infections or epistaxis. Evaluation should involve magnetic resonance imaging (MRI) or CT imaging because of the risk for intracranial communication.

ACQUIRED DISORDERS OF THE NOSE

Nasal Polyps

Nasal polyps are benign, inflammatory outgrowths of the nasal mucosa or sinuses leading to symptoms of postnasal drip, rhinorrhea, nasal obstruction, and anosmia. Associated impaired sinus drainage can lead to recurrent sinusitis. Development of nasal polyps is thought to be related to chronic inflammation, atopy, or recurrent infection. Nasal polyps rarely affect children younger than 10 years, unless they are associated with a chronic condition, most notably cystic fibrosis.

Nasal polyps appear as smooth, round growths on examination. Medical therapy (topical or oral corticosteroids) targets inflammation to reduce polyp size. Surgical excision is considered when symptoms do not improve with medical therapy.

Nasal Foreign Body

Nasal foreign bodies should be considered in toddlers presenting with nasal complaints. Foreign bodies are most commonly unilateral and right-sided (because of handedness). Most patients are asymptomatic and present to care because of witnessed foreign body insertion. Patients may complain of pain and unilateral, malodorous, nasal discharge.

Nasal foreign bodies can usually be visualized with anterior rhinoscopy. Intervention is not emergent, with the exception of magnets and batteries, which can cause severe soft tissue damage and septal perforation.

Removal of the nasal foreign body can be achieved with positive pressure applied to the mouth while the nonaffected nare is held closed, or by asking the child to blow forcefully from the affected nostril. If positive pressure is not successful, mechanical extraction can be attempted.

Nasal Trauma
Nasal Fractures

Nasal fractures are the most common facial fractures in children. Patients with a nasal fracture may present with epistaxis, soft tissue swelling, tenderness over the dorsum of the nose, bruising around the eyes, crepitus, step-offs, or obvious nasal deformity. The diagnosis of nasal fracture is clinical. Imaging is of limited utility and is not routinely recommended. CT scan should only be obtained if more extensive facial fractures are suspected. Children with suspected nasal fractures should be seen by an otorhinolaryngologist for reevaluation in 3 to 5 days, once the swelling has receded.

Septal Hematoma

Septal hematomas are collections of blood between the septal cartilage and perichondrium that develop 1 to 14 days after a nasal injury. Children may present with nasal obstruction, pain, or rhinorrhea. On examination, children may exhibit tenderness at the nasal tip, and internal examination will reveal boggy, compressible nasal mucosa. Swelling can be unilateral or bilateral. Once identified, emergent incision and drainage should be performed to prevent complications such as abscess formation and avascular necrosis of the septum.

Epistaxis

Epistaxis, or nasal bleeding, is a common complaint in children older than 2 years, with peak frequency occurring in children younger than 10 years.

In most cases, epistaxis is the result of mucosal irritation or digital trauma. Symptoms include mild, intermittent bleeding that resolves spontaneously or after holding brief, external pressure. Nasal bleeding that is profuse and difficult to control is suggestive of a more serious systemic or local pathologic condition, including platelet disorders, bleeding diatheses, hematologic malignancies, and vascular anomalies. These children often will have a history of recurrent nose bleeds that do not resolve with traditional measures. Detailed history and examination may offer additional clues suggestive of an underlying condition. Patients suspected of systemic illness should undergo a comprehensive hematologic workup with referral to the appropriate specialist.

The initial management of epistaxis is direct compression of the lower one-third of the lateral nasal wall for 10 to 15 minutes. If the bleeding cannot be slowed enough to identify a source, nasal packing should be considered. If a source is identified, topical lubricants or vasoconstrictors such as epinephrine, phenylephrine, or oxymetazoline can be applied. These agents should be used with caution in children younger than 6 years. Patients who fail attempts at local control should be referred to an otorhinolaryngologist for further management. Prevention should target the inciting agent and includes the use of water-based lubricants and humidified air to prevent crusting.

Rhinitis

Rhinitis occurs when the nasal mucosa becomes inflamed in response to an infectious, allergic, or nonallergic (vasomotor) trigger. Symptoms include nasal congestion, rhinorrhea, sneezing, and in some cases pruritus. In children, the most frequent cause is a viral upper respiratory tract infection (URI), most commonly rhinovirus. Nasal symptoms may be accompanied by cough, sore throat, fever, and headache. Treatment targets symptoms and varies based on the underlying cause.

Sinusitis

Sinusitis is a frequently diagnosed condition in pediatrics. Young children are estimated to have between six to eight colds per year, and 6% to 7% of those infections are thought to be complicated by acute bacterial rhinosinusitis (ABRS). Diagnosis can be difficult because the symptoms of sinusitis overlap with those of its predisposing conditions; however, it is a clinically important diagnosis because of the significant associated morbidity and potentially life-threatening complications.

Paranasal sinus development begins in utero and continues until adolescence. Development and pneumatization of the sinuses occurs throughout childhood and completes during adolescence (Fig. 74.1).

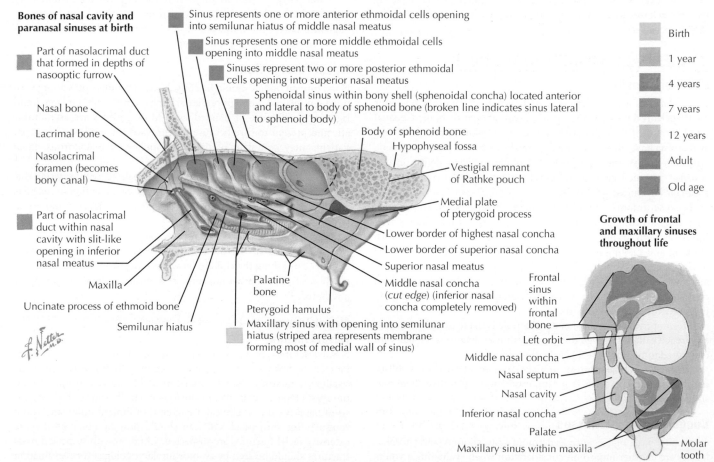

Fig. 74.1 Paranasal Sinuses: Changes With Age.

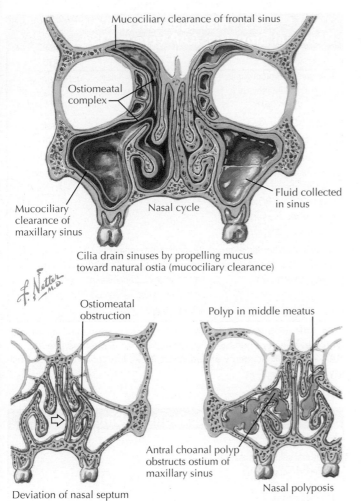

Fig. 74.2 Histology and Physiology of Nasal Cavity and Sinuses.

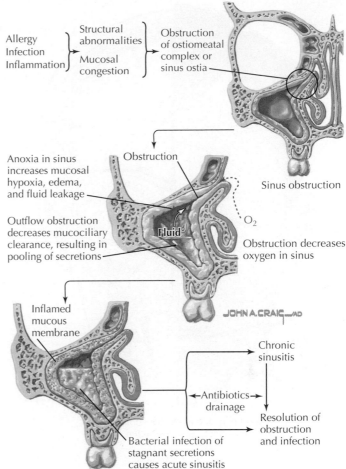

Fig. 74.3 Pathogenesis of Sinusitis.

The frontal, anterior ethmoid, and maxillary sinuses drain into the middle meatus of the nasal cavity through the ostiomeatal complex. Normally, sterility of the sinuses is maintained by the mucociliary apparatus, which mobilizes secretions and any bacteria toward the sinus ostia, and into the nasal cavity (Fig. 74.2). Mucociliary clearance is compromised when the sinus ostia become obstructed, which can be due to mechanical obstruction, inflammation, or impaired ciliary function. Impaired drainage leads to stasis of secretions, creating an ideal environment for bacterial overgrowth (Fig. 74.3).

The pathogens most commonly responsible for ABRS are the same as those for acute otitis media: *Streptococcus pneumoniae*, *Haemophilus influenzae*, and *Moraxella catarrhalis*. The clinical presentation of sinusitis compared with URI is reviewed in Table 74.1.

The diagnosis of uncomplicated ABRS is made clinically. Imaging cannot distinguish ABRS from a viral URI and thus is not recommended unless complications are suspected. Diagnosis is instead made by fulfilling the criteria for either persistent, worsening, or severe symptoms (Table 74.2). Evidence-based guidelines for diagnosis and management of ABRS have been put forth by both the American Academy of Pediatrics (AAP) and the Infectious Disease Society of America (IDSA) and are outlined in the following chart (Table 74.3). Clinicians should base their antibiotic choice and dosing on their local susceptibility patterns.

TABLE 74.1 Clinical Presentation of Sinusitis Compared With Upper Respiratory Infection

	Sinusitis	URI
Presenting symptoms	Persistent fever Rhinorrhea Nasal congestion Cough (commonly nocturnal) Headache Halitosis Facial pain (Fig. 74.4)	± Fever Rhinorrhea Nasal congestion Cough Headache Sore throat
Physical examination findings	Mucosal erythema and edema Purulent rhinorrhea ± Periorbital swelling ± Tenderness over frontal and maxillary sinuses (less common in children)	Mucosal erythema and edema Rhinorrhea (can be purulent)
Progression of illness	Persistent, worsening, or severe (Table 74.2)	Illness peaks at 3–5 days and then resolves by day 10 Fever resolves within the first 1–2 days

URI, Upper respiratory tract infection.

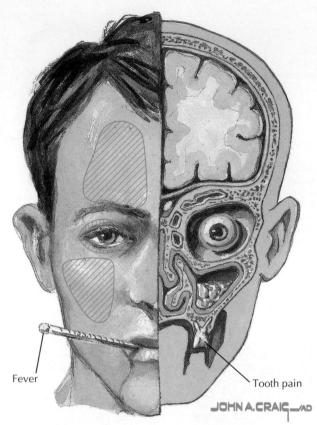

Fever

Tooth pain

JOHN A.CRAIG—AD

Areas of pain and tenderness (*green*). Pain caused by pressure in obstructed sinus

Fig. 74.4 Sinusitis.

TABLE 74.3   Management of Acute Bacterial Sinusitis: AAP Versus IDSA

	AAP	IDSA
Persistent symptoms in an otherwise healthy child older than 2 years	Observation for up to 3 days with initiation amoxicillin if symptoms persist or worsen[a]	High-dose amoxicillin-clavulanate
Severe onset or worsening course in any child	High-dose amoxicillin-clavulanate	High-dose amoxicillin-clavulanate
Persistent symptoms in a child who is younger than 2 years, in daycare, or has received antibiotics in the last 4 weeks	High-dose amoxicillin- clavulanate	High-dose amoxicillin-clavulanate
Children who are vomiting or unable to tolerate oral medications	Ceftriaxone intravenously or intramuscularly once or until able to tolerate transition to an oral antibiotic for completion of therapy	

[a]The AAP recommends standard-dose amoxicillin except in areas of high prevalence of nonsusceptible *Streptococcus pneumoniae*.
AAP, American Academy of Pediatrics; *IDSA,* Infectious Diseases Society of America.

BOX 74.1   Complications of Sinusitis

Orbital
- Orbital cellulitis/abscess
- Periorbital cellulitis

Intracranial
- Cavernous sinus thrombosis
- Epidural or subdural empyema
- Brain abscess
- Meningitis
- Encephalitis

Osseous
- Pott puffy tumor

TABLE 74.2   Diagnostic Criteria for Acute Bacterial Rhinosinusitis

Persistent symptoms	Respiratory symptoms lasting for more than 10 days without improvement
Worsening symptoms	Worsening symptoms or new onset of fever, nasal discharge, or cough after a period of improvement
Severe symptoms	Acute onset of fever greater than 102.2°F (>39°C) and purulent nasal discharge or facial pain for at least 3 days

Adjunctive therapy for symptomatic management may include intranasal corticosteroids (if history of allergic rhinitis), humidification, and intranasal saline irrigation. Antihistamines and decongestants are not recommended.

Patients who fail to improve within 72 hours after initial management, or who clinically worsen, should be evaluated for treatment failure. For these patients, it is reasonable to broaden antibiotic coverage and consider further evaluation for complications.

Complications of ABRS are characterized as orbital, intracranial, or osseous (Box 74.1) and when present warrant referral to the appropriate specialist. Any child presenting with worsening symptoms despite adequate treatment or exhibiting an abnormal neurologic examination should receive immediate evaluation for complications.

SUGGESTED READINGS

Available online.

75

Disorders of Dentition and Oral Cavity

Jeremy Jones and Morgan Congdon

 CLINICAL VIGNETTE

A 13-year-old boy is brought to the emergency department immediately after being struck in the mouth by a basketball after school. He is holding a cup with his right maxillary incisor submersed in milk. His mom states she read this can save the tooth and asks you if it can be reimplanted. You rinse the tooth with saline, place it in Hanks balanced salt solution, and page oral surgery. You reassure his mother that the prognosis for his tooth is better given her quick presentation to care.

DENTITION

Teeth originate from neuroectoderm beginning around 28 days after conception. The 20 primary teeth (deciduous or milk teeth) erupt between the ages of 6 and 30 months. During this process, known as teething, children acquire about 1 tooth per month. The expulsion of the primary dentition and the eruption of the 32 permanent teeth usually begin around age 6 years, with most children having lost all primary teeth by early adolescence (Fig. 75.1).

Normal Tooth Anatomy

The visible portion of the tooth (crown) protrudes from the gingiva. Its hard surface is an enamel made of hydroxyapatite crystals. The root connects the tooth to the maxillary and mandibular alveolar bones and has a hard covering called cement that attaches to the periodontal ligament, holding the root in place. Beneath the protective overlying enamel and cement, an innervated layer known as dentin provides the bulk of the body of the tooth. The dentin encases the pulp, which contains nerves, blood vessels, and connective tissue (Fig. 75.2).

Congenital Anomalies and Disorders of Tooth Eruption

Tooth eruption occurs when the tooth moves from the alveolar bone through the mucosa and into the oral cavity. This process may be impaired or lead to abnormal odontogenesis such as an impacted tooth that is impeded by overlying bone (malocclusion). Abnormal or delayed tooth entry can be a sign of inherited conditions such as trisomy 21 (Down syndrome) or Gaucher disease. Disorders such as congenital hypothyroidism can delay tooth development, and vitamin D deficiency may impair proper mineralization of the bone. Furthermore, immunodeficiencies such as leukocyte adhesion deficiency or Chediak-Higashi syndrome can lead to chronic periodontal infection and inflammation leading to premature loss of deciduous teeth.

Dental Trauma

The most common traumatic injuries in pediatric dentistry are luxation injuries to the incisors as a result of falls. This can range from simple concussive injury to avulsion of the tooth. A thorough examination should evaluate for evidence of soft tissue injury to the mouth, fracture of the teeth (with attention to whether enamel, dentin, or pulp is exposed), and loose, displaced, or missing teeth. Clinicians should consider the possibility of child abuse by evaluating for frenulum tears. Radiographic imaging may be appropriate to reveal fractures or locate missing tooth fragments, which may have been swallowed, aspirated, or completely intruded into the alveolar socket.

Management includes prevention of aspiration, infection, and damage to the permanent dentition. For most injuries to the primary teeth, there is no need for urgent dental care. For injuries to permanent teeth, maintaining the viability of the periodontal ligament is of paramount importance. For an avulsed tooth, the viability of the tooth is inversely proportional to the time to reimplantation. Parents should be advised to handle the tooth by the crown, gently rinse it with tap water or saline, place it back into the socket, and maintain pressure with a finger or by biting on gauze or a clean cloth to keep the tooth in place. Alternatively, transporting the tooth in milk or Hanks balanced salt solution will keep the tooth viable.

Dental Infections

Caries

Dental caries remains a highly prevalent disease, affecting five times as many children as asthma. The risk for early childhood caries is increased in babies who sleep with bottles, who graze (rather than eating at discrete mealtimes), and whose parents also have untreated caries. Bacteria, especially the *Streptococcus mutans* group, are typically transmitted from mother to infant soon after the eruption of the primary teeth. These bacteria colonize tooth surfaces and form plaques. Caries result when bacteria ferment sucrose from ingested dietary carbohydrate, producing organic acids on the tooth surface that cause the enamel to become more porous (Fig. 75.3). Areas of breakdown can erode through the enamel and dentin into the pulp, where an inflammatory response raises the pressure in the pulp chamber and can cause compression, and thus ischemia, of the pulp vessels. This is known as pulp necrosis, which can extend to form a periapical abscess that can erode the alveolar bone or involve other teeth and impair development of an underlying permanent tooth.

Caries prevention is centered on anticipatory guidance surrounding healthy dietary habits (limiting sugar-sweetened beverage intake, discontinuing bottle use at 1 year of age) and proper dental hygiene. From the first tooth eruption, parents should clean the child's teeth twice daily starting with only a smear of fluoride-containing toothpaste. Fluoride protects against caries by promoting enamel mineralization. If children live in an area without fluoride added to the local water system, they should start oral supplements.

Periodontal Infections

Gingivitis is an inflammatory response to bacteria that live in the sulcus between the enamel and the gingiva. The gingiva may be edematous

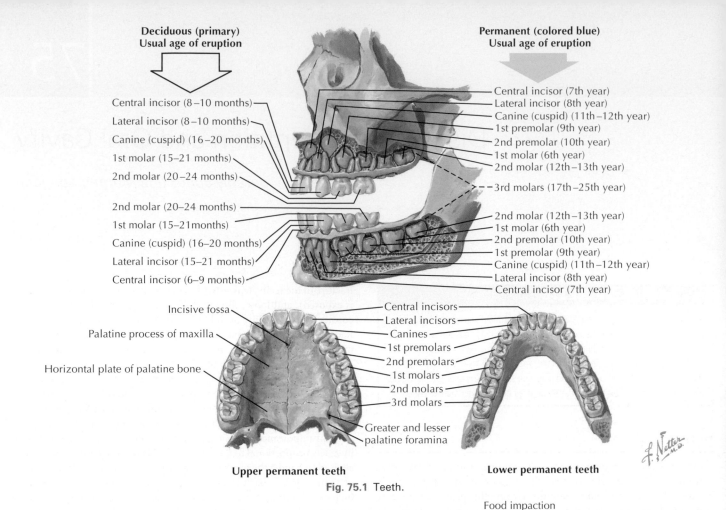

Deciduous (primary)
Usual age of eruption

Central incisor (8–10 months)
Lateral incisor (8–10 months)
Canine (cuspid) (16–20 months)
1st molar (15–21 months)
2nd molar (20–24 months)

2nd molar (20–24 months)
1st molar (15–21months)
Canine (cuspid) (16–20 months)
Lateral incisor (15–21 months)
Central incisor (6–9 months)

Permanent (colored blue)
Usual age of eruption

Central incisor (7th year)
Lateral incisor (8th year)
Canine (cuspid) (11th–12th year)
1st premolar (9th year)
2nd premolar (10th year)
1st molar (6th year)
2nd molar (12th–13th year)
3rd molars (17th–25th year)

2nd molar (12th–13th year)
1st molar (6th year)
2nd premolar (10th year)
1st premolar (9th year)
Canine (cuspid) (11th–12th year)
Lateral incisor (8th year)
Central incisor (7th year)

Incisive fossa
Palatine process of maxilla
Horizontal plate of palatine bone

Central incisors
Lateral incisors
Canines
1st premolars
2nd premolars
1st molars
2nd molars
3rd molars
Greater and lesser palatine foramina

Upper permanent teeth

Lower permanent teeth

Fig. 75.1 Teeth.

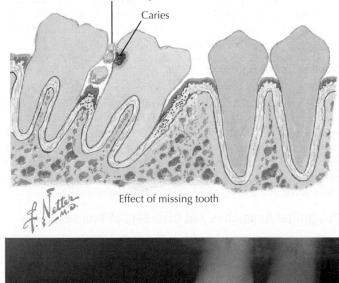

Food impaction
Caries

Effect of missing tooth

Fig. 75.3 Dental Caries.

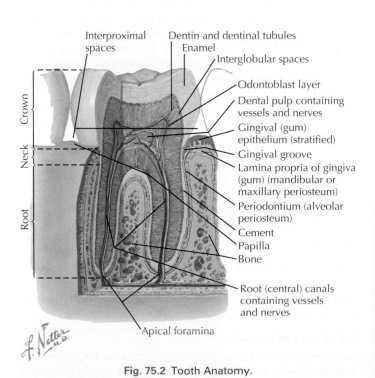

Interproximal spaces
Dentin and dentinal tubules
Enamel
Interglobular spaces
Odontoblast layer
Dental pulp containing vessels and nerves
Gingival (gum) epithelium (stratified)
Gingival groove
Lamina propria of gingiva (gum) (mandibular or maxillary periosteum)
Periodontium (alveolar periosteum)
Cement
Papilla
Bone

Crown
Neck
Root

Root (central) canals containing vessels and nerves

Apical foramina

Fig. 75.2 Tooth Anatomy.

Dental caries

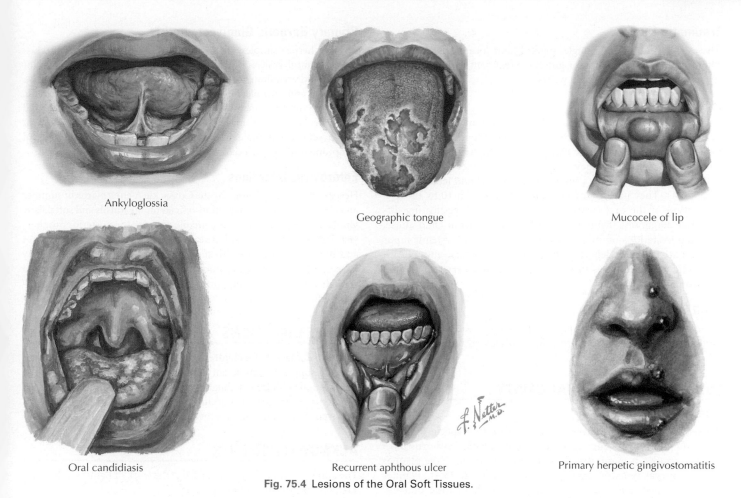

Ankyloglossia

Geographic tongue

Mucocele of lip

Oral candidiasis

Recurrent aphthous ulcer

Primary herpetic gingivostomatitis

Fig. 75.4 Lesions of the Oral Soft Tissues.

and may bleed and ulcerate. It is highly prevalent in children, usually because of poor dental hygiene.

Periodontitis evolves from gingivitis with destruction of the tooth's supportive structures. Several rare but aggressive forms exist in children. Clinical manifestations include loss of tooth attachment, gingival recession, and periodontal bone loss.

Tongue

The tongue is a highly mobile organ involved in many key functions. The root is anchored to the floor of the mouth and the lingual frenulum connects the anterior tongue to the lower jaw. For babies, the tongue is crucial for effective breastfeeding. Once a child is eating solid foods, the tongue helps press food against the palate to initiate breakdown and induces salivation by taste receptors. The tongue is also essential for speech and is able to perform over 20 different movements for sound production.

Ankyloglossia

Children may be born with a short lingual frenulum, known as ankyloglossia or "tongue-tie" (Fig. 75.4). Tongue movement may be restricted by close attachment of the frenulum to the tongue. The condition occurs in up to 10% children and is more prevalent in boys than in girls. It does not usually affect speech or feeding, and the frenulum often lengthens as the child grows. A frenulectomy may be required in the case of true disability.

Geographic Tongue

This benign condition is characterized by irregular red patches on the tongue (Fig. 75.4). The lesions typically spontaneously resolve

and then subsequently appear elsewhere (known as "migratory glossitis").

Macroglossia

Macroglossia refers to an excessively large tongue in relation to the oral cavity and can be associated with difficulty eating, airway obstruction, and challenges with speech. Macroglossia is associated with inherited disorders such as Down syndrome, Beckwith-Wiedemann syndrome, or primary amyloidosis. It also can be observed in infants with congenital hypothyroidism or chronic vitamin B_{12} deficiency. Rapid identification of the underlying cause and possible surgery are key to ensure normal development and speech.

COMMON SOFT TISSUE LESIONS OF THE ORAL CAVITY

Mucocele

This painless pseudocyst results from trauma to the duct of a minor salivary gland, usually in the lower lip or cheek (e.g., from lip biting). It is usually smooth, bluish to translucent, and filled with mucin from the damaged duct (Fig. 75.4). It may spontaneously drain; however, surgical excision may be required.

Ranula

This painless mucous cyst occurs on the floor of the mouth. Rarely, it may herniate through the mylohyoid muscle to involve the submandibular region and neck and require surgical excision.

Traumatic Ulcers

These lesions are usually single, painful, and located on the lateral tongue, buccal mucosa, lips, or gingiva. Treatment is supportive and the lesions resolve within 1 to 3 weeks.

Aphthous Ulcers

These recurrent and painful ulcers, also known as canker sores, occur in up to one-third of children. Their cause is unclear, but viruses, T-cell dysfunction, trauma, and genetic predisposition have been implicated. They appear as white necrotic areas surrounded by a red margin, usually on the buccal and labial mucosa (Fig. 75.4). They usually resolve completely within 10 to 14 days. Inspection of the oral cavity can be helpful in investigating differential diagnoses, including traumatic ulcers from child abuse, oral manifestations of inflammatory bowel disease, systemic lupus erythematosus, and Behçet disease, herpetic ulcers, and PFAPA (periodic fever, aphthous stomatitis, pharyngitis, cervical adenitis) syndrome.

Cleft Palate

Infants may be born with an opening in the lip or palate as a result of abnormal development in utero. This is discussed more in Chapter 66.

INFECTIONS OF THE ORAL CAVITY

Candidiasis

Thrush, caused by the overgrowth of *Candida* species (mostly *Candida albicans*), occurs in 2% to 5% of normal newborns until age 12 months. It manifests as pseudomembranous white plaques on the buccal mucosa, palate, and tongue (Fig. 75.4). Plaques may be wiped away to reveal painful, erythematous mucosa. Treatment with oral nystatin is usually effective; along with sterilization of pacifiers and nipples. For immunocompromised children or those with refractory thrush, systemic fluconazole should be considered.

Primary Herpetic Gingivostomatitis

Primary herpes simplex virus (HSV) infection manifests with clusters of painful vesicles, located on the gingiva, hard palate, anterior tongue, and vermilion border of the lips (Fig. 75.4). Vesicles may have a red halo and may ulcerate and become superinfected with bacteria. Systemic symptoms include fever, lymphadenopathy, arthralgia, and headache. Diagnosis is made by analysis of vesicular fluid. Treatment with acyclovir within 3 days of symptom onset shortens the length of symptoms and the period of viral shedding.

Enterovirus Infections

Herpangina, usually caused by the Coxsackie A enterovirus in summer and early fall, manifests as painful vesicles on the tonsils and soft palate. Unlike HSV stomatitis, it has a predilection for the posterior oropharynx. Hand, foot, and mouth disease, often caused by the Coxsackie A and B viruses, manifests with similar vesicles; however, children may have vesicles on the tongue, buccal mucosa, hands, feet, buttocks, and genitalia. Treatment is supportive, and resolution is usually spontaneous after 3 to 5 days.

FUTURE DIRECTIONS

Access to dental care for children is a challenge. Regular dental care and fluoride supplementation can dramatically reduce the prevalence of caries among children, highlighting the value of community outreach programs. Education surrounding acute response to dental trauma is important for families to prevent permanent damage to the teeth.

ACKNOWLEDGMENTS

The authors would like to acknowledge the work of Pamela A. Mazzeo, MD, on the previous edition chapter.

SUGGESTED READINGS

Available online.

76

Disorders of the Neck

Ayelet Rosen, Jessica Hills, and Melissa Patel

Kevin is a 7-year-old boy who presents with fever and odynophagia (pain with swallowing). His symptoms started a week ago, with fevers to 101.3°F (38.5°C), rhinorrhea, congestion, mild cough, and poor appetite. His rhinorrhea and congestion improved, but his fevers, odynophagia, and poor appetite have persisted. He has not had any difficulty breathing and has been able to drink but has not been eating solids. He has had decreased energy level and has been voiding at baseline. On examination, he is febrile to 102.5°F (39.2°C), tachycardic to 145 beats/min, with normal respiratory rate and oxygen saturation. He appears nontoxic, with moist mucous membranes, no signs of respiratory distress, and 2+ distal pulses with capillary refill less than 2 seconds. He has trismus (pain with opening his mouth). His oropharynx is erythematous and the left tonsil appears swollen. He has cervical lymphadenopathy with the left side significantly more affected than the right. When he speaks his voice sounds muffled and deeper than usual. He does not have lymphadenopathy elsewhere and the rest of his examination is reassuring.

His complete blood count shows leukocytosis with a neutrophilic predominance, and his C-reactive protein is elevated. A rapid strep test is negative. Computed tomography of the neck with intravenous contrast shows a 2-cm left peritonsillar abscess. He is diagnosed with peritonsillar abscess and given intravenous clindamycin based on local sensitivities. His fevers persist, and the abscess is drained the next day. After drainage, his symptoms improve and resolve within 2 days. He is discharged with oral clindamycin and has full recovery.

The neck is a complex location where many organ systems converge. Therefore, symptoms such as stridor, throat pain, and cervical lymphadenopathy can be caused by a variety of disease processes. Regardless of the cause, initial rapid assessment of airway, breathing, and circulation (ABCs) can be lifesaving in patients with neck pathologic conditions. Evaluating for severity of work of breathing, cyanosis, perfusion, hydration status, and responsiveness will guide further management.

STRIDOR

Stridor is a high-pitched sound reflecting passage of air through a narrowed airway. Although it is traditionally thought to be inspiratory, it also can be expiratory or biphasic. Stridor is a sign of upper airway obstruction, but it is not a diagnosis. When thinking about the causes of stridor, it is helpful to first understand the anatomy of the larynx (Fig. 76.1) and then to separate the causes of stridor into chronic and acute processes.

Chronic Stridor

Chronic stridor is more often the result of anatomic aberrations. The most common cause of chronic stridor is laryngomalacia. Table 76.1 details the differential diagnosis, pathophysiology, evaluation, and management of chronic stridor.

Acute Stridor

Viral croup (Fig. 76.2) is the most common cause of acute stridor and typically presents between ages 6 months to 3 years. Table 76.2 details the differential diagnosis, pathophysiology, evaluation, and management of acute stridor.

PHARYNGITIS

Pharyngitis is inflammation of the mucous membranes and submucosal structures of the pharynx, including the nasopharynx, oropharynx, and laryngopharynx (Fig. 76.3). Causes include infection, allergic rhinitis, environmental exposures, gastroesophageal reflux, and malignancy. The most common type of pharyngitis is acute infectious pharyngitis (Box 76.1). Viral infections account for 40% to 60% of pediatric pharyngitis and usually manifest as part of a larger viral syndrome. *Streptococcus pyogenes*, also known as group A β-hemolytic streptococci (GABHS), is the most common bacterial cause of pharyngitis. It accounts for 15% to 30% of pediatric pharyngitis and is important to identify because treatment is essential in reducing the risk for postinfectious complications.

Clinical Presentation

The most common findings in those with infectious pharyngitis include a history of fever, cervical lymphadenopathy, and oropharyngeal or tonsillar erythema, enlargement, or exudates (Fig. 76.4). Table 76.3 shows patterns of symptoms that correlate with particular pathogens.

Evaluation and Management

The workup and treatment of patients with pharyngitis differs based on the causative pathogen (Table 76.3). Testing for the common viruses is not

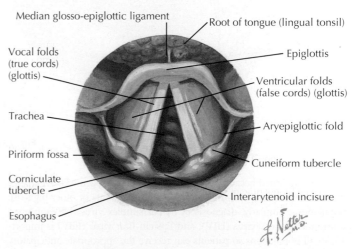

Fig. 76.1 Normal Larynx: Inspiration.

TABLE 76.1   Differential Diagnosis, Pathophysiology, Evaluation, and Management of Chronic Stridor

Cause/Presentation	Pathophysiology	Diagnostic Evaluation and Management
Laryngomalacia Accounts for 75% of neonatal stridor. Manifests from birth to 4 weeks, worsens when supine, crying, or feeding and improves when prone.	Immature cartilage in upper larynx collapses during inhalation	Direct laryngoscopy Resolves spontaneously by 2 years. Surgical intervention may be needed for significant obstruction or poor weight gain.
Vocal cord paralysis Second most common cause of neonatal stridor. Manifests as inspiratory stridor or weak or hoarse cry.	Congenital or iatrogenic as a result of injury to left recurrent laryngeal nerve during surgery or to vocal cords from intubation	Direct laryngoscopy or bronchoscopy Unilateral vocal cord paralysis usually resolves by age 2 years. Tracheostomy is often needed for bilateral vocal cord paralysis.
Subglottic stenosis Presents as inspiratory or biphasic stridor	May be congenital or acquired from prolonged intubation in the neonatal period	Radiograph can show airway narrowing Bronchoscopy is diagnostic Severe stenosis may require tracheostomy and surgical correction
Tracheomalacia Causes expiratory stridor or monophonic wheeze if the obstruction is intrathoracic	Can be congenital or acquired	Airway fluoroscopy or bronchoscopy Can spontaneously resolve Severe cases may require continuous positive airway pressure
Tracheal stenosis	Congenital formation of complete instead of the normally C-shaped tracheal rings	Bronchoscopy Requires surgical correction
Vascular ring See Chapter 30	Congenital abnormality of aortic arch compressing the airway	Computed tomography angiography or echocardiography are diagnostic
Airway hemangioma Typically develop symptoms at 6–12 weeks during the rapid growth phase. May have cutaneous hemangiomas in the "beard" distribution.	Vascular tumor that grows rapidly in infancy	Bronchoscopy Treated with propranolol

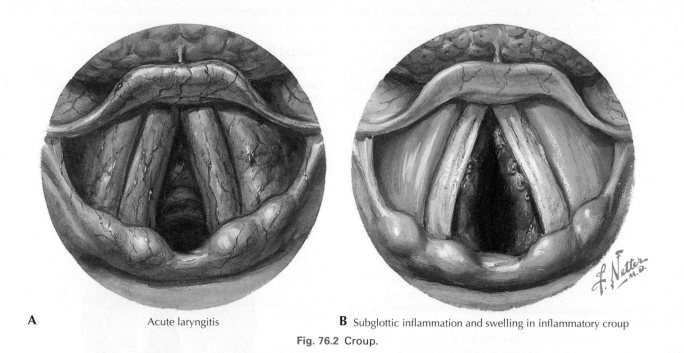

A   Acute laryngitis

B Subglottic inflammation and swelling in inflammatory croup

Fig. 76.2 Croup.

routinely indicated because identification of the pathogen will not change management except in immunocompromised patients or other high-risk populations. Similarly, diagnosis of herpes simplex virus (HSV), human immunodeficiency virus (HIV), and Epstein-Barr virus (EBV) is important in all populations so patients can receive the appropriate anticipatory guidance and treatment. GABHS is the only common form of pharyngitis for which antimicrobial therapy is definitively indicated to prevent complications of the illness, most importantly, acute rheumatic fever (Fig. 76.5). Antimicrobial treatment of GABHS also reduces the incidence of toxic shock syndrome, peritonsillar or retropharyngeal abscesses, cervical lymphadenitis, and mastoiditis. The one sequela that is not prevented by adequate treatment of GABHS pharyngitis is poststreptococcal glomerulonephritis.

TABLE 76.2 Differential Diagnosis, Pathophysiology, Evaluation, and Management of Acute Stridor

Cause/Presentation	Pathophysiology	Diagnostic Workup and Management
Croup or laryngotracheitis Harsh "barky" or "seal-like" cough Associated viral respiratory symptoms (fever, rhinorrhea) are common Stridor worse with crying	Classically caused by parainfluenza viruses but can be caused by any respiratory virus, such as respiratory syncytial virus influenza, or adenovirus	Usually a clinical diagnosis Lateral neck radiograph demonstrates subglottic narrowing (steeple sign) Symptoms self-resolve in about 7 days A single dose of oral or intramuscular dexamethasone improves upper airway inflammation and prevents return to medical care For patients in moderate to severe distress, nebulized racemic epinephrine gives temporary relief
Bacterial tracheitis High fever, toxic appearance, and respiratory distress after prodrome of viral upper respiratory infection symptoms	Rare bacterial superinfection in patients with a viral upper respiratory tract infection most frequently caused by *Staphylococcus aureus*, *Streptococcus pyogenes*, *S. pneumoniae*, *Haemophilus influenzae*, and *Moraxella catarrhalis*	May require intubation and admission to the intensive care unit Tracheal aspirate cultures guide antibiotic management Empiric coverage of *S. aureus* and respiratory pathogens Definitive diagnosis via bronchoscopy
Epiglottitis Classically manifests with the abrupt onset of high fever, stridor, drooling, "tripod" positioning, and toxicity	Traditionally caused by *H. influenzae* type B (Hib), now rare Causes include other strains of *H. influenzae*, streptococci, and *S. aureus*	Lateral neck radiograph demonstrates edematous epiglottis (thumbprint sign) Definitive diagnosis by direct laryngoscopy Requires empiric antibiotics May require intubation and admission to the intensive care unit
Retropharyngeal and peritonsillar abscess	See "Deep Neck Infections" section	
Anaphylaxis Acute onset stridor or wheeze, especially if accompanied by other typical symptoms	See Chapter 20, Anaphylaxis	
Foreign body aspiration Acute onset stridor in an unobserved toddler	Accidentally inhaled object such as a coin or small toy	Radiopaque foreign body can be seen on radiograph Inspiratory and forced expiratory or lateral decubitus chest radiographs may demonstrate hyperinflation and air trapping on the affected side Bronchoscopy is required for definitive diagnosis and foreign body removal

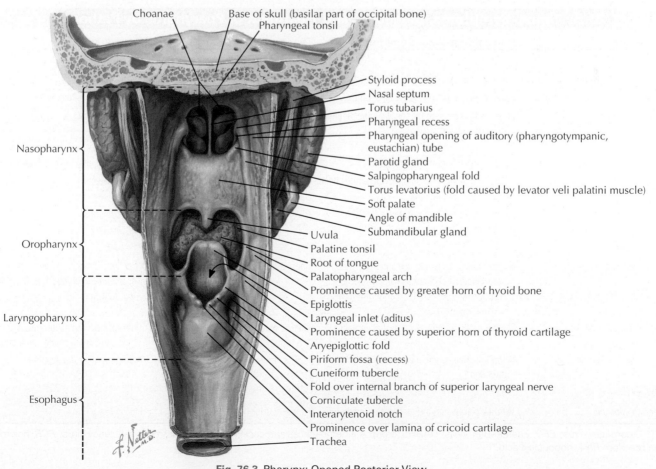

Fig. 76.3 Pharynx: Opened Posterior View.

BOX 76.1   Common Causes of Infectious Pharyngitis

Viral
- Adenovirus[a]
- Coronavirus[a]
- Cytomegalovirus
- Enterovirus
- Epstein-Barr virus
- Herpes simplex virus
- Human immunodeficiency virus
- Influenza[a]
- Parainfluenza[a]
- Respiratory syncytial virus[a]
- Rhinovirus[a]

Bacterial
- *Arcanobacterium haemolyticum*
- *Chlamydia pneumoniae*
- *Corynebacterium diphtheriae*
- Group A β-hemolytic streptococci (GABHS)[a]
- *Mycoplasma pneumoniae*
- *Neisseria gonorrhoeae*
- Non-GABHS (group C and G)[a]

Other Pathogens
- *Candida albicans*
- *Mycobacterium tuberculosis*

[a] Most common causes.

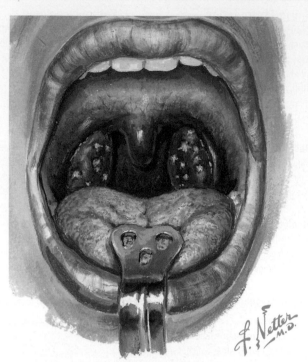

Acute follicular tonsilitis
Fig. 76.4 Tonsillitis.

TABLE 76.3   Signs, Symptoms, Diagnosis, and Treatment of Pharyngitis by Pathogen

Pathogen	Clinical Signs and Symptoms	Diagnostic Test	Treatment
Viral			
Rhinovirus, coronavirus, adenovirus	Fever, rhinorrhea, congestion, conjunctivitis	PCR	Supportive care
Influenza	Fever, myalgia, nonexudative pharyngitis	Rapid diagnostic testing, PCR	If indicated, oseltamivir
Epstein-Barr virus	Fever, malaise, posterior cervical lymphadenopathy, hepatosplenomegaly	Heterophile antibody, EBV serology, peripheral smear (atypical lymphocytosis), CMV antibody titers	Supportive care
Herpes simplex virus	Painful vesicles in anterior mouth	PCR	If indicated, acyclovir or valacyclovir
Coxsackievirus	Painful white vesicles on an erythematous base in posterior oropharynx	PCR	Supportive care
Human immunodeficiency virus	Aphthous ulcers, fatigue, fever, lymphadenopathy	HIV RNA or HIV antibody	Antiretrovirals
Bacterial			
Streptococcus pyogenes	Sudden onset, lack of cough and rhinorrhea, anterior cervical lymphadenopathy, headache, fever, palatal petechiae, scarlatiniform rash, nausea/vomiting	Rapid antigen detection, throat culture	First line: Penicillin or amoxicillin Second line: cephalexin, azithromycin, clindamycin
Neisseria gonorrhoeae	History of recent orogenital sexual contact	Nucleic acid amplification test, Thayer-Martin culture medium	Ceftriaxone (with azithromycin or doxycycline for chlamydia coinfection)
Mycoplasma pneumoniae	Nonproductive cough, lower respiratory tract infection	PCR or serology	Azithromycin or doxycycline
Fungal			
Candida albicans	Whitish plaques on the tongue and oropharynx	Fungal culture	Fluconazole

CMV, Cytomegalovirus; *EBV,* Epstein-Barr virus; *GABHS,* group A β-hemolytic streptococci; *HIV,* human immunodeficiency virus; *PCR,* polymerase chain reaction; *RNA,* ribonucleic acid.

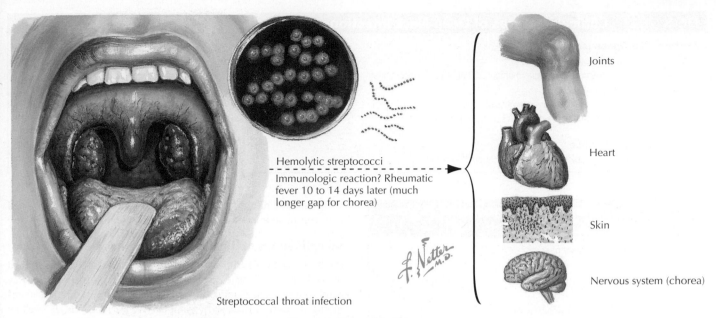

Hemolytic streptococci

Immunologic reaction? Rheumatic fever 10 to 14 days later (much longer gap for chorea)

Streptococcal throat infection

Joints

Heart

Skin

Nervous system (chorea)

Fig. 76.5 Rheumatic Fever.

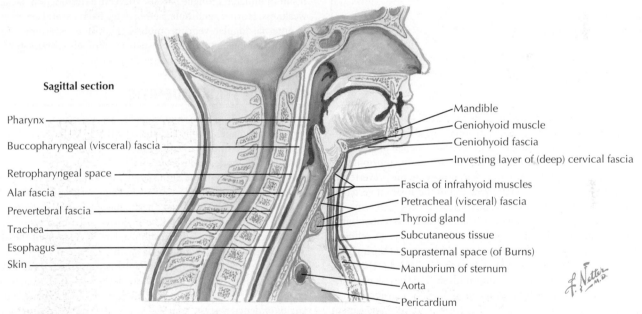

Sagittal section

Pharynx

Buccopharyngeal (visceral) fascia

Retropharyngeal space

Alar fascia

Prevertebral fascia

Trachea

Esophagus

Skin

Mandible

Geniohyoid muscle

Geniohyoid fascia

Investing layer of (deep) cervical fascia

Fascia of infrahyoid muscles

Pretracheal (visceral) fascia

Thyroid gland

Subcutaneous tissue

Suprasternal space (of Burns)

Manubrium of sternum

Aorta

Pericardium

Fig. 76.6 Major Fascial Spaces of the Neck.

DEEP NECK INFECTIONS

Multiple layers of cervical fascia encase the contents of the neck, creating three clinically important spaces: the peritonsillar area, retropharyngeal space, and parapharyngeal space (Fig. 76.6). Peritonsillar, retropharyngeal, and parapharyngeal infections are among a group of potentially life-threatening deep neck infections in children that can present significant diagnostic challenges. All of these infections have the potential to progress from cellulitis to organized phlegmon and then to mature abscess. Rapid assessment for upper airway obstruction is imperative in case there is a need for emergent airway management.

Clinical Presentation and Differential Diagnosis

The anatomy of deep neck spaces plays a role in the presenting signs, symptoms, and examination findings of these infections (Fig. 76.6,

Box 76.2). It can be difficult to differentiate between the early findings of peritonsillar, retropharyngeal, and parapharyngeal infections. Therefore, these diagnoses should be considered in the differential diagnosis of deep neck infections. A list of other differential diagnoses appears in Box 76.3.

Evaluation and Management

Laboratory evaluation is not necessary to make the diagnosis of deep neck infections, but it may help to assess the degree of illness and response to therapy. Leukocytosis with neutrophil predominance and elevated inflammatory markers are common, but nonspecific. Routine GABHS antigen test or throat culture should be done. Associated bacteremia is uncommon.

The diagnosis of peritonsillar abscess usually can be made clinically and is confirmed by a collection of pus at the time of drainage. A lateral

BOX 76.2   Clinical Features of Deep Neck Infections

Peritonsillar Space (see Fig. 76.6)
- Older school-age children and adolescents
- Fever, sore throat, trismus, dysphagia, muffled or "hot potato" voice, unilateral neck pain and swelling
- Asymmetric tonsils with fullness or fluctuance of superior pole of tonsil; uvula and tonsil may be deviated to the opposite side by the abscess

Retropharyngeal Space
- Preschool-age children (before retropharyngeal nodes atrophy)

- Typically, viral prodrome precedes abrupt onset of high fever, limited neck movement (especially resistance to extension), and occasionally stridor

Parapharyngeal (Lateral Pharyngeal) Space
- Infections often arise by contiguous spread from a peritonsillar or retropharyngeal abscess and manifest with fever, cervical lymphadenopathy, pain of ipsilateral neck and jaw, and parotid gland swelling

BOX 76.3   Differential Diagnosis of Deep Neck Infections

- Caustic burns of the posterior pharynx
- Cervical lymphadenitis
- Cervical osteomyelitis
- Cystic hygroma
- Epiglottis
- Foreign body
- Hemangioma
- Laryngotracheobronchitis
- Meningitis
- Penetrating pharyngeal trauma
- Retromolar abscess
- Tonsillopharyngitis

neck radiograph may be obtained initially to exclude epiglottis and retropharyngeal abscess. In the case of retropharyngeal and parapharyngeal abscess, a lateral neck radiograph may show widened prevertebral soft tissues and the presence of air-fluid levels within the retropharyngeal space. When retropharyngeal infection is present, the prevertebral soft tissue measures more than half the width of the adjacent vertebral body. The most useful imaging modality for deep neck infections is a computed tomography (CT) scan, which can define the extent of infection and determine whether there is abscess formation versus cellulitis or phlegmon. Magnetic resonance imaging (MRI) is another imaging option and avoids the radiation that accompanies CT scan. However, sedation is typically required for young children, and the risk of sedating a child with potential airway compromise must be considered.

There is a trend toward conservative early medical management with intravenous antibiotics for 24 to 48 hours when imaging is consistent with phlegmon, fluid collections are small, and there is no airway compromise. If there is worsening of clinical status or a suboptimal response to appropriate antibiotics, incision and drainage are necessary. Mature abscesses require surgical drainage. In the case of peritonsillar abscess, drainage is performed by either needle aspiration or incision and drainage.

Peritonsillar, retropharyngeal, and parapharyngeal abscesses tend to be polymicrobial, consisting of both aerobic and anaerobic organisms. Empiric therapy should include coverage for *S. pyogenes;* non–group A streptococcus; *Staphylococcus aureus;* and respiratory anaerobes such as *Prevotella, Bacteroides,* and *Peptostreptococcus* species. In areas where *S. aureus* remains susceptible to methicillin, ampicillin–sulbactam is appropriate. In areas with increased prevalence of community-associated methicillin-resistant *S. aureus* (CA-MRSA), antibiotic choices include clindamycin or vancomycin. Intravenous therapy should be continued until the patient is afebrile with improvement in

symptoms and resolution of any airway compromise. Appropriate oral regimens include amoxicillin-clavulanate, clindamycin, or linezolid.

Complications of Deep Neck Infections

If left untreated, a peritonsillar or retropharyngeal abscess can spread through the deep tissues and produce complications such as airway compromise, mediastinitis, thrombophlebitis, and aspiration pneumonia if rupture occurs. In parapharyngeal infections, if swelling occurs in the area of the larynx or epiglottis, stridor and respiratory distress may be present. Abscesses in the posterior compartment may result in unilateral tongue paresis, vocal cord dysfunction, facial nerve weakness, Horner syndrome, hemorrhage from carotid artery erosion, or internal jugular vein thrombosis (Lemierre syndrome). In addition, intracranial complications such as meningitis, brain abscess, and thrombosis of the cavernous sinus may occur.

CERVICAL LYMPHADENITIS

Almost all children have small palpable cervical lymph nodes, whereas cervical lymphadenopathy is defined by lymph nodes measuring more than 1 cm in diameter. Lymphadenitis refers specifically to inflammation of lymph nodes and is characterized by enlarged and tender nodes with warmth or erythema of the overlying skin. The cervical lymphatic system consists of a collection of both superficial and deep lymph nodes that protect the head, neck, nasopharynx, and oropharynx against infection (Fig. 76.7). The majority of lymphatics of the head and neck drain to the submandibular lymph nodes and the anterior and posterior cervical lymph node chains.

The cause of cervical lymphadenitis is most often viral, but many other organisms have been implicated (Box 76.4). Bacterial cervical lymphadenitis may be primary or result from direct extension of pharyngitis or dental abscess. *S. aureus* and GABHS are isolated in the majority of cases. More indolent causes of cervical lymphadenitis include mycobacterial infections, *Bartonella henselae,* and *Toxoplasma gondii.*

Clinical Presentation and Differential Diagnosis

The presentation of cervical lymphadenitis can be divided into three broad categories: (1) acute bilateral, (2) acute unilateral, and (3) subacute or chronic.

The most common causes of acute bilateral cervical lymphadenitis are viral upper respiratory tract (URI) infections followed by pharyngitis caused by GABHS. In general, the lymph nodes are small, soft, and mobile, without associated erythema, warmth, or significant tenderness.

Acute unilateral cervical lymphadenitis is caused by *S. aureus* and *S. pyogenes* in the majority of cases. The onset may be associated with a URI, pharyngitis, or periodontal disease, and associated fever is common. Typically, the onset is acute with development of large, tender, erythematous, and warm lymph nodes that may become fluctuant over a few days (Fig. 76.8). In addition, a cellulitis-adenitis syndrome

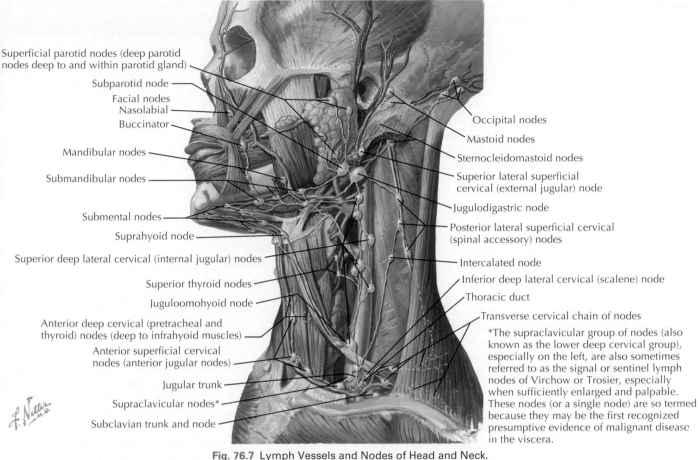

Superficial parotid nodes (deep parotid nodes deep to and within parotid gland)

Subparotid node

Facial nodes
Nasolabial
Buccinator

Mandibular nodes

Submandibular nodes

Submental nodes

Suprahyoid node

Superior deep lateral cervical (internal jugular) nodes

Superior thyroid nodes

Juguloomohyoid node

Anterior deep cervical (pretracheal and thyroid) nodes (deep to infrahyoid muscles)

Anterior superficial cervical nodes (anterior jugular nodes)

Jugular trunk

Supraclavicular nodes*

Subclavian trunk and node

Occipital nodes

Mastoid nodes

Sternocleidomastoid nodes

Superior lateral superficial cervical (external jugular) node

Jugulodigastric node

Posterior lateral superficial cervical (spinal accessory) nodes

Intercalated node

Inferior deep lateral cervical (scalene) node

Thoracic duct

Transverse cervical chain of nodes

*The supraclavicular group of nodes (also known as the lower deep cervical group), especially on the left, are also sometimes referred to as the signal or sentinel lymph nodes of Virchow or Trosier, especially when sufficiently enlarged and palpable. These nodes (or a single node) are so termed because they may be the first recognized presumptive evidence of malignant disease in the viscera.

Fig. 76.7 Lymph Vessels and Nodes of Head and Neck.

BOX 76.4 Infectious Causes of Cervical Lymphadenitis

Viruses
- Adenovirus
- Coronavirus
- Coxsackievirus
- Cytomegalovirus
- Enteroviruses
- Epstein-Barr virus
- Herpes simplex virus
- Human herpesvirus 6
- Human immunodeficiency virus
- Influenza
- Mumps
- Parainfluenza
- Parvovirus B19
- Respiratory syncytial virus
- Rhinovirus
- Varicella

Bacteria
- Anaerobes
- *Actinomyces israelii*

- Atypical *Mycobacterium*
- *Bacillus anthracis*
- *Bartonella henselae*
- *Brucella* species
- *Francisella tularensis*
- *Haemophilus* species
- *Leptospira interrogans*
- *Mycobacterium tuberculosis*
- *Mycoplasma pneumoniae*
- Nontuberculous *Mycobacterium*
- *Nocardia* species
- *Pasteurella multocida*
- *Salmonella typhi*
- *Staphylococcus aureus*[a]
- *Streptococcus pyogenes* (GABHS)[a]
- *Streptococcus agalactiae* (GBS)
- *Yersinia pestis*

Protozoa
- *Toxoplasma gondii*

[a] Most common bacterial cause.

Acute bacterial

Non-tuberculous mycobacterial

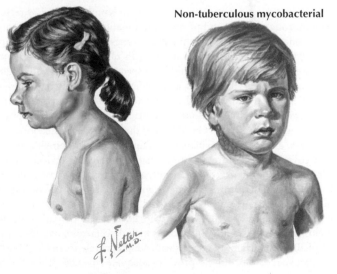

Fig. 76.8 Cervical Lymphadenitis.

caused by group B streptococcus in infants between 3 and 7 weeks of age is associated with irritability, fever, and unilateral facial or submandibular swelling with erythema and tenderness.

The most common causes of subacute or chronic lymphadenitis are mycobacterial infections, cat-scratch disease, and toxoplasmosis. Lymph node enlargement is typically gradual in onset and progresses over weeks to months. The most common manifestation of nontuberculous *mycobacterium* (NTM) disease in children is cervical lymphadenitis. The lymph nodes are large and indurated but nontender, and the overlying skin often becomes violaceous and thin (Fig. 76.8). Untreated lymphadenitis caused by NTM may resolve, but often it progresses to lymph node necrosis followed by fluctuance and spontaneous drainage. Cervical lymphadenitis caused by *Mycobacterium tuberculosis* has a similar presentation, but there are clinical and epidemiologic differences. Cat-scratch disease, caused by *B. henselae,* most commonly affects the axilla and cervical regions. Most patients have a history of recent contact with cats or kittens. Clinical manifestations begin with a papule or pustule that develops at the inoculation site a few days to weeks after a bite or scratch followed by lymphadenitis proximal to the site. Lymphadenitis is tender and erythematous and often associated with fever. Lymphadenitis typically persists for several weeks to months and may suppurate. Acquired *T. gondii* infection, when symptomatic, generally manifests as cervical lymphadenopathy and fatigue without fever. Lymphadenitis most frequently involves a solitary node in the head and neck region without systemic symptoms. Lymphadenitis secondary to toxoplasmosis tends to be nonsuppurative and may persist for many months.

Congenital cysts such as branchial cleft cysts, cystic hygromas, and thyroglossal duct cysts can mimic lymphadenitis, especially when infected. Malignancy should be considered in cases of indolent lymphadenopathy, especially with a history of weight loss, fevers, night sweats, or lymphadenitis that is unresponsive to antibiotic treatment. Other causes of cervical neck masses should be included in the differential diagnosis of cervical lymphadenitis (Box 76.5).

Evaluation and Management

The evaluation and management of cervical lymphadenitis is directed by a thorough history and physical examination. Patients with acute, small, bilateral nodes with minimal tenderness along with viral symptoms can be managed conservatively with observation and supportive care. A bacterial cause should be suspected in patients with acute, large, unilateral, erythematous, and tender nodes associated with fever. Antimicrobial therapy should be directed at GABHS and *S. aureus,* with cephalexin being a reasonable choice. Clindamycin is appropriate in areas with high rates of CA-MRSA. If there is an associated intraoral infection, amoxicillin-clavulanate or clindamycin will provide anaerobic coverage in addition to gram-positive coverage. Cervical lymphadenitis can be managed on an outpatient basis for most children. Hospital admission for intravenous antibiotics should be considered in infants, ill-appearing children, and children who have fluctuant nodes or associated cellulitis or who have failed outpatient treatment. Intravenous antibiotic choices include cefazolin, oxacillin, and ampicillin-sulbactam. In regions with a high prevalence of CA-MRSA, clindamycin or vancomycin provides adequate coverage. If there is no

> ### BOX 76.5 Noninfectious Causes of Cervical Lymphadenopathy
>
> **Congenital Cysts**
> - Branchial cleft cysts
> - Cystic hygromas
> - Thyroglossal duct cysts
>
> **Malignancies**
> - Lymphoma
> - Leukemia
> - Neuroblastoma
> - Rhabdomyosarcoma
>
> **Miscellaneous**
> - Castleman disease
> - Collagen vascular disease
> - Kawasaki disease
> - Kikuchi-Fujimoto disease (histiocytic necrotizing lymphadenitis)
> - Kimura disease
> - PFAPA (periodic fever, aphthous stomatitis, pharyngitis, and cervical adenitis)
> - Rosai-Dorfman disease (sinus histiocytosis with massive lymphadenopathy)
> - Sarcoidosis

response to antibiotic treatment within 48 to 72 hours or there is clinical worsening, evaluate for abscess formation. Ultrasound is useful to detect the presence and extent of an abscess, without radiation. CT provides detailed imaging before surgical intervention. Aspirated or drained material from a suppurative node should be sent for Gram stain and both aerobic and anaerobic bacterial culture. Acid-fast stain and culture for mycobacteria and fungi should be considered with the appropriate clinical picture. Purified protein derivative can be helpful in distinguishing tuberculous from NTM lymphadenitis. Serologic testing is available for *B. henselae, T. gondii,* EBV, and cytomegalovirus (CMV). Polymerase chain reaction (PCR) is the preferred diagnostic test for HIV. Toxoplasmosis and cat-scratch disease are typically self-limited infections that do not require treatment. For patients with systemic disease secondary to *B. henselae* infection, treatment with azithromycin is an option but remains controversial. With NTM lymphadenitis, excisional biopsy of the node can provide a definitive diagnosis and is the preferred treatment. If surgery is not feasible because of the location of involved nodes, clarithromycin or azithromycin with ethambutol or rifampin should be considered. When the cause of cervical lymphadenitis remains unclear after negative infectious workup results, patients should be monitored closely for systemic signs of disease. An excisional biopsy may be necessary to establish the diagnosis in cases of persistent lymphadenitis that do not respond to appropriate antibiotic treatment or when nodes are nontender and fixed to adjacent tissue suggestive of malignancy.

SUGGESTED READINGS

Available online.

Hematology

Char Witmer

77

Disorders of Red Blood Cells

Timothy T. Spear

✳ CLINICAL VIGNETTE

A 5-year-old boy with a history of neonatal hyperbilirubinemia presents with jaundice, fatigue, and dark urine. A thorough history reveals no infectious symptoms, recent travel, or new medications. The patient ingested fava beans about 48 hours before symptom onset. Physical examination is notable for scleral icterus and pallor. The patient is tachycardic, with a systolic flow murmur. Laboratory evaluation reveals a normocytic anemia (hemoglobin 4.2 g/dL, mean corpuscular volume [MCV] 85 femtoliters), with an elevated reticulocyte count, unconjugated bilirubin, and serum lactase dehydrogenase. Urinalysis is positive for urobilinogen. Red cell testing reveals a markedly low glucose-6-phosphate dehydrogenase (G6PD) enzyme activity.

The patient received a blood transfusion for his symptomatic anemia and received anticipatory guidance on oxidative stressors to avoid G6PD deficiency.

Red blood cells (RBCs) are nonnucleated cells composed of a cell membrane, complex surface glycoproteins, and hemoglobin (Hgb). Hgb, the major component of RBCs, facilitates oxygen transport from the lungs to tissue capillaries by reversible binding and releasing of oxygen, according to the characteristics of the oxyhemoglobin dissociation curve. As a result, RBC homeostasis is essential to prevent tissue hypoxia and maintain critical organ function. Anemia is not a disease itself, but rather a symptom of an underlying cause, and its diagnosis is determined using age- and sex-specific normal ranges.

Anemia can be classified into three pathologic causes, including blood loss, increased destruction, decreased production, or morphologic, using the RBC size to guide the differential. Anemias also can be considered as congenital versus acquired disorders. Congenital disorders include membrane defects, enzyme defects, disorders of hemoglobin (thalassemia, hemoglobinopathies), and marrow failure. Acquired disorders are broad and commonly include mechanical destruction, immune destruction, anemia of inflammation, nutritional deficiencies (i.e., deficiency of vitamin B_{12}, folate, iron), and aplasia. Various RBC disorders result in anemia with different clinical features, mechanisms of disease, diagnostic findings, and associated treatments.

ETIOLOGY AND PATHOGENESIS

Congenital Red Blood Cell Disorders
Membrane Defects
Defects in RBC membrane proteins induce abnormal, unstable membrane conformations, resulting in decreased membrane integrity, shorter lifespan, and increased susceptibility to cellular stress. Commonly affected RBC membrane proteins include ankyrin, band 3, and spectrin. The type of membrane defect influences the morphologic changes of the RBC.

Hereditary spherocytosis (HS) is the most common RBC membrane defect, affecting 1 in 5000 people of Northern European descent. Two-thirds of cases are inherited by autosomal dominant transmission, but de novo mutations can also occur. The most common defect in HS is in ankyrin. Membrane protein abnormalities in HS lead to an unstable RBC membrane that assumes a spherical shape rather than the biconcave disc shape found in normal RBCs. The spherical RBCs have poor deformability and cannot circulate freely through narrow capillaries. As a result, they become trapped in the spleen and are engulfed by macrophages, leading to a shortened RBC lifespan and signs of hemolysis. Clinical presentation can range from mild, well-compensated anemia to a severe hemolytic anemia. Laboratory evaluation shows an increased mean corpuscular hemoglobin concentration (MCHC) often paired with a decreased red cell distribution width (RDW) and the presence of spherocytes on peripheral smear. Confirmatory testing includes the osmotic fragility test or the eosin-5′-maleimide (EMA) binding assay. The EMA assay is favored secondary to a higher sensitivity and specificity. Genetic testing can confirm mutations in membrane protein genes.

Hereditary elliptocytosis (HE) is characterized by elliptical or oval-shaped RBCs on the peripheral blood smear, most commonly caused by mutations in α-spectrin and β-spectrin and less commonly band 4.1 and band 3. Unlike HS, HE is more common in people of African and Mediterranean ancestry. It is inherited mostly in an autosomal dominant fashion, with documented spontaneous mutations. Clinical manifestations are usually similar to those of HS, but phenotypic variations exist. Other rare inherited RBC membrane defects include hereditary stomatocytosis and hereditary xerocytosis, which involve abnormal ion channels, resulting in anemia with a wide range of clinical severity.

Enzyme Deficiencies
G6PD deficiency is an X-linked recessive disorder characterized by abnormally low or absent levels of the enzyme G6PD and is the most common enzyme deficiency worldwide. The highest prevalence of disease is among persons of African, Asian, and Mediterranean descent. G6PD is the rate-limiting enzyme of the pentose phosphate pathway, which is crucial for protecting RBCs from oxidative stress. In G6PD deficiency, damage by oxidant free radicals causes RBCs to hemolyze. Inciting culprits of stress-induced hemolysis include severe infection, certain drugs with oxidant properties, and fava beans.

Disease manifestation is generally an induced and episodic acute hemolytic anemia. The majority of individuals with G6PD have a moderate deficiency (10% normal activity), and at a steady state are hematologically normal. However, exposure to an oxidative stressor can induce acute hemolysis with resultant anemia, reticulocytosis, and hyperbilirubinemia. Patients with severe G6PD deficiency can exhibit a baseline mild hemolytic anemia. The degree of hemolysis is based on the type of oxidative exposure, the load ingested, and the severity of

TABLE 77.1 α-Thalassemia Gene Deletions

Number of α-Globin Genes Mutated	Syndrome	Clinical Features	Hemoglobin Electrophoresis
1 (−α/αα)	Silent carrier	Not anemic, normocytic	Normal levels of Hgb A2 and Hgb F. May have low amounts of Hgb Barts (γ4) on newborn screen.
2 (−/αα) or (−α/−α)	Thalassemia trait	Mild anemia, microcytosis, and hypochromia	Normal levels of Hgb A2 and Hgb F. Hgb Barts (γ4) on newborn screen (4%-6%).
3 (−α/−)	Hgb H disease	Moderate hemolytic anemia (Hgb 7–10 g/dL), splenomegaly, and hemolytic crisis with exposure to oxidant drugs and infections; not chronically transfusion dependent	Hgb H (β4) (5%-30%)
4 (−/−)	Hydrops fetalis	Death in utero induced by severe anemia; recent breakthroughs in intrauterine transfusions may rescue fetus as a bridge to stem cell transplant	Hgb H (β4)

Hgb, Hemoglobin.

the enzyme deficiency. Drugs that are oxidative stressors and should be avoided in patients with G6PD include sulfa-based medications, high-dose aspirin, methylene blue, and rasburicase. Other oxidative stressors to avoid include fava beans and naphthalene mothballs.

Pyruvate kinase (PK) deficiency is an inherited autosomal recessive metabolic disorder of the enzyme PK, which catalyzes the rate-limiting step in the glycolysis pathway. A deficiency of the enzyme PK compromises RBC adenosine triphosphate production and metabolic energy demand, leading to hemolysis. Clinically, patients have a moderate to severe hemolytic anemia, reticulocytosis (may be 40% to 70%), jaundice, and splenomegaly. The degree of hemolysis ranges but can be severe enough to necessitate chronic transfusions.

Thalassemia

Hemoglobin exists as a tetramer composed of four globin chains. The predominant adult Hgb A molecule is made up of two α-globin and two β-globin chains (α2β2). The thalassemias are a heterogeneous group of inherited disorders in which the normal ratio of α- to β-globin production is disrupted because of reduced or absent expression of either globin chain. A decrease in the production of either an α- or β-globin chain results in an excess of free globin chains that precipitate in the RBC, causing RBC membrane damage and resultant anemia from increased hemolysis and ineffective erythropoiesis.

There are four alleles encoding for α-globin located on chromosome 16. Usually, α- thalassemias are the result of large gene deletions, causing a reduction in α-globin production. The severity of disease is directly related to the number of genes involved (Table 77.1). α-Thalassemia is more commonly found in Southeast Asia, with up to 5% to 10% of the population carrying alleles for α-thalassemia.

β-Thalassemia is caused by absent (β0) or decreased (β+) expression of β-globin, encoded by two alleles on chromosome 11. Point mutations are the most common type of genetic mutation in β-thalassemia, rather than large gene deletions. β-Thalassemia trait occurs when only one gene is affected, resulting in a mild microcytic anemia. β-Thalassemia is more common in Mediterranean countries. The Hgb electrophoresis reveals an increased Hgb A2 or Hgb F level. In contrast, inheritance of two affected β-globin genes results in a broad spectrum of clinical disease, with severity determined by the residual amount of β-globin synthesis. The clinical phenotype ranges from transfusion dependence (thalassemia major) to a moderate anemia that does not necessitate chronic transfusions (thalassemia intermedia). Notably, β-thalassemia major is detected on newborn screen when only Hgb F is

present. Laboratory analysis reveals a moderate to severe microcytic anemia. Clinically, patients present with pallor, failure to thrive, hepatosplenomegaly, and bone deformities from marrow expansion.

Hemoglobinopathies

The hemoglobinopathies are a group of autosomal recessive inherited disorders characterized by synthesis of abnormal Hgb molecules (e.g., S, C, and E). The most common and severe hemoglobinopathy is sickle cell disease hemoglobin SS, in which only Hgb S is produced. Chapter 80 of this book is dedicated to the in-depth discussion of sickle cell disease.

Diamond-Blackfan Anemia

Diamond-Blackfan anemia (DBA) is a congenital bone marrow failure syndrome associated with pure RBC aplasia characterized by anemia, reticulocytopenia, and normocellular bone marrow with a paucity of erythroid precursors. The white blood cell count and platelets are usually normal. The anemia can be mildly macrocytic or normocytic and usually manifests in the first year of life. DBA is associated with various congenital abnormalities, most commonly short stature, craniofacial abnormalities, and thumb abnormalities (classically triphalangeal thumbs). It is also associated with an increased predisposition to cancer. Inheritance patterns vary, including dominant and recessive with the occurrence of spontaneous mutations. Approximately 50% of patients with DBA have a single mutation in a gene encoding for a ribosomal protein.

Other Congenital Bone Marrow Failure Syndromes

Inherited bone marrow failure syndromes include Fanconi anemia, Schwachman-Diamond syndrome, Pearson syndrome, dyskeratosis congenita, and amegakaryocytic thrombocytopenia. In contrast to DBA, these disorders affect multiple cell lines. Presentation can occur at a young age with symptoms of pancytopenia and congenital malformations, which differ by syndrome.

Acquired Red Blood Cell Disorders
Mechanical Red Blood Cell Destruction

In contrast to congenital RBC disorders in which hemolysis is induced by intrinsic RBCs defects, mechanical destruction involves hemolysis caused by extrinsic factors unrelated to the RBCs. Examples of nonimmune mechanical RBC destruction include cardiac valvular defects, vascular lesions (i.e., AVMs), and microangiopathic damage (i.e., hemolytic uremic syndrome or thrombotic thrombocytopenic purpura) caused by shear stresses. RBCs also can be destroyed by a variety of infections, drugs, toxins (the presentation of which can be exaggerated by additional intrinsic RBC defects), and the heat caused by severe burns.

Autoimmune Hemolytic Anemia

The most common immune-mediated extrinsic anemia is autoimmune hemolytic anemia (AIHA), in which circulating antibodies are directed against the patient's RBC antigens. AIHA can be primary or secondary to infection, drugs, or an underlying disease process such as lymphoma, systemic lupus erythematosus, or immunodeficiency. Primary AIHA occurs in the majority of children and often occurs after a viral illness. Pathogenic viral epitopes can look structurally similar to RBC antigen, inducing antibody production with host cross-reactivity. Certain infections can also alter the RBC membrane to appear immunogenically "foreign," eliciting an antigenic immune response. Other infections, including Epstein-Barr virus and *Mycoplasma pneumoniae*, induce agglutination with specific immunoglobulin M (IgM) antibodies. Certain drugs cause hemolysis by a "hapten" mechanism, binding to an RBC and mediating destruction in the spleen (penicillins and cephalosporins), or eliciting antibody-mediated clearance of drug-RBC antigen complexes (quinine, quinidine). Patients with AIHA require close monitoring because brisk hemolysis can result in a sudden decrease in Hgb that can be life-threatening. There are spherocytes on the peripheral smear.

Anemia of Inflammation

Anemia of inflammation is secondary to proinflammatory cytokine disruption of iron homeostasis by hepcidin. Inflammation induces liver-mediated production of hepcidin, a negative regulator of iron. Hepcidin binds the iron-transport channel ferroportin, facilitating its degradation. Lack of adequate transport channels prevents iron absorption in the small intestine and its release from macrophages. Additionally, proinflammatory cytokines stimulate the uptake of iron into macrophages, increasing the amount of iron stored as ferritin. An overall decrease in circulating iron reduces its availability for erythroid progenitor cells in the bone marrow. Anemia of inflammation is characterized by inadequate RBC production in the setting of low serum iron, iron-binding capacity, and transferrin with a concurrent elevated ferritin. The RBCs are usually normocytic but also can be microcytic.

Nutritional Deficiencies

Iron deficiency is the most common cause of anemia in the pediatric population, affecting approximately 9% of toddlers and 9% to 11% of adolescent females. The prompt diagnosis and treatment of this condition is important because clinical manifestations include poor academic achievement, reduced attention span, and growth retardation. Iron deficiency occurs when an insufficient amount of iron is available to meet the body's requirements. In toddlers, it is usually caused by inadequate dietary intake (picky eaters, excessive milk intake). Alternative causes include chronic blood loss (gastrointestinal or menstrual bleeding) or malabsorption (*H. pylori* infection, celiac disease, or inflammatory bowel disease). High-risk groups include premature infants (who receive less iron from the mother in the third trimester), infants consuming large amounts of cow's milk (>24 oz/day), and menstruating women. Iron-deficiency anemia is microcytic and hypochromic, with a low serum iron, iron saturation and ferritin, and an elevated transferrin and total iron-binding capacity. Physical examination findings may include pallor and in severe cases spoon nails and angular stomatitis. Treatment includes oral iron and treatment of the underlying cause.

Deficiencies of vitamin B_{12} (cobalamin) and folate lead to impaired DNA synthesis and subsequently decreased marrow production and dysmorphic RBCs. The anemia is macrocytic and megaloblastic and can be accompanied by leukopenia and thrombocytopenia. Deficiencies are caused by inadequate intake, primary malabsorption, infection (*H. pylori*, parasites), and, less commonly, inborn errors of metabolism. Dietary deficiencies of these vitamins are somewhat rare in the pediatric population. Animal products, such as meat and dairy, are the only dietary sources of vitamin B_{12}, so deficiencies can be seen in severely limited diets, though it may take many years to develop because of its long half-life. Folate is more widespread in the human diet and is found in cereal, fruits, vegetables, and meat. However, body stores of folate are more limited and deficiencies can occur sooner than vitamin B_{12}. Malabsorptive causes of vitamin B_{12} deficiency include defective B_{12} absorption from a failure to secrete intrinsic factor, a failure to absorb B_{12} in the small intestine, and congenital deficiencies in vitamin B_{12} transport or metabolism. Additional causes of folate deficiency include malabsorption, increased folate requirements in chronic hemolytic anemias, or congenital disorders of folic acid metabolism. Of note, certain drugs (i.e., methotrexate) interfere with folic acid metabolism and can cause folate deficiency. Uniquely, B_{12} deficiency is associated with neurologic manifestations (paresthesias, sensory defects, irritability, and developmental delay/regression). Treatment for either condition includes oral nutrient repletion or correction of underlying malabsorptive or metabolic causes.

Transient Erythroblastopenia of Childhood

Transient erythroblastopenia of childhood (TEC) is a disorder characterized by the temporary cessation of RBC production in previously healthy children. Despite the severity of anemia, patients usually present with slowly developing pallor without other symptoms. It is often incidentally found on routine screening. Laboratory workup reveals anemia and reticulocytopenia. In TEC, the anemia is transient (unlike DBA) and is not associated with dysmorphia. The mean age at diagnosis is 26 months; fewer than 10% are older than 3 years at diagnosis. The cause remains unknown, but a viral cause has been proposed. TEC generally is self-resolving. Some patients may require red cell transfusions until recovery.

Transient Red Blood Cell Aplasia From Parvovirus B19

Infection with parvovirus causes a reticulocytopenia for approximately 7 to 10 days. Patients with congenital RBC disorders with increased RBC turnover and decreased RBC lifespan are at greater risk for developing a significant anemia during the period of acquired reticulocytopenia. In addition, patients with immune disorders or receiving immunosuppression have trouble clearing a parvovirus infection and can develop anemia. Clinically, patients can present with pallor, headache, and a marked decrease in the Hgb level. The hallmark is a low reticulocyte count, indicating suppression of bone marrow activity and testing (PCR and/or serologies), indicating an active parvovirus infection. Blood transfusion is indicated in patients with significant symptomatic anemia.

CLINICAL PRESENTATION AND DIFFERENTIAL DIAGNOSIS

The clinical presentation of anemia varies greatly, depending on the severity of anemia (Hgb level compared with age- and sex-specific ranges; Table 77.2) and the time span in which it develops. Frequently, if it develops chronically over weeks to months, children can be asymptomatic with anemia incidentally found on routine screening of a complete blood count (CBC) because of their large physiologic reserve compared with adults. Generally, chronic compensated anemia manifests with fatigue, weakness, pallor, and a systolic flow murmur.

Conversely, individuals with acute onset of anemia can present with tachycardia, palpitations, shortness of breath, or even shock, if they are unable to compensate for acutely decreased oxygen-carrying capacity. The severity of these symptoms is generally inversely correlated with Hgb concentration.

The differential diagnosis of anemia is diverse. As mentioned earlier, physiologically, anemia can be divided into three categories: RBC loss, destruction, or underproduction. Physical examination findings can provide diagnostic clues, and causes can be further subdivided and identified using MCV, peripheral blood smear, reticulocyte index, markers of hemolysis, and newer methods of molecular testing (Fig. 77.1).

DIAGNOSTIC APPROACH

A thorough history, physical examination, and specific laboratory tests are often enough to determine the cause of anemia. Initial laboratory workup should include a CBC and reticulocyte count to help categorize anemia. All three cell lines on the CBC should be analyzed to determine whether the process causing the anemia is limited to erythroids or if other cell lines are affected. The MCV provides a quick, accurate, and readily available method of distinguishing the microcytic anemias (iron deficiency, thalassemia syndromes) from the normocytic (membrane disorders, enzyme deficiencies, AIHA, most hemoglobinopathies) or macrocytic (bone marrow or stem cell failure, disorders of vitamin B_{12}, and folic acid absorption or metabolism) anemias. The MCV varies with age, necessitating the use of age-adjusted normal values (see Table 77.2). The calculated reticulocyte index can help determine if anemia is caused by impaired RBC production or increased RBC destruction as reticulocyte index is often elevated in destruction or loss if the marrow is able to compensate, and inappropriately low for the degree of anemia if the etiology is underproduction. Serum lactate dehydrogenase (elevated), unconjugated bilirubin (elevated),

and haptoglobin (low) can be used to assess presence of hemolysis. Further diagnostic tests are available to help identify specific etiologies (Table 77.3). The peripheral blood smear can also provide additional

TABLE 77.2 Normal Hematologic Values for Age

Age	Hgb (g/dL) Mean (−2 SD)	HCT (%) Mean (−2 SD)	MCV (fL) Mean (−2 SD)
Birth (cord blood)	16.5 (13.5)	51 (42)	108 (98)
1–3 days	18.5 (14.5)	56 (45)	108 (95)
2 weeks	16.5 (12.5)	51 (39)	105 (86)
1 month	14.0 (10)	43 (31)	104 (85)
2 months	11.5 (9)	35 (28)	96 (77)
3–6 months	11.5 (9.5)	35 (29)	91 (74)
6 months–2 years	12.0 (10.5)	36 (33)	78 (70)
2–6 years	12.5 (11.5)	37 (34)	81 (75)
6–12 years	13.5 (11.5)	40 (35)	86 (77)
12–18 years			
Male	14.5 (13)	43 (37)	88 (78)
Female	14.0 (12)	41 (36)	90 (78)
18–49 years			
Male	15.5 (13.5)	47 (41)	90 (80)
Female	14.0 (12)	41 (36)	90 (80)

Hgb, Hemoglobin; *HCT,* hematocrit; *MCV,* mean corpuscular volume; *SD,* standard deviation.
Adapted from Orkin SH, Nathan D, Ginsburg D, et al., eds. *Nathan and Oski's Hematology of Infancy and Childhood.* 7th ed. Philadelphia, PA: Saunders; 2009:1774.

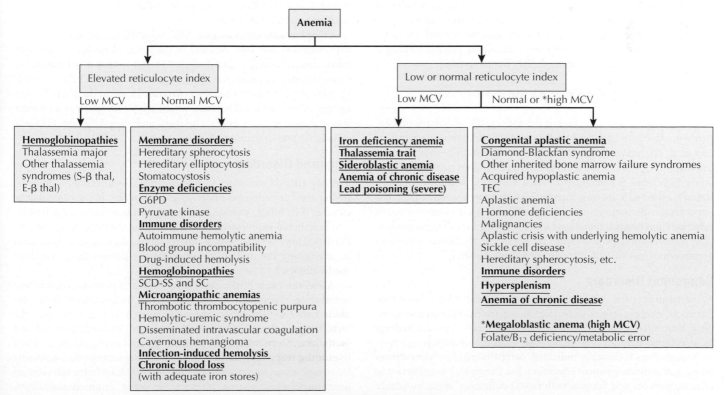

Fig. 77.1 Diagnostic Approach to Anemia.

TABLE 77.3 Diagnostic Tests for Evaluating Anemia

Diagnostic Test	Disease
DAT or Coombs test	AIHA
Hemoglobin electrophoresis	Sickle cell disease
	Thalassemia
RBC enzyme assays	G6PD deficiency
	PK deficiency
Osmotic fragility test	Hereditary spherocytosis
EMA binding assay	AIHA
Iron studies	Iron-deficiency anemia
Folate, vitamin B$_{12}$	Macrocytic or megaloblastic anemia
Bone marrow aspiration and biopsy	Myelodysplastic syndrome
	Aplastic anemia
	Malignancy
	Diamond-Blackfan anemia
ADAMTS13 activity and inhibitor level	TTP
Chromosomal breakage analysis	Fanconi anemia

AIHA, Autoimmune hemolytic anemia; *DAT,* direct antiglobulin; *EMA,* eosin-5'-maleimide; *G6PD,* glucose-6-phosphate dehydrogenase; *PK,* pyruvate kinase; *RBC,* red blood cell; *TTP,* thrombotic thrombocytopenic purpura.

morphologic clues (i.e., presence of spherocytes [HS or AIHA]), schistocytes (microangiopathic hemolytic anemia), bite cells (G6PD deficiency), sickled cells (sickle cell disease), and hypochromic microcytes (iron deficiency, thalassemia, and anemia of inflammation).

A complete physical examination is also important to establish the cause of anemia. Growth parameters should be obtained in all anemic patients. Failure to thrive suggests a more chronic anemia. Jaundice or darkened urine usually indicates a significant hemolytic process.

Hepatosplenomegaly is an important finding present in extramedullary hematopoiesis or infiltrative disorders. Frontal bossing is another sign suggestive of extramedullary hematopoiesis.

MANAGEMENT AND THERAPY

Generally, the treatment for anemia depends on the underlying process. Acute management includes transfusion, discontinuation or neutralization of an offending agent, and mitigation of losses. The indication for transfusion depends on the severity of symptoms, not necessarily based on the Hgb value. In pediatric patients, 5 mL/kg of packed red cell transfusion is expected to increase the total Hgb by approximately 1 g/dL. It is important to discontinue or neutralize offending agents such as drugs or infections and prudent to mitigate sources of loss, including gastrointestinal (cauterization, proton pump inhibitors) or menstrual (estrogen). Treatment of specific RBC disorders is discussed later.

Congenital Disorders

Acute treatment for congenital disorders, including RBC membrane disorders, enzyme defects, or hemoglobinopathies, relies on discontinuing, neutralizing, and/or avoiding offending agents (i.e., certain drugs or infections) that can precipitate acute episodes of anemia, supportive transfusions if clinically indicated, determining chronic treatment plans, and providing patient education. For example, it is important to educate patients and families with G6PD deficiency about avoidance of oxidative stressors that can trigger hemolysis, including exposure

to certain drugs (i.e., sulfa-containing medications, high-dose aspirin, and rasburicase), naphthalene-containing mothballs, and fava beans. In hereditary spherocytosis, splenectomy is curative but is associated with surgical risks. After splenectomy there is an increased risk for infections and pulmonary hypertension. The procedure is generally reserved for severe cases. Indications for splenectomy include severe anemia (Hgb <8 g/dL), poor growth, chronic fatigue, or recurrent hemolytic episodes requiring frequent RBC transfusions.

The clinical phenotype of α- and β-thalassemias depends on the number of alleles affected and subsequently the amount of α-globin and β-globin produced. Generally, α-thalassemia does not require treatment unless three alleles are deleted or nonfunctional (Hgb H [HbH] disease; see Table 77.1). These patients generally are susceptible to oxidative stresses such as G6PD deficiency and may require intermittent, supportive transfusions during illness but are not transfusion dependent. Deletion of all four α-globin alleles causes profound anemia during fetal life and is incompatible with life without intervention. Intrauterine transfusions can rescue the fetus, but they have a severe blood disorder that is transfusion dependent and bone marrow transplantation is recommended.

Patients with β-thalassemia major are transfusion dependent, requiring transfusions every 3 to 5 weeks to maintain a nadir Hgb of 9 to 10 g/dL. Hematopoietic stem cell transplant (HSCT) has been the only cure for β-thalassemia major, but breakthroughs in gene therapy are promising for alternative curative treatments. Thalassemia intermedia exhibits moderately severe anemia but is not transfusion dependent. Hydroxyurea has also been used in β-thalassemia intermedia and reduces the risk for leg ulcers, pulmonary hypertension, and extramedullary hematopoiesis. Patients with β-thalassemia trait have a mild microcytic anemia and do not require long-term treatment.

Management of DBA includes initially chronic RBC transfusions followed by a corticosteroid trial. Up to 80% of patients may initially respond to steroid treatment and no longer require red cell transfusions, but nonresponders or those that subsequently become steroid-resistant are transfusion dependent. Allogenic HSCT is the only curative treatment at this time.

Complications from chronic RBC transfusions include iron overload, which causes iron deposits in the liver, endocrine organs, and heart, causing severe organ dysfunction and is fatal if left untreated. Currently, patients with iron overload are treated with chelators, medications that bind iron. Chelators currently in use in the United States include deferoxamine (Desferal), which is typically given as a 12-hour subcutaneous infusion or oral chelators, including deferasirox (Exjade or Jadenu) and deferiprone (Ferriprox).

Acquired Disorders

Treating anemia secondary to acquired RBC disorders relies on identifying and correcting the underlying abnormality. In nutritional deficiencies (i.e., folate, vitamin B$_{12}$, iron), treatment focuses on trialing oral nutritional supplementation and treating the underlying cause of the deficiency. With anemia of inflammation, the treatment is focused on addressing the underlying inflammatory process (i.e., infectious, rheumatologic).

AIHA can cause brisk, severe hemolysis, and patients require close monitoring. Treatment of primary AIHA includes methylprednisolone 1 to 2 mg/kg/day intravenously every 6 to 12 hours. After the Hgb stabilizes, the patient can be switched to 1 to 2 mg/kg/day of oral prednisone. Steroids are then gradually tapered over a period of weeks to months. RBC transfusion is indicated in the setting of cardiovascular compromise. Second-line therapy for AIHA includes intravenous immunoglobulin, plasma pheresis, or other immunomodulators, including rituximab, danazol, vincristine, or cyclophosphamide.

Treatment of patients with TEC or an aplastic crisis from parvovirus requires transfusion support and regular monitoring of CBCs until the anemia normalizes. For patients with immune compromise (congenital or medication induced), intravenous immunoglobulin is efficacious to facilitate parvovirus clearance.

FUTURE DIRECTIONS

Diagnostic and therapeutic approaches for RBC disorders are continually evolving. Advancement in molecular and genetic techniques facilitates conformational testing for known RBC disorders and provides important diagnostic information when the cause is unclear with conventional testing. Traditionally, HSCT has been the only curative treatment for β-thalassemia major. Established protocols have led to a high success of thalassemia-free survival; however, there are many long-term complications from transplant, and availability of allogeneic donors is limited. Recent breakthroughs in gene therapy are beginning to offer alternative curative options. Currently, a novel therapy offered is autologous stem cell transplant after genetic modification that induces the production of a novel Hgb variant. Gene transfer using lentiviral or retroviral vectors has shown experimental promise as a means to replace missing or mutated globin genes and correct erythropoiesis without transplant. Induced pluripotent stem cells are also an area of intense investigation. Additionally, intrauterine transfusions have been recently shown to help fetuses with four α-globin gene deletions survive through delivery. This approach is not without risks but allows for delivery with subsequent chronic transfusions as a bridge to HSCT. Currently, investigators are evaluating the feasibility of in utero stem cell transplantation as a cure before delivery.

SUGGESTED READINGS

Available online.

78

Disorders of White Blood Cells

Rebecca M. Sutherland

Leukocytes, or white blood cells (WBCs), are an essential component of both the innate and acquired (adaptive) immune systems. This chapter discusses quantitative and qualitative disorders of neutrophils and provides a brief discussion of disorders of eosinophils, basophils, and monocytes. Disorders of lymphocytes and the adaptive immune system are examined in detail in the immunology chapter (see Chapter 23).

ETIOLOGY AND PATHOGENESIS

All WBCs are derived from a common progenitor, the hematopoietic stem cell, found in bone marrow. The maturation of each subclass of WBC is induced by the presence of colony-stimulating factors (Fig. 78.1). Each cell type has a unique appearance under the microscope (Fig. 78.2). A complete blood count (CBC) and manual differential notes the total number of WBCs per microliter (µL) of sample as well as the percentages and absolute counts of each subset. Absolute counts for each WBC are more clinically meaningful than percentages. The expected overall number and balance of cell types vary by age. At birth, a newborn has a high total WBC count, up to 30,000/µL with a neutrophil predominance. Within the first week of life, this number will decrease to a range of 5000 to 21,000/µL. As childhood progresses, the WBC count will decrease to the adult average of 7500/µL. From 2 weeks of life through the age of 5 years, lymphocytes are the predominant cell type. Through the rest of childhood, neutrophils are predominant, comprising over 50% of WBCs in circulation. Other cell types, including monocytes, eosinophils, and basophils, make up smaller percentages of the total WBC count.

Neutrophils are a cornerstone of the body's innate immune system and the first line of defense against infectious microorganisms. Each neutrophil will circulate for about 6 to 12 hours after release from the bone marrow, migrating to sites of infection or inflammation. The neutrophil engages in phagocytosis, the process through which it engulfs and digests invading microorganisms. Mature neutrophils are found in high proportion in bone marrow and along the endothelial lining of blood vessels, where they are well positioned to respond to breaches in the host's immune defense system.

Neutropenia is defined as an absolute neutrophil count (ANC) less than 1500/µL with a three-tier severity categorization. Mild neutropenia is an ANC less than 1500/µL, moderate neutropenia 1000 to 500/µL and severe neutropenia is less than 500/µL. As the ANC decreases, host defense against infection is diminished such that the risk for infection is inversely proportional to ANC. Qualitative neutrophil defects, in which neutrophil cell numbers are within the expected range, but the cells themselves are unable to function properly, can lead to a similar infectious risk. Of note, the ANC is affected by ethnicity, approximately 5% of African Americans have a lower baseline ANC by 200 to 600/µL. This is likely secondary to decreased neutrophil release from the bone marrow and does not lead to a greater predisposition for infection.

CLINICAL PRESENTATION AND DIFFERENTIAL DIAGNOSIS

Patients with neutrophil disorders most often present with frequent infections, most commonly bacterial or fungal. Children with chronic neutropenia may present with recurrent cellulitis, deep tissue abscesses, pneumonia, or bacteremia, among others. In the absence of an appropriate neutrophil response, clinical signs of infection can be diminished.

Congenital Disorders of Neutrophils

Congenital neutropenia can be caused by an array of genetic disorders of myelopoiesis (Table 78.1). These rare disorders are present at birth and typically manifest with severe neutropenia (ANC <200). A selection of other genetic disorders associated with neutropenia can be found in Table 78.2. Many of these rare disorders are associated with abnormalities in multiple cell lineages.

Neutrophil Function Defects

The neutrophil is a phagocyte that consumes invasive microorganisms. Intact neutrophil function requires a multistep process involving cellular adhesion, chemotaxis, opsonization, phagocytosis, degranulation and oxidative metabolism. A disorder in which any of these functions is ineffective or absent results in increased host susceptibility to bacterial and fungal infections (Table 78.3). Various disease states can also lead to acquired defects in neutrophil chemotaxis, including diabetes mellitus, metabolic storage diseases, malnutrition, prematurity and burns.

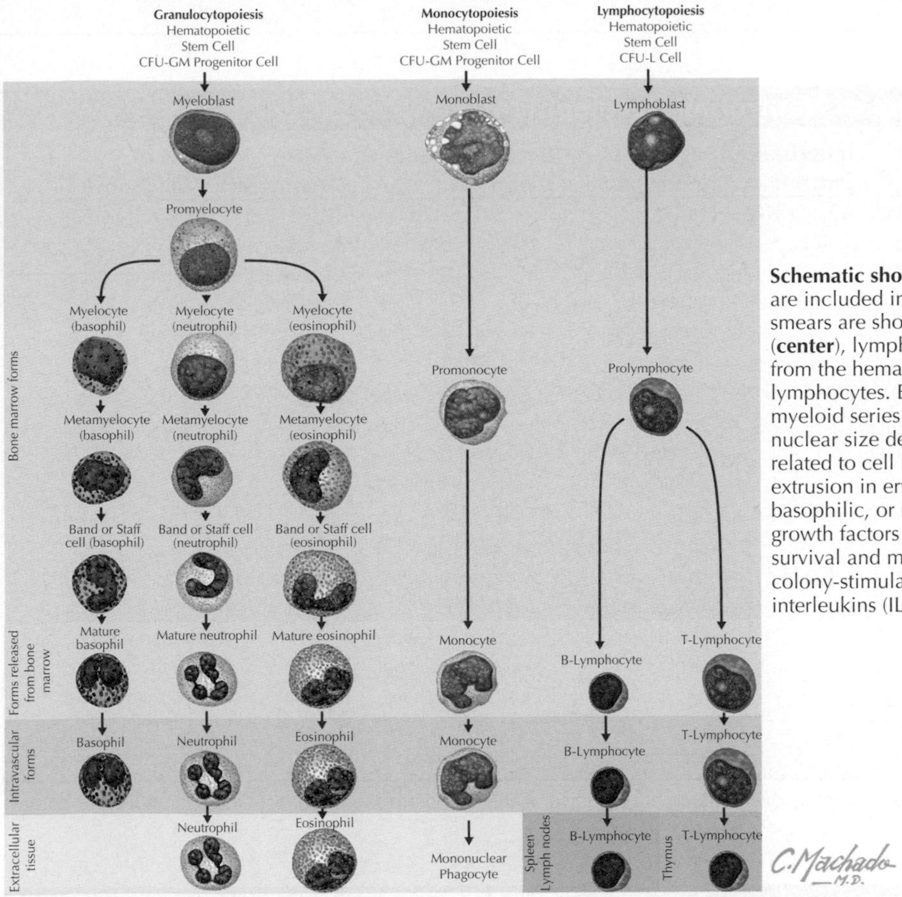

Granulocytopoiesis
Hematopoietic
Stem Cell
CFU-GM Progenitor Cell

Monocytopoiesis
Hematopoietic
Stem Cell
CFU-GM Progenitor Cell

Lymphocytopoiesis
Hematopoietic
Stem Cell
CFU-L Cell

Schematic showing stages of hematopoiesis. Although not all cells are included in each sequence, main cell types seen in bone marrow smears are shown in granulocytopoiesis (**left**), monocytopoiesis (**center**), lymphocytopoiesis (**right**). The various CFU cells that arise from the hematopoietic stem cell (not shown) closely resemble lymphocytes. Except for megakaryocytes, cells in erythroid and myeloid series as a rule get smaller during differentiation. Also, nuclear size declines, nuclear density increases, and special features related to cell lineage—such as hemoglobin production and nuclear extrusion in erythropoiesis, and specific granules (eosinophilic, basophilic, or neutrophilic) in granulocytopoiesis—appear. Various growth factors and cytokines mediate cell proliferation rate and survival and maturation of progenitor cells. Some of these are colony-stimulating factors, erythropoietin, thrombopoietin, interleukins (IL-1, IL-3, IL-6, IL-11), and stem cell factors.

Fig. 78.1 Stages of Hematopoiesis.

Features of Erythrocytes and Platelets in Wright-Stained Blood Smears

Cells	Diameter (μm)	Life span (days)	No. of cells/ L of blood	Shape and nucleus type	Cytoplasm	Functions
Erythrocyte (red blood cell) 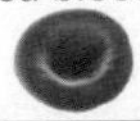	7–10	120	5×10^{12} in males; 4.5×10^{12} in females	Biconcave disc, anucleate	Pink because of acidophilia of hemoglobin; halo in center	Transports hemoglobin that binds O_2 and CO_2
Platelet (thrombocyte) 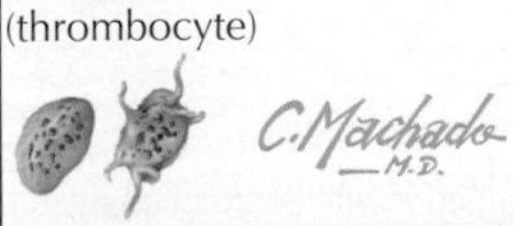	2–4	10	150 to 400×10^9	Oval biconvex disc, anucleate	Pale blue; central dark granulomere, peripheral less dense hyalomere	In hemostasis, promotes blood clotting; plugs endothelial damage

Features of Leukocytes in Wright-Stained Blood Smears (Total Number: 5–10 × 10⁹/L Blood)

Cells	Diameter (μm)	Differential count (%)*	Nucleus	Cytoplasm	Functions
Granulocytes					
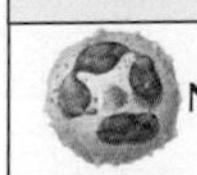 **Neutrophil**	9–12	60–70	Segmented, 3–5 lobes, densely stained	Pale, finely granular, evenly dispersed specific granules	Phagocytoses bacteria; increases in number in acute bacterial infections
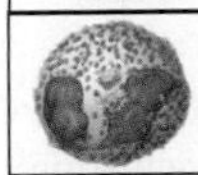 **Eosinophil**	12–15	1–4	Bilobed, clumped chromatin pattern, densely stained	Large homogeneous red granules that are coarse and highly refractile	Phagocytoses antigen-antibody complexes and parasites
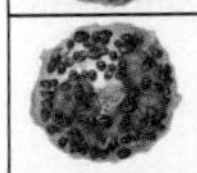 **Basophil**	10–14	0–1	Bilobed or segmented	Large blue specific granules that stain with basic dyes and often obscure nucleus	Involved in anticoagulation, increases vascular permeability
Agranulocytes					
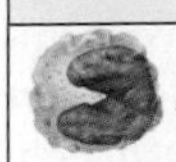 **Monocytes**	12–20	3–10	Indented, kidney shaped, lightly stained	Agranular, pale blue cytoplasm, with lysosomes	Is motile; gives rise to macrophages
Lymphocyte • Small • Medium to large	6–10 11–16	20–40	Small, round or slightly indented, darkly stained	Agranular, faintly basophilic, blue to gray	Acts in humoral (B cell) and cellular (T cell) immunity

*Note: Differential count (%) is based on adult values.

Fig. 78.2 Features of White Blood Cells in Wright-Stained Blood Smears.

TABLE 78.1 Congenital Disorders of Neutrophil Development

Disorder	Clinical Manifestations	Defect	Inheritance Pattern	Severity of Neutropenia	Evaluation and Diagnosis	Treatment	Risk of Malignancy
Severe congenital neutropenia (SCN) Kostmann syndrome (KS)	Life-threatening pyogenic infections in infancy	Maturational arrest of neutrophil precursors leading to impaired myeloid differentiation	AD (SCN), AR (KS)	ANC <200 since birth; associated mild anemia; occasional monocytosis and eosinophilia	Bone marrow demonstrates myeloid maturation arrest. SCN: *ELA2, GFL1*, other mutations; KS: *HAX1* mutations	GCSF Bone marrow transplant is curative	Increased risk for leukemia (AML) or myelodysplastic syndrome
Cyclic neutropenia	Cyclic fever, oral ulcers, gingivitis, periodontal disease, recurrent bacterial infections	Stem cell regulatory defect resulting in defective maturation	Sporadic or AD	<200 for 3–7 days every 3 weeks (range, 15– to 35–day cycle)	CBC two or three times a week for 6–8 weeks to document cycles and nadir; *ELA-2* mutation in 80%-90%	±GCSF	No increased risk for malignancy
Shwachman-Diamond syndrome	Neutropenia, exocrine pancreas insufficiency, and skeletal abnormalities	May have defects in neutrophil mobility, migration, and chemotaxis in addition to neutropenia	AR	Variable severity; may be associated with anemia and thrombocytopenia	Neutropenia, low serum trypsinogen, elevated fecal fat excretion, metaphyseal dysostosis, rib cage abnormalities, short stature; *SBDS* mutation in 90%	±GCSF, pancreatic enzyme replacement	Increased risk for myelodysplastic syndrome or leukemia; screened with yearly bone marrow biopsy/aspirate

AD, Autosomal dominant; *AML,* acute myelogenous leukemia; *AR,* autosomal recessive; *CBC,* complete blood count; *GCSF,* granulocyte colony-stimulating factor.

TABLE 78.2 Additional Congenital Disorders Associated With Neutropenia

Disorder	Clinical Manifestations
Cartilage-hair hypoplasia	Lymphopenia, short limbed dwarfism, metaphysical chondrodysplasia, abnormally fine hair
Myelokathexis with dysmyelopoiesis (WHIM syndrome)	Marrow retention of neutrophils, recurrent bronchopulmonary infections; WHIM syndrome: warts, hypogammaglobulinemia, infections, myelokathexis
Dyskeratosis congenita	Bone marrow failure syndrome; dystrophic changes in nails, skin (hyperpigmentation), and mucous membranes (leukoplakia)
Fanconi anemia	Bone marrow failure syndrome; genitourinary and skeletal abnormalities, increased chromosome fragility
Organic acidemias (propionic, methylmalonic)	Initially well at birth, then toxic encephalopathy
Osteopetrosis	Defective bone turnover with resultant hematopoietic insufficiency and bone fragility
Reticular dysgenesis (congenital aleukocytosis)	Absent WBC, hypogammaglobulinemia, thymic hypoplasia, severe infection and death in infancy
Immunodeficiencies (severe combined immunodeficiency, common variable immunodeficiency, hyper-IgM, IgA deficiency)	Abnormal levels of immunoglobulins; frequent infections, failure to thrive, hepatosplenomegaly
Glycogen storage disease type 1b (von Gierke disease) and other inborn errors of metabolism	Neutropenia and functional neutrophil defect, hepatosplenomegaly

Acquired Disorders of Neutrophils

Acquired neutropenia is significantly more common than congenital neutropenia. The pathophysiology is secondary to impaired bone marrow production, peripheral destruction, or splenic sequestration.

Infection-Associated Neutropenia

Acute infection often causes a transient reactive leukocytosis, which manifests with an increased number of WBCs seen on a CBC. Within a few days of illness, however, many viruses can cause neutropenia that lasts for 1 to 6 weeks. Common viral culprits include human immunodeficiency virus, parvovirus B19, Epstein-Barr virus, cytomegalovirus, hepatitis A and B, influenza A and B, respiratory syncytial virus, and varicella. Potential mechanisms of infection-associated neutropenia include decreased bone marrow production, depleted marrow reserves, increased neutrophil margination resulting in decreased circulating neutrophils, or antineutrophil antibody formation leading to peripheral destruction.

Drug-Induced Neutropenia

Myelosuppression, or suppression of bone marrow function, is a common and expected side effect of many of the cytotoxic agents used for cancer treatment. These drugs cause not only severe neutropenia but also anemia and thrombocytopenia. Other medications associated with drug-induced neutropenia are listed in Table 78.4. Drug-induced neutropenia may be caused by decreased bone marrow production or by the production of antineutrophil antibodies. The neutropenia typically resolves with discontinuation of the offending drug.

TABLE 78.3 **Congenital Disorders of Neutrophil Function**

Disorder	Clinical Manifestations	Functional Defect	Evaluation and Diagnosis	Frequency	Inheritance Pattern	Treatment	Prognosis
Leukocyte adhesion deficiency (types I–III)	Delayed separation of umbilical cord (≥3 weeks), recurrent and severe bacterial and fungal infections without the accumulation of pus, poor wound healing, periodontal disease	Adhesion: neutrophils have diminished adhesion to surfaces and cannot migrate out of blood vessels	Neutrophilia ≤100,000/μL, especially during infection; flow cytometry for absence of CD11/CD18 cell surface adhesive glycoproteins (LAD I) or sialyl Lewis X (LAD II)	Very rare	AR	Prophylactic antibiotics; HSCT	Depends on severity of deficiency, may die in infancy or have infrequent life-threatening infections
Hyperimmunoglobulin E syndrome (hyper-IgE, Job syndrome)	Severe eczema; bacterial infections, especially of the skin and lower respiratory tract; pneumatoceles; fungal infections	Chemotaxis	Elevated serum IgE (>2500 international units/mL), eosinophilia; *STAT3* (AD) or *DOCK8* (AR) mutation analysis	Very rare	Sporadic, AD or AR	Supportive, prophylactic antibiotics	Good
Chediak-Higashi syndrome	Partial oculocutaneous albinism; peripheral and cranial neuropathies; neutropenia, recurrent pyogenic infections; accelerated HLH phase leads to death	Ineffective granulopoiesis; defects in chemotaxis and degranulation	Giant granule formation in neutrophils and other granulocytes, neutropenia, *CHS1* and *LYST* gene analysis	Very rare	AR	HSCT is curative; prophylactic antibiotics	Few patients survive to the third decade of life
Myeloperoxidase deficiency	Usually clinically silent; rarely, disseminated candidiasis or fungal disease, usually in the setting of diabetes mellitus	Oxidative metabolism: H_2O_2-dependent killing not potentiated by myeloperoxidase	Flow cytometry for neutrophils with peroxidase activity; histochemical staining of neutrophils for peroxidase	1:4000 (complete deficiency), 1:2000 (partial)	AR with variable expression	None if asymptomatic; aggressive treatment of fungal disease in setting of infection	Excellent
Chronic granulomatous disease	Recurrent purulent infections with fungal or bacterial catalase-positive organisms[a] usually starting in infancy; chronic inflammatory granulomas	Oxidative metabolism: decreased or absent generation of superoxide (toxic to microbes) by NADPH oxidase	Nitroblue tetrazolium test; dihydrorhodamine fluorescence positive; genotyping for known mutations	1:250,000	Primarily X-linked recessive, rarely AR	Prophylactic antibiotics and antifungals, IFN-γ ± HSCT	Good prognosis with aggressive management of infection

[a]Catalase-positive organisms include *Staphylococcus aureus*, *Aspergillus* species, *Escherichia coli*, *Klebsiella* species, *Salmonella* species, *Serratia marcescens*, and *Burkholderia cepacia*.
AD, Autosomal dominant; *AR*, autosomal recessive; *HSCT*, hematopoietic stem cell transplant; *HLH*, hemophagocytic lymphohistiocytosis; *IFN*, interferon; *LAD*, leukocyte adhesion deficiency; *NADPH*, nicotinamide adenine dinucleotide phosphate.

Autoimmune Neutropenia

AIN can occur as a primary disease process or as a secondary result of other autoimmune disorders, drugs, infections, or immune dysregulation. Primary AIN is the most common cause of neutropenia in infancy and childhood and is often discovered incidentally in children between the ages of 8 months and 3 years. Patients are typically asymptomatic at presentation. It is rare for there to be a history of severe infections because the bone marrow is able to respond to stressors and appropriately increase granulocyte output. A monocytosis is often present. Antineutrophil immunoglobulin G (IgG) antibodies may be identified in these patients. Primary AIN is a self-limiting disorder with a median duration of 9 months; 95% resolve within 2 years of diagnosis.

Neonatal Alloimmune Neutropenia

Neonatal alloimmune neutropenia (NAIN) develops during the first 2 weeks of life as a result of maternal antineutrophil IgG antibodies against paternally inherited neutrophil antigens present on fetal neutrophils. Rarely, the antibody is secondary to maternal AIN. Transplacental antibody transfer results in neutropenia; this process is similar to the anemia caused by Rh-group incompatibility seen in hemolytic disease of the newborn. These babies present clinically with infections ranging from omphalitis to pneumonia and sepsis; however, many cases of NAIN are discovered incidentally with neutropenia noted on CBC, and it is likely that even more cases are clinically silent and never detected on laboratory work. NAIN will self-resolve within 3 to 6 months.

TABLE 78.4 Drugs (Commonly Used in Pediatrics) Associated With Neutropenia

Drug Class	Drugs
Antimicrobial	Trimethoprim-sulfamethoxazole, sulfonamides, macrolides, cephalosporins, semisynthetic penicillins (vancomycin), quinine, chloroquine, amphotericin B
Antiinflammatory	Nonsteroidal antiinflammatory drugs (ibuprofen, naproxen)
Antipsychotic	Clozapine, olanzapine, phenothiazines
Anticonvulsant	Carbamazepine, valproate, phenytoin
Antithyroid	Methimazole, propylthiouracil
Cardiovascular	Antiarrhythmics, diuretics
Toxins	Benzene
Chemotherapeutic agents	Cytotoxic drugs

TABLE 78.5 Additional Causes of Acquired Neutropenia

Conditions	Causes
Malignancies and bone marrow failure	Leukemia, lymphoma, preleukemic states, myelodysplastic syndromes, aplastic anemia
Nutritional deficiency	Vitamin B_{12}, folate, copper, or starvation
Other	Splenomegaly, complement activation, hemodialysis

Additional Causes of Acquired Neutropenia

Neutropenia can often occur in the setting of conditions that affect the entire bone marrow. In cases such as malignancies and marrow infiltrative processes, multiple cell lines are commonly affected and neutropenia is seen in conjunction with anemia and/or thrombocytopenia. Additional causes of acquired neutropenia are listed in Table 78.5.

Leukocytosis

Leukocytosis, or elevated number of circulating WBCs, usually indicates a systemic response to infection or inflammation. In children, the most common cause of elevated WBC is reactive leukocytosis in response to an infection, which will return to normal after resolution of the inciting event. Significantly elevated WBC counts (>100,000 cells) should immediately raise suspicion for oncologic processes such as leukemia. Microscopic evaluation of a peripheral blood smear may reveal atypical lymphocytes (suggestive of a viral process) or lymphoblasts (strongly associated with bone marrow infiltration from leukemia). Chronic inflammatory states can also cause leukocytosis, including autoimmune and rheumatologic disorders such as systemic lupus erythematosus (SLE), juvenile idiopathic arthritis (JIA), and inflammatory bowel disease (IBD).

Neutrophilia

Elevated levels of neutrophils in the bloodstream can occur in both acute and chronic conditions. The bone marrow can be induced to make more cells, neutrophils can be spurred from the marrow into circulation, and clearance can be impaired in the setting of splenic dysfunction. Disorders affecting almost any organ system can be associated with neutrophilia (Table 78.6).

TABLE 78.6 Causes of Neutrophilia

Infectious	Bacterial, viral
Rheumatologic	JIA, Kawasaki disease
Asplenia	Surgical or functional
Gastrointestinal	Liver failure, IBD
Endocrine	Diabetic ketoacidosis
Neutrophil function disorders	CGD, LAD (see Table 78.3)
Drugs	Corticosteroids, epinephrine
Stressors	Shock, trauma, burns, surgery, hemorrhage, hypoxia
Malignancy	Clonal expansion, leukemia, myeloproliferative disorders
Trisomy 21 (Down syndrome)	Defective proliferation and maturation of myeloid cells

CGD, Chronic granulomatous disease; *IBD,* inflammatory bowel disease; *JIA,* juvenile idiopathic arthritis; *LAD,* leukocyte adhesion deficiency.

Monocytosis

Monocytes are macrophage precursor cells derived, like neutrophils, from myeloblasts. Monocytes develop more rapidly than neutrophils and therefore a monocytosis may herald an impending rise in neutrophil count. Increased monocyte counts are found in cases of tuberculosis, syphilis, typhoid fever, and brucellosis. Monocytosis also can be found in chronic inflammatory states such as rheumatologic disorders (SLE, JIA), IBD, and Langerhans cell histiocytosis.

Basophilia

Basophils are involved in immediate hypersensitivity disease states and may play a role in defense against bacterial infections. Basophilia, however, is often nonspecific. An absolute basophil count greater than 120 cells can be seen in acute hypersensitivity reactions and in chronic inflammatory states, including JIA, chronic sinusitis, IBD, and malignancies.

Eosinophilia

Eosinophils have multiple functions, including mediating allergic responses and defending against metazoan parasite infections through toxic degranulation. The differential for persistent eosinophilia includes familial versus acquired disorders. Acquired eosinophilia is subdivided into primary versus secondary eosinophilia (Fig. 78.3). A thorough history, including allergies, medications, review of systems, travel, and animal exposures, is important to narrow this broad differential. Mild eosinophilia, with an absolute eosinophil count (AEC) between 600 and 1500/μL, is most commonly associated with allergic disorders. The elevated cell count is usually transient and resolves with treatment of the underlying process. *Toxocara* infection is a common cause of eosinophilia in children.

EVALUATION AND MANAGEMENT

If isolated neutropenia is found incidentally on a routine screening CBC, investigation should begin with a thorough history and physical examination. A recent history of fever, symptoms of upper respiratory tract infection, or diarrhea, may suggest a preceding viral illness. A complete history of infections, including the type and frequency, is important if there is concern for recurrent infections. Recent medication exposures should be reviewed. Additionally, a dietary history may

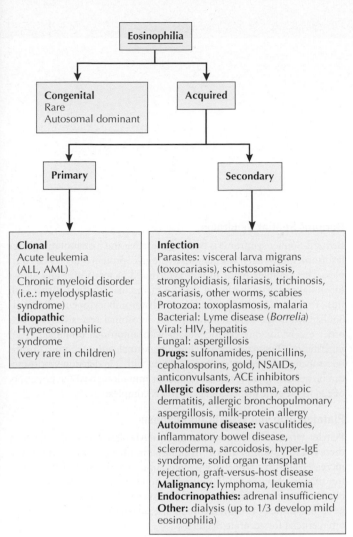

Fig. 78.3 Causes of Eosinophilia.

important to evaluate for hepatosplenomegaly and lymphadenopathy. If history and physical examination are unrevealing after thorough evaluation, and the child is otherwise healthy, a repeat CBC should be obtained in 2 to 3 weeks.

Persistent neutropenia on three separate occasions over 8 weeks in an otherwise well child should prompt a more extensive workup. Any drugs associated with neutropenia should be discontinued. Further testing should be determined based on the patient's age, physical examination, and clinical presentation.

As described at the beginning of this chapter, patients with persistent severe neutropenia are susceptible to bacterial and fungal infection. A fever may be the only manifesting symptom of a life-threatening infection. All patients with prolonged periods of neutropenia should follow strict fever precautions (defined as a temperature greater than 101.3°F [38.5°C]). Patients should immediately present for evaluation including a blood culture and CBC with differential. Additional infectious workup should be guided based on age and physical examination findings. In the setting of severe neutropenia (ANC <500) and fever, patients are treated empirically with broad-spectrum antibiotics for at least 24 hours, often in an inpatient hospital setting. Pending results of initial infectious studies, antibiotics may then be narrowed or discontinued.

In some cases, it is appropriate to treat the underlying neutropenia. Recombinant granulocyte colony-stimulating factor (GCSF) can effectively increase neutrophil counts. GCSF is the standard of treatment for severe congenital neutropenia, some cases of cyclic neutropenia, and AIN if infectious complications are severe. Hematopoietic stem cell transplants are a potentially curative option for some disorders, with a goal of reconstituting normal neutrophil number or function.

FUTURE DIRECTIONS

Ongoing research continues to improve diagnostic and therapeutic options for both known and yet-undiscovered disorders of white blood cells. Gene therapy is a promising potential treatment for congenital disorders such as severe congenital neutropenia and cyclic neutropenia, with the potential to cure or significantly alter the natural history of these diseases, with fewer inherent risks relative to hematopoietic stem cell transplantation.

SUGGESTED READINGS

Available online.

allude to potential nutritional deficiencies, such as folate or vitamin B_{12}. Family history should be elicited; unexplained deaths or known abnormalities of parental blood counts may suggest an inherited disorder. On physical examination, one may note the presence or absence of phenotypic abnormalities associated with particular disorders. It is

79

Platelet Disorders

Ajibike Lapite

 CLINICAL VIGNETTE

A 5-year-old previously healthy girl presented with sudden onset of a rash and bruising. Her parents denied known trauma or exposures. Aside from a recent viral illness, she has been well.

On physical examination, she is well-appearing and playful. A diffuse petechial rash is present on her extremities. She has a 4- × 2-cm palpable bruise on her right shin. There is no evidence of hepatosplenomegaly, lymphadenopathy, or other manifestations of bleeding on examination.

Initial laboratory assessment was notable for a platelet count of 10,000/μL; the remaining cell lines and peripheral blood smear were normal. Her clinical history, physical examination, and laboratory test results are consistent with a diagnosis of immune thrombocytopenia (ITP). Because of a lack of significant mucosal bleeding (i.e., epistaxis, wet purpura, hematuria, or blood in the stool), therapeutic intervention was not indicated. She had spontaneous normalization of her platelet count 4 months after initial presentation.

Hemostasis, the physiologic response to stop bleeding at the site of injury, is divided into two stages: primary and secondary hemostasis. Platelets play a key role in primary hemostasis. Platelets are small anucleate cell particles (5 to 7 μL) produced by megakaryocyte fragmentation in the bone marrow. Thrombopoietin (TPO) is a hormone produced in the liver that regulates platelet formation. Platelets circulate for 7 to 10 days before removal by the reticuloendothelial system.

In the setting of vascular injury, circulating platelets adhere to the site of injury with the help of von Willebrand factor and ultimately form a platelet plug. Signaling cascades activate platelets inducing structural changes necessary for platelet-fibrinogen interaction, platelet-platelet interaction, and release of platelet storage granules (Fig. 79.1). This process propagates the platelet plug and recruits procoagulant factors essential for secondary hemostasis. Disruption of this process can be clinically significant. Platelet disorders can be inherited or acquired and result in qualitative and/or quantitative defects. Platelet dysfunction results in abnormal/prolonged bleeding that is primarily mucosal.

ETIOLOGY AND PATHOGENESIS

Congenital Platelet Disorders

Congenital platelet disorders individually are rare but as a whole are more common than previously recognized. They are the result of either a qualitative or quantitative defect, and some can feature both. In general, children with congenital platelet disorders are more likely to have chronic mucosal bleeding symptoms that develop early in life. The bleeding can be mild to severe depending on the specific disorder. Refer to Table 79.1 for a list of inherited platelet disorders.

Bernard-Soulier Syndrome

Bernard-Soulier syndrome is both a qualitative and a quantitative platelet disorder secondary to mutations in the glycoprotein (GP) 1b/1X complex. This complex binds to von Willebrand factor (vWF) and allows for initial platelet adhesion at the site of vascular injury. Patients with this syndrome also have a variable macrothrombocytopenia. Bernard-Soulier syndrome is predominantly an autosomal recessive (AR) disorder except for one genetic variant with autosomal dominant (AD) inheritance. Heterozygotes are clinically normal, although mild thrombocytopenia has been described. Children with 22q deletion syndromes can be heterozygotes for Bernard-Soulier mutation given the proximity of 22q to the gene that encodes GP 1b/1X complex.

Platelet-Type von Willebrand Disease

Platelet-type von Willebrand disease is an AD platelet disorder in which there is a mutation in the GP Ib alpha subunit. This mutation leads to increased affinity between the platelet subunit and von Willebrand factor, thereby removing vWF multimers and platelet aggregates from the blood circulation. Clinical manifestations and laboratory findings can be similar to that of von Willebrand disease type 2B. Genetic analysis is often crucial for accurate diagnosis.

Storage Pool Defects

Defects in storage granules are associated with impaired primary and secondary hemostasis. Additionally, the role of platelet granules extends beyond hemostasis. Platelet granules belong to a family of lysosome-related organelles found in other cells such as cytotoxic T-lymphocytes, natural killer cells, and melanosomes. Disorders of platelet storage granules often accompany defects in processes mediated by other lysosome-related organelles. Of the disorders in this category, Chediak-Higashi syndrome is one of the most common. Chediak-Higashi syndrome is an AR disorder notable for platelet dysfunction, immune dysfunction, and oculocutaneous albinism. Hermansky-Pudlak is similar, autosomal recessive, and associated with platelet dysfunction, neutropenia, immune dysfunction, oculocutaneous albinism, pulmonary fibrosis, and granulomatous colitis.

Glanzmann Thrombasthenia

Glanzmann thrombasthenia is an autosomal recessive disorder with an incidence of 1 in 1 million. Platelet adhesion is dysfunctional because of an abnormality in the genes that encode either chain of the platelet αIIbβ3 integrin fibrinogen receptor. As a result, platelets cannot bind fibrinogen, resulting in a severe bleeding disorder. Screening laboratories will reveal a normal platelet count and size. Traditionally, children present within the first year of life with profound mucosal bleeding. Common clinical symptoms include easy bruising, gastrointestinal hemorrhage, persistent epistaxis, and abnormal uterine bleeding.

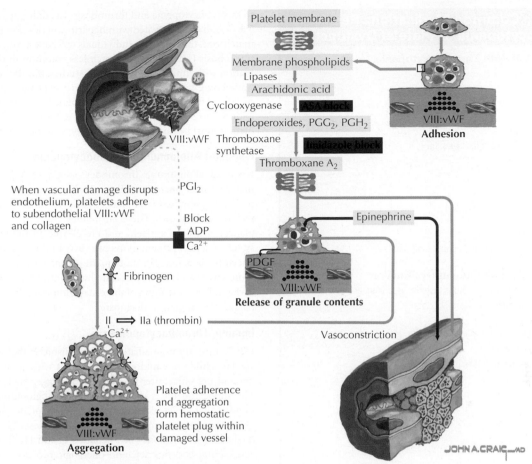

Fig. 79.1 Platelet Adhesion, Release, and Aggregation.

TABLE 79.1 Congenital Platelet Disorders

Disorder	Dysfunction	Mode of Inheritance
Bernard-Soulier syndrome	Qualitative ± Quantitative	AR (one AD variant)
Platelet-type von Willebrand disease	Qualitative ± Quantitative	AD
Chediak-Higashi syndrome	Qualitative	AR
Hermansky-Pudlak syndrome	Qualitative	AR
Glanzmann thrombasthenia	Qualitative	AR
Wiskott-Aldrich syndrome	Quantitative	X-linked recessive
MYH9-related disorders	Quantitative	AD
Congenital amegakaryocytic thrombocytopenia	Quantitative	AR
Thrombocytopenia absent radii	Quantitative	AR

AD, Autosomal dominant; *AR,* autosomal recessive.

Wiskott-Aldrich Syndrome

Wiskott-Aldrich syndrome is an X-linked recessive disorder notable for the triad of microthrombocytopenia, eczema, and recurrent infections secondary to immunodeficiency. Children often present with easy bruising in the neonatal period, eczema in infancy, and recurrent sinopulmonary infections throughout childhood.

MYH9-Related Disorders

The MYH9-related disorders are a group of AD inherited platelet disorders characterized by macrothrombocytopenia resulting from mutations in the cytoskeletal protein nonmuscle myosin heavy chain IIA. The macrothrombocytopenia is present at birth. The degree of thrombocytopenia and bleeding phenotype can vary. MYH9-related disorders encompass disorders previously thought to be unique, including May-Hegglin anomaly, Sebastian syndrome, Fechtner syndrome, and Epstein syndrome. MYH9-related disorders can be associated with cataract formation, nephropathy that can progress to end-stage renal disease, and sensorineural hearing loss.

Bone Marrow Failure Syndromes

Some inherited bone marrow failure syndromes present initially with thrombocytopenia, which can progress to marrow failure. Congenital amegakaryocytic thrombocytopenia is an autosomal recessive disorder characterized by the absence of megakaryocytes in the bone marrow. Thrombocytopenia is present at birth, and marrow failure develops later. It is fatal without bone marrow transplantation.

Thrombocytopenia–absent radii (TAR) is an autosomal recessive disorder characterized by thrombocytopenia and the absence of the bilateral radii. Some patients also may have cardiac or renal malformations. The thrombocytopenia is present at birth and typically resolves in the first year of life. Interestingly, cow's milk intolerance/allergy has been associated with TAR, and introduction to cow's milk may precipitate thrombocytopenic episodes.

BOX 79.1 Common Medications Resulting in Thrombocytopenia or Platelet Dysfunction

Drugs Associated With Thrombocytopenia
- Antibiotics
  - Linezolid
  - Penicillins
  - Quinine
  - Rifampin
  - Sulfa-containing antibiotics (Bactrim)
  - Vancomycin
- Antiepileptics
  - Carbamazepine
  - Phenytoin
  - Valproate
- Chemotherapeutics
- Anti-reflux medications (cimetidine and ranitidine)

Drugs Associated With Platelet Dysfunction
- Nonsteroidal antiinflammatory drugs (aspirin, ibuprofen, and ketorolac)
- Clopidogrel and ticlopidine
- Abciximab
- Antidepressants
  - Tricyclic antidepressants
  - Selective serotonin reuptake inhibitors
- Beta blockers
- Cholesterol medications
  - Statins
  - Fibrates
- Furosemide
- Ethanol
- Herbal supplements (garlic, ginger, ginseng, ginkgo biloba)

Acquired Platelet Disorders

Acquired platelet disorders are far more common than congenital and the most common cause is medication effect. Medications can induce thrombocytopenia or platelet dysfunction through (1) inhibition of bone marrow production, (2) creation of platelet antibodies, or (3) direct toxic effect on platelets. Refer to Box 79.1 for a list of common medications that result in thrombocytopenia and platelet function abnormalities.

Systemic disorders can cause thrombocytopenia due to increased destruction or decreased production of platelets. Some examples include disseminated intravascular coagulation, malaria, systemic lupus erythematosus, leukemia, lymphoma, viral infections, and human immunodeficiency virus. Thrombocytopenia is common in disorders associated with splenomegaly resulting from increased platelet sequestration. Profound uremia causes platelet dysfunction. The following is a discussion of clinically significant acquired platelet disorders.

Heparin-Induced Thrombocytopenia

Heparin-induced thrombocytopenia (HIT) is a process in which exposure to heparin results in the development of moderate thrombocytopenia and an increased risk for both arterial and venous thrombosis. Moderate thrombocytopenia (50 to 80,000/μL) develops 5 to 10 days after heparin exposure but can occur sooner if there has been prior heparin exposure. The pathophysiology is from heparin forming a complex with platelet factor 4 (PF4) on the surface of platelets. Antibodies against the heparin-PF4 complex bind and activate platelets leading

to thrombocytopenia and thrombosis. In adults, approximately 1% to 5% of individuals treated with heparin will develop HIT and approximately one-third of those individuals will have a course complicated by thrombosis (HITT). HIT is much less common in the pediatric population with limited epidemiologic studies. Similar to adults, children undergoing cardiac surgery with heparin exposure have increased rates of HIT. After cessation of heparin, platelet counts tend to up-trend within 2 to 3 days and normalize by 2 weeks. Nonheparin anticoagulation must be initiated concurrently with the cessation of heparin.

Neonatal Alloimmune Thrombocytopenia

Neonatal alloimmune thrombocytopenia (NAIT) is secondary to maternal-fetal incompatibility. Maternal antibodies form against paternally inherited fetal platelet antigens (common antigen: human platelet antigen 1a). These antibodies cross the placenta, coat fetal platelets with the antigen, and are cleared in the reticuloendothelial system. Clinical presentations can vary. In the first pregnancy, thrombocytopenia is mild; in subsequent pregnancies, thrombocytopenia is more severe and can be associated with intrauterine intracranial hemorrhage. Demonstration of maternal antibodies directed against paternal platelet antigens is diagnostic.

Immune Thrombocytopenia

ITP is an immune-mediated platelet disorder that affects 2 to 6 per 100,000 children. Children often present with acute thrombocytopenia and petechiae after an antecedent trigger such as a viral illness. Thrombocytopenia is secondary to immunoglobulin G (IgG) autoantibodies that target platelets and accelerate splenic clearance. Primary ITP is the most common. Secondary ITP is described and is related to medications, infections (i.e., hepatitis C and HIV) autoimmune diseases, immunodeficiency, and oncologic processes (i.e., lymphoma). Some pediatric syndromes such as Cornelia de Lange and DiGeorge have been associated with increased rates of ITP. For pediatric patients younger than 12 years of age, ITP is a self-limited illness, with 80% having spontaneous resolution within 6 months and 90% at 1 year. For patients older than 12 years of age at the time of the ITP diagnosis, there is an increased risk for developing chronic ITP.

Thrombotic Thrombocytopenic Purpura

Thrombotic thrombocytopenic purpura (TTP) is a microangiopathic hemolytic anemia characterized by platelet consumption secondary to thrombosis in small blood vessels and subsequent shearing of red blood cells. Clinically, TTP is a pentad of fever, hemolytic anemia, thrombocytopenia, renal insufficiency, and neurologic abnormalities. The underlying mechanism of TTP is related to low levels of ADAMTS13, an enzyme that cleaves multimers of von Willebrand factor (vWF) secondary to a congenital deficiency or acquired because of an IgG autoantibody. The absence of ADAMTS13 leads to an increased number of ultra-large vWF multimers that cause increased platelet aggregation and microvascular thrombosis particularly in the cardiac, neural, and renal vasculature.

Clinical Presentation

The spectrum of clinical presentation for platelet disorders is broad and depends on the degree of thrombocytopenia and/or platelet dysfunction. Some patients may be asymptomatic unless they face a hemostatic challenge such as surgery, dental extraction, or trauma. Most often, symptomatic patients present with mucocutaneous bleeding, which can manifest as epistaxis, easy or unexplained bruising, abnormal uterine bleeding, petechiae, purpura, gingival bleeding, or gastrointestinal or genitourinary bleeding (Fig. 79.2).

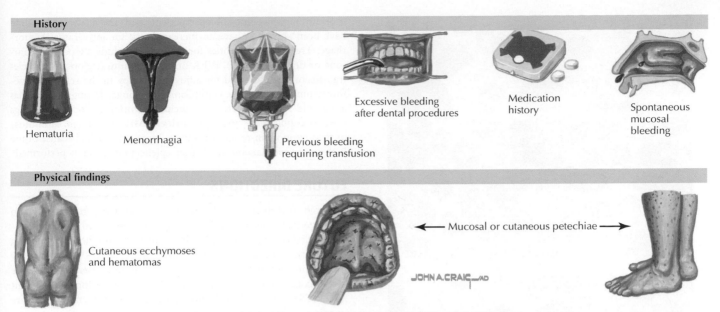

History

Hematuria

Menorrhagia

Previous bleeding requiring transfusion

Excessive bleeding after dental procedures

Medication history

Spontaneous mucosal bleeding

Physical findings

Cutaneous ecchymoses and hematomas

← Mucosal or cutaneous petechiae →

JOHN A.CRAIG—AD

Fig. 79.2 Clinical Presentation of Patients With Bleeding Disorders.

EVALUATION AND MANAGEMENT

A thorough history and physical examination are important in the initial evaluation of a patient with a suspected platelet disorder. It is important to elicit if there is a history of chronic or acute bleeding. It is worthwhile to ask targeted questions such as: "Do you ever have bruises that you're not sure where they came from?" "Do you ever have raised bruises?" "Do your gums bleed when you brush your teeth?" "Do you have nosebleeds? How often and how long does it take for the bleeding to stop?" Patients who menstruate should be asked about the volume and duration of their menses. Review prior hemostatic challenges. Also, ask about joint hyperflexibility and recurrent dislocations. A careful family history can be informative, specifically asking if there are any "bleeders" in the family. It is common in a family in which multiple members have an undiagnosed platelet disorder, for abnormal bleeding to be perceived as normative. A thorough medication history (including herbal supplements) should be completed to determine if the presentation is secondary to a medication side effect. On physical examination the skin should be observed carefully for the presence of petechiae and palpable bruising. In addition, carefully assess for lymphadenopathy and hepatosplenomegaly. Connective tissue disorders can have similar mucocutaneous bleeding symptoms, so assessment for joint flexibility is imperative. Dysmorphic features can provide a clue for a unifying syndrome.

Diagnostic Approach

The first set of laboratory studies should include at minimum a CBC and a peripheral blood smear. Additional coagulation testing can be sent based on the clinical history. The CBC will indicate the presence or absence of thrombocytopenia and whether other cell lines are affected; this will inform further laboratory assessments. An immature platelet fraction helps differentiate between decreased platelet production and increased destruction. The peripheral blood smear can be suggestive of the diagnosis in addition to the presence or absence of other hematologic abnormalities (Fig. 79.3). Coagulation studies will rule out other causes of bleeding. Platelet function assays are indicated if there is history suggestive of a platelet function defect. Genetic evaluation may be

necessary for patients for whom a genetic cause is under consideration. It is important to note that ITP is a diagnosis of exclusion. Although antiplatelet antibody testing is available, it is neither sensitive nor specific and is not recommended in the evaluation of a patient with thrombocytopenia.

Management

Prevention of bleeding is the initial and most important management step for platelet disorders. Counsel patients and families against the use of NSAIDs that can negatively affect platelet function. Avoidance of significant trauma is also important; participation in high-risk contact sports should be prohibited. Appropriate dental hygiene with routine dental care is important to prevent dental processes that would predispose to gingival bleeds or necessitate dental procedures. For patients with abnormal uterine bleeding, hormonal regulation is integral to management.

Therapeutic management for congenital platelet disorders may include desmopressin (DDAVP) or platelet transfusions for severe/life-threatening bleeds. Human leukocyte antigen–matched single-donor leukocyte-depleted platelets are preferred; due to potential formation of antibodies against transfused platelets. Use antifibrinolytics (such as tranexamic acid and aminocaproic acid) for mild/moderate mucosal bleeding. For severe platelet disorders, such as Glanzmann thrombasthenia, recombinant factor VIIa has been demonstrated to be efficacious, particularly for patients refractory to platelet transfusions. Bone marrow transplantation has been performed for patients with severe congenital platelet disorders.

In the case of acquired platelet disorders secondary to an underlying process or medication side effect, the focus of therapy is treatment of the disease process or cessation of the inciting agent. In the case of NAIT, treatment is indicated in the setting of severe thrombocytopenia and/or bleeding. Treatment can include intravenous immunoglobulin (IVIG) and platelet transfusions. Initial management for acquired TTP is plasmapheresis, followed by steroids ± rituximab in refractory TTP. Treatment of ITP depends on bleeding symptoms. For patients without symptoms or with mild symptoms (skin manifestations alone), observation is recommended. Treatment is needed only in the setting of mucosal bleeding (epistaxis, wet purpura, gastrointestinal or genitourinary bleeding) because patients with these sites of bleeding have been shown to have an increased risk for intracranial hemorrhage. Treatment modalities for acute ITP include steroids (prednisone or dexamethasone), IVIG, or anti-D immune globulin. Platelet transfusions are reserved for adjuvant therapy in the setting of life-threatening hemorrhage. For chronic ITP, longer-lasting options that are steroid-sparing are preferred, including immune-modulating drugs (i.e., mycophenolate, mercaptopurine (6MP), rituximab, sirolimus) or thrombopoietin-receptor agonists. In pediatric ITP, because of the high rate of spontaneous resolution, splenectomy is rarely performed.

FUTURE DIRECTIONS

Research to further characterize platelet disorders genetically and to optimize treatment is ongoing. Diagnosis of inherited platelet disorders is challenging in the pediatric population, and there are ongoing investigations to determine best laboratory practices. Bone marrow transplant continues to be explored as curative therapy for some severe congenital platelet disorders. Clinical trials for recombinant ADAMTS13 and anti-vWF molecules for management of TTP are ongoing.

SUGGESTED READINGS

Available online.

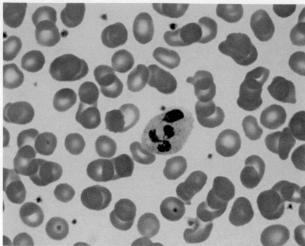

Normal*

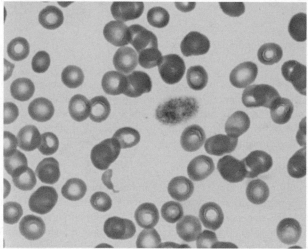

No platelets*

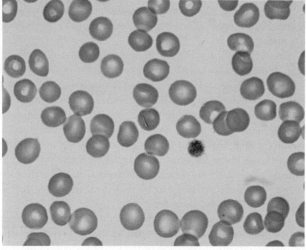

Giant platelet*

Pictures courtesy of Marybeth Helfrich

Fig. 79.3 Peripheral Blood Smears.

80

Sickle Cell Disease

Ajibike Lapite and Michael Triebwasser

CLINICAL VIGNETTE

A 7-month-old boy is brought to the emergency department by his foster mother because of inconsolability. She has noted that his eyes appear acutely yellow. She denies fever. He has had decreased oral intake and urine output. He has had rhinorrhea without other symptoms. She is uncertain about his birth or health history before fostering him a few months ago.

His vital signs are notable for tachycardia; he is afebrile. On physical examination, he is irritable and has scleral icterus and swelling of the dorsal surface of his bilateral hands and feet, which are tender to palpation. A systolic flow murmur is present. There is no evidence of hepatosplenomegaly on examination.

Initial studies include complete blood count, comprehensive metabolic panel, and C-reactive protein (CRP), which are notable for a hemoglobin (Hgb) of 7.5 g/dL with a normal mean corpuscular volume (MCV), reticulocyte count of 15%, elevated unconjugated bilirubin and aspartate aminotransferase, and CRP with mild elevation. Sickle cell forms are noted on the peripheral smear. Hgb electrophoresis is sent and consistent with sickle cell disease (SCD), type SS.

Although most patients with SCD are identified on newborn screen, there are circumstances in which this information is not available, including some children under foster care and children born outside of the United States. Hgb electrophoresis should be sent for patients who present with hemolytic anemia, clinical symptoms concerning for SCD (e.g., dactylitis, recurrent pain, splenomegaly), and an unknown newborn screen.

Sickle cell disease (SCD) is an inherited red blood cell (RBC) disorder secondary to abnormal Hgb with resultant chronic hemolysis. Approximately 70,000 to 100,000 Americans have SCD; the incidence is highest in the African American population (1/400). The carrier rate for African Americans is 8% (1/12). In the United States, there are approximately 75,000 hospitalizations, which costs approximately $900 million, each year. Worldwide, there are 3.2 million individuals with a diagnosis of SCD and 43 million with sickle cell trait.

ETIOLOGY AND PATHOGENESIS

Adult hemoglobin (Hgb A) consists of four subunits: two α-globin and two β-globin subunits. The difference between Hgb A and hemoglobin S (Hgb S) is a single amino acid substitution in the β-globin gene on chromosome 11 from glutamic acid to valine in position 6. SCD is an autosomal recessive disorder. The most common form of SCD is SCD-SS. Other variants of SCD are secondary to compound heterozygotes with one copy of Hgb S in addition to another β-globin variant such as Hgb C, β^+-thalassemia, or β^0-thalassemia. Clinical manifestations of SCD and the severity of these manifestations depend on the genotype. Although pathologic, Hgb S is resistant to *Plasmodium falciparum* (malaria), yielding a selective advantage for Hgb S in malaria-endemic regions.

In all forms of SCD the RBC containing the abnormal Hgb can assume an abnormal sickled shape, which predisposes the cells to impaired motility and hemolysis. The sickled RBC membrane more easily adheres to the capillary endothelium, resulting in occlusion of small capillaries and resultant reduction of perfusion to the peripheral tissues. The four specific processes leading to the pathogenesis of SCD include Hgb S polymerization (deoxygenated Hgb S polymerizes distorting the RBC into an abnormal sickle shape [Fig. 80.1]) vaso-occlusion, endothelial dysfunction, and inflammation. Vaso-occlusion that leads to ischemia is at the crux of vaso-occlusive episodes. Vaso-occlusion is the product of impaired blood flow; increased adhesion between erythrocytes, vascular endothelial cells, and inflammatory cells; and hemostatic activation. Endothelial dysfunction secondary to hemolysis increases reactive oxidative species formation and decreases nitric oxide bioavailability. Nitric oxide is imperative for vasodilation and adequate blood flow. Ischemia-reperfusion injury promotes inflammation.

CLINICAL PRESENTATION

Neonates with SCD are asymptomatic given the protection of fetal hemoglobin (Hgb F). The steady decline of Hgb F that reaches nadir around 6 months of life is often met with the onset of clinical manifestations. There is profound variability in clinical severity, which is related to genotype. Children with SCD-SS and Sβ^0 have the most severe phenotype.

Vaso-occlusive Episode

The most common clinical manifestation of SCD is a vaso-occlusive episode (VOE). In VOE, RBC sickling causes infarction, often of the bone and bone marrow and can occur anywhere. Pain is the principal feature of a VOE. Infants can present with a unique form of VOE, termed dactylitis, manifested by pain and swelling of the dorsal surface of the hands and/or feet. VOE must be distinguished from other pathologic conditions that cause pain; for example, an abdominal VOE can mimic acute appendicitis. Hypoxemia, dehydration, infection, and temperature variation have been identified as triggers for VOE. Many times no trigger is identified. The pain is notable for sudden onset and can last for up to a week. Patients with recurrent acute VOE can also develop chronic pain. Other potential sites of ischemic injury include the gastrointestinal tract, spleen, brain (see separate stroke section), eyes, and kidneys. Chronic renal ischemia leads to isosthenuria in children and later nephropathy and proteinuria in adults. Renal papillary necrosis can also occur, and patients present with gross hematuria.

Acute Chest Syndrome

Acute chest syndrome (ACS) is a common complication in SCD with peak incidence in children of 2 to 4 years of age. The most common

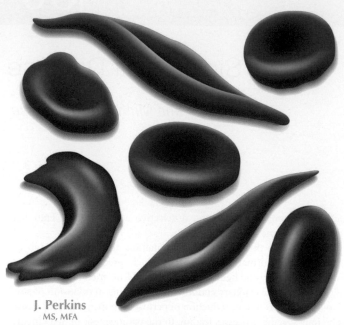

J. Perkins
MS, MFA

Fig. 80.1 Sickled Red Blood Cells.

symptoms at the time of presentation are fever, chest pain, and cough. Children with asthma and SCD have twice as many episodes of ACS than those without.

Bacterial Sepsis

Functional asplenia, decreased serum opsonic activity, and poor antibody response to the polysaccharide component of the bacterial capsule make children with SCD highly susceptible to serious bacterial infections. They are at highest risk for bacteremia resulting from encapsulated bacteria and have higher rates of osteomyelitis. In the United States, *Salmonella* and *Escherichia coli* are the most common pathogens for osteomyelitis. In sub-Saharan Africa and the Middle East, *Staphylococcus aureus* predominates.

Aplastic Crisis

RBC aplasia in the SCD population is due to parvovirus B19. Children with SCD will present with pallor, headache, and other symptoms consistent with profound anemia.

Splenic Sequestration

Splenic sequestration occurs at greatest frequency within the first 5 years of life. Patients have the onset of life-threatening anemia in the context of rapid spleen enlargement. Children who have an episode of splenic sequestration are at increased risk for recurrence.

Acute Stroke and Silent Cerebral Infarct

Children with SCD-SS are 200 to 300 times more likely to have a stroke compared with healthy children. Before screening interventions, approximately 10% of children with SCD experienced a stroke before the age of 20 years. The predominant cause is a large-vessel vasculopathy with proliferative intimal hyperplasia. Signs and symptoms are notable for focal neurologic deficits related to the site of injury that can include mild weakness to frank hemiparesis, visual and language disturbances, seizures, and/or altered mental status.

Silent cerebral infarct (SCI) is more common than overt stroke, found in up to 30% of patients with severe forms of SCD. It is thought to be secondary to small vessel disease and is not associated with overt stroke symptoms but is associated with long-term neurologic and cognitive decline. Patients with SCI are at higher risk for overt stroke than patients without SCI.

Priapism

Priapism is a sustained, painful penile erection. It is caused by vaso-occlusive obstruction of venous drainage from the penis. Recurrent episodes can lead to penile fibrosis and often impotence.

Additional Complications

Aside from the acute complications of SCD described earlier, patients with SCD may also develop cardiomyopathy, pulmonary hypertension, cholelithiasis, retinopathy, nephropathy, leg ulcers, and avascular necrosis.

EVALUATION AND MANAGEMENT

Diagnosis

In the United States, SCD testing is a part of the newborn screen. Patients with an abnormal newborn screen concerning for SCD should have confirmatory testing with Hgb identification. On newborn screen, all patients with SS, Sβ^0 thalassemia, and SC have no Hgb A present. Patients with Sβ^+ thalassemia will have some Hgb A, but the predominant Hgb is Hgb S. In patients with sickle cell trait, the newborn screening will reveal FAS, in which the predominant Hgbs are F and A (Table 80.1).

Acute Complications
Vaso-occlusive Episodes

At initial presentation, it is important to determine that VOE is the source of pain based on clinical history, physical examination, and laboratory and radiographic studies. Pain should be distinguished from other causes of discomfort (Table 80.2). Assessment of pain should include age-appropriate and developmentally appropriate tools. Uncomplicated VOE can be managed at home. Nonpharmacologic measures to help manage pain symptoms can be extremely helpful and include heat, massage, and distraction techniques (i.e., play activities). Pharmacologic management of VOE includes a combination of nonsteroidal antiinflammatory drugs (NSAIDs) such as ibuprofen or ketorolac and oral or intravenous analgesics (acetaminophen, oxycodone, morphine, hydromorphone).

Acute Chest Syndrome

ACS is a common complication in SCD and is defined by respiratory symptoms (i.e., cough, chest pain), fever, and evidence of a pulmonary infiltrate on chest radiography. Radiographic findings may lag behind initial symptoms. The pathophysiology of ACS in SCD is multifactorial and includes infection (bacterial or viral), in situ vaso-occlusion, pulmonary edema, fat embolism from bone infarction or thromboembolism. ACS commonly develops during a hospitalization for VOE, and use of incentive spirometry (10 times every 2 hours while awake), ambulation, and avoidance of overhydration can help prevent ACS. *Mycoplasma pneumoniae* and *Chlamydia pneumoniae*, as well as *Streptococcus pneumoniae*, are common bacterial causes of ACS, as are respiratory viruses. Antibiotic treatment should cover these bacterial causes and can include azithromycin and a cephalosporin/ampicillin, or levofloxacin monotherapy. Patients may develop an oxygen requirement, and close monitoring is essential to prevent significant morbidity, including respiratory failure necessitating intubation. Patients with hypoxemia and a falling Hgb can benefit from a simple blood transfusion. Exchange transfusion is indicated in the setting of respiratory failure.

TABLE 80.1 Sickle Hemoglobinopathies

Genotype	Newborn Screen Result	Hemoglobin Range (After 6 Months of Age)	MCV (After 6 Months of Age)	Reticulocyte Range
SS	FS	6–11 g/dL	Normocytic	2%–25%
SC	FSC	9–12 g/dL	Normocytic	1%–13%
Sβ⁺	FSA or FS[a]	9–12 g/dL	Microcytic	1%–7%
Sβ⁰	FS	6–10 g/dL	Microcytic	2%–25%

F, Hemoglobin F; S, hemoglobin S; C, hemoglobin C; A, hemoglobin A; MCV, mean corpuscular volume.
[a]The quantity of hemoglobin A at birth can be insufficient for detection.

TABLE 80.2 Location Based Differential Diagnosis for Pain in Sickle Cell Disease

Location of Pain	Differential	Studies to Consider
Head/Face	Hemorrhagic stroke Sinusitis Migraine Meningitis	MRI or MRA CT Lumbar puncture
Neck/Throat	Meningitis Torticollis Pharyngitis Tonsillitis	Lumbar puncture Throat culture
Chest	Acute chest syndrome Asthma exacerbation Costochondritis Cardiac pain Gastroesophageal reflux	Chest x-ray ECG ± echocardiogram
Abdomen	Appendicitis Cholelithiasis or chole- cystitis Pancreatitis Splenic sequestration Urinary tract infection Pyelonephritis	Abdominal ultrasound (appendix, RUQ, epi- gastric) Amylase and lipase Urinalysis and culture Renal bladder ultrasound
Limb/Joint	Osteomyelitis Septic joint Avascular necrosis	X-ray of the limb/joint Ultrasound ± joint fluid analysis MRI or MRA

Bacterial Sepsis

Febrile illness (>101.3°F [>38.5°C]) is an emergency in SCD, because it could be the first sign of life-threatening bacteremia and requires prompt medical evaluation and antibiotic administration. The evaluation should include a complete blood count (CBC), reticulocyte count, blood culture, physical examination, and pulse oximetry. Intravenous antibiotics should be given promptly and should have adequate coverage against S. pneumoniae and Haemophilus influenzae; ceftriaxone and ampicillin are frequently used. A chest radiograph should be considered in those with overlapping chest pain, cough, or hypoxia.

Transient Red Blood Cell Aplasia: Parvovirus B19

Infection with parvovirus causes reticulocytopenia for approximately 7 to 10 days. Because patients with severe forms of SCD have a decreased RBC lifespan of approximately 20 days (normal RBC lifespan is ~120 days), they develop significant anemia during the period of reticulocytopenia. Blood transfusion is indicated in patients with symptomatic anemia.

Splenic Sequestration

Splenic sequestration is defined by the sudden enlargement of the spleen and a drop in Hgb. Parental education helps establish early diagnosis, and prompt medical treatment decreases morbidity and mortality. Parents should be instructed on how to monitor for sequestration by spleen size palpation. Patients should be admitted and have an intravenous line and an active type and screen. The spleen size should be documented and monitored closely with serial examinations. The CBC and physical examination should be repeated at frequent intervals to assess the degree of sequestration and the potential need for RBC transfusion. Transfusion is indicated for severe anemia. Children who experience splenic sequestration are at risk for recurrent events. In children with recurrent events necessitating transfusion, splenectomy should be considered.

Acute Stroke

If a patient presents with concern for an acute ischemic event, they need prompt evaluation and treatment. After initial stabilization, patients should undergo noncontrast computed tomography of the brain to rule out hemorrhage or other nonischemic causes of symptoms followed by magnetic resonance imaging and magnetic resonance angiography. The treatment for patients with an acute stroke is erythrocytapheresis to rapidly decrease the percent of Hgb S to less than 30%. The Hgb should be kept below 11, because hyperviscosity is also a risk factor for stroke. After a stroke, patients are often maintained on chronic transfusion therapy to keep the Hgb S below 30% to prevent recurrence.

Priapism

Treatment should include hydration and pain control in consultation with urology. Prolonged episodes may require penile aspiration. Additional medications have also been used, including α-agonists (pseudoephedrine) and β-agonists (terbutaline). Chronic management can involve prophylaxis with either pseudoephedrine or sildenafil or arteriovenous (AV) fistula placement.

Routine Health Maintenance
Immunizations

Children with SCD should receive all routine childhood immunizations. In addition, patients should receive the 23-valent pneumococcal vaccine (Pneumovax) at ages 2 and 5. They should receive both doses of the meningococcal (MenACWY) vaccine before 2 years of age, and their meningococcal B (MenB) vaccine starting at 10 years of age (as compared with age 16 for children without SCD). They should also receive the influenza vaccine annually.

Stroke Screening

Cerebral blood flow velocity estimates from transcranial Doppler (TCD) ultrasonography of the distal internal carotid vessels correlates with stroke risk in patients with severe forms of SCD. Children with SCD type SS and Sβ^0 should start TCD surveillance at age 2 and obtain TCD annually until age 16 years. If the TCD velocity is abnormal, greater than 200 cm/sec, chronic transfusions should be started to reduce stroke risk.

Penicillin Prophylaxis

Penicillin prophylaxis for SCD was widely introduced after the Prophylactic Penicillin Study (PROPS) in Sickle Cell Disease found a significantly reduced incidence of pneumococcal infections in individuals younger than 5 years of age in those receiving prophylaxis. Prophylaxis should be started no later than 2 months of age with oral penicillin (125 mg twice daily for age younger than 3 years and 250 mg twice daily for age older than 3 years). Current National Institutes of Health (NIH) guidelines recommend discontinuation of penicillin prophylaxis after the age of 5 years if vaccinations are up to date, unless the patient has a history of bacteremia or splenectomy.

Folic Acid

Daily folic acid supplementation (1 mg/day) can be considered for patients with SCD. There is no high-quality evidence of benefit, but there remains a theoretical risk for folate deficiency given high RBC turnover.

Nutrition and Growth

Children with SCD may have deficiencies in fat-soluble vitamins or zinc. Additionally, patients can have a delay in growth likely related to increased caloric requirements caused by chronic anemia. Families should be encouraged to adopt healthy eating habits, and patients should be monitored closely for growth and development. Nutritional supplements should be initiated if there are concerns about growth delay. Patients can also take a daily multivitamin without iron.

Eye Examinations

All SCD patients should have ophthalmologic screening for SCD-associated retinopathy with a fundoscopic examination starting at 10 years of age. Individuals with a normal dilated retinal examination can be rescreened at 1- to 2-year intervals.

Chronic Issues

Transfusion, Iron Overload, and Iron Chelation Therapy

Chronic RBC transfusion is used in SCD to prevent disease-related complications, including stroke, ACS, and VOE. Prevention of neurologic complications is the most common reason for initiating a transfusion program. Transfusions help by decreasing the overall Hgb S percentage. However, there are risks associated with chronic transfusion, including alloimmunization (patients develop RBC antibodies) and iron overload. It is necessary to chelate excess iron in patients with transfusional iron overload; humans are unable to excrete excess iron. Chelators currently in use in the United States include deferoxamine (Desferal), which is typically given as a 12-hour subcutaneous infusion, or oral chelators, including deferasirox (Exjade or Jadenu) and deferiprone (Ferriprox).

In SCD, excess iron deposits primarily in the liver and can lead to significant organ dysfunction. This can be measured with MRI. Serum ferritin levels are also used to monitor iron overload, although ferritin measurements can be unreliable in patients with SCD because of their chronic inflammatory state.

Erythrocytapheresis (RBC exchange by removing a patient's RBCs and replacing with normal RBCs) is an alternative to simple transfusion and causes less iron loading because very little excess net blood is given. However, erythrocytapheresis does require more blood per procedure compared with simple transfusion, thus exposing patients to more donor units and theoretically increasing their risk for alloimmunization.

Hydroxyurea

Hydroxyurea is a therapeutic that increases fetal Hgb levels, thereby increasing oxygen-carrying capacity and decreasing RBC sickling with resultant decrease in morbidities related to chronic hemolysis. Hydroxyurea decreases the frequency of VOE and the need for transfusion. It is the current mainstay of treatment for sickle cell disease. Given potential for myelosuppression, patients on hydroxyurea are monitored closely. Current NIH recommendations are for patients with severe genotypes to start hydroxyurea at 9 to 12 months of age to prevent SCD complications.

Bone Marrow Transplant

Bone marrow transplantation (BMT) is the only curative therapy and can be considered for patients with severe SCD genotypes. The best outcomes are seen with matched sibling donors followed by a matched unrelated donor. Mismatched donors (unrelated and haploidentical) are controversial because of graft-versus-host disease and infection risks. Some centers offer reduced-intensity conditioning to decrease the morbidity of conditioning, but this increases the risk for graft failure. The decision to recommend BMT must be made carefully with input from the primary hematologist, transplant team, and family.

Avascular Necrosis

Avascular necrosis (AVN), also known as osteonecrosis, is a painful destruction of bone related to sickle vasculopathy, and most commonly affects the femoral and humeral heads. In pediatric patients, initial treatment is conservative and includes analgesics, NSAIDs, and physical therapy for weight-bearing recommendations. There is no preventive treatment. Joint-preserving surgical procedures can be used, including core decompression and osteotomy, or joint replacement (once growth has halted).

FUTURE DIRECTIONS

Gene therapy to supply non-sickle β-globin is currently under study. Use of a lentiviral vector to deliver the β-globin gene to a patient's own bone marrow cells ex vivo is currently under study in SCD. Gene-modified cells are returned to the patient after myeloablative conditioning, a form of autologous stem cell transplant. This therapy is approved by the European Medicines Agency for transfusion-dependent thalassemia (non-$\beta^0\beta^0$) but is still under investigation in SCD. An alternative approach is also currently under study in patients with SCDs, which uses gene editing to increase gamma globin levels. These methods also require return of gene-modified autologous cells after conditioning.

There are additional disease-modifying medications recently approved for SCD. Crizanlizumab is a monoclonal antibody to P-selectin that prevents RBC binding to endothelial cells. It reduces the frequency of VOE. Voxelotor is an oral small molecule that increases the oxygen affinity of Hgb, which prevents sickling of Hgb S. This has been shown to increase Hgb levels by reducing hemolysis and is being studied for the prevention of stroke.

SUGGESTED READINGS

Available online.

81

Disorders of Thrombosis and Hemostasis

Julianne McGlynn and Chelsea Kotch

 CLINICAL VIGNETTE

A 16-year-old girl presents for evaluation of abnormal uterine bleeding (AUB). Menses began 3 years ago, occurs every 28 days for 8 days duration. She saturates a feminine hygiene product every 1 to 2 hours. She reports she sometimes has palpable bruising. She has no significant medical history and takes no medication. Her prior surgical history is pertinent for wisdom tooth extraction, complicated by postprocedure bleeding. Her mother and older sister have heavy menses.

Physical examination is notable for scattered palpable bruising on the extremities and no hyperextensible joints. Her laboratory evaluation is diagnostic of type 1 von Willebrand disease (vWD). The prevalence of bleeding disorders in women with AUB is as high as 20%. In addition, AUB is a common manifesting symptom in women with vWD.

Hemostasis is the normal physiologic response to prevent and stop bleeding at sites of vascular injury. The process of thrombus formation and lysis is carefully balanced. Procoagulant factors and platelets interact to generate a clot to protect the vessel's integrity at sites of endothelial damage. Dynamic feedback loops prevent a hypercoagulable state by the activation of anticoagulant proteins, eventually leading to fibrinolysis. Decreased levels or function of procoagulant factors and platelets result in disordered bleeding, and anticoagulant protein dysfunction or deficiency promotes thrombosis.

EPIDEMIOLOGY

Bleeding Disorders

Pediatric bleeding disorders can be congenital or acquired, with age of presentation varying by disease severity and exposure to hemostatic challenges. The most common congenital bleeding disorders are von Willebrand disease (vWD), hemophilia A (factor VIII deficiency), hemophilia B (factor IX deficiency), and platelet disorders. Of these, the most common is type 1 vWD with an estimated prevalence of 1%. Hemophilia A affects 1 in 5000 male births and is six times more prevalent than hemophilia B. Both hemophilias are X-linked recessive and occur almost exclusively in males. However, females may present with hemophilia in the setting of Turner syndrome or unequal lyonization of the unaffected X chromosome. Up to 20% of female carriers will have a low factor level. Thirty percent of the time there is no family history of hemophilia secondary to spontaneous mutations or an unknown family history.

Thrombosis

Venous thromboembolism (VTE) is rare in children compared with adults, occurring in approximately 1 in 100,000 pediatric patients. The incidence is higher in hospitalized children, with up to 58 VTE events reported per 10,000 hospitalizations. This increase is due to several factors, including heightened awareness of pediatric VTE and growing use of central venous catheters (CVCs). There is a bimodal age distribution of pediatric VTE, peaking in neonates and adolescents. VTEs in neonates are most commonly associated with CVCs, whereas adolescent risk factors for VTE are similar to those in adults. VTE is associated with significant morbidity and mortality, including loss of venous access, pulmonary embolism, and postthrombotic syndrome.

ETIOLOGY AND PATHOGENESIS

Congenital Bleeding Disorders

vWD is characterized by impaired quality or quantity of von Willebrand factor (vWF), a plasma glycoprotein that promotes platelet adhesion and aggregation at sites of endothelial damage. Additionally, vWF stabilizes circulating factor VIII, prolonging its half-life. There are three main types of inherited vWD (Table 81.1). Type 2 variants are qualitative defects, whereas types 1 and 3 are quantitative defects. Type 1 vWD is the most common subtype, representing approximately 80% of vWD.

Hemophilia A and B are deficiencies of clotting factors VIII and IX, respectively. The absence of either factor significantly impairs the generation of thrombin, leading to delayed and impaired clotting (Fig. 81.1). Disease severity is stratified by baseline factor level concentration, which is determined by the genetic mutation and is stable over time. Hemostasis is achieved with a factor level of approximately 40% to 50%. Mild hemophilia corresponds to factor levels of 5% to 40%, moderate 1% to 5%, and severe less than 1%.

Congenital platelet disorders may affect platelet quantity, quality, or both. See Chapter 79 for further details.

Acquired Bleeding Disorders

Acquired bleeding disorders can occur in the setting of abnormalities of the liver, kidneys, or gastrointestinal (GI) tract, drug effect, or disseminated intravascular coagulation (DIC). Clotting factor production may be impaired in liver disease because of decreased synthesis. Uremia with chronic kidney disease leads to platelet dysfunction. Fat malabsorption syndromes and prolonged antibiotic use impair vitamin K absorption from the GI tract, which can lead to vitamin K deficiency. The vitamin K–dependent proteins include procoagulant factors II, VII, IX, X, and anticoagulant factors protein C and protein S. An important example of vitamin K–dependent bleeding is hemorrhagic disease of the newborn, which commonly includes intracranial and GI bleeding and can be life-threatening.

DIC most frequently occurs in the settings of sepsis, trauma, or malignancy. Coagulation mechanisms are overactivated in response to endothelial inflammation/damage, leading to extensive fibrin deposition, clot formation, and end-organ complications. This process leads to a consumptive coagulopathy with decreasing platelets and clotting factors resulting in paradoxical bleeding (Fig. 81.2).

TABLE 81.1   Classification of von Willebrand Disease

Type	Description	VW Antigen	VW Activity	Factor VIII Activity	Multimers	Inheritance
1	Partial quantitative deficiency	↓	↓	Nl to ↓	Normal	AD
2A	Decreased high-molecular-weight multimers resulting in impaired vWF platelet binding	↓	↓↓	Nl to ↓	Abnormal	AD
2B	Increased platelet and vWF binding	Nl to ↓	↓↓	Nl to ↓	Abnormal	AD
2M	Decreased vWF and platelet binding	↓	↓↓	Nl to ↓	Normal	AD or AR
2N	Impaired vWF binding to factor VIII	Nl to ↓	Nl to ↓	↓↓	Normal	AR
3	Complete quantitative deficiency	↓↓↓	↓↓↓	↓↓↓	Absent	AR

↓, Slightly decreased; ↓↓, moderately decreased; ↓↓↓, severely decreased; *AD,* autosomal dominant; *AR,* autosomal recessive; *Nl,* normal; *vWF,* von Willebrand factor.

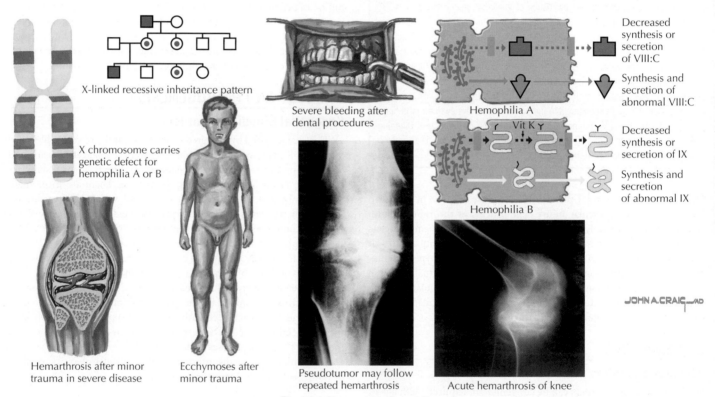

X-linked recessive inheritance pattern

X chromosome carries genetic defect for hemophilia A or B

Severe bleeding after dental procedures

Hemophilia A

Decreased synthesis or secretion of VIII:C

Synthesis and secretion of abnormal VIII:C

Vit K

Hemophilia B

Decreased synthesis or secretion of IX

Synthesis and secretion of abnormal IX

Hemarthrosis after minor trauma in severe disease

Ecchymoses after minor trauma

Pseudotumor may follow repeated hemarthrosis

Acute hemarthrosis of knee

JOHN A.CRAIG—AD

Fig. 81.1 Hemophilia A and B.

Thrombosis

The majority of VTE in children are provoked, with over 90% of children having at least one identifiable inherited or acquired prothrombotic risk factor. Inherited thrombophilias include factor V Leiden, prothrombin gene mutation, and anticoagulant protein deficiency (protein C, protein S, or antithrombin). Anatomic causes, such as May-Thurner syndrome or venous thoracic outlet syndrome, are less common (Fig. 81.3). Common acquired VTE risk factors include the presence of a CVC, immobility, inflammation, infection, estrogen-containing oral contraceptives, malignancy, and obesity. A CVC is the most common pediatric VTE risk factor accounting for up to 80% of all hospital-acquired VTE.

CLINICAL PRESENTATION

Congenital Bleeding Disorders

The clinical presentation of bleeding disorders varies by age and diagnosis. Excessive bleeding following circumcision, phlebotomy, or unexplained intracranial hemorrhage should prompt evaluation in a newborn. For infants with undiagnosed hemophilia, the first presenting symptoms may be raised bruising with onset of crawling or ambulation. In school-aged children, recurrent and prolonged epistaxis may indicate abnormal hemostasis. Adolescent females may present with abnormal uterine bleeding (AUB). Symptoms of AUB include saturating a feminine hygiene product every 1 to 2 hours, lasting longer than 7 days, passage of clots greater than 1 inch in size, and developing iron deficiency.

Platelet disorders and vWD manifest as mucocutaneous bleeding, including epistaxis, gingival bleeding, and AUB. The presentation of hemophilia A or B depends on the baseline factor activity. Bleeding may occur only after trauma or surgery (mild and moderate hemophilia) or spontaneously (severe hemophilia). Severe hemophilia A and B often manifest with extensive palpable bruising and/or bleeding into muscles and joints. Potentially fatal bleeds include intracranial hemorrhage, GI bleeding, or bleeding into the retropharyngeal space.

In children with an atypical bruising distribution, it is imperative to consider nonaccidental trauma. A bleeding disorder diagnosis does

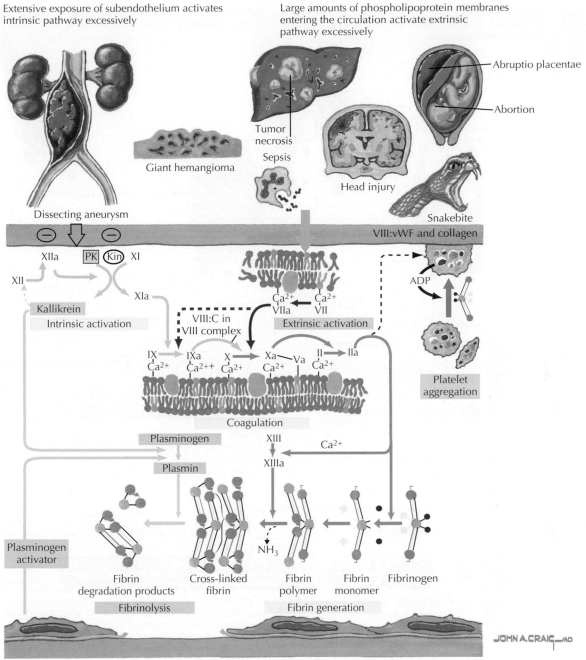

Extensive exposure of subendothelium activates intrinsic pathway excessively

Large amounts of phospholipoprotein membranes entering the circulation activate extrinsic pathway excessively

Abruptio placentae

Abortion

Tumor necrosis

Sepsis

Head injury

Giant hemangioma

Dissecting aneurysm

Snakebite

VIII:vWF and collagen

XIIa PK Kin XI

XII

Kallikrein

Intrinsic activation

XIa

VIII:C in VIII complex

Ca^{2+} VIIa Ca^{2+} VII

ADP

Extrinsic activation

IX Ca^{2+} IXa Ca^{2++} X Ca^{2+} Xa Ca^{2+} —Va II Ca^{2+} —IIa

Platelet aggregation

Coagulation

Plasminogen

Plasmin

XIII

XIIIa

Ca^{2+}

Plasminogen activator

NH_3

Fibrin degradation products

Cross-linked fibrin

Fibrin polymer

Fibrin monomer

Fibrinogen

Fibrinolysis

Fibrin generation

JOHN A. CRAIG—AD

Physiology and molecular events leading to DIC

Fig. 81.2 Disseminated Intravascular Coagulation.

not exclude concurrent nonaccidental trauma. Alternatively, bleeding symptoms also could be secondary to vasculitis, a connective tissue disorder (Ehlers-Danlos syndrome or scurvy), or abnormal blood vessels (hereditary hemorrhagic telangiectasia).

Thrombosis

Symptoms of VTE vary with the location and extent of thrombus. Deep venous thrombosis (DVT) in an extremity can manifest with unilateral edema, erythema, and warmth. Cerebral sinus thrombosis can have nonspecific neurologic symptoms and may manifest with headache, emesis, altered mental status, focal neurologic deficit, or seizure. Classic presenting symptoms of pulmonary embolism include tachycardia, tachypnea, hypoxia, and pleuritic chest pain. With CVC-associated VTE, the thrombus is typically located at the catheter site.

EVALUATION AND MANAGEMENT

Congenital Bleeding Disorder

A detailed history and physical examination comprise the initial evaluation of disordered bleeding. A detailed birth, family, and surgical history in addition to review of presenting symptoms is essential. Physical examination should include evaluation of the nasopharynx, trunk, buttocks, and extremities for abnormal bruising or vasculature. Initial laboratory evaluation should include a complete blood count (CBC), prothrombin time (PT), and partial thromboplastin time (PTT). Testing may also include fibrinogen to evaluate for afibrinogenemia or hypofibrinogenemia (Fig. 81.4).

For hemophilia A and B, laboratory evaluation demonstrates an isolated prolonged PTT and decreased factor VIII or IX levels, respectively.

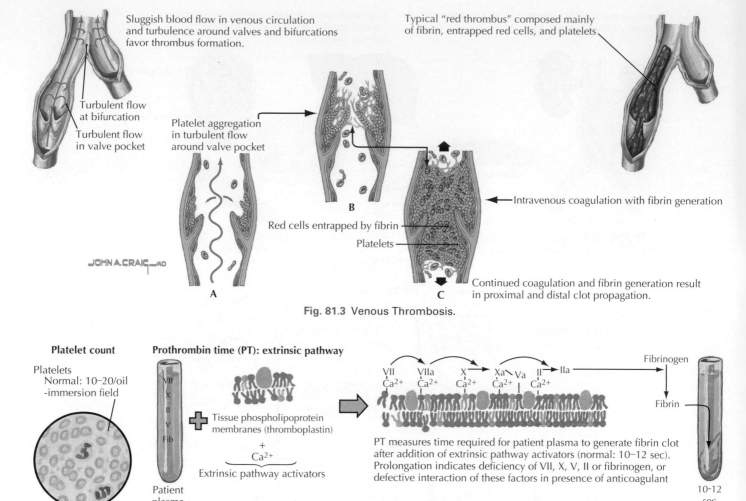

Sluggish blood flow in venous circulation and turbulence around valves and bifurcations favor thrombus formation.

Turbulent flow at bifurcation

Turbulent flow in valve pocket

Platelet aggregation in turbulent flow around valve pocket

Typical "red thrombus" composed mainly of fibrin, entrapped red cells, and platelets

Intravenous coagulation with fibrin generation

Red cells entrapped by fibrin

Platelets

Continued coagulation and fibrin generation result in proximal and distal clot propagation.

JOHN A.CRAIG—AD

A   B   C

Fig. 81.3 Venous Thrombosis.

Platelet count

Platelets
Normal: 10–20/oil-immersion field

Normal platelet count: 150,000–350,000/μL

Prothrombin time (PT): extrinsic pathway

VII
X
II
V
Fib

Patient plasma

Tissue phospholipoprotein membranes (thromboplastin)
+
Ca²⁺
Extrinsic pathway activators

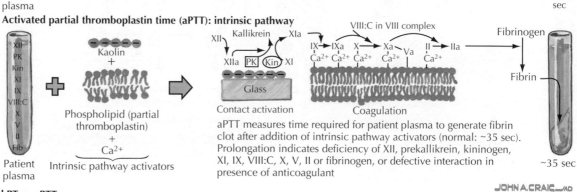

VII   VIIa   X   Xa   Va   II   IIa
Ca²⁺   Ca²⁺   Ca²⁺   Ca²⁺ Ca²⁺ Ca²⁺

Fibrinogen

Fibrin

PT measures time required for patient plasma to generate fibrin clot after addition of extrinsic pathway activators (normal: 10–12 sec). Prolongation indicates deficiency of VII, X, V, II or fibrinogen, or defective interaction of these factors in presence of anticoagulant

10-12 sec

Activated partial thromboplastin time (aPTT): intrinsic pathway

XII
PK
Kin
XI
IX
VIII:C
X
V
Fib

Patient plasma

Kaolin
+

Phospholipid (partial thromboplastin)
+
Ca²⁺
Intrinsic pathway activators

XII   Kallikrein   XIa
XIIa   PK   Kin   XI
Glass
Contact activation

VIII:C in VIII complex

IX   IXa   X   Xa   Va   II   IIa
Ca²⁺   Ca²⁺ Ca²⁺   Ca²⁺ Ca²⁺ Ca²⁺

Coagulation

Fibrinogen

Fibrin

aPTT measures time required for patient plasma to generate fibrin clot after addition of intrinsic pathway activators (normal: ~35 sec). Prolongation indicates deficiency of XII, prekallikrein, kininogen, XI, IX, VIII:C, X, V, II or fibrinogen, or defective interaction in presence of anticoagulant

~35 sec

JOHN A.CRAIG—AD

Mixing studies: prolonged PT or aPTT

Mixing factor-deficient patient plasma with normal plasma in 1:1 ratio corrects prolonged patient PT or aPTT

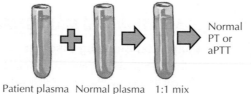

Patient plasma   Normal plasma   1:1 mix

Normal PT or aPTT

Mixing patient plasma containing anticoagulant with normal plasma in 1:1 ratio prolongs PT or aPTT of normal plasma

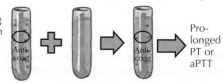

Patient plasma   Normal plasma   1:1 mix

Prolonged PT or aPTT

Fig. 81.4 Hemostasis Tests.

Coagulation studies are often normal in vWD; however, severe vWD may manifest with prolonged PTT because of decreased plasma factor VIII levels. The diagnosis of vWD is based on low levels of vWF antigen, vWF activity, and factor VIII. vWF multimers differentiate among subtypes. When testing for vWD it is important to be aware that multiple factors, such as significant distress from phlebotomy,

exogenous high-dose estrogen, inflammation, or pregnancy, can elevate vWF levels and not be reflective of the patient's baseline state.

Platelet disorders are diagnosed in the setting of thrombocytopenia, abnormal platelet function testing, or morphologic abnormality on peripheral blood smear. Medications, such as nonsteroidal antiinflammatory drugs, may affect platelet function testing results. Bleeding time is no longer recommended, given high interobserver variability and poor specificity.

Treatment of vWD is limited to prophylaxis for hemostatic challenges, such as surgical or dental procedures, and management of active bleeding. Desmopressin (DDAVP) is administered intranasally or intravenously and stimulates the release of endothelial stores of vWF and factor VIII, thus increasing VWF levels. The vWD subtypes respond heterogeneously to DDAVP administration; thus a DDAVP trial is recommended to determine efficacy before use. DDAVP is not recommended for types 2B or 3 vWD. As a vasopressin analog, DDAVP can lead to hyponatremia and water restriction is advised for 24 hours after administration. Tachyphylaxis occurs after three sequential DDAVP doses. When DDAVP is ineffective or prolonged treatment is needed, replacement therapy of plasma-derived vWF and factor VIII concentrate is used. Antifibrinolytic therapy may also be considered for mucocutaneous bleeding and AUB. Furthermore, hormonal therapy or intrauterine devices can be effective for AUB.

Hemophilia management is determined by severity. Until recently, the main treatment for hemophilia was limited to factor replacement that is either plasma derived or recombinant. Factor can be given on an as-needed basis to prevent or treat bleeding or on a routine basis to prevent bleeding (prophylaxis). For severe hemophilia, prophylactic factor replacement, started at a young age, is standard of care to prevent spontaneous bleeding and the associated morbidity and mortality. For hemophilia A, emicizumab was recently granted FDA approval for prophylaxis in patients with and without inhibitors.

Exogenous factor replacement may be complicated by the development of neutralizing inhibitors directed against the infused factor that render factor concentrate ineffective. The treatment of inhibitor development includes immune tolerance and emicizumab, which can concurrently be used to prevent bleeding.

Gene therapy for hemophilia A and B is currently under investigation, and results are encouraging. Longer term data regarding safety and duration of factor production are needed.

Acquired Bleeding Disorders

Acquired bleeding disorders secondary to vitamin K deficiency or liver disease manifest with a prolonged PT and, if severe, prolonged PTT. Factor V levels can distinguish between vitamin K deficiency and liver disease because it is synthesized by the liver but is not vitamin K dependent. Vitamin K deficiency is treated with oral or subcutaneous vitamin K. For acute bleeding, fresh frozen plasma is given to immediately replace clotting factors.

The clinical manifestation of DIC varies based on severity and underlying cause, but may be with petechiae, purpura, bleeding, thrombosis, and end-organ damage. There is no diagnostic test for DIC. Laboratory evaluation often demonstrates prolonged PT and PTT, thrombocytopenia, elevated D dimer, and low fibrinogen. Treatment includes supportive care such as product transfusions in the setting of bleeding and management of the underlying cause.

Thrombosis

For suspected VTE, initial diagnostic steps include physical examination and imaging. Although contrast venography is the traditional gold standard, it has lower utility in pediatrics given the invasiveness and potential need for sedation. Lower extremity, upper extremity, and jugular DVTs may be visualized with Doppler ultrasonography. To evaluate more proximal, internal, or intracranial thromboses, computed tomography (CT) or magnetic resonance venography is necessary. The gold standard to evaluate pulmonary embolism (PE) is CT angiography.

Laboratory studies for workup DVT and PE workup include the D-dimer assay. D-dimer has high sensitivity but low specificity, because it also can be elevated with malignancy, inflammation, and liver disease. Unlike in adults, the D-dimer has not been validated in pediatrics to be used in isolation to rule out a DVT or PE. In some pediatric VTE cases, it is appropriate to evaluate a child for a predisposing thrombophilia, including factor V Leiden and prothrombin G20210 mutation analyses, protein C and S activity, antithrombin, homocysteine, lipoprotein(a) levels, dilute Russell Venom time, anticardiolipin, and anti–β2-glycoprotein antibodies. In the setting of a central line–associated thrombosis a thrombophilia evaluation is not indicated.

Treatment options for VTE include observation, anticoagulation, or thrombectomy. The decision to treat is made by considering the risk of therapy versus the risk of complications from the thrombus such as clot propagation and/or embolization. Treatment decisions should be made in conjunction with a pediatric hematologist. Anticoagulation is generally initiated for patients with symptomatic VTE unless there is a high bleeding risk (Fig. 81.5).

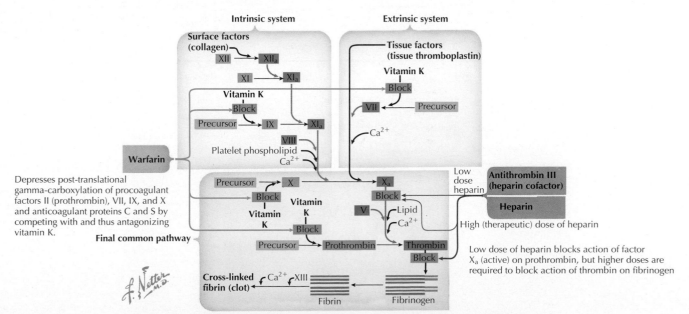

Fig. 81.5 Cascade of Clotting Factors and Sites of Action of Heparin and Warfarin.

In pediatrics, enoxaparin (a low-molecular-weight heparin [LMWH]) is the most commonly administered anticoagulant. Enoxaparin is generally preferred over unfractionated heparin (UFH) because of its subcutaneous administration, limited drug interactions, and ease of attaining therapeutic levels. Unfractionated heparin is favored for hospitalized patients with compromised kidney function or high bleeding risk because of its nonrenal clearance, short half-life, and reversibility.

Oral anticoagulant options in pediatrics are now expanding. Warfarin may be considered for maintenance therapy after establishing adequate anticoagulation with either UFH or LMWH. However, administration is often challenging because of age-related differences in vitamin K–dependent proteins, lack of liquid formulation, and frequent laboratory monitoring of therapeutic levels. The effects of warfarin may be reversed with vitamin K, prothrombin complex concentrate, or fresh frozen plasma. Direct oral anticoagulants (DOACs), such as direct thrombin inhibitors or direct factor Xa inhibitors, are now recommended over warfarin in adults for VTE treatment. DOAC benefits include fewer pharmacologic interactions, no dietary interactions, and no required laboratory monitoring. There is published pediatric phase 3 trial data for rivaroxaban demonstrating similar efficacy and a low bleeding risk as compared with standard anticoagulants. Targeted reversal agents for all DOACs have been developed, but the efficacy data are limited.

Anticoagulation duration depends on the clinical indication, including thrombus location and the presence of inherited or acquired thrombophilia. For provoked DVT, pediatric guidelines recommend a maximum of 12 weeks, although studies are examining shorter durations. The recommended duration of anticoagulation for unprovoked DVTs is 6 to 12 months. However, clinical factors such as inherited thrombophilia, life-threatening or recurrent unprovoked VTE may result in longer therapy.

Pharmacologic or mechanical thrombolysis should be considered in patients with life-, organ-, or limb-threatening thrombosis, such as an occlusive arterial clot with limb ischemia, cerebral sinovenous thrombosis with neurologic decompensation, bilateral renal vein thrombosis, or PE with hemodynamic instability. Thrombolysis carries a higher risk for bleeding than anticoagulation; thus risks and benefits must be weighed carefully.

FUTURE DIRECTIONS

The care of children with abnormal hemostasis continues to improve as knowledge gaps are addressed and new therapies emerge. Treatment options such as emicizumab have resulted in significant improvements in the quality of life of patients with severe hemophilia A. Gene therapy for hemophilia is still under investigation but has curative potential. Results from ongoing large-scale clinical trials evaluating oral anticoagulant use in pediatrics will provide guidance for use of these agents and will improve the care of these patients.

SUGGESTED READINGS

Available online.

Infectious Diseases

Julianne E. Burns

82

The Febrile Infant

Laura B. Goldstein and Allison M. Blatz

 CLINICAL VIGNETTE

An 8-day-old full-term male infant was brought to the emergency department for evaluation of fever to 102.9°F (39.4°C). His parents reported 1 day of increased sleepiness and poor oral intake. His presenting vital signs were notable for a temperature of 103.8°F (39.9°C) and pulse of 178 beats/min. On examination, he was sleepy with warm extremities and an open, flat fontanelle. No upper respiratory symptoms, rashes, or other infectious foci were noted.

He underwent an infectious evaluation with cultures obtained from blood, urine, and cerebrospinal fluid (CSF) and received empiric ampicillin, cefotaxime, and acyclovir. His blood culture grew group B streptococcus (GBS) at 16 hours of incubation, and urine culture, CSF culture, and herpes simplex virus (HSV) polymerase chain reaction (PCR) studies were negative. Cefotaxime and acyclovir were discontinued, and he completed a 10-day course of ampicillin for GBS bacteremia.

Fever, a common pediatric chief complaint, is most frequently suggestive of underlying infection. Whereas most pediatric infections are viral and self-limited, a minority, including urinary tract infection (UTI), bacteremia, and meningitis, are serious bacterial infections (SBIs).

Infants 3 months and younger, particularly neonates younger than 1 month, have the highest incidence of SBI among pediatric patients. It is particularly difficult to distinguish between viral infection and SBI in febrile infants because of nonspecific symptoms and a notoriously unreliable physical examination. However, early diagnosis and aggressive management of SBI are critical, because untreated neonatal sepsis carries a mortality rate of approximately 50%. Therefore, fever in a neonate is a medical emergency with a standardized approach to evaluation and management.

CAUSE, PATHOGENESIS, AND DIFFERENTIAL DIAGNOSIS

The differential diagnosis of neonatal fever can be broadly divided into viral versus bacterial infections. Although the literature estimates viral infections in more than 50% of febrile infants and SBI in 10% to 15% of febrile infants, precise distribution of infectious cause is difficult to determine. Reasons for this include inconsistent viral testing practices, inability of molecular viral testing to distinguish between prior asymptomatic disease and causative pathogens, and difficulty generalizing from older epidemiologic studies conducted before universal immunization with now-routine childhood vaccines (e.g., pneumococcal conjugate and *Haemophilus influenzae* type B vaccines), and/or before universal group B streptococcus (GBS) screening. These interventions have been associated with a decreased incidence of SBI over the past 3 decades. Neonates can acquire infection transplacentally, perinatally, and environmentally.

Serious Bacterial Infection Versus Viral Pathogens
Serious Bacterial Infection

Classification. SBI typically refers to UTI, bacteremia, and meningitis. UTIs account for almost three-quarters of all SBIs, with risk factors including lack of circumcision and underlying renal or urologic malformations. Bacteremia and meningitis account for a smaller proportion of SBIs but carry significant associated morbidity and mortality. Other bacterial infections not classically included in the definition of SBI but important to consider include pneumonia, bacterial enteritis, skin and soft tissue infections, osteomyelitis, omphalitis, and acute otitis media. Infants poorly compartmentalize infections, so pathogens may spread to other bodily compartments more easily than in an older child.

Bacterial pathogens. The most common pathogens implicated in neonatal SBIs are *Escherichia coli*, *Streptococcus agalactiae* (GBS), and *Listeria monocytogenes* (Fig. 82.1). *E. coli* causes a majority of neonatal UTIs and a significant proportion of cases of bacteremia and meningitis. GBS is commonly implicated particularly in bacteremia and meningitis (see later). *Listeria monocytogenes* remains an important cause of bacteremia and meningitis, though its overall prevalence is low. Infection classically occurs transplacentally after maternal exposure to contaminated dairy products or lunchmeat; premature and very young infants are at highest risk.

Additionally, infants 1 month or older also have a higher risk for SBI with typical childhood pathogens such as *Staphylococcus aureus*, *Streptococcus pneumoniae* (with prevalence decreasing because of the pneumococcal conjugate vaccine), *Neisseria meningitidis*, and *Haemophilus influenzae*. Other potential causes include *Salmonella* species, *Enterococcus* species, *Enterobacter cloacae*, *Moraxella catarrhalis*, and *Klebsiella* species.

Group B streptococcal infection. GBS infection is most often acquired perinatally. Infection with GBS is classified according to age of onset, with early-onset GBS occurring between birth and day 6 of life, late-onset GBS between 7 and 89 days of life, and very-late-onset GBS occurring at 90 days of life or older.

The primary risk factor for early-onset GBS is maternal genitourinary colonization, with prematurity, premature rupture of membranes, and chorioamnionitis all conferring additional risk. Universal maternal GBS screening and intrapartum antibiotic prophylaxis for colonized mothers have significantly decreased the incidence of early-onset GBS, though infection now skews toward preterm infants among whom morbidity and mortality are higher.

Early-onset GBS manifests most commonly as pneumonia, meningitis, or bacteremia. Late-onset GBS is thought to be acquired through exposure to colonized household contacts, and its incidence has been unaffected by maternal intrapartum antibiotic prophylaxis. It most frequently manifests as bacteremia or meningitis, though skin, soft-tissue, and bone infections also make up a significant proportion of

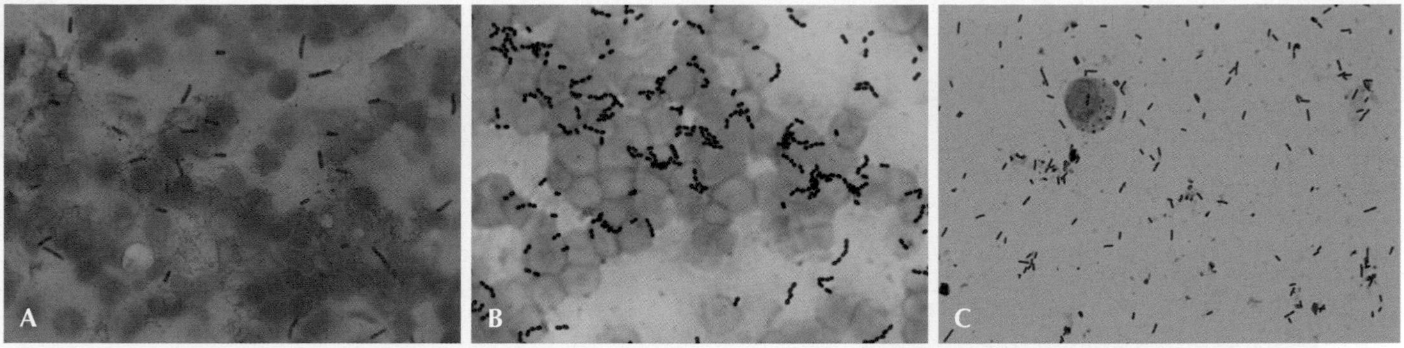

Fig. 82.1 Gram Stains of *Escherichia coli* (A), Group B Streptococcus (B), and *Listeria monocytogenes* (C). (Courtesy of Melissa Richard-Greenblatt, PhD.)

late-onset infections. Very-late-onset GBS typically occurs in extremely preterm or immunodeficient infants, and it most frequently manifests as bacteremia.

Viral pathogens. Viral infection is the most common cause of fever in young infants. Rhinovirus is the most frequently identified viral pathogen, and other common pathogens include respiratory syncytial virus, influenza, parainfluenza, adenovirus, enteroviruses, parechovirus, and herpes simplex virus (HSV). Some affected infants may be otherwise asymptomatic whereas others may exhibit upper respiratory symptoms or bronchiolitis.

Herpes simplex virus. Neonatal HSV infection carries particularly high morbidity and mortality. In most cases, HSV is transmitted perinatally by exposure to an infected maternal genitourinary tract. Risk for transmission is highest with primary HSV, prolonged rupture of membranes, use of fetal scalp monitoring, and vaginal (rather than cesarean) delivery; active maternal genital lesions are a contraindication to vaginal delivery, though most affected infants are born to mothers without known infection. Postnatal transmission may rarely occur by exposure to active HSV infection (e.g., cold sores or active HSV labialis infection).

HSV most frequently occurs during the first 6 weeks of life and can manifest as skin, eye, and/or mouth disease (SEM); infection of the central nervous system (CNS) with or without SEM; and disseminated disease. SEM is most common and can manifest with vesicular skin lesions, keratoconjunctivitis, and/or oral ulcerative lesions (Fig. 82.2). Outcomes are favorable early in the course of SEM, but if left untreated there is high risk for progression to CNS or disseminated disease. CNS disease, or HSV meningoencephalitis, occurs in one-third of cases, and disseminated HSV occurs in one-quarter of cases. Disseminated HSV is most common in the first 2 weeks of life and may manifest similarly to sepsis with multisystem organ dysfunction, particularly hepatitis.

CLINICAL PRESENTATION

The goal in evaluation of a febrile infant is to identify infants at high risk for SBI or HSV. Because history and physical examination in an infant with SBI may be nonspecific beyond the presence of fever, the approach to neonatal fever evaluation follows a standard algorithm.

Fever

Fever in an infant is defined as a temperature of 100.4°F (38°C) or greater. Neonates who are afebrile on presentation but have a reliable caregiver report of fever in the past 24 hours retain significant risk for SBI and should be fully evaluated. As poor temperature regulation in neonates may suggest sepsis, neonatal hypothermia

(temperature ≤96.8°F [≤36°C]) should elicit an identical management approach.

History

Although the history of present illness is frequently limited to fever, parents may report subtle behavioral changes suggestive of infection, including decreased feeding, irritability, lethargy, or increased/decreased sleeping. Associated signs and symptoms such as cough, congestion, rhinorrhea, respiratory distress, vomiting/diarrhea, eye or ear drainage, urinary frequency or foul-smelling urine, bloody stools, and rashes should be assessed. Seizure-like activity or abnormal movements are concerning for HSV meningoencephalitis or bacterial meningitis. Particular attention should be paid to the birth history, including gestational age, pregnancy and/or delivery complications, postnatal complications necessitating time in the neonatal intensive care unit, maternal GBS status, and maternal history of HSV. The social history should include exposures to ill contacts. Historical factors associated with SBI in febrile infants include young age (particularly younger than 28 days), history of high temperature (≥104°F [≥40°C]), lack of immunizations, prematurity, medical comorbidities, and recent antibiotic administration.

Physical Examination

A comprehensive physical examination is paramount, because findings may be subtle. Note any vital sign derangements suggestive of sepsis, including tachycardia, tachypnea, apnea, or hypotension. Irritability, inconsolability, decreased activity, or generalized ill-appearance should be noted, particularly as clinician assessment of ill-appearance has been associated with SBI in the literature. The fontanelle, a "pop-off valve" for increased intracranial pressure, should be assessed for bulging suggestive of meningitis (Fig. 82.3). Peripheral pulses and capillary refill should be assessed for evidence of circulatory compromise. A search for focal evidence of infection should be undertaken (including for rhinorrhea, congestion, adventitious lung sounds, conjunctival changes, signs of otitis media, rashes or foci of cellulitis/abscess, and abdominal distension or tenderness). A neurologic examination should include assessment of tone and strength of suck. Finally, in assessing for meningismus, note that nuchal rigidity and Kernig/Brudzinski signs are unlikely in this age group; instead, an infant with meningitis may exhibit paradoxical irritability (increased irritability when held, as body flexion stretches the meninges).

EVALUATION AND MANAGEMENT

Infectious Workup

The approach to evaluation can be stratified by age group, with separate guidance for neonates younger than 1 month versus older infants (between 1 and 2–3 months) detailed in the following section (Table 82.1).

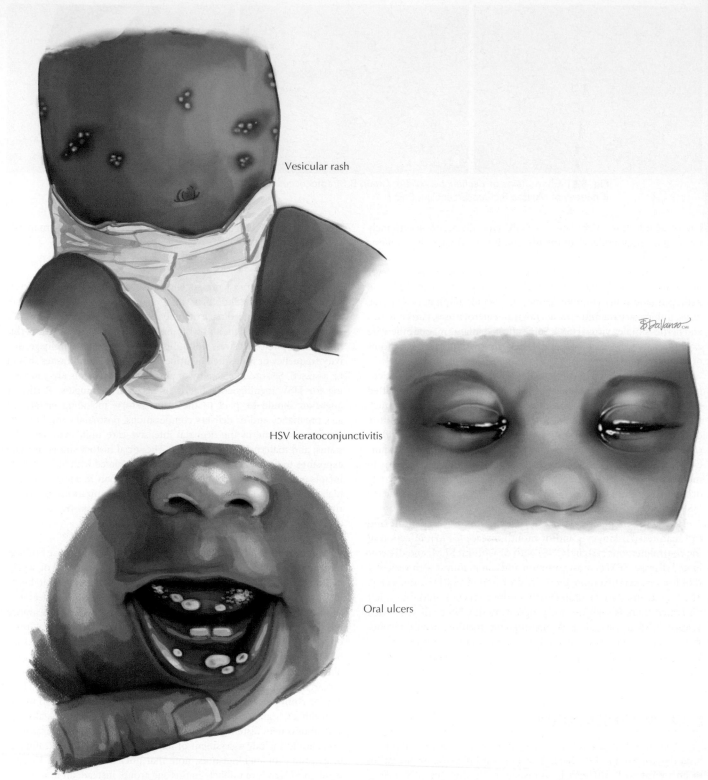

Vesicular rash

HSV keratoconjunctivitis

Oral ulcers

Fig. 82.2 Characteristic Findings in Neonatal Herpes Simplex Virus (HSV). (Vesicular Rash; HSV Keratoconjunctivitis; Oral Ulcers).

All febrile infants will require blood and urine evaluation, and neonates and/or those with particular risk factors for meningitis will require cerebrospinal fluid (CSF) evaluation. Ill-appearing infants with evidence of shock may require additional studies to assess for end-organ involvement, such as a comprehensive metabolic panel (CMP), coagulation studies, and serum lactate. Remaining workup should be dictated by any focal physical examination findings (e.g., chest radiograph for respiratory distress, stool studies for history of diarrhea).

Infants Younger Than 1 Month of Age

All neonates in this age group should undergo venipuncture for complete blood count (CBC) with differential and blood culture, bladder

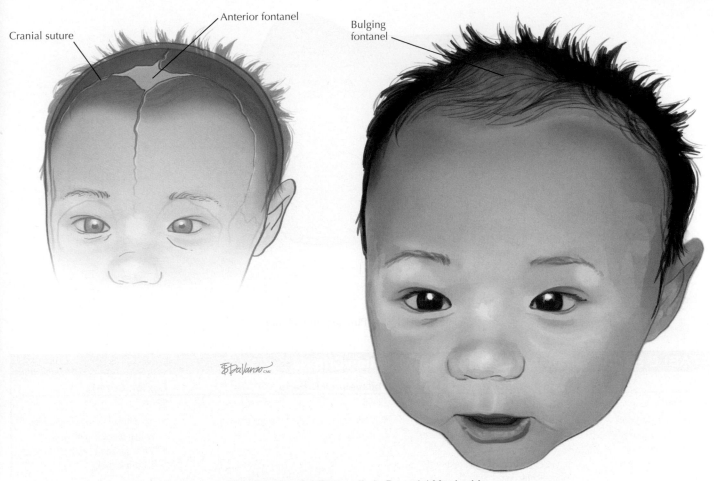

Fig. 82.3 Bulging Fontanelle in Bacterial Meningitis.

TABLE 82.1 Laboratory Evaluation of the Febrile Infant

Evaluation	Infant Characteristics	Laboratory Workup
SBI Evaluation	≤3 months	CBC with differential Blood culture Urinalysis Urine culture Inflammatory markers
Expanded SBI Evaluation	<1 month; 1–3 months with SBI risk factors or ill appearance	SBI evaluation, *plus* CSF Gram stain, culture, cell count, glucose, protein
HSV Evaluation	≤21 days or with HSV risk factors or ill appearance	HSV PCR from blood, CSF, any additional samples CMP Consider surface swabs + skin scrapings

CBC, Complete blood count; *CMP,* comprehensive metabolic panel; *CSF,* cerebrospinal fluid; *HSV,* herpes simplex virus; *SBI,* serious bacterial infection.

catheterization for urinalysis and urine culture, and lumbar puncture (Fig. 82.4) for CSF cell counts, glucose, protein, and culture (Table 82.1). HSV testing may be indicated and is discussed later; additional PCRs sent from the CSF may be considered based on seasonality and exposures. Other additional laboratory studies vary by institution and may include a CMP or inflammatory markers. Of note, neonates in this age group with confirmed viral infection or clinical bronchiolitis remain at high risk for concomitant SBI and require the same standardized approach to fever as those without a known virus.

Infants Ages 1 Month to 2–3 Months

Infants in this age group also require CBC with differential, blood culture, urinalysis, and urine culture. There is no universal consensus on indications for lumbar puncture, but multiple sets of criteria derived from large studies have sought to identify infants at low risk for SBI (Table 82.2). These commonly used guidelines consider comorbidities, clinical appearance, and initial blood and urine laboratory results, and they demonstrate similarly high negative predictive values (NPV) for SBI in febrile infants.

Herpes Simplex Virus Evaluation

HSV testing should be considered in infants 21 days or younger, or in older infants with ill appearance, neurologic changes and/or seizures, vesicular rash, hepatitis, history of known maternal primary HSV, or active maternal HSV lesions at delivery. HSV PCR should be sent from both serum and CSF. Infants with high clinical concern for HSV should also have surface swabs (from conjunctivae, mouth, nasopharynx, and rectum), scrapings of skin lesions, PCR evaluation of any additional available specimens (e.g., endotracheal aspirate in intubated infants), and CMP to evaluate for hepatitis and acute kidney injury.

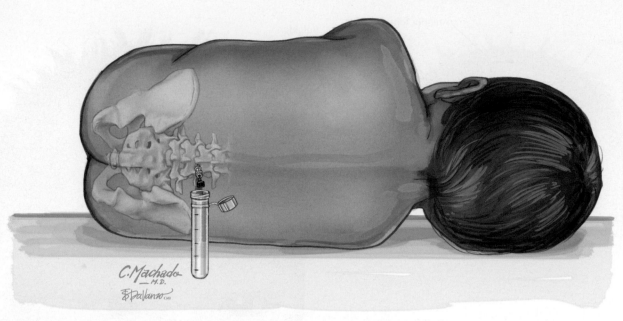

Fig. 82.4 Lumbar Puncture in an Infant.

TABLE 82.2	**Summary of Key Risk Stratification Criteria**		
	Rochester Criteria	**Philadelphia Criteria**	**Boston Criteria**
Age (days)	0–60	29–56	28–89
Low risk history and physical examination parameters	• Gestational age ≥37 weeks • Normal prenatal/postnatal course • No prior antibiotics • Well-appearing without signs of focal infection	• Well-appearing without signs of focal infection	• No antibiotics or immunizations within preceding 48 hours • Well-appearing without signs of focal infection
Low-risk laboratory parameters	• WBC: 5000–15,000/mm³ • Absolute bands: <1500/mm³ • UA: ≤10 WBC/HPF • Stool ≤5 WBC/HPF on smear[a]	• WBC: <15,000/mm³ • Ratio of immature to total neutrophils <0.2 • UA: <10 WBC/HPF • Negative urine Gram stain • CSF: <8 WBC/mm³ with negative Gram stain (modified Philadelphia criteria does not include routine CSF testing) • Chest radiograph: no infiltrate[a] • Stool: no blood, few or no WBCs on smear[a]	• WBC: <20,000/mm³ • UA: <10 WBC/HPF • CSF: <10 WBC/mm³ • Chest radiograph: no infiltrate[a]
Low risk management	• Discharge and follow-up within 24 hours if older than 28 days • No empiric antibiotics if older than 28 days	• Discharge and follow-up within 24 hours • No empiric antibiotics	• Discharge and follow-up within 24 hours • Ceftriaxone at discharge and again at 24-hour follow-up
High risk management	Hospitalize + empiric antibiotics	Hospitalize + empiric antibiotics	Hospitalize + empiric antibiotics
NPV of low-risk criteria (95% CI)	98.9% (97.2–99.6%)	100% (99–100%)	94.6% (92.2–96.4%)

[a]If clinically indicated and obtained.
CI, Confidence interval; *CSF,* cerebrospinal fluid; *HPF,* high-power field; *UA,* urinalysis; *WBC,* white blood cell.

Empiric Treatment

After obtaining cultures, it is critical to initiate empiric antimicrobial therapy promptly, as decreasing time to antibiotic administration reduces SBI mortality. If an infant with concern for sepsis is too unstable to undergo immediate lumbar puncture, empiric antimicrobial therapy should be started immediately; CSF cell counts remain interpretable even after several days of appropriate antibiotics. Empiric antimicrobials should cover the most common pathogens implicated in neonatal SBI at meningitic dosing and are stratified by patient age.

Infants Younger Than 1 Month Old

In neonates, an appropriate regimen includes a third-generation cephalosporin with CNS penetration (e.g., cefotaxime or ceftazidime) or gentamicin to cover *E. coli,* plus ampicillin to cover GBS and

L. monocytogenes. Ceftriaxone is contraindicated in infants 28 days or younger, because it can cause bilirubin displacement from albumin, precipitating kernicterus.

The addition of vancomycin can be considered if the infant is critically ill, has significant CSF pleocytosis, or has evidence of skin/soft tissue infection in a region with high community-acquired methicillin-resistant *S. aureus* prevalence. A carbapenem or cefepime should be considered for broader gram-negative coverage in infants with risk factors for infection with *Pseudomonas* species or other resistant gram-negative organisms, including immunodeficiency, prematurity, prior hospitalization, or indwelling hardware. Infants 21 days or younger or with HSV risk factors should receive empiric acyclovir. All antimicrobial choices should be guided by local antibiograms.

Infants Ages 1 Month to 2–3 Months

Older infants were historically treated with empiric ceftriaxone monotherapy, though recent evidence suggests adding ampicillin for improved coverage of GBS, *L. monocytogenes,* and *Enterococcus* species. Vancomycin, a carbapenem, or cefepime, and acyclovir should again be considered based on risk factors and degree of illness. In infants who are 1 month or older and meet low-risk criteria (Table 82.2), empiric antibiotics and/or hospital admission may be deferred after cultures are obtained, but there is significant institutional practice variation in this age group. In these permissively managed patients, it is critical to ensure excellent follow-up and provide specific return precautions.

Further Management

All infants younger than 1 month and older infants not meeting low-risk criteria should be admitted for continued parenteral antimicrobials while cultures are pending. If cultures become positive, antibiotics should be tailored to that organism, and length of treatment will vary based on organism and location of infection. Inpatient observation strategies vary among practitioners. Patients may require anywhere from 24 to 72 hours of negative cultures before discontinuing antimicrobials. Multicenter studies have shown that in infants with bacteremia, more than 90% will have positive blood cultures within 24 hours and more than 95% within 36 hours.

If cultures remain negative throughout the observation window and the patient is clinically improving with age-appropriate vital signs and adequate oral intake, it is reasonable to attribute the fever to a self-limited viral infection, discontinue antibiotics, and discharge with close pediatrician follow-up. It is important to counsel families on the natural history of viral infections, expected temperature parameters, and return precautions.

Since this chapter was originally written, the American Academy of Pediatrics (AAP) released the Clinical Practice Guideline: Evaluation and Management of Well-Appearing Febrile Infants 8 to 60 days Old, which updates the previous evaluation and management approaches discussed. The guidelines further stratifies evaluation and management based on age and emphasize the use of inflammatory markers, including procalcitonin, if available, among other practice recommendations.

FUTURE DIRECTIONS

Although risk criteria exist to support more permissive management of low-risk infants (Table 82.2), ongoing research is needed to further identify infants in whom LP and/or empiric antibiotics can be deferred. Some newer approaches rely on gene expression profiles and viral PCRs, though these approaches have yet to be validated.

SUGGESTED READINGS

Available online.

83

Fever of Unknown Origin

Brittany J. Van Remortel and Laura B. Goldstein

✳ CLINICAL VIGNETTE

A 4-year-old previously healthy boy presents to the emergency department with a 2-week history of daily fevers up to 101.8°F (38.8°C) and 1 day of abdominal pain. Previous outpatient evaluation has been largely unremarkable, aside from a minor rash on his left hand and a complete blood count notable for lymphocytosis. His mother reports a new pet kitten in the family.

Vital signs are significant for a temperature of 101.3°F (38.5°C) and heart rate of 136 beats/min. On examination, he is noted to have tender hepatomegaly and erythematous papules on the dorsal aspect of on his left hand. Repeat laboratory evaluation reveals elevated C-reactive protein, mildly elevated hepatic transaminases, and continued lymphocytosis. Abdominal ultrasound reveals multiple filling defects within the liver suggestive of granulomas. *Bartonella henselae* antibody titers are found to be elevated, and he is treated with a 10-day course of rifampin and azithromycin for disseminated cat-scratch disease.

Fever is one of the most common pediatric chief complaints, accounting for up to one-third of outpatient pediatrician visits. Although most pediatric febrile illnesses have an easily identifiable source, a minority of children have prolonged fevers with no clear cause. The term fever of unknown origin (FUO) is typically defined in children as at least 8 days of daily fevers above 100.4°F (38.0°C) with no identifiable cause after a thorough history, physical examination, and initial screening diagnostic evaluation. FUO must be distinguished from "fever without a source," which applies to children with fever for 7 days or less without an identified cause.

The goal in clinical evaluation of FUO is to identify illnesses with significant associated morbidity and mortality if left untreated. Reassuringly, FUO is often an uncommon presentation of a common illness, and outcomes are generally favorable.

ETIOLOGY AND PATHOGENESIS

The main causes of FUO are broadly divided into four main categories: infection, rheumatologic disorders, neoplasms, and miscellaneous. Each of these categories is discussed in detail later, with a comprehensive differential diagnosis summarized in Table 83.1. Globally, infectious causes of FUO account for approximately half of cases, rheumatologic disorders account for approximately 9%, neoplasms for 6%, and miscellaneous causes for 11%. In at least one-fourth of cases, the underlying cause for FUO is never determined, and fevers spontaneously resolve. It is important to rule out treatable and potentially life-threatening conditions, but establishing a final diagnosis is not always essential if fever has resolved and the patient has improved.

Notably, the proportion of undetermined FUO has increased over the last decade. As increasingly sophisticated diagnostic techniques allow for earlier identification of disease, fewer cases of fever progress to FUO altogether; thus, those that do become FUO are more difficult to diagnose.

Infection
Localized Infections

Localized infections, including urinary tract infections (UTIs), osteomyelitis, and upper respiratory tract infections, are common causes of pediatric FUO, particularly in developed countries. UTI has been identified by many studies as the most common cause of FUO in children worldwide, likely because of a notoriously unreliable history and physical examination, particularly in young and/or nonverbal children. Osteomyelitis is another common culprit, similarly related to difficulty with symptom localization in young children. Although older children with osteomyelitis may complain of pain or refuse to bear weight, very young and/or nonambulatory children may appear otherwise asymptomatic.

Infections of the upper respiratory tract and adjacent structures, including mastoiditis, sinusitis, otitis media, and tonsillopharyngitis, remain important causes of FUO in children, because localizing symptoms are common and may initially be dismissed as trivial. Similarly, soft tissue infections of the head and neck (peritonsillar abscess, cervical adenitis, and retropharyngeal infections) and lower respiratory tract infections may elude early diagnosis and manifest with prolonged fevers. Occult intraabdominal abscesses are also known to cause FUO and should be suspected if there is a history of abdominal disease, intraabdominal surgery, or abdominal pain.

Infective endocarditis (IE), while a rare cause of FUO, is an important entity to consider, given its significant associated morbidity and mortality; patients with existing cardiac lesions and central venous catheters are particularly at risk.

Generalized Infections

Generalized infections are another important cause of FUO, because they may manifest nonspecifically; distinguishing among individual infections requires a detailed exposure history and high clinical suspicion (Table 83.2).

Viral infections. Certain viral infections including Epstein-Barr virus (EBV), cytomegalovirus (CMV), human herpesvirus-6 (HHV-6), parvovirus, and adenovirus are common causes of FUO, as their symptoms are often nonspecific and variable. Less common viral causes include enteroviruses, human immunodeficiency virus (HIV), and arboviruses. Coinfection with multiple viruses is not uncommon in the school-aged child and should be considered in prolonged fever (Chapter 88).

Bacterial and parasitic infections. Systemic bacterial infections with indolent, nonspecific manifestations are another frequent cause of FUO. *Bartonella henselae*–associated cat-scratch disease is a particularly common infection, especially in developed countries. Cat-scratch disease may manifest classically with lymphadenitis or,

TABLE 83.1   Differential Diagnosis for Pediatric Fever of Unknown Origin[a]

Generalized infections	**Bacterial** • Actinomycosis • Anaplasmosis • Brucellosis • *Campylobacter* • **Cat scratch disease** • Ehrlichiosis • Leptospirosis • Lyme disease • Nontuberculous mycobacteria • Psittacosis • Q fever • Rat-bite fever (*Streptobacillus moniliformis*) • Rocky Mountain spotted fever • **Salmonellosis (typhoidal and nontyphoidal)** • Syphilis • Tick-borne typhus • **Tuberculosis (pulmonary and extrapulmonary)** • Tularemia **Viral** • **Atypical prolonged presentation of common viral illness** • **Adenovirus** • Arbovirus • **Cytomegalovirus (CMV)** • Enterovirus • **Epstein-Barr virus (EBV)** • Hepatitis viruses • Herpes simplex virus • **Human herpesvirus 6 (HHV-6)** • Human immunodeficiency virus (HIV) • Parvovirus B-19 **Other (fungal, parasitic)** • Babesiosis • Blastomycosis (extra-pulmonary) • Cryptosporidium • Coccidiomycosis (disseminated) • Histoplasmosis (disseminated) • Leishmaniasis • **Malaria** • Toxoplasmosis • Visceral larva migrans (*Toxocara*)	Lymphogranuloma venereum Meningitis **Osteomyelitis** **Pneumonia**, particularly due to *Mycoplasma pneumoniae* Septic arthritis Soft tissue infections of the head and neck: peritonsillar abscess, cervical adenitis, and retropharyngeal infections **Upper respiratory infection:** otitis media, pharyngitis, sinusitis, mastoiditis **Urinary tract infection/pyelonephritis**
	Rheumatologic diseases **Juvenile idiopathic arthritis** Sarcoidosis Systemic lupus erythematosus Undifferentiated connective disease Vasculitis: Behçet disease, granulomatosis with polyangiitis, polyarteritis nodosa, etc.
	Malignancies Atrial myxoma Bone tumors Hepatoma **Leukemia** **Lymphoma** Neuroblastoma Sarcoma Wilms tumor
Localized infections	Abscesses: abdominal, brain, dental, hepatic, pelvic, perinephric, rectal Infective endocarditis Liver infection: bacterial cholangitis, granulomatous hepatitis
	Miscellaneous Central nervous system dysfunction Cyclic neutropenia Diabetes insipidus **Drug fever** Ectodermal dysplasia Factitious fever Familial dysautonomia Granulomatous colitis Hemophagocytic lymphohistiocytosis Immunodeficiency Infantile cortical hyperostosis **Inflammatory bowel disease** **Kawasaki disease** Kikuchi-Fujimoto disease Langerhans cell histiocytosis Multisystem inflammatory syndrome in children (MIS-C) associated with COVID-19 Pancreatitis Periodic fever syndromes Sarcoidosis Serum sickness Thyrotoxicosis

[a]Common causes are in bold.

more rarely, as disseminated cat-scratch disease with hepatosplenic granulomatous invasion. Globally, tuberculosis (TB), both pulmonary and extrapulmonary, and malaria are important considerations in the differential diagnosis of FUO (Chapters 87 and 90). Malaria should be suspected in all patients with travel to endemic areas, even with a remote history of travel and appropriate prophylaxis.

Infection with *Salmonella* species by exposure to contaminated animal products is another common cause of FUO and can manifest with gastroenteritis or systemic typhoidal disease. Other zoonotic infections such as brucellosis, leptospirosis, toxoplasmosis, Q fever, and tularemia are important to consider, though they are less common overall and more likely to occur in developing countries. Tick-borne illnesses,

TABLE 83.2   Key Exposures Implicated in Generalized Infections in Fever of Unknown Origin

Condition	Causative Organism	Key Exposures
Babesiosis	*Babesia* species	Tick bite *(Ixodes scapularis)* Travel to endemic areas: northeast and midwest United States, northeast and southwest China
Brucellosis	*Brucella* species	Unpasteurized dairy Undercooked meat Farm animals
Cat-scratch disease	*Bartonella henselae*	Cats (particularly kittens)
Ehrlichiosis and anaplasmosis	*Ehrlichia* species	Tick bite (*Amblyomma americanum* and *Ixodes scapularis*)
Leptospirosis	*Leptospira* species	Animal urine Contaminated soil or water
Lyme disease	*Borrelia* species	Tick bite (*Ixodes* species) Travel to forested areas in United States, Europe, or Asia
Malaria	*Plasmodium* species: *falciparum > vivax, knowlesi, malariae*	Travel to endemic tropical areas
Psittacosis	*Chlamydia psittaci*	Contact with birds
Q fever	*Coxiella burnetii*	Farm animals
Rocky Mountain spotted fever	*Rickettsia rickettsii*	Tick bite Travel to endemic areas: southeast and south central United States, Canada, Mexico, Central America, parts of South America
Salmonellosis	Nontyphoidal *Salmonella* species	Poultry Raw eggs Reptiles
Toxoplasmosis	*Toxoplasma gondii*	Cat waste
Tuberculosis	*Mycobacterium tuberculosis*	Travel to endemic area Time in correctional facility, homeless shelter, or health care facility
Tularemia	*Francisella tularensis*	Rabbit carcasses Rabbit/squirrel meat consumption Insect bites
Enteric (typhoid) fever	*Salmonella enterica* serotypes	Travel to endemic area

including Lyme disease, Rocky Mountain spotted fever, anaplasmosis, and ehrlichiosis should be considered in endemic regions, particularly with exposure to wooded areas or after a known tick bite (Chapter 85).

Rheumatologic Disorders

Fever is a common presenting symptom in many connective tissue diseases. Among these disorders, systemic juvenile idiopathic arthritis (JIA) (Chapter 136) is most commonly implicated in FUO, because arthritis may not develop until much later. Additional rheumatologic considerations in FUO include systemic lupus erythematosus (SLE) (Chapter 139) and vasculitides (Chapter 138), though these diseases typically manifest with multiorgan involvement rather than isolated fever.

Malignancy

Although less common, malignancy remains an important diagnostic consideration for children with FUO, because prompt identification allows for earlier initiation of directed therapy. Most neoplasms manifest with additional signs and symptoms beyond fever, though isolated fever is possible. Leukemia and lymphoma are the most common malignancies to manifest as FUO (Chapters 123 and 124). Neuroblastoma, sarcomas, bony neoplasms, and Wilms tumor are less common causes of FUO but also potential culprits.

Miscellaneous

A broad array of miscellaneous conditions should also be considered in the evaluation of FUO.

Kawasaki disease (KD), a systemic pediatric vasculitis, should be considered early in the evaluation of all cases of FUO, because prompt recognition and treatment are essential in prevention of long-term cardiac sequelae from coronary artery aneurysms (Chapter 138). Incomplete KD, with fewer clinical stigmata, is more difficult to identify and requires high clinical suspicion. Although newly defined, the multisystem inflammatory syndrome in children (MIS-C) associated with COVID-19 should also be considered in cases of prolonged fever. MIS-C should be suspected in children presenting with a KD-like illness after recent COVID-19 infection or exposure (Chapter 138).

Another common but frequently overlooked cause of prolonged fevers in the well-appearing, asymptomatic child is drug fever. Commonly implicated drugs include sulfa drugs, antiepileptic medications, antiarrhythmic medications, sleep medications, and narcotics; however, fever can be precipitated by virtually any medication. Thus a detailed medication history, including inquiry into over-the-counter medications, illicit drugs, supplements, and complementary therapies, is critical. Once the offending agent is identified and discontinued, fevers typically resolve within 72 hours.

Inflammatory bowel disease (IBD) should be considered, particularly in adolescents. Patients with occult IBD may present with a history of prolonged isolated fever and growth failure with or without intestinal manifestations (Chapter 57).

Recurrent unexplained fevers may occur as part of a periodic fever syndrome. Most common among these is periodic fever with aphthous stomatitis, pharyngitis, and adenitis (PFAPA); although fevers are periodic by definition, they may be interpreted as prolonged, prompting FUO evaluation. Hereditary fever disorders including familial Mediterranean fever, hyperimmunoglobulin-D syndrome, and tumor necrosis factor receptor–associated periodic syndrome are rare but potential causes of recurrent fevers in children. In young children and especially infants with persistent or recurrent fevers, an underlying immunodeficiency, including HIV, should also be considered (Chapters 23 and 86).

A rare but life-threatening disorder that can manifest as FUO is hemophagocytic lymphohistiocytosis (HLH). Patients with HLH may present with hepatosplenomegaly, hyperferritinemia, and cytopenias but can rapidly progress to a severe sepsis-like syndrome and death, highlighting the importance of early recognition and intervention (Chapter 130).

Central nervous system (CNS) dysfunction characterized by damage to hypothalamic thermoregulatory centers may be associated with recurrent fevers; this entity is most commonly noted after severe brain damage. Diabetes insipidus, both central and nephrogenic, can also cause unexplained fevers and will manifest with evidence of free water loss.

Finally, factitious fever is a diagnosis of exclusion and should be considered only after a thorough evaluation for alternative causes. Factitious fever may range from less morbid (false reports of fever, tampering with temperature measurements) to highly morbid (true fever induced by the injection of infective or foreign material into the patient in cases of Munchausen by proxy [medical child abuse]).

CLINICAL PRESENTATION

The goal in FUO evaluation is to identify treatable conditions, as well as those with high morbidity and mortality. In a well-appearing, thriving child, evaluation may be performed in the outpatient setting; however, admission may be warranted for ill appearance, coordination of multiple diagnostic studies, or closer monitoring of fever pattern.

History

The clinical presentation of FUO varies widely based on underlying cause; therefore a thorough history is critical. Fever history should address how fevers were recorded, fever heights and temporal patterns, and whether fevers have been confirmed in a medical setting. Clinicians should note the exact timing of each fever to distinguish between true FUO and multiple serial illnesses with 24-hour intercurrent periods of defervescence, termed pseudo-FUO.

Associated signs and symptoms, such as infectious complaints, potential sources of pain, behavioral changes, and weight loss should be assessed, though review of systems may be unremarkable. A careful medication history and vaccination history can reveal risk factors for drug fever and occult infection, respectively. Family history should address ethnic background to assess for diseases with a genetic basis.

A detailed exposure history is key and should include inquiry into ill contacts, travel history, and TB risk factors. Zoonotic contact, including livestock, cats, rodents, and reptiles, should be investigated, and dietary history should include consumption of unpasteurized dairy products or raw meats. Sexual and drug histories may reveal risk factors for HIV and other sexually transmitted infections.

Physical Examination

A comprehensive physical examination is necessary in all patients with FUO, because findings may be subtle. Children should undergo serial examinations, as clinical presentation may evolve. It is useful to perform at least one examination while the patient is febrile. Any positive findings from the examination should be used to focus the diagnostic evaluation.

It is important to note vital sign derangements suggestive of acute illness or sepsis, including tachycardia, tachypnea, and hypotension. Growth parameters should be noted, because failure to thrive or weight loss may underlie chronic systemic processes such as IBD, rheumatologic disease, and malignancy. The child's overall state of health should be noted, with attention to general appearance, activity level, and behavior.

An ophthalmologic examination may reveal conjunctivitis, Roth spots, or uveitis. On oropharyngeal examination, it is important to note any oral mucous membrane changes. Ulcers may be suggestive of a viral syndrome, autoimmune disease, or PFAPA, and cracked lips may be noted in KD. A general search for focal evidence of infection should be undertaken, including for rhinorrhea, congestion, tonsillar abnormalities, dental infection, and signs of otitis media or its sequelae.

Chest examination may reveal a cardiopulmonary cause of FUO; adventitious lung sounds may suggest pneumonia, and a new murmur may suggest IE. An abdominal examination should include careful evaluation of the liver and spleen, because hepatomegaly and/or splenomegaly are concerning for certain systemic infections or malignancy. Any suprapubic and costovertebral tenderness should be elicited. A genitourinary examination should be performed. A rectal and perianal examination is indicated, particularly if there is concern for IBD.

The musculoskeletal examination should include observation of walking, if developmentally appropriate; refusal to bear weight, limited use of an extremity, or point tenderness may suggest underlying osteomyelitis or malignancy. All joints should be examined for effusions or arthritis, which may indicate infection or autoimmune disease.

Many important causes of FUO have associated dermatologic findings; thus careful skin examination is critical (Fig. 83.1). Some skin findings, such as the evanescent salmon-colored macules of systemic JIA, may appear with febrile episodes, whereas others, such as the malar rash of SLE or erythema migrans in Lyme disease, may be more fixed.

EVALUATION AND MANAGEMENT

Diagnostic Testing

The diagnostic workup for patients with FUO should proceed in a stepwise fashion, using the history and physical examination to guide testing.

Screening Evaluation

A screening laboratory evaluation is an appropriate first step. An abnormal complete blood count with differential may be revealing. An elevated white blood cell count is a nonspecific sign of inflammation, but the degree of elevation and type of cells that are prominent can be informative. Elevated neutrophils and immature neutrophils (a "left shift") suggest a bacterial infection, and lymphocytosis may suggest a viral infection; leukopenia also may be present in infection. Anemia can occur in the setting of chronic disease. Thrombocytosis is another nonspecific marker of inflammation, while thrombocytopenia may be present in sepsis and other severe illness. Suppression of multiple cell lines may occur in simple viral infections but also may indicate a rheumatologic or neoplastic process.

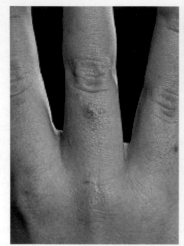

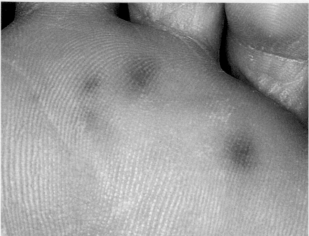

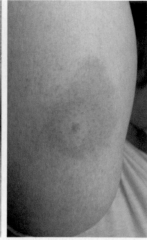

A. Cat scratch on finger of ipsilateral arm

B. Infective endocarditis: Janeway lesions

C. Lyme disease: erythema migrans

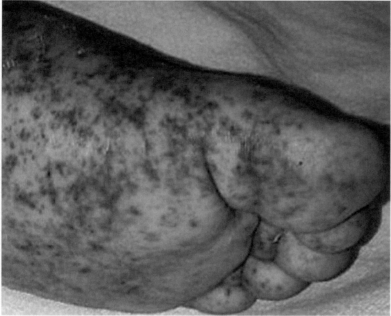

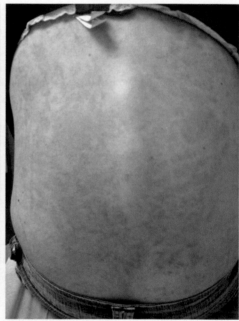

D. Rocky Mountain Spotted Fever: petechial rash involving palms and soles

E. Systemic juvenile idiopathic arthritis: evanescent macular salmon-colored rash

Fig. 83.1 Select Dermatologic Findings in Evaluation of Fever of Unknown Origin. (Photographs reused with permission. A, Stutchfield CJ, Tyrrell J. Evaluation of lymphadenopathy in children. *Paediatr Child Health.* 2012;22(3):98-102, Fig. 2; *B,* Beerman LB, Kreutzer J, Allada V. Cardiology. In: Zitelli BJ, McIntire S, Nowalk AJ, eds. *Zitelli and Davis' Atlas of Pediatric Physical Diagnosis.* 7th ed. Philadelphia, PA: Elsevier; 2017:136-170, Fig. 5.13; *C,* Michaels MG, Williams JV. Infectious diseases. In: Zitelli BJ, McIntire S, Nowalk AJ, eds. *Zitelli and Davis' Atlas of Pediatric Physical Diagnosis.* 7th ed. Philadelphia, PA: Elsevier; 2017:455-509, Fig. 13.50; *D,* Paddock CD, Alvarez-Hernández G. Rickettsia (Rocky Mountain spotted fever). In: Long SS, Prober CG, Fischer M, eds. *Principles and Practice of Pediatric Infectious Diseases.* 5th ed. Philadelphia, PA: Elsevier; 2018:952-957.e2, Figure 178.3; *E,* Torok K, Cassidy EL, Rosenkranza M. Rheumatology. In: Zitelli BJ, McIntire S, Nowalk AJ, eds. *Zitelli and Davis' Atlas of Pediatric Physical Diagnosis.* 7th ed. Philadelphia, PA: Elsevier; 2017:236-274, Fig. 7.7A.)

Inflammatory markers, including C-reactive protein (CRP) and erythrocyte sedimentation rate (ESR), are nonspecific but provide an overall impression of the level and chronicity of inflammation. Serial levels can be useful in tracking the course of illness; ESR rises more slowly and remains elevated for a longer time than CRP, making it more useful in chronic inflammation. There is currently inadequate evidence to support the use of procalcitonin in the screening evaluation of patients with FUO.

Urinalysis, urine culture, and blood culture should be obtained in all patients. A comprehensive metabolic panel (CMP) is helpful to assess for electrolyte derangements, hypoalbuminemia, kidney function, and elevated transaminases. Chest radiography is part of the universal initial evaluation and may identify parenchymal disease, lymphadenopathy, mediastinal masses, or cardiomegaly.

Additional Laboratory Testing

Further laboratory testing should be dictated by the history, physical, and screening evaluation, using less invasive testing preferentially. Common infections should be considered first, with early evaluation including EBV and *Bartonella* serologies and polymerase chain reaction (PCR) testing for adenovirus and enterovirus. PCR testing of multiple sources (e.g., blood, urine, respiratory secretions) raises the likelihood of identifying a given pathogen. PCR testing of EBV, CMV, and HHV-6 may be considered; however, positive results must be interpreted in clinical context and with serologies because of periodic asymptomatic reactivation. Serologies are the preferred test for parvovirus in immunocompetent patients due to prolonged viral shedding. A purified protein derivative (PPD) tuberculin skin test is indicated if risk factors for TB are identified.

Gastrointestinal symptoms should prompt stool studies, including culture and guaiac, and concern for endocarditis should prompt serial large-volume blood cultures. HIV immunoassay should be performed if any risk factors for HIV are identified. Targeted testing for zoonotic or geographically specific infections should be performed only if indicated by history. A low threshold should exist for performing lumbar puncture in patients with ill appearance, meningeal signs, or a history of CNS symptoms.

Antinuclear antibody testing is nonspecific and a poor screen for rheumatologic disease; it should be obtained only if there is particular concern for SLE. Testing for additional rheumatologic diagnoses should be performed in a more targeted manner. Lactate dehydrogenase, uric acid, ferritin, and hematologic smear should be considered if there is concern for malignancy or HLH. Finally, any concern for immunodeficiency should prompt a screening evaluation.

Diagnostic Imaging

The potential benefit of imaging studies in FUO should always be weighed against the degree of radiation exposure to the patient. Plain radiographs are appropriate in the initial evaluation of localized extremity pain. Ultrasound is another appropriate initial imaging modality, because it is noninvasive and lacks ionizing radiation. It should be considered in evaluation of joint effusions; skin or soft tissue abnormalities; and abdominal pain, palpable mass, or organomegaly. Echocardiography should be performed in patients with a concern for endocarditis, KD, or MIS-C.

Computer tomography (CT) and magnetic resonance imaging (MRI) can provide superior diagnostic information but should be used prudently, given concerns for high radiation exposure from CT and potential need for sedation during MRI.

CT may be useful in evaluation of the chest, abdomen, and pelvis for mass lesions, fluid collections, bowel wall abnormalities, or adenopathy. Although imaging is not recommended for the diagnosis of uncomplicated sinusitis, concern for orbital or intracranial complications should prompt CT with contrast of the brain, orbits, and sinuses. MRI is useful in the assessment of localized bony tenderness to assess for osteomyelitis, and it is the preferred imaging modality for CNS lesions. Whole-body MRI and positron emission tomography are occasionally considered when workup is otherwise unrevealing. However, there is currently insufficient evidence to support their use in the routine evaluation of children with FUO.

Invasive Testing

Invasive testing should be performed conservatively and in conjunction with expert consultation. Bone marrow biopsy is indicated when there is concern for hematologic malignancy, while a biopsy of other suspicious masses or lesions may be necessary. Concern for IBD may prompt endoscopy and/or colonoscopy.

Management

The management of FUO varies widely depending on the underlying cause. At minimum, nonessential medications should be sequentially discontinued to rule out drug fever. Empiric antimicrobials can delay diagnosis and confound testing; they should be avoided unless there is suspicion for life-threatening infection. Antipyretics can be used for symptomatic management, though families should be reassured that fever alone is not harmful.

FUTURE DIRECTIONS

Ongoing research is needed to improve diagnostic accuracy and decrease time to diagnosis in the evaluation of FUO. Some newer approaches rely on cytokine profiles or pathogen detection using metagenomic next-generation sequencing, though these approaches have yet to be validated.

SUGGESTED READINGS

Available online.

84

Fever in a Returning Traveler

Laurel Gabler and Katherine M. Laycock

 CLINICAL VIGNETTE

A 3-year-old boy presents to clinic with 5 days of fevers that have become higher each day. He also has nonbilious vomiting and nonbloody diarrhea. He returned 3 weeks ago from a month-long visit with family in Pakistan to attend his grandfather's funeral. Because the trip occurred on short notice, he did not receive pretravel vaccinations.

In the clinic, he is febrile to 103.6°F (39.8°C), appears ill, and has diffuse abdominal tenderness. He is referred to the local emergency department, where laboratory test samples, including blood and stool cultures, are collected. He is given empiric intravenous ceftriaxone and admitted to the hospital. The next day, his blood culture grows gram-negative bacilli identified as *Salmonella enterica* serovar Typhi, confirming the diagnosis of enteric fever. His fevers and abdominal symptoms resolve with antibiotic treatment over the next 4 days.

Enteric fever, a systemic bacterial infection that includes typhoid and paratyphoid fevers, is a common cause of febrile illness in international travelers. Positive blood or stool cultures are diagnostic, though stool cultures may be negative in early disease. Vaccines are available for travelers to endemic areas.

International travel has become increasingly common, with over 1.4 billion international tourist arrivals recorded globally in 2019. Many of these travelers are children and adolescents. The exposures that occur can place pediatric travelers at risk for a broad assortment of infectious diseases ranging in severity from mild and self-limited to potentially life-threatening, often with fever as the initial symptom. An approach to the pediatric patient who presents with fever after recent travel requires careful attention to symptomatology and exposures to reach a diagnosis. This chapter provides a framework for evaluation and describes key features of common travel-related infections.

ETIOLOGY

Children and adolescents travel for many reasons: to sightsee, visit friends and relatives, study or volunteer, or as refugees or adoptees. Travel-related illnesses, defined as any illness acquired en route or at the destination, vary just as widely. Although focus often goes to destination-specific infections, children can also acquire routine infections, such as acute otitis media and urinary tract infections, at any point during travel. Studies of children evaluated for fever after recent travel have identified cosmopolitan infections in over half of cases.

Some destination-specific infections result from a bite from an insect vector such as a mosquito (e.g., malaria, dengue) or tick (e.g., rickettsial diseases). Others result from exposure to a contaminated food or water source (e.g., enteric fever, leptospirosis, hepatitis A). Person-to-person transmission occurs with viral respiratory infections. For adolescent travelers, high-risk behaviors during travel may lead to exposure to sexually transmitted or bloodborne infections (e.g., human immunodeficiency virus [HIV], hepatitis C).

The reason for travel can inform a child's risk for acquiring a destination-specific infection. For example, a child who travels to a tourist destination, stays in a hotel with bed netting, eats only fully cooked food and drinks only treated water may be at lower risk for infection than an adventure traveler who stays in a camp with few amenities. Children who travel to visit friends and relatives face particular risk for destination-specific infections. More so than other travelers, these children tend to travel at younger ages, stay for longer periods, and assume the behaviors of the local population without the benefit of locals' potential immunity to some endemic infections.

Some children become ill during their time abroad, but many do not develop symptoms until they return home. The incubation period of most travel-related infections means that children generally become symptomatic within 30 days of travel. Some diseases have longer incubation periods; thus any travel within the previous 12 months should be considered when evaluating fever.

CLINICAL PRESENTATION

Fever is one of the most common chief complaints in children and adolescents who seek care for a travel-related illness. The nonspecific symptoms of systemic febrile illness, such as headache, myalgias, and malaise, occur with many travel-related illnesses, especially at the onset of illness; more specific symptoms and signs may not appear until later in the illness course. This overlap in symptoms makes diagnosis challenging. A thorough history that reviews any infectious exposures the child may have had during travel (Box 84.1) often provides the most useful information to narrow the differential diagnosis through a risk-based approach:

1. *Geographic risk:* Consider the infections that are endemic to areas where the patient traveled. Online public health reports provide up-to-date information on endemic diseases and outbreaks by country (Box 84.2).
2. *Activity risk:* Certain activities can increase a child's chance of exposure to specific diseases. The child's immunization history, including pre-travel vaccinations, and prophylactic medications taken during travel also provide important information.
3. *Incubation period risk:* Consider the timing of the patient's symptoms in relation to travel and the incubation periods of potential infections (Fig. 84.1). For example, dengue, which has an incubation period of up to 14 days, would be unlikely in a child who develops new fever 4 weeks after returning from a dengue-endemic area.

Although a comprehensive review of all potential travel-related infections is outside the scope of this chapter, Table 84.1 provides key information on many important infections. The next sections describe in greater detail the clinical findings, diagnostic considerations, and treatment for four febrile illnesses commonly identified in children after travel.

BOX 84.1   Key Elements of Exposure History During Travel

- Complete travel itinerary, including all stops
- Accommodation type—hotel, private home, camp
- Diet—raw foods, unpasteurized dairy, untreated drinking water
- Close contact with animals
- Insect exposures—mosquitoes, ticks, flies, fleas, lice, reduviid bugs
- Recreational activities
  - Safari
  - Hiking
  - Spelunking
  - Swimming in freshwater
  - Sexual contact
- Needle exposures—injection drug use, new tattoos or piercings
- Sick contacts, both during and after travel
- Pre-travel precautions
  - Pretravel immunizations
  - Antimalarial prophylaxis
- Medical care received while traveling
- Known outbreaks in the travel destination

BOX 84.2   Resources for Destination-Specific Infections

- Centers for Disease Control and Prevention (CDC) Travelers' Health Destination List: https://wwwnc.cdc.gov/travel/destinations/list
- CDC Yellow Book: https://wwwnc.cdc.gov/travel/page/yellowbook-home
- World Health Organization (WHO) Disease Outbreak News: https://www.who.int/emergencies/disease-outbreak-news

Timeframe	Disease	Typical Incubation Period (Range)
<14 days	Influenza	1 – 3 days
	Chikungunya	2 – 4 days (1 – 14 days)
	Yellow fever	3 – 8 days
	Zika virus	3 – 14 days
	Arboviral encephalitis (Japanese encephalitis, West Nile virus)	3 – 14 days (1 – 20 days)
	Spotted fever rickettsioses	3 – 21 days
	Dengue	4 – 8 days (3 – 14 days)
	Legionellosis	5 – 6 days (2 – 10 days)
14 days – 6 weeks	Malaria, *Plasmodium falciparum*	6 – 30 days
	Leptospirosis	7 – 12 days (2 – 30 days)
	Enteric fever	7 – 18 days (3 – 60 days)
	Acute HIV	7 – 28 days (3 days to 6 weeks)
>6 weeks	Malaria, *Plasmodium vivax*	8 days – 12 months
	Hepatitis E	26 – 42 days (2 – 9 weeks)
	Hepatitis A	28 – 30 days (15 – 50 days)
	Amebic liver abscess	Weeks – months
	Acute schistosomiasis (Katayama syndrome)	4 – 8 weeks
	Hepatitis B	90 days (60 – 150 days)
	Visceral leishmaniasis	2 – 10 months
	Tuberculosis	Primary, weeks; reactivation, years

Fig. 84.1 Incubation Periods of Travel-Related Diseases. *HIV*, Human immunodeficiency virus.

Malaria

Malaria is one of the most common and potentially serious causes of febrile illness in the returning child traveler. The disease is endemic throughout the tropics and subtropics (Fig. 84.2). The majority of cases diagnosed in the United States involve travel to sub-Saharan Africa. Children under 5 years of age are at highest risk for severe disease and death from malaria. Because of the potential for rapid disease progression, it is critical to exclude malaria as a cause of fever in any child with travel to an endemic region in the past 6 months.

Caused by the parasite *Plasmodium*, malaria spreads through the bite of the female *Anopheles* mosquito, which bites from dusk until dawn. Four main *Plasmodium* species cause disease in humans: *Plasmodium falciparum*, *P. vivax*, *P. ovale*, and *P. malariae*. See Chapter 90 for a detailed description of the *Plasmodium* life cycle in human hosts. People living in endemic regions develop partial immunity, but this immunity wanes quickly upon leaving the endemic area. *P. falciparum* is the most common species to infect humans and the most likely to cause fulminant disease. Most travelers infected with *P. falciparum* become ill within 2 months of departure from the malarious region.

Symptoms typically begin 1 to 2 weeks after a bite from an infected mosquito. Patients present with high fevers, which may occur every 3 to 4 days, along with headaches, chills, myalgias, nausea/vomiting, and abdominal pain. These symptoms may be mistaken for a viral syndrome. Altered mental status, seizures, acute kidney injury, acute respiratory distress syndrome, and coma are signs of severe disease and warrant urgent treatment. Physical examination may indicate hepatosplenomegaly or jaundice. Laboratory test results may demonstrate elevated inflammatory markers, anemia, thrombocytopenia, leukopenia with increased bands, or elevated liver enzymes. Hyponatremia and hypoglycemia are associated with more severe cases and occur more commonly in children.

Diagnosis is based on visualization of malaria parasites in thick and thin peripheral blood smears. A *thick smear* is a drop of blood on a slide and is most useful for detecting the presence of parasites and determining the level of parasitemia. A *thin smear* is a drop of blood that is spread across a large area of the slide and is more helpful in determining the specific species of parasite causing the infection. Rapid antigen detection tests can be useful in situations in which reliable microscopy is not available. Positive rapid antigen detection test results should always be confirmed as soon as possible using thick and thin smears to determine level of parasitemia and the *Plasmodium* species.

Prevention of infection involves avoidance and chemoprophylaxis; vaccines are in development but not widely available. All travelers to endemic regions should use DEET-containing insect repellants (30% to 50% DEET) on exposed skin, sleep under insecticide-impregnated mosquito nets, wear long sleeves and pants at night, and consider treating clothes with permethrin. Chemoprophylaxis with chloroquine, mefloquine, atovaquone-proguanil, or doxycycline is recommended. Drug resistance has made chloroquine and mefloquine ineffective in many regions.

Antimalarial treatment should begin promptly because delays can lead to more severe or fatal disease. Treatment options depend on the clinical severity, *Plasmodium* species, likelihood of drug resistance, and prior antimalarial prophylaxis. Because of the potential for rapid disease progression, children infected with *P. falciparum* require inpatient admission regardless of clinical status. Most uncomplicated infections can be treated with oral antimalarials. Children with complicated infections, including those with impaired consciousness, severe anemia (hemoglobin <7 g/dL), acute kidney injury, acidosis, acute respiratory distress syndrome, shock, jaundice, evidence of disseminated intravascular coagulation, or parasite density of 5% or greater, and children unable to tolerate oral medications require intravenous treatment with artesunate. Clinicians can contact the

TABLE 84.1 Select Travel-Related Infectious Diseases Associated With Fever[a]

Disease	Geographic Distribution	Route of Transmission	Incubation Period	Clinical Manifestations	Physical and Laboratory Findings	Diagnostic Testing	Management
West Nile virus	North America, Europe, Africa, Middle East, Asia	Mosquito bite	2–14 days	Fever, headache, myalgia, nausea, vomiting, abdominal pain, maculopapular rash. Meningitis, encephalitis, or acute flaccid paralysis occur in <1%[b]	CSF: lymphocytic pleocytosis (early neutrophil predominance)	Anti-WNV IgM antibodies in serum or CSF	Supportive care[c]
Leptospirosis	Worldwide	Direct contact with or ingestion of body fluids from infected animals	2–30 days	*Acute phase:* Fever, headache, myalgia, nausea, vomiting, non-purulent conjunctivitis *Immune-mediated phase:* Fever, jaundice, aseptic meningitis, uveitis, hemorrhage, arrhythmias[b]	Nonspecific	Anti-*Leptospira* IgM antibodies in serum. Contact local health department or CDC for confirmatory testing	Penicillin G, intravenous third-generation cephalosporin, or doxycycline[c]
Chikungunya	Central and South America, Caribbean, Africa, Asia, Australia, South Pacific	Mosquito bite	3–7 days	Fever, headache, polyarthralgia, myalgia, conjunctivitis, nausea, vomiting, maculopapular rash	Thrombocytopenia Lymphopenia Elevated liver transaminases	*<7 days from onset:* RT-PCR for chikungunya virus RNA in serum. *≥7 days from onset:* Anti-chikungunya IgM antibodies in serum	Supportive care[c]
Yellow fever	Central and South America, Africa	Mosquito bite	3–8 days	*Acute illness:* Fever, headache, myalgia, photophobia, vomiting *Progressive illness:* Jaundice, bleeding[b]	Thrombocytopenia Leukopenia *Progressive illness:* Elevated liver transaminases, prolonged blood coagulation, multisystem organ dysfunction	Contact local health department or CDC for testing	Supportive care Vaccine available[c]
Dengue	Central and South America, Caribbean, Africa, Asia, Australia, South Pacific	Mosquito bite	3–14 days	Fever, headache, myalgia, arthralgia, vomiting, abdominal pain, maculopapular rash, petechiae[b]	Thrombocytopenia Leukopenia Hyponatremia	*<7 days from onset:* RT-PCR for dengue virus antigen or immunoassay for nonstructural protein 1 (NS1) antigen *≥5 days from onset:* Anti-dengue virus IgM and IgG antibodies (compare acute and convalescent serologies)	Supportive care Avoid aspirin and other nonsteroidal anti-inflammatory drugs (NSAIDs) due to bleeding risk[c]
Zika	Central and South America, Caribbean, Africa, Asia, Australia, South Pacific	Mosquito bite	3–14 days	Fever, myalgia, conjunctivitis, maculopapular rash[b]	Thrombocytopenia Leukopenia Elevated liver transaminases	*<14 days from onset:* RT-PCR for Zika virus RNA in serum. *≥14 days from onset:* Anti-Zika IgM antibodies in serum	Supportive care[c]
Rickettsial diseases (spotted fever rickettsioses, scrub typhus, anaplasmosis, ehrlichiosis)	Worldwide	Tick, flea, louse, or mite bite	3–21 days	Fever, headache, nausea, vomiting, abdominal pain, rash (maculopapular, vesicular, or petechial)	Eschar at site of bite in some species Lymphadenopathy Hepatosplenomegaly Meningeal irritation Thrombocytopenia Hyponatremia	Acute and convalescent antibodies (IgM and IgG) in serum. RT-PCR for *Anaplasma* or *Ehrlichia* in serum. Contact CDC to test for species not endemic to the United States	Doxycycline Treatment recommended before confirmatory test results are available[c]
African trypanosomiasis (African sleeping sickness)	Sub-Saharan Africa	Tsetse fly bite	3–21 days	See Chapter 90 for details			

TABLE 84.1   Select Travel-Related Infectious Diseases Associated With Fever[a]—cont'd

Disease	Geographic Distribution	Route of Transmission	Incubation Period	Clinical Manifestations	Physical and Laboratory Findings	Diagnostic Testing	Management
Enteric fever (typhoid and paratyphoid fever)	Worldwide in developing areas, especially South Asia	Fecal-oral	3–60 days	Fever, headache, vomiting, diarrhea, constipation, abdominal pain, transient maculopapular rash (rose spots)	Nonspecific Hepatosplenomegaly (second week of illness)	Blood cultures Stool cultures	Ceftriaxone, azithromycin, fluoroquinolone, or carbapenem (consider antimicrobial resistance patterns at travel destination) Vaccine available[c]
Japanese encephalitis	Asia, South Pacific	Mosquito bite	5–15 days	Fever, headache, vomiting, acute encephalitis[b]	Leukocytosis Anemia Hyponatremia *CSF:* lymphocytic pleocytosis, elevated protein, and normal glucose	Anti-JE IgM antibodies in serum or CSF. Contact local health department or CDC for confirmatory testing	Supportive care Vaccine available
Malaria	Africa, Asia, South Pacific, Central and South America, Caribbean	Mosquito bite	6 days to months	Fever, headache, cough, nausea, vomiting, diarrhea, abdominal pain, altered mental status, seizures, shock, coma	Pallor Jaundice Hepatosplenomegaly Anemia Thrombocytopenia Hypoglycemia	Thick and thin blood smears Rapid antigen diagnostic test	Atovaquone-proguanil, chloroquine, mefloquine, artesunate (consider antimicrobial resistance patterns at travel destination). Assistance available at all hours through the CDC Malaria Hotline (770-488-7788)[c]
Acute HIV	Worldwide	Bloodborne or sexual	3 days to 6 weeks	Fever, headache, sore throat, myalgia	Diffuse lymphadenopathy Hepatosplenomegaly	Antigen/antibody combination testing Serum HIV RNA or DNA PCR	Combination antiretroviral therapy[c]
American trypanosomiasis (Chagas disease)	Southern United States, Mexico, Central and South America	Direct contact with feces of infected triatomine insects ("kissing bugs")	1–2 weeks	See Chapter 90 for details			
Hepatitis A	Worldwide	Fecal-oral	15–50 days	Fever, nausea, anorexia, jaundice; only 30% of children younger than 6 years of age are symptomatic	Jaundice Elevated liver transaminases	Anti-HAV IgM and IgG antibodies in serum	Supportive care Vaccine available[c]
Acute schistosomiasis (Katayama fever)	Africa, South America, Middle East, China, Southeast Asia	Direct contact with larvae in freshwater	4–8 weeks	See Chapter 90 for details			
Visceral leishmaniasis (kala-azar)	Central and South America, Southern Europe, Africa, Middle East, Asia	Sand fly bite	2–8 months or longer	See Chapter 90 for details			

Continued

TABLE 84.1   Select Travel-Related Infectious Diseases Associated With Fever[a]—cont'd

Disease	Geographic Distribution	Route of Transmission	Incubation Period	Clinical Manifestations	Physical and Laboratory Findings	Diagnostic Testing	Management
Tuberculosis	Worldwide, especially Eastern Europe, sub-Saharan Africa, Asia	Airborne from adolescent or adult with contagious disease	Weeks to years	*Pulmonary disease:* fever, cough, weight loss, delayed growth, night sweats. *Extrapulmonary disease:* vary by patient age and disease location	Variable depending on disease location. Can affect any organ. Disseminated disease more likely in infants and immunocompromised patients	Tuberculin skin test, interferon-γ release assay, chest radiograph	Multidrug treatment regimen in consultation with infectious diseases specialist and local health department. Family members with cough should be isolated and evaluated for pulmonary TB[c]

[a]Infections are ordered from shortest to longest incubation period.
[b]Most infections are asymptomatic.
[c]Nationally notifiable disease.

CDC, Centers for Disease Control and Prevention; *CNS,* cerebrospinal fluid; *DNA,* deoxyribonucleic acid; *HAV,* hepatitis A virus; *HIV,* human immunodeficiency virus; *IgG,* immunoglobulin G; *IgM,* immunoglobulin M; *JE,* Japanese encephalitis; *NSAIDs,* nonsteroidal antiinflammatory drugs; *PCR,* polymerase chain reaction; *RNA,* ribonucleic acid; *RT-PCR,* reverse transcription polymerase chain reaction; *TB,* tuberculosis; *WNV,* West Nile virus.

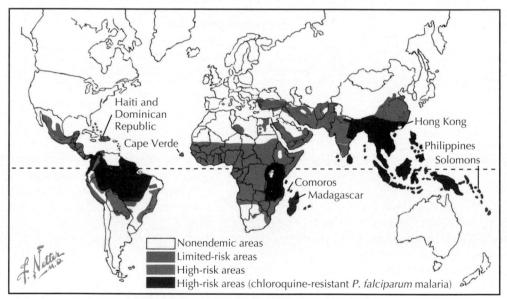

Fig. 84.2 Geographic Distribution of Malaria.

Centers for Disease Control and Prevention (CDC) Malaria Hotline (770-488-7788) at all hours for management assistance.

Dengue

Endemic throughout the tropics and subtropics, dengue is a common cause of fever in travelers returning from Latin America, the Caribbean, and Southeast Asia. Dengue is caused by infection with one of four strains of dengue virus, which is transmitted by day-biting *Aedes* mosquitoes. Symptomatic disease occurs in approximately 1 in 4 infected people, and 1 in every 20 cases progresses to severe disease.

Most symptomatic infections begin abruptly 5 to 7 days after exposure. In the acute febrile phase, symptoms include high fevers, headache, retro-orbital pain, myalgias, and arthralgias. Patients may have maculopapular rash or minor hemorrhagic manifestations (petechiae,

bleeding gums, positive tourniquet test). Fever subsides after 2 to 7 days as patients enter the critical phase, a 48-hour period of increased vascular permeability. Most patients improve at this point and enter the convalescent phase. Some patients instead develop severe disease, heralded by persistent emesis, abdominal pain, altered consciousness, worsening thrombocytopenia, increasing hematocrit, and hemorrhage with progression to shock. Children are more likely than adults to develop plasma leakage and shock but less likely to develop major bleeding complications. Prior infection with any one dengue virus type predisposes to more severe disease from the remaining strains.

Initial diagnosis is often clinical. Serologic assays or detection of viral ribonucleic acid or antigen in the blood can confirm infection.

No specific antiviral treatments exist, and vaccines are not widely available. As a result, prevention with mosquito control and

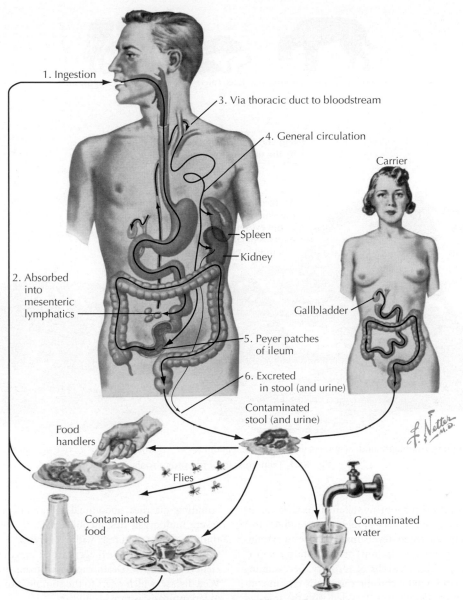

1. Ingestion

3. Via thoracic duct to bloodstream

4. General circulation

Carrier

Spleen

Kidney

2. Absorbed into mesenteric lymphatics

Gallbladder

5. Peyer patches of ileum

6. Excreted in stool (and urine)

Contaminated stool (and urine)

Food handlers

Flies

Contaminated food

Contaminated water

Fig. 84.3 Transmission of Enteric Fever

DEET-containing repellants is key. Supportive care focuses on hydration and avoidance of salicylates and nonsteroidal antiinflammatory drugs, which increase bleeding risk.

Enteric Fever (Typhoid and Paratyphoid Fever)

Enteric fever is caused by bacteremia with *Salmonella enterica* serovars Typhi or Paratyphi A, B, or C. Infection can be severe and potentially life-threatening. Young children are particularly vulnerable. In the United States, most cases occur in travelers returning from South Asia (Bangladesh, India, and Pakistan); infections have also been reported in travelers from the African continent and Southeast Asia. Transmission occurs through consumption of water or food contaminated by feces of either an infected person or a chronic, asymptomatic carrier (Fig. 84.3). The incubation period is typically 1 to 2 weeks but can be as long as 60 days.

Typhoid and paratyphoid infections are clinically indistinguishable febrile illnesses. Fevers tend to increase in a step-wise fashion before becoming sustained at 102.6°F to 105.1°F (39.2°C to 40.6°C). Additional symptoms include abdominal pain, diarrhea, and cough. Some children present with constipation and do not develop diarrhea until the second or third week of illness. Some children may have rose spots, transient maculopapular blanching lesions, on the trunk or legs. Hepatomegaly or splenomegaly can develop in the second week of illness. Children tend not to have the relative bradycardia seen in adults. Gastrointestinal bleeding or perforation occur rarely in children with severe or prolonged illness.

Diagnosis is made by obtaining a positive culture from blood, stool, or bone marrow. Stool cultures are often negative initially. Bone marrow cultures are the most sensitive but rarely performed because of their invasiveness. The Widal serology test should not be used given high rates of false positive results.

Oral and intramuscular typhoid vaccines exist but are not fully protective, so enteric fever should still be considered in those who received pre-travel vaccination. Frequent handwashing and safe food and water precautions can also help prevent disease.

Because of emerging antibiotic resistance, empiric treatment with azithromycin or intravenous ceftriaxone is recommended.

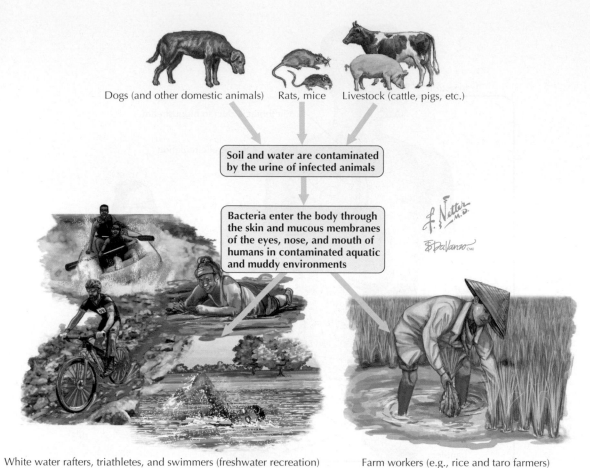

Dogs (and other domestic animals)   Rats, mice   Livestock (cattle, pigs, etc.)

Soil and water are contaminated by the urine of infected animals

Bacteria enter the body through the skin and mucous membranes of the eyes, nose, and mouth of humans in contaminated aquatic and muddy environments

White water rafters, triathletes, and swimmers (freshwater recreation)   Farm workers (e.g., rice and taro farmers)

Fig. 84.4 Transmission of Leptospirosis

Ciprofloxacin, amoxicillin, or trimethoprim-sulfamethoxazole can be used to treat susceptible infections. Fevers should improve after 3 to 5 days of antibiotic treatment. Persistent fevers may indicate an extraluminal infection (i.e., abscess or bone infection) or antibiotic resistance. Some patients may relapse within 4 weeks of recovery, necessitating additional antibiotics. Asymptomatic chronic carriage is rare in children. To limit disease spread, people who traveled with the infected patient should also have stool cultures performed and should receive treatment if positive.

Leptospirosis

Although a less common cause of fever in the returning child traveler, leptospirosis is one of the most widespread zoonoses. *Leptospira* species, the causative agent of leptospirosis, is a spirochete that infects many species of wild and domestic animals, including rodents, dogs, cats, and livestock. Rats are the main source of human infection. Infected animals shed spirochetes in their urine, and humans become infected through contact with contaminated soil or water when the spirochete enters open cuts in the skin, the conjunctiva, or mucous membranes (Fig. 84.4). As a result, people who come in contact with animals or undertake recreational activities involving freshwater lakes, rivers, or canals are most likely to develop infection. *Leptospira* occurs worldwide and is endemic in tropical regions. Infections are more common during times of flooding.

Most infections are asymptomatic or self-limited. Symptomatic patients typically present 5 to 14 days after exposure with an acute febrile illness with associated headache, photophobia, conjunctival suffusion, severe myalgias (usually in the calves and lower back), nausea,

vomiting, diarrhea, abdominal pain, and cough. Illness progresses to severe multiorgan dysfunction in 5% to 10% of cases. This second immune phase manifests with recurrence of fevers, aseptic meningitis, renal failure, hemorrhage, cardiac arrythmias, pulmonary insufficiency, and shock. Death can occur from multisystem organ failure. Weil disease, which refers to the combination of renal and liver failure in leptospirosis, is rare in children.

Lack of specific symptoms and laboratory findings makes early diagnosis difficult. Serologic testing performed on acute and convalescent samples provides the diagnosis. Confirmatory testing is available through the CDC. Culture is insensitive and requires long incubation times using special media. Because antibiotic therapy provides the greatest benefits early in infection, therapy should be initiated before definitive diagnosis. Intravenous penicillin or ceftriaxone is preferred for severe disease. Oral doxycycline can be given for mild disease. Treatment can lead to a Jarisch-Herxheimer reaction soon after initiation.

EVALUATION AND MANAGEMENT

Initial evaluation should focus on the standard assessment and appropriate resuscitation of a febrile child. Two routine laboratory tests, complete blood count (CBC) and blood culture, best predict the presence of a serious travel-related infection. For this reason, a CBC and blood culture should be obtained on every febrile returning traveler. Every febrile child returning from a malaria-endemic region should also have parasite smears and, if available, a rapid diagnostic test for malaria. Other laboratory tests, such as stool cultures, respiratory viral testing, lumbar puncture, or HIV testing, and imaging should be considered based on the child's history and clinical presentation. Diagnostic tests for specific infections of concern are listed in Table 84.1. Many of these specific laboratory tests are expensive and have limited performance with long turnaround times, so a routine battery of expansive testing is not recommended. Cases of diagnostic uncertainty or high suspicion for a serious infection may warrant hospital admission for further management in consultation with an infectious diseases specialist. Many travel-related infections are nationally notifiable diseases that should be reported to the local health department.

Families planning international travel benefit from pre-travel consultation with a pediatrician or infectious diseases specialist to help minimize the risk for infection during travel. The pre-travel visit, ideally performed at least 2 months before travel to allow time for immunizations, can be used to review food and water safety, update routine childhood immunizations, and provide destination-specific prevention such as typhoid vaccination and malaria chemoprophylaxis.

FUTURE DIRECTIONS

As globalization continues, children will remain at risk for febrile illnesses associated with travel. Vaccines in development show promise against dengue and malaria, and advances in insect control may limit the burden of vector-borne diseases. At the same time, emerging antimicrobial resistance presents a challenge for disease control worldwide.

SUGGESTED READINGS

Available online.

85

Tick-Borne Illness

Anna Costello and Sanjeev K. Swami

✳ CLINICAL VIGNETTE

An otherwise healthy 5-year-old girl presents to the emergency department for fever and rash. Her parents report daily fevers for 7 days. She subsequently developed a rash that started on her forearms and spread to the rest of her body. She reports headache, myalgias, and several episodes of emesis and diarrhea. Her parents noticed that she is becoming increasingly tired and is not acting like herself. Her family recently returned from a camping trip in Maine, and she attends an outdoor camp in New Jersey. She has no known tick bites and no other animal exposures.

On physical examination, she is febrile to 102.6°F (39.2°C) and is ill-appearing. She is very irritable and rolls around the bed, though she is able to follow commands. Her skin has red pinpoint papules and petechiae on her arms, legs, and torso. The rash is also present on her palms and soles. She has no lymphadenopathy or hepatosplenomegaly. Her complete metabolic panel shows a sodium of 131 mmol/L, a creatinine of 0.2 mg/dL, alanine aminotransferase (ALT) of 65 U/L, and aspartate aminotransferas (AST) of 82 U/L. Her complete blood count shows a white blood cell (WBC) count of 3.5 K/μL without bandemia, hemoglobin of 11.5 g/dL, and platelet count of 76 10^3/μL. Her C-reactive protein (CRP) is 17.6 mg/dL, and her erythrocyte sedimentation rate (ESR) is 35 mm/hr. On admission, she is started on vancomycin, ceftriaxone, and doxycycline. The following day, brain magnetic resonance imaging (MRI) is performed and is normal. A nontraumatic lumbar puncture shows a WBC count of 3 cells/μL. Blood cultures and cerebrospinal fluid (CSF) cultures grow no organisms. Several days later, Rocky Mountain spotted fever (RMSF) serologic result is positive, with an RMSF IgG of 1:64 and an IgM of 1:1024. She clinically improves and is discharged home with a diagnosis of RMSF to complete a 7-day course of doxycycline.

This patient's clinical presentation with fever, petechial rash, and altered mental status is highly concerning for meningitis or a tick-borne illness such as RMSF. This patient's laboratory findings were notable for hyponatremia, leukopenia, thrombocytopenia, and mild elevation of ALT/AST, which appropriately raised the clinician's suspicion for tick-borne illnesses. In addition to broad-spectrum antibiotics, the clinicians astutely started empiric treatment with doxycycline and did not await confirmatory testing to start therapy. It is also important to note that this patient's potential tick exposures were in New Jersey and Maine, which are not areas classically associated with RMSF. Clinicians must maintain a high level of suspicion for tick-borne illnesses as the geographic ranges in which these diseases are found have been expanding.

The incidence of tick-borne illnesses in the United States has been steadily rising. These illnesses can have a wide variety of clinical manifestations, including severe multisystem organ dysfunction. Of note, empiric broad-spectrum antibiotics used to cover bacterial diseases in critical illness do not provide adequate coverage of tick-borne infections. Thus, it is important that clinicians consider tick-borne causes in severe illness and treat empirically if necessary. Most patients who present with a tick-borne illness have no recollection of a tick bite; therefore clinicians must maintain a high index of suspicion for tick-borne illnesses.

DIAGNOSTIC CONSIDERATIONS

The clinical presentation of tick-borne illnesses vary, but fever, rash, and flu-like symptoms such as headache and myalgias are common. Serology is the most common method to diagnose tick-borne infections. While awaiting serologic testing, laboratory findings that are suggestive of these illnesses include hyponatremia, leukopenia, thrombocytopenia, and mild elevations of alanine aminotransferase (ALT) and aspartate aminotransferase (AST).

Lyme Disease
Etiology and Pathogenesis

Lyme disease is caused by *Borrelia burgdorferi*, a spirochete carried by the *Ixodes scapularis* or blacklegged tick (Fig. 85.1). It is the most common vector-borne illness in the United States, and cases are most commonly contracted in the Northeast, mid-Atlantic, and Upper Midwest. Peak infections occur in the summer months between May and September.

Clinical Presentation

The most common form of Lyme disease is early localized disease. In early localized disease, a rash called erythema migrans (EM) appears at the site of the tick bite. EM is classically an erythematous, targetoid or "bull's eye" rash that expands in size over several days (Fig. 85.2). However, the appearance of the rash can vary and can lack central clearing. The EM rash is often accompanied by flu-like symptoms such as fevers, headache, and myalgias. These symptoms typically occur about 7 to 14 days after a bite from an infected tick.

Some patients with Lyme disease never develop any signs or symptoms of early localized disease and may present with early disseminated disease. This occurs weeks to months after the infection was contracted. The most common manifestations are neurologic and include meningitis, cranial neuropathies, and radiculopathies. Cranial nerve 7 (CN VII) palsy is the most frequent neurologic complication of Lyme disease. Both unilateral and bilateral nerve palsies are seen. Cardiac complications, including atrioventricular block and myocarditis also can be seen. This is the rarest form of Lyme disease and affects less than 1% of patients. Patients with early disseminated Lyme can also present with multiple EM lesions. They may have systemic symptoms (fever, myalgias, arthralgias) in addition to the more specific signs and symptoms of Lyme disease.

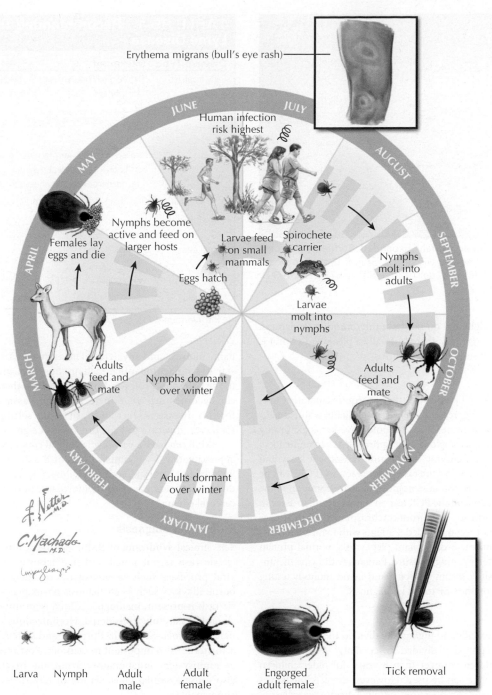

Erythema migrans (bull's eye rash)

Human infection risk highest

Nymphs become active and feed on larger hosts

Females lay eggs and die

Larvae feed on small mammals

Spirochete carrier

Eggs hatch

Nymphs molt into adults

Larvae molt into nymphs

Adults feed and mate

Nymphs dormant over winter

Adults feed and mate

Adults dormant over winter

Larva   Nymph   Adult male   Adult female   Engorged adult female

Tick removal

Fig. 85.1 Spirochetal Infections: Lyme Disease.

The late disseminated form of Lyme disease typically develops months to years after the infection was contracted. The most common late complication is Lyme arthritis. Lyme arthritis typically affects the larger joints, most commonly the knee. It usually is a monoarticular nonmigratory arthritis that classically manifests with a large effusion that is less painful than it appears.

After an episode of early localized Lyme disease, patients may not have lasting immunity and reinfection with Lyme disease is possible. This is rare in patients who develop later manifestations of Lyme disease. There is no evidence for a chronic form of Lyme disease, and there is no clinical indication for long-term antibiotic use after a Lyme infection.

Differential Diagnosis

The differential diagnosis for EM includes cellulitis, spider bite, viral exanthem, or urticaria multiforme. Lyme meningitis is similar in presentation to viral meningoencephalitis. Patients with Lyme meningitis are usually not as ill as those with bacterial meningitis. The CN VII palsy seen in Lyme disease can be misdiagnosed as Bell's palsy, which is an idiopathic CN VII palsy. The 7th nerve palsy caused by Lyme disease can be bilateral, which can help distinguish between the diagnoses. When a pediatric patient presents with Lyme arthritis, the differential includes septic arthritis, postviral arthritis, poststreptococcal arthritis, juvenile idiopathic arthritis, or other autoimmune processes. Lyme arthritis is typically much less painful than septic arthritis, and therefore patients

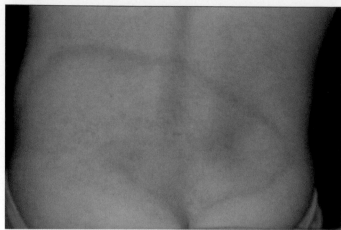

Fig. 85.2 Classic Targetoid Widely Expanded Erythema Migrans Rash. (From Stanek G, Wormser GP, Gray J, Strle F. Lyme borreliosis. *Lancet.* 2012;379(9814):461-473. doi:10.1016/S0140-6736(1160103-7). PMID: 21903253, Figure 4.)

TABLE 85.1	Recommended Treatment of Lyme Disease
Disease Type	**Treatment**
Early localized, erythema migrans	Amoxicillin 50 mg/kg/day PO, divided three times a day for 14 days *OR* Doxycycline 4.4 mg/kg/day PO, divided twice daily for 10 days
Arthritis	Oral agent as per early localized disease, for 28 days. If arthritis recurs, repeat a 28-day course (amoxicillin is recommended for patients younger than 8 years)
Atrioventricular block, carditis	Oral agent as per early localized disease, for 14–21 days *OR* Ceftriaxone 50–75 mg/kg IV, daily for 14–21 days
Meningitis	Doxycycline for 14–21 days *OR* Ceftriaxone 50–75 mg/kg IV, daily for 14–21 days
Facial palsy	Doxycycline for 14–21 days

IV, Intravenously *PO,* orally.

can usually still bear weight and do not have micromotion tenderness. If an arthrocentesis is performed, there is usually a pleocytosis, but it is rarely as dramatic as that seen in septic arthritis.

Evaluation

Cutaneous presentations of Lyme disease do not require laboratory testing, and patients should be treated empirically. Patients with extracutaneous manifestations of Lyme disease should have serologic testing performed. A two-tiered serologic testing approach is recommended. Clinicians should order an enzyme-linked immunosorbent assay and a confirmatory Western blot. Polymerase chain reaction (PCR) can be performed, but false positive and false negative tests are common in the serum. It is appropriate to send the PCR test on synovial fluid to assist in the diagnosis of Lyme arthritis. PCR from cerebrospinal fluid (CSF) has poor sensitivity and is not recommended. Patients with Lyme meningitis usually have a mononuclear predominant pleocytosis, normal protein and glucose, and elevated opening pressure. Patients with Lyme meningitis should have a positive serum serology, and Lyme antibody testing can also be performed on the CSF to aid in diagnosis.

Management

Treatment is with amoxicillin 50 mg/kg/day divided three times daily or doxycycline 4.4 mg/kg/day divided twice daily. Amoxicillin is recommended for children younger than 8 years; for older children amoxicillin or doxycycline can be used. However, doxycycline is recommended for neurologic complications of Lyme disease regardless of age. The duration of therapy varies based on the clinical manifestations as seen in Table 85.1.

Rocky Mountain Spotted Fever
Etiology and Pathogenesis

Rocky Mountain spotted fever (RMSF) is caused by *Rickettsia rickettsii*, an obligate intracellular gram-negative coccobacillus transmitted by the American dog tick, Rocky Mountain wood tick, and the brown dog tick. It targets the endothelial cells of blood vessels and causes a small-vessel vasculitis. *Rickettsia rickettsii* has now been found throughout the United States, though it is most common in the southeastern and south central regions. Almost all infections occur between April and September.

Clinical Presentation

Clinical symptoms of RMSF typically develop within 3 and 12 days of the tick bite. Early symptoms include fever, headache, abdominal pain, nausea, and myalgias. The rash tends to develop later and starts as a maculopapular rash on the wrists and ankles that spreads to the palms and soles and subsequently to the trunk (Fig. 83.1E). It can become purpuric or petechial. The classic clinical presentation for this disease is fever and rash in the setting of a tick exposure. However, it is rare to have this triad of signs at presentation.

RMSF can have a very severe clinical course with a mortality rate of approximately 5%. Complications of the disease are widespread and include shock physiology, renal failure, altered mental status, myocarditis, pulmonary edema or hemorrhage, intracranial hemorrhage, or cerebral edema.

Differential Diagnosis

The clinical syndrome of RMSF can be relatively nonspecific if the classic rash is not noted. Other diagnostic considerations include viral processes such as enterovirus or adenovirus and other tick-borne illnesses such as ehrlichiosis or anaplasmosis. When the classic rash is present, meningococcemia is an important mimicker that should be carefully considered. Noninfectious causes such as malignancy, Henoch-Schönlein Purpura, and systemic juvenile idiopathic arthritis are also important to consider. Postinfectious processes such as multisystem inflammatory syndrome in children (MIS-C) can also cause a similar constellation of rash, fever, and laboratory test abnormalities.

Evaluation

Diagnostic testing for RMSF is serologic. Often both acute and convalescent titers are required to make the diagnosis. A fourfold increase in titers is considered diagnostic. Serologic testing is often negative during the acute presentation. Therefore in the correct clinical context, treatment should be started while awaiting test results and continued even if acute serologies are negative. Other laboratory findings suggestive of RMSF include leukopenia, thrombocytopenia, hyponatremia, and an elevated ALT and AST. Some patients will present with a leukocytosis rather than leukopenia. An elevated creatinine is common. When CSF is obtained, a pleocytosis is often observed.

Management

Treatment is doxycycline 4.4 mg/kg divided twice daily for a minimum of 5 to 7 days or at least 2 to 3 days after the patient has defervesced. Patients should receive doxycycline regardless of age. The risk for teeth discoloration is very low with a short course of therapy. Chloramphenicol can be used in patients with a doxycycline allergy. If there is clinical concern for RMSF, doxycycline should be started urgently and clinicians should not await confirmatory testing.

Ehrlichiosis and Anaplasmosis
Etiology and Pathogenesis

Human monocytic ehrlichiosis (HME) is caused by *Ehrlichia chaffeensis*. This obligate intracellular gram-negative organism is transmitted by the lone star tick or the American dog tick, with deer serving as a reservoir. Human granulocytic anaplasmosis (HGA) is caused by *Anaplasma phagocytophilum*, also an obligate intracellular gram-negative organism but transmitted by *Ixodes scapularis* or *Ixodes pacificus*, with deer and white-footed mice serving as a reservoir. Because the *Ixodes* tick also carries other tick-borne illnesses, coinfection with Lyme disease or babesiosis is possible. Infections now can be seen throughout the United States, but HME is most common in the southeastern, south central, and northeastern United States. HGA is most commonly seen in the upper midwest and the northeast. Both infections are most commonly seen in the summer months.

Clinical Presentation

HME is associated with fever, rash, headache, myalgias, and anorexia. Gastrointestinal symptoms are common in children. The rash can be maculopapular or petechial. HGA manifests similarly with fever, headache, and myalgias. Rash is much less commonly noted.

Both illnesses can be very severe and lead to mortality. HME is more likely to cause severe complications, including renal failure, acute respiratory distress syndrome, coagulopathy, multisystem organ failure, meningoencephalitis, or hemophagocytic lymphohistiocytosis.

Both HME and HGA can also cause very mild disease, and serology studies in endemic regions suggest that many cases are never diagnosed because patients are likely asymptomatic or have very mild courses.

Differential Diagnosis

The clinical syndrome associated with ehrlichiosis includes rash, fever, and cytopenias. This constellation of findings also can be seen in numerous other infections, including viral processes such as enterovirus or Epstein-Barr virus. Other tick-borne illnesses such as RMSF are also important considerations. MIS-C can also manifest with hyponatremia, thrombocytopenia, rash, and fever and should be considered in the setting of the COVID-19 pandemic.

Evaluation

In both HME and HGA, elevated liver function tests, thrombocytopenia, and hyponatremia are seen. In HME, lymphopenia is characteristic, whereas in HGA, neutropenia is more likely. If CSF is obtained, a mild pleocytosis can be observed. Serologic testing is commonly used for diagnosis. Serologic testing results are often negative during the acute infection, and convalescent titers should be drawn 2 to 4 weeks after the illness to confirm the diagnosis. PCR testing is becoming more common and is a more reliable way of making a diagnosis during acute illness. However, PCR testing can have a negative result if it was performed after the initiation of antibiotic therapy.

Management

Treatment is doxycycline 4.4 mg/kg divided twice daily for a minimum of 5 to 7 days or at least 2 to 3 days after the patient has defervesced. Rifampin can be used in the setting of drug allergy or pregnancy. If there is high clinical concern for ehrlichiosis or anaplasmosis, doxycycline should be started urgently, and clinicians should not await confirmatory testing.

Other Tick-Borne Illnesses
Babesiosis

Babesiosis is caused by *Babesia microti*, a protozoan that targets erythrocytes. It is transmitted by *Ixodes scapularis* and can be seen as a coinfection with Lyme disease or anaplasmosis. Babesiosis is rare in pediatric patients, but, when seen, it can cause a clinical syndrome similar to malaria. It manifests with cyclic fevers, fatigue, headache, and myalgias. It can cause intravascular hemolysis leading to jaundice and anemia. It can be diagnosed on peripheral smear where *Babesia microti* rings are seen within erythrocytes. PCR testing also can be performed. Patients with babesiosis should be treated for 7 to 10 days with atovaquone plus azithromycin or clindamycin plus quinine.

Tularemia

Tularemia is caused by *Francisella tularensis*, a gram-negative coccobacillus that can be transmitted by several tick species in addition to other animal vectors such as rabbits. This illness is endemic to the south central United States. The ulceroglandular form of the disease is characterized by a pustular, ulcerated lesion that develops at the site of the tick bite. Patients can subsequently develop fever, headache, and regional lymphadenopathy. Antibody testing can be used to establish the diagnosis and patients can be treated with 7 to 10 days of streptomycin or gentamycin.

PREVENTION

Prevention of all tick-borne illnesses involves avoiding tick bites and removing any ticks as quickly as possible. Key steps in tick bite prevention include wearing long sleeves and long pants and using DEET-containing insect repellant when at risk for tick exposures.

FUTURE DIRECTIONS

With the increasing prevalence and larger geographic range of tick-borne illnesses, clinicians are likely to see more cases of tick-borne illness in pediatric patients. This will enable better powered studies to understand optimal antibiotic duration, disease complications, and other aspects of these illnesses. In addition, several new rickettsial species have been identified that cause disease. Further research is needed to better understand these emerging tick-borne pathogens.

SUGGESTED READINGS

Available online.

86

Human Immunodeficiency Virus

Elizabeth D. Lowenthal and Hannah R. Ford

 CLINICAL VIGNETTE

After receiving scant prenatal care, a woman vaginally delivers a healthy appearing infant. The mother's rapid human immunodeficiency virus (HIV) immunoassay result is positive, and her confirmatory HIV viral load is 10,000 copies/mL. The infant is given presumptive HIV therapy. Her mother is counseled on safe feeding practices. The mother and infant are discharged on antiretroviral therapy (ART) with close follow-up. HIV is detectable in the infant's blood from a sample taken shortly after birth and the baby's HIV viral load at the first outpatient follow-up visit is confirmed to be high. Her HIV viral load is suppressed below the limit of detection over her first few months of life. She is closely monitored as she ages, increasing antiretroviral doses as needed based on her growth. In addition to routine medical care, she and her family receive support and counseling for ART adherence and maintaining her health.

Worldwide, there are approximately 1.8 million children younger than 15 years of age infected with human immunodeficiency virus (HIV). Untreated HIV infection leads to a complex immunosuppressive state that increases the risk for serious morbidities and mortality. A few decades ago, the diagnosis of HIV was thought to be a death sentence. In contrast, children born with HIV today can grow into healthy adulthood with a manageable chronic infection. Children who are living with HIV require the long-term administration of antiretroviral therapy (ART). Effective ART must be combined with a holistic approach that considers the functioning and quality of life of the child and family.

PATHOGENESIS

HIV is a lentivirus that infects humans chronically, progressively damaging the hosts' immune systems. Two viral types have been characterized in humans: HIV type 1 (HIV-1) and HIV type 2 (HIV-2). Based on viral genetic sequences, HIV-1 isolates have been classified into three groups (M, N, and O). The majority of HIV-1 strains identified belong to group M ("major group"), which is further classified into a number of subtypes *(clades)* designated by letters A through K.

After entry into the human body, HIV begins its life cycle when it binds to CD4 receptors and one of two coreceptors (CCR5 or CXCR4) on CD4$^+$ T-lymphocytes and other receptor-containing cells and fuses with the host cell. The virus releases single-stranded viral RNA and three enzymes essential to its replication: reverse transcriptase, integrase, and protease. Reverse transcriptase is a "low-fidelity," or error-prone, enzyme that converts the single-stranded RNA into double-stranded deoxyribonucleic acid (DNA). On average, it inserts the "wrong" base into the growing complementary DNA (cDNA) chain at least every 4000 bases, producing mutated viral quasispecies. The existence of drug-resistant quasispecies often creates therapeutic challenges.

After reverse transcription, the double-stranded DNA enters the host cell's nucleus, where integrase facilitates its integration into the host DNA. The integrated HIV DNA is referred to as a *provirus* and can remain inactive for years. Activation of the cell induces transcription of proviral DNA into messenger ribonucleic acid (mRNA). The mRNA migrates into the cytoplasm, where viral proteins are produced by the host cell. Protease cleaves the large viral proteins into smaller pieces to create the infectious virus. Two viral RNA strands and the replication enzymes are then surrounded by a capsid of core proteins. The viral capsid acquires a glycopeptide-studded envelope during budding from the host cell. These HIV glycoproteins are necessary for the virus to bind to CD4 receptors and co-receptors. The process of viral replication leads to death of the host cell.

As many as 10 billion HIV virions are produced daily in a single human host. Untreated children typically have 10^3 to 10^6 virions per milliliter of plasma. The concentration of virus in lymph nodes is usually two to three orders of magnitude higher than in plasma. The amount of virus in the plasma is measured using quantitative HIV RNA polymerase chain reaction (PCR) tests, also called "viral loads." ART aims to halt HIV replication and reduce the viral load to undetectable levels.

CLINICAL MANIFESTATIONS OF HIV INFECTION

The process of HIV replication leads to depletion of CD4$^+$ T lymphocytes. The degree of immunologic suppression is classified based on the number and percent of CD4$^+$ T lymphocytes present in the bloodstream. Age-specific CD4$^+$ T lymphocyte count ranges are used to determine the degree of immune suppression. CD4$^+$ T lymphocyte percentages vary less with age and can be used instead of absolute counts to classify the degree of immune suppression in children living with HIV (Table 86.1).

Along with depletion of CD4$^+$ T lymphocytes, HIV infection leads to functional defects in existing CD4$^+$ T lymphocytes and defects in B cell function. These combined immunosuppressive processes lead to a wide variety of clinical manifestations. The most severe and common of these manifestations are outlined in Table 86.2. Opportunistic infections, cancers, hematologic aberrations, and other noninfectious manifestations are among the most severe acquired immunodeficiency syndrome (AIDS)-defining conditions.

TABLE 86.1   Immunologic Categorization Based on Age-Specific CD4⁺ T-Lymphocyte Counts and Percent of Total Lymphocytes

Immunologic Category	Age <1 Year	Age 1–5 Years	Age 6–12 Years
1: No evidence of suppression	≥1500 cells/μL	≥1000 cells/μL	≥500 cells/μL
	≥34%	≥30%	≥26%
2: Moderate suppression	750–1499 cells/μL	500–999 cells/μL	200–499 cells/μL
	26%-33%	22%-29%	14%-25%
3: Severe suppression	<750 cells/μL	<500 cells/μL	<200 cells/μL
	<26%	<22%	<14%

TABLE 86.2   Selected Clinical Manifestations of HIV Infection

Manifestation	Description
Severe Manifestations	
Pneumocystis jiroveci pneumonia	Definitive diagnosis via microscopy of induced sputum or BAL
Multiple or recurrent serious bacterial infections	Septicemia, pneumonia, meningitis, bone or joint infection, internal organ infections
Kaposi sarcoma	Characterized by pink or purple lesions on the skin and soft tissues; diagnosis confirmed with biopsy
Lymphoma	Cerebral or B cell non-Hodgkin lymphoma
Mycobacterial infections	Extrapulmonary mycobacterium tuberculosis infection and nontuberculous mycobacterial infections
HIV encephalopathy	Failure to attain or loss of developmental milestones or loss of intellectual ability, impaired brain growth, or acquired symmetric motor deficits lasting for >2 months without a cause other than HIV
HIV wasting syndrome	Unexplained severe wasting, stunting, or severe malnutrition not adequately responding to standard therapy
Severe herpes simplex infections	Bronchitis, pneumonitis, esophagitis (or mucocutaneous ulcer persisting >1 month)
Severe candidiasis	Esophageal or pulmonary (including bronchi and trachea)
Moderately Severe Manifestations	
Single episode of serious bacterial infection	Septicemia, pneumonia, meningitis, bone or joint infection, internal organ infections
Lymphoid interstitial pneumonitis	Definitive diagnosis by biopsy but characterized by chronic bilateral reticulonodular interstitial pulmonary infiltrates and hypoxemia
Recurrent or chronic diarrhea	Persistent ≥14 days
Anemia, neutropenia, or thrombocytopenia persisting ≥30 days	Anemia: hemoglobin <8 g/dL Neutropenia: ANC <1000 cells/mm³ Thrombocytopenia: platelets <100,000 cells/mm³
Herpes zoster	At least two distinct episodes or more than one dermatome
Herpes simplex virus	Recurrent stomatitis (more than two episodes in 1 year)
Complicated varicella	Disseminated or severe chickenpox
Candidiasis	Oropharyngeal lasting for longer than 2 months
Mild Manifestations	
Lymphadenopathy	≥0.5 cm at more than two sites
Recurrent or persistent upper respiratory tract infections	Including sinusitis or otitis media
Hepatosplenomegaly	Unexplained, persistent
Mucocutaneous lesions	Extensive wart virus infection, extensive molluscum contagiosum, popular pruritic eruptions, recurrent oral ulcers

ANC, Absolute neutrophil count; *BAL,* bronchoalveolar lavage.

DIAGNOSIS

Within 6 to 12 weeks of infection with HIV, people produce HIV-specific antibodies detectable by commercially available assays. Adults and children older than 18 months of age can be tested for HIV with antibody-based assays such as rapid HIV immunoassays ("rapid test" or enzyme immunoassay [EIA]) and enzyme-linked immunosorbent assay (ELISA) or with HIV-1/2 antigen/antibody immunoassays. A positive rapid test or ELISA result can be confirmed with a Western blot test. These antibody tests are positive in virtually all HIV-infected individuals after the first 3 months of infection. The period during which the person is HIV infected but does not have detectable antibodies is referred to as the *window period.* With the currently available antibody

TABLE 86.3   Expected Diagnostic Test Results for Children by Age

Diagnostic Test	HIV-Infected Infant	HIV-Exposed Uninfected Infant	Infected Adolescent During Window Period	Infected Adolescent After Window Period	HIV-Exposed Uninfected Adolescent
Antibody-based tests	Positive	Positive	Negative	Positive	Negative
DNA PCR	Positive	Negative	Positive	Positive	Negative
RNA PCR (viral load)	Positive (high viral load)	Negative	Positive (high viral load)	Positive	Negative

PCR, Polymerase chain reaction.

assays, antibodies to HIV are usually detectable by 4 to 6 weeks after infection. Combined antigen/antibody tests allow for detection earlier, usually by about 2 weeks after infection.

Infants born to mothers with HIV are considered to be HIV-exposed and need to undergo testing for HIV. HIV-exposed infants will have positive HIV antibody test results, even if the infants are not HIV-infected, because maternal anti-HIV immunoglobulin G (IgG) antibodies cross the placenta. On average, maternal antibodies to HIV persist for the first 9 to 18 months of life. Therefore virologic tests, most commonly HIV DNA PCR or HIV RNA PCR, are used to confirm the presence of HIV infection in infants who are younger than 12 months of age. Negative DNA or RNA PCR test results done at 1 month and 4 months of age can rule out HIV infection in perinatally HIV-exposed infants who are not breastfeeding. HIV viral culture and p24 antigen assays may also be done for diagnosis but are considered less sensitive and specific than RNA and DNA PCR tests. Early negative HIV virologic test results can be confirmed by obtaining a negative antibody-based test after 12 months of age.

Table 86.3 summarizes the expected results of HIV diagnostic tests for HIV-exposed and HIV-infected infants and adolescents. Children who have lost their maternal antibodies would have the same test results as adolescents in the same infection or exposure category.

TREATMENT

Before antiretroviral drugs were available, care for children with HIV focused on prevention and management of HIV-related complications and palliative care. When the first antiretroviral drugs became available in the early 1990s, significant clinical and immunologic benefits were seen. Combinations of at least three drugs from two different drug classes traditionally were recommended for HIV treatment to avoid the development of viral resistance. Some potent two-drug regimens have recently proven to provide durable viral suppression. Excellent adherence to appropriate ART regimens is necessary to sustain viral suppression, immunologic recovery, reduction in opportunistic infections and other disease manifestations, and improve survival.

Currently available ARTs target various points in the HIV life cycle (Fig. 86.1). The four main classes of antiretroviral drugs are nucleoside/nucleotide reverse transcriptase inhibitors (NRTIs), nonnucleoside reverse transcriptase inhibitors (NNRTIs), protease inhibitors (PIs), and integrase inhibitors (INSTI). NRTIs are drugs whose chemical structure is a modified version of a natural nucleoside or nucleotide and interfere with the action of reverse transcription by causing premature termination of the proviral DNA chain. NNRTIs are noncompetitive inhibitors of the HIV-1 reverse transcriptase that bind to the reverse transcriptase catalytic site. PIs block protease from cleaving HIV protein precursors, preventing formation of new infectious virions. INSTIs inhibit integration or proviral DNA into the human genome. Less commonly used antiretroviral drugs include drugs that inhibit viral fusion with the cell membrane and cell entry.

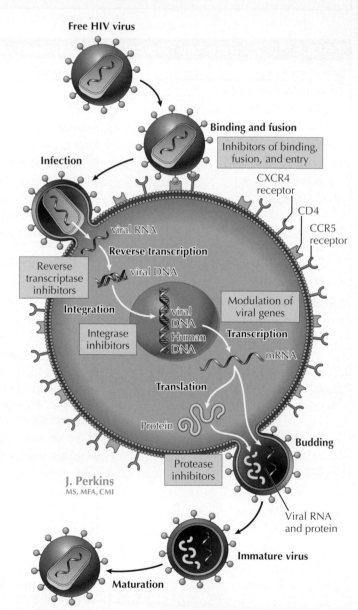

Fig. 86.1 Life Cycle of HIV and Targets of Antiretroviral Medications.

For antiretroviral-naïve children, ART consisting of two NRTIs plus either an INSTI, an NNRTI, or a PI two NRTIs is recommended. In the United States and other high-resource settings, therapy choices are usually guided by viral resistance testing. For adolescents, several single-tablet formulations that combine commonly used ART drugs simplify treatment adherence.

Table 86.4 describes key features of the antiretroviral medications used for treatment of children with HIV. To maintain

TABLE 86.4   Antiretroviral Medications Available for Children

	Pediatric Indication	Main Side Effects	Special Considerations
Nucleoside/Nucleotide Reverse Transcriptase Inhibitors (NRTI)			
Abacavir (ABC)	≥3 months	Potentially fatal hypersensitivity reaction in ≈5% of people	Genetic testing (HLA B*5701) for susceptibility to hypersensitivity is available.
Didanosine (ddI)	Yes (now rarely used)	Lipoatrophy, peripheral neuropathy, lactic acidosis	Delayed-release formulation allows for once-daily dosing in older children. Other formulation must be given on an empty stomach.
Emtricitabine (FTC)	Yes	Relatively well tolerated	Also active against hepatitis B. Should not be given with 3TC.
Lamivudine (3TC)	Yes	Relatively well tolerated	Also active against hepatitis B. Should not be given with FTC.
Stavudine (d4T)	Yes (now rarely used)	Lipoatrophy, peripheral neuropathy, hyperlipidemia, lactic acidosis	Should not be given with AZT because of antagonism. Should not be given with ddI because of overlapping side effects.
Tenofovir Disoproxil fumarate (TDF)	≥2 years	Reduced bone mineral density, nephrotoxicity	Also active against hepatitis B (nucleotide analog; NRTI).
Tenofovir Alafenomide (TAF)	≥25 kg	Better side effect profile than TDF	Also active against hepatitis B (nucleotide analog; NRTI).
Zidovudine (AZT)	Yes	Bone marrow suppression	Given to infants to help prevent MTCT of HIV.
Non-Nucleoside Reverse Transcriptase Inhibitors (NNRTI)			
Efavirenz (EFV)	≥3 years	Neuropsychiatric side effects are common	Prior concerns about potential teratogenicity have not been supported by large studies.
Etravirine (ETR)	≥2 years	Hepatoxicity, GI distress; potentially severe rashes or Stevens-Johnson syndrome	Must be taken with food.
Nevirapine (NVP)	Yes	Hepatoxicity; potentially severe rashes or Stevens-Johnson syndrome	Long half-life and single-point mutation causes high-level resistance to this and EFV.
Rilpivirine (RPV)	≥12 years	Hepatoxicity, depression, rash	Combined with DTG to make an effective two-drug regimen. Long-acting injectable formulation is being studied.
Protease Inhibitors (PI)			
Atazanavir (ATV)	≥3 months	Indirect hyperbilirubinemia, prolonged PR interval	Commonly administered with low-dose ritonavir to boost doses.
Darunavir (DRV)	≥3 years	May cause less GI distress than other PIs	Sometimes used in children with highly resistant virus. May maintain activity when resistance to other PIs has occurred.
Lopinavir/ritonavir (LPV/r)	≥2 weeks	GI distress	Lopinavir and ritonavir are co-formulated as a single liquid or tablet.
Fusion Inhibitor			
Enfuvirtide (T-20, fusion)	Yes	Local injection site reactions	Subcutaneous injections. Rarely used.
CCR5 Receptor Blocker			
Maraviroc (MVC)	Yes	Nausea, vomiting, hepatotoxicity	Need to do a Trofile assay prior to using – for use in CCR5-trophic virus only.
Integrase Inhibitor (INSTI)			
Bictegravir	≥6 years; ≥25 kg	Diarrhea, nausea, headache	Adult dosing recommended when minimum age and weight requirements reached
Dolutegravir (DTG)	≥4 weeks	May increase depressive symptoms	Recommended first-line therapy for people with high baseline viral loads
Raltegravir (RAL)	Yes	GI distress, headache	Frequent dose changes needed in infancy because of rapid changes in metabolism

GI, Gastrointestinal; *HLA*, human leukocyte antigen; *MTCT*, mother-to-child transmission.

TABLE 86.5	**Primary Prophylaxis of Opportunistic Infection in HIV**	
Infection	**Indications for Prophylaxis**	**Prevention Strategy**
Pneumocystis jiroveci pneumonia	<1 year: HIV infection or HIV exposure with uncertain HIV infection status 2–5 years: CD4 <500 cells/μL or <15% >5 years: CD4 <200 cells/μL or <15%	TMP-SMX daily (dapsone or pentamidine are alternative regimens)
Tuberculosis	Positive TB skin test result (≥5 mm) and no evidence of active TB disease	Isoniazid daily for 9 months (potential for drug-drug interactions between rifamycin regimens and ART)
Mycobacterium avium complex	<1 years: CD4 <750 cells/μL 1–2 years: CD4 <500 cells/μL 2–5 years: CD4 <75 cells/μL ≥6 years: CD4 <50 cells/μL	Azithromycin given weekly
Vaccine-preventable illnesses	All children with HIV	All routine recommended childhood immunizations; additional pneumococcal vaccinations added to routine childhood schedule; defer live vaccines (varicella and MMR) if CD4 <15% or <200

ART, Antiretroviral therapy; *MMR,* mumps, measles, and rubella; *TB,* tuberculosis; *TMP-SMX,* trimethoprim-sulfamethoxazole.

long-term effectiveness, these drugs must be given in appropriate combinations and adherence to therapy must be excellent. Adherence is sometimes complicated by drug side effects. The PIs often cause gastrointestinal distress, particularly early in therapy, that makes medication tolerance challenging. Many of the drugs commonly used in the past have significant long-term effects, including hyperlipidemia, body habitus changes, and peripheral neuropathy. Newer drug options have better tolerability and side effect profiles, but many available antiretroviral drugs do not have pediatric formulations or studies to guide dosing of the smallest children. Careful monitoring by physicians who are experienced in the treatment of HIV allows for early detection of problems and appropriate adjustment of regimens to help ensure long-term therapeutic success.

For children with severe HIV-related immunosuppression, prophylactic medications should also be given to help prevent opportunistic infections. Common infections in children without HIV are also seen in children with HIV but frequently are more severe. Therefore routine vaccination of HIV-infected children is essential. Table 86.5 outlines recommended strategies for primary prevention of infectious complications in children with HIV. After treatment of an opportunistic infection, long-term secondary prophylaxis is often given to prevent recurrence of disease, regardless of immunologic recovery.

Comprehensive care of children living with HIV must include psychosocial support to facilitate excellent lifelong adherence to therapy and overall health. Age-appropriate counseling regarding the child's HIV status and strategies to maintain health are essential. Counseling and support must be extended to the child's entire family to ensure that the child's environment will support medication adherence and help the child achieve his or her life goals.

PREVENTION

One of the greatest successes in HIV medicine has been the development of therapies to prevent the mother-to-child transmission (MTCT) of HIV. Without intervention, approximately 40% of infants born to breastfeeding women who are living with HIV will be infected with HIV. When comprehensive preventive methods are adopted, the MTCT risk can be reduced to less than 1%.

Prevention of HIV infection in neonates begins with early identification of HIV infection in pregnant women. HIV testing during the first prenatal visit should be part of routine prenatal care. This allows for early initiation (<28 weeks of gestation) of ART. Repeat HIV testing during the third trimester is recommended in many settings because a mother's acquisition of HIV during pregnancy puts the child at especially high risk for peripartum infection. After delivery, perinatally HIV-exposed babies typically are given zidovudine (AZT) for prophylaxis. Additional antiretroviral drugs are given to the infant when the risk for perinatal infection is considered high (e.g., when the mother received no preventive therapy before delivery).

For women who are living with HIV who do not have an undetectable viral load at the time of delivery, a number of nonpharmacologic interventions have proven to be valuable for the prevention of MTCT. Avoiding instrumentation (e.g., forceps and fetal scalp monitors) during deliveries decreases MTCT risk. Cesarean section deliveries are recommended when the maternal HIV viral load is greater than 1000 copies/mL at the time of delivery and resources are available for safe cesarean sections. Treating other sexually transmitted diseases (e.g., active herpes lesions) also decreases HIV transmission risk. Breastfeeding is another important mode of HIV transmission. Infants born to women living with HIV are usually recommended to formula feed in settings such as the United States when it can be made affordable, feasible, accessible, safe, and sustainable. However, a nonjudgmental approach to parental education and feeding choices is important so that ongoing strategies to minimize the risk of infection through breastfeeding can be implemented when parents choose to breastfeed.

Prevention of new HIV infections among adolescents is also a challenge in pediatrics. Although abstinence is a sure way to avoid sexual transmission of HIV, abstinence-only education has proven to be an unsuccessful preventive approach. The consistent use of condoms is important for avoiding the spread of HIV and other sexually transmitted diseases among sexually active individuals. Preexposure prophylaxis (PrEP) with antiretrovirals can greatly decrease the risk for transmission in adolescents engaging in risky sexual behavior or using injection drugs. Male circumcision has also proven to be useful for decreasing the risk for HIV transmission.

SUMMARY

HIV is a major cause of pediatric morbidity and mortality worldwide. Available therapies allow children who are born with HIV to maintain their health well into adulthood. Effective strategies for the prevention of MTCT of HIV are also available. Unfortunately, these prevention strategies are not yet reaching many women living with HIV worldwide. Preventive measures for adolescents at risk for acquiring HIV are also not available for or used by a large proportion of those who need them. Thus new pediatric HIV infections are still common.

FUTURE DIRECTIONS

A great deal of work needs to be done to expand prevention and treatment options in low-resource settings where the HIV prevalence is highest. New antiretroviral drugs and pediatric formulations of existing drugs are being developed to make long-term effective treatment easier to tolerate. Vaccine development is also a key area of research. The rapid mutation of HIV and its skill at evading antibodies and other immune responses makes it a particularly difficult target for preventive vaccines. Many researchers are also trying to create therapeutic vaccines that would improve the body's ability to fight HIV, augmenting currently available ARTs for individuals already infected with the virus.

SUGGESTED READINGS

Available online.

87

Tuberculosis

Hannah K. Mitchell and Torsten A. Joerger

 CLINICAL VIGNETTE

A 4-year-old girl is seen in clinic for a well-child examination and you examine her growth curve. At 2 years of age she was 50th percentile for weight, but her growth chart today shows she has only gained 1 kg and is now 10th percentile for her weight. On further questioning, her mother also thinks that she has felt warm most days over the last several months, although they do not have a thermometer at home. She also reports they had been living in a homeless shelter until 3 months ago. Her initial vital signs show she is febrile to 101.3°F (38.5°C) and tachycardic to 120 beats/min, with a normal blood pressure. On examination she has reduced breath sounds at her right lung base. On evaluation, a complete blood count shows a mild anemia to 10.5 g/dL and chest radiograph shows right sided hilar enlargement with atelectasis of the right lower lobe. An interferon-γ (IFN-γ) release assay is ordered. She does not have a productive cough, so she is admitted to the hospital, and three samples of early morning gastric aspirates are sent for smear, culture, and GeneXpert. The IFN-γ release assay is positive. The GeneXpert is positive for TB but negative for rifampin resistance. Given her fever, weight loss, and chest radiograph findings, you diagnose active pulmonary tuberculosis. You initiate the child on rifampin, isoniazid, pyrazinamide, and ethambutol after getting vision screening and a human immunodeficiency virus (HIV) test, and you report the diagnosis to the local public health department.

Always consider a diagnosis of TB in the child who has a history of failure to thrive, chronic cough, and fevers. All cases of confirmed or suspected TB should be reported to the local public health department. Children are frequently infected by adult family members, and additional cases of TB can often be identified through contact tracing.

Tuberculosis (TB) refers to the spectrum of illness caused by the organism *Mycobacterium tuberculosis*. TB is a common illness globally with a quarter to a third of the world's population estimated to be infected. The World Health Organization estimates that annually there are 1.5 million deaths from TB, including over 200,000 deaths in children. Pediatric cases are likely to be underreported given challenges in obtaining appropriate testing in children. It is estimated that only 35% of pediatric cases are actually reported.

TB has become much less common in high-resource countries over the last century with advances in socioeconomic conditions, public health, and the introduction of drugs treating TB in the 1940s. The United States has a lower incidence and prevalence of TB compared with many other countries. According to the Centers for Disease Control and Prevention there are up to 13 million people living with latent TB infection in the United States. In 2018 there were 9000 cases of TB reported in the United States, and 4% of these were in children under the age of 15. Among the entire population, the majority of cases of tuberculosis in the United States occur in foreign-born individuals; however, among children, only 25% of cases occur in children born outside of the United States.

ETIOLOGY AND PATHOGENESIS

TB is caused by *M. tuberculosis*, a slow-growing bacillus. *M. tuberculosis* is described as being "acid fast." This refers to the ability of the bacteria to retain the stain of arylmethane dyes after treatment with mineral acid or acid alcohol solution. This leads to its characteristic appearance under a microscope (Fig. 87.1).

Manifestations of TB can be broken down into exposure, infection, and disease. Contact with a person with active pulmonary TB leads to exposure through respiratory droplets or by direct contact. Infection occurs after mycobacteria are inhaled and survive in lung and hilar lymph nodes. The typical incubation period from exposure to infection is 3 weeks to 3 months. Patients infected with the mycobacterium can develop either overt disease or latent infection with no symptoms.

Patients who have latent infection will be asymptomatic, and the only evidence that they are infected with the disease is a positive tuberculin skin test (TST) or interferon-γ (IFN-γ) release assay (IGRA). The typical time from exposure to TB to a positive TST or IGRA is 2 to 10 weeks.

A primary complex can form where the *M. tuberculosis* bacteria enter the body. The bacteria initially multiply in the alveoli and are then taken up by macrophages; some of the bacteria survive intracellularly and then spread to local lymph nodes. These foci of infection become encapsulated with the bacteria inside surviving intracellularly for many years. The typical appearance of tissue infected with TB is of granulomatous inflammation with a caseating "cheese-like" necrosis in the center.

Latent infection with *M. tuberculosis* can progress to overt disease. In immunocompetent adults, 5% to 10% of untreated TB infections will progress to active disease; this risk is much higher in younger children, with around 40% of infants with latent infections progressing to clinical disease. In contrast to adults, children have a higher chance of having extrapulmonary disease, with around one-quarter of cases in children being extrapulmonary.

An immunodeficient state, for example, human immunodeficiency virus (HIV) infection, increases susceptibility to TB and increases the rate of progression from latent to active TB. Around one-eighth of TB cases globally are thought to be in HIV-positive people.

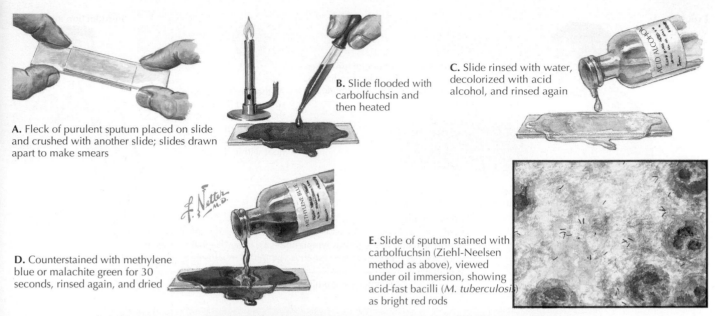

A. Fleck of purulent sputum placed on slide and crushed with another slide; slides drawn apart to make smears

B. Slide flooded with carbolfuchsin and then heated

C. Slide rinsed with water, decolorized with acid alcohol, and rinsed again

D. Counterstained with methylene blue or malachite green for 30 seconds, rinsed again, and dried

E. Slide of sputum stained with carbolfuchsin (Ziehl-Neelsen method as above), viewed under oil immersion, showing acid-fast bacilli (*M. tuberculosis*) as bright red rods

Fig. 87.1 Staining of *Mycobacterium tuberculosis* Specimens.

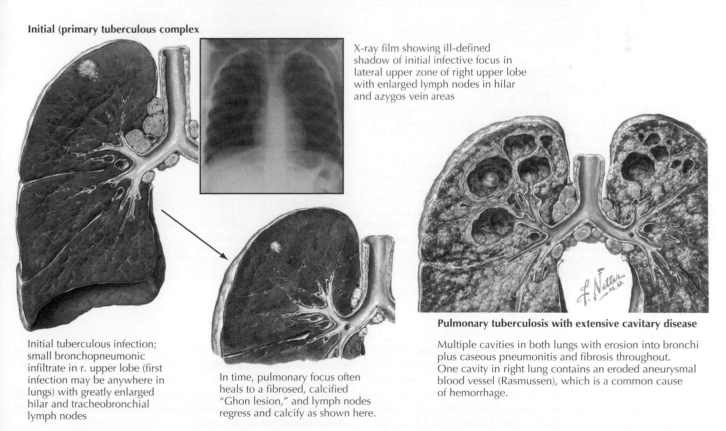

Initial (primary tuberculous complex

X-ray film showing ill-defined shadow of initial infective focus in lateral upper zone of right upper lobe with enlarged lymph nodes in hilar and azygos vein areas

Initial tuberculous infection; small bronchopneumonic infiltrate in r. upper lobe (first infection may be anywhere in lungs) with greatly enlarged hilar and tracheobronchial lymph nodes

In time, pulmonary focus often heals to a fibrosed, calcified "Ghon lesion," and lymph nodes regress and calcify as shown here.

Pulmonary tuberculosis with extensive cavitary disease

Multiple cavities in both lungs with erosion into bronchi plus caseous pneumonitis and fibrosis throughout. One cavity in right lung contains an eroded aneurysmal blood vessel (Rasmussen), which is a common cause of hemorrhage.

Fig. 87.2 Appearance of Lungs in Tuberculosis.

CLINICAL PRESENTATION

TB can manifest in a variety of different ways in children. Approximately 75% of cases of *M. tuberculosis* disease are pulmonary (Fig. 87.2). Extrapulmonary sites of infection include lymph nodes, pleura, central nervous system (CNS), kidney, eye, skin, vertebrae, joint, bone, abdomen, and pericardium.

Pulmonary TB can be difficult to distinguish from other pulmonary diseases. The classic manifestation will be with fever, cough, and weight loss or delayed growth. Children can have systemic symptoms such as fatigue, malaise, and poor appetite. On physical examination, children may have focal lung findings, for example, crackles, wheeze, or reduced air entry to affected parts of the lung.

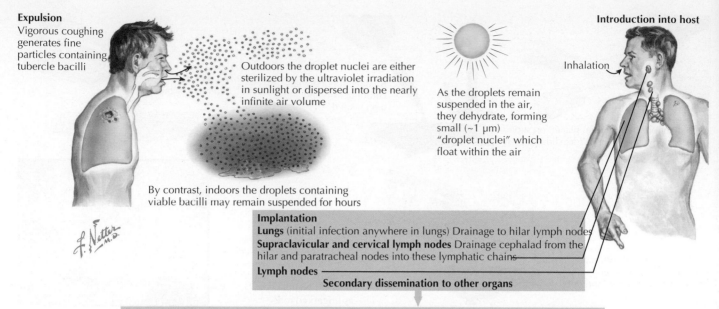

Expulsion
Vigorous coughing generates fine particles containing tubercle bacilli

Outdoors the droplet nuclei are either sterilized by the ultraviolet irradiation in sunlight or dispersed into the nearly infinite air volume

By contrast, indoors the droplets containing viable bacilli may remain suspended for hours

As the droplets remain suspended in the air, they dehydrate, forming small (~1 μm) "droplet nuclei" which float within the air

Introduction into host
Inhalation

Implantation
Lungs (initial infection anywhere in lungs) Drainage to hilar lymph nodes
Supraclavicular and cervical lymph nodes Drainage cephalad from the hilar and paratracheal nodes into these lymphatic chains
Lymph nodes
Secondary dissemination to other organs

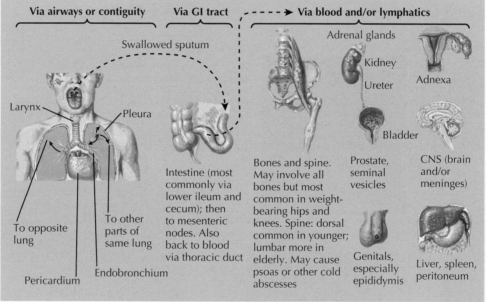

Via airways or contiguity   **Via GI tract**   **Via blood and/or lymphatics**

Swallowed sputum

Larynx
Pleura
To opposite lung
To other parts of same lung
Pericardium
Endobronchium

Intestine (most commonly via lower ileum and cecum); then to mesenteric nodes. Also back to blood via thoracic duct

Adrenal glands
Kidney
Ureter
Adnexa
Bladder

Bones and spine. May involve all bones but most common in weight-bearing hips and knees. Spine: dorsal common in younger; lumbar more in elderly. May cause psoas or other cold abscesses

Prostate, seminal vesicles

CNS (brain and/or meninges)

Genitals, especially epididymis

Liver, spleen, peritoneum

Fig. 87.3 Extrapulmonary Spread of Tuberculosis.

The most common extrapulmonary site for *M. tuberculosis* disease in children is in the lymph nodes. This will typically manifest with an enlarged lymph node, most commonly in the neck. The enlarged lymph nodes are usually unilateral. The node can slowly enlarge over a period of months. On examination a firm, mobile, nontender nodule can be found, with or without induration of overlying skin. Sometimes ulceration of the overlying skin can occur.

CNS disease includes tuberculous meningitis, brain abscess, or tuberculoma. Symptoms are usually gradual in onset. The initial symptoms may be subtle with irritability and mild systemic symptoms. Following this, symptoms of raised intracranial pressure and cerebral vasculitis occur, with altered mental status, neck stiffness, vomiting, convulsions, and cranial nerve palsies (typically CN III, VI, and VII). Finally, illness may progress to coma with unstable vital signs.

In pleural disease, children may present with pleuritic chest pain, dyspnea, and fever and have signs of a pleural effusion (reduced air entry and dullness to percussion) on examination. In pericardial

disease, children may present with systemic symptoms such as fever or weight loss. An echocardiogram or electrocardiogram may show evidence of pericarditis.

The most commonly affected bones in *M. tuberculosis* infection are the vertebrae. Patients may complain of pain that is worse at night, and gibbus deformity may be present.

Miliary disease occurs when there is wide dissemination of *M. tuberculosis* in the body by the bloodstream. The presentation of miliary disease can vary from an asymptomatic patient found by contact tracing to severe onset. Patients may have systemic symptoms, tachypnea, fatigue, and features of CNS TB. Chest radiography will show evidence of disseminated disease (Fig. 87.3).

Congenital TB infection is uncommon but can occur through lymphohematogenous spread or through infected endometrium.

Children are most commonly infected after exposure to a household contact with TB. Additional risk factors for TB include:
• Being born in a high TB prevalence area
• Having a parent who is born in a high TB prevalence country

TABLE 87.1	Differential Diagnosis of *Mycobacterium tuberculosis* Disease	
Pulmonary tuberculosis		Bacterial, viral, or fungal pneumonia, bronchiectasis, primary or secondary lung malignancy, sarcoidosis, pulmonary infarct, congenital cyst
Extrapulmonary tuberculosis	Lymph node	Bartonella, brucellosis, toxoplasmosis, bacterial lymphadenitis, lymphoma, sarcoid, nontuberculous mycobacterium, branchial cleft cyst, cystic hygroma
	Pleura	Malignancy, heart failure, renal failure, parapneumonic effusion, empyema
	Meninges	Bacterial meningitis, fungal meningitis, viral meningitis, encephalitis, space occupying lesion
	Joint/bone	Bacterial osteomyelitis, rheumatoid arthritis, malignancy, avascular necrosis

- Living in a high TB prevalence area for more than 2 months
- Contact with residents of prisons, nursing homes, and homeless shelters
- History of residence in a homeless shelter

DIFFERENTIAL DIAGNOSIS

See Table 87.1.

EVALUATION AND MANAGEMENT

TB is challenging to diagnose in children and a microbiologic diagnosis is ultimately obtained in a minority of children; negative cultures do not rule out a diagnosis of TB. Clinical examination and imaging are important parts of making a diagnosis of TB. It often can be hard to obtain samples to send for culture in children if they cannot expectorate sputum.

Diagnostic workup should begin with a screening test for children with risk factors for infection with *M. tuberculosis* and then pursuing microbiologic tests and imaging to make a definitive diagnosis.

Screening

TST and IGRA are the two most commonly available screening tests. The TST involves injecting a purified protein derivative of TB (antigen) intradermally. The skin is examined 48 to 72 hours later for evidence of reaction, with induration being indicative of TB infection (Fig. 87.4). Interpretation of TST results depends on epidemiologic and clinical risk factors.

The TST may be falsely positive if the child has a nontuberculous mycobacterium or has previously had the bacillus Calmette-Guérin (BCG) immunization. It cannot distinguish between latent and current infection and there is a high false negative rate.

IGRA is as sensitive as TST but more specific. The IGRA involves taking a blood sample that is then tested for IFN-γ production by T lymphocytes in response to *M. tuberculosis* antigens. It is not falsely positive with BCG vaccination. If both tests are available, IGRA should be used as the first line except in children younger than 2 years. TST is an acceptable alternative if IGRA is not available. Both tests can be performed simultaneously to increase sensitivity. It is important to note that if there is strong suspicion for TB, a negative TST or IGRA does not rule out infection.

Children with HIV are at substantially higher risk for being infected with TB and should be screened annually. Children who have had an organ transplant have a higher risk for TB. Screening for TB is often done before initiating certain immunosuppressive medications such as tumor necrosis factor-α inhibitors.

Microbiologic Tests

In suspected TB disease, microbiologic samples should be sent. If a child is able to expectorate, a sputum sample can be sent. For children who are not able to produce a sputum sample, early morning

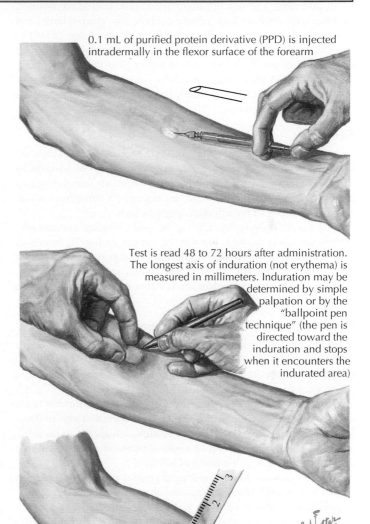

0.1 mL of purified protein derivative (PPD) is injected intradermally in the flexor surface of the forearm

Test is read 48 to 72 hours after administration. The longest axis of induration (not erythema) is measured in millimeters. Induration may be determined by simple palpation or by the "ballpoint pen technique" (the pen is directed toward the induration and stops when it encounters the indurated area)

Diameter of marked indurated area measured in transverse plane.
Reactions 5 mm or greater are considered positive in children suspected to have TB disease or who are immunosuppressed. Reactions 10 mm or greater are considered positive in children at increased risk of disease, and 15 mm or greater in children without any risk factors. Less than 5 mm of induration is regarded as negative

Fig. 87.4 Tuberculin Skin Test.

gastric aspirates obtained from a nasogastric tube or an induced sputum sample should be obtained. For suspected TB meningitis, a sample of cerebrospinal fluid (CSF) should be sent for culture. Of note, other characteristic CSF features of TB meningitis include elevated protein, decreased glucose, and moderately elevated CSF lymphocytes. Tissue samples from biopsy of the area of concern (e.g., lymph node) can also be obtained. Initially microscopy is done looking for acid-fast bacilli, and then the sample is cultured. *M. tuberculosis* is a slow growing organism, so positive cultures may take 3 to 6 weeks to give a result. Examination of three samples can improve sensitivity. Molecular diagnostic tools such as nucleic acid amplification tests (e.g., GeneXpert) are becoming more widely available and can be used in conjunction with culture to accelerate diagnosis, increase sensitivity, and detect rifampin resistance.

In cases with a pleural effusion, pleural fluid should be obtained. Samples typically have high protein content, low glucose levels, and elevated white cell counts. Elevated adenosine deaminase (ADA) in pleural or pericardial fluid is suggestive of TB. Pathologic examination and culture of the pleural lining is of higher yield than pleural fluid. The role of ADA levels, urine mycobacterial cell wall glycolipid lipoarabinomannan (urine LAM assay), and detection of TB in stool are currently being investigated.

Radiology

Imaging can increase suspicion for TB if characteristic findings are present. On chest radiograph, a primary complex or hilar adenopathy may be seen. In miliary TB, multiple small lesions are seen throughout the lung fields. Less specific signs, for example, a consolidation that does not improve with antibiotics, might be seen.

Computed tomography (CT) can be used to further evaluate adenopathy or chest findings, but this should not be used to screen an asymptomatic child. Neuroimaging can be important in suspected CNS infection and may show tuberculomas, infarction, or hydrocephalus. Basal ganglia involvement is a characteristic finding of CNS infection.

Other Laboratory Tests and Management

Workup for underlying susceptibility to TB infection, for example HIV testing, also should be performed. TB drugs are associated with high toxicity rates. Baseline assessment of liver and renal function and vision assessment is recommended.

Management differs depending on whether the patient has latent tuberculosis or active tuberculosis disease. Consultation with an infectious disease specialist or referral to a TB clinic is highly recommended. Latent TB can be treated with 12 weeks of isoniazid and rifapentine, 4 months of rifampin, or 9 months of isoniazid.

For tuberculosis disease, prolonged courses of quadruple therapy (typically isoniazid, rifampin, ethambutol, and pyrazinamide) are used. Typically, 6 months of rifampin and isoniazid are used with pyrazinamide and ethambutol used for the first 2 months. Treatment courses are longer for extrapulmonary disease. For multidrug-resistant (MDR) or extensively drug-resistant (XDR) TB, second-line therapies include fluoroquinolones. Multidrug-resistant TB was first described in the 1990s and is prevalent in areas with poor TB treatment infrastructure.

Tuberculosis drugs are associated with toxicity:

- Isoniazid—peripheral neuritis and hepatitis
- Rifampicin—leukopenia and thrombocytopenia, hepatitis
- Pyrazinamide—hepatotoxicity, gastrointestinal upset
- Ethambutol—optic neuritis, decreased red-green color discrimination

Therapeutic drug monitoring may be warranted in children with severe disease or concerns about drug metabolism.

Adjunctive treatment with corticosteroids in tuberculous meningitis is recommended because it reduces mortality and neurologic impairment after infection. Patients can still receive immunizations while being treated for TB unless they have other contraindications. Optimization of a child's nutritional status is also essential.

Typically, young children do not transmit TB. Transmission can occur in older adolescents and young adults who can forcefully cough and often have more adult-type disease with cavities. These patients should be placed under airborne precautions. Patients are unlikely to transmit TB after several weeks of appropriate antimicrobials. Documentation of negative cultures is also reassuring.

The course of treatment for TB is long, and supporting families with medication adherence, such as through directly observed therapy (DOT), is an important part of management. Reduced rates of relapse, treatment failure, and drug resistance are seen with DOT.

Public health measures are essential in management of TB, and contact tracing should be done to look for the likely source case of the child's TB. In the United States, all cases of TB must be reported.

Treating children with HIV and active TB is challenging and should be undertaken only by a provider experienced with these diseases. Issues include interactions with HIV and TB medications and immune reconstitution inflammatory syndrome. Mortality from TB in HIV-positive children is high and increases with decreasing CD4 count.

FUTURE DIRECTIONS

Even in high-resource settings, the majority of children do not obtain a microbiologic diagnosis. Difficulty with diagnosis has important implications in the management of TB. This also makes it challenging to accurately estimate the true prevalence of TB. Advancing diagnostics is central to the future of TB research.

Only three new drugs have been approved by the US Food and Drug Administration for TB between 1980 and 2020. Multidrug-resistant TB is becoming increasingly problematic worldwide, making drug development a priority for TB research.

The BCG vaccine was developed in the 1920s and is not routinely given to children in the United States. It has a protective effect of around 70% against the most severe forms of TB. Development of a more effective vaccine would be instrumental in reducing the global burden of TB.

SUGGESTED READINGS

Available online.

88

Viral Infections

Bryn Carroll and Yasaman Fatemi

✳ CLINICAL VIGNETTE

An 18-month old girl presents to the pediatrician with 3 days of fever associated with a runny nose, decreased appetite, and fatigue. She has also developed a rash on her chest. She has no chronic conditions and is up-to-date on vaccinations.

On examination, the child is febrile to 101.5°F (38.6°C) and tired-appearing. Her examination is notable for minimal clear rhinorrhea, shotty cervical lymphadenopathy, and an erythematous macular rash on her trunk. She is well-perfused without respiratory distress, hepatosplenomegaly, petechiae, or purpura.

This child's presentation encompasses some of the nonspecific features that characterize many of the common viral infections in childhood. A careful history and detailed physical examination can reveal distinguishing characteristics. In many cases, diagnosis of a viral infection can be made clinically without the need for diagnostic testing. Although no specific antiviral therapy exists for many childhood viruses, most cause acute, self-limited illness. Fortunately, for several viruses that cause significant pediatric morbidity, immunizations have been developed.

MEASLES

Etiology and Pathogenesis

Measles is an RNA virus in the Paramyxoviridae family that is spread by aerosolized respiratory droplets that come in contact with the respiratory tract or conjunctivae of susceptible individuals. It is highly contagious, and in a fully-susceptible population, an infected person can, on average, spread the virus to 12 to 18 others, compared with 2 or 3 others for the influenza virus. It has an incubation period up to 1 to 2 weeks. The virus causes necrosis of epithelium and a small vessel vasculitis of skin and oral mucosa.

Clinical Presentation

The clinical presentation of measles is defined by four phases: incubation, prodromal phase, exanthematous phase, and recovery. The prodromal period is characterized by symptoms of fever and one or more of the three "Cs": cough, conjunctivitis, and coryza. In some cases, it is also characterized by the appearance of pathognomonic Koplik spots, which are blue-white macules or plaques on the buccal mucosa (Fig. 88.1). The prodromal phase is followed about 3 to 4 days later by the exanthematous period, which is characterized by onset of a maculopapular rash that spreads from head to toe and typically resolves in 1 week. Histologically, the rash contains perivascular, lymphocytic infiltrates.

Acute infectious complications of measles include otitis media, pneumonia, and gastroenteritis. Pneumonia accounts for the majority of measles-associated morbidity and mortality and can be due to the virus itself, referred to as Hecht giant cell pneumonia, or a secondary bacterial infection. Central nervous system (CNS) complications include acute disseminated encephalomyelitis (ADEM), measles inclusion body encephalitis, and subacute sclerosing panencephalitis (SSPE). SSPE is a delayed complication that may not develop until 5 to 10 years after acute infection and is characterized by seizures, progressive motor and cognitive deterioration, and death.

Differential Diagnosis

Other viral infections to consider include rubella, parvovirus B19, human herpesvirus 6 (HHV-6), adenovirus, enterovirus, and Epstein-Barr virus (EBV). Bacterial processes that can cause a similar rash include *Mycoplasma pneumoniae* infections, group A streptococcus (GAS), and rickettsial infections (including Rocky Mountain spotted fever). Noninfectious causes include drug reactions or vasculitides such as Kawasaki disease or systemic juvenile idiopathic arthritis (JIA).

Prevention, Evaluation, and Management

Measles can be prevented by administration of a live-attenuated vaccine, most often in combination with the mumps and rubella vaccines as part of a two-dose series first given at 12 to 15 months and then again at 4 to 6 years old. The measles vaccine also can be given as postexposure prophylaxis within 72 hours of an exposure with up to 90% efficacy. For individuals who cannot receive live-attenuated vaccines, immune globulin is an alternative option.

Measles is most often diagnosed clinically, but immunoglobulin M (IgM) serology from a serum or plasma sample can be used for confirmation. Viral reverse transcription–polymerase chain reaction (RT-PCR) testing from blood, the nasopharynx, or urine also can be performed early in the course before antibody development. Measles is an immunosuppressive infection, and laboratory test results obtained during acute infection may show lymphopenia.

Management is largely supportive. Vitamin A supplementation has been associated with improved mortality in developing countries and so is recommended by the World Health Organization for all children. In the United States, where vitamin A deficiency may be less prevalent, the American Academy of Pediatrics (AAP) has modified this recommendation for vitamin A supplementation to be applicable only for patients with severe disease.

Future Directions

As measles continues to be detected globally, more investigation into the potential for point-of-care diagnostic testing is needed. Likewise, physician advocacy and partnership with patients and families is needed to increase vaccine uptake in the wake of social media campaigns propagating fears about vaccine safety.

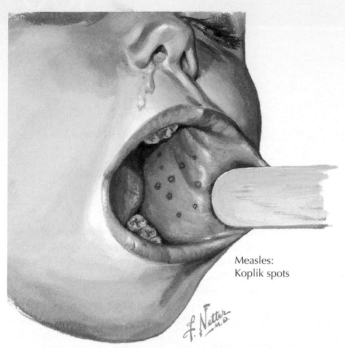

Measles:
Koplik spots

Fig. 88.1 Koplik Spots.

MUMPS

Etiology and Pathogenesis

Mumps is an RNA virus in the Paramyxoviridae family that causes acute, self-limited illness. It is spread by direct contact, respiratory droplets, or fomites and has an incubation period of approximately 2 to 3 weeks.

Clinical Presentation

The hallmark presentation of mumps is parotitis, which is painful and bilateral and develops after a brief prodromal period of fever and flu-like symptoms. Orchitis is an important potential complication for pubescent males and is not associated with an increased risk for sterility. Other complications of mumps include pancreatitis, aseptic meningitis, and sensorineural deafness.

Differential Diagnosis

Other viruses that can cause parotitis include influenza, parainfluenza, adenovirus, EBV, cytomegalovirus (CMV), and human immunodeficiency virus (HIV). Bacteria, most commonly *Staphylococcus aureus*, can also cause parotitis. However, the clinical presentation of bacterial parotitis is usually unilateral, whereas viral parotitis typically manifests bilaterally. Noninfectious causes of parotid swelling include malignancy or cyst, salivary gland stones, or Sjögren syndrome.

Prevention, Evaluation, and Management

A live-attenuated vaccine is available to help prevent mumps. In most countries, it is administered as part of the two-dose measles-mumps-rubella (MMR) combination vaccine series given at 12 to 15 months and 4 to 6 years of age. Use of the two-dose series has been associated with a 99% or greater reduction in the incidence of mumps.

Mumps can be diagnosed clinically, especially in the setting of large outbreaks. In more complicated cases, isolation of the virus or viral RNA or IgM serology can be used to diagnose. Serum amylase is usually elevated in cases of parotitis or pancreatitis.

Cerebrospinal fluid (CSF) studies from patients with mumps meningitis tend to have an elevated lymphocyte count. Management is supportive.

Future Directions

Given outbreaks in the 21st century, particularly in congregate settings such as college campuses, recent studies have evaluated the efficacy of providing an additional vaccine booster during outbreaks. More research is needed to determine if these populations require a modified vaccine schedule and to define an optimal postexposure prophylaxis regimen.

HERPES SIMPLEX VIRUS

Etiology and Pathogenesis

Herpes simplex virus (HSV) is a ubiquitous double-stranded DNA virus. There are two clinically significant serotypes of the virus: HSV-1, which is primarily associated with infections of the mouth, face, and CNS, and HSV-2, which is more commonly associated with infections of the anogenital region. Both forms are spread primarily by direct contact with mucus membranes or cutaneous surfaces and have an incubation period of 2 days to 2 weeks. Transmission is greatest at the time of primary infection, but viral shedding can occur even once a patient is asymptomatic. Once HSV has entered an infected person, it invades and remains latent in the sensory ganglia of the autonomic nervous system with the capacity to reactivate in the context of stress, illness, or immune suppression (Fig. 88.2).

Clinical Presentation

HSV usually manifests in a self-limited fashion but can be severe, especially in neonates (Chapter 82) and immunocompromised persons. Often preceded by prodromal symptoms of fever, myalgias, and fatigue, the classic findings for HSV infection include a cluster of monomorphous vesicles on an erythematous base that evolve into painful ulcers or crusted papules over a period of 1 to 3 days. The most common mucocutaneous manifestations of HSV-1 include herpes labialis (colloquially known as fever blisters or cold sores), gingivostomatitis, herpes gladiatorum (infection on face, ear, or trunk typically seen in wrestlers), herpetic whitlow (vesicular eruption on distal end of finger), and eczema herpeticum (febrile herpetic superinfection of eczematous skin) (Fig. 88.2). The most common mucocutaneous manifestation of HSV-2 is genital herpes. Development of erythema multiforme has been associated with HSV infections. CNS manifestations include herpetic keratoconjunctivitis and HSV encephalitis, with the latter usually affecting the temporal lobes most prominently. Either primary infection or reactivation can be asymptomatic.

Differential Diagnosis

Other infections to consider in a patient suspected to have HSV-1 skin infection include varicella zoster, coxsackievirus, and impetigo. In the oral or perioral region, HSV tends to affect the anterior oropharynx, gingiva, and vermillion border, while coxsackievirus tends to affect the posterior oropharynx. Noninfectious differential for vesicular lesions, particularly of the oral or perioral region, include drug eruptions, Stevens-Johnson syndrome, and mycoplasma-induced rash and mucositis. For patients with genital ulcers suspected to be due to HSV-2, the differential includes infections such as syphilis or chancroid and noninfectious causes such as Behçet syndrome. Consideration for periodic fever, aphthous stomatitis, pharyngitis, adenitis (PFAPA) and extraintestinal manifestations of inflammatory bowel disease should be made in the appropriate clinical setting.

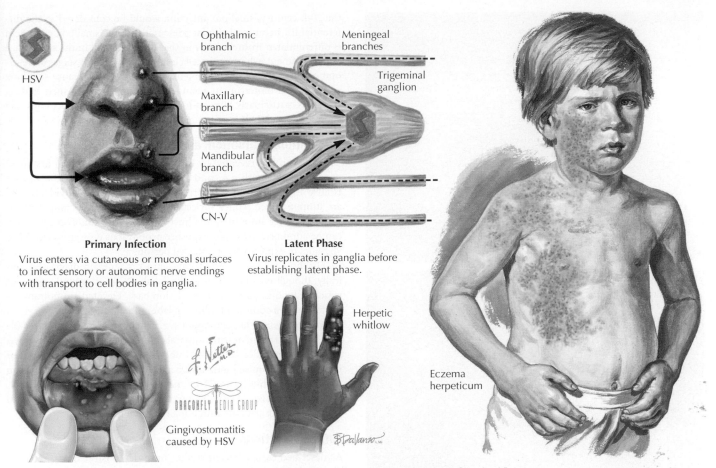

Fig. 88.2 Pathogenesis and Clinical Presentation of Herpes Simplex Viruses.

Evaluation and Management

Although viral culture of a herpetic ulcer is the gold standard for diagnosis, immunohistochemistry or viral PCR has become the more common diagnostic practice. Viral PCR is particularly useful for detecting HSV in CSF samples. The Tzanck smear is a historic diagnostic method that involved staining cells obtained from a vesicle base and evaluating them for characteristic findings, including multinucleated giant cells; however, this technique is no longer routinely performed given the development of immunohistochemistry and molecular techniques.

In disseminated forms of HSV infection, laboratory studies often show elevated aminotransferase levels. CSF studies for patients with encephalitis tend to show pleocytosis with lymphocyte predominance and red blood cells in the fluid. Electroencephalographic studies classically exhibit a pattern of periodic lateralizing epileptiform discharges.

Acyclovir (or prodrugs valacyclovir and famciclovir) is used as primary treatment for HSV infection and tends to be most helpful when started early (i.e., within the first 72 hours) in a patient's course. Topical formulations are ineffective and not recommended. Parenteral formulations are preferred over enteral therapy for treatment of neonates, immunocompromised hosts, and patients with eczema herpeticum and HSV encephalitis. Consultation with an ophthalmologist is recommended for co-management of children with HSV keratoconjunctivitis. Although effective in shortening the duration of symptoms and preventing complications, these antiviral medications do not eradicate the virus. Nonetheless, when taken chronically as suppressive therapy to prevent recurrent reactivation episodes, these medications can be effective in patients with a history of frequent outbreaks (typically more than six episodes per year).

Future Directions

Recent studies have demonstrated a lower incidence of herpes simplex virus among children since the implementation of the varicella vaccine program. However, development of a vaccine specific for HSV has not yet been produced.

VARICELLA-ZOSTER VIRUS

Etiology and Pathogenesis

Varicella-zoster is a globally widespread, double-stranded DNA virus that is spread by respiratory droplets, direct contact with fluid from skin lesions, or from aerosolization of skin lesion contents. It has an incubation period of about 2 weeks, with a range of 10 to 21 days. Like HSV, it remains latent in sensory neurons of the dorsal root ganglia after primary infection and can reactivate to cause recurrent infections.

Clinical Presentation

Varicella, or chickenpox, is the hallmark clinical manifestation associated with primary varicella-zoster infection, typically affecting children between 1 and 9 years of age. Chickenpox is characterized by fever and prodromal malaise, followed by onset of widespread macules and papules that evolve into pruritic, vesicular lesions that appear in various stages of healing (Fig. 88.3). These lesions have been described as "dewdrops on a rose petal" because of the characteristic presence of a vesicle with clear fluid overlying a small rim of erythematous base. Infected persons remain contagious until all skin lesions are crusted and healed. Lesions usually fully heal and resolve in 1 to 2 weeks but may leave hypopigmented scars.

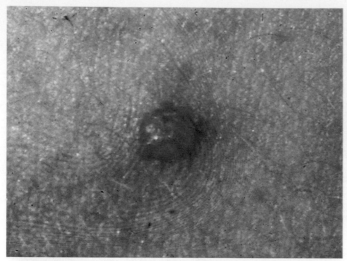

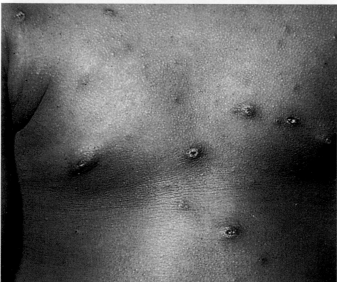

Fig. 88.3 Varicella (Chickenpox). (From Michaels MG, Williams JV. Infectious diseases. In: Zitelli BJ, McIntire S, Nowalk, AJ, eds. *Zitelli and Davis' Atlas of Pediatric Physical Diagnosis.* 7th ed. Philadelphia, PA: Elsevier; 2017;455-509, Fig. 13.13AB.)

Complications of primary varicella infection include superinfection of skin lesions with GAS or *S. aureus,* which can lead to invasive infections such as bacteremia or osteomyelitis. Other complications include varicella pneumonia and CNS complications, including acute cerebellar ataxia and meningoencephalitis. Varicella infection can be fatal, especially in older and immunocompromised populations. In pregnant women, primary infection in the first or second trimester can result in congenital varicella syndrome. Reye syndrome may occur in children given aspirin as antipyretic or analgesic therapy while infected with varicella.

Herpes zoster is the hallmark clinical manifestation of reactivated varicella virus. It is characterized by acute to subacute onset of pain and paresthesias, followed by an outbreak of vesicular lesions, in a unilateral dermatomal distribution.

Differential Diagnosis

The differential diagnosis for varicella infection includes HSV and enteroviral infections. Skin infections such as bullous impetigo with *S. aureus* may manifest similarly. Additionally, before eradication in

the 20th century, smallpox infection would be considered in the differential list because of similar presentation. The smallpox exanthem is differentiated from varicella in that lesions are all in the same stage of development, whereas varicella lesions are at various stages of development. It is important to remember this contrast because smallpox is a potential bioterrorism agent. Noninfectious causes such as drug reactions, particularly Stevens-Johnson syndrome, or insect bites also could be considered.

Prevention, Evaluation, and Management

Varicella can be prevented by live-attenuated vaccine given first at 12 months of age, with a second dose at 4 to 6 years old. The vaccine is 80% to 85% effective in preventing disease. For individuals who are unimmunized, either varicella vaccine, if immunocompetent, or varicella-zoster immune globulin (VZIG), if immunocompromised, can be administered as postexposure prophylaxis if given within 72 to 96 hours of exposure to an infected person.

For those who are infected, chickenpox is generally diagnosed clinically, though it can be diagnosed officially by PCR or viral culture of vesicular lesions, particularly the lesion base. Elevated aminotransferase levels are a common finding on laboratory studies.

Management is largely supportive. Chickenpox is a self-limited illness, and so treatment with antivirals such as acyclovir or valacyclovir is not recommended by the AAP for use in uncomplicated cases. For immunocompromised individuals and those at higher risk, initiation of acyclovir within 24 to 72 hours of symptom onset is most effective and beneficial. Acyclovir is excreted renally and should be dosed appropriately in patients with impaired renal function.

Future Directions

As described earlier, recent studies have demonstrated a lower incidence of HSV among children since the implementation of the varicella vaccine program. Additional research is needed to explore if there are causative factors for this observation. As the first generation to receive the varicella vaccine during childhood enters adulthood, research is also needed to monitor the rates of herpes zoster in this population.

HUMAN HERPESVIRUS 6

Etiology and Pathogenesis

HHV-6 is a ubiquitous, double-stranded DNA virus that infects up to 95% of children by 2 years of age. The primary clinically relevant strain is HHV-6B. It is spread primarily by saliva or respiratory secretions. Its primary target cell is the CD4$^+$ T lymphocyte. After primary infection, it remains latent in the salivary glands of affected individuals.

Clinical Presentation

The classic presentation of HHV-6 is known as "roseola" or "sixth disease" and is an acute, self-limited, undifferentiated febrile illness characterized by several days of high-spiking fevers without other localizing symptoms. Defervescence tends to be associated with subsequent onset of full-body erythematous, macular rash (Fig. 88.4). Roseola most commonly manifests in infants 6 to 9 months old. HHV-6 infections have been associated with incidence of febrile seizures, including febrile status epilepticus, in up to 30% of patients.

Differential Diagnosis

Similar infections to consider in children with febrile illness and rash include measles, rubella, enterovirus, adenovirus, and scarlet fever. Noninfectious causes to consider include drug reactions or vasculitides such as Kawasaki disease.

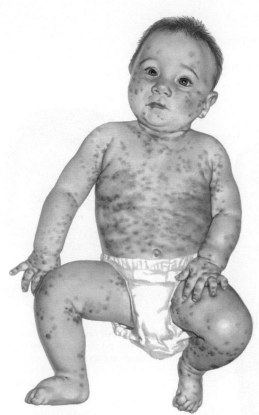

Rose-colored maculopapular rash seen in roseola.

Fig. 88.4 Human Herpes Virus-6 (Roseola).

Evaluation and Management

Diagnosis of HHV-6 is generally a clinical one. Viral culture is the gold standard for diagnosis of HHV-6, though PCR also can be used. However, because HHV-6 establishes latency after initial acquisition, PCR cannot differentiate between new infection or asymptomatic shedding. Because of the ubiquitous nature of HHV-6, serologic tests tend not to be clinically useful. Management is supportive.

Future Directions

Although HHV-6 generally causes an acute, self-limited illness in young children, it does remain latent in infected individuals for a prolonged period. There have been reports of viral reactivation and association with more severe presentations, such as encephalitis and graft rejection, in immunocompromised and organ transplant patients, though the pathogenesis is not fully understood. Similarly, HHV-6 infection has been associated with autoimmune conditions, such as multiple sclerosis and Hashimoto thyroiditis, though again evidence for a causative link is lacking.

EPSTEIN-BARR VIRUS

Etiology and Pathogenesis

EBV is a double-stranded DNA virus in the herpesvirus family that is globally distributed, with estimates that more than 95% of the world's adult population has been infected. It is spread via oral secretions and sexual intercourse. Its primary cellular target is the B lymphocyte, though it does become disseminated throughout the lymphoreticular system, including the liver and spleen. It has an incubation period of 30 to 50 days and establishes lifelong latency in infected hosts.

Clinical Presentation

In children 4 years of age and younger, primary infection with EBV is usually asymptomatic. In children school-aged and older, EBV is responsible for more than 90% of cases of infectious mononucleosis, a self-limited illness characterized by fever, fatigue, exudative pharyngitis, generalized lymphadenopathy (particularly cervical), and hepatosplenomegaly. Dermatologic manifestations include "ampicillin rash," a macular rash that develops in patients with acute EBV infection who are exposed to penicillins, and Gianotti-Crosti, a papular rash affecting cheeks and extensor surfaces that develops as a hypersensitivity response to EBV (Fig. 88.5). Neurologic manifestations are less common but can include a phenomenon called metamorphopsia or "Alice in Wonderland syndrome," in which individuals exhibit distorted perceptions of size, shape, and spatial relationships.

Complications of EBV infection include hemolytic anemia and spleen rupture. EBV is also associated with development of lymphoproliferative diseases, including hemophagocytic lymphohistiocytosis and posttransplant lymphoproliferative disease, and was the first virus to be associated with malignancies, including nasopharyngeal carcinoma, Burkitt lymphoma, and Hodgkin lymphoma.

Differential Diagnosis

Other infections to consider in a patient presenting with infectious mononucleosis-type symptoms include CMV, HIV, adenovirus, and toxoplasmosis. Bacterial infections to consider include GAS pharyngitis, especially because the posterior oropharyngeal findings of GAS can be indistinguishable from those observed in EBV. However, hepatosplenomegaly is not usually detected in patients with GAS pharyngitis.

Evaluation and Management

Typical laboratory test findings in acute EBV infection include leukocytosis with an elevated number of atypical lymphocytes, mild thrombocytopenia, and elevated aminotransferase levels.

Diagnosis can be made serologically with either the Monospot test or EBV-specific antibodies. The Monospot is a heterophile antibody test that detects IgM antibodies known as Paul-Bunnell antibodies. Up to 25% of Monospot tests can be negative in the first week of infection, but sensitivity increases in week 2 and beyond. The test is also less sensitive in younger children so is not recommended for diagnostic use in children younger than 4 years. EBV can also be detected by serologic examination (Table 88.1). In the acute phase, there is a rapid IgM and IgG response to viral capsid antigen and IgG to early antigen. Positive antibody to EBV nuclear antigen indicates past infection because this is not usually present until several weeks to months after initial infection.

Management of EBV infection is largely supportive. Activity restriction and avoidance of contact sports for 2 to 4 weeks is recommended for individuals with hepatosplenomegaly to decrease the risk for splenic rupture. Steroids have been used sporadically to manage tonsillar hypertrophy and pharyngitis, though data supporting the efficacy of this practice are lacking.

Future Directions

Given its link with lymphoproliferative diseases and malignancies, further research is needed to investigate antiviral regimens and vaccination for EBV.

PARVOVIRUS B19

Etiology and Pathogenesis

Parvovirus B19 is a single-stranded DNA virus that is globally distributed. It commonly affects children ages 5 to 15 years and occurs most frequently in winter and spring months. It is transmitted primarily by

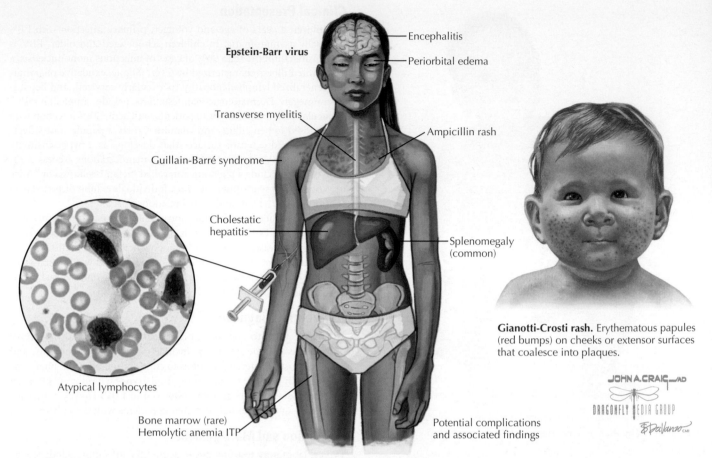

Epstein-Barr virus

Encephalitis

Periorbital edema

Transverse myelitis

Ampicillin rash

Guillain-Barré syndrome

Cholestatic hepatitis

Splenomegaly (common)

Atypical lymphocytes

Bone marrow (rare) Hemolytic anemia ITP

Potential complications and associated findings

Gianotti-Crosti rash. Erythematous papules (red bumps) on cheeks or extensor surfaces that coalesce into plaques.

Fig. 88.5 Clinical Presentation of Epstein-Barr Virus.

TABLE 88.1	Antibodies in Epstein-Barr Virus Infection			
Infection	Viral Capsid Antigen Immunoglobulin G	Viral Capsid Antigen Immunoglobulin M	Early Antigen Immunoglobulin G	EBV Nuclear Antigen Immunoglobulin G
No previous infection	−	−	−	−
Acute infection	+	+	±	−
Recent infection	+	±	±	±
Past infection	+	−	±	+

EBV, Epstein-Barr virus.
From American Academy of Pediatrics; Kimberlin DW, Brady MT, Jackson MA, Long SS, eds. *Red Book: 2018 Report of the Committee on Infectious Diseases*. Itasca, IL: American Academy of Pediatrics; 2018. Copyright 2018.

respiratory droplets but also can be transmitted by blood. The virus' primary cellular target is erythroid progenitor cells, and infection of these cells can result in transient arrest of red blood cell production.

Clinical Presentation

Most people infected with parvovirus B19 are asymptomatic. Erythema infectiosum, or "fifth disease," is the most common presentation of parvovirus B19 infection and is a manifestation of the body's immune response to the virus. It is characterized by a "slapped cheek" appearance with a lacy, reticular rash on an individual's trunk and extremities (Fig. 88.6). Arthralgias also may be present, particularly in older children and adults. Because the virus persists best in erythroid progenitor cells, other acute signs of parvovirus B19 infection include transient red cell aplasia or transient aplastic crisis in individuals with chronic hemolysis. When perinatal transmission occurs, nonimmune fetal

hydrops can result. Parvovirus B19 also has been implicated in the development of "papular-purpuric gloves and socks syndrome" and has been associated with myocarditis.

Differential Diagnosis

The differential diagnosis for parvovirus B19 includes rubella, measles, and enterovirus. Drug reactions should be considered. For children with arthralgias or arthritis, JIA or serum sickness could be considered.

Evaluation and Management

Erythema infectiosum can usually be diagnosed clinically without further evaluation, but in ambiguous or complicated clinical situations, parvovirus B19 can be detected by serologic studies, with IgM antibodies present by day 3 of illness. Viral PCR is typically not

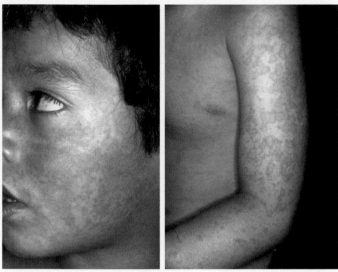

Fig. 88.6 Erythema Infectiosum Secondary to Parvovirus B19. (From Viral diseases. In: James WD, Elston DM, Treat JR, Rosenbach MA, Neuhaus IM, eds. *Andrews' Diseases of the Skin.* 13th ed. Philadelphia, PA: Elsevier; 2020:362-240.e8, Fig. 19.40.)

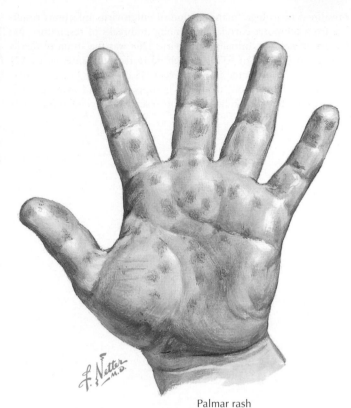

Palmar rash

Fig. 88.7 Hand, Foot, and Mouth Disease.

recommended because it may not represent acute infection but can be useful in immunocompromised hosts. Management is largely supportive, though packed red blood cell transfusions may be required for patients with aplastic crises. IVIG can be considered for treatment in immunocompromised patients.

Future Directions

Screening for parvovirus B19 in blood products may help prevent complications in immunocompromised children, but currently there is insufficient evidence to recommend universal testing. A protective vaccine has been developed but distribution has been delayed because of lack of commercial interest.

ENTEROVIRUS (NONPOLIOVIRUS)

Etiology and Pathogenesis

Commonly referred to as the "summer viruses," the nonpolio enteroviruses are globally detected viruses whose incidence peaks in warmer months. The name "enterovirus" reflects the prominence of the gastrointestinal (GI) tract, particularly the mucosal M cells, as the key site of invasion, replication, and transmission for these viruses. Enterovirus, coxsackievirus, and echovirus are representative members of this group and are transmitted by respiratory or fecal-oral routes. The incubation period for acute infection is typically 3 to 6 days, but viral shedding in the GI tract can persist for 2 to 3 months. There may be two stages of viremia, and thus a biphasic pattern can be seen.

Clinical Presentation

The most common presentation for this group of viruses is a nonspecific, acute, febrile illness characterized by fever, headache, and malaise, mild upper respiratory symptoms, or GI symptoms. More specific presentations include (1) herpangina, which is caused by coxsackievirus and consists of fever, pharyngitis, and painful ulcers on the tonsils and in the posterior oropharynx; and (2) hand-foot-and-mouth disease (HFM), which produces oral lesions similar to herpangina on the buccal mucosa in addition to vesicles and papules on the hands, feet, and buttocks (Fig. 88.7). Acute hemorrhagic conjunctivitis is another

mucocutaneous manifestation of enteroviruses and is most often caused by enterovirus 70. Systemically, enteroviruses are implicated in up to one-third of myopericarditis cases, are the leading viral cause of aseptic meningitis, and have been associated with cases of acute flaccid myelitis (AFM).

Differential Diagnosis

Given the nonspecific presentations of most enterovirus infections, the differential diagnosis is quite broad and can include many other common viruses. Regarding the enteroviral exanthems and enanthems, herpangina tends to affect the posterior oropharynx whereas HSV gingivostomatitis and herpes labialis affect the anterior oropharynx, gingiva, and vermillion border. HFM disease can be distinguished from varicella infection by the localized nature of HFM lesions, which do not spread diffusely.

Evaluation and Management

For children with nonspecific illness, a precise diagnosis may not be indicated. Likewise, for children with classic manifestations of HFM or herpangina, diagnosis can be made clinically. For more severe infections, especially those affecting the myocardium or CNS, PCR detection of viral RNA is more useful than detection by viral culture. Additional molecular testing can be pursued if serologic typing is clinically indicated.

Management is largely supportive. Use of IVIG has been used in severe infections, including those affecting the CNS, though definitive data on the effectiveness are limited.

Future Directions

Since 2014, there have been outbreaks of the neurologic condition AFM occurring approximately every other summer. AFM is a presumed neurologic manifestation of enterovirus infections resulting from temporal correlations among outbreaks of respiratory and GI manifestations. Initially enterovirus D68 was the strain primarily implicated in cases of AFM, though more recently, enterovirus A71 also has been implicated in both recent US outbreaks and prior outbreaks globally. Current treatment is supportive, and many patients require long-term rehabilitation. More research is needed to determine the pathophysiology of and risk factors for AFM, establish efficient surveillance and diagnostic procedures, and evaluate therapeutic options.

SUGGESTED READINGS

Available online.

89

Fungal Infections

William R. Otto and Torsten A. Joerger

CLINICAL VIGNETTE

A 4-year-old boy presents to your clinic with a scalp lesion. The lesion initially manifested as red pustules. You had seen the patient in your office at that time and treated him empirically with cephalexin. The lesion continued to worsen, so you changed the child's antibiotics to clindamycin, without any improvement. He remains well and has not had fever. His examination shows a 2- × 3-cm, raised, tender, erythematous lesion with some overlying yellow crust. The area around the lesion is boggy and swollen, and there is localized alopecia. Occipital lymphadenopathy is noted as well.

This child is suffering from tinea capitis with a kerion, an inflammatory response to a dermatophyte infection of the scalp. Tinea capitis can manifest with diffuse scaling, pustule formation, or patchy hair loss. The presence of black dots, or well-demarcated areas of hair loss with short broken hairs, is common. Diagnosis is made by skin scraping and fungal culture. Prolonged systemic antifungal therapy is necessary to treat tinea capitis as topical antifungals will not penetrate the hair shaft.

Fungi are eukaryotic organisms that are classified morphologically based on their appearance in culture or tissue. Development of fungal disease is largely mediated by the status of the host immune system. Immunocompromised children are at increased risk for fungal infection. Premature infants are also at increased risk for fungal infection because of immature barrier functions of the immune system and frequent use of medical devices.

This chapter discusses the most clinically significant fungal infections in childhood, including infections with yeast, molds, dimorphic fungi, and dermatophyte infections.

INFECTIONS WITH YEASTS

Yeasts are unicellular fungi that reproduce by budding. They are ubiquitous in the environment. Some yeasts, such as *Candida* species or *Cryptococcus* species, are opportunistic pathogens that cause disease in humans.

Candida Species

Candida species are a frequent cause of infections in neonates and children, causing both superficial infections and invasive disease. *Candida albicans* remains the most common species identified in infections.

Clinical Manifestations

Superficial candidiasis of the skin or mucosal surfaces is a common infection of children. Diaper dermatitis, characterized by a beefy red, confluent rash with satellite lesions, frequently occurs in infants younger than 12 months of age. Thrush is another common condition in infants and is characterized by thick white plaques on the buccal mucosa, tongue, or palate. Thrush can cause an uncomfortable, burning sensation that may lead to decreased oral intake. Vulvovaginitis secondary to *Candida* species occurs commonly and will manifest with vaginal discharge, irritation, or pruritus.

Risk factors for invasive candidiasis include exposure to broad-spectrum antibiotics, presence of a central venous catheter, or receipt of parenteral nutrition. The most common form of invasive candidiasis is candidemia, a *Candida* bloodstream infection. Symptoms of candidemia are nonspecific. Neonates may present with temperature instability, lethargy, respiratory distress, or feeding intolerance, whereas older children present with fever or a systemic inflammatory response.

Invasive candidiasis can also occur after hematogenous dissemination of *Candida* organisms (Fig. 89.1). Dissemination to the brain, eyes, liver, spleen, kidneys, musculoskeletal system, or skin has been described. Central nervous system (CNS) involvement can manifest with meningitis or parenchymal disease such as granulomas, microabscesses, or vasculitis. *Candida* urinary tract infections include candiduria, cystitis, pyelonephritis, or urinary tract fungal balls. Bones and joint involvement may manifest days to weeks after clearance of blood cultures.

Diagnosis

Growth of *Candida* species on culture or identification of fungal organisms on histopathology are the gold standards for diagnosis. *Candida* species will grow in standard blood cultures and do not require fungal blood cultures. The beta-D-glucan biomarker assay detects (1, 3)-beta-D-glucan, a cell wall component found in numerous fungal organisms. However, there is no specific cutoff for a positive result in children, and its use is not routinely recommended in pediatric patients.

Evaluation for dissemination using clinical examination and diagnostic imaging should be part of the diagnostic evaluation. All patients with candidemia should undergo a dilated ophthalmological examination because of concern for ocular infection. Neonates with candidemia should also undergo ultrasonography of the head and abdomen, lumbar puncture, and an echocardiogram. For older children, diagnostic imaging of the abdomen and genitourinary tract, as well as an echocardiogram, is recommended if persistent candidemia occurs.

Treatment

Superficial infections are treated with topical agents. Thrush is commonly treated with oral nystatin suspension. *Candida* diaper dermatitis is treated with topical nystatin or miconazole. *Candida* vulvovaginitis is treated with topical antifungal formulations or oral azoles. Systemic therapy may be needed for refractory disease.

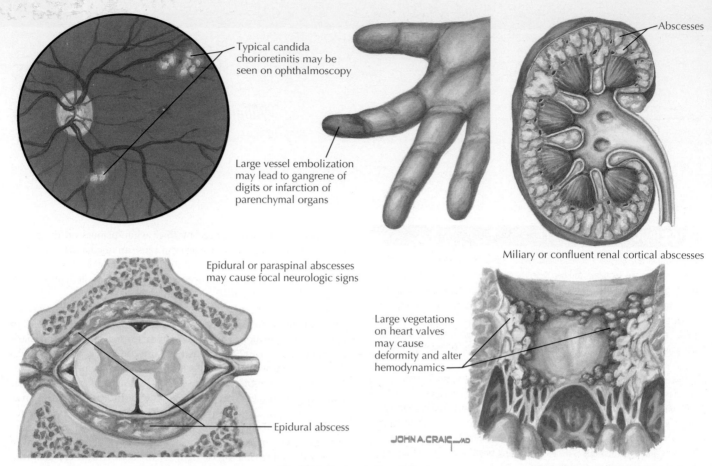

Typical candida chorioretinitis may be seen on ophthalmoscopy

Large vessel embolization may lead to gangrene of digits or infarction of parenchymal organs

Abscesses

Miliary or confluent renal cortical abscesses

Epidural or paraspinal abscesses may cause focal neurologic signs

Large vegetations on heart valves may cause deformity and alter hemodynamics

Epidural abscess

JOHN A.CRAIG—AD

Fig. 89.1 Systemic Candidiasis.

Recommended treatment of systemic candidiasis includes echinocandins, amphotericin B, or triazole antifungals. Candidemia should be treated with an echinocandin, such as caspofungin. Treatment is continued for 2 weeks after clearance of blood cultures; removal of central venous catheters should be considered. For invasive candidiasis in other organs, the exact medication and duration of therapy is determined by the location of disease and any underlying conditions.

Cryptococcus Species

Cryptococcus species are encapsulated yeasts found in temperate climates in soil contaminated by bird droppings. Humans acquire infection after inhalation of fungal spores, and major risk factors for infection include immunodeficiencies such as human immunodeficiency virus (HIV)/acquired immunodeficiency syndrome (AIDS), malignancy, or transplantation. *Cryptococcus neoformans* and *Cryptococcus gattii* are the most common species worldwide.

Clinical Manifestations

Pulmonary infection is the most frequently encountered infection (Fig. 89.2). In immune competent individuals, infections are frequently asymptomatic. Patients may have fever, respiratory symptoms, or constitutional symptoms such as weight loss. Immunocompromised patients may present with a life-threatening pneumonia with acute respiratory distress syndrome. Disseminated infection with skin lesions can occur in immunocompromised individuals.

Subacute meningitis is the most common manifestation of disseminated cryptococcosis. Symptoms may be subtle, with the only presenting signs being headache, behavioral change, or signs of increased intracranial pressure. Focal neurologic signs are rarely present.

Diagnosis

Cryptococcus species can grow in standard microbiologic media, and culture of blood or cerebrospinal fluid (CSF) may reveal the organism. Cryptococcal antigen tests can be performed on blood or CSF and are extremely accurate, with greater than 90% sensitivity and specificity. Classically, diagnosis of cryptococcal meningitis was made by staining CSF with India ink to visualize encapsulated yeast, though that is less common now.

Treatment

For patients with CNS disease or other disseminated disease, induction therapy with amphotericin B and flucytosine for at least 2 weeks is recommended, followed by consolidation therapy with fluconazole. Those with localized pulmonary infection can be treated with fluconazole alone. Treatment should extend for at least 3 to 12 months and should be guided by clinical response.

INFECTION WITH MOLDS

Molds, including *Aspergillus* species and the Mucorales order, possess hyphae and reproduce via the formation of large numbers of spores.

Aspergillus Species

Aspergillus species are found in the soil and on decaying plants. Exposure occurs commonly by inhalation of spores. *Aspergillus* species

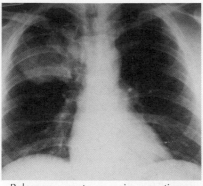

Pulmonary cryptococcosis presenting as a large mass-like lesion, easily mistaken for carcinoma

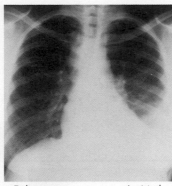

Pulmonary cryptococcosis. Mediastinal lymph nodes enlarged and pleural effusion on left

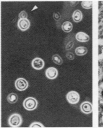

India ink preparation showing budding and capsule

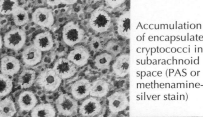

Accumulation of encapsulated cryptococci in subarachnoid space (PAS or methenamine-silver stain)

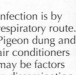

Infection is by respiratory route. Pigeon dung and air conditioners may be factors in dissemination.

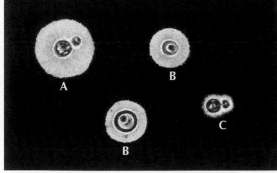

India ink preparation showing *C. neoformans*
A. Budding organism with thick capsule
B. Nonbudding organisms
C. Unencapsulated

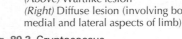

Skin lesions on foot and ankle
(Above) Wartlike lesion
(Right) Diffuse lesion (involving both medial and lateral aspects of limb)

Fig. 89.2 Cryptococcus.

then colonize the respiratory tract. Children who are immunocompromised or have underlying respiratory conditions have the highest risk for disease. *Aspergillus fumigatus* is the most common species isolated clinically.

Clinical Manifestations

The most common site of invasive aspergillosis is the respiratory tract (Fig. 89.3). Upper respiratory tract disease occurs predominantly as rhinosinusitis, with facial pain or numbness, soft tissue swelling, or even eye pain. Pulmonary disease often manifests with nonspecific clinical findings, such as fever, cough, difficulty breathing, chest pain, or even hemoptysis. Patients may be asymptomatic, and the diagnosis may be made based on the presence of pulmonary nodules or other radiographic findings.

Direct inoculation through the skin is another common method of primary infection. Patients may have a history of trauma, occlusive tape, or surgery. Cutaneous aspergillosis can manifest as a solitary erythematous nodule that progresses to a hemorrhagic or necrotic lesion.

Aspergillus species are known for angioinvasion, with dissemination to the eyes, gastrointestinal (GI) tract, liver, kidneys, or bones. Cutaneous disease that results from hematogenous dissemination manifests with multiple lesions. Dissemination to the brain can result in abscesses, meningoencephalitis, or vasculitis, and patients present with altered mental status or seizures.

Allergic bronchopulmonary aspergillosis (ABPA) is a chronic immunoglobulin E (IgE)-mediated hypersensitivity reaction to *Aspergillus*. It occurs most commonly in patients with asthma or cystic fibrosis. Mucosal colonization with *Aspergillus* species leads to an exaggerated allergic response, resulting in recurrent bronchospasm and transient pulmonary infiltrates. Patients present with increased cough or wheezing, exercise intolerance, increased sputum, or decrease in pulmonary function.

Diagnosis

Diagnostic imaging plays a large role in the diagnosis of invasive aspergillosis. Imaging should focus on the common sites of infection: the sinuses and the lungs. There are no specific sinus imaging findings that are diagnostic for *Aspergillus* rhinosinusitis. Characteristic imaging signs of pulmonary aspergillosis include the halo sign or the air crescent sign, though an aspergilloma, consolidations, or fungal nodules may be seen.

The beta-D-glucan and galactomannan assays are frequently used in the diagnosis of invasive aspergillosis. As noted previously, the beta-D-glucan is limited by poor specificity and sensitivity. The *Aspergillus* galactomannan assay detects the galactomannan component of the *Aspergillus* cell wall. The galactomannan assay has variable sensitivity and specificity in children, and routine use of the galactomannan assay is not widespread.

Tissue biopsy for culture and histopathology remains the gold standard for the diagnosis of invasive aspergillosis. Growth on culture media allows for species identification and antifungal susceptibility testing. Histopathologic study may demonstrate tissue invasion by fungal organisms. Molecular testing can be performed if organisms do not grow in culture but are seen on histopathologic examination.

Diagnosis of ABPA requires fulfillment of multiple criteria, including (1) reversible episodic bronchial obstruction; (2) immediate

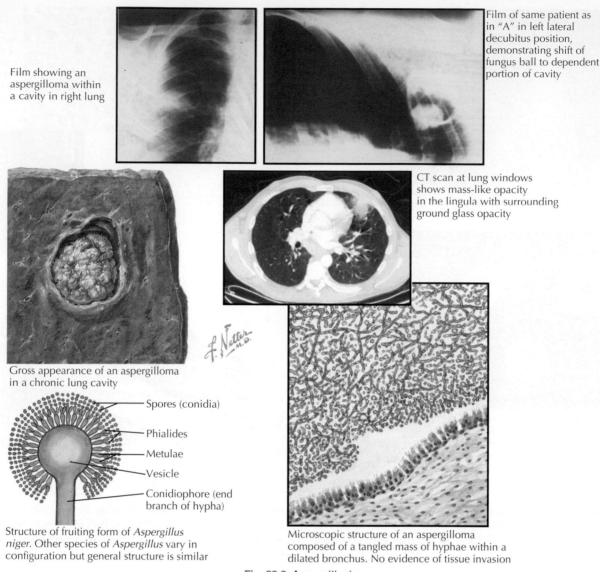

Film showing an aspergilloma within a cavity in right lung

Film of same patient as in "A" in left lateral decubitus position, demonstrating shift of fungus ball to dependent portion of cavity

CT scan at lung windows shows mass-like opacity in the lingula with surrounding ground glass opacity

Gross appearance of an aspergilloma in a chronic lung cavity

Spores (conidia)
Phialides
Metulae
Vesicle
Conidiophore (end branch of hypha)

Structure of fruiting form of *Aspergillus niger*. Other species of *Aspergillus* vary in configuration but general structure is similar

Microscopic structure of an aspergilloma composed of a tangled mass of hyphae within a dilated bronchus. No evidence of tissue invasion

Fig. 89.3 Aspergillosis.

scratch test reactivity to *Aspergillus* antigens, (3) elevated total serum IgE, (4) peripheral blood eosinophilia, and (5) precipitating IgG serum antibodies to *A. fumigatus*.

Treatment

Voriconazole is the drug of choice for the treatment of invasive aspergillosis. Therapeutic drug monitoring should be employed when voriconazole is administered, because it improves outcomes and decreases toxicity. Amphotericin B products or echinocandins can be used as alternative treatment agents if voriconazole cannot be tolerated.

Treatment of ABPA focuses on reducing acute symptoms and generally includes administration of corticosteroids. Current guidelines recommend concomitant use of antifungal therapy, predominantly itraconazole, because antifungal therapy has been shown to reduce corticosteroid use and improve pulmonary function.

Mucorales Molds

Members of the Mucorales order have broad, nonseptate hyphae that branch at right angles. With the exception of cases of severe trauma, mucormycosis occurs almost exclusively in immunocompromised individuals. *Rhizopus*, *Mucor*, and *Rhizomucor* are commonly identified genera.

Clinical Manifestations

Mucormycosis classically manifests as one of five clinical entities: rhinocerebral disease, pulmonary disease, cutaneous disease, gastrointestinal disease, or disseminated disease. Symptoms depend on the site of infection. All infections can spread rapidly because of a predilection for angioinvasion, which leads to dissemination.

Diagnosis

The gold standard for diagnosing mucormycosis is culture and histopathologic analysis of a tissue sample. Diagnostic imaging is used in a similar fashion to the diagnostic process for invasive aspergillosis. Nonculture diagnostic methods such as beta-D-glucan or galactomannan assays do not detect the Mucorales molds.

Treatment

Treatment of mucormycosis is reliant on administration of appropriate antifungals, surgical resection when possible, and restoration of immune function. Amphotericin B products remain the cornerstone of treatment of mucormycosis. The triazole antifungals posaconazole and isavuconazole have also been used with some success.

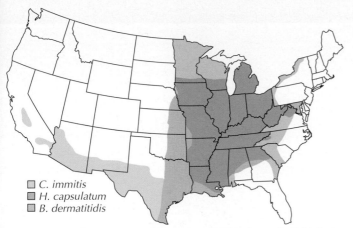

Fig. 89.4 Distribution of the Major Geographic Areas in Which the Endemic Mycoses Are Found in the United States.

☐ *C. immitis*
☐ *H. capsulatum*
☐ *B. dermatitidis*

INFECTION WITH DIMORPHIC FUNGI

Dimorphic fungi are infrequent causes of fungal infection in children. The most common dimorphic fungi are known as the endemic mycoses, which include *Histoplasma capsulatum*, *Blastomyces dermatitidis*, and the causative agents of coccidioidomycosis, *Coccidioides immitis* and *Coccidioides posadasii*. These fungi each have a defined geographic distribution (Fig. 89.4), and knowing a patient's likelihood of exposure is important when considering these pathogens.

Clinical Manifestations

For immunocompetent children, these infections generally manifest as asymptomatic or self-limiting pulmonary infections. Rarely, extrapulmonary or disseminated disease may occur. Immunocompromised patients frequently will have severe pneumonia, with extrapulmonary disease involving the CNS, abdominal organs, or bone and joints.

Diagnosis

Detection of fungal antigen in blood, urine, or CSF is the most common way that endemic mycoses are diagnosed; there are specific assays for histoplasmosis, blastomycosis, and coccidioidomycosis. Serum antibody testing can be performed. Tissue biopsy for culture, histopathology, and molecular testing also can be performed.

Treatment

Treatment of histoplasmosis or blastomycosis begins with 1 to 2 weeks of treatment with amphotericin B products, followed by prolonged therapy with itraconazole. Azole antifungals such as fluconazole or itraconazole are the preferred therapy for coccidioidomycosis.

DERMATOPHYTE INFECTIONS

Dermatophytes, including *Trichophyton* and *Microsporum* species cause superficial infections of the hair, skin, or nails that are collectively known as tinea. The specific condition is generally named after the body site involved.

Clinical Manifestations

Tinea capitis is discussed in the clinical vignette. Tinea corporis, known as ringworm, is a dermatophyte infection of skin. Lesions are well demarcated, circular, and slightly erythematous, with a scaly, pustular, or vesicular border (Fig. 89.5). Tinea pedis, or athlete's foot, is a superficial infection of the feet. It presents with pruritic vesiculopustular or vesicular lesions

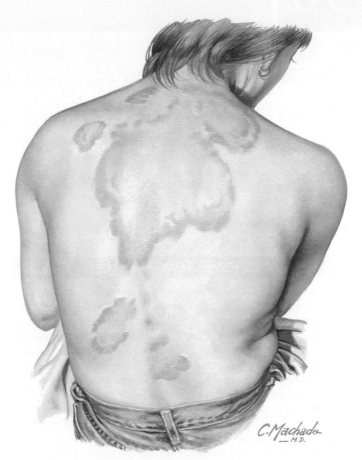

Fig. 89.5 Tinea Corporis.

with fissuring and scaling between the toes. Tinea cruris, is also known as jock itch. Affected skin is erythematous and scaly with a bilateral distribution. Pruritus is a common symptom with all forms of tinea.

Diagnosis

Diagnosis of these infections is largely clinical, but the diagnosis is confirmed by the visualization of fungal hyphae in a preparation of skin scrapings with potassium hydroxide. Fungal culture can also be performed.

Treatment

Treatment depends on the location of infection. Topical therapy with miconazole, clotrimazole, or terbinafine is usually effective. Persistence of lesions after 4 weeks of therapy may indicate treatment failure with topical therapy.

FUTURE DIRECTIONS

As therapies for cancer and autoimmune conditions continue to improve, it is likely that there will be an increasing population of children at risk for invasive fungal infections. Research is needed to improve understanding of the utility of serum biomarkers and molecular testing for the diagnosis of invasive fungal disease in children. Finally, as novel antifungal drugs are developed, trials should be performed in pediatric cohorts to provide needed information about effectiveness for children.

SUGGESTED READINGS

Available online.

90

Parasitic Diseases

Alexandra R. Linn and Katherine M. Laycock

A 10-year-old girl presented to the emergency department (ED) with 3 days of fevers. She returned 2 weeks ago from visiting family in Senegal. She describes the fevers as intermittent with associated headache, nausea, abdominal pain, fatigue, chills, and myalgias. She did not take malaria prophylaxis and received multiple mosquito bites during her trip. On arrival to the ED, she has a temperature of 101.3°F (38.5°C) and heart rate of 130 beats/min. She appears ill and uncomfortable but interacts appropriately. Laboratory tests are ordered, including a rapid malaria antigen test and blood smears. Her rapid malaria test is positive. Small, thin ring structures are visualized within her erythrocytes on Giemsa-stained thick and thin smears, consistent with *Plasmodium falciparum* malaria infection. The laboratory reports that she has 6% parasitemia. She is admitted to the hospital and treated with intravenous artesunate. Her fever and other symptoms resolve over the next 48 hours.

Malaria is a common cause of fever in children worldwide and should be considered in travelers who return from endemic areas. Malaria is caused by the parasite *Plasmodium*. It manifests with nonspecific symptoms that can be confused with other infectious causes, including dengue fever, tuberculosis, and viral illnesses. Thick and thin blood smears for direct visualization of the parasite are the gold standard for diagnosis; rapid antigen testing is also available. Choice of antimalarial treatment depends on the severity and the geographic location of infection.

Parasitic diseases are a major cause of illness and death in children globally. Although many parasites have a worldwide distribution, the morbidity of parasitic disease disproportionately affects resource-limited regions. Malaria causes the largest number of deaths, killing approximately 405,000 people each year, most of them young children in sub-Saharan Africa.

A parasite is an organism that relies on a host organism for survival, with some compromise to the host. A parasite may take different forms and require multiple hosts to complete its life cycle. Parasites that infect humans are classified as endoparasites or ectoparasites. Endoparasites are further broken down into protozoa and helminths. Protozoa are single-celled organisms that live and multiply inside the host's body. Helminths, or worms, are large, multicellular organisms that only multiply within human hosts in their nonadult form. Ectoparasites are blood-sucking arthropods that interact with the host's skin or hair.

This chapter provides an overview of important parasitic diseases with a specific emphasis on malaria because of its global impact. The chapter is organized into environmentally derived parasites (i.e., those acquired by ingestion or environmental exposure), arthropod vector–borne parasites, and ectoparasites. Of note, *Trichomonas* species is the most common cause of parasitic infections in the United States, with 7.4 million infections each year; this is described separately in Chapter 19.

ENVIRONMENTALLY DERIVED PARASITES

Protozoa

Etiology and Pathogenesis

Various environmental exposures, including ingestion of contaminated food or water and contact with infected animals, can transmit parasites to humans. Humans can also acquire infection by swimming or bathing in fresh water. A careful history with particular attention to travel, water activities, and food and water intake is valuable when assessing a patient for parasitic diseases.

Environmentally derived parasites typically infect the intestines. The most common intestinal parasites that cause disease in children in the United States are *Entamoeba histolytica*, *Giardia lamblia*, and *Cryptosporidium parvum*. Helminths, a specific subsection of intestinal environmentally derived parasites, are discussed later. Parasitic infections acquired via ingestion of raw or undercooked meat include *Trichinella* and *Toxoplasma gondii*. Life cycles vary by parasite and are described in Table 90.1 and Fig. 90.1.

Clinical Presentation and Differential Diagnosis

Children with intestinal parasites typically present with diarrhea and abdominal pain. *E. histolytica* infection produces characteristic dysentery, and *G. lamblia* infection causes greasy, malabsorptive stools. Immunocompromised hosts with *Cryptosporidium* species infection can present more severely with intractable diarrhea, fever, anorexia, and vomiting. Intestinal parasitic infections cause loss of essential electrolytes and nutrients in stool, which can lead to dehydration and failure to thrive. Examination often shows a distended abdomen. Liver abscesses caused by *E. histolytica* can lead to hepatomegaly and jaundice (Table 90.1).

The differential diagnosis for intestinal parasite infections includes invasive and noninvasive gastroenteritis caused by viruses and bacteria. Appendicitis can also manifest with diarrhea, abdominal pain and fever. Anemia and failure to thrive caused by intestinal parasites can be misdiagnosed as iron-deficiency anemia, inflammatory bowel disease, or celiac disease.

Evaluation and Management

Laboratory evaluation for environmentally derived parasitic infections starts with a complete blood count and electrolyte profile. Patients often have anemia from blood loss in the stool and electrolyte derangements from significant gastrointestinal losses. Stool

TABLE 90.1   Environmentally Derived Parasites Found Worldwide: Protozoa

Parasite	Mode of Infection/Life Cycle	Clinical Presentation	Treatment
Acanthamoeba	Free-living amoeba found in water (freshwater, salt water, and treated water) Infects the cornea (especially contact lens wearers) or enters through nasal passages	Keratitis: severe ocular pain in immunocompetent contact lens wearers Granulomatous amebic encephalitis (GAE): slowly progressive neurologic disease in immunocompromised hosts	Keratitis: topical chlorhexidine GAE: combination antiparasitic therapy
Entamoeba histolytica	Fecal-oral Ingested cysts become trophozoites in host gut, attach to colonic mucosa and form ulcers. Can migrate to portal circulation or form ameboma in intestinal wall	Bloody diarrhea (dysentery); liver abscess; bowel obstruction from ameboma in intestinal wall	Paromomycin or diloxanide furoate; add metronidazole for extraluminal disease
Cryptosporidium species *Microsporidia* species	Fecal-oral Oocysts resist chlorine treatments	Nonbloody diarrhea (prolonged in immunocompromised hosts)	Nitazoxanide *(Cryptosporidium)* or albendazole (Microsporidia); antiretroviral therapy (ART) if HIV positive
Giardia lamblia	Fecal-oral See Fig. 90.1	Acute or chronic diarrhea (may be asymptomatic)	Metronidazole, tinidazole, or nitazoxanide; may be self-limited
Naegleria fowleri	Free-living amoeba found in warm freshwater and soil Enters the nose during swimming or diving and migrates to the brain through the cribriform plate	Primary amebic meningoencephalitis: rapidly progressive, often fatal in healthy patients. CSF chemistry resembles that of bacterial infection with motile amoebas visible on microscopy.	Amphotericin B
Toxoplasma gondii	Ingestion of oocysts (undercooked meats or contaminated food/water) or vertical transmission Cats are definitive hosts and shed oocysts in stool	Congenital infection: chorioretinitis, cerebral calcifications, hydrocephalus Acute infection: Lymphadenopathy (local or generalized), flulike illness, chorioretinitis Immunocompromised hosts: Severe disseminated disease with encephalitis, myocarditis, pneumonitis	Pyrimethamine and sulfadiazine Often self-limited in immuno-competent hosts

microscopy to look for ova (eggs) and parasites (O&P analysis) is diagnostic. A single stool sample can have low yield, so multiple stool samples should be collected over a few days. Standard O&P testing cannot identify *Cryptosporidium* and *Microspora* species; therefore, PCR-based stool testing is increasingly used. Immunoassay detection of *Cryptosporidium, G. lamblia,* and *E. histolytica* antigens is a common method of diagnosis. Treatment involves supportive care with oral rehydration therapy, which is discussed in Chapter 63. Directed antiparasitic therapy varies by organism (Table 90.1).

Helminths

Helminths are a subset of environmentally derived intestinal parasites that can be further divided into four categories: (1) intestinal nematodes, (2) tissue nematodes (filaria), (3) trematodes (flukes), and (4) cestodes (tapeworms). Nematodes are also known as roundworms. Helminth infections are most common in areas with poor water sanitation. Helminths often cause intestinal symptoms of bloating, abdominal pain, and bloody stool. *Enterobius vermicularis* (pinworm), the most common helminth of industrialized nations, causes pruritus ani. Schistosomiasis infects approximately 200 million people worldwide and is an important cause of bladder cancer.

Helminth infections are diagnosed by direct visualization of worms. The Scotch tape test, in which tape is pressed to the anus to pick up eggs excreted at night, diagnoses pinworms. Treatment varies based on species, but the majority of helminths can be treated with albendazole. For this reason, many endemic countries administer albendazole

to children multiple times a year in mass deworming efforts. The life cycle, clinical presentation, and treatment considerations are described in Table 90.2 and Fig. 90.2.

VECTOR-BORNE PARASITES

Parasites also can be transmitted to human hosts by the bite of an arthropod vector. Within the host, the parasite may pass through various life cycle stages until transmission to another insect vector by a blood meal repeats the cycle. Common vector-borne parasitic diseases include malaria (by mosquito), leishmaniasis (by sand fly), trypanosomiasis (by tsetse fly in Africa or reduviid bug in America), and babesiosis (by tick). These diseases have varied clinical presentations. Diagnosis generally occurs through direct microscopic visualization of the parasite. Treatment varies based on parasite. Details of common vector-borne parasitic diseases are described in Table 90.3, and a detailed description of malaria follows.

Malaria
Etiology and Pathogenesis

Malaria is caused by the protozoa *Plasmodium,* which is transmitted by nighttime-feeding female *Anopheles* mosquitoes. Four main species of *Plasmodium* infect humans: *P. falciparum, P. ovale, P. vivax,* and *P. malariae.* These species occupy different but overlapping geographic ranges throughout the tropics. *P. falciparum,* the most prevalent species, dominates in sub-Saharan Africa. *P. vivax* malaria occurs in Asia,

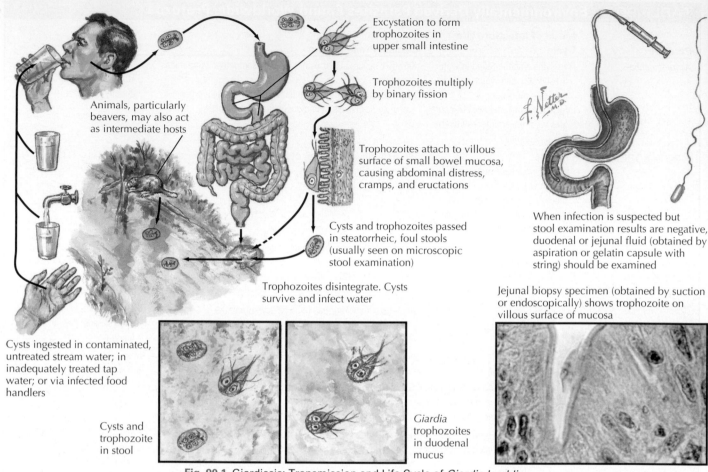

Excystation to form trophozoites in upper small intestine

Trophozoites multiply by binary fission

Animals, particularly beavers, may also act as intermediate hosts

Trophozoites attach to villous surface of small bowel mucosa, causing abdominal distress, cramps, and eructations

Cysts and trophozoites passed in steatorrheic, foul stools (usually seen on microscopic stool examination)

Trophozoites disintegrate. Cysts survive and infect water

When infection is suspected but stool examination results are negative, duodenal or jejunal fluid (obtained by aspiration or gelatin capsule with string) should be examined

Jejunal biopsy specimen (obtained by suction or endoscopically) shows trophozoite on villous surface of mucosa

Cysts ingested in contaminated, untreated stream water; in inadequately treated tap water; or via infected food handlers

Cysts and trophozoite in stool

Giardia trophozoites in duodenal mucus

Fig. 90.1 Giardiasis: Transmission and Life Cycle of *Giardia lamblia*.

Eastern Europe, and South America. *P. ovale* malaria occurs in Western Africa. Infection with *P. falciparum* is the most clinically devastating, causing an estimated 1 to 2.7 million pediatric deaths annually. The typical incubation period ranges from 7 days to months after infection. Although malaria is no longer endemic in the United States, cases are often seen in returning travelers.

Plasmodium transitions through multiple stages during its life cycle. The mosquito releases sporozoites into the human bloodstream during a blood meal. Sporozoites travel to the liver, where they grow and multiply over 7 to 14 days. In contrast to *P. falciparum*, *P. vivax*, and *P. ovale* may remain in the liver stage as hypnozoites for months before reactivation. Once mature, the parasite reenters the bloodstream to invade and multiply within erythrocytes (the blood stage). Infected erythrocytes eventually lyse releasing daughter parasites, or merozoites, that infect new erythrocytes. This release causes the clinical symptoms of malaria. Some merozoites mature into gametocytes (male and female sexual forms), which can be taken up by a new mosquito during a subsequent blood meal. In the mosquito gut, gametocytes mate and produce a sporozoite that migrates to the mosquito salivary glands to start a new cycle.

Humans can develop acquired immunity to malaria after multiple infections. Those with acquired immunity have milder presentations and may be asymptomatic. Immunity is short-lived. As a result, cases of severe malaria often occur in travelers who return to endemic areas after a significant amount of time away. In areas with high prevalence of *P. falciparum*, maternal antibodies protect infants from infection following birth. Genetic factors also protect against severe disease: heterozygotes for sickle cell disease have partial protection against *P. falciparum*, and those negative for the Duffy group antigen have resistance to *P. vivax*.

Clinical Presentation and Differential Diagnosis

Uncomplicated malaria manifests with nonspecific symptoms including fever, chills, headache, vomiting, diarrhea, myalgias, sweats, and fatigue. Fevers are classically described as periodic, correlating with lysis of erythrocytes during the blood stage of the parasite's life cycle. In clinical practice, fevers are often less formulaic. Physical examination findings are also nonspecific but can include jaundice and hepatosplenomegaly. Complicated (severe) malaria causes end-organ damage. Symptoms of severe malaria include altered mental status, seizures, respiratory distress, pulmonary edema, kidney injury, hypoglycemia, disseminated intravascular coagulation, shock, and coma.

Severe malaria, including cerebral malaria, occurs most often with *P. falciparum* infections. *P. falciparum* uniquely causes erythrocytes to become sticky and malformed by inducing budding proteins on the erythrocyte surface. These abnormal erythrocytes then cause stasis and thrombosis in capillary beds, leading to manifestations of end-organ damage in the kidneys, liver, and brain. Severe malaria is a medical emergency requiring prompt diagnosis and treatment.

The differential diagnosis for malaria is broad and described further in Chapter 84.

TABLE 90.2 Environmentally Derived Parasites: Helminths

Name	Life Cycle and Geographic Distribution	Clinical Presentation	Diagnosis/Treatment
Intestinal Nematodes			
Strongyloides	Female worms produce eggs in gut; larvae in feces then penetrate host skin, migrate to lungs, and are swallowed Worldwide	Abdominal pain, vomiting, diarrhea, serpiginous rash; severe disseminated disease in immunocompromised hosts	Visualization of larvae in stool Ivermectin
Enterobius vermicularis (pinworm)	Ingested eggs hatch in intestine; adult females live in colon and lay eggs on the perineum Worldwide	Pruritus ani	Scotch tape test Albendazole once, repeat in 2 weeks; pyrantel alternative Empiric treatment of contacts recommended
Ascaris	See Fig. 90.2 Worldwide	Asymptomatic or mild abdominal discomfort Lung phase: cough, hemoptysis Severe disease: failure to thrive, intestinal obstruction	Visualization of eggs or worms in stool Albendazole
Trichinella	Ingestion of larvae in undercooked contaminated meats (pigs, boar, bear) Larvae are released in the stomach, enter bloodstream, and infect host skeletal muscle Worldwide	Nausea, fatigue, abdominal pain, then myalgias and periorbital edema with eosinophilia	Serologic studies, muscle biopsy Albendazole and corticosteroids
Tissue Nematodes (filaria)			
Loa loa; onchocerciasis; *Wuchereria*	Insect vector transmits larvae to host; adult worms mature in host lymphatics or tissues Tropics worldwide	*Loa loa*—eye and skin swelling Onchocerciasis (river blindness)—subcutaneous nodules, ocular lesions *Wuchereria*—elephantiasis	Microscopy with filaria on blood smear Diethylcarbamazine Onchocerciasis: ivermectin (diethylcarbamazine contraindicated)
Trematodes (flukes)			
Schistosoma	Snails release parasite into slow-moving freshwater. Parasite penetrates host skin and migrates in bloodstream to lungs, then liver, then bladder or intestines to release eggs Worldwide except North America	Acute (Katayama fever): Fever, cough, abdominal pain within 1–2 months of infection Chronic infection: liver disease; bladder cancer; hematuria; neurologic disease	Identify eggs in the urine (*S. haematobium*) or feces (*S. japonicum, S. mansoni*) Praziquantel
Cestodes (tapeworms): ***Taenia, Echinococcus***			
Taenia solium (pork tapeworm) and *Taenia saginata* (beef tapeworm)	Taeniasis: ingested larval cysts (cysticerci) from undercooked meat mature in intestines Cysticercosis: ingested eggs from tapeworm carrier invade tissues (*T. solium* only) Worldwide	Taeniasis: asymptomatic or mild abdominal discomfort Cysticercosis: major cause of seizures	Visualization of eggs or worms in stool or tissue CNS imaging Praziquantel or albendazole
Echinococcus	Dogs are definitive hosts. Ingested eggs from canine feces hatch in human intestine and disseminate in bloodstream to form cysts in tissues. Worldwide	Single or multiple slow-growing cysts, usually in liver (>65%) or lung (25%), asymptomatic until large enough to cause mass effect Cyst rupture causes anaphylaxis	Imaging detects cysts. Serologic study often negative if cyst intact Albendazole or surgical removal

Evaluation and Treatment

Diagnosis of malaria is made by Giemsa-stained thick and thin blood smears (Fig. 90.3). Parasite density on the slide can indicate disease severity, though patients with no prior exposure to malaria may exhibit severe symptoms even with lower parasitemia. Highly sensitive and specific rapid antigen detection tests also exist and are used widely endemic areas. If positive, a rapid test should be confirmed with blood smears to visualize the parasite and determine parasite density. A complete blood count and metabolic profile are also helpful to identify evidence of severe malaria with markers of hemolysis and end-organ malperfusion.

Antimalarial treatment should begin immediately. Drug choice depends on the *Plasmodium* species, local drug susceptibilities, and the patient's clinical status and history of antimalarial use. The risk for malaria infection is much lower but not zero in those taking antimalarial prophylaxis. See Chapter 84 for more information on malaria treatment and prevention.

ECTOPARASITES

An ectoparasite is a parasite that lives on the outside of the host. The most common ectoparasites in children are lice and scabies.

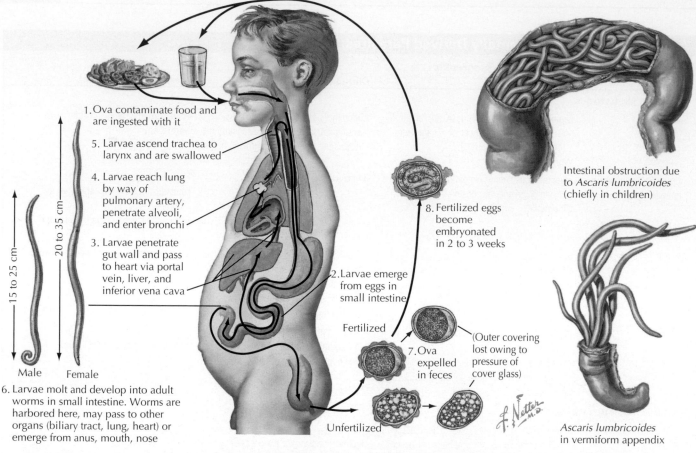

1. Ova contaminate food and are ingested with it

5. Larvae ascend trachea to larynx and are swallowed

4. Larvae reach lung by way of pulmonary artery, penetrate alveoli, and enter bronchi

3. Larvae penetrate gut wall and pass to heart via portal vein, liver, and inferior vena cava

8. Fertilized eggs become embryonated in 2 to 3 weeks

2. Larvae emerge from eggs in small intestine

Fertilized

7. Ova expelled in feces

(Outer covering lost owing to pressure of cover glass)

Unfertilized

15 to 25 cm

20 to 35 cm

Male   Female

6. Larvae molt and develop into adult worms in small intestine. Worms are harbored here, may pass to other organs (biliary tract, lung, heart) or emerge from anus, mouth, nose

Intestinal obstruction due to *Ascaris lumbricoides* (chiefly in children)

Ascaris lumbricoides in vermiform appendix

Fig. 90.2 Ascariasis: Transmission and Life Cycle of *Ascaris lumbricoides*.

TABLE 90.3 Vector-Borne Parasitic Diseases

Vector	Parasite	Life Cycle and Geographic Distribution	Clinical Presentation	Diagnosis/Treatment
Sand fly	*Leishmania* species	Female sand flies transmit by bite. Infect macrophages to become intracellular amastigotes. 20 species of *Leishmania* cause human disease. Rodents and dogs are intermediate hosts. Central and South America, Southern Europe, the Middle East, Africa, and Asia	Cutaneous leishmaniasis—skin ulcers. Mucosal leishmaniasis—mucous membrane sores, disseminated from cutaneous disease. Visceral leishmaniasis (kala-azar)—fever, massive splenomegaly, hepatomegaly, pancytopenia	Microscopic parasite identification in tissue; antibody blood testing. Cutaneous leishmaniasis often self-limited, may scar or disseminate. Visceral leishmaniasis treated with Amphotericin B; often fatal if untreated
Reduviid bug ("kissing bug")	*Trypanosoma cruzi*	Insect releases trypomastigotes in its feces near area of bite. Parasite enters host through the bite wound or local mucosa (conjunctiva), then invades cells. Can be transmitted congenitally, in blood transfusions, and in transplanted organs. Mexico and Central and South America	Chagas disease: Acute—fever and local swelling (chagoma) followed by asymptomatic stage. Chronic—develops in 20%–30%; esophageal/colon dysmotility, dilated cardiomyopathy	Microscopic parasite identification in thick and thin blood smears (acute). Chronic disease diagnosed via clinical findings/history. Nifurtimox, benznidazole
Tsetse fly	*Trypanosoma brucei gambiense, Trypanosoma brucei rhodesiense*	Flies inject trypomastigotes into the skin of the host. Parasite multiplies in bloodstream and bodily fluids; remains extracellular. Sub-Saharan Africa	African sleeping sickness. Acute stage (1–3 weeks)—fever, headache and malaise. Second stage—meningoencephalitis, often fatal	Microscopic parasite identification in bodily fluid. Pentamidine for *gambiense*, suramin for *rhodesiense*
Tick	*Babesia* species	White-footed mouse passes parasite to *Ixodes* tick via a blood meal. Tick then infects human host via bite. Sporozoites then infect erythrocytes. Can be transmitted in blood transfusions. North America and Europe	Often asymptomatic. May cause fever and flulike symptoms. Severe disease with hemolytic anemia if immunocompromised or asplenic.	Microscopic parasite identification in thick or thin blood smear (may see intraerythrocytic "Maltese cross"). Clindamycin and quinine; or atovaquone and azithromycin

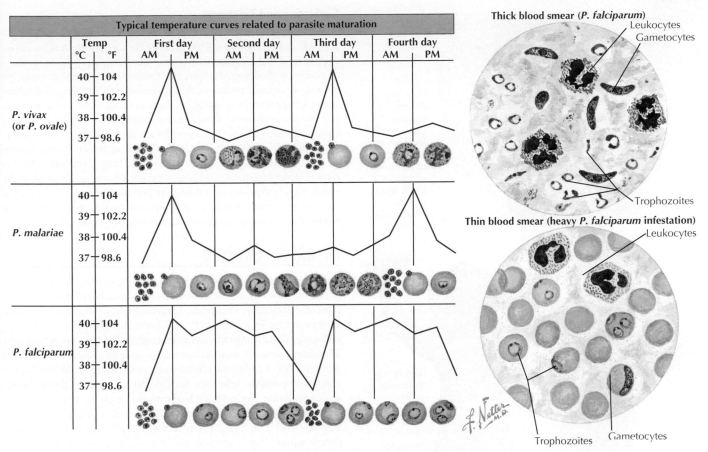

Fig. 90.3 Malaria Clinical Course and Diagnosis.

Lice

Clinical Manifestations and Pathophysiology

Head lice is caused by *Pediculus humanus capitis*. Head lice is found worldwide and affects 6 to 12 million people per year in the United States, with highest prevalence among children. Transmission occurs by direct contact or by fomites on hats and scarves. Daycare centers and schools are at high risk for lice infestation.

Adult female lice lay nits (eggs) on the hair shaft close to the scalp. Nits are small, oval-shaped and yellow or white. They typically hatch within 9 days producing a nymph (immature louse). Nymphs feed on blood and mature into adults within 12 days. Adult lice survive on the head up to 30 days but can only survive for 24 hours away from the scalp.

Clinical Presentation and Differential Diagnosis

Patients typically present with pruritus of the scalp or with sores on the head caused by scratching. Posterior cervical lymphadenopathy also may be seen. When involving the body, patients may have widespread dermatitis, similar to a viral exanthem. The differential diagnosis for lice includes scabies and noninfectious dermatologic conditions such as eczema.

Evaluation and Treatment

Lice is diagnosed by visualization of nits, nymphs, or adult lice on examination. A magnifying glass or fine-toothed comb can aide in identification. Close contacts also should be screened.

Treatment is available over the counter with formulations that incorporate pyrethrin and permethrin. Prescription medications include benzyl alcohol lotion and ivermectin lotion. Prevention of lice is critical. Louse inspections in schools or camps and community education during outbreaks can be effective in identifying infested patients before spread to close contacts.

Scabies

Etiology and Pathophysiology

Human scabies is caused by the mite *Sarcoptes scabiei* var. *hominis*. About 300 million cases of scabies occur yearly worldwide. Scabies is acquired by direct skin-to-skin contact and is common in areas with overcrowding and poor hygiene. Outbreaks occur in group centers such as daycare facilities, prisons, shelters, and nursing homes.

Mites burrow under the skin to live and lay eggs. Adult mites lay 2 to 3 eggs daily. These eggs hatch after 3 to 4 days, releasing larvae that migrate to the skin surface. Larvae molt to produce nymphs, which mature into adult mites. Adults mate when adult males penetrate the female's molting patch. Females are then fertile for the rest of their lifetime, continuing the life cycle.

Clinical Presentation and Differential Diagnosis

Scabies manifests with an intensely pruritic skin rash that is caused by an allergic reaction to the mite's feces. Patients exposed to scabies for the first time often do not develop symptoms for 4 to 8 weeks but are still infectious to others. Symptoms typically begin with itching at night; rash develops shortly after. The characteristic rash is papular, scaly, and concentrated in skinfolds of extremities (Fig. 90.4). In infants and young children, the scalp, face, neck, and palms/soles are often involved.

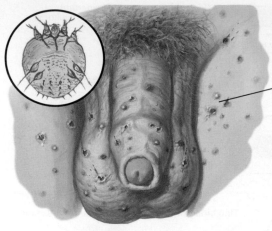

Scabies (*Sarcoptes scabiei* in circle)

Inflammatory excoriated papules (note penile involvement). Involvement of genitalia, umbilicus, and finger webs is characteristic for scabies.

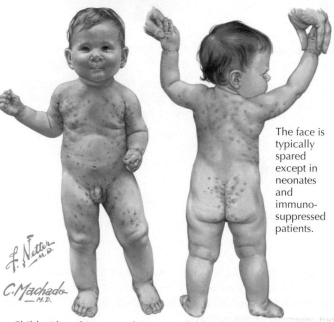

The face is typically spared except in neonates and immuno-suppressed patients.

Child with scabies, ventral view   Child with scabies, dorsal view

Fig. 90.4 Scabies.

Scratching and introduction of bacteria can lead to overlying infection. Superimposed impetigo with *Staphylococcus aureus* and β-hemolytic streptococcus is often seen.

The differential diagnosis list for scabies infection is similar to that for lice, as described earlier.

Evaluation and Treatment

Scabies is diagnosed on physical examination with evidence of the characteristic rash. Diagnosis can be confirmed by identification of the mites, eggs, or fecal material by microscopy of skin scrapings from burrows.

Scabies is often treated empirically if suspected. Permethrin cream 5% is the most common treatment, though ivermectin is an effective oral alternative. Cream should be applied to the entire body from the neck down. For infants, application should also include the face, scalp, and neck. Cream should be left on for at least 8 hours and reapplied in 7 to 10 days.

All household, sexual, or close contacts of patients with scabies should be empirically treated. Clothing, bed linens, and soft toys also require decontamination through washing or sealing in an air-tight plastic bag. Symptoms of scabies may persist after treatment because the rash is allergen-mediated. If symptoms persist more than 2 to 4 weeks after treatment, a repeat treatment may be required.

FUTURE DIRECTIONS

To decrease the global burden of parasitic infections, integrated programs are working to improve access to clean water, safe food supplies, and sanitation worldwide. Mass drug administration campaigns have prevented infections such as schistosomiasis, onchocerciasis, and soil-transmitted helminthiasis in some regions but have not yet reached all endemic areas. A new vaccine shows promise against malaria, and development of additional effective vaccines is urgently needed to prevent other parasitic infections such as trypanosomiasis. Other large-scale prevention strategies are beginning to target the transmission of endemic parasites from domestic animals, with efforts to implement dog deworming campaigns to reduce echinococcosis and to vaccinate sheep against *Taenia* species. Vector surveillance programs are also expanding to track the geographic distribution of disease-transmitting insects like sand flies and tsetse flies, which may shift to new regions under the influences of insecticide resistance and climate change, and to implement novel vector control approaches. Key next steps in diagnosis and treatment, particularly for highly morbid infections like leishmaniasis and trypanosomiasis, include the development of effective, affordable point-of-care diagnostic tests and of safe, low-cost, oral medications with pediatric formulations. Intensive public health efforts have led to the recent elimination of some devastating parasitic infections from some regions, but much work remains.

SUGGESTED READINGS

Available online.

Neonatal Medicine

Joanna Parga-Belinke

91

Newborn Examination

Leora Lieberman and Kristin McKenna

The vast majority of term infants have a normal postnatal transition. Late preterm (35 to 36 weeks gestational age) infants are generally well, but at higher risk for respiratory distress, hyperbilirubinemia, hypoglycemia, temperature instability, and poor feeding. The physical examination is a pivotal screening method for discernment of imminent versus innocuous findings. This quick assessment will let a family know if reassurance or escalation is warranted. Additionally, it establishes the foundation of the family-pediatrician relationship, allowing the pediatrician to build rapport. Clinicians need a systematic approach to avoid missing key elements and overlooking critical findings.

CLINICAL PRESENTATION

General Appearance

Observation alone can provide a wealth of initial information about a neonate. Generally, normal findings include an easily arousable, consolable, vigorous when stimulated, and well-perfused (pink) infant. Arms and legs should be flexed with symmetric movement of the extremities, and breathing should be unlabored.

Growth Parameters

Three growth parameters are measured in infants—weight, length, and head circumference. Small for gestational age (SGA, <10th percentile), appropriate for gestational age (AGA), and large for gestational age (LGA, >90th percentile) are determined according to where weight plots on standardized growth charts. The cause of SGA or LGA may warrant further evaluation.

Ideally, fetal growth results in a proportional infant when comparing weight, length, and head circumference. Intrauterine growth restriction (IUGR) can be symmetric or asymmetric. Symmetric IUGR affects all three growth parameters and raises concerns for genetic conditions. Asymmetric IUGR spares head growth and is generally thought to be secondary to some degree of placental insufficiency. These neonates have a relatively large head circumference (head sparing) compared with weight and length.

Vital Signs

Please see Table 91.1 for normal vital signs in the newborn.

Head

The head examination includes head circumference, suture palpation, and fontanelle number, size, and character. Newborns present with varying head shapes, often associated with fetal presentation and mode of delivery. An infant engaged in the vaginal canal during labor commonly presents with head elongation or molding and/or overriding sutures.

Open sutures allow for skull malleability and should form two soft spots known as the anterior and posterior fontanelles (Fig. 91.1). Fontanelles should be palpated with the infant upright and should reveal flat, nonbulging anterior and posterior fontanelles measuring approximately 3 cm or less.

The birth process may cause extracranial head trauma, including caput succedaneum (crosses suture lines), cephalohematoma (does not cross suture lines), or the most clinically concerning, subgaleal hematoma (dependent swelling) (Fig. 91.2). A cephalohematoma increases the risk for hyperbilirubinemia, and presence of a subgaleal hematoma requires prompt assessment given the risk for hemorrhage into the subgaleal space. A delivery with forceps increases the risk for head trauma, including facial nerve palsy, (observed as the inability to close an eye, loss of the nasolabial fold, or asymmetric crying with lateral mouth drooping).

Accurate measurement of head circumference should circle from the supraorbital ridges to the occiput and may be falsely enlarged in extracranial head trauma, or falsely small with molding. Aberrant measurements should be rechecked. Macrocephaly is defined by head circumference greater than the 97th percentile or two standard deviations above the mean for age and sex, and microcephaly is defined by head circumference less than the 3rd percentile or two standard deviations below the mean for age and sex.

TABLE 91.1 **Normal Vital Sign Ranges for the Term Newborn**	
Heart rate	120–160 (beats/min)
Respiratory rate	40–60 (breaths/min)
Blood pressure	50–70 mm Hg (systolic)
	30–60 mm Hg (diastolic)

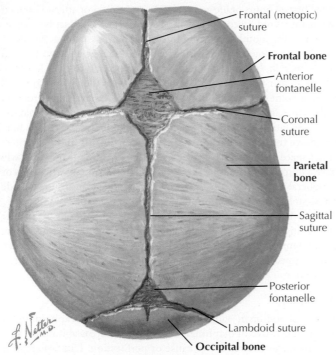

Fig. 91.1 Superior View of Newborn Skull Showing Fontanelles.

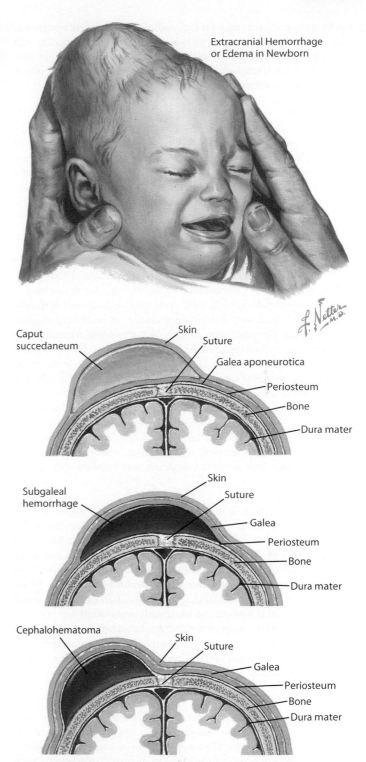

Fig. 91.2 Extracranial Head Bleeds in Newborns.

Eyes

Examination of the eyes is best performed holding the neonate slightly upright in a dimly lit environment. This facilitates spontaneous eye opening, allowing for assessment of the eye.

Most babies are born with dark gray-blue or gray-brown irises. The surrounding eye should be white. Scleral icterus, or a yellow hue, before 24 hours of life is abnormal. Blue-tinged sclera may be a normal finding, but a more pronounced hue may require investigation. Subconjunctival hemorrhages or ruptured blood vessels in the eye can be a sequela of delivery. They appear as a bright red band around the iris, and can be unilateral or bilateral. Disconjugate gaze, discoordination of eye movements and malalignment due to immature extraocular muscles, is common. Transient nystagmus is also common.

An ophthalmoscope assesses the red reflex, the light reflection off the retina. A normal red reflex is symmetric, ranging from pale yellow to orange to dark red. Without dilation, comprehensive evaluation of the eye is difficult, thus limiting assessment for abnormalities such as congenital cataracts, retinoblastoma, or coloboma. Abnormal findings, such as no reflex, white spots, or black spots, require evaluation by an ophthalmologist.

Ocular discharge may be noninfectious or infectious. Unilateral, clear discharge with ipsilateral swelling lateral to the nose may be secondary to dacryostenosis, a narrowed or blocked lacrimal duct. Normal appearance of the conjunctiva separates dacryostenosis from ophthalmia neonatorum, or neonatal conjunctivitis.

This manifests early in life as conjunctival injection and eyelid edema and requires antibiotic therapy generally in the form of an ointment.

Ears

To assess ear position, a diagonal, imaginary line should be drawn from the lateral canthus of the eye to the superior helix of the ear pinna, and a perpendicular line should be drawn against this initial line. Low-set ears will fall below the first line, whereas rotated ears will lie posterior to the second. Preauricular ear tags and ear pits are often benign, but may be associated with renal pathology if found in conjunction with additional dysmorphisms, a family history of renal anomalies, or congenital deafness. Variations in the shape and folding of the helix, pinna, and tragus are common and generally benign in isolation.

Nose

Because neonates are obligate nose breathers, normal anatomy of the nares is essential for air exchange. With the infant sucking on a gloved finger or pacifier, each nare should be occluded separately. If the infant exhibits respiratory distress or opens the mouth, consider choanal stenosis or atresia. A feeding tube can be passed through the nares to assess patency. A normal nasal septum should be midline, and dislocation (not corrected with depression of the nasal tip) may result from in utero malpositioning.

Mouth

Cleft lip and palate may be isolated findings or associated with a genetic syndrome. A submucosal or complete cleft palate can be palpated or directly observed. A bifid uvula may be associated with submucosal clefts and may warrant surveillance for additional midline abnormalities. The palate may show 1- to 3-mm white accumulations on the median palatal raphe called Epstein pearls, which resolve spontaneously. Bohn nodules, similar in appearance although on the gums, are salivary gland remnants and also resolve spontaneously. Natal teeth may require removal if they pose an aspiration risk (if loose) or disrupt feeding. Jaw abnormalities, such as micrognathia (small mandible) or retrognathia (retroverted mandible), pose risk to the aerodigestive systems. Ranulas, purple/red mucus retention cysts on the mouth floor, often require surgical removal. Ankyloglossia, a short lingual frenulum, prevents protrusion of the tongue and may interfere with feeding.

Neck

The neck examination should assess for congenital torticollis, sternocleidomastoid swelling, clavicular fracture, and webbing. Assess for symmetric neck rotation. Webbing of the neck can be associated with Turner syndrome. Sternocleidomastoid palpation should assess for masses. Cystic hygroma is the most common neck mass characterized by redundant skinfolds posterior to the sternocleidomastoid. Other neck masses include branchial clefts (found laterally) and thyroglossal duct cysts (found at midline and move with swallowing).

The clavicle is the most commonly fractured bone during delivery and presents as decreased or absent arm movement, gross deformity of the clavicle, tenderness or crepitus appreciated with palpation, and an asymmetric or absent Moro reflex.

Chest Wall and Lungs

Chest wall abnormalities, such as pectus excavatum (concavity) and carinatum (convexity), can be asymptomatic or cause alteration in cardiorespiratory mechanics. They may occur in isolation or in conjunction with connective tissue disorders. A small thorax may be associated with pulmonary hypoplasia, whereas a bell-shaped chest may signal dwarfism or neurologic abnormalities. Estrogen exposure in pregnancy may cause transient breast budding, and supernumerary nipples are common and appear along the milk line. Nipples should sit near the midclavicular line, and if widely spaced, may be associated with a genetic abnormality.

Given the immaturity of neural respiratory centers, newborns exhibit physiologic, periodic breathing, characterized as pauses every 5 to 10 seconds without other associated vital sign changes. This response is magnified in preterm infants, manifested as apnea and bradycardia. To account for this, it is important to count breaths for a full 60 seconds to accurately measure respiratory rate. Although mild work of breathing may reflect postnatal transitioning, persistent, progressive, or significant respiratory distress after 1 hour of life, manifested as tachypnea, retractions, nasal flaring, grunting, or cyanosis, should be investigated. A normal chest examination includes symmetric chest rise with clear breath sounds to the lung bases bilaterally.

Cardiovascular

Acrocyanosis, peripheral blue discoloration of the hands and feet, should be distinguished from central cyanosis. Acrocyanosis is normal in the first 24 hours of life as circulation normalizes or after 24 hours if the infant is cold. In contrast, central cyanosis, which describes discoloration of the mouth, head, and torso, is abnormal and may be reflective of poor oxygenation. Neonatal heart rates range between 120 and 160 beats/min, but special attention should be paid to rates less than 100 or greater than 170 beats/min. Palpation of the precordium will reveal a point of maximal impulse at the left lower sternal border, as right ventricular hypertrophy is common because of fetal physiology.

Auscultation should occur at the right and left upper sternal border, down the left sternal border and between the fifth and sixth intercostal space at the midclavicular line. Roughly 60% of neonates will have a murmur, commonly the result of a closing ductus arteriosus or peripheral pulmonic stenosis. Features of pathologic murmurs include holosystolic, diastolic, continuous, harsh, and grade of 3 or greater.

Both femoral pulses should be palpated and should be regular and strong; weak pulses signify poor cardiac output, and bounding pulses signify high cardiac output. Assess for a brachial-femoral delay, accompanied by four extremity blood pressures, to screen for aortic coarctation.

Abdomen

A normal abdomen will have slight roundedness. Scaphoid abdomen is suggestive of diaphragmatic hernia, whereas abdominal distension suggests obstructive cause or perforation. Diastasis recti is a benign outpouching at the midline of the abdomen common in neonates.

The umbilical stump should have two arteries and one vein. Umbilical drainage suggests omphalitis, a patent urachus, or patent omphalomesenteric duct remnants and requires evaluation. Umbilical hernias can manifest in varying sizes and do not require intervention. The umbilical cord should dry and fall off within approximately 10 days. If the cord remains attached for more than 2 weeks, further evaluation may be warranted.

Auscultation should reveal bowel sounds in all four quadrants. Palpation of the abdomen should start in the lower quadrant and work up on both the left and right so as not to miss hepatosplenomegaly or masses. In neonates, a normal liver edge can be felt 1 to 2 cm below the right costal margin.

GENITOURINARY

The transient manifestations of maternal estrogen in newborns include genital swelling and vaginal discharge. Voiding should occur within the first 24 hours of life, and meconium passage should occur within 48 hours of life. Delayed stool transit is concerning for conditions such as Hirschsprung disease or cystic fibrosis. The anus should be inspected for position and presence of the anal reflex, in which the external anal sphincter contracts after the surrounding skin is stroked. Absence of the anal reflex suggests a lumbar spine pathologic condition.

Male genitalia should be inspected for penile length, intact foreskin, urethral positioning, and bilateral testicle descension. Urethral abnormalities include hypospadias, in which the urethra

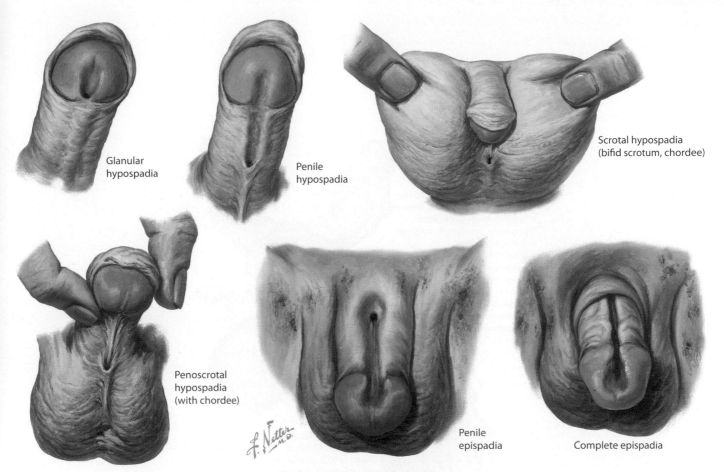

Glanular hypospadia

Penile hypospadia

Scrotal hypospadia (bifid scrotum, chordee)

Penoscrotal hypospadia (with chordee)

Penile epispadia

Complete epispadia

Fig. 91.3 Hypospadia, Epispadia.

is ventrally displaced, and epispadias, in which the urethra is dorsally displaced (Fig. 91.3). Importantly, micropenis, urethral malpositioning, and bilateral cryptorchidism are contraindications to circumcision. Inguinal hernias are present in 3% to 5% of full-term neonates and 30% of preterm neonates and should easily reduce.

Female genitalia should show distinct labia majora and labia minora. Clitoral lengthening indicates virilization, seen with congenital adrenal hyperplasia. Vaginal obstruction or mass may be seen with imperforate hymen. Benign findings include hymenal skin tags, which spontaneously resolve.

Back

In the prone position, the spine should be assessed for abnormal curvature. Simple, sacral dimples occur at midline, within 2.5 cm of the anus, and have an easily visualized base that is less than 0.5 cm deep. Spinal imaging (ultrasound) is warranted when dimples do not meet these criteria or when a cleft, skin tag, hair tuft, mass, or hemangioma is present in the spinal or paraspinal region.

Extremities

The hands and feet should show 10 fingers, 10 toes, and symmetric extremities with normal muscle bulk and full range of motion. Extra digits, or polydactyly, may occur preaxially, on the radial side, or postaxially, on the ulnar side. Preaxial polydactyly is associated with underlying syndromes, whereas postaxial is a common, isolated finding. Syndactyly, abnormal fusion of the digits, may be sporadic or genetic. The palms should be inspected for a single palmar crease, which may be found with some genetic abnormalities such as trisomy

21. Swelling of the hands and feet may be secondary to lymphedema and may be associated with Turner syndrome

Trauma to the roots of the fifth cervical to first thoracic spinal nerves may result in a brachial plexus injury/palsy. Erb-Duchenne palsy, the most common, affects the fifth and sixth cervical roots, presenting with arm adduction and internal rotation, absent Moro, and intact grasp. Klumpke palsy affects the seventh and eighth cervical and first thoracic root. It manifests with hand paralysis, absent wrist movement, and absent grasp and may be associated with an ipsilateral Horner syndrome.

The hips should be examined with special maneuvers, the Barlow, Ortolani, and Galeazzi (Fig. 91.4), to screen for developmental dysplasia of the hip. Neonatal feet should be supine with slight adduction that easily abducts beyond neutral position. Abnormalities in foot positioning include metatarsus adductus (when the foot cannot abduct past neutral position) and clubfoot (Fig. 91.5). Extensive limb deformities can be seen after teratogenic exposures or secondary to intrauterine amniotic bands.

Neurologic

The neurologic examination includes assessment of mental status (response to stimuli), suck, and primitive and postural reflexes. Irritability or lethargy is abnormal. Primitive reflexes include the startle (Moro), asymmetric tonic neck (Fencer), trunk incurvation (Galant), body extension (Perez), palmar grasp, plantar grasp, and rooting. As neuronal myelination matures, these reflexes disappear cephalocaudally and from the core outward in accordance with myelination and motor developmental milestones.

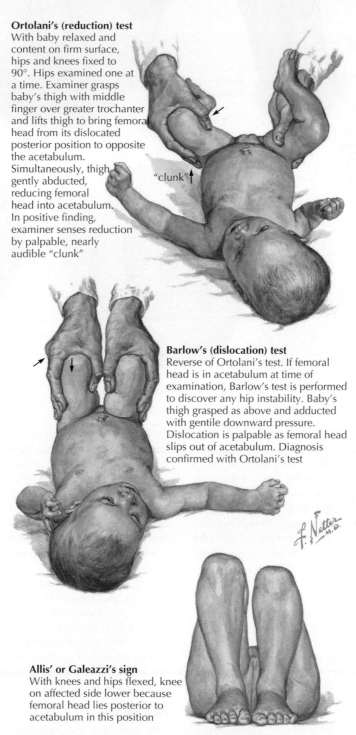

Ortolani's (reduction) test
With baby relaxed and content on firm surface, hips and knees fixed to 90°. Hips examined one at a time. Examiner grasps baby's thigh with middle finger over greater trochanter and lifts thigh to bring femoral head from its dislocated posterior position to opposite the acetabulum. Simultaneously, thigh gently abducted, reducing femoral head into acetabulum. In positive finding, examiner senses reduction by palpable, nearly audible "clunk"

"clunk"↑

Barlow's (dislocation) test
Reverse of Ortolani's test. If femoral head is in acetabulum at time of examination, Barlow's test is performed to discover any hip instability. Baby's thigh grasped as above and adducted with gentile downward pressure. Dislocation is palpable as femoral head slips out of acetabulum. Diagnosis confirmed with Ortolani's test

Allis' or Galeazzi's sign
With knees and hips flexed, knee on affected side lower because femoral head lies posterior to acetabulum in this position

Fig. 91.4 Physical Examination of the Thigh and Hip.

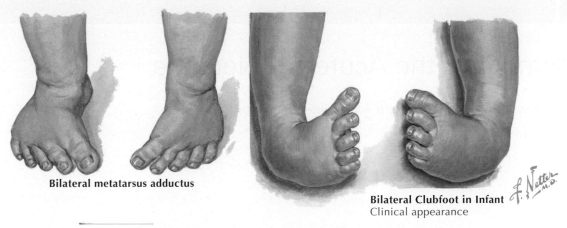

Bilateral metatarsus adductus

Bilateral Clubfoot in Infant
Clinical appearance

Fig. 91.5 Physical Examination of the Foot and Ankle.

Skin

At delivery, term infants are covered with a thick, white, lipid-rich substance called vernix caseosa, which promotes barrier immunity and decreases insensible heat losses. Dry, flaky, or peeling skin is common, especially in postterm neonates, but underlying erythema, edema, or fissuring is abnormal. Early or significant jaundice warrants checking serum bilirubin levels. Newborns display many benign skin findings (Chapter 97).

SUMMARY

Many findings on the neonatal physical examination require only reassurance and anticipatory guidance. Concerning findings necessitate prompt investigation, intervention, and escalation of care in consultation with neonatologists or appropriate pediatric subspecialists. Thus nuanced experience with the neonatal physical examination is critical. All findings, even benign, should be detailed in the medical record for longitudinal monitoring by the primary care physician.

SUGGESTED READINGS

Available online.

92

Assessment of the Acutely Ill Neonate

Robin Chin, Carolyn M. McGann, and Michelle-Marie Peña

CLINICAL VIGNETTE

The pediatrics team is called to the delivery of a 39-weeks' gestation infant with meconium-stained amniotic fluid. A brief history reveals the birth parent had a positive group B streptococcus culture and was febrile to 102°F (38.9°C). They are treated with ampicillin and gentamicin 1 hour before delivery for suspected chorioamnionitis. The infant is delivered vaginally and emerges limp with no respiratory effort. The infant dried and stimulated but remains apneic, so the team initiates positive pressure ventilation (PPV). Initial heart rate on auscultation is less than 100 but greater than 60 beats/min. After several PPV breaths, the heart rate has not changed and the infant has poor chest movement. The team repositions the mask and head to a "sniffing" position with improvement in chest rise. After 2 minutes of PPV, the infant's heart rate increases to greater than 100 beats/min with an oxygen saturation of 75%. The infant begins to cry with regular, labored respirations. The baby is transitioned to continuous positive airway pressure (CPAP) and admitted to the neonatal intensive care unit. An evaluation for infection is performed, and broad spectrum antibiotics are started.

Pediatric practitioners must be familiar with the assessment and management of the critically ill neonate. Approximately 4% to 10% of term and late preterm infants will require some form of respiratory support at birth, and less than 1% will require chest compressions. Recognition of neonatal distress and timely, standardized care using the Neonatal Resuscitation Program is critical in avoiding serious perinatal complications or death. This infant responded to adequate PPV with adjustments. Given chorioamnionitis and perinatal depression, infection rule out and antibiotics were warranted.

ETIOLOGY AND PATHOGENESIS

Fetal circulation optimizes placental gas exchange through adaptive mechanisms, including a relatively low systemic blood pressure, right-to-left cardiac shunting, and elevated pulmonary vascular resistance (PVR). Oxygenated blood from the placenta returns to the fetus by the umbilical vein and largely bypasses the liver via the ductus venosus. Blood is then shunted away from the lungs by the foramen ovale and the ductus arteriosus (Fig. 92.1). The fetal circulatory system is characterized by lower partial oxygen pressures (average 20 to 30 mm Hg).

The neonate undergoes a series of rapid physiologic shifts after delivery to transition from fetal circulation to mature postnatal circulation and gas exchange conducted by the lungs. Before the onset of labor, an unknown trigger slows the production of fetal lung fluid. Labor itself stimulates the absorption of fetal lung fluid into the pulmonary interstitium in preparation for postnatal breaths.

After delivery, several external stimuli trigger spontaneous respiration. These include umbilical cord clamping, tactile stimulation, and warming. Initial breaths taken by the infant are responsible for clearing the remaining fetal lung fluid by high inspiratory and expiratory pressures. As the lung tissue is aerated, surfactant is released, which reduces alveolar surface tension. Ventilation corrects the mild hypoxia and metabolic acidosis sustained during labor, which contributes to a decrease in PVR and a rise in systemic vascular resistance. This partially reverses the right-to-left shunting by closure of the foramen ovale. The increase in partial oxygen pressure prompts closure of the ductus arteriosus over subsequent days.

There are many fetal and maternal medical conditions and prenatal, perinatal, and postnatal events that may lead to disruption of the normal neonatal transition (Table 92.1). These factors may lead to metabolic acidosis, delayed transition, and neonatal distress. When metabolic acidosis is severe, the neonate may present with bradycardia (<100 beats/min), hypotonia, apnea, or gasping after delivery. Regardless of the cause, resuscitation should proceed using standardized Neonatal Resuscitation Program (NRP) guidelines.

EVALUATION AND MANAGEMENT OF THE NEWBORN IN THE DELIVERY ROOM

It is critical for the care team to perform an assessment of neonatal risk factors before delivery and an evaluation after birth. A complete discussion on the routine newborn examination can be found in Chapter 91.

When called to the delivery of an at-risk infant, the pediatric provider should ask four pre-birth questions: (1) gestational age, (2) color of the amniotic fluid, (3) any additional risk factors (including pregnancy risk factors, labor course, or significant prenatal ultrasound findings), and (4) if there is an established management plan for the umbilical cord (e.g., delayed cord clamping or immediate clamping).

Upon delivery of the infant, the clinician should rapidly assess three clinical factors: (1) term versus preterm, (2) tone, and (3) respiratory effort or cry. If a term infant emerges vigorous with good tone and spontaneous respiratory effort or strong cry, he or she may remain with the birth parent for routine care upon the discretion of the pediatric and obstetrics providers. If the infant appears vigorous, the obstetrics provider can perform delayed cord clamping (30 to 60 seconds) and proceed with routine postnatal care, which includes placing the infant on the birth parent's chest ("skin-to-skin") and initiating early breastfeeding or bottle feeding based on family preference and birth parent medical history. Delayed cord clamping has been associated with a decreased risk for several neonatal complications, including intraventricular hemorrhage (IVH), anemia requiring transfusion, and necrotizing enterocolitis; these benefits are particularly pronounced among

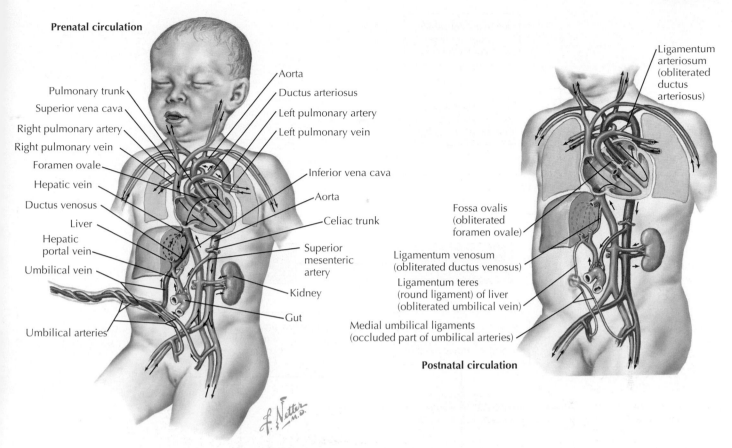

Prenatal circulation

Pulmonary trunk
Superior vena cava
Right pulmonary artery
Right pulmonary vein
Foramen ovale
Hepatic vein
Ductus venosus
Liver
Hepatic portal vein
Umbilical vein
Umbilical arteries

Aorta
Ductus arteriosus
Left pulmonary artery
Left pulmonary vein
Inferior vena cava
Aorta
Celiac trunk
Superior mesenteric artery
Kidney
Gut

Ligamentum arteriosum (obliterated ductus arteriosus)

Fossa ovalis (obliterated foramen ovale)
Ligamentum venosum (obliterated ductus venosus)
Ligamentum teres (round ligament) of liver (obliterated umbilical vein)
Medial umbilical ligaments (occluded part of umbilical arteries)

Postnatal circulation

Fig. 92.1 Prenatal and Postnatal Circulation.

TABLE 92.1	**Conditions Predisposing to Neonatal Asphyxia or Depression**
Maternal	Uterine malformations, rupture
	Chorioamnionitis, other infection
	Diabetes
	Hypertension, preeclampsia
	Substance use
	Opioid administration
	Magnesium administration for preeclampsia/ eclampsia
Placental/umbilical	Uteroplacental insufficiency
	Abruption
	Previa
	Cord compression/prolapse
Fetal	Hydrops
	Poly/oligohydramnios
	Malformations
	Multiple gestations, twin-twin transfusion
Delivery	Precipitous
	Prolonged labor/rupture of membranes
	Meconium
	Poor fetal tracing

preterm neonates. If the infant demonstrates poor tone or respiratory effort, the umbilical cord should be immediately clamped, and the infant should be transferred to the pediatric provider for further assessment and resuscitation.

NEONATAL RESUSCITATION

Efficient, timely resuscitation practiced in a standardized manner is critical to reduce neonatal morbidity and mortality. The American Heart Association and American Academy of Pediatrics established an algorithm for the resuscitation of infants (Fig. 92.2). NRP places emphasis on ventilation as the primary mechanism of resuscitation with the understanding that the vast majority of neonates in distress suffer from respiratory failure rather than circulatory collapse. NRP is applied in cycles of 60 seconds, with frequent reassessments and opportunities to adjust, escalate and deescalate interventions. NRP may be applied across all delivery scenarios, including births of preterm infants, multiples, or infants with cardiac and surgical diagnoses (e.g., omphalocele, congenital diaphragmatic hernia). Special considerations for preterm infants are described in the following text.

Equipment Check

Before delivery, the pediatrics team should perform a thorough equipment check. The resuscitation area should include a radiant warmer, towels or blankets, temperature probe, stethoscope, pulse oximeter, electrocardiogram (ECG) monitor, bulb and suction catheter, and oxygen and bag-mask ventilation device adjusted to be ready to deliver positive pressure ventilation (PPV) if needed. PPV may be applied using a self-inflating bag, a flow-inflating bag, or a T-piece resuscitator. An appropriately sized mask should be selected to cover the nose and mouth with a tight seal; alternative sizes should be readily available. Advanced airway supplies should be available at all deliveries (including laryngeal mask, laryngoscope and endotracheal tubes), as should central venous/arterial access kits.

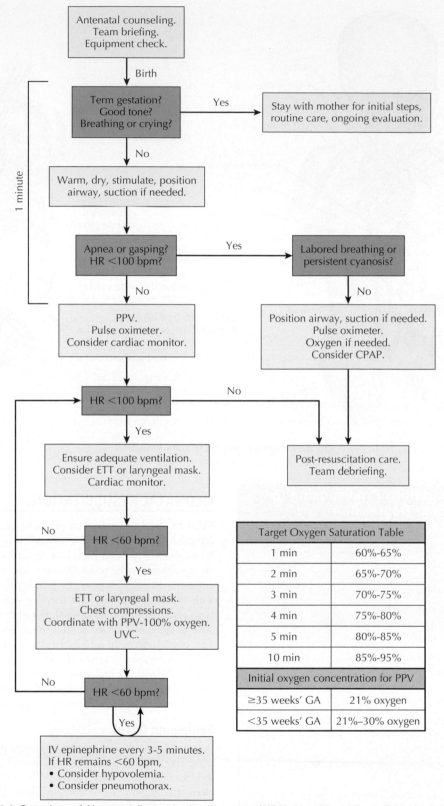

Fig. 92.2 Overview of Neonatal Resuscitation Program (NRP) Algorithm. (From Zaichkin J, Kamath-Rayne BD, Weiner G. The NRP 8th Edition: Innovation in Education. *Neonatal Netw.* 2021;40(4):251-261. Figure 1, Springer Publishing Company. DOI: 10.1891/11-T-756.)

BOX 92.1 Basic Components of Positive Pressure Ventilation

- Applied if infant is apneic or gasping or if heart rate is less than 100 beats/min after initial Neonatal Resuscitation Program steps
- Goal initiation within 60 seconds of life (including time spent during delayed cord clamping)
- Rate: 40 to 60 breaths/min
- Peak inspiratory pressure (PIP): initiate at 20 to 25 cm H_2O
- Positive end-expiratory pressure (PEEP): 5 cm H_2O
- Fraction of inspired oxygen (FiO_2): 21% (if <35 weeks' gestation, FiO_2 21%-30%, according to hospital guidelines)
- Infant placed in neutral or slightly extended neck position ("sniffing position")
- Rapid impact on heart rate if applied successfully
- Can be coordinated with compressions (ratio 3:1 compressions to breaths)

TABLE 92.2 Expected Preductal Oxygen Saturations by Minute(s) of Life

Minute of Life	Targeted Preductal Oxygen Saturations
1 minute	60%–65%
2 minutes	65%–70%
3 minutes	70%–75%
4 minutes	75%–80%
5 minutes	80%–85%
10 minutes	85%–95%

TABLE 92.3 Corrective Ventilation Steps: MR. SOPA

Acronym	Corrective step	Actions
M	Mask adjustment	Apply mask over mouth and bridge of nose. Check mask size. Consider a two-handed grip with assistant. Apply jaw thrust.
R	Reposition head and neck	Place infant in "sniffing" position. Consider neck roll.
Try PPV and Reassess Chest Movement		
S	Suction mouth then nose	Use a bulb syringe or suction catheter
O	Open mouth	Open the mouth and lift the jaw forward
Try PPV and Reassess Chest Movement		
P	Pressure increase	Increase PIP by increments of 5–10 mm H_2O, not to exceed 40 mm H_2O
Try PPV and Reassess Chest Movement		
A	Alternative airway	Place an endotracheal tube or laryngeal mask

PIP, Peak inspiratory pressure; *PPV*, positive pressure ventilation.
Reused from Weiner GM, Zaichkin J, Kattwinkel J, et al. *Textbook of Neonatal Resuscitation*. 7th ed. Elk Grove Village, IL: American Academy of Pediatrics; 2016.

Assessment

In the initial assessment, the obstetrics and pediatric teams collaborate to evaluate the neonate in the first seconds of life before umbilical cord clamping. If the infant emerges limp or has apnea/irregular breathing, the cord should be immediately clamped and the clinician should initiate resuscitation.

Once the infant is brought to the warmer, drying and stimulation should be performed. For neonates with mild respiratory distress or hypoxia, this noninvasive care may be enough to stimulate spontaneous respirations and successful extrauterine transition. While drying occurs, the clinician should monitor respiratory effort and auscultate the heart rate.

If the infant continues to be apneic, has irregular or gasping breaths, or has a heart rate below 100 beats/min, PPV should be initiated within the first minute of life, which includes the time spent during delayed cord clamping. While respiratory support is initiated, a team member should place the pulse oximeter, ECG leads (as available), and temperature probe on the infant.

Positive Pressure Ventilation

Adequate ventilation is the most important component of neonatal resuscitation; thus the ability to provide effective PPV is a critical skill to be mastered by all pediatric clinicians (Box 92.1). PPV may be administered by a single practitioner using a one-handed mask hold, but is easier with an assistant and two-handed mask hold. The infant should be placed in a neutral or slightly extended neck position (the "sniffing" position). Overextension or flexion of the neck will occlude the airway and impair effective ventilation. PPV should be initiated with a peak inspiratory pressure (PIP) of 20 to 25 cm H_2O and positive end-expiratory pressure (PEEP) of 5 cm H_2O. Ventilation should be applied at a rate of 40 to 60 breaths/min. Hyperoxygenation should be avoided because of an associated risk for altering cerebral blood flow and increased incidence of bronchopulmonary disease. The oxygen blender should be set to 21% to start for term infants.

After PPV is initiated, it is essential to monitor heart rate, chest rise, and respiratory effort, because these provide immediate feedback on the quality and effectiveness of ventilation. If PPV is effective, the heart rate should respond promptly within the first 15 seconds. Oxygen saturations should be monitored as an indicator of successful PPV. Note that normal oxygen saturation changes by each minute of life (Table 92.2), with full saturation (85% to 95%) reached by 10 minutes. If the heart rate or oxygen saturations fail to normalize, or if chest rise is not observed, the team should take corrective measures.

Positive Pressure Ventilation Corrective Techniques

The most common causes of ineffective ventilation are mask leak and airway obstruction. The following corrective techniques aid in achieving successful delivery of PPV: mask adjustment, repositioning the airway, suctioning of the mouth and nose, opening the mouth, pressure increase, and considering an alternative airway. The pneumonic "*MR. SOPA*" (Table 92.3) can be used to remember the steps and the order in which they should be applied.

If the team is able to achieve adequate ventilation with appropriate heart rate response, PPV is continued until the infant has sustained spontaneous respirations with a heart rate greater than 100 beats/min. PPV may then be transitioned to CPAP, nasal cannula or even room air.

Advanced Resuscitation

If no improvement is noted or heart rate remains less than 60 beats/min after all corrective steps have been taken and the infant is intubated, chest compressions should be initiated and the fraction of

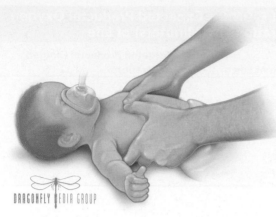

External cardiac compressions in an infant using the two-handed thumb technique. The compressor's hands encircle the patient's chest to provide countertraction, while the two thumbs are placed over the lower half of the patient's sternum to compress the chest.

Fig. 92.3 Neonatal Chest Compressions.

TABLE 92.4	**APGAR Score**		
		SCORE	
Sign	**0**	**1**	**2**
Heart rate	None	<100 beats/min	>100 beats/min
Respiration	None	Irregular, slow, gasping	Vigorous, crying
Muscle tone	Limp	Some flexion	Active motion
Reflex irritability	None	Grimace	Cough, sneeze, pulls away
Color	Blue or pale	Pink body, pale or blue extremities	Completely pink

inspired oxygen (FiO_2) should be adjusted to 100% (Fig. 92.3). Three compressions should be given for every PPV breath administered. The chest should be compressed by one-third to half the anteroposterior diameter using a two-thumbed technique. If the heart rate fails to respond after 30 seconds of chest compressions, epinephrine should be administered by the endotracheal tube, umbilical venous catheter, peripheral intravenous or intraosseous access. Epinephrine can be readministered every 3 to 5 minutes as needed.

If the infant still does not respond, alternative diagnoses such as pneumothorax or hypovolemic shock should be considered. Other medications to consider include crystalloid fluid boluses or packed red blood cells.

Other Care

Throughout the duration of resuscitation, it is vital to avoid hypothermia and maintain temperatures between 97.7°F and 99.5°F (36.5°C and 37.5°C) by drying the infant properly and using a radiant warmer. Hypothermia is associated with poor outcomes and elevated risk for complications such as IVH, sepsis, and hypoglycemia.

Apgar scores should be assigned at 1 and 5 minutes of life, then repeated every 5 minutes until the Apgar score is 7 or greater. Resuscitation should not be paused or delayed for Apgar scoring (Table 92.4).

SPECIAL CIRCUMSTANCES

Prematurity

Infants with low birth weight (<1500 g) or extremely low birth weight (<1000 g) are treated with the same resuscitation algorithm as term infants, with special attention given to respiratory support, fluid status, temperature regulation, and risk for IVH. Premature infants are at higher risk for respiratory distress and failure because of immature lung tissue and inadequate surfactant production. In previous decades, many premature infants were automatically intubated at birth because of concern for respiratory failure. Current practice favors a trial of noninvasive ventilation if the infant has spontaneous respirations. Evidence indicates that noninvasive ventilation is associated with superior outcomes, specifically a decreased risk for developing bronchopulmonary dysplasia. For infants younger than 30 weeks' gestation, the team should immediately apply CPAP if the infant is spontaneously breathing. For deliveries of infants of less than 35 weeks, the oxygen blender should be set to 21% to 30% FiO_2, according to local guidelines.

Premature infants are also at risk for severe hypothermia due to a relatively high surface area to volume ratio and, based on their weight at birth, may require a thermal mattress or wrapping in a polyethylene plastic bag rather than drying. Rapid fluid administration and rapid changes in carbon dioxide levels may cause shifts in cerebral perfusion and place premature infants at an increased risk for IVH. Fluids should be administered cautiously, and ventilation should be closely monitored. Most premature infants will require placement of a central venous catheter by the umbilical vein to allow for administration of intravenous medications and parenteral nutrition administration. An arterial catheter inserted via the umbilical artery is useful for unstable infants or infants of very low gestational ages for monitoring blood pressure and frequent laboratory blood draws.

Meconium Aspiration

Infants born through meconium-stained amniotic fluid (MSAF) are at increased risk for meconium aspiration syndrome. Management of neonatal care in the setting of MSAF has shifted to a less invasive approach after research studies indicated little to no benefit associated with routine deep suctioning of the oropharynx or endotracheal intubation with tracheal suctioning among stable, vigorous infants. Nonvigorous infants should undergo routine resuscitation per the NRP algorithm, with consideration of using a meconium aspirator if the infant requires intubation.

Hypoxic-Ischemic Injury

Therapeutic hypothermia within 6 hours of a sentinel hypoxic event improves long-term neurodevelopmental outcomes and should be considered in the resuscitation of neonates with suspected hypoxic ischemic encephalopathy. Therapeutic hypothermia is thought to reduce hypoxic ischemic injury by decreasing cerebral metabolism and cellular apoptosis. See Chapter 98 for more details.

POSTRESUSCITATIVE CARE

In the postnatal period, infants who require resuscitation should be monitored for symptoms of underlying disease or infection. An abbreviated list of common neonatal diseases and corresponding "red flag" symptoms can be found in Table 92.5.

TABLE 92.5	"Red Flag" Symptoms by Organ Systems in Ill Neonates	
Organ System	**Diagnoses and Associated "Red Flag" Findings**	**Further Evaluation**
Neurologic	**HIE:** irritability or lethargy/obtunded, hypotonia or hypertonia, abnormal posturing, incomplete or absent Moro, weak or absent suck, constricted or dilated pupils **IVH:** asymptomatic seizures, decerebrate posturing, weakness, bulging fontanelle, acute anemia, acute metabolic acidosis **NAS/NOWS:** irritability, poor feeding, diarrhea, sneezing, sweating, tremors, hypertonicity	EEG Brain ultrasound Brain MRI Drug screening, NAS scoring
Pulmonary	**RDS/TTN:** tachypnea, grunting, nasal flaring, retractions **Pneumothorax:** respiratory distress, chest asymmetry, unilateral breath sounds, hypotension or hypoxemia **MAS:** meconium-stained amniotic fluid/skin/nails/vernix, respiratory distress, barrel-shaped chest	Transillumination of chest Chest x-ray Blood gas Needle decompression
Cardiac	**Shock:** tachycardia, hypotension, hyperthermia or hypothermia, cool/mottled extremities, lethargy, metabolic acidosis **Ductal-dependent CHD:** cyanosis, hypoxemia, shock, failure to thrive, feeding intolerance **Pulmonary hypertension:** loud S_2, respiratory distress, gallop, right to left ductal shunting, pre-/post-ductal oxygen saturation differential, hypotension	Chest x-ray Preductal/postductal Blood gas Extremity blood pressure ECG, echocardiogram Cardiac catheterization
Gastrointestinal	**Necrotizing enterocolitis:** feeding intolerance, increased abdominal girth, bilious vomiting, diarrhea, hematochezia, lethargy, shock, apnea **Spontaneous intestinal perforation:** abdominal distension with blue hue **Malrotation with volvulus:** bilious emesis, may or may not have abdominal distension **Hirschsprung disease:** failure to pass meconium within the first 48 hours of life	Abdominal x-ray Abdominal ultrasound Upper GI Barium enema
Hematologic	**Hyperbilirubinemia/kernicterus:** jaundice, pallor, encephalopathy, lethargy, seizure	Bilirubin (conjugated and unconjugated), blood typing, CBC, DAT
Infectious	**Early-onset sepsis:** fever/hypothermia, vital sign instability, lethargy, poor feeding, respiratory distress, apnea and bradycardia events, hemolysis, shock	Blood, urine and/or CSF cultures Chest x-ray
Endocrinologic	**Hypoglycemia:** jitteriness, difficulty feeding, lethargy **Adrenal insufficiency:** hyponatremia, hyperkalemia, hypotension **Hypothyroidism:** lethargy, difficulty feeding, macroglossia, hernia, enlarged fontanelles, low tone, hypothermia	Newborn screening TSH, T_4 Serial blood glucose testing

CBC, Complete blood count; *CHD,* congenital heart disease; *CSF,* cerebrospinal fluid; *DAT,* direct antiglobulin test; *ECG:* electrocardiography; *HIE,* hypoxic ischemic encephalopathy; *IVH,* intraventricular hemorrhage; *MAS,* meconium aspiration syndrome; *NAS/NOWS,* neonatal abstinence syndrome/neonatal opioid withdrawal syndrome; *RDS,* respiratory distress syndrome; T_4, thyroxine; *TSH,* thyroid-stimulating hormone; *TTN,* transient tachypnea of the newborn.

SUGGESTED READINGS

Available online.

93

Disorders of the Respiratory System

Alyssa R. Thomas and Kathryn M. Rubey

 CLINICAL VIGNETTE

An infant born by elective repeat cesarean delivery is evaluated in the newborn nursery at 1 hour of life by the pediatrician. There was no active labor, and the amniotic fluid was clear. The infant had routine delivery room care. On examination, there are mild subcostal retractions, tachypnea with respiratory rate of 80 breaths/min, and coarse lung sounds. A chest radiograph shows perihilar streaking and fluid in the horizontal fissure of the right lung. The infant is started on continuous positive airway pressure by nasal mask using room air. Twelve hours later, the infant is able to breathe comfortably without respiratory support.

Transient tachypnea of the newborn is a common disorder of term infants that develops early after birth, classically after cesarean delivery without labor. The symptoms improve and resolve over time. If symptoms persist beyond 72 hours, or there is significant hypoxemia or respiratory failure, other diagnoses should be considered.

Advancements in the field of neonatal medicine have significantly reduced infant mortality in the United States. However, morbidity among infants with respiratory disorders remains high. Despite important progress in management of these disorders, they are still associated with prolonged hospital stays and need for advanced respiratory support. With increased survival of extremely premature infants, rates of certain pulmonary disorders have even increased.

ETIOLOGY AND PATHOGENESIS

The transition from fetal to extrauterine life requires a series of highly coordinated steps to ensure that adequate ventilation and oxygenation is established. The infant must breath spontaneously, clear amniotic fluid from the lungs, produce surfactant, and allow increased blood to flow to the lungs by decreasing pulmonary vascular resistance. Respiratory distress in the neonate can be caused by complications at any of these crucial points from an acquired disorder or a congenital anomaly. Nonpulmonary causes of respiratory distress include congenital heart disease (CHD), infection, central nervous system or neuromuscular disease, metabolic disorders, temperature instability, and anemia or polycythemia (Table 93.1). This chapter focuses on pulmonary disorders causing neonatal respiratory distress.

Transient Tachypnea of the Newborn

Transient tachypnea of the newborn (TTN) is a common respiratory disorder resulting from delayed or incomplete clearance of fetal alveolar fluid from the airways resulting in pulmonary edema. This alveolar fluid is secreted from lung epithelial cells throughout gestation. Several days before delivery, ion channels shift from chloride secretion to sodium resorption by epithelial sodium channels (ENaCs). Passive fluid absorption resulting from the squeezing through the birth canal is thought to play only a minor role. Risk factors that increase the likelihood of TTN include: planned cesarean delivery without labor, prematurity, male sex, small or large for gestational age, multiple gestation, or a maternal history of asthma, diabetes, or nulliparity. The risk for TTN in the setting of cesarean delivery increases in the absence of labor before delivery, and with delivery before 39 weeks.

Respiratory Distress Syndrome

Respiratory distress syndrome (RDS), previously known as hyaline membrane disease, is due to a relative surfactant deficiency. The surfactant deficiency decreases lung compliance, which promotes alveolar atelectasis and prevents newborns from developing a normal functional residual capacity. The most significant risk factor for RDS is prematurity. Surfactant production begins between 24 and 28 weeks' gestation and is not complete until at least 35 weeks' gestation. The incidence of RDS increases with decreasing gestational age. Nearly all infants born at 22 to 24 weeks have RDS. Other RDS risk factors include male sex, European descent, early-onset sepsis, perinatal hypoxia-ischemia, and maternal diabetes mellitus. There is increasing evidence of some inheritable forms of RDS occurring as a result of pathogenic gene mutations.

Meconium Aspiration Syndrome

Meconium aspiration syndrome (MAS) is respiratory distress and hypoxemia in a newborn born through meconium-stained amniotic fluid (MSAF). In utero passage of meconium results in MSAF and occurs mostly in term or postterm neonates. With fetal distress there is relaxation of the fetal anal sphincter, which can lead to the release of meconium. Aspirated meconium causes tissue damage throughout the lung. Airway obstruction leads to distal lung collapse. Surfactant inactivation decreases lung compliance. Inflammation or pneumonitis causes damage to the respiratory epithelium and a predisposition to serious bacterial infections. The mechanism of pulmonary vasoconstriction in this presentation is not clear, but severe MAS can be associated with persistent pulmonary hypertension of the newborn (PPHN).

Approximately 10% of pregnancies experience MSAF. Of infants born through MSAF, 2% to 10% will have symptoms of MAS. Risk

TABLE 93.1   Differential Diagnosis of Neonatal Respiratory Distress

System	Category	Specific Examples
Respiratory	Upper airway disorders	Laryngomalacia
		Subglottic stenosis
		Subglottic hemangioma
		Tracheomalacia
		Tracheoesophageal fistula
		Pierre-Robin sequence
		Choanal atresia
		Vascular ring or sling
	Parenchymal diseases	*Congenital*
		Congenital lobar emphysema
		Congenital pulmonary airway malformation (CPAM)
		Bronchopulmonary sequestration (BPS)
		Pulmonary hypoplasia
		Acquired
		Transient tachypnea of the newborn
		Respiratory distress syndrome
		Pneumonia
		Meconium aspiration syndrome
		Persistent pulmonary hypertension of the newborn
	Diaphragm disorders	Congenital diaphragmatic hernia
		Phrenic nerve injury
	Air leak syndromes	Pneumothorax
Cardiac	Acyanotic lesions	Patent ductus arteriosus
		Coarctation of the aorta, aortic stenosis, and interrupted aorta
	Cyanotic lesions	Transposition of the great arteries
		Tetralogy of Fallot
		Tricuspid atresia
		Ebstein anomaly
		Pulmonary atresia
		Total anomalous pulmonary venous return
Neurologic	CNS disorders	Hypoxic-ischemic encephalopathy
		Seizure disorder
		Apnea
		Intraventricular or intracranial hemorrhage
		Meningitis
		Exposure to sedating medications
	Neuromuscular disease	Neuromuscular weakness
Metabolic		Hypoglycemia
		Hypocalcemia
		Inborn error of metabolism
Hematologic		Anemia
		Polycythemia
Other	Infection	Sepsis
	Thermoregulation	Hypothermia, hyperthermia

factors for MSAF include fetal distress, uteroplacental insufficiency, cord compression, intrauterine growth restriction, and postterm dates (gestational age >41 weeks). The incidence of MAS has decreased with decreasing postterm deliveries.

Persistent Pulmonary Hypertension of the Newborn

PPHN is a condition of elevated pulmonary vascular resistance and failed transition from fetal to postnatal circulation. In the fetus, pulmonary pressures are high to shunt oxygenated blood from the placenta to the body, bypassing the lungs. Postnatally, pulmonary vascular resistance drops immediately after birth, allowing increased pulmonary blood flow. In PPHN, the persistently elevated pulmonary pressures cause continued low blood flow to the lungs and right-to-left shunting of blood through a patent ductus arteriosus or intracardiac shunt. This leads to hypoxemia and cyanosis in the neonate. There are multiple causes of PPHN, including MAS, TTN,

RDS, hypoxic-ischemic injury, maternal selective serotonin reuptake inhibitor or nonsteroidal antiinflammatory drug use, and infection. In addition, PPHN can develop in infants with pulmonary hypoplasia such as congenital diaphragmatic hernia or rarer causes, such as alveolar capillary dysplasia. Pulmonary hypertension can also develop as a long-term consequence of bronchopulmonary dysplasia (BPD) in premature neonates.

Bronchopulmonary Dysplasia

BPD is an important respiratory complication of prematurity. The prevalence of BPD is inversely related to birth weight and gestational age. The definition of BPD includes factors such as need for positive pressure ventilation, oxygen use, age at birth, and corrected gestational age. BPD occurs when a constellation of pathogenic factors converge on immature lungs of extremely premature infants. Inflammation from infection, barotrauma from mechanical ventilation, oxygen toxicity, and pulmonary overcirculation from a patent ductus arteriosus are all thought to contribute to lung injury in BPD.

The clinical picture of BPD has changed as neonatal care has evolved. In "classic" BPD, the progression was from RDS to severe chronic lung disease with a high risk for heart failure and death. Current management has helped create less severe presentations of BPD, with many preterm infants discharged without respiratory support. More severe forms of BPD may require home supplemental oxygen or even tracheostomy placement. Strategies used to prevent or mitigate BPD have inconclusive evidence, including antenatal steroid use. BPD may be complicated by pulmonary hypertension, impaired growth due to increased nutritional demands, and poor feeding. Infants with a history of BPD are also at increased risk for wheezing disorders, and all infants with BPD should receive Synagis (palivizumab) for prophylaxis against respiratory syncytial virus.

Pneumothorax and Air Leak Syndromes

Air leak syndromes result from the rupture of alveolar sacs, with subsequent flow of gas outside of the air spaces of the lungs. In term infants, pneumothorax is the most common result of an air leak, occurring in 1% of all deliveries. Pneumothorax can occur spontaneously, from positive pressure ventilation with high peak inspiratory pressures (>20 to 25 mm Hg) or in the setting of air-trapping in MAS.

CLINICAL PRESENTATION

On physical examination, infants generally present with tachypnea (respiratory rate >60 breaths/min), apnea, intercostal or subcostal retractions, grunting, nasal flaring, or cyanosis. On auscultation, breath sounds may be coarse, diminished, or even absent in the case of pneumothorax. The liver or spleen can be palpable if there is lung hyperinflation as a result of air trapping. Attempting to pass a suction catheter or nasogastric tube may raise concern for choanal atresia or a tracheoesophageal fistula. Birth history, including gestational age, mode of delivery, maternal diabetes, MSAF, and Apgar scores, can narrow the differential. The timeline of symptoms is another clue. TTN and MAS manifest shortly after birth, with TTN self-resolving within 72 hours and RDS symptoms progressing over the first 48 to 96 hours.

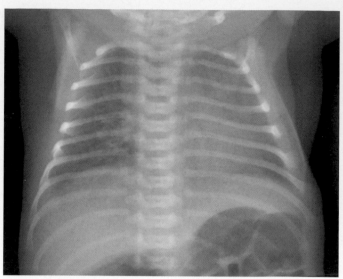

Fig. 93.1 Chest Radiograph With Findings of Transient Tachypnea of the Newborn. (Courtesy Dr. Misun Hwang and Dr. Luis O. Tierradentro-Garcia, Children's Hospital of Philadelphia.)

EVALUATION AND INITIAL MANAGEMENT

Pulse oxygen saturation (SpO_2) should be obtained early using a noninvasive pulse oximeter placed on the right hand (preductal). In any condition with impaired gas exchange, infants may have a low SpO_2. In PPHN, the right upper extremity may have a higher SpO_2 compared with the lower extremities because of shunting of blood.

Chest radiography also can aid in diagnosis. In TTN, chest radiographs characteristically show fluid in the interlobar fissure, as well as perihilar streaking, which represents fluid in the perihilar lymphatic system (Fig. 93.1). In RDS, there is a uniform "ground-glass" opacification from alveolar atelectasis, with superimposed peripheral air bronchograms (Fig. 93.2). Hyperinflation, patchy atelectasis and infiltrates, and pneumothorax may be noted in an infant with MAS (Fig. 93.3). Pneumothorax appears as hyperlucency or lung collapse (Fig. 93.4).

Arterial blood gases help differentiate types of respiratory failure. Elevated carbon dioxide indicates ventilation failure and a need for increased respiratory support. Low arterial partial pressure of oxygen (PaO_2) can indicate either severe lung disease or CHD with mixing physiology. Metabolic acidosis usually indicates poor end-organ perfusion, but can also indicate an inborn error of metabolism. Infants with metabolic acidosis can become tachypneic in an effort to decrease carbon dioxide levels to compensate for an acidotic pH. Finally, additional evaluation will depend on the infant's particular risk factors based on history and physical examination and may include screening and treatment for sepsis, blood glucose testing, and echocardiography.

Disease-Specific Management

Supportive care is provided for TTN. Prolonged or severe tachypnea (>60 breaths/min), supplemental oxygen requirement greater than 40% FiO_2, or deteriorating clinical status should prompt further evaluation for concurrent or alternative diagnoses, such as sepsis or RDS.

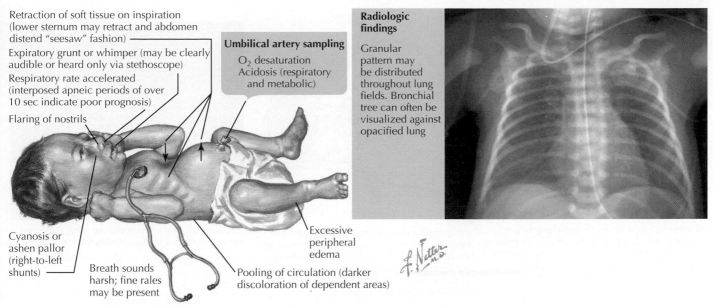

Retraction of soft tissue on inspiration (lower sternum may retract and abdomen distend "seesaw" fashion)

Expiratory grunt or whimper (may be clearly audible or heard only via stethoscope)

Respiratory rate accelerated (interposed apneic periods of over 10 sec indicate poor prognosis)

Flaring of nostrils

Umbilical artery sampling

O_2 desaturation
Acidosis (respiratory and metabolic)

Radiologic findings

Granular pattern may be distributed throughout lung fields. Bronchial tree can often be visualized against opacified lung

Cyanosis or ashen pallor (right-to-left shunts)

Breath sounds harsh; fine rales may be present

Excessive peripheral edema

Pooling of circulation (darker discoloration of dependent areas)

Fig. 93.2 Manifestations of Respiratory Distress Syndrome in the Newborn and Chest Radiograph Findings. (Radiology image courtesy Dr. Misun Hwang and Dr. Luis O. Tierradentro-Garcia, Children's Hospital of Philadelphia.)

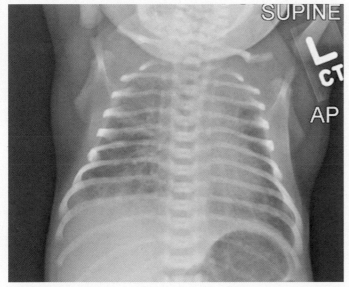

Fig. 93.3 Chest Radiograph With Findings of Meconium Aspiration Syndrome. (Courtesy Dr. Misun Hwang and Dr. Luis O. Tierradentro-Garcia, Children's Hospital of Philadelphia.)

Corticosteroids given at least 24 to 48 hours before delivery have been shown to decrease the incidence and severity of RDS in premature infants. Surfactant replacement therapy has had the greatest effect on the outcomes of newborns with RDS. Exogenous surfactant is instilled into the lungs to reduce surface tension in the alveoli and improve lung compliance, functional residual capacity, and oxygenation. Continuous positive airway pressure is a mainstay of respiratory management of infants with RDS, though some may require intubation.

Current Neonatal Resuscitation Program (NRP) guidelines state that nonvigorous infants born through MSAF should be managed with drying, stimulation, and bag-mask ventilation if there is poor respiratory effort. Routine endotracheal intubation for suctioning of the meconium from the trachea is no longer recommended. Infants with MAS may be treated with antibiotics until infection is ruled out. The infant with severe MAS may require a high level of respiratory support. Inhaled nitric oxide may be used in cases complicated by pulmonary hypertension. The development of pulmonary hypertension increases the risk of mortality. Extracorporeal membrane oxygenation (ECMO) may be indicated for severe cases.

It is crucial to differentiate PPHN from cyanotic CHD in a hypoxemic neonate. An echocardiogram should be obtained to definitively rule out CHD. Supplemental oxygen should be given for hypoxemia in PPHN, both to increase oxygen delivery to the brain and tissues and to improve pulmonary vasodilation. In severe cases, inhaled nitric oxide may be used and refractory cases may progress to ECMO. Infants who survive moderate to severe PPHN are at risk for neurodevelopmental impairment and should have long-term multidisciplinary follow-up after discharge.

Tension pneumothorax should be emergently managed with needle aspiration, followed by consideration of definitive treatment with chest tube placement.

FUTURE DIRECTIONS

Preterm infants with RDS requiring surfactant administration currently undergo intubation. A technique known as less invasive surfactant administration delivers the surfactant using a thin catheter rather than endotracheal tube, to minimize exposure to mechanical ventilation. Emerging research on surfactant administration by nebulization aims to deliver this medication even less invasively.

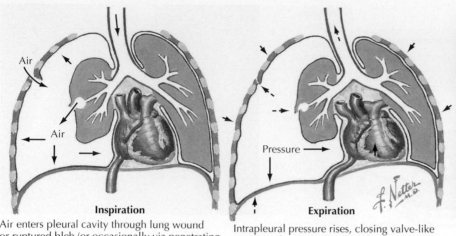

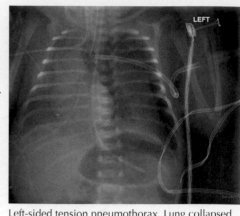

Inspiration

Air enters pleural cavity through lung wound or ruptured bleb (or occasionally via penetrating chest wound) with valve-like opening. Ipsilateral lung collapses and mediastinum shifts to opposite side, compressing lung.

Expiration

Intrapleural pressure rises, closing valve-like opening, thus preventing escape of pleural air. Pressure is thus progressively increased with each breath. Mediastinal and tracheal shifts are augmented, diaphragm is depressed, and venous return is impaired.

Left-sided tension pneumothorax. Lung collapsed, mediastinum and trachea deviated to opposite lung.

Fig. 93.4 Chest Radiograph and Schematic Demonstrating Left-Sided Tension Pneumothorax With Mediastinal Shift. (Radiology image courtesy Dr. Misun Hwang and Dr. Luis O. Tierradentro-Garcia, Children's Hospital of Philadelphia.)

SUGGESTED READINGS

Available online.

94

Disorders of the Gastrointestinal Tract

Evelyn Ruth Wang and Emily Echevarria

CLINICAL VIGNETTE

A 3-week-old infant born at 29 weeks' gestation has apneic and bradycardic events and a bilious gastric residual. The baby has reached full enteral formula feeds and is on noninvasive ventilation.

On examination, the infant is gray and lethargic with labored breathing. His abdomen is tender and distended. An abdominal radiograph reveals pneumatosis intestinalis and portal venous gas. He is intubated. His feeds are stopped, an orogastric tube is placed, and intravenous fluids started. Blood cultures are drawn, and he is started on antibiotics.

The initial presentation of necrotizing enterocolitis (NEC) in a premature infant may be nonspecific. The cause of NEC is multifactorial, and the pathophysiologic process is not fully understood. Diagnosis can be made from examination and radiographic evidence of pneumatosis intestinalis, portal venous gas, or pneumoperitoneum. Stopping feeds, decompressing the abdomen, and covering with antibiotics for intestinal flora are mainstays of treatment.

Gastrointestinal (GI) disorders can affect preterm and full-term infants. Many of the signs and symptoms of a GI disorder are shared across gestational ages. Some conditions can be managed with medical therapies, whereas others require a pediatric surgical team. With a complete history, physical examination, and targeted imaging studies, a pediatric clinician can create a narrowed differential diagnosis. Knowing when to surgically intervene in these disorders is of key clinical importance.

PREMATURE INFANTS: NECROTIZING ENTEROCOLITIS AND SPONTANEOUS INTESTINAL PERFORATION

Clinical Presentation

Early signs of necrotizing enterocolitis (NEC) and spontaneous intestinal perforation (SIP) are nonspecific. They include feeding intolerance, abdominal distension, lethargy, apnea, hypoglycemia, temperature instability, and red/blue/black abdominal discoloration. Later findings in NEC include hematochezia and fulminant sepsis. SIP generally occurs at several days of life, while NEC occurs at several weeks of life with the infant on full feeds.

Necrotizing Enterocolitis
Etiology and Pathogenesis
NEC is a complex disease and common GI condition complicating up to 7% of neonatal intensive care unit (NICU) admissions of infants

born 500 to 1500 g. It is rarely seen in full-term infants. Rates of NEC have been largely stable in recent years as a result of increased survival of infants born at earlier gestational ages. Mortality associated with NEC remains significant, with overall mortality rising to over 50% in infants with extremely low birth weight (born at <1000 g).

The pathogenesis of NEC is multifactorial and incompletely understood. The risk for NEC is inversely related to the degree of prematurity, with increased incidence at earlier gestational ages. Other factors involved in the development of disease include intestinal immaturity, type of enteral feeds, intestinal microbiome, inflammation, and ischemic injury. The association of NEC with feed initiation and osmolarity suggests immature gut mucosa allows for intestinal bacterial translocation. This results in a systemic inflammatory response and shock. Bacteria isolated from infants affected by NEC include *Klebsiella pneumoniae*, *Pseudomonas aeruginosa*, *Escherichia coli*, and *Enterobacter* species.

Evaluation and Management

Initial evaluation of infants with suspected NEC includes abdominal radiography. This may show bowel loop distension or the classic sign of pneumatosis intestinalis, the presence of gas within the intestinal wall (Fig. 94.1). Portal venous gas also may be seen on plain film. In the most severe cases, pneumoperitoneum is evident. Ultrasound (US) shows promise for evaluating infants with NEC; in addition to pneumatosis intestinalis and portal venous gas, it can assess for peristalsis and intestinal wall thickness and perfusion. Common laboratory findings include neutropenia, thrombocytopenia, metabolic acidosis with rising lactate, hyponatremia, and hypoglycemia.

The majority of infants affected by NEC are initially managed medically. Feeds are held, the abdomen is decompressed with an orogastric tube, and intravenous fluids are initiated. Blood cultures are drawn, and infants are treated with broad-spectrum antibiotics. Infants should be followed closely for disease progression with serial examinations and radiographs. Bowel rest and antibiotics are indicated for 7 to 14 days. Around half of patients with NEC require surgical intervention. Indications for surgical management are intestinal perforation or progressive clinical deterioration. Surgical management includes peritoneal drainage or exploratory laparotomy with resection of necrotic bowel.

Recurrence of disease is seen in approximately 6% of NEC survivors. The most common complication is intestinal stricture, presenting with feeding intolerance several weeks after resolution of the initial illness. NEC survivors are at increased risk for neurodevelopmental delays. Surgical NEC resulting in intestinal resection is the most common cause of short gut syndrome.

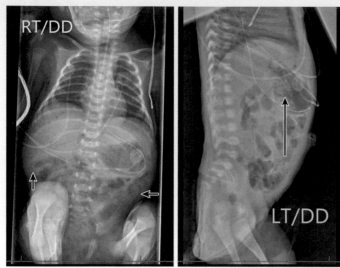

Fig. 94.1 Pneumatosis Intestinalis on Abdominal Radiograph in Necrotizing Enterocolitis (NEC). Note air trapped in the intestinal wall and a soapy/bubbly appearance on the lateral film. The *arrows on the left* show two areas of extensive pneumatosis where air is seen outlining the bowel wall. On the right, the *arrow* highlights a soap bubble appearance, also characteristic of pneumatosis. (Courtesy Dr. Luis O. Tierradentro-Garcia, Children's Hospital of Philadelphia.)

Spontaneous Intestinal Perforation

SIP is an isolated intestinal perforation in preterm infants, with case reports in term infants. Perforation is typically found in the terminal ileum with an incidence of up to 7% in preterm populations. The cause of SIP remains unclear, but studies have shown thinning or absence of the muscularis propria at the perforation site. Pneumoperitoneum is seen on radiographs without pneumatosis or portal venous air. Management includes bowel rest, abdominal decompression, and surgical intervention with peritoneal drains or an exploratory laparotomy to look for the perforated segment of bowel.

INTESTINAL OBSTRUCTION

Etiology and Pathogenesis

Intestinal obstruction is possible at any point along the GI tract. Mechanical obstructions result from failure of normal GI tract development and include intestinal and anal atresias, malrotation, and pyloric stenosis. Functional obstructions are the result of impaired peristalsis and include meconium plug syndrome, Hirschsprung disease, and small left colon syndrome.

Clinical Presentation

Intestinal obstruction in a neonate often manifests with common signs and symptoms: vomiting or feeding intolerance, abdominal distension, and failure to pass meconium. Subtle differences in presentation can localize the obstruction (Table 94.1).

Evaluation and Management

Evaluation should proceed quickly. After stabilizing the patient, the presence of obstruction should be confirmed with imaging, and consultation arranged with pediatric surgery specialist. Initial management includes stopping enteral feeds, intravenous fluid resuscitation, correcting metabolic abnormalities, and placing a nasogastric (NG) or orogastric (OG) tube to decompress the abdomen. Some diseases may be associated with genetic syndromes and should prompt complete evaluation for potential associated

TABLE 94.1   Localizing Features of Intestinal Obstruction

Sign or Finding	Proximal or Distal	Specific Site (When Applicable)
Nonbilious vomiting	Proximal	Proximal to the ampulla of Vater
Bilious vomiting	Proximal or distal	Distal to the ampulla of Vater
Scaphoid abdomen	Proximal	Often preduodenal
Distended abdomen	Distal	
Maternal polyhydramnios	Proximal	

TABLE 94.2   Site of Obstruction and Associated Genetic Syndromes

Type of Obstruction	Genetic Association
Esophageal atresia	VACTERL
Duodenal atresia	Trisomy 21
Colonic atresia	Eye, heart, and abdominal wall anomalies
Meconium ileus	Cystic fibrosis
Small left colon syndrome	Diabetic mother

VACTERL, Vertebral anomalies, anal atresia, cardiovascular anomalies, tracheoesophageal fistula, esophageal atresia, renal or radial anomalies, and limb defects.

conditions (Table 94.2). The specific diagnostic options and management steps to consider based on the underlying cause are discussed below.

Cause, Pathogenesis, Evaluation, and Management of Intestinal Obstructions

Esophageal Atresia

The esophagus can be obstructed in the form of esophageal atresia (EA), which occurs when the esophagus fails to separate from the trachea during normal development. EA generally coexists with tracheoesophageal fistula (TEF). A standard classification scheme describes the relationship between the atresia and the coexistent TEF (Fig. 94.2). The most common combination is a blind proximal esophageal pouch with distal TEF (type C). Pure EA with no TEF is rare. The most difficult to diagnose is "H-type," which refers to isolated TEF without EA.

EA presents early in the newborn period with feeding intolerance and copious oral secretions. Infants display nonbilious emesis, choking, and coughing with initial feeds. Infants with H-type TEF often tolerate feeds without significant difficulty, and present with more subtle signs of tachypnea or recurrent pneumonia from feed aspiration.

Inability to pass an NG/OG tube into the stomach is diagnostic of EA with or without TEF. Initial radiographs will reveal the NG/OG tube curled in the esophagus. In patients without a connection between the trachea and distal esophagus, abdominal radiographs will reveal a gasless abdomen. In contrast, the stomach and abdomen will be distended with air in the presence of a distal TEF. When H-type TEF is suspected, a dedicated upper GI radiography series may be required to confirm diagnosis as plain films may be unrevealing.

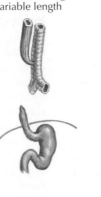
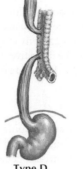

Type C

Most common form (90% to 95%) of tracheo-esophageal fistula. Upper segment of esophagus ending in blind pouch; lower segment originating from trachea just above bifurcation. The two segments may be connected by a solid cord

Type B

Upper segment of esophagus ending in trachea; lower segment of variable length

Type D
Double fistula

Type E or Type H
Fistula without esophageal atresia

Type A
Esophageal atresia without fistula

Fig. 94.2 Tracheoesophageal Fistula.

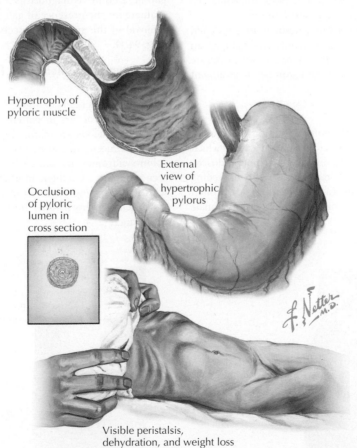

Hypertrophy of pyloric muscle

Occlusion of pyloric lumen in cross section

External view of hypertrophic pylorus

Visible peristalsis, dehydration, and weight loss

Fig. 94.3 Hypertrophic Pyloric Stenosis.

Treatment consists of surgical anastomosis of the esophageal segments. In the presence of a TEF, the fistula should be repaired early in the hospital course to prevent ongoing pulmonary aspiration. In premature infants and infants with other congenital anomalies, surgical repair may be delayed or performed in several stages to allow for growth.

Hypertrophic Pyloric Stenosis

Hypertrophic pyloric stenosis (HPS) is an acquired thickening of the pyloric sphincter muscles causing gastric outlet obstruction (Fig. 94.3). Approximately 1 in 500 infants develop HPS during the first month of life. The classic presentation is a 3- to 4-week-old infant with persistent, nonbilious, projectile emesis after feeds and poor weight gain.

Risk factors include first-born, male gender, White race, and use of erythromycin as a neonate. On examination, infants with HPS appear irritable and hungry and may have a palpable olive-shaped mass in the right upper quadrant (hypertrophic pyloric sphincter). Immediately after feeding, a reverse peristaltic wave may be seen just before vomiting. The abdomen may appear scaphoid, as air and feeds are unable to pass beyond the pylorus.

Initial stabilization of infants with HPS includes fluid resuscitation and imaging. Hypochloremic hypokalemic metabolic alkalosis is commonly associated with HPS as a result of recurrent emesis of acidic gastric contents. Abdominal ultrasound is the definitive diagnostic test and will reveal a thickened and elongated pylorus. Treatment is with surgical pyloromyotomy.

Intestinal Atresias and Stenosis

Intestinal atresias and stenosis are possible at any point along the GI tract. Jejunoileal atresia is the most common, followed by duodenal then colonic atresia. Duodenal and jejunal atresias generally present with bilious emesis. Although more distal obstructions may manifest with emesis as well, their presentation is often insidious and characterized by subtle symptoms of feeding intolerance. Another key to diagnosing the location of an atresia is a prenatal history of polyhydramnios, more common in proximal obstructions impeding the absorption of amniotic fluid by the proximal small intestine.

The initial resuscitation for infants with intestinal atresia should proceed as described earlier. In addition to abdominal radiography, an upper GI series with small bowel follow-through or barium enema are needed to identify the level of intestinal obstruction before treatment with surgical repair.

Malrotation and Volvulus

Malrotation refers to a disruption of the normal rotation and fixation of the bowel during embryogenesis. This creates a stalk around which the gut can twist (volvulize), leading to bowel obstruction and ischemia. Malrotation without volvulus can manifest as reflux or feeding intolerance. Malrotation with volvulus is a surgical emergency. It often manifests as bilious emesis in the first month of life. There is a 2:1 male predominance.

When an infant presents with bilious emesis, an upper GI series must be performed emergently. Rapid recognition of volvulus saves bowel from ischemic injury. Malrotation is diagnosed when an upper GI demonstrates an abnormal point of attachment of the ligament of Treitz. Surgical management with a Ladd procedure is required to release the mesentery and straighten the bowel.

Hirschsprung Disease

Hirschsprung disease results from incomplete neural crest cell migration and ganglion cell development in the myenteric plexus of the colon, which leads to dysfunctional peristalsis. There is a wide range of severity. Mildly affected infants often have failure to pass meconium by 24 hours of life or a history of intractable constipation. Severe cases may present with signs of obstruction or enterocolitis and a sepsis-like picture with fever, vomiting, diarrhea, and abdominal distension necessitating fluid resuscitation and antibiotics. On examination, the abdomen is often nontender but distended. There may be an expulsion of gas and stool after rectal stimulation because of temporary relief of the obstruction.

Patients with Hirschsprung disease often have abdominal radiographs with dilated bowel loops or stool in the colon. A barium enema may show a transition point, where the colon becomes aganglionic. Definitive diagnosis is made with a suction rectal biopsy to evaluate for the presence of ganglion cells. Surgical repair involves removal of the aganglionic section of bowel to restore peristalsis (Fig. 94.4).

Meconium Ileus, Meconium Plug Syndrome, and Small Left Colon Syndrome

Meconium ileus refers to impaction of the distal ileum by inspissated meconium. It occurs in patients with cystic fibrosis (CF) because abnormal mucous secretion and lack of pancreatic enzyme activity cause the meconium to be viscous. Meconium plug and small left colon syndromes are caused by poor gut motility. Both are often seen in infants of diabetic mothers, but can also be seen in patients with Hirschsprung disease. Infants generally present with abdominal distension shortly after birth followed by symptoms of feeding intolerance.

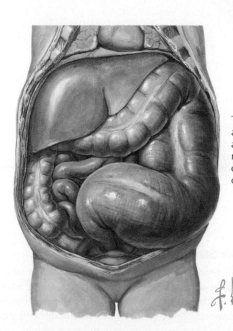

Tremendous distension and hypertrophy of sigmoid and descending colon; moderate involvement of transverse colon; distal constricted segment

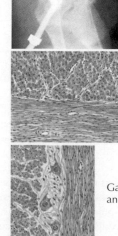

Barium enema; characteristic distal constricted segment

Ganglion cells absent

Ganglion cells present between longitudinal and circular muscle layers

Fig. 94.4 Hirschsprung Disease.

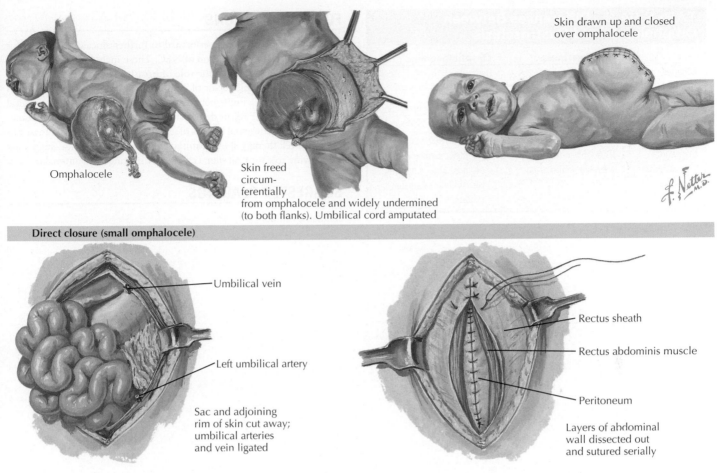

Skin drawn up and closed
over omphalocele

Omphalocele

Skin freed
circum-
ferentially
from omphalocele and widely undermined
(to both flanks). Umbilical cord amputated

Direct closure (small omphalocele)

Umbilical vein

Left umbilical artery

Sac and adjoining
rim of skin cut away;
umbilical arteries
and vein ligated

Rectus sheath

Rectus abdominis muscle

Peritoneum

Layers of abdominal
wall dissected out
and sutured serially

Fig. 94.5 Omphalocele.

These entities have a similar diagnostic workup. Abdominal radiography will reveal intestinal distension proximal to the site of obstruction. Contrast enemas may be used to better localize the obstruction and is also often therapeutic. If contrast enema fails to relieve the obstruction, surgical intervention is indicated. Because of the specificity of meconium ileus for CF, genetic testing should be pursued.

Imperforate Anus

Imperforate anus results from abnormal development of the hindgut. The presence of imperforate anus can be readily apparent on physical examination. Cases that are not obvious will have failure to pass meconium from the rectum, abdominal distension, and other symptoms of obstruction. Imperforate anus may be associated with congenital anomalies such as VACTERL (vertebral anomalies, anal atresia, cardiovascular anomalies, tracheoesophageal fistula, esophageal atresia, renal or radial anomalies, and limb defects) association.

In patients with imperforate anus, the distance from the end of the large intestine to the perineum dictates the complexity of surgical repair. This can be assessed with radiography where a lead marker on the anal dimple can reveal the length to the distal intestinal air bubble. A contrast enema can be used in patients with a perianal fistula to further elucidate the severity of disease. A diverting colostomy may be required to allow the patient to grow before definitive surgical repair.

ABDOMINAL WALL DEFECTS

Etiology and Pathogenesis

The two most common abdominal wall defects in neonates are omphalocele and gastroschisis, with prevalences of 2 and 4 per 10,000 live births, respectively. Both result from incomplete embryologic abdominal wall closure after extraabdominal development and rotation of the GI tract.

Clinical Presentation

Gastroschisis and omphalocele are often diagnosed prenatally on ultrasound and are readily apparent on physical examination (Fig. 94.5). Omphalocele is characterized by its midline location with an overlying membrane. Gastroschisis is displaced to the right of the umbilicus without an overlying membrane (Table 94.3).

Evaluation and Management

After infant delivery, the defect should be covered and kept moist. Infants often require additional fluids given their higher-than-normal insensible losses. Both require surgical correction when able. Omphalocele has a high association with genetic syndromes, therefore a careful physical examination and genetic evaluation are indicated.

TABLE 94.3 **Differences Between Omphalocele and Gastroschisis**

	Gastroschisis	Omphalocele
Location	Right side	Center
Covering sac	Absent	Present
Description	Free intestinal loops	Intestine, liver (commonly), spleen, colon, bladder (occasionally)
Congenital anomalies	10%–15%; intestinal atresia, malrotation	40%–80%; trisomy syndromes, cardiac defects, Beckwith-Wiedemann syndrome

FUTURE DIRECTIONS

Ongoing research is being performed to further elucidate strategies for early detection and prevention of NEC. These include identifying NEC biomarkers and evaluating the role of breastmilk and probiotics. Since the first thoracoscopic repair of TEF in 2000, there has been increased development and implementation of minimally invasive surgical approaches for TEF repair demonstrating success and improved cosmesis. Finally, experimental models of gastroschisis treated with transamniotic stem cell therapy showed mitigated bowel wall damage, suggesting an evolving role for fetal stem cell therapy in congenital anomalies.

SUGGESTED READINGS

Available online.

95

Hematologic Disorders of the Neonate

Leah Downey and Morgan Elise Hill

 CLINICAL VIGNETTE

A male infant born at 39 weeks gestation by uncomplicated vaginal delivery presents hours after birth with petechiae and mucocutaneous purpura. The pregnancy was notable for normal prenatal laboratory tests results and a benign course. This was the birth parent's first pregnancy. She has an unremarkable medical history. Vitamin K was administered. The nursery team was called to assess the infant after development of a petechial rash and bruising in a whole-body distribution. Other than skin findings, the physical examination was unremarkable. A CBC was obtained with a normal leukocyte count and hemoglobin and a platelet count of 23 $\times 10^9$/L. The infant was transferred to the neonatal intensive care unit for further workup and treatment of isolated thrombocytopenia. Blood cultures were drawn and remained negative. Coagulation studies were normal. Head ultrasound was normal. He required several platelet transfusions over the following week to maintain a minimum platelet count of 50 $\times 10^9$/L. He remained well appearing and vigorous, with a normal neurologic examination. Maternal serum was tested for antiplatelet antibodies, and the infant was diagnosed with neonatal alloimmune thrombocytopenia (NAIT).

NAIT is an uncommon cause of thrombocytopenia. Maternal immunoglobulin G antibodies directed against fetal platelet antigens are passed to the baby through the placenta. These infants tend to be symptomatic and are at risk for severe bleeding. Monitoring in the neonatal intensive care unit and therapy with platelet transfusion are often warranted.

ANEMIA

Etiology and Pathogenesis

After birth, the infant's source of oxygen transitions from placenta to lungs. This abrupt change in oxygen tension and increase in oxygen delivery causes erythropoietin (EPO) production to decrease and reticulocytosis to slow. All neonates demonstrate a decline in hemoglobin in the weeks after birth, falling until a physiologic nadir at 8 to 12 weeks. Additionally, red blood cells (RBCs) have a shorter life span in the neonate versus adults. This further contributes to the physiologic anemia of infancy. Hemoglobin levels recover once relative tissue hypoxia promotes increased EPO.

Pathologic anemia in the neonate, however, can be divided into three potential causes: blood loss, inadequate production of RBCs, or increased RBC destruction (Fig. 95.1).

Inadequate Production

RBC production can be compromised by several pathologic causes. Infections (parvovirus B19) or inherited syndromes (Diamond-Blackfan anemia) can cause total marrow suppression or selectively target RBC production with other cell lines relatively spared. Nutritional anemias such as iron deficiency can be observed if iron stores are depleted without supplementation and occurs earlier in preterm infants than full-term infants.

Blood Loss

Blood loss in the neonate is rare but can happen before, during, or after birth and may be acute or chronic. Common obstetric causes of anemia include placental abruption, placenta previa, and cord or placental trauma during delivery. Other causes of blood loss include twin-twin transfusion, internal hemorrhage (intracranial, subgaleal, cephalohematoma, adrenal, subcapsular hepatic), or iatrogenic blood loss from frequent blood draws in the neonatal intensive care unit (NICU).

Increased Destruction

Hemolysis is a process that shortens the RBC's lifespan. Hemolytic anemias can stem from either intrinsic or extrinsic causes. Intrinsic causes of hemolysis include hereditary RBC disorders. These include enzyme deficiencies, such as glucose-6-phosphate dehydrogenase (G6PD) or pyruvate kinase deficiency, RBC membrane defects such as hereditary spherocytosis, or hemoglobinopathies such as α-thalassemia. Extrinsic causes include neonatal infections and immune-mediated hemolysis. Immune-mediated hemolysis caused by Rhesus factor (Rh), ABO, or minor blood group incompatibilities can cause significant morbidity in infants.

ABO incompatibility primarily occurs in blood group O mothers with fetuses who have blood group A or B. All group O individuals have anti-A and anti-B antibodies that are produced as a result of immune stimulation by the A or B antigens contained in food and bacteria. Interactions between these maternal isoantibodies and fetal RBCs result in hemolysis. Fifteen percent of pregnancies are ABO incompatible, yet disease is found in only 3% of pregnancies, with 1% requiring exchange transfusions (ETs). This is because ABO hemolytic disease tends to occur in newborns whose mothers have high levels of immunoglobulin G (IgG) antibody. Although anti-A and anti-B antibodies are found in the plasma as IgA, IgM, and IgG, only the latter can cross the placenta and interact with fetal RBCs.

Rh incompatibility affects 1 in 15 pregnancies and causes a wide variety of symptoms in the fetus, ranging from mild anemia to hydrops fetalis. Sensitization to the Rh (D) antigen is the result of exposure of an Rh-negative mother to Rh-positive blood. Possible exposures include prior pregnancy with an Rh-positive fetus, feto-maternal hemorrhage, and obstetric procedures (e.g., amniocentesis, chorionic villus sampling, abortion). Unlike A or B antigens, which are expressed on a number of different tissues, Rh antigens are expressed only on RBCs.

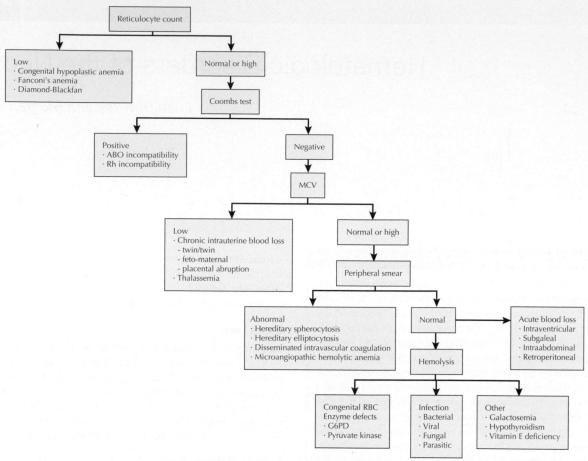

Fig. 95.1 Differential Diagnosis of Neonatal Anemia. (Modified from Blanchette VS, Zipursky A. Assessment of anemia in newborn infants. *Clin Perinatol.* 1984;11[2]:489-510.)

Thus maternal anti-Rh (anti-D) IgG antibodies (Rh-negative mother) cross the placenta and interact with a greater number of fetal RBCs (Rh-positive infant), resulting in significant fetal hemolysis.

Clinical Presentation

Anemias manifest in myriad ways depending on severity and degree of compensation. As in older children and adults, signs of anemia include pallor, tachycardia, tachypnea, and increased fraction of inspired oxygen (FiO_2) requirement. Severe anemia may cause metabolic acidosis. In the neonate, additional signs include apnea, lethargy, poor feeding, and hepatosplenomegaly as a result of extramedullary hematopoiesis and splenic sequestration. Both ABO incompatibility and Rh disease are associated with jaundice within the first 24 hours of life. In severe hemolytic disease, fetuses may present with signs of hydrops fetalis, including ascites, pleural or pericardial effusions, and edema (Fig. 95.2).

Of the hemoglobinopathies, α-thalassemias are generally the most severe. The switch from fetal ($\alpha_2\gamma_2$) to adult ($\alpha_2\beta_2$) hemoglobin occurs during the first year of life. As a result, defects in α-globin synthesis manifest in utero, whereas defects in β-globin synthesis become apparent in late infancy. Deletion of three (hemoglobin H disease) or four (hemoglobin Barts) α-globin genes can cause significant hemolytic anemia and manifest as hydrops fetalis. Newborn screening enables early detection and treatment of infants with major hemoglobinopathies and therefore reduces the mortality and morbidity associated with these conditions.

Diagnosis

Family history, ethnicity, and a detailed pregnancy history, including medications and diet, can uncover potential causes of anemia. The infant's gestational age, chronologic age, and dietary history is also important. Studies should be tailored to the history and physical examination. Initial laboratory tests include a complete blood count with smear and a reticulocyte count. In certain infants presenting with jaundice total and direct bilirubin levels should be obtained, and a blood type and screen with a direct antiglobulin test may be useful. Coagulation studies should be considered for an infant presenting with bleeding. Further studies such as hemoglobin analysis, bone marrow biopsy, or infectious screening, can be based on results of initial testing. Ultrasound is ideal for initial evaluation if concern for internal hemorrhage (head, abdomen) arises, or as an initial evaluation for hepatosplenomegaly.

Management

Management depends on the cause and severity of the anemia. Initial steps include ensuring hemodynamic stability, including packed RBC transfusion if necessary. If severe symptomatic anemia is present, care must be taken to treat slowly by serial small-volume transfusions (aliquoted from one unit so as to avoid several donor exposures), so as not to overwhelm the circulatory system. Studies are ongoing to determine the ideal transfusion thresholds for infants. If the infant is clinically stable, an underlying cause should be investigated and targeted. Laboratory tests should be limited when possible so as to avoid iatrogenic anemia.

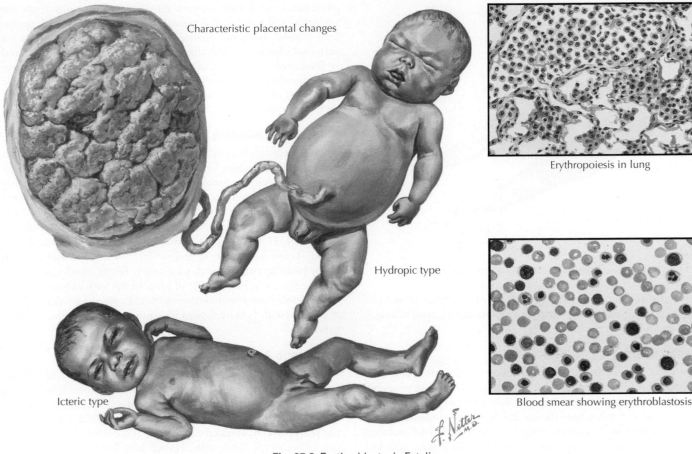

Characteristic placental changes

Erythropoiesis in lung

Hydropic type

Icteric type

Blood smear showing erythroblastosis

Fig. 95.2 Erythroblastosis Fetalis.

Phototherapy and ET are the primary modes of treatment for infants with hemolytic disease. In Rh incompatibility, intensive phototherapy should be started immediately after birth and might prevent the need for ET (Chapter 96). Efforts to reduce perinatal mortality and the need for ET have led to the development of several prenatal care strategies, including RhoGAM, Doppler ultrasound to monitor fetal anemia, and intrauterine blood transfusions. The use of RhoGAM (anti-D prophylaxis) in Rh-negative women has led to a marked decline in Rh sensitization and hemolytic disease of the newborn. In developed countries, a high proportion of clinically significant hemolytic disease is now caused by antibodies to antigens other than D (e.g., anti-C, anti-E, or anti-Kell).

Intravenous immunoglobulin (IVIG) is a supplemental therapy that may be effective in reducing the need for ET in infants with immune-mediated hemolytic disease. In isoimmune hemolysis, RBCs are destroyed by an antibody-dependent cytotoxic process directed by Fc receptor–bearing cells of the reticuloendothelial system. IVIG's mechanism of action is postulated to be attributable to nonspecific blockade of Fc receptors. Potential benefits of IVIG over ET include relative ease of administration, reduced invasiveness, and improved safety profile. However, meta-analyses have found no obvious benefit to IVIG for hemolytic disease of the newborn and therefore it is not recommended for routine treatment at this time.

POLYCYTHEMIA

Etiology and Pathogenesis

Polycythemia can be subdivided into three categories: (1) increased RBC mass and plasma volume (e.g., maternal diabetes, delayed cord clamping, twin–twin, or maternal–fetal transfusion); (2) increased RBC mass and normal plasma volume related to a congenital syndrome (trisomies 13, 18, and 21); and (3) increased RBC mass and normal or decreased plasma volume caused by intrauterine growth restriction, placental insufficiency, maternal hypertension, or smoking. The incidence of polycythemia is 1% to 5% in all neonates, versus 10% to 15% in neonates who are small for gestational age.

Clinical Presentation

Polycythemic infants appear ruddy and plethoric with sluggish capillary refill and poor peripheral perfusion. Hyperviscosity of blood results in increased resistance to blood flow and decreased oxygen delivery. Although most neonates with polycythemia are asymptomatic, it can cause abnormalities in central nervous system function (lethargy, apnea, tremors or jitteriness, poor feeding, and hypotonia), hypoglycemia, decreased renal function (oliguria, proteinuria, and hematuria), cardiorespiratory distress (tachypnea, cyanosis, and cardiomegaly), and coagulation disorders with complications such as renal vein thrombosis and cerebral sinovenous thrombosis. Rare complications include strokes, seizures, congestive heart failure, disseminated intravascular coagulation (DIC), and necrotizing enterocolitis (NEC). Studies have also noted associations between hyperviscosity and long-term motor and neurodevelopmental disorders.

Diagnosis

Polycythemia is defined as a venous hematocrit above 65%. In neonates, hematocrit (Hct) levels peak at 2 hours of life because of fluid shifts and then progressively decrease, stabilizing by 6 to 24 hours of life. Capillary Hct values are significantly higher than venous values,

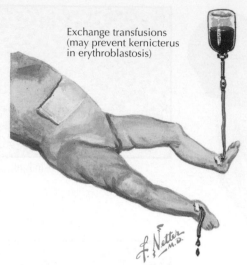

Exchange transfusions
(may prevent kernicterus
in erythroblastosis)

Fig. 95.3 Blood Management in an Exchange Transfusion.

and arterial and umbilical vessel values are generally lower. Infants also should be monitored for hypoglycemia, hypocalcemia, hyperbilirubinemia, and thrombocytopenia.

Management

Symptomatic polycythemia is first treated with hydration and close observation. If symptoms of polycythemia are progressive or severe, partial exchange transfusion is used to lower Hct and the associated hyperviscosity. Studies have shown that it reduces pulmonary vascular resistance and increases cerebral blood flow. Partial exchange transfusion should be performed in symptomatic infants with Hct greater than 65%, or asymptomatic infants with Hct greater than 75%. The data are limited for the use of partial exchange transfusion in asymptomatic neonates. The volume to be exchanged is based on the observed and desired Hct (generally 50% to 55%). Total blood volume is estimated to be 80 to 90 mL/kg. The equation is as follows: Exchange volume (mL) = Blood volume × (Observed Hct – Desired Hct)/Observed Hct. During this procedure, blood is removed using a central venous or arterial line and replaced with fluid infused by a peripheral intravenous line. Crystalloid (normal saline) is favored over colloid (albumin or fresh frozen plasma) because the extra proteins in colloid can contribute to viscosity. Complications of partial exchange transfusion are thought to be similar to a single- or double-volume ET (Fig. 95.3).

PLATELET DISORDERS AND COAGULOPATHIES: THROMBOCYTOPENIA

Etiology and Pathogenesis

Thrombocytopenia is diagnosed in 1% to 5% of newborns, with 22% to 35% of infants admitted to NICUs. The most frequent cause of early-onset thrombocytopenia (<72 hours of life) is reduced megakaryopoiesis secondary to chronic fetal hypoxia from maternal diabetes, pregnancy-induced hypertension (PIH), or intrauterine growth restriction. Late-onset thrombocytopenia (>72 hours of life) is caused by sepsis (e.g., bacterial infection with group B β-hemolytic streptococci, *Escherichia coli*, *Enterococcus* species) or NEC in more than 80% of cases. The differential also includes drug-included or catheter-related thrombosis.

Less common disorders manifesting with thrombocytopenia at birth include congenital infections (e.g., cytomegalovirus, perinatal asphyxia, aneuploidy (e.g., trisomies 13, 18, and 21), and neonatal alloimmune thrombocytopenia (NAIT). NAIT results from the transplacental passage of maternal IgG antibodies directed against fetal platelet antigens inherited from the father and absent on maternal platelets. NAIT affects 1 to 2 per 1000 pregnancies and is associated with the transplacental passage of maternal platelet autoantibodies in mothers with idiopathic thrombocytopenic purpura (ITP) or an autoimmune disease such as systemic lupus erythematosus.

Clinical Presentation and Differential Diagnosis

Affected neonates may be asymptomatic. Those with symptoms can present with petechiae or purpura or have bleeding. Early-onset thrombocytopenia is generally mild to moderate and self-limiting (usually resolves within 10 days). Late-onset thrombocytopenia develops rapidly over 1 to 2 days, can be severe (platelets <30 × 10⁹/L) depending on the cause, and may take several weeks to recover. NAIT often occurs in the first pregnancy (almost 50% of cases), is extremely severe (platelets <20 × 10⁹/L), and may result in major bleeding (intracranial, pulmonary, renal). Intracranial hemorrhage is seen in 10% to 20% of pregnancies with untreated NAIT versus fewer than 1% of mothers with ITP. Bleeding risk is highest in patients with NAIT followed by sepsis or NEC and chronic fetal hypoxia.

Diagnostic Approach

Thrombocytopenia is defined as a platelet count below 150 × 10⁹/L. Neonates with thrombocytopenia secondary to chronic fetal hypoxia have additional hematologic abnormalities, including transient neutropenia, increased circulating nucleated RBCs with or without polycythemia, elevated EPO levels, and evidence of hyposplenism (spherocytes, target cells, Howell-Jolly bodies). The diagnosis of NAIT is made by demonstrating platelet antigen incompatibility between the mother and baby serologically or by polymerase chain reaction.

Management and Therapy

Platelet transfusion is the only specific therapy for neonatal thrombocytopenia. Clear indications for transfusion include active bleeding in association with thrombocytopenia, neonates in the first week of life with platelets below 50 × 10⁹/L, and severe thrombocytopenia (platelets <30 × 10⁹/L). Recent randomized controlled trials, however, suggest liberal thresholds (receiving more platelet transfusions) may result in a higher rate of death or major bleeding in preterm infants.

Infants of mothers with autoimmune disease should have their platelet counts determined at birth. In those with thrombocytopenia, a platelet count should be repeated after 2 to 3 days (time of platelet nadir). If severe thrombocytopenia develops, treatment with IVIG (1 g/kg) for 2 days is usually effective. Corticosteroids can also be used as an adjunctive therapy.

HEMORRHAGIC DISEASE OF THE NEWBORN

Etiology and Pathogenesis

Hemorrhagic disease of the newborn (HDN) is caused by low plasma levels of vitamin K–dependent clotting factors (II, VII, IX, X), which are synthesized in the liver. Concentrations of these factors in neonates are 30% to 60% of those in adults. In the absence of prophylactic vitamin K, HDN occurs in 1 in 200 to 400 infants. Although placental transfer of vitamin K does occur, it is limited. As a result, infants with insufficient enteral intake of vitamin K can quickly become deficient. Breast milk contains lower amounts of vitamin K than formula, thus increasing the risk for vitamin K deficiency.

TABLE 95.1 Normal Values for Coagulation Tests in Healthy Full-Term and Premature Infants

Coagulation Test	Full-Term Infant	Premature Infant	Older Child
Platelets (per μL)	150,000–400,000	150,000–400,000	150,000–400,000
Prothrombin time (seconds)	10.1–15.9	10.6–16.2	10.6–11.4
Partial thromboplastin time (seconds)	31.3–54.5	27.5–79.4	24–36
Thrombin clotting time (seconds)	19–28.3	19.2–30.4	19.8–31.2
Fibrinogen (mg/dL)	167–399	150–373	170–405
Fibrin degradation products (μg/mL)	<10	<10	<10
Factor VIII (U/mL)	0.50–1.78	0.50–2.13	0.59–1.42
Factor IX (U/mL)	0.15–0.91	0.19–0.65	0.47–1.04
von Willebrand factor (U/mL)	0.50–2.87	0.78–2.10	0.60–1.20

From Cantor AB. Developmental hemostasis: relevance to newborns and infants. In: Orkin SH, Fisher D, Look AT, et al., eds. *Nathan and Oski's Hematology of Infancy and Childhood*. 7th ed. Philadelphia, PA: Saunders; 2009, Table 16-2.

Clinical Presentation and Differential Diagnosis

Classic HDN is observed on days 1 to 7 of life and is associated with bleeding from the gastrointestinal (GI) tract, cutaneous sites (e.g., circumcision), and nasal passages. Late HDN occurs during weeks 2 to 12. Common sites of bleeding include intracranial, cutaneous, and GI.

Diagnostic Approach

Vitamin K deficiency results in a prolonged prothrombin time (PT) and an international normalized ratio (INR) above 1. PT depends on various clotting factors, several of which are vitamin K dependent. INR compares the blood coagulation status of an individual to that of the normal population. Thus an INR greater than 1 indicates that coagulation is slower than in the control group (Table 95.1).

Management and Therapy

A single dose (1 mg) of intramuscular vitamin K after birth is effective in preventing classic and late HDN. The safety of intramuscular vitamin K has been questioned, but studies have shown no association between a single dose of IM vitamin K and childhood cancers such as leukemia.

Oral vitamin K prophylaxis has been shown to improve indices of coagulation status at 1 to 7 days; however, a universal dosing regimen has not been established. Oral vitamin K has been shown to protect against early and classic HDN at rates similar to those with intramuscular vitamin K, although it may not protect as effectively against late HDN. Oral vitamin K also requires a reliable absorption mechanism, so neonates with impaired fat-soluble vitamin absorption (e.g., cystic fibrosis, biliary atresia, diarrhea) are at considerably higher bleeding risk. Oral vitamin K is therefore not a recommended treatment for HDN at this time. Because it takes approximately 2 hours for systemically administered vitamin K to increase levels of vitamin K–dependent factors, infants with bleeding secondary to vitamin K deficiency should also be treated with plasma.

LEUKOCYTE DISORDERS: NEUTROPENIA

Etiology and Pathogenesis

When evaluating neonates with neutropenia, it is important to first determine whether the cytopenia results from a defect in cellular production or peripheral destruction or is of mixed etiology (Box 95.1). The most common causes of neonatal neutropenia are maternal PIH, sepsis, and congenital viral infections. Infants with severe and prolonged neutropenia should be evaluated for immune-mediated conditions and inherited genetic mutations.

BOX 95.1 Causes of Neonatal Neutropenia

Decreased Production
- Bone marrow failure syndromes
  - Kostmann syndrome
  - Cartilage-hair hypoplasia
  - Reticular dysgenesis
  - Shwachman-Diamond syndrome
- Maternal pregnancy-induced hypertension
- Viral infections
- Copper deficiency
- Organic acidemias
- Glycogen storage disease type 1b

Increased Destruction
- Alloimmune
- Maternal autoimmune
- Fetal or neonatal autoimmune

Mixed Causes
- Prematurity
- Drug-induced neutropenia
- Necrotizing enterocolitis
- Bacterial or fungal sepsis

Clinical Presentation and Differential Diagnosis

The neutropenia of maternal PIH and sepsis is generally transient, rarely persisting for more than 72 hours. In contrast, infants with immune-mediated and inherited disorders show evidence of severe neutropenia for many weeks to months and can have recurrent bacterial infections. Clinical signs of neutropenia in this population include ulcerations of the oral mucosa or gingival inflammation. Otitis media, skin infections (cellulitis, pustules, abscesses), adenitis, pneumonia, and bacterial sepsis can also occur. The most common organisms are *Staphylococcus aureus* and gram-negative bacteria derived from the child's skin or bowel flora.

Diagnostic Approach

Normal values for the absolute neutrophil count (ANC) vary by age, particularly during the first weeks after birth. The lower limit of normal is 6000/μL during the first 24 hours after birth, 5000/μL for the first week, 1500/μL during the second week, and 1000/μL between 2 weeks and 1 year of age. Severe neutropenia is defined as an ANC of less than 500/μL.

The initial evaluation of an infant with severe neutropenia should include a thorough history and physical examination. It is critical to know whether there is a family history of neutropenia or associated congenital anomalies suggestive of an inherited syndrome. If additional evaluation is warranted, antineutrophil antibody titers (elevated in immune-mediated neutropenias) and immunoglobulin quantification (decreased levels in underlying immunodeficiency) may be performed. Neonates with severe and prolonged neutropenia should be referred to a hematologist for bone marrow examination and possible genetic testing.

Management and Therapy

Infants with fever and severe neutropenia should be hospitalized and started on parenteral broad-spectrum antibiotics. If recovery from neutropenia is not expected, as in inherited syndromes, granulocyte colony-stimulating factor (G-CSF) administration or stem cell transplantation may be necessary. G-CSF has been shown to mobilize preformed neutrophils from the bone marrow, promote neutrophil precursor proliferation, and enhance phagocytic bactericidal function. However, there is currently insufficient evidence to support the use of G-CSF in neutropenic neonates with systemic infection, or as prophylaxis to prevent systemic infection in high-risk neonates.

SUGGESTED READINGS

Available online.

Hyperbilirubinemia

Katherine E. Schwartz

 CLINICAL VIGNETTE

A 4-day-old boy born at 39 4/7 weeks' gestational age by vaginal delivery presents to the emergency department (ED) from his pediatrician's office for elevated bilirubin levels. Parents report the baby received approximately 24 hours of phototherapy in the well-baby nursery, and his bilirubin level on day 2 of life was 10.8. He has been breastfeeding with formula supplementation and voiding and stooling appropriately. Parents report no symptoms of illness but describe jaundice and sleepiness. Mother's blood type is B+, antibody-screen negative.

The baby's total bilirubin in the ED is 29, with a conjugated bilirubin of 3.2. The baby's blood type is B+, and he is Coombs negative. The baby receives peripheral access, a normal saline bolus, and phototherapy and is transferred to the neonatal intensive care unit (NICU). On admission to the NICU, the baby is noted to be lethargic, with posturing and intermittent tongue smacking. A low-lying umbilical venous catheter is placed. The baby undergoes two double-volume exchange transfusions for hyperbilirubinemia, and phototherapy is reinitiated. He subsequently has a drop in his bilirubin levels. The baby's newborn screen later results positive for glucose-6-phosphate dehydrogenase (G6PD) deficiency.

Physical examination findings in infants with severe hyperbilirubinemia can be subtle. The degree of jaundice cannot be assessed by examination alone, and confirmation with bilirubin measurements is warranted. Despite adequate follow-up with the pediatrician, this baby developed severe unconjugated hyperbilirubinemia because of G6PD deficiency.

Unconjugated hyperbilirubinemia is seen frequently in neonates. It can be physiologic as opposed to pathologic, and screening newborns for jaundice is part of typical well-baby nursery care. Making the determination between physiologic and pathologic jaundice requires a thorough history, physical examination, and laboratory evaluation looking for signs of hemolysis.

Conjugated hyperbilirubinemia is always pathologic and requires investigation and consultation with an appropriate pediatric subspecialty service.

ETIOLOGY AND PATHOGENESIS

Bilirubin is produced from the breakdown of heme (Fig. 96.1). Heme is released from hemoglobin in the red blood cells (RBCs), metabolized to an intermediate product called biliverdin and metabolized further into unconjugated bilirubin. This circulates in the bloodstream primarily bound to albumin. Unconjugated bilirubin is then taken up by the liver, where it is bound to glucuronic acid by the enzyme uridine diphosphate glucuronyl transferase (UDPGT), creating water-soluble conjugated bilirubin. This complex can then be excreted into the gastrointestinal (GI) tract through the bile ducts. When stool has a delayed transit time, conjugated bilirubin can be broken down in the GI tract and

reabsorbed into the bloodstream, a process known as enterohepatic circulation.

Unconjugated Hyperbilirubinemia

Jaundice refers to a yellow discoloration of skin, eyes, and mucous membranes. Most infants have a transient increase in their unconjugated bilirubin levels in the first week of life known as physiologic jaundice. This is attributable to low activity of UDPGT at birth, large RBC mass, and the short duration of survival of newborn RBCs. Physiologic jaundice develops after 24 hours of life, and generally peaks during the first week of life. Bilirubin levels in physiologic jaundice rarely require treatment.

Unconjugated hyperbilirubinemia is considered pathologic when it develops in the first 24 hours of life, is associated with rapidly rising or extremely elevated bilirubin levels or lasts beyond the first 2 to 3 weeks of life in term infants. The causes of pathologic jaundice are typically divided into two primary categories of increased production or decreased clearance of bilirubin (Box 96.1).

Increased Production

Increased bilirubin production can occur due to increased RBC breakdown or elevated total-body RBCs (i.e., polycythemia). The causes of increased RBC breakdown can be grouped into immune and nonimmune causes. Hemolytic disease of the fetus and newborn (HDFN) is the primary immunologic cause for hyperbilirubinemia. In HDFN, maternal immunoglobulin G antibodies are transmitted to the fetus by the placenta, and lead to immune-mediated RBC breakdown. Examples include maternal-fetal ABO incompatibility, when a rhesus (Rh)-negative pregnant parent is carrying an Rh-positive fetus, or when the pregnant parent has another blood-related antibody. Notable antibodies include Anti-C, anti-c, or anti-Kell. Nonimmune mediators of increased RBC breakdown include RBC defects (G6PD, hereditary spherocytosis/elliptocytosis), hemoglobinopathies (particularly thalassemia), and RBC sequestration (cephalohematomas, subgaleal hemorrhage, intracranial hemorrhage).

Decreased Clearance

Decreased bilirubin clearance can occur in the setting of decreased conjugation or increased enterohepatic circulation. Two common causes in this group are breastfeeding jaundice and breast milk jaundice. Breastfeeding jaundice is an exaggeration of physiologic jaundice by inadequate intake because of insufficient maternal milk production or poor milk transfer. In contrast, breast milk jaundice typically peaks during the second week of life and may take several more weeks to resolve completely. Prolonged jaundice may be seen in 20% to 30% of all breastfed infants. The mechanism of this process is not entirely understood but may involve components of breast milk inhibiting hepatic conjugating enzymes or increasing enterohepatic circulation.

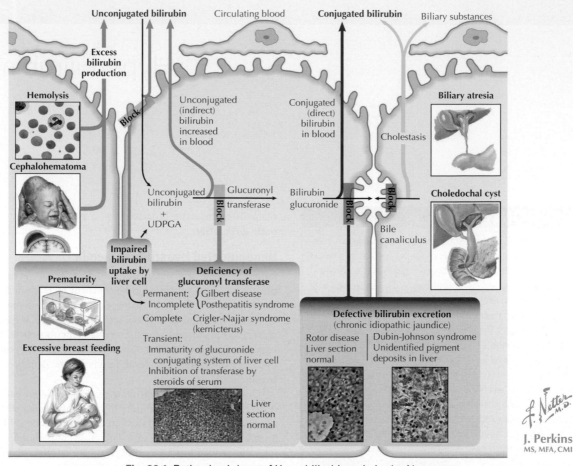

Fig. 96.1 Pathophysiology of Hyperbilirubinemia in the Neonate.

Less common causes include hereditary syndromes (Gilbert syndrome, Crigler-Najjar), congenital hypothyroidism, and drug exposure (sulfa drugs, ceftriaxone, ibuprofen, and others).

Conjugated Hyperbilirubinemia

Conjugated hyperbilirubinemia (cholestasis) is inherently pathologic and can be diagnosed either with absolute elevation of conjugated bilirubin when total bilirubin is low or by relative elevation, making up more than 20% of the total bilirubin level if high (greater than 5 mg/dL). The differential diagnosis of neonatal cholestasis is vast, and includes anatomic, metabolic, and infectious causes (see Fig. 96.1 and Box 96.1). Common anatomic causes of cholestasis include biliary atresia and choledochal cysts (Fig. 96.2) and require prompt subspecialty evaluation by pediatric gastroenterologists and surgeons. Metabolic causes include α-1 antitrypsin deficiency, galactosemia, tyrosinemia, and mitochondrial disorders. Other causes of neonatal cholestasis include Alagille syndrome, infections (cytomegalovirus, herpes simplex virus, bacterial sepsis, urinary tract infections), ischemic injury (asphyxia, hypoxia, severe metabolic acidosis, or shock), and prolonged parenteral nutrition.

CLINICAL PRESENTATION

Unconjugated Hyperbilirubinemia

Jaundice is the most common manifesting symptom of unconjugated hyperbilirubinemia and often the only symptom in mild cases. Jaundice is classically first evident in the face (including the sclera and intraoral mucous membranes) nend moves caudally as bilirubin levels increase. Estimation of bilirubin levels based on extension and intensity of jaundice are unreliable and require verification with direct measurement. Particular attention should be paid to jaundice in the first 24 hours of life and extensive jaundice that is rapidly worsening. It is recommended all neonates get screened for hyperbilirubinemia 24 to 48 hours after birth.

Although jaundice is the primary symptom of mild-to-moderate unconjugated hyperbilirubinemia, other physical examination findings may point to exacerbating or underlying conditions. Signs and symptoms consistent with hemolytic anemia are tachycardia and pallor. Cephalohematomas and ecchymoses should be documented as a source of RBC breakdown. Evidence of dehydration such as tacky mucous membranes or a sunken fontanelle may increase suspicion for breastfeeding jaundice. Infection can cause hyperbilirubinemia and vital sign instability.

The primary toxicity of bilirubin results from unconjugated bilirubin crossing the blood-brain barrier. Neurotoxicity appears to be closely related to the amount of free or unbound bilirubin in the bloodstream, but risk for neurotoxicity is increased by factors associated with an altered blood-brain barrier, including asphyxia, sepsis, acidosis, and prematurity. The chronic neurologic sequala of severe hyperbilirubinemia is called kernicterus. It is caused when bilirubin is deposited in the brain, typically in the basal ganglia, brainstem nuclei, and cerebellum. Development of kernicterus should be suspected when an infant shows early symptoms of acute bilirubin encephalopathy: lethargy, hypotonia, high-pitched cry, and poor feeding. This is followed by irritability, hypertonia, retrocollis, and opisthotonus in the intermediate stages and apnea, coma, seizures, and death in advanced cases. Kernicterus is a pathologic or radiographic diagnosis. Clinical characteristics are athetoid cerebral palsy, cognitive and developmental

BOX 96.1 Selected Differential Diagnosis of Unconjugated and Conjugated Hyperbilirubinemia

Unconjugated Hyperbilirubinemia
Physiologic Increased Bilirubin Production
- Hemolytic anemia
  - ABO incompatibility
  - Rh disease
  - G6PD deficiency
- Polycythemia
  - IDM
- Blood extravasation
  - Cephalohematoma
  - Caput succedaneum

Decreased Bilirubin Clearance
- Defects of conjugation
  - Crigler-Najjar, Gilbert syndromes
- Increased enterohepatic circulation
  - Breastfeeding jaundice
  - Breast milk jaundice

Decreased Albumin Binding Capacity
- Medications
- Comorbid conditions

Conjugated Hyperbilirubinemia
Structural
- Biliary atresia
- Choledochal cyst
- Alagille syndrome
- Neonatal sclerosing cholangitis

Toxins
- Parenteral nutrition

Endocrinopathy
- Hypothyroidism

Genetic Disorders
- Trisomy 21
- Cystic fibrosis
- Dubin-Johnson, Rotor syndrome
- α-1 Antitrypsin deficiency

Metabolic Diseases
- Galactosemia
- Tyrosinemia
- Vascular disorders
- Neonatal asphyxia
- Budd-Chiari syndrome

Infection
- TORCH infections
- Sepsis
- Urinary tract infection

Neoplastic Disease
—

G6PD, Glucose-6-phosphate dehydrogenase; *IDM,* infant of a diabetic mother; *TORCH,* toxoplasmosis or *Toxoplasma gondii,* other infections, rubella, cytomegalovirus, and herpes simplex virus.

delays, behavioral and psychiatric disorders, auditory disturbances, impaired upward gaze, and dysplasia of the primary teeth (Fig. 96.3).

Conjugated Hyperbilirubinemia

Conjugated bilirubin does not cross the blood-brain barrier. The primary clinical concern is not kernicterus but rather the risks associated with a significant underlying disease. Patients with neonatal cholestasis may present with prolonged jaundice, pale or acholic stools, and dark urine. Pertinent findings on physical examination may include jaundice, hepatomegaly, abnormal neurologic examination caused by infectious or metabolic causes, or dysmorphisms suggestive of an underlying syndrome or intrauterine infection. The patient may also exhibit evidence of coagulopathy as a result of underlying liver disease. Patients with conjugated hyperbilirubinemia who undergo phototherapy can develop a typically benign and self-limiting discoloration of the skin termed bronze baby syndrome.

EVALUATION AND MANAGEMENT

Unconjugated Hyperbilirubinemia

Many patients with neonatal hyperbilirubinemia are identified through recommended routine screening in the newborn nursery. Transcutaneous or serum bilirubin levels should be measured in all jaundiced infants. A high level obtained through transcutaneous measurement should be confirmed with a serum sample. The patient's bilirubin level should be compared with nomograms to determine whether the level requires intervention (Fig. 96.4). Important historical information in a newborn with jaundice includes feeding and stooling patterns, family history, prenatal and perinatal course, and maternal laboratory

results. For prevention of hyperbilirubinemia, breastfeeding mothers should nurse their infants at least 8 to 12 times daily for the first several days of life. Supplementation with formula should be discussed with a pediatrician in cases of excessive weight loss or signs of dehydration.

Infants born earlier than 38 weeks of gestational age, of East Asian descent, exclusively breastfed, with asphyxia or bruising from delivery, or with a sibling with a history of neonatal hyperbilirubinemia are at increased risk. The mother's prenatal laboratory study results, including blood type and antibody testing, are useful. G6PD deficiency and blood disorders such as hereditary spherocytosis and thalassemia cause increased hemolysis after birth and might be noted in the family history. Infant blood type, direct Coombs testing, a complete blood count with smear, and reticulocyte count should be performed in patients requiring phototherapy to evaluate for the possibility of a hemolytic process. If hemolysis is suspected in a male infant, G6PD testing also should be considered. A basic metabolic panel can be helpful in a child with associated clinical concern for dehydration. A type and screen and an albumin level should be obtained if there is a possibility that the infant needs an exchange transfusion.

For unconjugated hyperbilirubinemia, the infant's total bilirubin level should be plotted according to hour of life (see Fig. 96.4). This nomogram determines the age-specific bilirubin level at which phototherapy or exchange transfusion should be initiated in infants who are 35 weeks' gestational age or greater. The treatment threshold is based on hour of life, total serum bilirubin level, and presence of additional risk factors. The conjugated bilirubin level should not be subtracted from the total bilirubin level when using the nomogram, but if conjugated bilirubin exceeds 20% of the total bilirubin, evaluation for conjugated hyperbilirubinemia is advised.

Bile duct atresia; extrahepatic

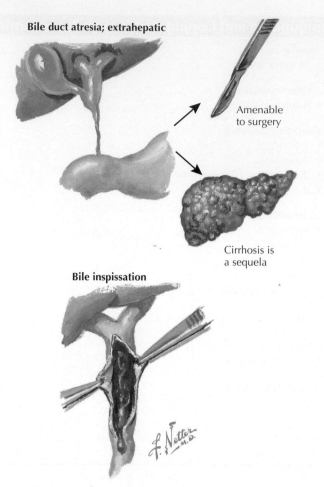

Amenable to surgery

Cirrhosis is a sequela

Bile inspissation

Fig. 96.2 Abnormal Biliary Tree as a Concern for Conjugated Hyperbilirubinemia and Cholestasis.

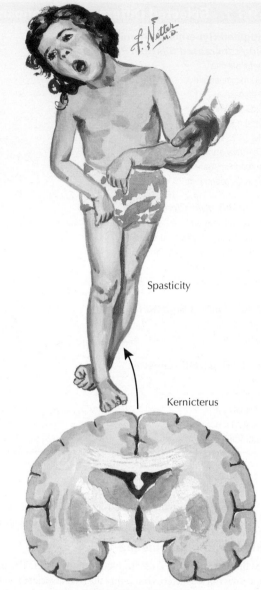

Spasticity

Kernicterus

Fig. 96.3 Kernicterus.

Treatment with phototherapy aids in clearance of bilirubin through photoisomerization of unconjugated bilirubin into a water-soluble form that can be excreted in the bile and urine without further conjugation. Phototherapy is most effective with appropriate wavelengths of light (ideally 460 to 490 nm), appropriate distance and irradiance, and maximal skin exposure. Phototherapy can be toxic to the immature retina, requiring protective eye shields during treatment (Fig. 96.5). Phototherapy can be delivered by overhead banks of lights or a portable blanket placed under the neonate. Although most neonates currently receive phototherapy in the hospital setting, blanket devices are available for use in the home.

Exchange transfusion is initiated at severe levels of hyperbilirubinemia based on the infant's hour of life and in any infant exhibiting signs of acute bilirubin encephalopathy. In a double-volume exchange transfusion (DVET) for hyperbilirubinemia, two times the estimated circulating blood volume of the neonate are simultaneously withdrawn and replaced with an equivalent volume of donor blood (see Fig. 96.5). Severe hyperbilirubinemia requiring DVET should be treated as a medical emergency and requires immediate admission to an intensive care unit. Intravenous immunoglobulin (IVIG) may be considered in infants with isoimmune hemolytic disease who are approaching the exchange transfusion threshold. IVIG works by binding antibodies causing hemolysis.

In addition to these specific treatments for hyperbilirubinemia, it is important to respond appropriately to any concomitant issues, such as dehydration or sepsis. If hyperbilirubinemia is determined not to require treatment at the time of evaluation, it is important to determine when the total serum bilirubin level should next be obtained, to provide the patient's parents with education about jaundice, and to ensure appropriate follow-up.

Conjugated Hyperbilirubinemia

Conjugated hyperbilirubinemia is defined as conjugated bilirubin greater than 1 mg/dL or greater than 20% of the total bilirubin level if total bilirubin is greater than 5 mg/dL. Initial evaluation entails a thorough history and physical examination as well as fractionated bilirubin levels and liver function tests. Evaluation should proceed in a stepwise fashion, focusing first on disease processes requiring urgent treatment such as sepsis, urinary tract, and TORCH infections (see Chapter 99), hypothyroidism, and metabolic disorders. Next, imaging studies should be considered to evaluate for anatomic causes of hyperbilirubinemia. Ultrasound can provide useful information about the gallbladder and biliary tree; hepatobiliary scintigraphy, however, has better sensitivity for biliary atresia. If no cause is found, consultation with a pediatric gastroenterologist and additional evaluation for other specific causes, such as cystic fibrosis and α-1 antitrypsin deficiency, may be helpful.

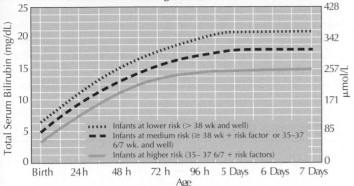

Guidelines for phototherapy in hospitalized infants of 35 or more weeks' gestation.

Infants at lower risk (> 38 wk and well)
Infants at medium risk (≥ 38 wk + risk factor or 35–37 6/7 wk. and well)
Infants at higher risk (35–37 6/7 + risk factors)

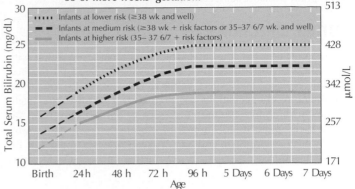

Guidelines for exchange transfusion in infants of 35 or more weeks' gestation.

Infants at lower risk (≥38 wk and well)
Infants at medium risk (≥38 wk + risk factors or 35–37 6/7 wk. and well)
Infants at higher risk (35– 37 6/7 + risk factors)

· Use total bilirubin. Do not subtract direct reacting or conjugated bilirubin.
· Risk factors = isoimmune hemolytic disease, G6PD deficiency, asphyxia, significant lethargy, temperature instability, sepsis, acidosis, or albumin < 3.0 g/dL (if measured).
· For well infants 35–37 6/7 wk can adjust TSB levels for intervention around the medium risk line. It is an option to intervene at lower TSB levels for infants closer to 35 wk and at higher TSB levels for those closer to 37 6/7 wk.
· It is an option to provide conventional phototherapy in hospital or at home at TSB levels 2–3 mg/dL (35-50 mmol/L) below those shown, but home phototherapy should not be used in any infant with risk factors.

· The dashed lines for the first 24 hours indicate uncertainty due to a wide range of clinical circumstances and a range of responses to phototherapy.
· Immediate exchange transfusion is recommended if infant shows signs of acute bilirubin encephalopathy (hypertonia, arching, retrocollis, opisthotonos, fever, high-pitched cry) or if TSB is ≥5 mg/dL (85 μmol/L) above these lines.
· Risk factors - isoimmune hemolytic disease, G6PD deficiency, asphyxia, significant lethargy, temperature instability, sepsis, acidosis.
· Measure serum albumin and calculate B/A ratio.
· Use total bilirubin. Do not subtract direct reacting or conjugated bilirubin.
· If infant is well and 35–37 6/7 wk (median risk) can individualize TSB levels for exchange based on actual gestational age.

Fig. 96.4 Management of Hyperbilirubinemia in the Newborn Infant 35 or More Weeks' Gestation. (From American Academy of Pediatrics Subcommittee on Hyperbilirubinemia. Management of hyperbilirubinemia in the newborn infant 35 or more weeks of gestation. *Pediatrics*. 2004;114[1]:297-316. https://doi.org/10.1542/peds.114.1.297. Erratum in: *Pediatrics*. 2004;114[4]:1138. PMID: 15231951, Figures 3 and 4.)

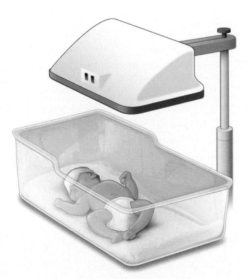

Jaundiced infant under phototherapy (with eye protection)

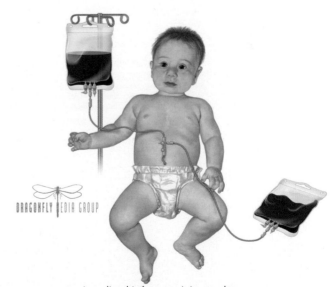

Jaundiced infant receiving exchange transfusion (through umbilical lines)

Fig. 96.5 Treatments for Unconjugated Hyperbilirubinemia.

Therapy for neonatal cholestasis varies depending on the underlying cause. Sepsis requires antibiotic therapy, and inborn errors of metabolism may require dietary modification or enzyme supplementation. Biliary atresia requires urgent surgical treatment with a Kasai procedure because prognoses are markedly better when surgery occurs within the first 60 days of life (see Fig 96.2). In contrast, treatment of patients with other causes focuses more on supportive care such as nutritional support with caloric and fat-soluble vitamin supplementation. Ursodeoxycholic acid can be used for symptomatic treatment to enhance bilirubin excretion and may reduce associated pruritus.

Further management should be conducted in consultation with the appropriate pediatric subspecialist.

FUTURE DIRECTIONS

Clear guidelines for term and near-term infants presenting with unconjugated hyperbilirubinemia are available based on the best current evidence and expert opinion. Less consensus remains in treatment recommendations for premature and low-birth-weight infants, making further study necessary to optimize treatment for these at-risk populations. Improving our ability to use noninvasive testing such as brainstem auditory evoked responses to monitor for bilirubin-induced neurotoxicity will further enhance our targeting of therapy. Phototherapy has long been considered a benign treatment, but recent evidence has surfaced of associations with infantile cancer and childhood seizures in males. The mechanism is as yet unknown, and it remains unclear whether the increased risks are clinically significant. In addition to refining current guidelines for treatment as more evidence becomes available, it is important to ensure that these guidelines are translated into universal clinical practice to maximize prevention of the permanent consequences of severe hyperbilirubinemia.

SUGGESTED READINGS

Available online.

97

Neonatal Dermatology

Leah Downey and Sandy Johng

CLINICAL VIGNETTE

A term female infant is born by uncomplicated spontaneous vaginal delivery to a healthy 33-year-old G1P1 birth parent with a normal pregnancy and normal prenatal laboratory test results. She presents on day of life 3 to her first pediatric appointment with a rash noted after hospital discharge that concerns the parents. The baby's first physical examination in the newborn nursery was notable for a few scattered erythematous macules over the trunk but was otherwise normal. The parents report the rash has been changing since their discharge from the hospital. In the office, the infant is vigorous and well appearing with an eruption over her trunk of erythematous macules, papules, and pustules on the trunk and extremities. The lesions do not appear vesicular, candidal, nor impetiginous, and a diagnosis of erythema toxicum neonatorum is made. The parents are given anticipatory guidance that this eruption is common, benign, and self-limited and to expect a shifting appearance until resolution, which usually happens within 2 weeks.

Maturation of neonatal skin is still occurring after delivery as the infant transitions from being surrounded by amniotic fluid to air. Without a well-developed skin barrier, babies are at risk for skin breakdown and infection. However, there are a host of typical and benign skin lesions in infancy that are well described and do not require intervention. Prompt recognition and reassurance of these skin manifestations for families is a key feature of general pediatric care.

Skin functions as the first defense against infection, contributes to thermoregulation, and helps control insensible losses. These functions are immature in neonatal skin, especially in premature infants. Neonatal skin is thinner; it has fewer sweat and sebaceous glands and fewer intercellular connections, leading to epidermal fragility. The outermost layer of the epidermis, the stratum corneum, develops in the third trimester of pregnancy alongside a greasy, waxy protective substance called vernix caseosa. After exposure to the extrauterine environment, maturation of the skin and stratum corneum takes 2 to 4 weeks.

Infants also have a higher ratio of surface to body weight relative to older children and adults. Given these properties of neonatal skin, infants are at risk for developing toxicity because of systemic absorption of chemicals and topical medications. Sun exposure is also more likely to burn neonates, because melanin production begins in utero but continues to develop after birth. Of note, different skin tones can manifest common neonatal rashes in different ways. Health care professionals should familiarize themselves with the presentation of these rashes on lighter and darker skin. This chapter serves as an overview of some common skin findings in the neonate (Table 97.1).

CLINICAL PRESENTATIONS

Extrauterine Transition

Peeling

Desquamation is a common finding in the days to weeks after birth, particularly if an infant is born at greater than 40 weeks' gestation, or is small for gestational age. The skin can appear dry and flaky, or be overtly peeling. In these instances, the epidermal barrier remains intact and no intervention is required. Physiologic desquamation is important to distinguish from conditions such as congenital ichthyoses or scaling.

Cutis Marmorata

Cutis marmorata, or mottling, appears as a blanching, lacy, reticulated erythema on any part of the body. It occurs as a result of vasomotor instability and transient shifts in skin blood flow and can be particularly prominent if the infant is cold. Cutis marmorata usually resolves with rewarming and may occur beyond 1 month of age in infants with genetic abnormalities (i.e., trisomy 21, trisomy 18, Cornelia de Lange syndrome).

Noninfectious Papules, Pustules, and Vesicles
Erythema Toxicum Neonatorum

The cause of erythema toxicum neonatorum, or erythema toxicum, is unknown. It may be related to hair follicle formation because it tends to occur in areas of hair distribution in the neonate. It occurs in approximately 50% of newborns and manifests within the first 3 to 14 days of life. The lesions are painless papules and pustules with an erythematous base (Fig. 97.1). The diagnosis is most often made clinically; however, if cultured and stained, the pustules would have an eosinophilic predominance. The area of distribution is commonly the face, trunk, back, and extremities, sparing the palms and soles.

Transient Pustular Melanocytosis

Transient pustular melanocytosis (TPM) is a benign eruption affecting up to 4% of neonates, predominantly those with abundant skin pigmentation. TPM typically manifests as small pustules without surrounding erythema. Ruptured pustules leave a hyperpigmented macule with a crust or collarette of scale (Fig. 97.2). Pustular fluid is sterile and would reveal predominantly neutrophils on Wright stain.

The pattern of distribution for TPM is commonly the forehead, chin, neck, and trunk; however, it can affect any body area, including the palms and soles. This eruption is self-limited and resolves without treatment. Hyperpigmented macules may take up to 3 to 6 months to fade.

Milia

Milia are small (1 to 2 mm) cysts containing keratin, which become trapped in the epidermis. They are frequently found on the face (cheek, eyelids, nose, chin), scalp, and trunk, but may also arise in the mouth on the palate (Bohn nodules) and mucosa (Epstein pearls). Milia usually self-resolve by 1 to 2 months of life. They are often confused with sebaceous gland hyperplasia and miliaria.

TABLE 97.1   Common Skin Findings in the Newborn

Milia	Small (<2 mm), white, papules; present at birth, commonly on the face and scalp.
Neonatal acne	Occurs at birth or early in life; inflammatory, erythematous papules and pustules, located on the cheeks, face, or scalp.
Sebaceous gland hyperplasia	Follicular, smooth white-yellow papules grouped into plaques on the nose and upper lip.
Nevus simplex	Capillary malformation presenting as erythematous macules and patches over the occiput, eyelids, glabella, nose, or upper lip.
Erythema toxicum neonatorum	Presents in first days of life as a yellowish papule or pustule with an irregular macular flare or erythema. Lesions wax and wane.
Transient neonatal pustular melanosis	Develops in utero, presents in three different stages: (1) superficial vesico-pustules, 2–10 mm, (2) collarette of scale around resolving pustule, and (3) hyperpigmented brown macules at site of the prior pustule.
Miliaria	Caused by immature, blocked sweat ducts, manifesting as diffuse, small, clear vesicles.
Congenital dermal melanocytosis	Present at birth as blue-gray or black macules found over the buttocks and sacrum.
Café au lait spots	Circumscribed, flat, round to oval, tan to brown macules located anywhere on the body. Most are present at birth or in the first few months, but may increase in number and size with age (require further workup if six or more that are ≥5 mm in diameter).

Fig. 97.1 Erythema Toxicum Neonatorum. (From Weston WL, Morelli JG, Lane AT. *Color Textbook of Pediatric Dermatology.* 4th ed. Philadelphia, PA: Mosby; 2007:386, Figure 21.13.)

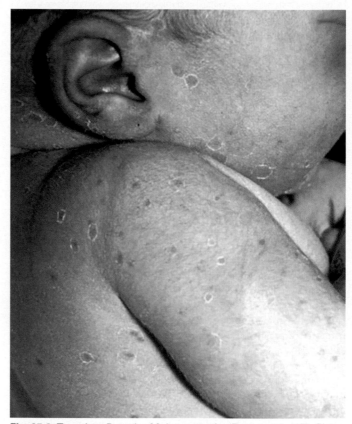

Fig. 97.2 Transient Pustular Melanocytosis. (From James WD, Elston DM, Neuhaus IM, Rosenbach M, Treat J, eds. *Andrews' Diseases of the Skin: Clinical Dermatology.* Edinburgh: Elsevier; 2020:862-880, Figure 36.8.)

Sebaceous Gland Hyperplasia

Sebaceous gland hyperplasia appears as a cluster of small, yellowish papules. It is a very common neonatal skin finding related to maternal androgen stimulation. Clusters tend to occur around the nose and midface (Fig. 97.3). Sebaceous hyperplasia is benign and regresses within the first few weeks of life.

Miliaria

Miliaria results from obstruction of the eccrine sweat ducts leading to leakage and trapping of sweat in the skin. There are three subtypes of miliaria: crystallina, rubra, and profunda. Miliaria crystallina is a superficial obstruction within or below the stratum corneum, and presents as 1- to 2-mm fragile vesicles that are easily wiped away (Fig. 97.4). Miliaria rubra appears as erythematous papules and pustules and occurs when the eccrine duct is obstructed in the epidermis, often because of overheating. Miliaria profunda is rare in neonates and infants and occurs with dermal–epidermal junction occlusion of eccrine ducts, producing a deeper, firmer, flesh-colored papular eruption. Miliaria occurs on the forehead, upper trunk, and intertriginous areas, or under clothing, bandages, or monitor leads. Although benign, miliaria can be prevented by avoiding overdressing infants, sustained high temperatures, and widespread use of thick emollients that block eccrine ducts.

Seborrheic Dermatitis

Seborrheic dermatitis, also known as "cradle cap," is characterized by waxy or greasy yellow scale overlying patches of erythema. Although the cause of seborrheic dermatitis is unknown, some studies point to an interplay between maternal androgens stimulating sebaceous

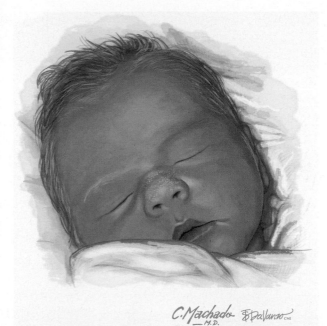

Fig. 97.3 Sebaceous Gland Hyperplasia.

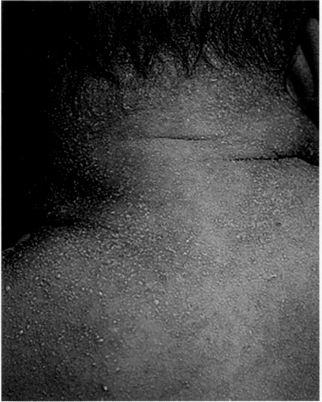

Fig. 97.4 Miliaria Crystallina. (From Lucky AW. In: Eichenfield LF, Frieden IJ, Mathes EF, Zaenglein AL, eds. *Neonatal and Infant Dermatology.* London: Saunders; 2015:65-76, Figure 7.4.)

gland activity, individual susceptibility, and presence of *Malassezia*, a common genus of yeast. Its distribution is most often found on the scalp, forehead, and nasolabial folds; however, it can also affect the diaper area and other intertriginous zones. This self-limited eruption

presents in the first several months of life and generally resolves by 1 year.

Seborrheic dermatitis can be observed or treated with mineral oil or baby oil to comb or brush out scale, with daily shampooing. Persistent cases can be treated with a topical antifungal or low-potency corticosteroid cream.

Neonatal Cephalic Pustulosis

Neonatal acne, or neonatal cephalic pustulosis, manifests as erythematous papules and pustules on the face, scalp, and neck of infants. It is not true acne, in that the eruption is not comedonal. It is thought instead to be related to an inflammatory reaction to *Malassezia* species. It usually manifests by 3 to 4 weeks of life and resolves over weeks to months.

Neonatal cephalic pustulosis does not require treatment. Topical antifungal or low-potency corticosteroid preparations may speed its clearance.

Sucking Blister

Sucking blisters are usually solitary lesions from fetal sucking in utero. They manifest as tense bullae on areas accessible to an infant's mouth, such as on the hands or forearms. They may also manifest as erosions if previously ruptured. No workup is required for these solitary bullae. Extensive blistering or clusters of bullae should raise concern for neonatal herpes simplex virus infection and would require culturing and consultation with Infectious Disease (Chapter 99).

Vascular Lesions

Nevus simplex, nevus flammeus, and hemangiomas are important to recognize in infants and are discussed in more depth in Chapter 40.

Disorders of Pigmentation
Café au Lait Macules

Café au lait spots or macules (CALMs) are well-demarcated light to dark brown macules and patches that can manifest either at birth or in early childhood, and grow in size with the child. Up to 35% of children may have a single CALM; however, presence of large or segmental lesions or multiple CALMs may indicate an associated syndrome and should be referred for additional workup (McCune-Albright syndrome or neurofibromatosis type 1, respectively).

Harlequin Sign

The harlequin color change, or harlequin sign, appears as an infant is placed on one side. The dependent half appears erythematous whereas the upper half appears pale, separated by a sharp midline demarcation (Fig. 97.5). It is most commonly observed in the days after birth, especially in low-birth-weight infants, and typically improves after several minutes or with repositioning, muscle activity, or crying. The harlequin sign is most likely caused by an immature autonomic regulatory system. It is transient and benign.

Congenital Dermal Melanocytosis

Congenital dermal melanocytosis is the most common pigmented lesion in newborns, frequently observed in Black, Latinx, Asian, and Native American infants. It is a benign finding and can present as one or more blue-gray, brown, or greenish patches with ill-defined borders over the lumbosacral area and can additionally be found on the back, shoulders, or extremities (Fig. 97.6). It is important to note them at birth and distinguish them from bruising by following them over time, as bruising would fade within days to weeks, while congenital dermal melanocytosis would persist. These patches usually fade somewhat by puberty but may persist through life.

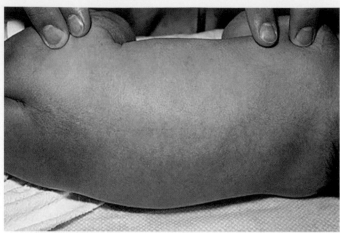

Fig. 97.5 Harlequin Sign. (From Lucky AW. In: Eichenfield LF, Frieden IJ, Mathes EF, Zaenglein AL, eds. *Neonatal and Infant Dermatology.* London: Saunders; 2015:65-76, Figure 7.30.)

SUMMARY

Neonates can experience a broad range of common and uncommon skin findings, a few of which are discussed in this chapter. Although some of the most common eruptions and lesions are benign and self-limited, some findings may require further workup and management. The provider must use a keen eye and perform a thorough physical examination to discern innocuous from worrisome.

SUGGESTED READINGS

Available online.

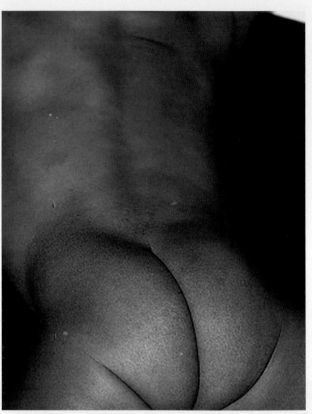

Fig. 97.6 Congenital Dermal Melanocytosis. (From Lucky AW. In: Eichenfield LF, Frieden IJ, Mathes EF, Zaenglein AL, eds. *Neonatal and Infant Dermatology.* London: Saunders; 2015:65-76, Figure 7.19.)

98

Disorders of the Nervous System

Laura M. McGarry and Katharine Press Callahan

 CLINICAL VIGNETTE

A male infant is born at 39 weeks gestation to a 29-year-old G2P1 birth parent. Prenatal laboratory test results were unremarkable, and pregnancy was uneventful. She presented in labor with vaginal bleeding and was diagnosed with placental abruption and underwent immediate cesarean delivery. At birth, the infant had no spontaneous respiratory effort and an initial heart rate of 100 beats/min. Positive pressure ventilation was initiated. Occasional spontaneous respiratory effort was noted by 90 seconds, and sustained respiratory effort at 3 minutes of life. Apgar scores were 1 at 1 minute of life, 3 at 5 minutes of life, and 5 at 10 minutes of life. The infant demonstrated inconsistent respiratory effort and was intubated and placed on mechanical ventilation. Cord blood gas showed significant acidosis with a pH of 6.8. Neurologic examination was concerning for encephalopathy with lethargy, extremities in extension, hypotonia, weak suck, absent Moro reflex, and pupils sluggishly reactive to light. Therapeutic hypothermia was initiated at 3 hours of life with video electroencephalography (EEG) and frequent laboratory monitoring. Video EEG revealed severe diffuse cerebral dysfunction with clinical and subclinical seizures. Seizure control was achieved with phenobarbital and fosphenytoin. Head ultrasound was performed on first day of life with no evidence of hemorrhage. The infant was extubated on the second day of life and gradually rewarmed after 72 hours of cooling. Neurologic examination findings improved, with increased spontaneous movements, extremities in mild distal flexion with improved tone, and present suck and Moro reflexes. MRI of the brain at 1 week of life showed T1 hyperintensities with diffusion restriction in the basal ganglia and thalamus consistent with hypoxic-ischemic injury. The infant was discharged home at 2 weeks of life with referral to early intervention and neurology specialist follow-up.

Hypoxic-ischemic encephalopathy in term infants requires rapid recognition by the pediatrics team in the delivery room or immediately after birth. The initial assessment of HIE includes delivery history, physical examination, Apgar scores, and cord blood gases. Infants with suspected HIE should undergo therapeutic hypothermia within 6 hours of delivery. Failure to identify the risk factors and sequalae of HIE could place neonates at risk for increased morbidity and mortality.

The neonatal period is an important time for development of the nervous system. Interruption of normal development through disease or injury often leads to permanent neurologic sequelae. As our ability to care for critically ill neonates improves, neurologic disorders continue to be a significant cause of morbidity and mortality. It is crucial to identify neonates at risk for neurologic disorders through careful history taking and physical examination so that problems can be prevented or treated early.

ETIOLOGY AND PATHOGENESIS

Hypoxic-Ischemic Encephalopathy

With dramatic advances in neonatal critical care, hypoxic-ischemic encephalopathy (HIE) has emerged as a primary cause of neurologic morbidity in the newborn period. It can occur in both premature and term neonates. HIE is a consequence of poor oxygen delivery to the brain, with hypoxia and ischemia leading to anaerobic metabolism, energy failure, and oxidative stress. Much of the injury actually occurs during subsequent reperfusion of the ischemic brain, which exacerbates oxidative stress and excitotoxic injury. Although white matter is more vulnerable in preterm neonates, both term and preterm infants can have white matter and gray matter injury. HIE can result from both maternal and fetal events that disrupt blood flow to the fetal brain, including chorioamnionitis, placental abruption, tight nuchal cord, cord prolapse, preeclampsia, fetal arrhythmia, and postnatal cardiac or respiratory arrest. Many identified antecedent events occur immediately before or after birth; it is unclear if earlier prenatal insults can increase the risk for HIE. Infants with HIE are also vulnerable to seizures, and preterm infants are at increased risk for intraventricular hemorrhage (IVH).

Intraventricular Hemorrhage

The premature cerebrovasculature has little ability to autoregulate outside the norms of blood pressure. This predisposes the brain to ischemic injury and hemorrhage. The periventricular germinal matrix of the premature brain is at especially high risk for hemorrhagic injury because of a rich but relatively immature capillary network. This region is critical because it harbors the neural stem and progenitor cell population that provides precursors necessary for future myelination and brain development. The germinal matrix involutes between 26 and 32 weeks' gestation, which reduces susceptibility to IVH (Fig. 98.1).

Neonatal Seizures

Neonatal seizures are often a manifestation of underlying neurologic disease or injury (Table 98.1). Metabolic or structural abnormalities cause disorganized electrical activity that can lead to epileptogenic foci.

Neonatal Brachial Plexus Injury

The brachial plexus sits in the infant's shoulder, and injury occurs during the birthing process. The brachial plexus comprises the nerve roots of C5 to T1, sensory and motor nerves that innervate the upper extremity. The most common injury is neurapraxia, stretch without tearing of the nerve, but tearing and rupture are also possible. Avulsion, tearing of nerve from the spinal cord, occurs in about 10% of cases. A palsy also can be due to compression by a neuroma where the injured nerve scars during the healing process.

Known risk factors include birthweight greater than 3500 g, infants of diabetic mothers, shoulder dystocia, and forceps vaginal delivery. Cesarean-delivery single births carry the lowest risk. However, approximately half of all infants with brachial plexus injury have no known risk factor.

CLINICAL PRESENTATION

Hypoxic-Ischemic Encephalopathy

HIE is diagnosed by clinical signs of neonatal encephalopathy, laboratory evidence of oxygen deprivation, and history of a peripartum or intrapartum event causing disruption of oxygen delivery to the infant. Encephalopathy in the neonate can manifest with changes in tone, reflexes, and consciousness, as well as seizures and irregular breathing or apnea. Depending on the severity of the brain injury, the presentation may range from lethargy with depressed tone and spinal cord reflexes to coma with loss of central reflexes. Although HIE is a common cause of neonatal encephalopathy, there are more rare causes that should be considered when there is not a clear antecedent event or the course is progressive or associated with other systemic problems. Other causes include inborn errors of metabolism, genetic disorders, and toxin exposure.

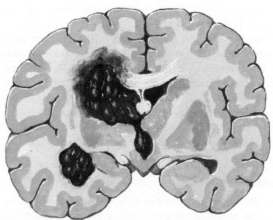

Unilateral periventricular-intraventricular hemorrhage.
Originating in germinal center over head of caudate nucleus, distending frontal and temporal horns of lateral ventricle, and
passing through interventricular foramen (of Monro) into 3rd ventricle

Fig. 98.1 Intraventricular Hemorrhage in a Newborn.

Intraventricular Hemorrhage

In a premature baby the majority of IVH occurs in the first 72 hours. IVH may be clinically silent or characterized by subtle signs such as apnea or decreased activity. A catastrophic bleed may manifest as a dramatic change in mental status along with cardiovascular collapse. Hydrocephalus is a common sequela of IVH and manifests clinically as increasing head circumference with neurologic signs such as apnea. Consultation with a neurosurgery specialist and shunt placement is needed for progressive hydrocephalus after IVH.

Neonatal Seizures

The newborn brain remains immature, particularly with regard to myelination. This immature anatomic organization makes neonatal seizures difficult to recognize, classify, and treat. Healthy newborns often exhibit unusual movements confounding the diagnosis of seizures. With these difficulties, neonatal seizures experience a paradoxical combination of overevaluation and underdiagnosis. Neonatal seizures have a variety of manifestations and a variety of normal mimickers. Phenotypically seizures can be clonic, tonic, or generalized.

Clonic seizures can be focal or multifocal and are repetitive high-amplitude, low-frequency jerking movements. Tonic seizures are constant stiffening of a portion of the body, and may be focal or generalized. Myoclonic seizures include sudden extension or flexion of part of the body. Subtle seizures encompass small abnormal movements that do not fit into the previously listed seizure types, including eye deviation, lip smacking, and tongue thrusting, among others. Subtle seizures and generalized tonic seizures often do not have electroencephalographic (EEG) correlates and are thought to emanate from deeper subcortical brain regions. Generalized tonic-clonic seizures are not possible in neonates because of immature myelination.

Several other unusual newborn movements are in the differential diagnosis of seizures. These may occur in normal infants or may suggest other underlying disease. Jitteriness is a hypersensitivity to stimulus and may suggest underlying abnormalities—for example, drug withdrawal, hypoxic-ischemic injury, and metabolic diseases such as hypoglycemia. Benign myoclonus is a sudden, brief, jerking movement of the extremities occurring during sleep in many normal infants. Opisthotonus, a tonic stiffening of the body often resulting in arching of the back, may be associated with gastroesophageal reflux. Apnea may sometimes accompany seizures, but it is frequently an independent clinical event in premature infants.

TABLE 98.1	Common Causes of Neonatal Seizures			
Vascular Injuries	**Structural Malformations**	**Infections**	**Metabolic Disorders**	**Genetic Epilepsy Syndromes**
Hypoxic-ischemic encephalopathy	Neuronal migration defects	Meningitis	Transient	Benign familial neonatal convulsions
Intraventricular hemorrhage	Neurocutaneous syndromes	Encephalitis	• Hyponatremia	Idiopathic benign neonatal seizures
Perinatal arterial stroke	Tumors		• Hypoglycemia	
Sinus venous thrombosis	Vein of Galen malformations		• Hypocalcemia	Early myoclonic encephalopathy
Subdural hemorrhage			• Hypomagnesemia	Ohtahara syndrome
Subarachnoid hemorrhage			Persistent	
			• Inborn errors of metabolism	
			• GLUT-1 deficiency	
			• Pyridoxine-dependent epilepsy	

GLUT-1, Glucose transporter protein type 1.

Neonatal Brachial Plexus Injury

Brachial plexus injuries manifest on a spectrum from weakness to complete paralysis of the upper extremity from birth. Examination findings depend on which nerves are affected. The Narakas classification system is commonly used to describe the relation between examination findings and affected nerve roots (Table 98.2). As peripheral nerve injuries, all findings are ipsilateral to the side of the injury.

Erb-Duchenne palsy is injury to the upper brachial plexus (C5 and C6 roots) and is the most common (Fig. 98.2). In a total palsy there is avulsion of the nerve roots from the spinal cord. In Horner syndrome the sympathetic chain is also injured and the infant will have ptosis, miosis, and anhidrosis ipsilaterally. Klumpke palsy, which refers to injury of lower brachial plexus (C8 and T1 roots), is a very rare birth injury in isolation; if these roots are affected, it is likely a full plexus injury. Klumpke palsy may occur when the hand or arm is the initial presenting fetal part. In this palsy there will be weakness of arm and hand. The infant's arm is supinated with elbow flexed and wrist extended.

EVALUATION AND MANAGEMENT

History and Physical Examination

Many neurologic disorders share a common set of symptoms in the neonatal period, and the tools for evaluating these infants are similar. A thorough history and physical examination should be performed initially. The history must encompass the pregnancy, including gestational age and the results of any prenatal testing. Details of any previous pregnancies are helpful. Frequent pregnancy losses could suggest the presence of an underlying genetic abnormality or a hypercoagulable disorder that may cause placental insufficiency. Method of delivery and birth complications may raise concern for birth injury.

The neonatal neurologic examination is difficult to master, but it is of value for both localization of pathology and prognosis. The clinician should measure the head circumference and examine the fontanelles, sutures, and general shape of the head. Molding of the skull, overlapping sutures, and extracranial hemorrhages, including caput succedaneum and cephalohematomas, do not portend underlying brain anomalies. A tense fontanelle and widely patent sutures are suggestive of hydrocephalus or infection. Testing of cranial nerves should focus on pupillary responses, extraocular movements, sucking, and swallowing. The motor examination includes assessment of overall tone and spontaneous movements and primitive reflexes. Hypotonic infants often appear in a frog-leg posture with hips abducted and knees flexed when lying supine and show fewer spontaneous movements (Fig. 98.3). Useful physical examination maneuvers to test for hypotonia are traction and prone suspension (Fig. 98.4). The next step

TABLE 98.2 Classification of Neonatal Brachial Plexus Injuries

Narakas Group	Affected nerve roots	Presentation
Group 1 (Erb-Duchenne palsy)	C5, C6	Weakness of deltoid and bicep. Intact wrist and hand strength. Adduction and internal rotation of shoulder with extended and pronated elbow.
Group 2 (intermediate palsy)	C5, C6, C7	Weakness of deltoid, bicep, wrist extension and finger extension. Intact wrist and finger flexion.
Group 3 (total brachial plexus palsy)	C5–T1, sympathetic chain	Weakness throughout upper extremity
Group 4 (total brachial plexus palsy, Horner syndrome)	C5–T1, sympathetic chain	Weakness throughout upper extremity with ptosis, miosis, and anhidrosis.

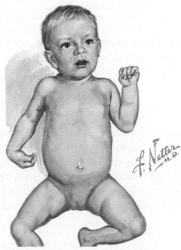

Infant with Erb palsy on right side. Muscles of shoulder and upper arm chiefly affected. Elbow extended and wrist flexed, but grasp normal

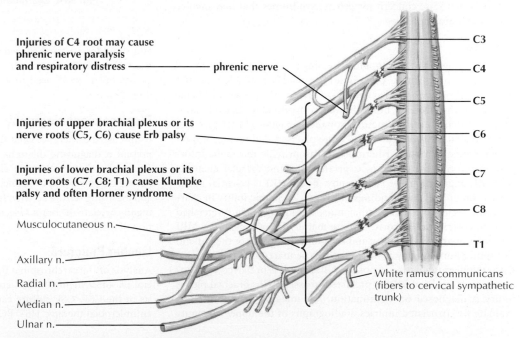

Injuries of C4 root may cause phrenic nerve paralysis and respiratory distress — phrenic nerve

Injuries of upper brachial plexus or its nerve roots (C5, C6) cause Erb palsy

Injuries of lower brachial plexus or its nerve roots (C7, C8; T1) cause Klumpke palsy and often Horner syndrome

Musculocutaneous n.

Axillary n.

Radial n.

Median n.

Ulnar n.

C3
C4
C5
C6
C7
C8
T1

White ramus communicans (fibers to cervical sympathetic trunk)

Fig. 98.2 Brachial Plexus and Clinical Presentation of Erb Palsy.

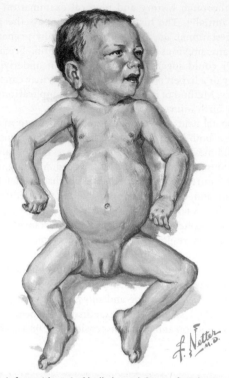

Infant with typical bell-shaped thorax, frog-leg
posture, and "jug-handle" position of upper limbs

Fig. 98.3 Clinical Presentation of Neonatal Hypotonia.

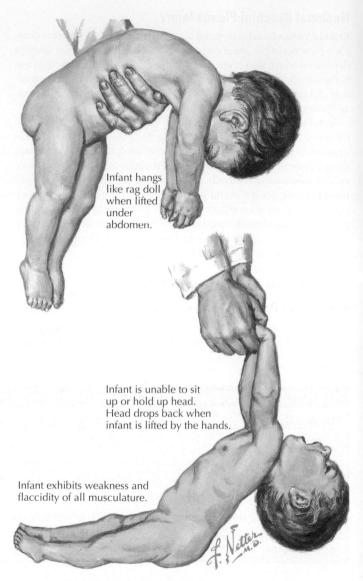

Infant hangs
like rag doll
when lifted
under
abdomen.

Infant is unable to sit
up or hold up head.
Head drops back when
infant is lifted by the hands.

Infant exhibits weakness and
flaccidity of all musculature.

Fig. 98.4 Examination Findings of Hypotonia.

in the motor examination is to assess the primitive reflexes, including Moro, grasp, and asymmetric tonic neck (fencing) reflex. An asymmetric Moro reflex can alert the examiner to more subtle weakness of the upper extremity. Primitive reflexes should be present by 28 weeks' gestation but become stronger as the infant nears term. The sensory examination should describe the type of stimulus and characterize the response. For example, whereas flexion of an extremity to a painful stimulus may be a reflex response, crying and specific withdrawal to such stimuli indicate intact cortical processing of pain. Dysmorphic features often raise concern for genetic syndromes that may involve structural brain anomalies.

Imaging

Neuroimaging is a crucial tool for assessing neonatal brain injuries or structural abnormalities. Ultrasound is a readily available tool, and imaging can be performed at bedside to identify the presence of hemorrhage in the neonatal brain; however, it provides relatively poor anatomic definition. Magnetic resonance imaging (MRI) provides excellent anatomic resolution and more precisely defines the location of pathologic lesions. Furthermore, it can provide metabolic information through the use of MR spectroscopy and vascular anatomy with MR angiography or venography. Brain MRI is essential in the evaluation of HIE, with findings of hypoxic-ischemic injury in characteristic regions such as the thalamus, basal ganglia, and watershed areas of cortex and subcortical white matter. The ability to use MRI can be limited by availability and the clinical stability of the patient. Computed tomography is rarely used in neonates as it is associated with significant radiation exposure. Ultrasound is preferred to evaluate hemorrhage, and MRI is preferred to assess HIE. Brachial plexus injury is diagnosed on examination, but imaging may be used to evaluate for associated injuries. Radiographs of the upper extremity

and shoulder are used to evaluate for fractures. Ultrasound may be used when there is concern for joint subluxation. MRI is rarely necessary, but may be used to evaluate for avulsion of nerve roots in severe injury.

Electroencephalography

As discussed earlier, neonatal seizures are difficult to identify and thus present a diagnostic dilemma for clinicians. EEG, which measures electrical activity with scalp electrodes, is critical for distinguishing between seizures and nonepileptic movements, as well as quantifying and localizing seizure activity. It can be combined with video monitoring to correlate the brain's electrical activity with the clinical presentation of the patient.

Lumbar Puncture

Analysis of the cerebrospinal fluid (CSF) is an important test for several reasons. Meningitis and encephalitis are indicated by a pleocytosis in the CSF. CSF culture can help identify a pathogen and direct antimicrobial therapy. HSV PCR should always be sent as part of the infectious work-up. Blood in the CSF that does not clear can demonstrate the presence of a subarachnoid hemorrhage.

Additional Testing

Additional more rarely used studies include genetic tests, nerve conduction tests, and tissue biopsies. Genetic and metabolic studies can help identify inherited disorders. The proliferation of chromosomal microarray and whole exome sequencing has been helpful in this regard, although if specific disorders are suspected, targeted gene studies are helpful. Typical metabolic screening tests include plasma amino acids, lactate, pyruvate, ammonia, and urine organic acids. CSF also can be analyzed with these studies. Nerve conduction studies and electromyography can be performed to help localize the source of hypotonia. Finally, nerve and muscle biopsies can be helpful to identify particular myopathies and metabolic disorders.

DISEASE SPECIFIC MANAGEMENT

Hypoxic-Ischemic Encephalopathy

Early identification of neonates at risk for HIE is important to optimize management. Hypothermia is a neuroprotective treatment that should be offered to all infants at greater than 36 weeks' gestation with evidence of moderate to severe HIE. Criteria for cooling vary across institutions, but typically include cord or blood gas acidosis, 10-minute Apgar score less than 5, and evidence of moderate to severe encephalopathy. Cooling must be initiated within 6 hours of delivery. Other management issues focus on supportive care. Seizure management may provide protection against further injury by reducing metabolic demand and excitotoxic injury. Careful management of fluids and blood pressure are important because volume overload and hypertension can exacerbate cerebral edema. MRI performed around a week after warming can help prognostication. Long-term outcomes range from mild cognitive effects and developmental delays to profound cognitive disability and cerebral palsy. Some infants may develop epilepsy or cortical blindness. Early initiation of physical therapy, occupational therapy, and speech therapy is essential to optimize future neurodevelopment.

Intraventricular Hemorrhage

Little can be done to change prognosis after significant IVH has occurred, so prevention is key. Antenatal management associated with reduced risk for IVH in premature neonates includes maternal corticosteroids and avoiding infant transport by transporting the mother before delivery. At delivery, delayed cord clamping and careful management of temperature, blood pressure, and ventilation in the neonate decrease the risk for IVH.

If a baby develops IVH, acute management is focused on supporting the baby through any physiologic instability. Because IVH is often clinically silent, screening ultrasound should be performed in neonates with gestational age younger than 32 weeks within the first 3 to 7 days after birth. If IVH is present, ultrasound is repeated at 2 weeks to grade the extent of hemorrhage (Table 98.3). Infants with IVH must be monitored closely for the development of hydrocephalus over the ensuing weeks by serial head circumference measurements and intermittent cranial ultrasound. Severe cases of hydrocephalus may necessitate placement of a ventricular shunt to divert the flow of CSF. Infants with grade III and IV IVH are at significant risk for neurodevelopmental impairment. As with HIE, physical therapy, occupational therapy, and speech therapy are important long-term treatments.

TABLE 98.3	Classification of Intraventricular Hemorrhage	
Grade	**Area of Hemorrhage**
I	Germinal matrix only
II	Involvement beyond germinal matrix without ventricular dilation
III	With ventricular dilation
IV	Periventricular infarct

Neonatal Seizures

Although there has been robust growth in the number of antiepileptic agents available to pediatric patients, the treatment of neonatal seizures has been comparatively slow to evolve. The difficulty of accurately identifying neonatal seizures and the risk associated with many antiepileptic medications fueled past controversy regarding how aggressive clinicians should be in treating neonatal seizures. Accumulating evidence suggests, however, that repeated seizures in the neonatal period are independently associated with poor neurologic outcomes, so early therapy is warranted.

Treatment of neonatal seizures should always focus on correction of the underlying cause if possible. Transient metabolic disturbances should be addressed. In the absence of such abnormalities, phenobarbital continues to be the mainstay of treatment for neonatal seizures. Second-line agents include phenytoin or its preferred precursor fosphenytoin and benzodiazepines. The most significant risks associated with these drugs are sedation, respiratory depression, and hypotension, and neonates should be monitored closely during initiation of these therapies. Clearance of these drugs from the neonatal system is notoriously variable, and infants must be closely monitored for signs of toxicity with clinical observation and drug levels. Although there are concerns about the impact of these antiepileptic drugs on development of the neonatal brain, newer antiepileptics such as levetiracetam with fewer adverse effects in older children have not been as effective in controlling neonatal seizures in neonates. It is also important to consider some of the rarer causes of refractory seizures in neonates, particularly if there are no identifiable risk factors. Some of these disorders respond to alternative therapies such as pyridoxine or the ketogenic diet, although in-depth discussion of these topics is beyond the scope of this text.

Neonatal Brachial Plexus Injury

Physical and occupational therapy is the first-line treatment for brachial plexus injury. Approximately 10% to 20% of children with brachial plexus injury will have some degree of permanent neurologic functional impairment. In neurapraxic injuries, infants usually recover spontaneously or with occupational and physical therapy. If the nerve is ruptured or there is a neuroma, infants may require surgery to repair or release the nerve. For children with palsies not resolved by therapy, referral should be made to a pediatric neurologist or neurosurgeon by 3 months of age.

FUTURE DIRECTIONS

Basic science has provided extraordinary information regarding the nervous system in recent decades, and clinicians have seen tremendous benefit in terms of diagnostic potential. Much of this information has yet to be translated into therapeutic interventions. Neuroprotection is an active area of research, with current studies investigating the optimal timing and duration of hypothermia, as well as expanding to earlier gestational ages or using adjunctive therapies such as sedation and erythropoietin. Regenerative medicine is a rapidly developing area as well, and research on neural stem cell physiology will hopefully yield therapies targeted to improve development in neonates after neurologic injury. Genetic medicine holds promise for inherited disorders.

SUGGESTED READINGS

Available online.

99

Neonatal Infections

David M. Rub and Dustin D. Flannery

CLINICAL VIGNETTE

A 1-day-old neonate born at 38 weeks' gestation after an unremarkable pregnancy exhibits poor feeding. On examination, the neonate is afebrile, tachypneic, and lethargic. Delivery was complicated by prolonged rupture of membranes 18 hours before delivery and maternal fever to 102°F (38.9°C) just before delivery. The mother received broad-spectrum antibiotics. The neonate is transferred to the intensive care nursery, undergoes evaluation for sepsis, and receives empiric antibiotic therapy. The following morning, the laboratory reports the blood culture is growing group B streptococci.

The differential for a full-term neonate with tachypnea is broad. Given the neonate's lethargy, poor feeding, and maternal risk factors of prolonged rupture of membranes and fever, sepsis leads the differential diagnosis list. Appropriate next steps are to transfer the neonate to the intensive care nursery, draw blood cultures, and start empiric antibiotics. For the patient in the vignette, once the blood culture becomes positive, additional blood cultures should be drawn and a lumbar puncture should be performed to evaluate for meningitis. Antibiotic therapy should be narrowed to penicillin for group B streptococci.

Neonates are at increased risk for bacterial, viral, and fungal infections because of immature immune systems and perinatal exposures. These infections may occur in the prenatal or postnatal period. Given the associated risk for significant morbidity and mortality, early diagnosis and treatment are critical. This chapter will review a wide range of neonatal infections, with a focus on newborns in the hospital setting.

NEONATAL SEPSIS

Clinical Presentation

Neonatal sepsis is defined as blood or cerebrospinal fluid (CSF) culture growing a pathogenic bacterial or fungal species. Viruses are not consider to be classical forms of neonatal sepsis and will be discussed later under TORCH infections. This sepsis definition is in contrast to pediatric and adult sepsis, which are typically defined by a set of clinical criteria. Neonatal sepsis is further classified into early- and late-onset based on age of the neonate at diagnosis. The pathophysiology, microbiology, and management of early- and late-onset neonatal sepsis differ and are discussed separately.

Evaluation and Management
Early-Onset Neonatal Sepsis
Early-onset sepsis (EOS) is defined as blood or CSF culture–confirmed infection within the first 7 days after birth for a term neonate, or the first 72 hours after birth for a continuously hospitalized neonate. EOS has a reported incidence of 0.5 per 1000 live births for term neonates, 3 per 1000 for preterm neonates (<37 weeks' gestational age), and 11 per 1000 for neonates with very low birth weight (VLBW; <1500 g). The

estimated mortality for EOS is 11% to 16%, with the majority of deaths occurring in preterm infants.

EOS is most commonly caused by colonization of the infant from the translocation of maternal genitourinary and gastrointestinal bacteria after rupture of amniotic membranes, or during delivery by the vaginal canal. The most common organisms include group B streptococci (GBS) and *Escherichia coli*. Less common organisms include other gram-positive and gram-negative bacteria and fungi. Of note, *Listeria monocytogenes*, although an uncommon cause of EOS, is usually transmitted by the transplacental hematogenous route.

The clinical presentation of EOS is variable and may be subtle and nonspecific. Possible signs include respiratory distress, temperature instability, apnea, bradycardia, hypoglycemia, poor feeding, and lethargy, among others. Given the wide range of nonspecific signs, a low threshold should be used to evaluate for sepsis.

Evaluation of all neonates begins with a thorough maternal, pregnancy, and delivery history. Maternal risk factors to assess include indication for and mode of delivery, duration of rupture of membranes, GBS colonization, temperature during labor, intrapartum antibiotic treatment, and siblings with prior GBS infection. Notably for GBS, pregnant women are screened for vaginal-rectal colonization at 36 0/7 to 37 6/7 weeks' gestation. Intrapartum antibiotic prophylaxis is indicated for colonized women. Risk assessment strategies based on maternal and delivery characteristics are useful in identifying neonates at higher risk for infection.

Symptomatic and asymptomatic neonates at high risk for infection should undergo a sepsis evaluation. This includes blood cultures and initiation of empiric antibiotics for at least 24 to 48 hours. The sensitivity and specificity of inflammatory markers, such as white blood cell count and C-reactive protein, are poor. The empiric antibiotic regimen includes ampicillin and gentamicin, which cover the most common pathogens. Additional broad-spectrum antimicrobials should be considered for critically ill newborns until culture results are known. Lumbar puncture should be considered.

Neonates with culture-confirmed bacteremia should be treated for 7 to 10 days. Antibiotic course is extended for meningitis. Antibiotic coverage should be narrowed after bacterial speciation and antibiotic susceptibilities.

Late-Onset Sepsis

Late-onset sepsis (LOS) refers to culture-confirmed blood, urine, or CSF infection affecting hospitalized neonates more than 72 hours after birth. LOS often affects premature neonates with prolonged hospital stays and intravascular catheters. The primary clinical findings of LOS are similar to those of EOS, but LOS is usually acquired from the surrounding hospital environment. The most common bacterial pathogens include coagulase-negative staphylococci, *Staphylococcus aureus*, and *E. coli*. Other gram-positive and gram-negative bacteria, as well as *Candida* fungal species, may be implicated.

Neonates with concern for LOS should have cultures sent from blood, urine, and CSF. Empiric antibiotic therapy should be started and cover a broad range of both gram-positive and gram-negative organisms based on the center's typical pathogen profile and antibiogram. Antifungal therapy should be considered for at-risk neonates, particularly those who are preterm with intravascular catheters. Duration of antibiotic therapy depends on the results of CSF cultures. The empiric antibiotic regimen should be narrowed accordingly following after bacterial speciation and antibiotic susceptibilities.

TORCH INFECTIONS

Clinical Presentation

TORCH infections refer to a group of congenital infections acquired during gestation or at the time of delivery, and include *toxoplasmosis*, "*other*" infections, *rubella*, *cytomegalovirus* (CMV), and *herpes* simplex virus (HSV). The "other" category has expanded since the initial description of TORCH infections in the 1950s. In this section, varicella-zoster virus (VZV), human immunodeficiency virus (HIV), syphilis, hepatitis B, and Zika virus will be discussed.

TORCH infections have many overlapping signs and symptoms. Therefore keeping a broad differential is important when evaluating a neonate for vertically transmitted infectious disease.

Evaluation and Management
Toxoplasmosis

Toxoplasmosis is caused by the parasite *Toxoplasma gondii*. Cats are the primary host, and maternal infection is typically a result of oocyte

ingestion by contaminated food or water (Fig. 99.1). Congenital toxoplasmosis is most commonly a result of transplacental transmission after a primary infection during pregnancy.

The classic triad associated with congenital toxoplasmosis consists of chorioretinitis, scattered cerebral calcifications, and hydrocephalus. This triad is present in less than 10% of affected neonates. The majority of neonates are asymptomatic at birth or have nonspecific findings of rash, lymphadenopathy, or hepatosplenomegaly. If untreated, congenitally infected neonates may present in the second or third decade of life with visual, auditory, or learning impairments.

In neonates with suspected toxoplasmosis, both serologic testing (immunoglobulin A [IgA], IgG, IgM) and DNA polymerase chain reaction (PCR) testing should be performed. IgM testing is known to be particularly susceptible to false positive results; therefore close discussion with an infectious disease specialist is needed when interpreting test results. Infected neonates require ophthalmologic, auditory, and neurology screening. This may include lumbar puncture, brain imaging, and audiology testing.

Antimicrobial treatment of neonates with toxoplasmosis includes pyrimethamine, sulfadiazine, and folic acid. Symptomatic neonates require 12 months of treatment, and asymptomatic neonates require 3 months of treatment.

Varicella-Zoster Virus

VZV may be transmitted during gestation or delivery or postpartum. Phenotype depends on the mode of transmission.

Primary maternal infection in the first 20 weeks of pregnancy results in transplacental transmission in approximately 2% of cases,

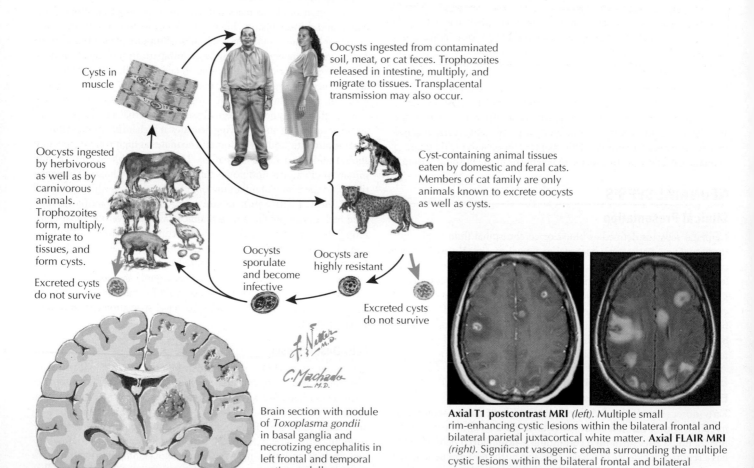

Oocysts ingested from contaminated soil, meat, or cat feces. Trophozoites released in intestine, multiply, and migrate to tissues. Transplacental transmission may also occur.

Cysts in muscle

Oocysts ingested by herbivorous as well as by carnivorous animals. Trophozoites form, multiply, migrate to tissues, and form cysts.

Excreted cysts do not survive

Cyst-containing animal tissues eaten by domestic and feral cats. Members of cat family are only animals known to excrete oocysts as well as cysts.

Oocysts sporulate and become infective

Oocysts are highly resistant

Excreted cysts do not survive

Brain section with nodule of *Toxoplasma gondii* in basal ganglia and necrotizing encephalitis in left frontal and temporal corticomedullary zones

Axial T1 postcontrast MRI (*left*). Multiple small rim-enhancing cystic lesions within the bilateral frontal and bilateral parietal juxtacortical white matter. **Axial FLAIR MRI** (*right*). Significant vasogenic edema surrounding the multiple cystic lesions within the bilateral frontal and bilateral parietal juxtacortical white matter.

Fig. 99.1 Life Cycle of Toxoplasmosis and Brain Manifestations.

causing fetal death or a constellation of symptoms known as congenital varicella syndrome: scarring skin lesions, ocular defects, limb abnormalities, and central nervous system (CNS) defects. Treatment is supportive.

More commonly, transmission occurs during the peripartum period as a result of exposure to maternal VZV lesions, leading to a clinical syndrome called neonatal varicella. Clinical features vary, ranging from mild, chickenpox-like illness to severe disseminated disease; mortality approaches 30%. The primary risk factor for severe infection is lack of placental transfer of maternal IgG antibodies. Therefore primary maternal infection from 5 days before to 2 days after delivery and prematurity (most IgG antibody transfer occurs in the third trimester) are significant risk factors for morbidity and mortality.

Postexposure prophylaxis with varicella immunoglobulin is indicated for infants born to mothers who are symptomatic at delivery and for preterm infants with significant VZV exposure. Additionally, neonates born to mothers with active VZV lesions should be isolated until the mother is noninfectious.

HIV

Mother-to-child transmission (MTCT) of HIV may occur in utero, during labor and vaginal delivery, or postpartum while breastfeeding. Risk for MTCT correlates directly to maternal viral load. Before the availability of antiretroviral treatment (ART), transmission was as high as 25% in the United States. In recent years, with pregnancy screening, ART for infected women, cesarean delivery, and neonatal prophylaxis, MTCT has decreased to less than 1%.

Clinical manifestations of perinatally acquired, untreated HIV may include fever, lymphadenopathy, hepatosplenomegaly, failure to thrive, recurrent bacterial or fungal infections, HIV encephalopathy, and other AIDS-defining illnesses.

Neonates with perinatal HIV exposure should undergo PCR testing PCR testing at 14 to 21 days, 1 to 2 months, and 4 to 6 months. A neonate is considered infected if two samples from two separate timepoints are positive. Antibody testing should be avoided until 24 months of age because of placental maternal antibody transfer.

The treatment regimen for neonates with perinatal HIV exposure depends on transmission risk, defined as "low" or "higher" risk, and is determined by antepartum ART and sustained maternal viral suppression near delivery. Low-risk neonates are treated with zidovudine for 4 weeks. Higher-risk neonates should receive ART for 6 weeks. Neonates who test positive for HIV will require lifelong ART treatment.

Additionally, HIV may be transmitted by breastfeeding. Therefore in environments in which safe, human-milk alternatives exist, breastfeeding should be avoided by HIV-infected mothers. If families still choose to breastfeed, risk mitigation strategies should be followed to minimize transition. The risk of transmission via breast milk in a mother with an undetectable viral load in a monitored and treated infant is less than 1% and requires support and multidisciplinary care coordination.

Zika

Zika virus is primarily transmitted by the *Aedes aegypti* mosquito. Initially discovered in Uganda, Zika has spread to Asia and the Americas, with its most significant outbreak in 2015 to 2016, affecting Brazil, Puerto Rico, and parts of Florida and Texas.

Children and adults are generally asymptomatic. Congenital Zika virus infection may lead to serious developmental defects and fetal loss. A common finding is microcephaly (Fig. 99.2). Brain and ocular anomalies and congenital contractures are also reported.

Zika testing is recommended for neonates born to mothers with possible exposure to, or positive testing for, Zika virus during pregnancy. Testing is also recommended for all neonates with symptoms concerning for congenital Zika. Laboratory testing includes serum, urine, and

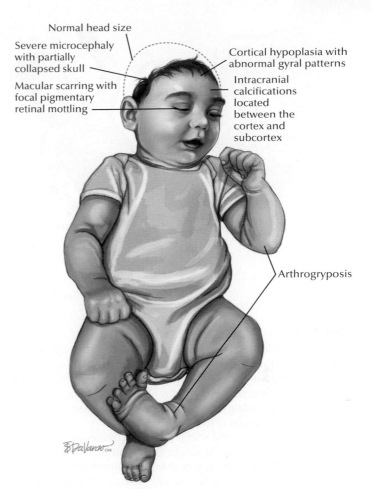

Normal head size

Severe microcephaly with partially collapsed skull

Macular scarring with focal pigmentary retinal mottling

Cortical hypoplasia with abnormal gyral patterns

Intracranial calcifications located between the cortex and subcortex

Arthrogryposis

Fig. 99.2 Clinical Features of Congenital Zika Virus.

CSF RNA, as well as serum and CSF IgM antibodies. Testing should occur as soon as possible after birth. Treatment is strictly supportive.

Syphilis

Congenital syphilis (Fig. 99.3) is caused by transplacental transmission of the spirochete *Treponema pallidum* at any time during pregnancy. Approximately 40% of intrauterine acquired syphilis results in stillbirth or hydrops fetalis, and 50% of survivors suffer significant morbidities. Early manifestations of disease, within the first 2 months of life, involve all organ systems and may include copious nasal secretions ("snuffles"), mucocutaneous lesions, rash involving palms and soles, pneumonia, hepatosplenomegaly, hemolytic anemia, and bone abnormalities such as osteochondritis or periostitis. If left untreated, at 2 years of age children may develop "late" manifestations of disease from chronic tissue inflammation. These include CNS, bone, teeth, skin, and eye abnormalities such as interstitial keratitis, eighth cranial nerve deafness and notched teeth, known as the Hutchinson triad.

T. pallidum diagnosis relies on either direct visualization of spirochetes from an active lesion or through indirect treponemal or nontreponemal testing. Pregnant women in the United States are routinely screened with nontreponemal testing (rapid plasma reagin [RPR]). If this screen is positive, diagnosis is confirmed with a treponemal test and appropriate treatment with penicillin should be administered. Neonates born to mothers with positive screens should receive a nontreponemal test, such as the RPR. If neonatal RPR titers are four times the maternal titers, or if maternal treatment is unknown or inadequate, the neonate should undergo full evaluation, including complete blood count, CSF studies, and long-bone radiographs. Treatment is a 10-day course of parenteral penicillin.

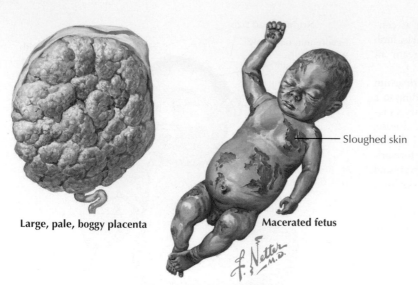

Large, pale, boggy placenta   Macerated fetus

— Sloughed skin

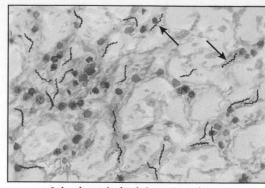

Spirochetes in fetal tissue (Levaditi stain)

Fig. 99.3 Transplacental Transmission of Syphilis.

Hepatitis B

Neonatal hepatitis B infection most commonly occurs through vertical transmission during delivery. There were 20 reported cases of neonatal hepatitis B infection in the United States in 2018. Perinatally acquired hepatitis B manifests around 2 months of age with a range of hepatic manifestations, including self-limited hepatitis, fulminant hepatitis, or cirrhosis and progression to liver failure.

Neonates born to mothers with positive or unknown hepatitis B surface antigen status should receive the hepatitis B vaccine within 12 hours after birth. If mom is positive, hepatitis B immunoglobulin (HBIG) should be administered with vaccine. If maternal status is unknown and the neonate is term, HBIG should be administered within the first 7 days after birth pending results of maternal testing. If the neonate weighs less than 2 kg, HBIG should be administered within the first 12 hours of life even if maternal testing is pending.

Rubella

Congenital rubella syndrome (CRS) results from the transplacental transmission of rubella virus during pregnancy. CRS is rare in the United States as a result of widespread vaccination. However, 80,000 neonates are born with CRS annually in countries without universal vaccination protocols.

Development of CRS after maternal rubella infection is largely dependent on the gestational age when infection occurred. Maternal infection in the first trimester poses the highest risk for vertical transmission (80% to 90%).

CRS is a severe and debilitating disease resulting in ocular defects (cataracts, chorioretinitis, microphthalmia), radiolucent bone disease, thrombocytopenia, growth restriction, dermal erythropoiesis or blueberry muffin rash (Fig. 99.4), congenital heart disease, and death.

Diagnosis of CRS may be made clinically and is commonly confirmed with rubella IgM antibody testing in the first 6 months of life. Serologic testing in the first year is critical, as serologic testing is difficult to interpret after vaccination. Treatment for CRS is supportive.

Cytomegalovirus

CMV is the most common congenital viral infection in the United States, affecting up to 40,000 neonates annually, and the most common cause of acquired sensorineural hearing loss. Maternal infection may occur through sexual contact, exposure from transplanted organs and blood transfusions, or contact with infected young children.

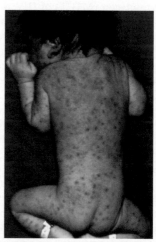

Fig. 99.4 Dermal Erythropoiesis or "Blueberry Muffin" Rash Seen in TORCH infections, most often congenital rubella and CMV. (From Jong E, Stevens D. *Netter's Infectious Diseases.* Philadelphia, PA: Saunders; 2010, Fig. 12.1.)

Congenital CMV infection after transplacental transmission may manifest with a variety of symptoms; however, 90% of neonates are asymptomatic at birth. Symptomatic neonates may have hepatosplenomegaly, direct hyperbilirubinemia, microcephaly, periventricular calcifications, hearing loss, chorioretinitis, and/or thrombocytopenia with petechiae/purpura.

Diagnosis of CMV requires viral DNA PCR identification from urine, respiratory secretions, stool, and/or CSF in the first 3 weeks after birth. In suspected cases, head imaging should be performed to screen for periventricular calcifications. Hearing screening may not identify associated sensorineural hearing loss until several months after birth; therefore repeated screens throughout infancy and childhood are recommended in suspected and confirmed cases.

Treatment of congenital CMV is reserved for symptomatic neonates and consists of 6 months of oral valganciclovir, which improves audiologic and neurodevelopmental outcomes at 2 years of age. Neutropenia is a common complication of valganciclovir therapy and absolute neutrophil counts should be monitored.

Herpes Simplex Virus

In the United States, the incidence of neonatal HSV infection is 1 in 2000 to 3000 live births. Unlike the other TORCH infections,

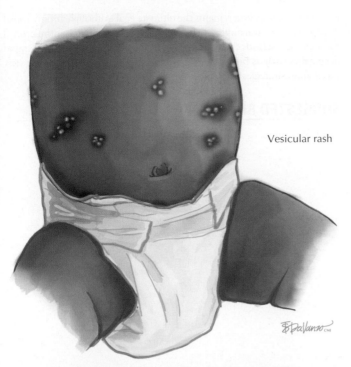

Vesicular rash

Fig. 99.5 Neonatal Herpes Simplex Virus Vesicles.

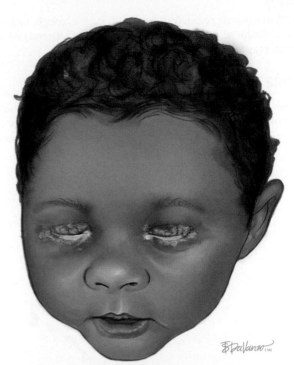

Fig. 99.6 Neonatal Gonococcal Conjunctivitis.

transmission of neonatal herpes usually occurs during the intrapartum period; however, prenatal transmission is still possible and leads to severe disease. Transmission is thought to be primarily caused by exposure to lesions associated with HSV-1 or HSV-2 during delivery. The highest risk for transmission occurs during primary active maternal infection, with transmission rates as high as 50%. Prior maternal infection with HSV reduces rate of transmission to less than 2% because of passage of maternal antibody during gestation.

Clinical manifestations are stratified based on organ involvement. The three categories are disseminated disease, localized CNS disease, and skin, eye, and/or mouth (SEM) disease. Approximately 25% of cases are disseminated, 30% localized CNS, and 45% SEM disease. Notably, up to 70% of SEM disease will progress to disseminated disease if left untreated.

SEM disease consists of localized grouped vesicles on an erythematous base affecting the skin, eyes, or mouth (Fig. 99.5). Associated CNS findings may include irritability, lethargy, bulging fontanelle, poor feeding, temperature instability, and seizures. Seizures in particular are associated with significant long-term morbidity. Finally, disseminated neonatal HSV tends to affect the lungs and liver, leading to liver failure with associated coagulopathies and hemorrhagic pneumonitis. Skin findings may or may not be present in both the localized CNS and disseminated forms of neonatal herpes.

Diagnosis of neonatal herpes is confirmed with HSV PCR testing. Samples should be collected from unroofed vesicles, if skin lesions are present, blood, and CSF. Head imaging with ultrasound, computed tomography, or magnetic resonance imaging (preferred) and ophthalmologic examination should be obtained.

Intravenous acyclovir is the treatment of choice. Duration of treatment is 14 days for SEM disease and 21 days for CNS or disseminated disease. Oral acyclovir should be continued for 6 months.

CONJUNCTIVITIS

Clinical Presentation

Neonatal conjunctivitis, or ophthalmia neonatorum, refers to conjunctival infection within the first 4 weeks after birth. Age at onset of

symptoms is the most important factor in determining the etiologic agent. The two organisms contrasted in this section are *Neisseria gonorrhoeae* and *Chlamydia trachomatis*.

Evaluation and Management
Gonorrhea

N. gonorrhoeae classically causes conjunctivitis that appears 2 to 5 days after birth. This infection is acquired from exposure to infectious vaginal secretions. Gonococcal conjunctivitis is profoundly mucopurulent (Fig. 99.6), and if left untreated can destroy local ocular structures leading to blindness and disseminated infection, most notably meningitis. All neonates, especially those born to women with gonorrhea infection, should receive topical erythromycin ophthalmic ointment as prophylaxis immediately after birth.

Evaluation of the neonate with suspected gonococcal conjunctivitis should include an ophthalmology consult, Gram stain and culture of purulent drainage, and evaluation for systemic disease. Neonates with gonococcal conjunctivitis should be treated with a parenteral third-generation cephalosporin. Treatment with a macrolide for presumed chlamydial coinfection should be considered as well.

Chlamydia

Chlamydial conjunctivitis typically presents between days 5 and 14. Similar to its gonococcal counterpart, chlamydial infection is also acquired from exposure to vaginal secretions during delivery. However, unlike *N. gonorrhoeae*, *C. trachomatis* colonizes the sinuses, therefore making topical prophylaxis or treatment ineffective. Additionally, chlamydial conjunctivitis tends to be less purulent and less dangerous to the ocular structures.

Evaluation is similar to gonococcal conjunctivitis and should include an ophthalmology consult and Gram stain and culture of the purulent drainage. Because of sinus colonization, treatment is with a systemic macrolide antibiotic.

Neonates with history of chlamydial conjunctivitis or born to women with chlamydia infection should be monitored for the development of chlamydia pneumonia. This manifests around 4 to 12 weeks of age with nonspecific respiratory symptoms such as cough, tachypnea, and nasal discharge. Typical chest x-ray findings of bilateral interstitial infiltrates may be seen.

FUTURE DIRECTIONS

Neonates are at risk for exposure to a wide range of pathogens in both the prenatal and postnatal periods. Rapid identification and treatment of infection is of paramount importance to prevent morbidity and mortality.

Prevention of infection remains the ultimate goal. Although antimicrobial therapy is often warranted, the development of neonatal antimicrobial resistance is a serious threat. Advances in infection risk assessment, rapid diagnostics such as biomarkers, and prevention measures including new vaccination strategies will contribute to this rapidly evolving field.

SUGGESTED READINGS

Available online.

Nephrology and Urology

Benjamin L. Laskin

100

Hematuria and Proteinuria

Mohammed A. Shaik and Madhura Pradhan

⁂ **CLINICAL VIGNETTE**

A 3-year-old boy with no medical history presents to the emergency department (ED) with acute onset of bloody diarrhea, nonbloody nonbilious emesis, and dehydration. He is afebrile, mildly tachycardic, tired-appearing, and fussy and has diffuse abdominal tenderness. He is given intravenous fluids and discharged home after being able to tolerate oral intake. His laboratory test results show a normal hemoglobin, normal platelet count, BUN of 6 mg/dL, and a serum creatinine of 0.2 mg/dL. His bloody diarrhea resolves 2 days later. One week later he again presents to the ED with decreased urine output, and repeat laboratory test values are notable for anemia to 7.1 g/dL, thrombocytopenia to 53,000, an increased BUN of 38 mg/dL, and a serum creatinine of 1.0 mg/dL. He is monitored closely as an inpatient and receives several red blood cell transfusions, and his urine output gradually increases over the next few days. At follow-up in clinic 1 week later his serum creatinine has improved to 0.5 mg/dL and his urinalysis shows continued hematuria and proteinuria. The patient developed hemolytic-uremic syndrome (HUS), which is typified by microangiopathic hemolytic anemia, thrombocytopenia, and acute kidney injury. Shiga toxin–producing *Escherichia coli* (STEC) is the most common cause of HUS; 6% to 9% of STEC infections are complicated by HUS, which typically develops 5 to 10 days after the onset of diarrhea. In addition to hematologic and kidney involvement, HUS can also affect the central nervous system, causing altered mental status and seizures. Treatment of STEC-HUS is mainly supportive and includes management of anemia with transfusions, close monitoring of fluid balance, and the use of dialysis if needed for significant fluid overload or electrolyte abnormalities. Most patients recover completely from the acute phase of HUS though microscopic hematuria may persist, and some patients develop chronic kidney disease with manifestations including hypertension and proteinuria.

HEMATURIA

Hematuria refers to the presence of blood in the urine. Gross hematuria manifests with visible discoloration of urine; brown, burgundy, cola, or tea colored urine suggests hematuria of glomerular origin, whereas bright red or pink urine suggests a lower urinary tract source. Red or brown urine can also result from hemoglobinuria without hematuria; myoglobinuria; urinary pigmentation from ingestion of various drugs, foods, and dyes; and the presence of urinary metabolites resulting from other clinical conditions (e.g., porphyria). A urinary dipstick test for blood provides a highly sensitive colorimetric indicator for the presence of hemoglobin (or myoglobin). A positive dipstick test for hematuria must be confirmed by microscopic analysis of 10 to 15 mL of freshly voided and centrifuged urine. Hematuria is defined as the presence of more than 5 red blood cells per high power field (RBC/HPF).

Etiology and Pathogenesis

Box 100.1 provides a comprehensive list of causes of hematuria, and Table 100.1 lists history, physical examination, and urinalysis features that distinguish glomerular and nonglomerular hematuria. Common causes of gross hematuria include urinary tract infections (UTIs),

trauma, and irritation of the perineal area or urethral meatus. Some causes are described in further detail later. Glomerulonephritis is reviewed in Chapter 102.

Trauma

Traumatic injury to the urogenital tract is frequently seen with blunt force trauma. The presence of hematuria with minimal traumatic injury is highly suggestive of anatomic abnormalities of the kidney such as polycystic kidney disease. Hematuria associated with kidney trauma requires evaluation by computed tomography, magnetic resonance imaging, or bedside renal ultrasound. Urologic evaluation should be obtained before placement of a urinary catheter in cases of lower urinary tract trauma. Most kidney contusions or lacerations can be managed conservatively. However, significant lacerations of the kidney or injury to the collecting system or lower urinary tract may require emergent surgical intervention.

Hypercalciuria and Urolithiasis

Hypercalciuria can occur with low, normal, or high serum calcium levels. In normocalcemic patients, the most common causes are idiopathic, immobilization, Cushing syndrome, distal renal tubular acidosis, and Bartter syndrome. Disorders associated with hypercalcemia include hyperparathyroidism, vitamin D intoxication, hypophosphatasia, and tumors. Rare familial abnormalities of renal calcium channels are the cause of hypercalciuria with hypocalcemia. Hypercalciuria is the most common cause of stone disease. Idiopathic hypercalciuria typically manifests with asymptomatic microscopic hematuria. Patients with stones can present in a variety of ways, including with dysuria, gross hematuria, and renal colic (Fig. 100.1). Renal ultrasound or CT should be considered. Radiographs can detect radiopaque stones but not those formed by uric acid. The initial screening test for hypercalciuria is a urine calcium-to-creatinine ratio on a random urine sample. A ratio of greater than 0.2 in older children and adults is highly suggestive of hypercalciuria, with higher normal values in infants and young children. Confirmation should be obtained by a 24-hour urine collection, with an excretion of more than 4 mg/kg in 24 hours indicating hypercalciuria. Urine from this collection should be tested for cystine, citrate, oxalate, phosphorus, and uric acid excretion. Serum chemistries, including calcium, phosphorus, magnesium, uric acid, creatinine, and bicarbonate should also be ordered. A detailed family history for stone disease, diet history, and evaluation of medications and nutritional supplements should be sought. Recovery of a stone should be attempted for analysis. Stones caused by infection are rare in children. Management of these patients is twofold. Pain management should be optimized. Surgical intervention or lithotripsy is indicated in cases of urinary obstruction or recurrent stones with superimposed UTI. After the cause has been determined, therapy to prevent stone recurrence, including increased fluid intake to ensure dilute hypotonic urine, dietary manipulation, and drug therapy in some cases, can be implemented.

BOX 100.1 Differential Diagnosis of Hematuria

Nonglomerular Conditions

- Urinary tract infections
  - Bacterial, viral, parasites, tuberculosis
- Structural abnormalities
  - Congenital anomalies
  - Polycystic kidneys
  - Trauma
  - Vascular anomalies: angiomyolipomas, arteriovenous malformations
  - Tumors
- Hematologic
  - Sickle cell trait or disease
  - Coagulopathies: von Willebrand disease, renal vein thrombosis
- Hypercalciuria and nephrolithiasis
- Exercise
- Medications
  - Penicillins, polymyxin, sulfa-containing agents, anticonvulsants, warfarin, aspirin, colchicine, cyclophosphamide, busulfan, indomethacin, gold salts
- Others
  - Loin pain: hematuria syndrome
  - Urethrorrhagia

Glomerular Conditions

- IgA nephropathy
- Alport syndrome
- Benign familial hematuria
- Acute postinfectious glomerulonephritis
- Lupus nephritis
- Membranoproliferative glomerulonephritis
- Henoch-Schönlein purpura
- Membranous nephropathy
- Focal segmental glomerulosclerosis
- Rapidly progressive glomerulonephritis

Hematologic Causes

Hematuria commonly occurs with sickle cell hemoglobinopathy due to sickling of red blood cells in the renal medulla. Typically painless, it can be precipitated by trauma, exercise, dehydration, or infection. Papillary necrosis is also seen with severe dehydration and renal infarction. Coagulopathies can be a cause of hematuria, although this is rare. Nevertheless, coagulopathies should be investigated in patients without another source for painless, gross hematuria and a history of bruising or bleeding, or a family history of a bleeding diathesis.

Malignancy

Wilms tumor is the most common childhood malignancy of the kidney and can manifest with microscopic or gross hematuria. Tumors of the bladder are also a cause of hematuria, although these are rare in children.

Medications

Microscopic hematuria can be caused by medications, including cyclophosphamide and busulfan. Other medications, including antibiotics, can cause the urine to appear red or orange-colored but do not cause overt hematuria.

Benign Familial Hematuria

This disorder is defined by usually autosomal dominant transmission of persistent hematuria without proteinuria, hearing loss, or progressive kidney disease. It is a diagnosis of exclusion based on family history. Hematuria detected in the parents' or siblings' urine can support the diagnosis. Biopsy shows thin basement membranes in most patients.

Clinical Presentation

A complete history is essential to the diagnostic evaluation of hematuria. The focus of questions should be on previous episodes of gross hematuria or UTI; the pattern of hematuria in relation to the urinary stream (initial, terminal); history of recent upper respiratory tract infections, sore throat, or impetigo; and dysuria, frequency, and voiding patterns. Additional questions include the presence of fever, weight loss, abdominal or flank pain, skin lesions, trauma or foreign

TABLE 100.1 Distinguishing Features of Glomerular and Nonglomerular Hematuria

Feature	Glomerular	Nonglomerular
History		
Burning on micturition	No	Urethritis, cystitis
Systemic complaints	Edema, fever, pharyngitis, rash, arthralgia	Fever with UTIs, pain with calculi
Family history	Deafness in Alport syndrome, end-stage kidney disease	Usually negative except with calculi
Physical Examination		
Hypertension	Often	Unlikely
Edema	Sometimes present	No
Abdominal mass	No	Wilms tumor, polycystic kidneys
Rash, arthritis	SLE, HSP	No
Urinalysis		
Color	Brown, tea, or cola colored	Bright red or pink
Clots	No	Yes
Proteinuria	Often	No
Dysmorphic RBCs	Yes	No
RBC casts	Yes	No
Crystals	No	May be informative

HSP, Henoch-Schönlein purpura; *RBC,* red blood cell; *SLE,* systemic lupus erythematosus; *UTI,* urinary tract infection.

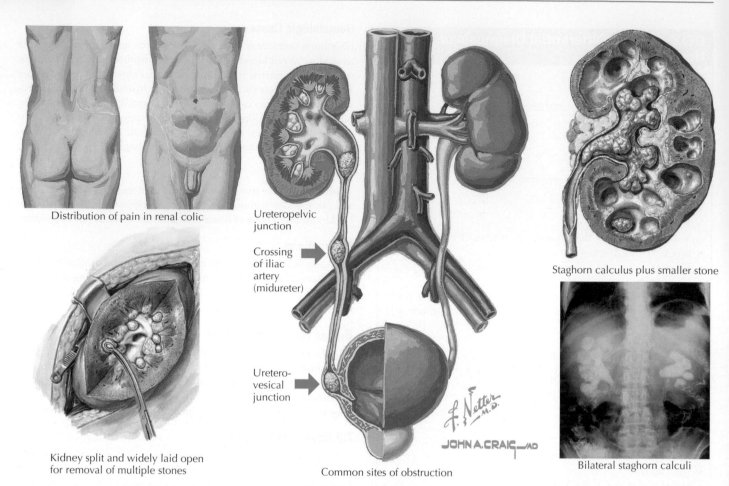

Distribution of pain in renal colic

Kidney split and widely laid open for removal of multiple stones

Ureteropelvic junction

Crossing of iliac artery (midureter)

Uretero-vesical junction

Common sites of obstruction

Staghorn calculus plus smaller stone

Bilateral staghorn calculi

Fig. 100.1 Kidney Stones.

body exposure, and drug, dietary, and vitamin or nutritional supplements. A family history of kidney disease including dialysis and transplant, hematuria, urolithiasis, sickle cell disease, coagulation disorders, or hearing loss may provide clues to the cause of hematuria. A history of international travel may uncover rare, infectious causes of hematuria. The physical examination of the patient should focus on blood pressure; edema assessment; the presence of rash, purpura, or arthritis; and a careful abdominal examination looking for masses.

Evaluation and Management

The diagnostic evaluation of hematuria depends on findings on history and physical examination as noted earlier and shown in Fig. 100.2. Laboratory assessment should be focused and includes urinalysis with microscopic examination of sediment for RBCs, crystals, and casts. Blood work includes serum electrolytes, BUN, creatinine, calcium, phosphorus, uric acid, and a complete blood count with platelets. Further studies may include complement, antistreptolysin O titers, antinuclear antibody, urine culture, ratio of urine calcium to creatinine, or 24-hour urine calcium excretion. Patients with concerns for kidney stones should be evaluated with urinary excretion of calcium, cystine, oxalate, citrate, and urate. Radiographic imaging is indicated for evaluation of gross hematuria in the absence of RBC casts and proteinuria. Ultrasound evaluation of the kidneys and bladder should be part of the initial evaluation of hematuria unless the patient has isolated microhematuria. Magnetic resonance urography can delineate the anatomic

structure of the collecting systems and elucidate functional obstructions. Additional studies such as nuclear scans, cystoscopy, angiography, or kidney biopsy should be considered in consultation with a subspecialist. The treatment of hematuria is driven by the underlying etiology and is usually conservative. Hematuria with concurrent proteinuria, hypertension, acute kidney injury, trauma, or severe hemorrhage may indicate the need for more extensive investigation and therapy.

PROTEINURIA

Proteinuria, the presence of excessive protein in the urine, is a common finding in children. Up to 10% of children have proteinuria (>30 mg/dL on urine dipstick) at any given time. Its prevalence increases with age and peaks during adolescence. Although most proteinuria is transient or intermittent, it is the most common laboratory finding indicative of progressive kidney disease. Pathologic proteinuria can be difficult to distinguish from physiologic proteinuria. Normal urinary protein excretion in adults is less than 150 mg/day and in children is less than 4 mg/m²/hr.

Etiology and Pathogenesis
Transient Proteinuria

Transient proteinuria is unrelated to kidney disease and resolves when the inciting factor disappears. Febrile proteinuria usually appears with the onset of fever and resolves in 10 to 14 days. Proteinuria that occurs after exercise usually abates within 48

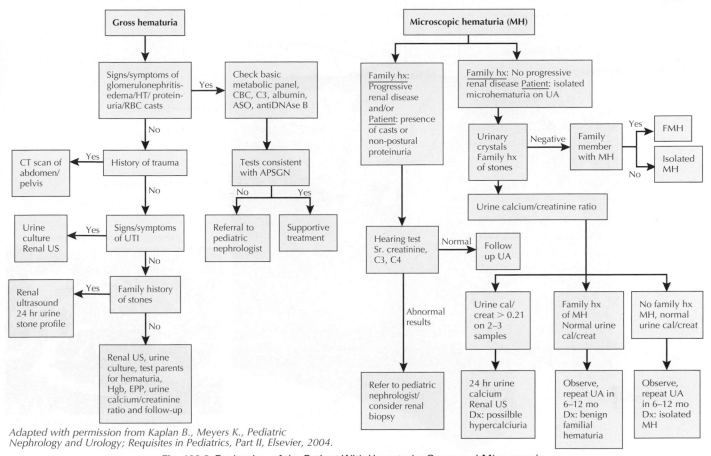

Adapted with permission from Kaplan B., Meyers K., Pediatric Nephrology and Urology; Requisites in Pediatrics, Part II, Elsevier, 2004.

Fig. 100.2 Evaluation of the Patient With Hematuria: Gross and Microscopic.

hours. Transient proteinuria seen with fever or exercise is caused by hemodynamic alterations in kidney blood flow that increases the passage of proteins across the glomerular basement membrane (Fig. 100.3).

Orthostatic (Postural) Proteinuria

Orthostatic proteinuria is elevated protein excretion that occurs only when the patient is upright. It is most likely the result of excessive glomerular filtration of protein. Orthostatic proteinuria is fairly common, accounting for 60% of all causes of childhood proteinuria. The prevalence is even higher among teenagers. Orthostatic proteinuria is an incidental finding. There are no specific clinical features (e.g., edema) and no known cause.

The diagnosis of orthostatic proteinuria is made by doing a first morning urinalysis, which should be negative for protein or by comparing the urine protein-to-creatinine ratio in urine collected in recumbent and upright positions or by 24-hour urine collection separated into daytime and nighttime collections. Total protein excretion is generally less than 1 g/day.

Persistent Asymptomatic Isolated Proteinuria

Persistent asymptomatic isolated proteinuria is defined as persistent proteinuria (>3 months) in an otherwise healthy child detected in more than 80% of the urine specimens tested, including recumbent samples. It is usually less than 1 g/day and is never associated with edema. Studies have reported divergent results with a significant number of patients having glomerulopathies, such as focal sclerosis, but others having normal histology or mild

glomerular abnormalities. It is reasonable, in the absence of other findings, to consider a kidney biopsy if proteinuria progresses to greater than 1 g/day or persists for more than 12 months. Children with persistent isolated proteinuria form a heterogeneous group and should be monitored over time for the development of kidney disease.

Glomerulonephritis and Nephrotic Syndrome

Proteinuria occurs in most glomerular diseases. Glomerulonephritis and nephrotic syndrome are reviewed in Chapters 102 and 103, respectively. In brief, nephrotic syndrome is defined by the presence of proteinuria, edema, hypercholesterolemia, and hypoalbuminemia. Nephrotic syndrome can be primary (isolated to the kidney) or secondary (part of a systemic disease, such as systemic lupus erythematosus). Glomerulonephritis can occur with or without nephrotic syndrome and can manifest with gross hematuria, edema, hypertension, and acute kidney injury.

Tubular Diseases

Proteinuria caused by tubular disease can be from either congenital causes (dysplasia, polycystic kidney disease, Fanconi syndrome) or acquired ones (acute tubular necrosis, interstitial nephritis).

Clinical Presentation

The differential diagnosis of proteinuria is shown in Box 100.2. Patients with proteinuria can present with edema, or it can be detected incidentally in an otherwise asymptomatic child. The history should focus on recent infections (pharyngitis, impetigo), UTIs, oliguria or

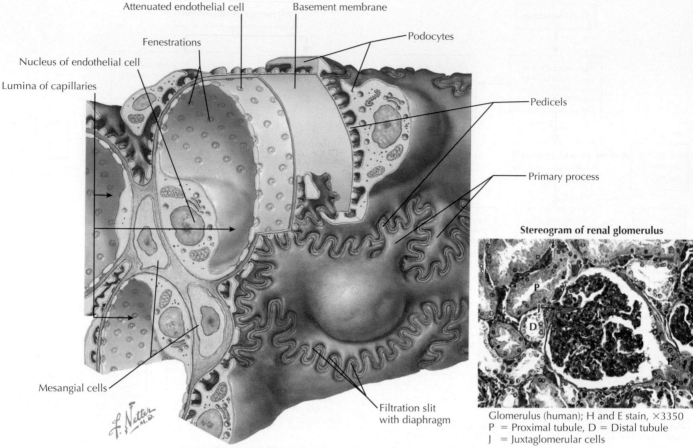

Attenuated endothelial cell

Basement membrane

Podocytes

Fenestrations

Nucleus of endothelial cell

Lumina of capillaries

Pedicels

Primary process

Stereogram of renal glomerulus

Mesangial cells

Filtration slit
with diaphragm

Glomerulus (human); H and E stain, ×3350
P = Proximal tubule, D = Distal tubule
J = Juxtaglomerular cells

Fig. 100.3 Histology and Fine Structure of Kidney Corpuscle.

BOX 100.2   Differential Diagnosis of Proteinuria

- Transient proteinuria
  - Fever
  - Dehydration
  - Exercise
  - Cold exposure
  - Seizures
- Isolated proteinuria
  - Orthostatic proteinuria
  - Persistent asymptomatic isolated proteinuria
- Glomerular disease
  - Minimal change nephrotic syndrome
  - Focal segmental glomerulosclerosis
  - Postinfectious glomerulonephritis
  - Membranoproliferative glomerulonephritis
  - Membranous nephropathy
  - IgA nephropathy

- Henoch-Schönlein purpura
- Hemolytic uremic syndrome
- Hereditary nephritis
- Systemic lupus erythematosus
- Diabetes mellitus
- Sickle cell disease
- HIV-associated nephropathy
- Tubulointerstitial disease
  - Reflux nephropathy
  - Pyelonephritis
  - Interstitial nephritis
  - Fanconi syndrome: cystinosis, tyrosinemia, Lowe syndrome
  - Toxins: drugs (aminoglycosides, penicillins, heavy metals)
  - Ischemic tubular injury
  - Renal hypoplasia or dysplasia
  - Polycystic kidney disease

---

hematuria, and family history of kidney disease. The physical examination should evaluate for hypertension (glomerulonephritis), edema (nephrotic syndrome), rash or arthritis (vasculitis), and short stature (chronic kidney disease).

Evaluation and Management

Laboratory investigations should always include a urine dipstick (random and first morning), a urinalysis including microscopic examination if there is hematuria, and a protein-to-creatinine ratio. The dipstick measures the concentration of protein in urine. A urine sample is considered positive for protein if it measures 1+ or greater when the specific gravity of urine is less than 1.015 or 2+ or greater when the specific gravity is greater than 1.015. Persistent proteinuria is defined as a positive dipstick for protein in two of three random urine samples collected at least 1 week apart. The following can cause false positive results on dipstick analysis: alkaline urine (pH >7.0), prolonged immersion, placing the strip directly in the urine stream, cleansing of the urethral orifice with quaternary ammonium compounds before collecting the sample, pyuria, and bacteriuria. False negative results can occur when the urine is too dilute (i.e., the specific gravity is <1.005) or when the patient excretes abnormal amounts of proteins other than albumin. A timed urine collection for protein quantification is essential to establish the degree of proteinuria. A 24-hour urine collection can be done by asking the child to void as soon as he or she wakes up and discarding the specimen; then every void should be collected for the next 24 hours, including the first void the next morning. In clinical practice, it is difficult to obtain timed urine collections in children. Therefore a spot urine specimen can be analyzed for protein and creatinine concentration and used to estimate the 24-hour total protein content. Additional diagnostic considerations are summarized in Fig. 100.4. Indications for kidney biopsy in a child with persistent proteinuria include strong family history of glomerulonephritis, systemic symptoms concerning for vasculitis or lupus, abnormal kidney function, and nonresponse to steroids in a patient with nephrotic syndrome. Management of proteinuria depends on the underlying cause and may include antiproteinuric therapy with angiotensin-converting enzyme inhibitors, angiotensin receptor blockers, or immunosuppression, including corticosteroids.

FUTURE DIRECTIONS

It remains unknown if persistent proteinuria is an early sign of glomerular disease, such as focal sclerosis in some patients. Advances in home urine monitoring may allow more frequent tracking of patients by providers. Novel antifibrotic and antiinflammatory agents may offer treatment advances in addition to or in combination with angiotensin-converting enzyme inhibitors and angiotensin receptor blockers and may prevent or slow the progression of chronic kidney disease.

SUGGESTED READINGS

Available online.

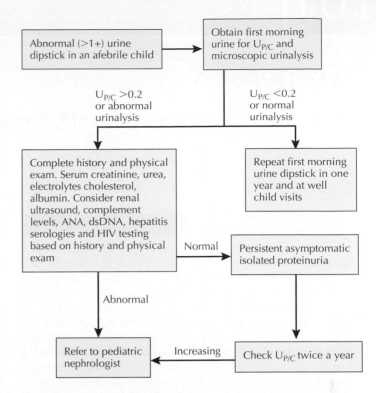

Adapted with permission from Kaplan B., Meyers K., Pediatric Nephrology and Urology; Requisites in Pediatrics, Part II, Elsevier, 2004.

Fig. 100.4 Suggested Approach for the Evaluation of Proteinuria.

101

Hypertension

Rushelle Byfield, Michael L. O'Byrne, and R. Thomas Collins II

 CLINICAL VIGNETTE

A 5-year-old boy was referred to nephrology clinic for evaluation of elevated blood pressure (BP) that was first noted at a routine well-child visit. He is overweight but otherwise healthy. His medical history is unremarkable except for a one-time episode of gross hematuria after falling from a swing. He was born full-term, and there were no complications during the pregnancy or delivery. His family history is notable for hypertension in his father and paternal grandparents. In the clinic his BP is 126/90 mm Hg (>95th percentile for age, sex, and height) in the upper extremity and 142/95 mm Hg in the lower extremity. The remainder of his physical examination is unremarkable. A random urinalysis has a specific gravity of 1.008 with no blood or protein. Laboratory studies show normal kidney function and normal electrolytes. Given his history of gross hematuria, a renal bladder ultrasound is performed and demonstrates bilateral macrocysts in the renal cortex and medulla. Given suspected autosomal dominant polycystic kidney disease, both parents obtain screening ultrasounds and the child's father is found to have bilateral renal cysts as well, confirming the diagnosis. The child is started on an angiotensin-converting enzyme inhibitor and is counseled on weight loss, healthy diet, and exercise; BPs at follow-up visits have been normal. Secondary causes for hypertension should always be considered in children, especially those presenting at younger than 6 years of age. Perinatal and family history can often offer clues to the underlying diagnosis.

Hypertension is a known risk factor for cardiovascular morbidity and mortality in the adult population. Over the last two decades, there has been an increase in the prevalence of childhood hypertension, which is now estimated to affect 3.5% of children and adolescents. This trend has been linked to obesity and lifestyle factors such as high-calorie, high-sodium diets and decreased physical activity. Those with hypertension in childhood have an increased risk for hypertension in adulthood, with its accompanying cardiovascular risks and burden on the health care system.

ETIOLOGY AND PATHOGENESIS

Physiology

Blood pressure (BP) is determined by both cardiac output (CO) and systemic vascular resistance (SVR). Factors increasing output or resistance can result in hypertension. CO in turn is determined by heart rate (HR) and stroke volume (SV). The relationship between BP and CO is summarized by the following equations:

$$BP = CO \times SVR$$

$$CO = HR \times SV$$

Conditions that increase the HR, SV, or SVR can lead to an increase in BP. Considering these fundamental factors in BP elevation can guide the therapeutic approach for a given patient.

Definitions

In adults, hypertension classifications are based on risk for end-organ damage using large epidemiologic cohort studies. Because of the lack of such large-scale cohorts in the pediatric population, classification of pediatric hypertension is based on normative data. The American Academy of Pediatricians published updated pediatric hypertension guidelines in 2017. These guidelines include new normative data based on 50,000 children and adolescents and were updated from the previous 2004 "Fourth Report." Normal BP is defined as an average systolic or diastolic BP below the 90th percentile for sex, age, and height. Elevated BP is defined as systolic or diastolic BPs between the 90th and 95th percentiles. Stage 1 hypertension is defined as a BP between the 95th and 95th + 12 mm Hg percentile or 130/80 to 139/89 mm Hg (whichever is lower). Stage 2 hypertension is above 95th + 12 mm Hg percentile or above 140/90 mm Hg (whichever is lower). Additionally, these new guidelines distinguish adolescents 13 years and older from younger children, using a threshold of 120/80 mm Hg to define hypertension regardless of sex to align with adult guidelines for the detection of elevated BP (Table 101.1). In patients with stage 2 hypertension, it is important to immediately screen for signs and symptoms of end-organ damage. Hypertensive urgency refers to high BP without evidence of end-organ damage. Hypertensive emergency is defined as having acute end-organ dysfunction, such as neurologic symptoms, vision changes, cardiac chest pain, or acute kidney injury in the setting of marked hypertension. Hypertensive urgency and emergency require immediate intervention to safely control BP.

White coat hypertension is defined as having elevated BP in the clinic but being normotensive outside of the clinic setting. This diagnosis usually requires ambulatory blood pressure monitoring (ABPM) for confirmation. White coat hypertension is diagnosed by ABPM when the systolic and diastolic loads are less than 25%, where load is defined as the percentage of ABPM measurements above the 95th percentile for age, sex, and height. It is estimated that up to half of children who are evaluated for elevated office BP have white coat hypertension confirmed by ABPM. Masked hypertension occurs when patients have normal office BPs but elevated BP on ABPM. Masked hypertension is particularly prevalent in patients with chronic kidney disease, including those with a transplanted kidney.

Hypertension has many causes (Fig. 101.1). Whereas high BP for which a clear cause can be determined is described as secondary hypertension, hypertension without a clear cause is referred to as primary or essential hypertension. This is a diagnosis of exclusion.

CLINICAL PRESENTATION

In the United States, primary hypertension is now the prevailing diagnosis for children referred for hypertension. Some general features of children with primary hypertension include older age (6 years and

TABLE 101.1	Blood Pressure Classifications	
BP Classification	**Children Aged 1 to 12 Years (Percentile)**	**Everyone 13 Years and Older (mm Hg)**
Normotensive	<90th and <120/80 mm Hg	<120/<80
Elevated blood pressure	≥90th or ≥120/80 mm Hg (lower) to <95th	120–129/<80
Stage 1 hypertension	≥95th to <95th + 12 mm Hg or 130/80–139/89 mm Hg (lower)	130–139/80–89
Stage 2 hypertension	≥95th + 12 mm Hg or ≥140/90 mm Hg (lower)	≥140/90

From Guzman-Limon M, Samuels J. Pediatric hypertension: diagnosis, evaluation, and treatment. *Pediatr Clin North Am.* 2019;66(1):45-57. https://doi.org/10.1016/j.pcl.2018.09.001. PMID: 30454750. Data from Flynn JT, Kaelber DC, Baker-Smith CM, et al. Clinical practice guideline for screening and management of high blood pressure in children and adolescents. *Pediatrics.* 2017;140(3):ii:e20171904; and Whelton PK, Carey RM, Aronow WS, et al. 2017 ACC/AHA/AAPA/ABC/ACPM/AGS/APhA/ASH/ASPC/NMA/PCNA guideline for the prevention, detection, evaluation, and management of high blood pressure in adults: executive summary. A report of the American College of Cardiology/American Heart Association Task Force on Clinical Practice Guidelines. *Hypertension.* 2018;71(6):1269-1324.

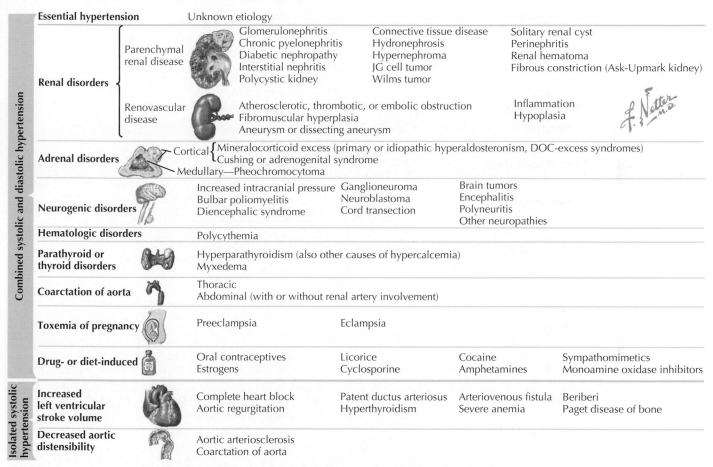

Fig. 101.1 Causes of Secondary Hypertension. *DOC,* 11-Deoxycorticosterone.

older), positive family history, and being overweight. Some studies suggest that systolic rather than diastolic hypertension may be more predictive of primary hypertension. Secondary hypertension is more common in the pediatric population than in adults. Diastolic hypertension tends to be more predictive of a secondary cause. There will often be clues in the family history or physical examination that can lead to the diagnosis (Table 101.2).

EVALUATION AND MANAGEMENT

Measurement of Blood Pressure

Accurate and consistent measurement of BP is essential for appropriate medical management. BP measurements, even when performed correctly, demonstrate significant variability. As a result, the arithmetic mean of three or more BP measurements on separate occasions is used to diagnose hypertension. The mean BP of multiple measurements most closely approximates those obtained by ABPM. The measured BP should be compared against BP tables that are normalized for sex, age, and height percentile.

Accepted epidemiologic statistics for BP are based on measurements made by auscultation. Despite this, automated oscillometric measurements of BP are increasingly used because of their ease of use. Oscillometric "measurements" of systolic and diastolic BP are based on proprietary algorithms that extrapolate the presented values from measured mean BPs. These estimates have been shown to be consistently at least 5 to 10 mm Hg higher than those measured by auscultation. Because of this, high BP derived from oscillometric measurements should always be confirmed by auscultation.

TABLE 101.2 **Examples of Physical Examination Findings and History Suggestive of Secondary Hypertension or Related to End-Organ Damage Secondary to Hypertension**

Body System	Finding, History	Possible Etiology
Vital signs	Tachycardia	Hyperthyroidism
		PCC
		Neuroblastoma
	Decreased lower extremity pulses; drop in BP from upper to lower extremities	Coarctation of the aorta
Eyes	Proptosis	Hyperthyroidism
	Retinal changes	Severe HTN, more likely to be associated with secondary HTN
Ear, nose, throat	Adenotonsillar hypertrophy	SDB
	History of snoring	Sleep apnea
Height, weight	Growth retardation	Chronic renal failure
	Obesity (high BMI)	Cushing syndrome
	Truncal obesity	Insulin resistance syndrome
Head, neck	Elfin facies	Williams syndrome
	Moon facies	Cushing syndrome
	Thyromegaly, goiter	Hyperthyroidism
	Webbed neck	Turner syndrome
Skin	Pallor, flushing, diaphoresis	PCC
	Acne, hirsutism, striae	Cushing syndrome
		Anabolic steroid abuse
	Café-au-lait spots	Neurofibromatosis
	Adenoma sebaceum	Tuberous sclerosis
	Malar rash	Systemic lupus
	Acanthosis nigricans	Type 2 DM
Hematologic	Pallor	Renal disease
	Sickle cell anemia	
Chest, cardiac	Chest pain	Heart disease
	Palpitations	
	Exertional dyspnea	
	Widely spaced nipples	Turner syndrome
	Heart murmur	Coarctation of the aorta
	Friction rub	Systemic lupus (pericarditis)
		Collagen vascular disease
	Apical heave	LVH
Abdomen	Abdominal mass	Wilms tumor
		Neuroblastoma
		PCC
	Epigastric, flank bruit	RAS
	Palpable kidneys	Polycystic kidney disease
		Hydronephrosis
		Multicystic dysplastic kidney
Genitourinary	Ambiguous or virilized genitalia	Congenital adrenal hyperplasia
	Urinary tract infection	Renal disease
	Vesicoureteral reflux	
	Hematuria, edema, fatigue	
	Abdominal trauma	

TABLE 101.2 Examples of Physical Examination Findings and History Suggestive of Secondary Hypertension or Related to End-Organ Damage Secondary to Hypertension—cont'd

Body System	Finding, History	Possible Etiology
Extremities	Joint swelling	Systemic lupus
		Collagen vascular disease
	Muscle weakness	Hyperaldosteronism
		Liddle syndrome
Neurologic, metabolic	Hypokalemia, headache, dizziness, polyuria, nocturia	Reninoma
	Muscle weakness, hypokalemia	Monogenic HTN (Liddle syndrome, GRA, AME)

AME, Apparent mineralocorticoid excess; *BMI,* body mass index; *BP,* blood pressure; *DM,* diabetes mellitus; *GRA,* glucocorticoid-remediable aldosteronism; *HTN,* hypertension; *LVH,* left ventricular hypertrophy; *PCC,* pheochromocytoma; *RAS,* renal artery stenosis; *SDB,* sleep-disordered breathing.
From Flynn JT, Kaelber DC, Baker-Smith CM, et al; Subcommittee on Screening and Management of High Blood Pressure in Children. Clinical practice guideline for screening and management of high blood pressure in children and adolescents. *Pediatrics.* 2017;140(3):e20171904. https://doi.org/10.1542/peds.2017-1904. Erratum in *Pediatrics.* 2017;30. Erratum in *Pediatrics.* 2018;142(3): PMID: 28827377, Table 14.

TABLE 101.3 Technique for Blood Pressure Measurement

Ideal Conditions	1. No stimulant medications or foods before measurement. 2. Blood pressure should be measured in a relaxed environment. 3. Allow a 5-minute rest period before measurement.
Positioning	1. Patient should be seated with back supported. 2. Feet on the floor. 3. Right arm supported. 4. Antecubital fossa at the level of the heart.
Method	1. Perform measurement by auscultatory method. 2. Stethoscope should be placed over the brachial artery pulse, proximal and medial to the cubital fossa, below the bottom edge of the cuff.
Cuff	1. Cuff should be applied to bare skin. 2. Bladder width should be 40% of arm circumference. 3. Bladder length should cover 80%–100% of the arm circumference.
Confirm	1. Take blood pressure in all four limbs. 2. Recheck blood pressure on repeated visits. 3. Consider ambulatory blood pressure monitoring.

From Guzman-Limon M, Samuels J. Pediatric hypertension: diagnosis, evaluation, and treatment. *Pediatr Clin North Am.* 2019;66(1):45-57. https://doi.org/10.1016/j.pcl.2018.09.001. PMID: 30454750, Table 1.

Cuff size can dramatically affect BP measurement. Cuffs that are too small overestimate BP and excessively large cuffs may underestimate BP. However, the range of the underestimation with a large cuff is generally smaller in magnitude than errors from very small cuffs. The correct cuff size can be obtained by ensuring that the inflatable bladder has (1) a width that is approximately 40% of the arm circumference at the point midway between the olecranon and acromion and (2) enough length to cover 80% to 100% of the arm circumference (Table 101.3).

For appropriate auscultation, the stethoscope should be placed over the site of the brachial pulse proximal and medial to the cubital fossa below the distal border of the cuff. Measurement using the bell (instead of the diaphragm) produces superior discrimination of the Korotkoff sounds. The systolic BP corresponds to the pressure at which the first Korotkoff sound is audible, and the diastolic BP corresponds to the pressure at which the fifth Korotkoff sound is audible or

with obliteration of the last sound. If sounds are still heard at 0 mm Hg, a repeat BP should be attempted with less pressure on the stethoscope head.

An ABPM consists of a BP cuff attached to a small box that records BP periodically over 24 hours (usually every 15 to 20 minutes during the day and every 20 to 30 minutes during sleep). These data are later downloaded for analysis. Current data suggest that ABPM may be superior to clinic BP in predicting cardiovascular morbidity and mortality in adults. The use of ABPM in the pediatric population is becoming more common to confirm the diagnosis and severity of hypertension and assess for abnormal circadian variation in BP (blunted dipping or nocturnal hypertension).

Diagnosis

Before making a diagnosis of hypertension, it is important to rule out immediate causes of transient BP elevations such as acute pain, anxiety, or short-term medication exposure. After such causes have been ruled out, the diagnostic approach in a patient with hypertension can be organized as follows: (1) define the degree of hypertension, (2) evaluate for possible causes of secondary hypertension, and (3) investigate for end-organ damage (Fig. 101.2).

Management

The goal of antihypertensive therapy is to reduce the BP to diminish the risk for accumulating short- and long-term end-organ damage without incurring excessive side effects. Current recommendations are to reduce the BP below the 90th percentile or less than 130/80 mm Hg in adolescents older than 13 years of age, if no other risk factors are present or below the 50th percentile if other risk factors, such proteinuria or chronic kidney disease, are present.

The first-line therapy for stage 1 hypertension and prehypertension is therapeutic lifestyle change. Data supporting the efficacy of these modifications are limited; however, based on data from studies in adult groups, weight reduction in obese patients, increased intake of vegetables and fruits, increased physical activity, and reduction in dietary sodium intake are all recommended.

Indications for pharmacologic intervention include insufficient response to therapeutic lifestyle modifications, severe hypertension, and identification of secondary hypertension, which cannot be corrected otherwise. There is no consensus regarding the choice of antihypertensive medication in children, although dihydropyridine calcium channel blockers such as amlodipine are frequently first-line medications in many groups because of the low risk for side effects and ease of dosing. Treatment choice is empiric and generally guided by the cause of the

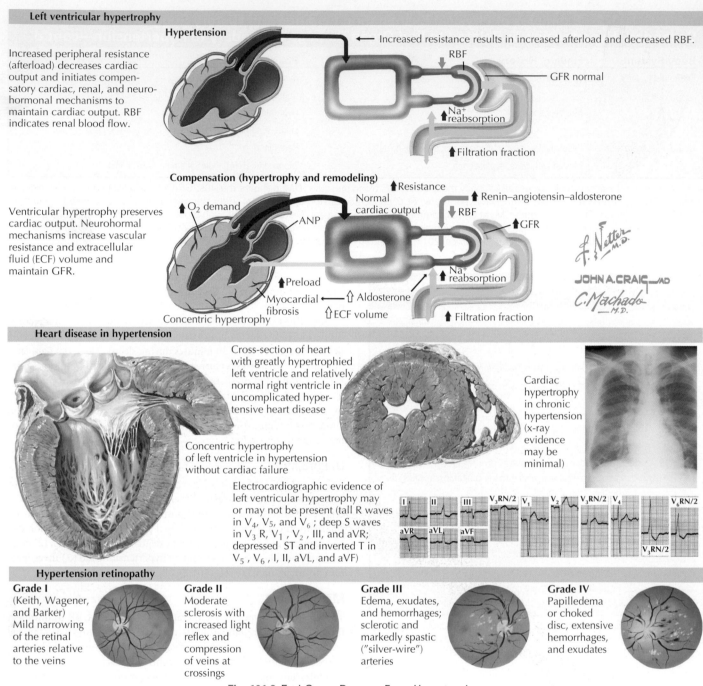

Left ventricular hypertrophy

Hypertension

Increased peripheral resistance (afterload) decreases cardiac output and initiates compensatory cardiac, renal, and neurohormonal mechanisms to maintain cardiac output. RBF indicates renal blood flow.

Increased resistance results in increased afterload and decreased RBF.

RBF

GFR normal

Na+ reabsorption

Filtration fraction

Compensation (hypertrophy and remodeling)

Ventricular hypertrophy preserves cardiac output. Neurohormal mechanisms increase vascular resistance and extracellular fluid (ECF) volume and maintain GFR.

O$_2$ demand

ANP

Preload

Myocardial fibrosis

Concentric hypertrophy

Resistance

Normal cardiac output

Renin–angiotensin–aldosterone

RBF

GFR

Na+ reabsorption

Aldosterone

ECF volume

Filtration fraction

Heart disease in hypertension

Cross-section of heart with greatly hypertrophied left ventricle and relatively normal right ventricle in uncomplicated hypertensive heart disease

Concentric hypertrophy of left ventricle in hypertension without cardiac failure

Electrocardiographic evidence of left ventricular hypertrophy may or may not be present (tall R waves in V$_4$, V$_5$, and V$_6$; deep S waves in V$_3$R, V$_1$, V$_2$, III, and aVR; depressed ST and inverted T in V$_5$, V$_6$, I, II, aVL, and aVF)

Cardiac hypertrophy in chronic hypertension (x-ray evidence may be minimal)

Hypertension retinopathy

Grade I
(Keith, Wagener, and Barker)
Mild narrowing of the retinal arteries relative to the veins

Grade II
Moderate sclerosis with increased light reflex and compression of veins at crossings

Grade III
Edema, exudates, and hemorrhages; sclerotic and markedly spastic ("silver-wire") arteries

Grade IV
Papilledema or choked disc, extensive hemorrhages, and exudates

Fig. 101.2 End-Organ Damage From Hypertension.

hypertension, especially in secondary hypertension. Medication classes include calcium channel blockers, β-blockers, angiotensin-converting enzyme inhibitors, angiotensin receptor blockers, and diuretics. Other agents such as clonidine, prazosin, and minoxidil are primarily used by subspecialists in patients with refractory hypertension (Fig. 101.3). Data regarding pediatric dosing of most antihypertensive medications are expanding. When considering the choice of medication, secondary benefits, in addition to BP control, are often warranted. As just a few examples, patients with proteinuria may benefit from angiotensin-converting enzyme inhibitors or angiotensin receptor blockers, patients taking systemic corticosteroids may benefit from diuretics, and patients with concern for central hypertension may benefit from clonidine.

The management of hypertensive urgency and emergency should be considered separately. Therapy should be initiated immediately while the diagnostic workup is ongoing. The goal of pharmacologic intervention in hypertensive urgency is to reduce the BP to an appropriate level within 24 to 48 hours. In the setting of hypertensive emergency, the goal is to reduce the mean arterial pressure by no more than 25% (within minutes to 2 hours). The BP should then be lowered slowly to a normal level over the next 48 hours. A trial of oral agents may be attempted in the setting of hypertensive urgency. However, in hypertensive emergency, intravenous medications should be used. Intravenous antihypertensive agents, such as calcium channel blockers and β-blockers can be given by bolus or continuous infusion, are titratable, and have shorter times to onset. Any patient with a hypertensive emergency or those with hypertensive urgency requiring a continuous infusion should be admitted to a pediatric intensive care unit or other facility with staffing and equipment necessary for close BP monitoring.

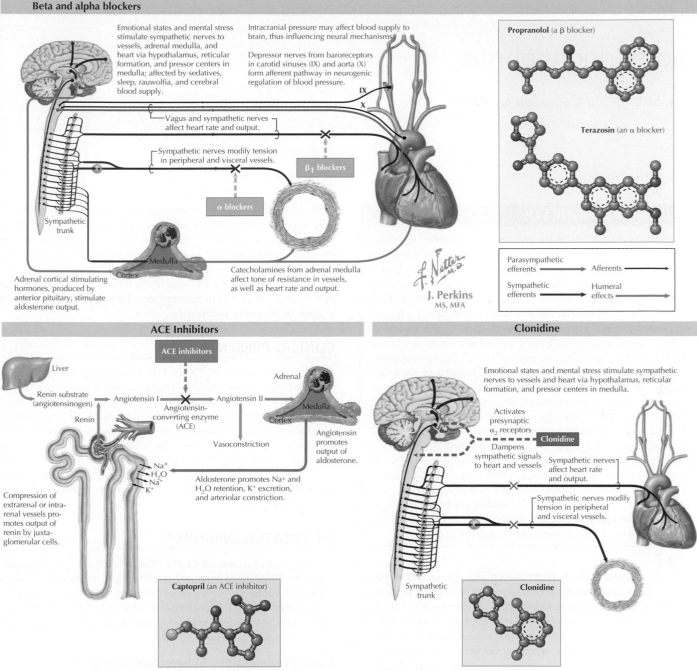

Beta and alpha blockers

Emotional states and mental stress stimulate sympathetic nerves to vessels, adrenal medulla, and heart via hypothalamus, reticular formation, and pressor centers in medulla; affected by sedatives, sleep, rauwolfia, and cerebral blood supply.

Intracranial pressure may affect blood supply to brain, thus influencing neural mechanisms.

Depressor nerves from baroreceptors in carotid sinuses (IX) and aorta (X) form afferent pathway in neurogenic regulation of blood pressure.

Vagus and sympathetic nerves affect heart rate and output.

Sympathetic nerves modify tension in peripheral and visceral vessels.

β₁ blockers

α blockers

Sympathetic trunk

Medulla
Cortex

Adrenal cortical stimulating hormones, produced by anterior pituitary, stimulate aldosterone output.

Catecholamines from adrenal medulla affect tone of resistance in vessels, as well as heart rate and output.

Propranolol (a β blocker)

Terazosin (an α blocker)

| Parasympathetic efferents | Afferents |
| Sympathetic efferents | Humeral effects |

J. Perkins
MS, MFA

ACE Inhibitors

ACE inhibitors

Liver

Renin substrate (angiotensinogen) → Angiotensin I → Angiotensin II

Renin

Angiotensin-converting enzyme (ACE)

Vasoconstriction

Adrenal
Medulla
Cortex

Angiotensin promotes output of aldosterone.

Na⁺
H₂O
Na⁺
K⁺

Aldosterone promotes Na⁺ and H₂O retention, K⁺ excretion, and arteriolar constriction.

Compression of extrarenal or intra-renal vessels pro-motes output of renin by juxta-glomerular cells.

Captopril (an ACE inhibitor)

Clonidine

Emotional states and mental stress stimulate sympathetic nerves to vessels and heart via hypothalamus, reticular formation, and pressor centers in medulla.

Activates presynaptic α₂ receptors

Clonidine

Dampens sympathetic signals to heart and vessels

Sympathetic nerves affect heart rate and output.

Sympathetic nerves modify tension in peripheral and visceral vessels.

Sympathetic trunk

Clonidine

Fig. 101.3 Management of Hypertension.

Arterial access for continuous BP monitoring also may be necessary. In patients who are hypertensive secondary to severe volume overload, aggressive diuresis or even temporary hemodialysis may be effective interventions.

FUTURE DIRECTIONS

Hypertension is a growing chronic health issue in the pediatric population. Acute cardiac events are rare in children and adolescents; thus much of our knowledge about the long-term sequelae of hypertension is extrapolated from adult data. There remains a need for longitudinal studies to determine how childhood hypertension informs adult risk for cardiovascular mortality.

SUGGESTED READINGS

Available online.

102

Glomerulonephritis

Amy Strong and Benjamin L. Laskin

 CLINICAL VIGNETTE

A 6-year-old previously healthy boy presents to the emergency department after an episode of visible blood in the urine. The urine color is described as appearing brown and red and almost like iced tea. His urine output has been a bit less than usual. There is no pain with urination. He is well appearing and acting like himself; however, his parents note that he seems to be a bit "puffy" around the eyes. He was previously a very healthy child, presenting to medical attention only for well care and colds. He was last seen by a doctor about 2 weeks ago for a sore throat and was treated with 10 days of amoxicillin for streptococcal pharyngitis. His vital signs are notable for a blood pressure of 125/92 mm Hg, heart rate of 134 beats/min, and oxygen saturation of 94% on room air. On examination he has trace edema in the lower extremities and slight abdominal fullness with mild periorbital edema. Urinalysis was obtained, which showed 3+ blood and 3+ protein with microscopy, revealing red blood cells too numerous to count. The urine was negative for leukocyte esterase or nitrites. Blood work was performed and notable for slightly elevated serum creatinine to 0.6 mg/dL with otherwise normal electrolytes. Complement levels show a depressed C3 and normal C4. Diagnosis of postinfectious glomerulonephritis was made. He is admitted for 24 hours of observation and monitoring of his BP. His hematuria resolves within the next few days. He is followed for 2 months, after which his laboratory results have normalized but his microscopic hematuria has persisted for 1 year.

Glomerulonephritis (GN) is a term used to describe an inflammatory injury to the renal glomeruli. A clinical pattern of hematuria, proteinuria, hypertension, azotemia, oligoanuria, and edema occurs in various combinations. The inciting process varies depending on the specific cause and can be infectious, immunologic, autoimmune, or hereditary. Prompt recognition of GN is imperative because it can lead to hypertensive emergency, heart failure, pulmonary edema, hyperkalemia, or other electrolyte derangements. In addition, the early diagnosis of GN permits prompt medical treatment of severe subtypes that can cause long-term kidney damage. Supportive care consists of strict attention to fluid and electrolyte management and blood pressure (BP) control. Certain types of GN require medical management to combat renal inflammation. An understanding of the diagnosis and management of GN ensures the best chance at reducing immediate morbidity and mortality as well as decreasing the likelihood of progression to chronic kidney disease (CKD).

ETIOLOGY AND PATHOGENESIS

Most glomerulonephritides result from either circulating immune complex deposition within the glomerulus or in situ immune complex formation. Both will activate the complement cascade, as well as the cellular and humoral pathways of inflammation. Within the

glomerulus, there can be endothelial, epithelial, and/or mesangial inflammation leading to hypercellularity, thickening or duplication of the glomerular basement membrane, and necrosis. This injury results in loss of capillary integrity and obstruction of blood flow through the glomerular capillary loops, thus leading to the clinical findings outlined below. The underlying cause of the GN is often not known but may involve risk factors including family history, genetics, infectious triggers, or idiopathic mechanisms.

CLINICAL PRESENTATION

The clinical presentation of acute GN is variable. Some children are asymptomatic and are found by screening, and others present to the emergency department with hypertensive emergency, edema, and acute kidney injury and failure. On history, the child's urine may be described as the color of cola or iced tea and there will generally be no report of associated dysuria. The child's face, abdomen, or legs may look swollen. One-third of patients will complain of cough, sore throat, fever, or headache. The most common physical examination findings are any combination of hypertension, edema, and gross hematuria (Fig. 102.1)

DIFFERENTIAL DIAGNOSIS

The two most common causes of GN in children are acute postinfectious GN (APIGN) and immunoglobulin A (IgA) nephropathy (IgAN). Other less common but important causes of GN include Henoch-Schönlein purpura (HSP), membranoproliferative GN (MPGN), antineutrophilic cytoplasmic antibody (ANCA)-positive vasculitis, and systemic lupus erythematosus (SLE).

Acute Postinfectious Glomerulonephritis

APIGN is presumed to be caused by nephritogenic forms of group A streptococci. In most cases, there is clinical or laboratory evidence of antecedent streptococcal infection. APIGN must be confirmed or ruled out before looking for less common causes of postinfectious GN, although many infections can lead to an APIGN. APIGN is characterized by sudden onset and variable presentation of hypertension, periorbital, or lower extremity edema, oliguria, and painless gross hematuria, typically several weeks after a streptococcal infection. The glomerular damage in APIGN is immune mediated, with antigen-antibody reactions occurring in the circulation or in situ within the glomeruli. These antigen-antibody reactions activate the alternative complement pathway, thus leading to a reduction in the serum C3 concentration. By light microscopy, findings in APIGN include glomerular enlargement, mesangial cell expansion and proliferation, and neutrophil exudation. Electron microscopy (EM) reveals discrete subepithelial deposits (Fig. 102.2).

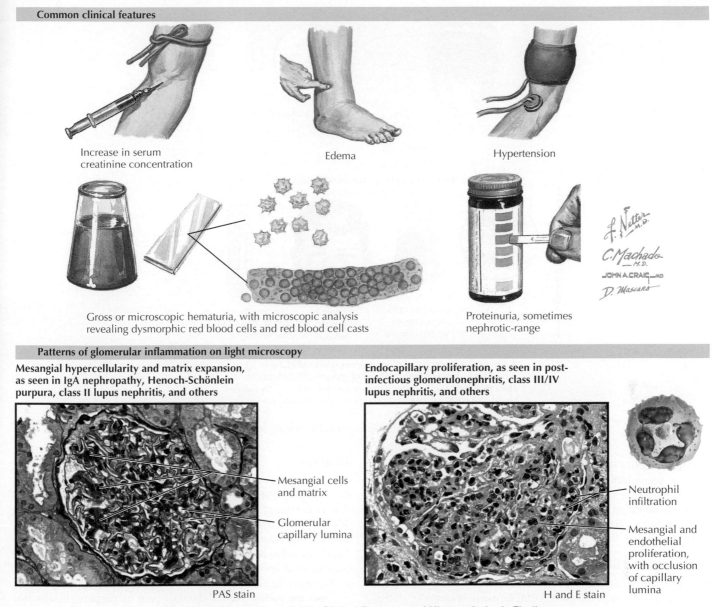

Fig. 102.1 Glomerulonephritis: Clinical Features and Histopathologic Findings.

Immunoglobulin A Nephropathy

IgAN is an immune complex–mediated GN. Its course is highly variable and can range from asymptomatic microhematuria to recurrent episodes of gross hematuria to hypertensive crisis and acute kidney injury. Although many children with IgAN present at the beginning or same time as an upper respiratory tract infection, no infectious cause has been identified. Most IgAN is sporadic, although some studies have suggested rare genetic forms. When obtained, an abnormally glycosylated IgA1 can be found in the circulation and in deposits in the skin and mesangium of the kidneys. The deposition of IgA within the mesangium causes activation of cytokines and growth factors, leading to mesangial expansion and extracellular matrix deposition. Light microscopy findings show cellular and matrix expansion of the mesangium with deposition of IgA seen by immunofluorescence. EM reveals electron-dense deposits within the mesangium that may extend along capillary loops.

Henoch-Schönlein Purpura Nephritis

HSP nephritis is a small vessel vasculitis caused by IgA deposition within the glomeruli. This is seen in the context of systemic HSP with rash, joint pain, and abdominal pain. Recently the nomenclature has changed to reflect the considerable overlap with IgAN and is referred to as IgA vasculitis (IgAV). Renal manifestations may appear weeks after the onset of other HSP features and is rarely the first sign in this syndrome. Pediatric nephrology centers report that 50% of children with IgAV have some evidence of hematuria and proteinuria and 8% have acute GN, 13% have nephrotic syndrome, and 29% have a mixed nephritic and nephrotic syndrome. The treatment for HSP nephritis is controversial because of the high rate of spontaneous remission and the lack of rigorous studies regarding treatment.

Membranoproliferative Glomerulonephritis

MPGN is another form of GN with a variable presentation that ranges from asymptomatic proteinuria and hematuria to acute

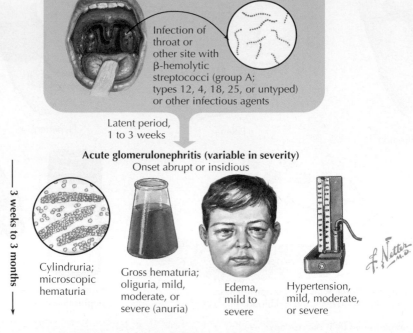

Acute post-streptococcal glomerulonephritis (APSGN)
is caused by nephritogenic strains of group A streptococcus.
The child seen with acute glomerulonephritis classically has red
blood cell casts, gross hematuria, periorbital edema, and
hypertension.

Fig. 102.2 Acute Poststreptococcal Glomerulonephritis.

nephritis. MPGN is a histologic diagnosis and can be either primary or secondary to other disorders. It is an important diagnosis to consider in cases of presumed acute post-streptococcal glomerulonephritis (APSGN) in which the serum C3 concentration does not revert to normal within 6 to 8 weeks after the initial presentation.

Pauci-immune Glomerulonephritis

Pauci-immune glomerulonephritis, small-vessel vasculitides, include granulomatosis with polyangiitis (GPA; formerly Wegener's), microvascular polyangiitis (MPA), and Churg-Strauss syndrome. The pathogenesis involves the formation of antimyeloperoxidase (c-ANCA) and antiserinase 3 (p-ANCA) anti-neutrophil cytoplasmic autoantibodies. These patients may present with night sweats, fever, weight loss, cough, and hemoptysis. More than 50% present with a pulmonary-renal syndrome. The GN associated with ANCA can be severe, with rapid progression to end-stage renal failure.

Rapidly Progressive Glomerulonephritis

Rapidly progressive glomerulonephritis (RPGN) may be idiopathic or secondary to any of the aforementioned glomerulonephritides. It is associated with rapidly deteriorating renal function, and these patients should undergo an urgent renal biopsy to determine therapy. Renal biopsy histologic examination will often reveal crescentic changes indicating significant disease activity and damage.

EVALUATION AND MANAGEMENT

Performing a directed patient history and physical examination focused toward the major causes of GN and targeted use of laboratory tests will help the practitioner with diagnosis.

History

It is important to elicit a history of any recent illnesses or exposures. For example, APIGN often occurs after a group A streptococcal infection of the throat (7 to 21 days later) or skin (14 to 28 days later). It is important to ask if there have been any skin infections (impetigo, infected bug bites, cellulitis) within the past month. In IgAN, gross hematuria often begins concurrently or within 1 to 2 days following the start of an upper respiratory tract infection.

Questions to ask in the review of systems include:
- Does the patient have abdominal pain or purpuric lesions that would suggest HSP nephritis?
- Is there a malar rash, pleuritic chest pain, neurologic changes, or other stigmata of SLE?
- Is there any hemoptysis or sinusitis that could suggest ANCA vasculitis?
- Does the child have any hearing loss that would suggest a diagnosis of Alport syndrome?

In a child with suspected GN, it is also important to obtain a detailed family history, focusing on inherited forms of GN such as Alport syndrome (also known as hereditary nephritis). Important questions include:
- Has anyone else in the family ever had gross or microscopic hematuria?
- Does the mother of the child have any brothers? Are they healthy?
- Is there any hearing loss in the family?
- Is there a history of kidney disease, dialysis, or renal transplant?

Physical Examination

In acute GN, the most important feature of the physical examination is determining the degree of intravascular volume overload. Other physical examination findings may also give clues as to the underlying cause

TABLE 102.1 Physical Examination Findings in Acute Glomerulonephritis

Disease	Findings
Postinfectious glomerulonephritis	Healing or healed impetigo
Immunoglobulin A nephropathy	Coryza, congestion, pharyngitis, cough
Henoch-Schönlein purpura	Abdominal tenderness, joint tenderness, palpable purpura
Systemic lupus erythematosus	Malar or discoid rash, painless oral ulcers, neurologic changes, arthritis, serositis
Pauci-immune glomerulonephritis	Weight loss, fever, myalgias, sinusitis, hemoptysis (pulmonary-renal syndrome)

TABLE 102.2 Laboratory Studies to Consider in Acute Glomerulonephritis

Disease	Laboratory Evaluation
Postinfectious glomerulonephritis	C3 (low), antistreptolysin titer, rapid streptococcal or throat culture
Immunoglobulin A nephropathy	C3 (normal) and kidney biopsy
Systemic lupus erythematosus	C3, C4, antinuclear antibodies, anti-Smith, anti–double-stranded DNA, and kidney biopsy
Pauci-immune glomerulonephritis	Antineutrophil cytoplasmic antibody titers: anti–serine protease 3 and antimyeloperoxidase, and kidney biopsy
Membranoproliferative glomerulo-nephritis	C3, C4, kidney biopsy
Alport syndrome	Genetic test for mutations in type IV collagen gene *COL4A5* and kidney biopsy

of the GN (Table 102.1). It is important to determine the degree of fluid overload and whether it may be compromising the child's cardiorespiratory status. Intravascular volume overload can be suggested by weight gain, an elevated BP, jugular venous distension, gallop rhythm, reduced oxygenation by pulse oximetry, increased work of breathing, rales, crackles, hepatomegaly, and/or peripheral edema. The edema in acute GN varies in severity. Hypertensive children may present with seizures, but headache and nonspecific behavioral changes are more commonly seen.

Studies

Laboratory evaluation is required to assess for the presence of GN and to determine the cause of the glomerular inflammation. The presence of red blood cell casts in a fresh urine specimen examined by microscopy will help confirm the diagnosis of GN. Electrolytes and kidney function should be assessed as well, with particular attention being paid to the potassium concentration, because hyperkalemia can be life threatening. The serum C3 concentration can help differentiate among the many causes of GN. For example, a low serum C3 concentration is present in APIGN and MPGN. Patients with SLE generally have low serum concentrations of both C3 and C4. In those with IgAN, Alport syndrome, and HSP nephritis, both the serum C3 and C4 levels are generally normal. The serum C3 concentration should return to normal in 6 to 8 weeks in children with APIGN. If this does not occur and the patient remains symptomatic, a biopsy should be considered to evaluate for MPGN. Studies used to differentiate among the glomerulonephritides are detailed in Table 102.2. Renal ultrasonography can show nonspecific echogenicity. Chest radiograph may be valuable to show evidence of fluid overload or features of vasculitis. The most definitive way to diagnose and to guide therapy in GN is with a percutaneous renal biopsy, although this is not always necessary. Using a combination of light microscopy, immunofluorescence, and electron microscopy, the underlying GN type can often be discerned (Fig. 102.3).

Management

Management of fluid balance, control of hypertension, and correction of electrolyte abnormalities are the most acute considerations in the treatment of GN. After these have been addressed, use of other agents that may modify the disease course are used. For patients with oliguria, fluid administration should be limited to insensible fluid losses plus replacement of urine output. Insensible losses can be estimated at one-third of daily maintenance requirements. Children who are volume overloaded also can be given intravenous diuretics. Over time, as the child's urine output improves, fluid intake can be liberalized. Ongoing evaluation of daily weights and the physical examination for signs of volume overload help to guide total daily fluid requirements. Hypertension associated with GN is caused by intravascular fluid retention secondary to decreased glomerular filtration as well as nitrous oxide–endothelin imbalance. Loop diuretics and calcium channel blockers should be used as initial therapy. Hyperkalemia can be life threatening, especially in the presence of acidosis, hemolysis, and anuria. The acute management of hyperkalemia focuses on the administration of calcium to stabilize the myocardium. Measures to shift the potassium intracellularly (insulin/glucose or bicarbonate administration) and diuretics and potassium resin binders can be used to remove potassium from the body. Dialysis, in some instances, may ultimately be required if conservative measures do not work. In patients requiring immunosuppression, therapeutic options include corticosteroids, cyclophosphamide, calcineurin inhibitors, mycophenolate mofetil, and plasmapheresis.

FUTURE DIRECTIONS

Progress is being made in improving the evaluation and management of GN. Current studies focus on earlier detection of glomerular injury and directed therapy specific to each underlying cause of GN. Finally, research continues in understanding how to prevent, halt, or reverse the chronic renal damage that can be caused by the various glomerulonephritides.

SUGGESTED READINGS

Available online.

Electron microscopic findings

Epithelial cell swollen

Electron-dense "hump" γ
globulin (IgG) and immune bodies)

Basement membrane usually normal

Foot processes only focally fused

Erythrocyte and proteinaceous
deposits in urinary (Bowman) space

Polymorphonuclear leukocyte

Swollen endothelial cell
bulging into capillary lumen

Mesangial cell proliferation thickening
lobular stalk and narrowing capillary lumen

Mesangial matrix deposited in stalk

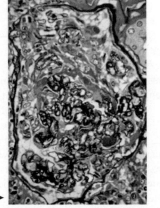

**Rapidly progressive
glomerulonephritis**

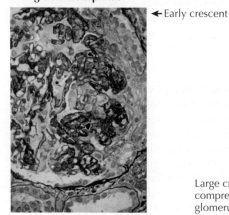

◄ Early crescent

**Rapidly progressive
glomerulonephritis**

Acute diffuse glomerulonephritis

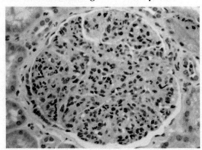

Glomerulus. Greatly increased cellularity and
mesangial matrix and almost complete obliteration
of capillary lumina. The cells are chiefly mesangial,
with some polymorphonuclear leukocytes and a
few eosinophils.

Large crescent
compressing
glomerular tuft ➤

Fig. 102.3 Acute Glomerulonephritis.

103

Nephrotic Syndrome

Rebecca R. Scobell and Michelle Denburg

 CLINICAL VIGNETTE

A 3-year-old previously healthy boy presented with swollen eyes for several days, worse in the morning and improved throughout the day. He was treated with antihistamine medication for presumed seasonal allergies, but swelling worsened so his mother brought him to the emergency department (ED). He was well appearing with normal vital signs, but weight was 2 kg higher than baseline. Examination revealed bilateral periorbital edema, moderate ascites, and 1+ pitting edema of his lower extremities. Laboratory workup was notable for 3+ protein on urine dipstick, serum creatinine 0.3 mg/dL, albumin 2.3 g/dL, hemoglobin 14.8 g/dL, and elevated triglycerides and total cholesterol. He was diagnosed with nephrotic syndrome and started on 2 mg/kg of prednisolone with nephrology follow-up planned. However, he returned to the ED 1 week later with fever, abdominal pain, and vomiting for 2 days. On arrival, he was febrile to 102.6°F (39.2°C), tachycardic, and ill-appearing. His abdomen was diffusely tender to palpation. He received a bolus of normal saline and was admitted to the hospital on intravenous antibiotics for presumed bacterial peritonitis. The next day his blood culture grew *Streptococcus pneumoniae*.

Nephrotic syndrome is a clinical diagnosis defined by four clinical and laboratory findings: proteinuria, hypoalbuminemia, edema, and hyperlipidemia. This clinical syndrome is a manifestation of many underlying disease processes in the kidney that lead to massive protein loss in the urine as a result of a defect in the glomerular filtration barrier. Commonly, pediatric nephrotic syndrome is idiopathic, meaning that no secondary cause is identified. Idiopathic nephrotic syndrome (INS) affects 4.7 (range 1.2 to 16.9) of 100,000 children worldwide with substantial variability in ethnic background and geographic location.

ETIOLOGY AND PATHOGENESIS

There are a variety of ways to classify nephrotic syndrome (Box 103.1), and a patient's classification may change over time. It is important to consider a patient's age, family history, and comorbidities in discerning their risk for an underlying genetic cause for nephrotic syndrome (Table 103.1). Secondary causes such as infections, drugs or toxins, malignancy, and rheumatologic conditions also should be considered (Table 103.2). Nephrotic syndrome may be a feature of several glomerulonephritides, such as lupus nephritis, membranoproliferative glomerulonephritis (MPGN), and immunoglobulin A (IgA) nephropathy. Similarly, some patients with nephrotic syndrome may have nephritic features (hypertension, hematuria, and decreased kidney function). This chapter will focus on nephrotic syndrome without prominent nephritic features.

The frequent association of both onset and relapse of INS with viral illness, as well as the response to immunosuppressive therapy, suggests that it is immunologically mediated. The exact pathophysiology remains unknown, but the unifying pathologic process in all causes of nephrotic syndrome is alteration of the glomerular filtration barrier made up of the glomerular basement membrane and a complex network of podocyte foot processes. In INS, light microscopy may show no abnormalities (minimal change disease [MCD]) (Fig. 103.1), focal segmental glomerulosclerosis (FSGS), or membranous nephropathy (rare in pediatrics). Immunofluorescent staining is generally negative. On electron microscopy, there is effacement of the epithelial foot processes. Although the histopathologic examination is important, the response to corticosteroid therapy is the most important predictor of clinical disease course.

CLINICAL PRESENTATION

The evaluation of a child with nephrotic syndrome includes a history and physical examination targeted at identifying secondary causes (see Table 103.2) and complications of the disease. It is also important to get an accurate assessment of the patient's intravascular volume status and degree of fluid overload to guide initial management.

History and Physical Examination

The age of presentation of nephrotic syndrome influences the most likely underlying cause. Children presenting at younger than 1 year of age most commonly have a genetic cause, but congenital infection should be considered especially in those younger than 3 months. Some monogenic forms of nephrotic syndrome manifest later, and more pathogenic mutations have been identified with the increased availability of genetic testing. Patients with an identified pathogenic mutation most often have steroid-resistant disease. INS most commonly presents between 2 and 8 years of age. Most children presenting in this age range (up to 80% to 90%) will respond to an initial course of steroids and are presumed to have MCD. FSGS becomes more common as age of presentation approaches adolescence, and these patients are more likely to be steroid-resistant. Steroid-resistant nephrotic syndrome is more common in Black and Hispanic children and has an increased likelihood of progressing to end-stage kidney disease (ESKD).

Edema is the main manifesting feature of nephrotic syndrome, and its onset may be rapid or insidious. The pathophysiologic process of edema in nephrotic syndrome is multifaceted, but it is important to conceptualize in order to understand the laboratory abnormalities and approach to fluid management (Fig. 103.2). The edema is gravity dependent; thus it is often most noticeable in the periorbital region in the morning and is sometimes misdiagnosed and treated as allergies. Edema may fluctuate with positional changes and activity, with lower extremity swelling being more noticeable later in the day. Scrotal, penile, and labial edema can be particularly distressing and uncomfortable. Pleural effusions are generally asymptomatic, but if large may cause respiratory compromise. Ascites can lead to umbilical or inguinal hernias, and bowel wall edema may cause abdominal pain or diarrhea.

Children with MCD may have mild elevations in blood pressure, but significant hypertension can suggest underlying FSGS or glomerulonephritis. Despite total body fluid overload, patients with nephrotic syndrome may have profound intravascular volume depletion. Tachycardia, orthostatic blood pressure changes, and hemoconcentration are indicative of intravascular hypovolemia. Patients with nephrotic syndrome are often oliguric, and the urine appears concentrated and foamy. Gross hematuria or cola-colored urine should raise concern for glomerulonephritis.

Complications

The most important acute complications of nephrotic syndrome are infections and thromboembolic events. Common serious infections include pneumonia, spontaneous bacterial peritonitis, and cellulitis. Several factors contribute to impaired immunity and increased risk for infection: (1) defective opsonization through complement and IgG loss in urine, (2) changes in T cell function, (3) edema as a medium

for bacterial growth, and (4) immunosuppressive treatment. Children with nephrotic syndrome are at higher risk for infection with encapsulated organisms, especially *Streptococcus pneumoniae*.

The prothrombotic state of nephrotic syndrome is also multifactorial, resulting from a combination of disproportionate urinary loss of anticoagulant factors (antithrombin III, protein C, protein S), increased production of clotting factors, thrombocytosis, increased blood viscosity resulting from intravascular volume depletion, and hyperlipidemia. This state may be exacerbated by diuretic therapy, venous catheters, and immobilization. Pulmonary embolus should be considered in a nephrotic patient with respiratory distress, hemoptysis, or pleuritic chest pain. Asymmetric extremity swelling should prompt evaluation for a deep venous thrombosis. Rarely, patients may present with gross hematuria and flank pain in the setting of renal vein thrombosis.

Patients with nephrotic syndrome are at risk for acute kidney injury related to intravascular volume depletion. This can be exacerbated by diuretic therapy, infection, or other medications used to treat nephrotic syndrome (angiotensin-converting enzyme [ACE] and calcineurin inhibitors).

BOX 103.1 Classification Schemes for Nephrotic Syndrome

- Age of presentation: congenital (birth to 3 months of age), infantile (4 to 12 months), childhood (older than 1 year)
- Idiopathic versus secondary
- Genetic versus acquired
- Histologic appearance: minimal change disease (MCD), focal segmental glomerulosclerosis (FSGS), membranous nephropathy
- Steroid sensitive versus steroid resistant

EVALUATION AND MANAGEMENT

Laboratory Testing and Workup

The initial evaluation should establish the diagnosis of nephrotic syndrome and screen for secondary causes and complications. A urinalysis with microscopy, basic metabolic panel, albumin, complete blood count, lipid panel, and complement levels (C3, C4) should be considered (Table 103.3). The diagnosis of nephrotic syndrome can be made in a patient with edema who has nephrotic-range proteinuria, hypoalbuminemia, and hyperlipidemia. Nephrotic-range proteinuria is characterized by urine

---

TABLE 103.1 Examples of Genetic Causes of Steroid-Resistant Nephrotic Syndrome

Gene (protein)	Diagnosis or Syndrome	Typical Age of NS Onset (Inheritance)	Additional Clinical Features
NPHS1 (nephrin)	Finnish-type congenital nephrotic syndrome	Birth to 3 months (AR)	↑ Maternal serum AFP, large placenta, prematurity, Often develop ESKD in early childhood
NPHS2 (podocin)		1 month to early childhood (AR)	Progression to ESKD average ~7 years old
PLCE1 (phospholipase C epsilon 1)		1 month to early childhood (AR)	
WT1 (Wilms tumor protein = transcription factor)	Denys-Drash syndrome	3–6 months (germline)	Urogenital abnormalities (ambiguous genitalia in XY patients) Risk for Wilms' tumor Hypertension Histology: diffuse mesangial sclerosis
	Frasier syndrome	Early childhood to adolescence (AD)	Male pseudohermaphroditism: XY Karyotype, female external genitalia, streak for gonadoblastoma Histology: FSGS
LAMB2 (laminin β2-chain)	Pierson syndrome	Birth to 3 months (AR)	Eye abnormalities: microcoria, retinal changes, blindness Developmental delay
WDR73 and others	Galloway-Mowat syndrome	Birth to 3 months (AR)	Neurologic abnormalities: microcephaly, seizures, developmental delay Hiatal hernia
ACTN4 (α-actinin-4) TRPC6 (transient receptor potential 6)	Autosomal dominant isolated SRNS	Late childhood to adolescence or adulthood (AD)	Variable age of diagnosis and progression to ESKD Histology: FSGS

AD, Autosomal dominant; *AFP*, α-fetoprotein; *AR*, autosomal recessive; *ESKD*, end-stage kidney disease; *FSGS*, focal segmental glomerulosclerosis; *NS*, nephrotic syndrome; *SRNS*, steroid-resistant nephrotic syndrome.

TABLE 103.2 Secondary Causes of Nephrotic Syndrome

Category	Examples
Infections	Hepatitis B, hepatitis C, HIV, malaria, congenital infections (toxoplasmosis, CMV, syphilis)
Drugs/toxins	Penicillamine, NSAIDs, pamidronate, interferon, heroin, lithium, heavy metals (gold, mercury)
Malignancy	Leukemia, lymphoma
Rheumatologic disease	Systemic lupus erythematosus, IgA vasculitis (Henoch-Schönlein purpura)
Glomerular hyper-filtration	Sickle cell disease, morbid obesity

CMV, Cytomegalovirus; *HIV,* human immunodeficiency virus; *IgA,* immunoglobulin A; *NSAIDs,* nonsteroidal antiinflammatory drugs.

protein excretion greater than 40 mg/m²/hr on a 24-hour urine collection or a random ratio of urinary protein to creatinine (UPCR) greater than 2, but often 3+ proteinuria on dipstick in the presence of other laboratory findings is sufficient. Antinuclear antibody (ANA) and viral testing (human immunodeficiency virus [HIV], hepatitis B, hepatitis C) should be considered in older children or adolescents. A kidney biopsy should be performed in patients with steroid-resistant disease or in patients with findings suggestive of a condition other than MCD. Genetic testing is most useful in patients younger than 1 year at presentation, those with syndromic features, or those with a family history of nephrotic syndrome. However, genetic testing is increasingly used in children with steroid-resistant disease because if a monogenic cause is identified, immunosuppressive treatment is less likely to benefit the patient.

Approach to Therapy

The standard initial treatment for patients with presumed or biopsy-proven MCD or FSGS without an identified genetic cause is oral

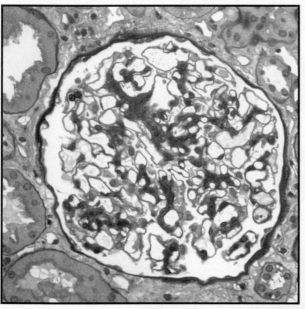

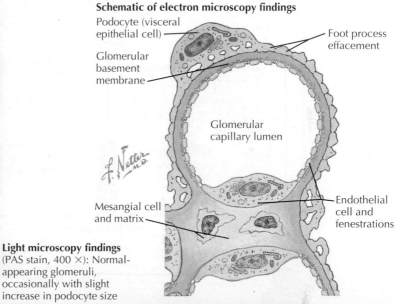

Schematic of electron microscopy findings

Podocyte (visceral epithelial cell)
Glomerular basement membrane
Glomerular capillary lumen
Foot process effacement
Endothelial cell and fenestrations
Mesangial cell and matrix

Light microscopy findings (PAS stain, 400 ×): Normal-appearing glomeruli, occasionally with slight increase in podocyte size

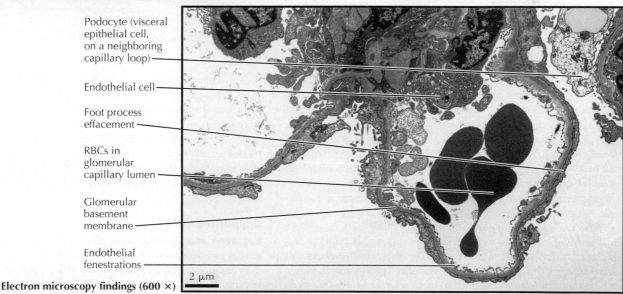

Podocyte (visceral epithelial cell, on a neighboring capillary loop)
Endothelial cell
Foot process effacement
RBCs in glomerular capillary lumen
Glomerular basement membrane
Endothelial fenestrations

2 μm

Electron microscopy findings (600 ×)

Fig. 103.1 Histopathologic Findings of Minimal Change Disease. (Micrographs reused from Landman J, Kelly CR. *The Netter Collection of Medical Illustrations. Vol. 5, Urinary System.* 2nd ed. Philadelphia, PA: Saunders; 2012.)

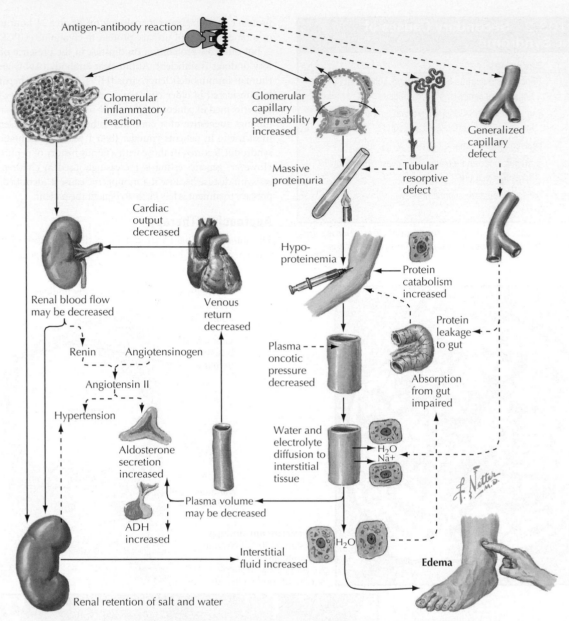

Fig. 103.2 Pathophysiologic Factors in Etiology of Nephrotic Edema. *ADH,* Antidiuretic hormone.

corticosteroid therapy: prednisone 2 mg/kg or 60 mg/m² (maximum 60 to 80 mg) daily for 4 to 6 weeks followed by 1.5 mg/kg or 40 mg/m² (maximum 40 mg) on alternate days for 4 to 6 weeks. The first morning urine sample should be monitored daily by urine dipstick. Remission is defined as 3 consecutive days of negative or trace urine protein. Approximately 95% of patients with MCD (compared with 20% to 25% of those with FSGS) will respond to prednisone within 6 weeks. Patients who do not respond are labeled as steroid resistant.

Long-term prognosis is good for patients who are responsive to steroids, but approximately 80% of patients will have at least one relapse and 50% to 60% will develop a steroid-dependent pattern (relapse while weaning steroids or within 2 weeks of stopping therapy) or frequently relapsing pattern (more than two relapses within 6 months of initial therapy or four or more relapses in any 1-year period). Home urine monitoring is recommended to catch relapses before the development of clinically apparent edema. Relapses are treated with reinitiation of 2 mg/kg or 60 mg/m² prednisone daily with variable taper once remission is achieved. For patients with frequent relapses, especially if

there are significant steroid side effects, a variety of agents are used to prevent relapses and minimize the need for steroid therapy. Options include oral cyclophosphamide, calcineurin inhibitors (cyclosporine, tacrolimus), mycophenolate mofetil (MMF), and rituximab.

Steroid-resistant patients with MCD or FSGS on biopsy are often treated with a calcineurin inhibitor along with an ACE inhibitor (ACE-I) or angiotensin II receptor blocker (ARB). Those who are refractory to treatment have a greater than 50% risk for progression to ESKD within 5 years.

Supportive Care

Regardless of underlying cause, all patients with nephrotic syndrome should receive education on a low-sodium diet (<2 g/day) to minimize fluid retention and decrease the risk for steroid-induced hypertension. Because the majority of children will have normal kidney function, additional dietary restrictions are generally not necessary. Diuretic therapy may be indicated in patients with symptomatic edema, but should be prescribed with caution in patients with evidence

TABLE 103.3	Laboratory Findings in Nephrotic Syndrome	
Laboratory Test	**Findings in Nephrotic Syndrome**	**Notes**
Urinalysis	3+ proteinuria *or* UPCR >2	
Albumin	Often <2.5 mg/L	
Lipid panel	↑ Cholesterol, ↑ triglycerides	↑ Synthesis in liver
BMP	↓ Sodium (often 120–130 mEq/L)	↑ ADH resulting from intravascular volume depletion
	↑ BUN and/or creatinine	Result of ↓ renal perfusion
	↓ Calcium	Result of ↓ albumin (ionized calcium usually normal)
CBC	↑ Hemoglobin	Hemoconcentration resulting from intravascular volume depletion
Complement levels	Normal in MCD or FSGS	Low C3 and C4 in lupus, low C3 in postinfectious glomerulonephritis or MPGN
Vitamin D 25-OH	Low because of urinary loss of vitamin D binding protein	Requires supplementation in patients with a prolonged nephrotic state

ADH, Antidiuretic hormone; *BMP,* basic metabolic panel; *BUN,* blood urea nitrogen; *CBC,* complete blood count; *FSGS,* focal segmental glomerulosclerosis; *MCD,* minimal change disease; *MPGN,* membranoproliferative glomerulonephritis.

of intravascular volume depletion. Patients may require admission to the hospital for administration of 25% intravenous albumin in conjunction with diuretic medications. Children with nephrotic syndrome should receive pneumococcal vaccination to protect against *S. pneumoniae,* as well an annual influenza vaccination. Families should be advised of the short-term side effects (gastrointestinal irritation, increased appetite, sleep, and mood disturbance) and long-term complications of glucocorticoids.

FUTURE DIRECTIONS

Increased availability of genetic testing has led to an improved understanding of the genetic contribution to nephrotic syndrome. Ongoing research attempts to integrate genetic, molecular, and clinical data to better understand the disease cause and improve therapeutic decision-making and outcome prediction. For patients with steroid-sensitive disease requiring the addition of a steroid-sparing medication, there is a need for a better understanding of which patients will respond to which classes of medication. Finally, there is a need to develop novel therapies for steroid-resistant disease to prevent or slow progression to ESKD.

SUGGESTED READINGS

Available online.

104

Hemolytic-Uremic Syndrome

Clement Lee

 CLINICAL VIGNETTE

A 5-year-old girl presents with abdominal pain, vomiting, and bloody diarrhea after returning from a family trip to a local farm. Given the inability to tolerate oral hydration, she was taken to the emergency department and discharged after being given intravenous fluids. Over the next several days, her abdominal pain and diarrhea improved, but she gradually developed periorbital and lower extremity edema. She presented to her pediatrician, who ordered laboratory studies revealing a hemoglobin of 6.0 g/dL, platelet count of 30,000/μL, and a serum creatinine of 2.2 mg/dL. Urinalysis showed 2+ blood and 3+ protein. Schistocytes were noted on a peripheral blood smear. She was admitted to the hospital for further management of hemolytic-uremic syndrome (HUS). This case highlights the vigilance clinicians must have in detecting HUS, including the need for ordering bloodwork in patients with a history of bloody diarrhea. During admission, the patient requires close monitoring of fluids and electrolytes and potential renal replacement therapy.

Hemolytic-uremic syndrome (HUS) describes the constellation of microangiopathic hemolytic anemia, thrombocytopenia, and acute kidney injury (AKI). HUS is primarily seen in children; while the overall annual incidence of the condition is 1 to 2 cases per 100,000, the incidence in children under 5 years is 6 cases per 100,000. Since Conrad von Gasser's initial description of five children with HUS in 1955, it has become increasingly evident that the syndrome can be caused by several conditions that converge in the final expression of the clinical triad of anemia, thrombocytopenia, and AKI. Research has linked the disease to many genetic defects of the complement system and has deepened our comprehension of HUS.

ETIOLOGY AND PATHOGENESIS

The pathologic correlate of HUS is thrombotic microangiopathy (TMA), characterized by fibrin and platelet thrombi deposition in the small vessels of organs, most notably in the kidney (Fig. 104.1). This leads to capillary damage and splitting of the glomerular basement membrane with double-contouring of the capillary walls on light microscopy. Cortical necrosis can be seen in severe cases associated with chronic kidney disease. Kidney injury can result in endothelial swelling and laminar proliferation with intimal thickening, muscular hypertrophy ("onion skin" appearance), and subsequent luminal narrowing. Trapped erythrocytes are seen inside fibrin thrombi, fragmented as a result of mechanical hemolysis. These sheared erythrocytes are also evident on blood smears. Finally, mesangial involvement may lead to hypercellularity, mesangiolysis, and, with chronic injury, sclerosis. Notably, there is an absence of immune complexes on electron microscopy. Besides the kidney, other affected organs can include the brain, pancreas, heart, lungs, and gastrointestinal tract.

HUS results from various processes affecting the interaction between endothelial cells and platelets. Classically, these diseases have been classified as typical (with diarrheal prodrome, or D+, as shown in the case vignette) or atypical (without diarrheal prodrome, or D–). HUS can also be categorized as infection-induced, hereditary, or secondary to coexisting diseases.

Infection-Induced Hemolytic-Uremic Syndrome

Infections can lead to HUS through many pathways. Most frequent and well-known, accounting for 85% to 90% of the syndrome, is Shiga toxin–producing *Escherichia coli* (STEC). Shiga toxin (Stx) is also known as verotoxin, named after its ability to lyse Vero cells, a lineage of primate kidney epithelial cells. Accordingly, the virulence of Shiga toxin stems from its predilection for destroying cells lining the kidney (Fig. 104.2). Older children and adults may develop antibodies against Shiga toxin, possibly explaining proclivity for the disease in young children who are less protected.

Several bacteria produce Shiga toxin, including *Escherichia coli* serotypes O157:H7 and O26:H11, as well as *Shigella dysenteriae* type 1. Historically, O157:H7 caused most cases of HUS worldwide, though non-O157 STEC now causes as many cases as O157:H7 in North America and Europe. O157:H7 still predominates in Latin America, where HUS is endemic, with up to 17 cases per 100,000 children annually. *S. dysenteriae* type 1 primarily affects resource-limited countries in Asia, South America, and Africa and is associated with a more fulminant course and chronic kidney disease. HUS develops in 5% to 10% of patients with sporadic STEC-gastroenteritis and the incidence can increase to 20% in the setting of outbreaks.

Shiga toxin–producing bacteria are transmitted through contact with food, animals, or humans. With O157:H7, foodborne illness is most prevalent, traditionally through undercooked ground beef, though cases involving unpasteurized dairy, fresh produce, poultry, pork, nuts, and contaminated water or apple juice have all been described. Cattle serve as reservoirs for STEC and shed the bacteria into feces, explaining the increased prevalence of HUS in rural areas. Shedding patterns in cattle are complex, influenced by the environment, lactation, farm management, and animal health, and culminates in high rates of shedding in summer months, correlating with the summer and early fall peaks of HUS. With non-O157:H7 STEC, person-to-person transmission is most common. Of note, most cases of HUS are sporadic, not linked to any outbreak.

Infection with *Streptococcus pneumoniae* can also lead to endothelial cell injury, accounting for 5% of HUS. The mechanism of injury is not fully elucidated, but studies have shown that *S. pneumoniae* surface proteins Tuf and PspC bind human plasminogen, generating

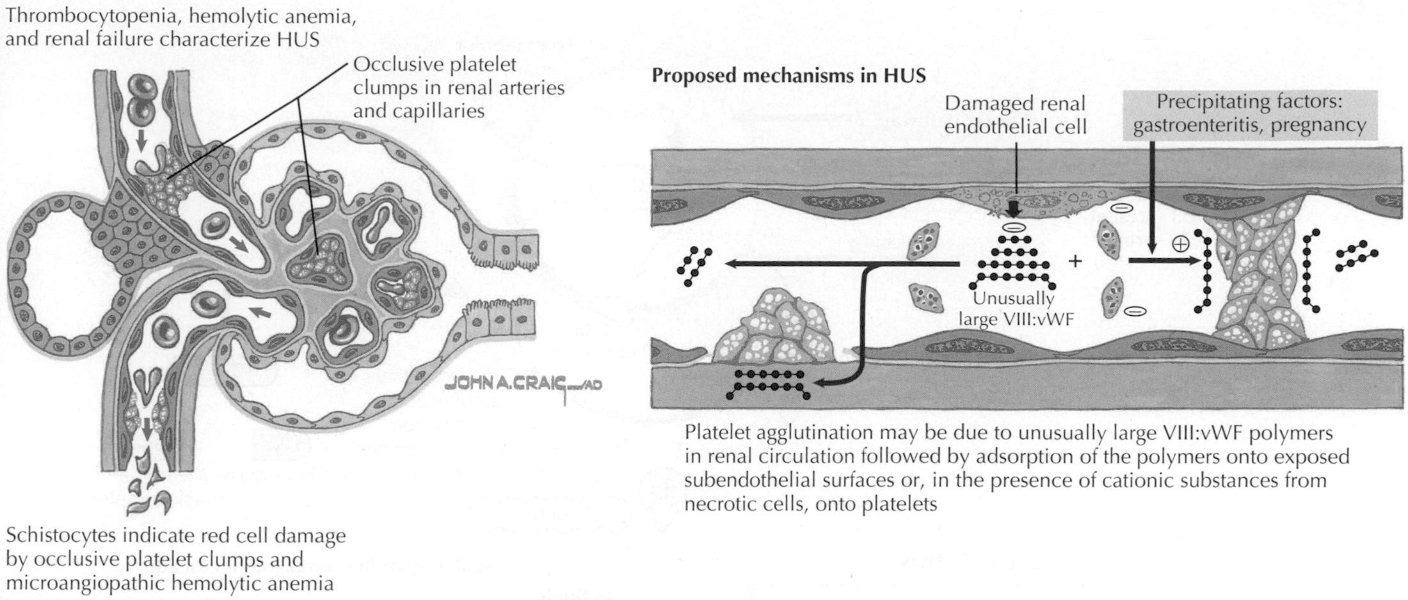

Thrombocytopenia, hemolytic anemia, and renal failure characterize HUS

Occlusive platelet clumps in renal arteries and capillaries

JOHN A. CRAIG—MD

Schistocytes indicate red cell damage by occlusive platelet clumps and microangiopathic hemolytic anemia

Proposed mechanisms in HUS

Damaged renal endothelial cell

Precipitating factors: gastroenteritis, pregnancy

Unusually large VIII:vWF

Platelet agglutination may be due to unusually large VIII:vWF polymers in renal circulation followed by adsorption of the polymers onto exposed subendothelial surfaces or, in the presence of cationic substances from necrotic cells, onto platelets

Fig. 104.1 Proposed Mechanisms in Hemolytic-Uremic Syndrome.

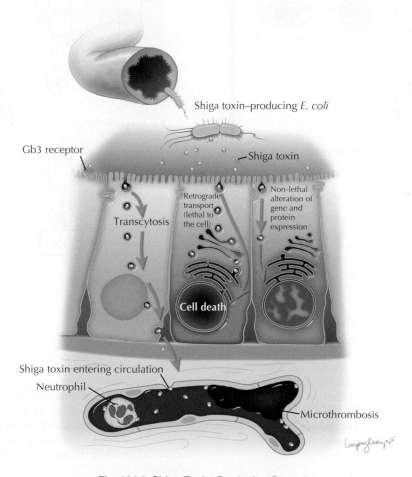

Shiga toxin–producing *E. coli*

Gb3 receptor

Shiga toxin

Transcytosis

Retrograde transport (lethal to the cell)

Non-lethal alteration of gene and protein expression

Cell death

Shiga toxin entering circulation

Neutrophil

Microthrombosis

Fig. 104.2 Shiga Toxin–Producing Bacteria.

plasmin and activating thrombogenesis in the endothelium. In some patients, *S. pneumoniae* infection can activate the complement cascade similar to certain genetic forms of HUS. Older hypotheses involved the exposure of Thomsen-Friedenreich antigen (TA), though detection of this antigen turned out to be neither sensitive nor specific for pneumococcal-associated HUS. Most cases of pneumococcal-associated HUS present as pneumonia, with pericardial effusion and meningitis being less common triggers. There have also been reports of HUS associated with influenza H1N1, though this may reflect an associated secondary pneumococcal pneumonia after influenza infection.

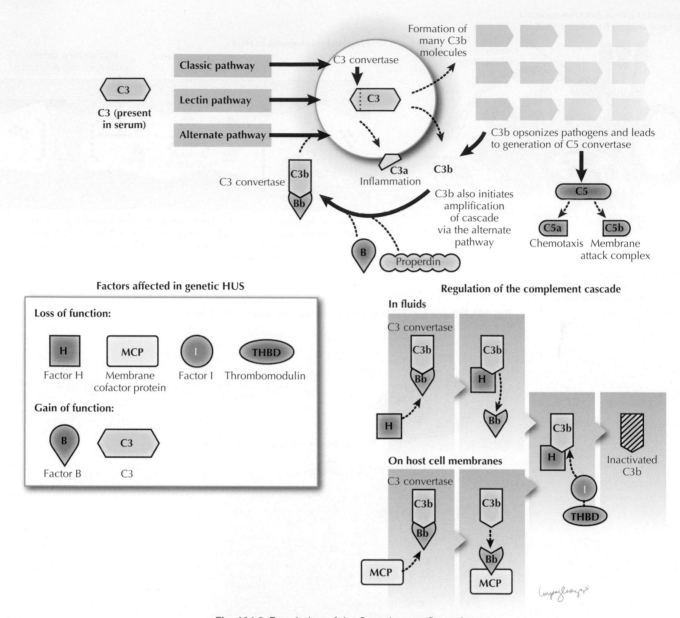

Fig. 104.3 Regulation of the Complement Cascade.

Human immunodeficiency virus (HIV) is another infection reported to cause HUS. Multiple factors in HIV-infected patients can contribute to endothelial cell damage, including medications, opportunistic infections, and HIV-associated malignancies. Furthermore, the HIV-specific p24 antigen has been isolated from the epithelial cells of a patient with HIV-associated TMA, suggesting direct viral cytotoxicity. Histologically, HIV-associated TMA is notable for a striking paucity of inflammation and increased epithelial cell apoptosis. HUS related to HIV has decreased in incidence after the introduction of antiretroviral therapies.

Hereditary Hemolytic-Uremic Syndrome

The genetic forms of HUS mainly involve defects in the complement cascade, coagulation pathway, or cobalamin metabolism. These mutations account for fewer than 10% of all cases of HUS, with diarrhea-positive cases remaining the most common. The most commonly identified genetic causes of hereditary HUS (atypical HUS) are mutations in the complement cascade, accounting for up to 60%

of non-STEC disease. These include mutations in complement factors B, H, and I (*CFB, CFH,* and *CFI*), membrane cofactor protein (*MCP*), thrombomodulin (*THBD*), and C3 (Fig. 104.3). *CFH* mutations are most commonly identified and may be associated with a low C3 concentration. In a normal endothelial cell, all of the factors work together to prevent membrane attack complex (MAC) formation; CFH and MCP bind to C3b to allow cleavage by CFI, enhanced by THBD. This prevents C3b from binding to CFB and forming C3 convertase and eventually the MAC. Gain- or loss-of-function mutations anywhere along the pathway can lead to abnormal complement activation.

DGKE mutations (encoding diacylglycerol kinase ε) can account for up to 27% of non-STEC HUS presenting before the age of 1 year. Affected individuals present during infancy and demonstrate persistent hypertension leading to chronic kidney disease. DGKE normally inactivates diacylglycerols that participate in the thrombosis cascade, so it is hypothesized that *DGKE* mutations lead to HUS through the abnormal promotion of thrombosis.

Intravascular coagulation, hemolytic-uremic syndrome, and thrombotic microangiopathy

Common electron microscopic findings: Deposits (D) and mesangial cell cytoplasmic processes (M) in the subendothelial space; endothelium (E) swollen; both mesangial (MC) and endothelial cells (EN) contain many vacuoles and dilated rough endoplasmic reticulum; lumen (L) narrowed (may be slit-like); red blood cells (RC) may or may not be present; basement membrane (B) often wrinkled; epithelial foot processes (F) partly fused

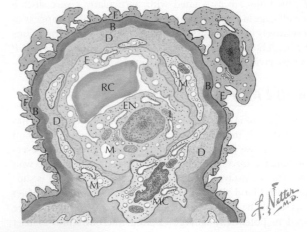

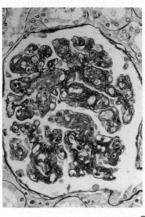

◀ Glomerulus showing thickening of capillary walls and partial capillary collapse (PAS stain, ×160)

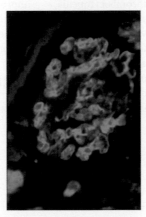

▶ Fibrinogen deposition along capillary walls of glomerulus (immuno-fluorescent preparation, tagged anti-fibrinogen serum, ×100)

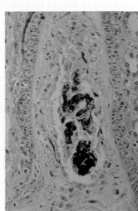

▶ **Small artery in kidney obstructed by fibrin thrombus.** (stained purple) (phosphotungstic acid, hematoxylin stain, ×100)

Fig. 104.4 Microangiopathic Hemolytic Anemia and Thrombotic Microangiopathy.

A third major category of genetic HUS is cobalamin C–related disease resulting from mutations in *MMACHC*. This manifests as abnormal vitamin B_{12} metabolism, organic aciduria, homocystinuria, neurocognitive symptoms, and HUS.

Secondary Hemolytic-Uremic Syndrome

HUS can occur in association with many systemic illnesses, including bone marrow and solid organ transplantation, adenocarcinomas, autoimmune disorders (e.g., systemic lupus erythematosus), medications (e.g., calcineurin inhibitors), malignant hypertension, and pregnancy. A complete discussion of these rare forms of HUS is beyond the scope of this chapter.

CLINICAL PRESENTATION

The classic presentation of Shiga toxin–associated HUS is bloody diarrhea followed by the sudden onset of irritability, pallor, oliguria, edema, and frank hematuria 1 to 2 weeks later. In pneumococcal-associated disease, these symptoms may be preceded by a respiratory illness instead. Genetic cases may manifest without diarrhea but are often triggered by illness. Patients with hereditary disease can, however, still present with gastrointestinal symptoms. The presentation of nondiarrheal disease is often more insidious and nonspecific.

Hematologic manifestations of HUS include thrombocytopenia, Coombs-negative hemolytic anemia, and schistocytes on peripheral blood smear. Biopsy is rarely indicated but shows thrombotic microangiopathy (Fig. 104.4). Markers of hemolysis may be elevated, including lactate dehydrogenase, reticulocytes, aspartate aminotransferase, and unconjugated bilirubin. Haptoglobin is expectedly low. In most cases,

there is no active bleeding, and coagulation study results are within normal limits. The ADAMTS13 level may be low, but not as low as in thrombotic thrombocytopenic purpura, in which its activity is less than 10%. There is no correlation between the severity of thrombocytopenia and kidney injury of HUS, and the hematologic abnormalities often precede kidney damage.

Kidney manifestations of HUS can range from mild kidney injury to anuric kidney failure. Microscopic or macroscopic hematuria is seen, occasionally with red blood cell casts. Hyperkalemia as a result of kidney failure may be insidious because of initial hypokalemia from gastrointestinal losses in the cases of diarrhea-associated disease. Hypertension often occurs and is rarely accompanied by hypertensive emergency. Because blood transfusions are often required as supportive care for anemia and thrombocytopenia, oliguric patients tend to become edematous, with potential congestive heart failure and pulmonary vascular congestion. Up to 50% of children will require renal replacement therapy (RRT), though fewer than 25% sustain long-term kidney sequelae from the disease.

Other manifestations of HUS include pancreatitis, cholecystitis, thrombosis, toxic megacolon or colonic necrosis, seizures, purpura fulminans, acute respiratory distress syndrome (ARDS), and hearing loss. Purtscher retinopathy is a rare complication of HUS and complement activation leading to acute vision loss. Pneumococcal-associated HUS is marked by a longer period of thrombocytopenia, higher requirement for RRT and for a longer duration, and worse long-term kidney function and survival. Interestingly, Coombs testing has been reported to be positive in the majority of pneumococcal-associated cases. Genetic HUS is associated with common relapses during illness, as well as graft failure after kidney transplantation. Specifically, *CFB* and *CFH* mutations are associated with particularly severe disease leading to end-stage kidney disease, whereas *MCP* mutations appear to portend a relatively benign course. Similarly, *CFB* and *CFH* mutations tend to have high rates of relapse after kidney transplant, whereas *MCP* mutations have favorable transplant outcomes.

EVALUATION AND MANAGEMENT

Early identification of HUS is crucial because prompt intervention has been associated with improved outcomes. Early volume expansion with intravenous fluids is potentially linked to decreased disease severity, though fluid overload should be avoided, especially in patients who are oliguric. The mainstay of typical Shiga toxin–related HUS is supportive care with blood transfusions and fluid management. Platelet transfusions should be used sparingly, because circulating platelets are hypothesized to potentially enlarge existing microthrombi. Platelet transfusions should be limited to those with severe thrombocytopenia, patients with active bleeding, and prophylaxis for invasive procedures.

Antibiotics are discouraged because they have been linked to increased toxin production. Exceptions include patients with concern for sepsis and with invasive *S. pneumoniae*. In patients with mutations in the complement cascade, eculizumab is an option for therapy. Eculizumab is a humanized monoclonal immunoglobulin G that inhibits complement formation by binding to complement protein C5. Because of its effect on the complement system, patients receiving eculizumab therapy must be vaccinated against meningococcus and continued on antibiotic prophylaxis while on therapy. There is some evidence that the therapy even benefits patients with atypical HUS without known complement mutations. In the rare case of anti-CFH antibodies leading to HUS, plasma exchange and immunosuppression may be trialed. Finally, kidney transplant was historically a more commonly employed treatment modality for HUS. With the advent of targeted genetic testing, it is now clear that certain genes confer a higher risk of relapse after transplant (e.g. *CFH, C3, CFB*), so this must be weighed in decision-making.

FUTURE DIRECTIONS

Advances in the understanding of complement pathways and associated disease will lead to novel complement-targeted therapies to improve outcomes for patients with refractory disease. In patients with infection-related HUS, research is needed to determine which patients will need targeted therapies to prevent the need for RRT and multisystem organ dysfunction.

SUGGESTED READINGS

Available online.

105

Acute Kidney Injury and Chronic Kidney Disease

Leonela Villegas, Olivera Marsenic Couloures, and H. Jorge Baluarte

 CLINICAL VIGNETTE

A previously healthy 2-year-old boy presents to the emergency department with a 5-day history of bloody diarrhea, fatigue, and decreased oral intake. The frequency of his stools have decreased in the past 24 hours, but he has had three episodes of emesis. Parents report that he has been having fewer wet diapers, but difficult to discern from his stools. He does not take any medications. New exposures include a visit to a petting zoo 1 week ago. On initial evaluation, he is febrile, tachycardic, and hypotensive (80/40 mm Hg). His weight is 11 kg, although he was 12 kg at his pediatrician visit last week. Examination was notable for a thin, tired-appearing boy, tacky mucous membranes, and normal respiratory and abdominal examination, with no signs of edema. Initial laboratory test results showed hemoglobin of 14.6 g/dL, platelet count of 250,000, blood urea nitrogen of 40 mg/dL, serum creatinine of 1.2 mg/dL, and normal liver enzymes. Urinalysis showed granular casts, 1+ protein, 1+ blood, and specific gravity greater than 1.030. Based on his initial physical examination and vitals, he has clinical signs of dehydration and requires initial resuscitation with isotonic fluids. Further workup includes inpatient monitoring of kidney function, hemoglobin, platelets, complement levels, stool studies, and a renal bladder ultrasound.

ACUTE KIDNEY INJURY

Acute kidney injury (AKI), previously referred to as acute renal failure, is defined as an abrupt reduction in kidney function diagnosed by a decline in glomerular filtration rate (GFR) or urine output. AKI is characterized by a disturbance of renal physiologic functions, including reduced excretion of nitrogenous waste products, dysregulation of electrolytes, and disruption of fluid homeostasis. The incidence and prevalence of AKI in children depends on the study population and the staging and definition of AKI. The overall incidence of AKI is rising because of advances in pediatric medical technology such as bone marrow and solid organ transplantation, corrective surgeries for congenital heart disease, and in the care of neonates with very low birth weight.

Etiology and Pathogenesis

The causes of AKI can be related to any process that interferes with the structure or function of the glomeruli, renal tubules, interstitium, vasculature, or urinary tract. The causes of AKI are typically categorized as prerenal, intrarenal, and postrenal.

Prerenal

Prerenal AKI results from either volume depletion or decreased effective blood volume, which precipitates a reduction in renal perfusion. Volume depletion causes include bleeding (surgery), gastrointestinal (vomiting, diarrhea), urinary (diuretics, diabetes insipidus), and cutaneous losses (burns). Decreased effective blood volume can be seen in cases of decreased cardiac output (heart failure, cardiac tamponade) or decreased intravascular volume (shock, sepsis). In prerenal AKI, the kidneys are intrinsically normal, and it is reversible after renal blood flow is restored by correcting the underlying disturbance. However, prolonged prerenal injury results in intrarenal AKI.

Intrarenal

Intrarenal AKI is the result of disorders that involve the renal vascular, glomerular, or tubular–interstitial compartments. The most common cause is acute tubular necrosis (ATN) that results from prolonged ischemia caused by decreased renal perfusion or injury from tubular nephrotoxins (Fig. 105.1). All causes of prerenal AKI can progress to ATN if renal perfusion is not restored or nephrotoxins are not withdrawn.

Nephrotoxic AKI is mostly caused by toxic tubular injury by medications, including aminoglycosides, contrast agents, amphotericin B, chemotherapeutic agents (ifosfamide, cisplatin), and antivirals. Toxic tubular injury also can be induced by the release of heme pigments, as occurs from myoglobinuria caused by rhabdomyolysis and hemoglobinuria caused by intravascular hemolysis. Uric acid nephropathy and tumor lysis syndrome (TLS) are causes of AKI in children with newly diagnosed cancer. During chemotherapy, a rapid breakdown of tumor cells causes increased release and subsequent excretion of uric acid, resulting in precipitation of uric acid crystals in the tubules and renal microvasculature. Hyperphosphatemia in TLS results in precipitation of calcium phosphate crystals in the tubules.

Acute interstitial nephritis most commonly results from hypersensitivity reactions to drugs, including penicillin analogs (e.g., methicillin), cimetidine, sulfonamides, rifampin, nonsteroidal antiinflammatory drugs, and proton pump inhibitors but can also be idiopathic. Glomerulonephritis of any cause (including those caused by vasculitis, systemic lupus erythematosus, or anti–glomerular basement membrane disease) may manifest with AKI, with postinfectious glomerulonephritis being the most common cause of AKI in this group. Rapidly progressive glomerulonephritis manifests as the most severe degree of any form of glomerulonephritis. Vascular causes of AKI include cortical necrosis (mostly caused by hypoxic or ischemic injury in newborns), renal artery or vein thrombosis, and hemolytic-uremic syndrome (HUS).

Postrenal

Postrenal AKI is caused by bilateral urinary tract obstruction or unilateral obstruction of a solitary kidney. Examples of congenital disorders causing obstruction and AKI are posterior urethral valves (PUVs), bilateral ureteropelvic junction obstruction, and bilateral ureteroceles. Examples of acquired causes of obstruction and AKI include kidney stones, clots, urethral pathologic conditions, and tumors.

Clinical Presentation

A careful history and physical examination can frequently identify the underlying etiology for AKI.

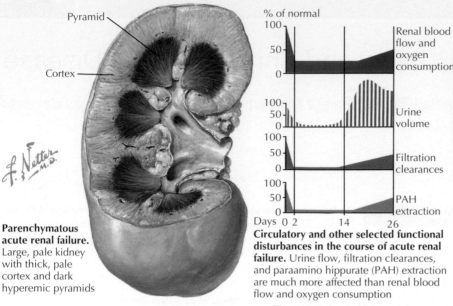

Parenchymatous acute renal failure. Large, pale kidney with thick, pale cortex and dark hyperemic pyramids

Circulatory and other selected functional disturbances in the course of acute renal failure. Urine flow, filtration clearances, and paraamino hippurate (PAH) extraction are much more affected than renal blood flow and oxygen consumption

Biopsy section. Glomerulus normal; distal convoluted tubules dilated, with flattened epithelium, "pretzel-like" distortion, and containing heme casts (H and E stain)

Fig. 105.1 Acute Kidney Injury.

- Vital signs, specifically heart rate and blood pressure, are important in determining a patient's volume status: hypovolemic, euvolemic, or hypervolemic.
- Physical examination findings can help narrow the differential diagnosis. An AKI from prerenal causes or ATN can be depicted by dry mucous membranes, sunken eyes, and decreased skin turgor.
- A history of vomiting, diarrhea, hemorrhage, or decreased oral intake resulting in hypovolemia associated with decreased urine output can be associated with prerenal AKI or ATN.
- Nephrotic syndrome, heart failure, and liver failure can cause prerenal AKI because of a decrease in effective intravascular volume present with edema.
- In the hospital, a history of hypotension (caused by sepsis or intraoperative events), administration of nephrotoxic agents, or recent use of chemotherapy may cause AKI.
- History of the use of medications that are known to cause a hypersensitivity reaction, together with a rash, fever, and arthralgias, suggests AKI caused by acute interstitial nephritis.
- Clinical presentation that includes hypertension, edema, and gross hematuria is likely caused by AKI attributable to a glomerulonephritis. A history of pharyngitis or impetigo a few weeks before the onset of gross hematuria suggests post-infectious glomerulonephritis.
- History of bloody diarrhea and pallor and petechiae on physical examination are associated with HUS.
- Skin findings, such as purpura, malar rash, or petechiae or joint pain favor a diagnosis of vasculitis, such as systemic lupus erythematosus or Henoch-Schönlein purpura.
- Anuria or oliguria in a newborn suggests a congenital malformation (i.e., PUVs) or bilateral renal venous thrombosis.

Evaluation and Management

In addition to a thorough history and physical examination, the initial evaluation includes laboratory studies. AKI is diagnosed by an increase in serum creatinine concentration, which implies a decrease in the GFR. However, the serum creatinine concentration is insensitive and a delayed measure of decreased kidney function after an acute insult. Creatinine is dependent on muscle mass and can be affected by medications (sulfamethoxazole-trimethoprim, cimetidine, and

tyrosine kinase inhibitors). Research biomarkers that may detect AKI earlier include neutrophil gelatinase-associated lipocalin (NGAL), interleukin-18, and kidney injury molecule-1 (KIM-1). A standardized classification of AKI has evolved culminating in the development of the Kidney Disease: Improving Global Outcomes (KDIGO) classification system.

Urine Studies

Urinalysis is an important noninvasive test in the diagnostic evaluation because characteristic findings on microscopic examination of the urine sediment strongly suggest certain diagnoses. A normal or near-normal urinalysis result, characterized by few cells with no casts or proteinuria, suggests prerenal disease or urinary tract obstruction. Muddy brown granular casts and epithelial cell casts are highly suggestive of ATN. The finding of red blood cell (RBC) casts is diagnostic of glomerulonephritis, and heavy proteinuria is indicative of glomerular disease, both suggesting AKI caused by glomerulonephritis. The presence of pyuria with white blood cell (WBC), granular, or waxy casts is suggestive of tubular or interstitial disease or urinary tract infection. The urine specific gravity can help differentiate between early stages of ATN given loss of concentrating ability and concentrated urine in the setting of prerenal disease.

Measurement of the urine sodium concentration is helpful in distinguishing ATN (urine sodium >40 mEq/L) from prerenal AKI (urine sodium <20 mEq/L). In ATN, there is tubular damage impairing maximal reabsorption of sodium. Meanwhile, the kidney is actively retaining sodium in an effort to sustain an effective circulating volume in prerenal AKI. To note, urinary sodium levels are affected by diuretics and saline-containing intravenous fluids.

The fractional excretion of sodium (FENa) is a direct measurement of renal tubular handling of filtered sodium and eliminates the effect of variations in urine volume on Na excretion in AKI. It can help differentiate between prerenal AKI and ATN in children as follows:

$$FENa = \left[\frac{(U_{Na} \times P_{Cr})}{P_{Na} \times U_{Cr}} \right] \times 100$$

U_{Cr} and P_{Cr} are the urine and serum creatinine concentrations, respectively.

- Maintenance of electrolyte and fluid balance
- Adequate nutritional support
- Avoidance of life-threatening complications
- Treatment of the underlying cause

U_{Na} and P_{Na} are the urine and serum sodium concentrations, respectively.

- Less than 1% suggests prerenal disease.
- A value of 1% to 2% can be attributable to either disorder.
- Greater than 2% indicates ATN.

Fractional excretion of urea (FEUrea) is a diagnostic tool to allow measurement of a filtered molecule (i.e., urea) without being affected by diuretics. Patients with prerenal AKI typically have an FEUrea less than 35% and ATN has an FEUrea greater than 50%. The test is limited by institution and availability.

AKI can manifest with decreased (oliguria), absent (anuria), normal, or increased (nonoliguric) urine output. The urine output is classically low in prerenal AKI because of the combination of sodium and water avidity. Oliguria is defined as urine output less than 500 mL/24 h in older children, less than 0.5 mL/kg/h in younger children, and less than 1 mL/kg/h in infants. Oliguria or anuria is likely to occur in AKI because of hypoxic/ischemic insults, HUS, glomerulonephritis or urinary tract obstruction. Nonoliguric AKI is commonly associated with acute interstitial nephritis and nephrotoxic renal insults.

Serologic and Biochemical Abnormalities

Hyperkalemia and hyperphosphatemia occur in AKI because of the decreased renal excretion. Hypocalcemia can occur secondary to hyperphosphatemia and decreased calcium absorption in the gastrointestinal tract because of inadequate renal production of 1,25-vitamin D. Elevated phosphorus and potassium levels with associated hypocalcemia can also occur with TLS. Acidosis seen in AKI results from decreased urinary excretion of hydrogen ions.

A compete blood count is helpful to determine if there is hemoconcentration in the setting of hypovolemia. Microangiopathic hemolytic anemia associated with thrombocytopenia in the setting of AKI confirms the diagnosis of HUS. Severe hemolysis, whether drug induced or secondary to hemoglobinopathies, may also result in ATN caused by massive hemoglobinuria. Eosinophilia may be associated with interstitial nephritis caused by a hypersensitivity reaction.

Additional Studies

Renal ultrasonography should be considered in children with AKI. It can document the presence of one or two kidneys, determine renal size (often enlarged in those with AKI), assess the renal parenchyma, and diagnose urinary tract obstruction or occlusion of the major renal vessels. A renal biopsy is performed if diagnosis cannot be established by other noninvasive tests or if the initial presentation is suggestive of rapidly progressive glomerulonephritis.

Management

Despite extensive research, there are no validated medications to prevent or treat AKI. Hence, the basic principles of management include supportive measures while addressing fluid balance and electrolyte abnormalities (Box 105.1). General measures to help prevent AKI include close monitoring of serum levels of nephrotoxic drugs, adequate fluid repletion in patients with hypovolemia, and hydration before chemotherapy. Unless contraindicated, a child with a history of fluid loss (vomiting and diarrhea), a physical examination consistent with hypovolemia (hypotension and tachycardia), or oliguria requires immediate intravenous fluid therapy in an attempt to restore renal function and prevent ischemic renal injury. Commonly used fluids are crystalloid solutions, such as normal saline (20 mL/kg) administered over 20 to 30 minutes, which may be repeated as clinically indicated. If urine output does not increase and renal function fails to improve, invasive monitoring may be required to adequately assess the child's fluid status and help guide further therapy.

Hyperkalemia is a life-threatening complication of AKI that may result in a fatal cardiac arrhythmia. For cardiac cell membrane stabilization, an intravenous infusion of calcium is used, which decreases the risk for arrhythmias. Hyperkalemia can be treated by shifting potassium from the intravascular to the intracellular space using intravenous glucose and insulin, β-agonists (albuterol), and bicarbonate. Other methods of removing potassium include diuretics, enteric exchange resins (i.e., polystyrene sulfonate), and renal replacement therapy (RRT).

Acid (H^+) generated by diet and intermediary metabolism is excreted by the kidney. In AKI, acid excretion is decreased, resulting in metabolic acidosis. Acidosis can be treated with intravenous or oral sodium bicarbonate or oral sodium citrate solutions.

Given that the kidney plays a major role in phosphorus regulation, it can be disrupted in patients with kidney injury leading to hyperphosphatemia. It is treated with dietary phosphorus restriction and phosphorus binders. These agents bind phosphorus in the gastrointestinal system and prevent absorption. A complication from hyperphosphatemia and decreased production of 1,25-vitamin D is hypocalcemia. In the setting of acidosis, less calcium is bound to albumin, and more calcium is free in its ionized form. With the use of bicarbonate therapy for correction of acidosis or hyperkalemia, more calcium binds to albumin, and there is less free ionized calcium, which may exacerbate the degree of hypocalcemia. Therefore, if hypocalcemia is severe or bicarbonate therapy is necessary, intravenous calcium gluconate or calcium chloride should be given.

Hypertension in AKI may be related to volume overload or alterations in vascular tone (i.e., renin-mediated). Volume-mediated initial therapy with a diuretic can be attempted depending on the clinical scenario. If unable to use diuretics, fluid removal with dialysis or hemofiltration may be required. For severe hypertension, intravenous infusion therapies with nicardipine, labetalol, or sodium nitroprusside are indicated. After the blood pressure has been appropriately controlled, oral long-acting agents can be initiated. Angiotensin-converting enzyme inhibitors (ACEIs) and angiotensin receptor blockers (ARBs) should be used with caution in AKI because they reduce intraglomerular filtration pressure and cause potassium retention.

AKI can be associated with severe anorexia and subsequent malnutrition. Proper nutrition is essential in the management of children with AKI. At a minimum, daily maintenance calories should be provided, although calorie needs may be higher because of a catabolic state. If the gastrointestinal tract is intact and functional, enteral feedings with formula should be instituted in children as soon as possible. Based on electrolyte abnormalities and trajectory of renal function, substitution with a lower phosphorus/potassium diet may be used. If unable to feed enterally, parenteral nutrition may be necessary.

RRT in children with AKI should be initiated for the indications listed in Box 105.2. Three dialysis modalities are available: peritoneal dialysis (PD), hemodialysis (HD), and continuous renal replacement therapy (CRRT). The choice of modality is influenced by the clinical presentation of the child, the availability of vascular access, adequacy of the peritoneal membrane (necessary for PD), presence or absence of multiorgan failure, and the overall goal of the dialysis. For example,

---

BOX 105.2 **Initiation of Renal Replacement Therapy**

- Signs and symptoms of uremia
  - Pericarditis, altered mental status, vomiting, peripheral neuropathy, platelet dysfunction
- Severe fluid overload state
  - Hypertension
  - Pulmonary edema
  - Heart failure
- Severe electrolyte abnormalities (that are refractory to supportive medical therapy)
  - Hyperkalemia
  - Acidosis
  - Hypocalcemia secondary to refractory hyperphosphatemia
  - Intoxication (e.g., salicylate, ethylene glycol, methanol)
  - Inborn errors of metabolism (e.g., hyperammonemia)
  - Need for intensive nutritional support in a child with oliguria/anuria

---

HD is most efficient in rapid correction of electrolyte and other solute abnormalities and CRRT is appropriate for hemodynamically unstable patients.

Future Directions

Several biomarkers of AKI (cystatin C, NGAL, interleukin-18, KIM-1) have been identified, but the utility of these biomarkers is largely confined to research studies, whereas widespread clinical applicability is limited.

CHRONIC KIDNEY DISEASE

Chronic kidney disease (CKD) is defined as the presence of kidney damage, either structural or functional, or by a decline in GFR less than 60 mL/min/1.73 m^2 that is present for longer than 3 months. The term CKD has replaced the clinical terms of chronic renal failure and chronic renal insufficiency. The stages of CKD for children are based on estimated GFR and are aimed at promoting early detection and treatment of CKD.

The annual incidence and prevalence of CKD is challenging to estimate given limited data. However, there are population-based studies that show an estimated 11.9 cases per million of age-related population of children with stage 3 to 5 CKD in Europe and 2.8 to 15.8 cases per million in Latin America. The annual incidence and prevalence in end-stage renal disease (ESRD) is reported as less than 4 to 14.8 per million children in different countries. The variability in the worldwide incidence of CKD is thought to be affected by genetic and environmental factors, as well as the ability to detect CKD and provide care to children with significant renal impairment. In North America, the incidence of CKD is greater in African American than White children. The incidence and prevalence of CKD are greater in boys than girls because of the higher incidence of congenital anomalies of the kidney and urinary tract, including obstructive uropathy, renal dysplasia, renal hypoplasia, and prune belly syndrome, in boys.

Etiology and Pathogenesis

Based on the registry of the North American Pediatric Renal Trials and Collaborative Studies (NAPRTCS), the causes of CKD are as follows:

- Congenital renal anomalies are present in 57% of cases (obstructive uropathy, renal aplasia, hypoplasia, or dysplasia, reflux nephropathy, and polycystic kidney disease)

- Glomerular disease is present in 17% of cases, with focal segmental glomerulosclerosis (FSGS) being the most common glomerular disorder (9% of all CKD cases; African American children are three times more likely to develop FSGS than White children).
- Other causes accounted for 25% of cases and included hemolytic uremic syndrome, genetic disorders (e.g., cystinosis, oxalosis, hereditary nephritis), and interstitial nephritis.
- In a large number of cases (18%), the primary disease is unknown because patients present in late stages of CKD. Unlike in adults, diabetic nephropathy and hypertension are rare causes of CKD in children (Fig. 105.2).

After initial injury to the kidney, there is continued progression of renal disease and functional impairment that can lead to stage 5 CKD. This can be a result of repeated, chronic insults to the renal parenchyma leading to permanent damage or to the adaptive hyperfiltration response of the remaining nephrons in the kidney compensating for the loss of nephrons from the initial injury. Over time, the enhanced transglomerular ultrafiltration and glomerular pressure leads to glomerular damage and leakage of protein, resulting in interstitial inflammation and fibrosis. The rate of progression of CKD is usually greatest during the two periods of rapid growth, infancy and puberty, when the sudden increase in body mass results in an increase in the filtration demands of the remaining nephrons. Other factors associated with acceleration of the progressive CKD include hypertension, obesity, dyslipidemia, proteinuria, anemia, intrarenal precipitation of calcium and phosphate, metabolic acidosis, and tubular interstitial disease. Some of these factors are modifiable, and timely therapeutic interventions may result in a reduced rate of deterioration of renal function.

Clinical Presentation

The clinical presentation of CKD depends on the severity of renal disease and the underlying disorder. Stage 1 and 2 CKD are usually asymptomatic. As CKD progresses, patients begin to exhibit clinical features, with growth impairment being the most common. Other signs and symptoms of CKD include changes to urine output (polyuria or oliguria), edema, hypertension, proteinuria, and hematuria. Polyuria may be an early presenting symptom as congenital anomalies of the kidney and urinary tract (e.g., obstructive uropathy), inherited disorders (e.g., nephronophthisis), and tubulointerstitial disorders caused by impairment in renal concentrating ability, which generally precedes a significant reduction in GFR. More severe symptoms and signs of CKD begin to appear with stage 3 disease and worsen with stages 4 and 5.

A moderate to severe loss of GFR (stages 3 to 5 of disease) is associated with a number of complications resulting in disorders of fluid and electrolytes, acid-base homeostasis, metabolic bone disease, anemia, hypertension, endocrine abnormalities, and growth retardation.

- Normal kidneys can adapt to a wide range of sodium and water intake, and these homeostatic mechanisms are usually maintained until the GFR decreases to advanced stages of CKD. Fluid abnormalities result in fluid retention and hypertension (particularly with glomerular diseases) or dehydration and hyponatremia (caused by polyuria with decreased renal-concentrating ability in nephronophthisis, congenital renal disorders, and obstructive uropathy).
- Hyperkalemia develops primarily because of decreased potassium excretion with reduced GFR as a result of decreased delivery of sodium to the distal tubule (type IV renal tubular acidosis). Contributing factors include dietary potassium intake, metabolic acidosis, and hypoaldosteronism (administration of ACEIs or ARBs).
- Metabolic acidosis is a result of decreased ability of the kidney to excrete hydrogen ions (impaired ammoniagenesis), and in addition, there is a reduction of titratable acid excretion and bicarbonate reabsorption.

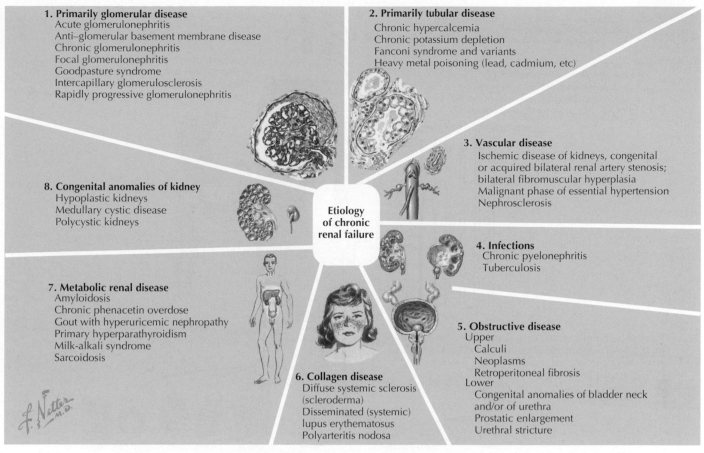

1. Primarily glomerular disease
Acute glomerulonephritis
Anti–glomerular basement membrane disease
Chronic glomerulonephritis
Focal glomerulonephritis
Goodpasture syndrome
Intercapillary glomerulosclerosis
Rapidly progressive glomerulonephritis

2. Primarily tubular disease
Chronic hypercalcemia
Chronic potassium depletion
Fanconi syndrome and variants
Heavy metal poisoning (lead, cadmium, etc)

3. Vascular disease
Ischemic disease of kidneys, congenital
or acquired bilateral renal artery stenosis;
bilateral fibromuscular hyperplasia
Malignant phase of essential hypertension
Nephrosclerosis

8. Congenital anomalies of kidney
Hypoplastic kidneys
Medullary cystic disease
Polycystic kidneys

Etiology of chronic renal failure

4. Infections
Chronic pyelonephritis
Tuberculosis

7. Metabolic renal disease
Amyloidosis
Chronic phenacetin overdose
Gout with hyperuricemic nephropathy
Primary hyperparathyroidism
Milk-alkali syndrome
Sarcoidosis

5. Obstructive disease
Upper
  Calculi
  Neoplasms
  Retroperitoneal fibrosis
Lower
  Congenital anomalies of bladder neck
  and/or of urethra
  Prostatic enlargement
  Urethral stricture

6. Collagen disease
Diffuse systemic sclerosis
(scleroderma)
Disseminated (systemic)
lupus erythematosus
Polyarteritis nodosa

Fig. 105.2 Etiology of Chronic Kidney Disease.

- Metabolic bone disease includes abnormalities in mineral metabolism and bone structure, which are common findings in stage 3 CKD (Fig. 105.3). There is retention of phosphate because of decreased GFR and decreased renal production of 1,25-dihydroxy vitamin D. This leads to decreased serum calcium levels and subsequent elevation of serum parathyroid hormone (PTH). This secondary hyperparathyroidism results in reabsorption of calcium from bone leading to bone disease that manifests with difficulty in walking, bone pain, skeletal deformities, and fractures.
- Anemia of CKD is initially normocytic and normochromic and is caused by reduced renal erythropoietin production. Nutritional deficiencies, including iron deficiency (most common), vitamin B_{12}, or folate may contribute to the anemia. This results in progressive fatigue and weakness.
- Hypertension is caused by volume expansion or activation of the renin-angiotensin system. It can be present in the earliest stages of CKD. Cardiovascular abnormalities found in CKD include left ventricular hypertrophy (caused by hypertension) and evidence of early atherosclerosis (coronary artery calcification, increased aortic stiffness).
- Dyslipidemia results from abnormal lipid metabolism in CKD, causing an increase in triglyceride-rich lipoproteins and low high-density lipoproteins (HDL) cholesterol levels. This increases the risk for having cardiovascular disease.
- Endocrine dysfunction in CKD is reflected in disorders of growth hormone metabolism (end-organ resistance to growth hormone caused by increased levels of insulin growth factor binding proteins), thyroid dysfunction known as "sick euthyroid syndrome" (low total and free T_4 and T_3, normal thyroid-stimulating hormone

and normal thyrotropin-releasing hormone), and reduced gonadal hormones, resulting in delayed puberty and anovulation.
- In children with CKD, risk factors for impaired growth include metabolic acidosis, decreased caloric intake, metabolic bone disease, anemia, and electrolyte abnormalities. After early childhood, it is primarily caused by alterations in growth hormone metabolism, specifically insulin-like growth factor-I (IGF-I).
- Uremia represents a constellation of symptoms and signs present in the final stage of CKD (Fig. 105.4). These include anorexia, nausea, vomiting, growth retardation, platelet dysfunction (abnormal platelet adhesion and aggregation), pericardial disease (pericarditis and pericardial effusion), neurologic abnormalities (peripheral neuropathy, lethargy, seizures, coma, and death), and altered cognitive development (loss of concentration and poor school performance).

Evaluation and Management

The history should focus on signs and symptoms of CKD and factors that may place that patient at higher risk for CKD.
- Medical history: diagnosis of congenital anomaly of the kidney or urinary tract, history of urinary tract infection, urologic abnormalities
- Family history of renal disease or hypertension
- Poor growth and/or development, history of fractures
- Urinary symptoms: gross hematuria, polyuria, daytime/nighttime enuresis
- Elevated blood pressures, blurry vision, headaches
- Presence of uremic symptoms: weakness, fatigue, anorexia, vomiting

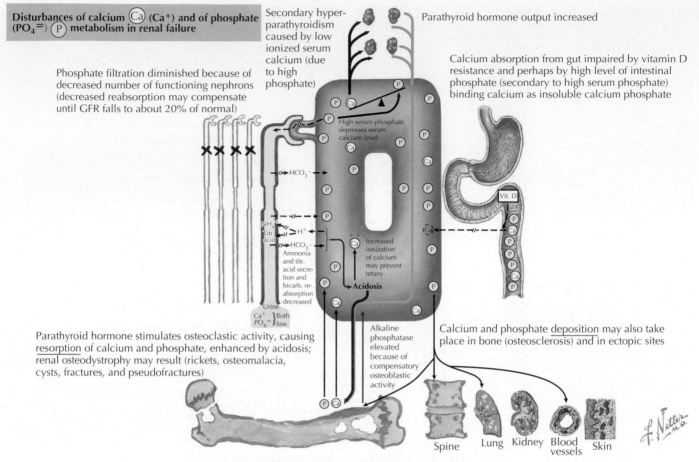

Fig. 105.3 Renal Failure: Calcium and Phosphorus Metabolism.

- Systemic symptoms: fever, rash, arthralgia, joint swelling

The examination should include measurements of growth parameters (weight, height) and vital signs, specifically blood pressure with the correct cuff size. The general assessment should include overall appearance, including volume status. CKD can affect every organ system and can be evaluated as follows:

- General: pallor, fatigue
- Respiratory: dyspnea, diminished breath sounds (edema)
- Cardiovascular: pericardial rub, diminished heart sounds
- Abdomen: abdominal pain (related to nausea)
- Neuro: decreased sensation (peripheral neuropathy), motor strength (weakness), confusion
- Skin: pallor, nonpitting/pitting edema, pruritus, changes in skin pigmentation
- Musculoskeletal: bone pain

There is no single pattern of laboratory abnormalities that characterizes pediatric CKD, but some abnormalities are commonly present. Serum creatinine is the most commonly used test to estimate the GFR (creatinine clearance indirectly represents the GFR) using the Schwartz formula: GFR = k × L/SCr, where k is a constant that varies with age and sex, L is length (cm), and SCr is serum creatinine in mg/dL. As cystatin C is becoming more widely used, there have been adaptations to obtain a more accurate GFR with combined equations. The GFR is then used to determine the stage of CKD (Table 105.1). Normal levels of GFR vary with age and height (Table 105.2). GFR increases with maturation from infancy and approaches adult mean value by 2 years of age.

Urinalysis as described for AKI can identify the underlying cause of both AKI and CKD. Proteinuria is an important biomarker associated with CKD because it may contribute to CKD progression and early signs of hyperfiltration injury.

Renal ultrasonography is the most widely used imaging modality and is noninvasive. It assesses the renal size and structure. It may also identify the cause of CKD such as detecting cystic kidney disease. Other imaging studies such as voiding cystourethrography, computed tomography, and magnetic resonance imaging are used in specific clinical settings.

Kidney biopsy (percutaneous ultrasound guided) provides diagnosis of the underlying renal disorder that caused CKD, and the possibility of recurrence after kidney transplantation. The results also serve to guide therapy and provide information about disease severity, including whether the findings may be reversible, and the degree of renal scarring.

Management

The general management of a patient with CKD includes treatment of reversible renal dysfunction (some renal function may be recovered if treatment is initiated early), prevention of progression, supportive treatment of complications, and identification of renal replacement therapy.

Slowing the progression of CKD is achieved by treating hypertension, decreasing proteinuria, and addressing metabolic acidosis because these are known to accelerate the progression of CKD. As far as low protein restriction in children is concerned, the current consensus is to provide the age-appropriate recommended daily allowance of protein to maximize nutritional status.

Sodium and water retention occur as GFR becomes severely decreased in stages 4 and 5 CKD. This is treated with dietary sodium restriction and diuretics. Some children with obstructive uropathy or

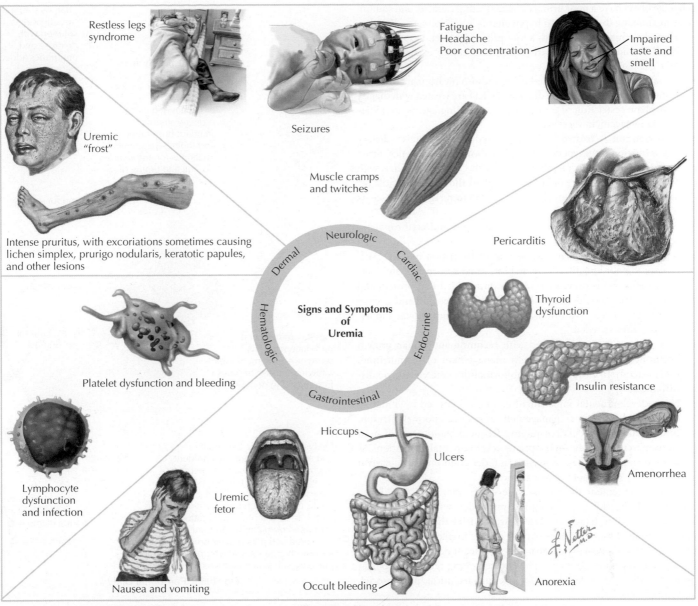

Fig. 105.4 Uremia.

TABLE 105.1	**Stages of Chronic Kidney Disease for Children Older Than 2 Years of Age**
Stage	**Glomerular Filtration Rate**
1	Normal (≥90 mL/min/1.73 m²)
2	60–89 mL/min/1.73 m²
3	30–59 mL/min/1.73 m²
4	15–29 mL/min/1.73 m²
5	<15 mL/min/1.73 m² or end-stage renal disease

TABLE 105.2 Estimated Glomerular Filtration Rate Equations

Types of Equations (Year)	eGFR Equation
Bedside Schwartz equation (2009)	$0.413 \times (height/Scr)$
Cystatin C–based Equation (2012)	$70.69 \times (cysC)^{-0.931}$
Creatinine–Cystatin C–based Equation (2012)	$39.8 \times (ht/Scr)^{0.456} \times (1.8/cysC)^{0.418}$ $\times (30/BUN)^{0.079} \times (1.076)^{male}$ $(1.00)^{female} \times (ht/1.4)^{0.179}$

BUN, Blood urea nitrogen; *cysC,* cystatin C; *GFR,* glomerular filtration rate; *ht,* height (cm); *SCr,* serum creatinine.
Calculators available on the National Kidney Foundation website (https://www.kidney.org). In the equations, male = 1, 1.076 and female = 1, 1.0.

renal dysplasia have a poor urinary concentrating capacity and sodium wasting, making them prone to hypovolemia and hyponatremia.

- Hyperkalemia is treated with a low-potassium diet, loop diuretics, alkali therapy (sodium bicarbonate), and cation exchange resins (Kayexalate).
- Metabolic acidosis is corrected using sodium bicarbonate therapy.
- Bone metabolism and bone disease of CKD are treated with dietary phosphate restriction, use of phosphate binding agents, and vitamin D replacement therapy.
- Hypertension is treated with weight reduction, exercise, dietary salt reduction, antihypertensive medications, and diuretics. Strict blood pressure control in all children with CKD is necessary, with a target blood pressure of at least less than the 90th percentile for age, gender, and height and less than 120/80 mm Hg for adolescents with CKD.
- Anemia is treated with iron supplementation and erythropoietin replacement therapy.
- Nutrition should be managed so that malnutrition of CKD (secondary to poor appetite, decreased intestinal absorption, and metabolic acidosis) is prevented. It is recommended that protein and caloric intake should be at least 100% of the recommended daily allowance for age. Nutritional support using nutritional supplements is often needed.
- Growth impairment is treated with recombinant human growth hormone (GH) therapy and with management of malnutrition, renal osteodystrophy, acid–base abnormalities, and electrolyte disturbances.
- Neurodevelopmental impairment can be minimized by initiating dialysis and by optimal management of anemia and malnutrition. Infants and young children require frequent monitoring of head circumference and age-appropriate developmental evaluations. A more formal assessment is needed in older children, particularly if they have poor school performance.

Renal replacement therapy is achieved by PD, HD, and kidney transplantation. RRT is generally recommended with GFR less than 15 mL/min/1.73 m² (stage 5 CKD). However, RRT therapy in children may be initiated sooner if there is poor calorie intake resulting in failure to thrive, symptomatic uremia, and significant delay in psychomotor and cognitive development. The choice among renal replacement options is dictated by family preference and technical, psychosocial, and compliance issues.

- PD is more common in infants and younger children because of challenges with vascular access in these age groups and it is able to provide gentle fluid removal (Fig. 105.5). A PD catheter is surgically placed into the peritoneal space and is typically used after 2 weeks to allow for appropriate healing. PD fluid is instilled into the peritoneal space. The peritoneal membrane serves as a "filter" through which waste products and water are cleared from blood that circulates through blood vessels of the peritoneal membrane. Waste products and water are transferred to the PD fluid in the peritoneal space by processes of diffusion and osmosis. This fluid is then drained out of the peritoneal space. PD can be performed by parents at home overnight with a cycling machine that allows the least disruption of home life, school, and work attendance.
- HD is more commonly used in older children (Fig. 105.6). HD requires vascular access such as placement of an arteriovenous fistula, arteriovenous graft, or central venous catheter. Blood is pumped from the vascular access into the dialyzer, which contains an artificial membrane that serves as a filter through which waste products and water are cleared from the blood into the dialysis fluid by processes of diffusion, convection, and ultrafiltration. Dialysis fluid flows through the dialyzer countercurrent to the blood. HD is performed

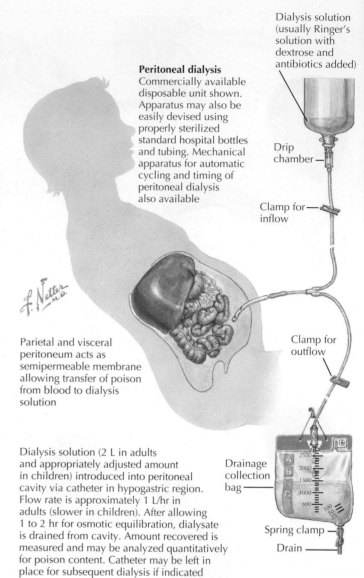

Peritoneal dialysis
Commercially available disposable unit shown. Apparatus may also be easily devised using properly sterilized standard hospital bottles and tubing. Mechanical apparatus for automatic cycling and timing of peritoneal dialysis also available

Dialysis solution (usually Ringer's solution with dextrose and antibiotics added)

Drip chamber

Clamp for inflow

Clamp for outflow

Parietal and visceral peritoneum acts as semipermeable membrane allowing transfer of poison from blood to dialysis solution

Dialysis solution (2 L in adults and appropriately adjusted amount in children) introduced into peritoneal cavity via catheter in hypogastric region. Flow rate is approximately 1 L/hr in adults (slower in children). After allowing 1 to 2 hr for osmotic equilibration, dialysate is drained from cavity. Amount recovered is measured and may be analyzed quantitatively for poison content. Catheter may be left in place for subsequent dialysis if indicated

Drainage collection bag

Spring clamp

Drain

Fig. 105.5 Peritoneal Dialysis.

in specialized HD centers using a HD machine and requires at least three weekly treatments that are each 3 to 5 hours long.

- Renal transplantation is performed using a deceased or living (related or unrelated) kidney donor. It can be performed in stage 5 CKD before dialysis begins (preemptive kidney transplantation). Renal transplantation is accepted as the optimal therapy of choice because transplantation not only ameliorates uremic symptoms but also allows for significant improvement, and often correction, of delayed skeletal growth, sexual maturation, cognitive performance, and psychosocial functioning.

FUTURE DIRECTIONS

There are ongoing studies, including the Chronic Kidney Disease in Children Study (CKiD), that provide information on children with CKD to identify incidence, prevalence, risk factors, and the impact of CKD on growth, cognition, and the risk for cardiovascular disease. Recognition of the overestimation of GFR that regularly occurs when using the current estimating formulas has prompted studies on the development and implementation of more accurate formulas.

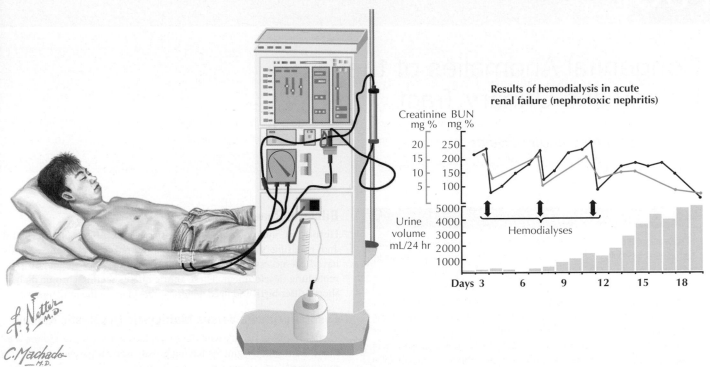

Fig. 105.6 Hemodialysis.

SUGGESTED READINGS

Available online.

106

Congenital Anomalies of the Kidney and Urinary Tract

Eloise C. Salmon and Ulf H. Beier

 CLINICAL VIGNETTE

A male infant is delivered at 35 weeks' gestation with a prenatal course notable for bilateral hydronephrosis and low amniotic fluid levels. He shows respiratory effort and requires noninvasive ventilation not typically expected based on gestational age. Postnatal imaging confirms dilation of the urine collecting system and identifies posterior urethral valves as the cause. A catheter provides urinary drainage until valve ablation by a pediatric urology surgeon. The infant has a strong urine stream postoperatively. The serum creatinine trends downward, but remains elevated for age. Otherwise, the postnatal course includes gradual weaning of respiratory support to room air and good weight gain with electrolytes remaining in normal range on breastmilk. At discharge, a plan is made for close nephrology and urology follow-up.

Impaired kidney function in utero can occur for a variety of reasons, including obstruction. Regardless of cause, overall postnatal prognosis depends significantly on the degree of pulmonary hypoplasia secondary to oliguria and anuria. The subsequent trajectory of kidney function during childhood varies. A pediatric nephrologist provides regular monitoring for chronic kidney disease.

Congenital and inherited anomalies of the kidney and urinary tract (CAKUT) are frequent causes of kidney failure in children, accounting for more than 30% of end-stage kidney disease (ESKD). CAKUT can be subdivided into three categories based on the primary abnormality in embryologic development (Fig. 106.1). The first category refers to failure to form a functional nephron, leading to renal parenchyma malformations, such as agenesis or cystic dysplasia. The second group of anomalies relates to failure of the developing kidney to migrate to its appropriate destination. This may lead to renal ectopy (e.g., pelvic kidney) or fusion abnormalities (e.g., horseshoe kidney). The third category describes variations in the urinary collecting system, such as double ureters or posterior urethral valves. Here, changes of the renal parenchyma (e.g., dysplasia) often are secondary to obstructive uropathy or vesicoureteral reflux (VUR). Inherited conditions such as polycystic kidney diseases (PKD) result from specific genetic mutations that may manifest with detectable renal abnormalities at birth or later in life. The following sections detail exemplary conditions representative of these subcategories.

ETIOLOGY AND PATHOGENESIS

Unilateral Renal Agenesis (Single Kidney)

Single kidney occurs in approximately 1 in 2000 births. Data on expected lifetime course remains incomplete, but may not be as benign as originally thought, with one cohort study demonstrating 50% of children developing hypertension, albuminuria, or decreased glomerular filtration rate (GFR) by age 18.

Bilateral Renal Agenesis

Historically incompatible with life because of absent amniotic fluid and resulting pulmonary hypoplasia, some centers more recently have had success with amniotic infusions during pregnancy to promote lung development. These anuric infants require chronic dialysis shortly after birth and need a kidney transplant in the long term.

Cystic Dysplasia Versus Multicystic Dysplastic Kidney

Cystic dysplasia occurs when cysts replace one or more kidney segments with other segments having grossly normal parenchyma. If the number of cystic segments is small, prognosis is good. In contrast, multicystic dysplastic kidney (MCDK) lacks normal parenchyma and occurs in roughly 1 in 4000 births.

Horseshoe Kidney

Horseshoe kidney is the most prevalent fusion abnormality of the kidney. The fusion occurs commonly at the lower poles with two separate excretory urinary systems maintained (Fig. 106.2). The reported incidence is 1 in 400 to 1600. The isthmus may contain actual parenchyma or a fibrous band. The kidneys cannot complete their ascension toward the dorsolumbar position as the inferior mesenteric artery holds the isthmus and prevents further rostral migration. Consequently, the blood supply of the fused kidney is variable and may come from the iliac arteries, aorta, or even hypogastric and middle sacral arteries. Horseshoe kidney can occur in isolation or as part of a syndrome, including Turner and trisomies 13, 18, and 21. It occasionally is associated with other genitourinary findings, such as bicornuate or septate uterus in girls, and hypospadias and undescended testis in boys.

Double Ureter

Double ureters are part of a duplicated collecting system complex (defined as two pyelocaliceal systems within one renal unit) and are relatively common, present in 0.2% of live births and in more than 10% of persons who have an affected first-degree relative. They occur when two ureteral buds arise from the Wolffian duct and can be associated with a variety of congenital genitourinary tract anomalies. The ureters may drain separately or jointly over a single orifice into the bladder. Most patients are asymptomatic, with double ureters detected incidentally on imaging studies. In cases of complete duplication, the lower renal unit typically drains into the normal ureteric insertion, and the ureter of the upper renal unit inserts ectopically in the bladder, urethra, or elsewhere.

Ureteropelvic Junction Obstruction

Ureteropelvic junction (UPJ) obstruction is the most common cause of antenatally detected hydronephrosis, found in 1 in 500 live births. It is more common in boys and more often on the left than right side. UPJ diameter enlarges as a result of partial restriction of urinary flow,

Failure to form a functional nephron

The distal ends of the collecting ducts connect with the tubule system of the nephron developing from the metanephric mesoderm. The nephron extends from the collecting duct to the renal corpuscle.

The tubule lengthens, coils, and begins to dip down toward the renal pelvis, as Henle loop; one area of the tubule remains close to the glomerular mouth, as the future macula densa.

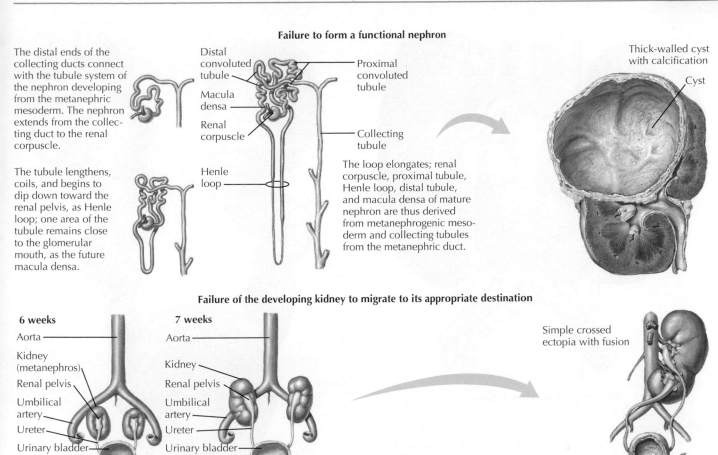

Distal convoluted tubule

Macula densa

Renal corpuscle

Henle loop

Proximal convoluted tubule

Collecting tubule

The loop elongates; renal corpuscle, proximal tubule, Henle loop, distal tubule, and macula densa of mature nephron are thus derived from metanephrogenic meso-derm and collecting tubules from the metanephric duct.

Thick-walled cyst with calcification

Cyst

Failure of the developing kidney to migrate to its appropriate destination

6 weeks

Aorta

Kidney (metanephros)

Renal pelvis

Umbilical artery

Ureter

Urinary bladder

Frontal view

7 weeks

Aorta

Kidney

Renal pelvis

Umbilical artery

Ureter

Urinary bladder

Frontal view

Simple crossed ectopia with fusion

Defects of the urinary collecting system

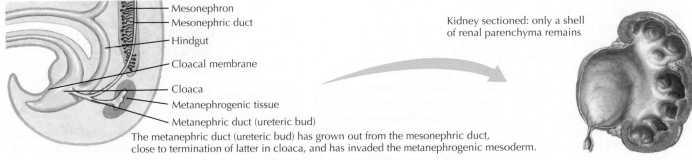

Mesonephron

Mesonephric duct

Hindgut

Cloacal membrane

Cloaca

Metanephrogenic tissue

Metanephric duct (ureteric bud)

Kidney sectioned: only a shell of renal parenchyma remains

The metanephric duct (ureteric bud) has grown out from the mesonephric duct, close to termination of latter in cloaca, and has invaded the metanephrogenic mesoderm.

Fig. 106.1 Congenital Anomalies Categories.

resulting in hydronephrosis. The hydronephrosis may progress, arrest, or improve spontaneously.

Posterior Urethral Valves

Posterior urethral valves (PUVs) are the most common cause of lower urinary tract obstruction in male neonates (Fig. 106.3). The reported incidence ranges from 1 in 8000 to 25,000 live births. The cause of PUV remains disputed. The posterior urethra is formed by the cloacae and the urogenital sinus, and its lining contains transitional epithelium. One theory is that abnormal integration of the Wolffian ducts into the posterior urethra ultimately creates a congenital obstructing posterior urethral membrane (COPUM). The valves classically seen on ultrasound and voiding cystourethrography (VCUG) occur as a result of perforation of the COPUM by a Foley catheter.

Polycystic Kidney Disease

PKDs are a group of inherited conditions in which replacement of renal parenchyma by cyst formation (Fig. 106.4) can occur anytime from fetal life to adulthood. The two major forms are autosomal recessive PKD (ARPKD) and autosomal dominant PKD (ADPKD) (Table 106.1). They share ciliary dysfunction as a common principle in their pathogenesis.

ARPKD typically manifests early in life, commonly detected on routine prenatal ultrasound. Severe cases may result in Potter sequence (i.e., oligohydramnios with lung hypoplasia and characteristic limb and facial abnormalities from decreased intraamniotic space). ARPKD has a reported incidence of 1 in 20,000. The phenotype is variable. At least 20% of identified patients do not survive the neonatal period, mainly because of respiratory insufficiency. Of those who survive infancy, approximately one-third will need chronic renal replacement therapy

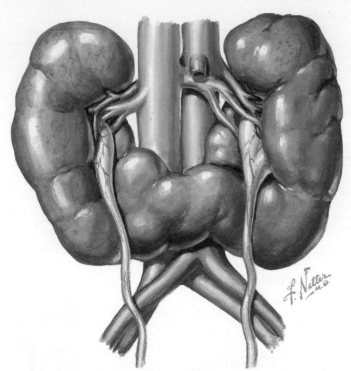

Fig. 106.2 Horseshoe Kidney.

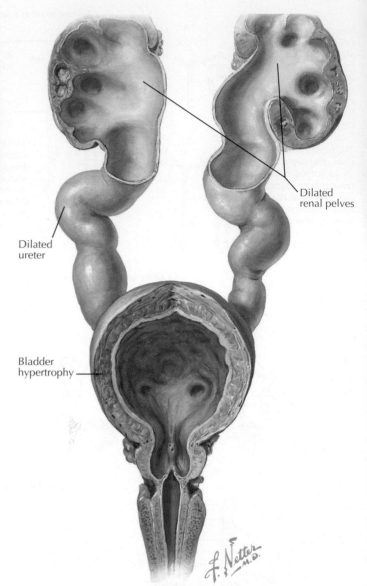

Dilated ureter

Dilated renal pelves

Bladder hypertrophy

Fig. 106.3 Urethral Congenital Valve.

(RRT). Cystic biliary dysgenesis is another hallmark of ARPKD. It can result in congenital hepatic fibrosis and may manifest later in childhood or even adulthood. Hepatic fibrosis may lead to portal hypertension, gastrointestinal bleeding from esophageal varices, cholangitis, and hepatic failure. The gene identified with ARPKD encodes fibrocystin (polyductin), a protein expressed on the cilia of renal and bile duct epithelial cells and thought critical to maintenance of normal tubular architecture in these systems.

In contrast to ARPKD, ADPKD usually is diagnosed in adulthood, although it may be detected at any age, including prenatally. With an estimated incidence from 1 in 400 to 1000, it is one of the more common genetic disorders. There is considerable phenotypic variation, ranging from infants presenting in renal failure to asymptomatic elderly patients with adequate renal function. In the United States, roughly 5% of adult patients requiring RRT have ADPKD. Morphologically, both kidneys show progressive bilateral development and enlargement of focal cysts. ADPKD is a systemic disease, with cysts occurring in the liver, pancreas, and vasculature. In contrast to ARPKD, hepatic failure is rare. Other extrarenal manifestations are uncommon in children; intracranial aneurysms and male fertility problems can occur in adulthood. Two genes have been identified with ADPKD. The *PKD1* gene encodes polycystin 1 and accounts for 85% of all ADPKD cases. *PKD2* encodes for polycystin 2. Both proteins are involved with the ciliary apparatus. A small number of cases are not linked to either gene, suggesting involvement of other genes.

CLINICAL PRESENTATION

Patients with CAKUT can be diagnosed prenatally, incidentally when imaging for another indication is obtained, or when presenting with electrolyte abnormalities or symptoms, including gross hematuria, urinary tract infection (UTI), or hypertension. A screening ultrasound of the kidneys and bladder is the most efficient initial examination, offering detailed anatomy without the risks of radiation or invasive procedures.

Historically, a single kidney was noted incidentally on imaging for other causes or uncovered during evaluation for concern of renal dysfunction. Now, many individuals receive the diagnosis prenatally. Most patients with horseshoe kidney are asymptomatic and diagnosed incidentally by ultrasonography. Some patients may present with pain, hematuria, obstruction, or UTIs. Hydronephrosis can occur in up to 80% of children with horseshoe kidneys as a result of VUR, obstruction of the collecting system by external ureteric compression (e.g., blood vessels), or UPJ obstruction from a relatively high insertion of ureters. Twenty percent of patients have urolithiasis.

In girls, urinary dribbling or incontinence may be the manifesting sign of a double ureter if there is insertion into the vagina, urethra, or uterus. Otherwise, symptoms may result from reflux into the ureter of the lower renal unit or obstruction of the upper ureter (Fig. 106.5), which increases the risk for UTI. It is noteworthy that up to 80% of ureteroceles are associated with double ureters. In duplex kidneys, ureteroceles are usually an outgrowth of the ectopic ureter. Most patients with UPJ obstruction are asymptomatic. Occasionally, newborns present with abdominal masses or renal insufficiency if the obstruction is bilateral. Older children may present with pain, vomiting, or hypertension.

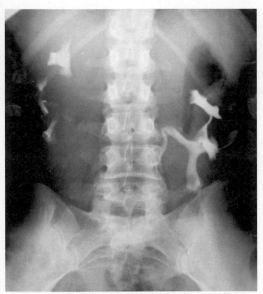

Intravenous pyelogram. Bilateral polycystic disease

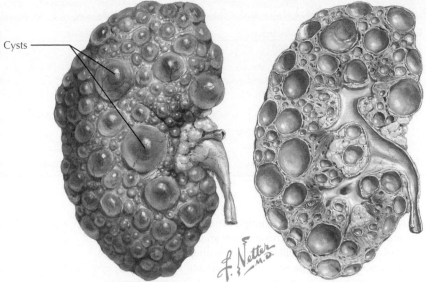

Cysts

Polycystic kidney. Surface aspect   Polycystic kidney sectioned

Fig. 106.4 Renal Cystic Diseases.

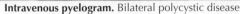

TABLE 106.1 Autosomal Recessive Polycystic Kidney Disease Versus Autosomal Dominant Polycystic Kidney Disease

	Autosomal Recessive Polycystic Kidney Disease	Autosomal Dominant Polycystic Kidney Disease
Gene	Chromosome 6p21.2-p12.2	Chromosome 16p13.3, chromosome 4q22.1
Protein	Fibrocystin	Polycystin 1, polycystin 2
Age of presentation	Commonly prenatally, childhood, adolescence	Highly variable
Renal cysts	Radial pattern	Anywhere in kidney, varying size
Extrarenal manifestations	Biliary obstruction, hepatic fibrosis with portal hypertension, liver failure	Liver cysts, pancreas cysts, vascular cysts ("berry aneurysms")

PUV has a wide spectrum of clinical presentation depending largely on the initial degree of obstruction. The associated morbidity is not limited to renal abnormalities; impaired lung development in utero (Potter sequence), bladder wall thickening and dilatation, hydroureters, and urinomas also occur. The obstructive uropathy may result in renal dysplasia, chronic kidney disease, and ESKD. Up to 15% of patients undergoing renal transplantation in childhood have PUV as the underlying condition. The widespread use of prenatal ultrasound has resulted in diagnosis of most cases in the fetal or neonatal period. In cases manifesting later in life, a voiding history is important because patients with PUV usually have a diminished or abnormal urinary stream.

ARPKD can be detected prenatally or after birth in patients presenting with hypertension. As costs have declined, genetic testing has become the gold standard for diagnosis. Historically, diagnosis depended on radiographic features (large kidneys, increased echogenicity of the parenchyma, loss of corticomedullary differentiation, radially oriented cysts) and one or more of the following: (1) absence of renal

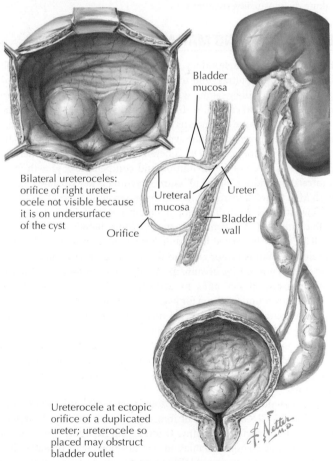

Bilateral ureteroceles: orifice of right ureterocele not visible because it is on undersurface of the cyst

Bladder mucosa

Ureteral mucosa

Orifice

Ureter

Bladder wall

Ureterocele at ectopic orifice of a duplicated ureter; ureterocele so placed may obstruct bladder outlet

Fig. 106.5 Ureterocele.

cysts in both parents, (2) a previously affected sibling, (3) consanguinity, or (4) hepatic fibrosis. Children with ADPKD may be asymptomatic or present with flank pain, hematuria, renal colic, UTIs, or hypertension. ADPKD can be diagnosed by renal ultrasound, computed tomography,

TABLE 106.2   **Syndromes Associated With Kidney Manifestations**

Gene (Inheritance)	Syndrome	Manifestations	Other Organ Involvement
CHD7 (AD) *SEMA3E* (AD)	CHARGE	Dysplasia	Coloboma, heart defects, choanal atresia, genital and ear anomalies
EYA1 (AD) *SIX1* (AD)	Branchio-oto-renal syndrome	Hypoplasia	Hearing impairment, abnormal structures of outer middle or inner ear, branchial cyst
HNF1B (AD)	Renal cysts and diabetes	Cystic or hypoplastic kidneys	Diabetes
JAG1 (AD) *NOTCH2* (AD)	Alagille syndrome	Dysplasia	Cholestasis, failure to thrive, heart defects, characteristic facies, butterfly vertebra
PAX2 (AD)	Renal coloboma syndrome	Cystic or hypoplastic kidneys	Optic nerve dysplasia

AD, Autosomal dominant.

or magnetic resonance imaging. Multiple renal parenchymal cysts generally are visible and usually increase in size and number with age. The finding of a single cyst in a child may merit further observation. In general, the combination of a parent with ADPKD and more than one cyst in a child is considered diagnostic. Rarely, ADPKD may arise sporadically. Diagnosing ADPKD in a presymptomatic, otherwise healthy child may not be desirable given the financial and psychosocial implications. Because of the complexities of these issues, pediatric practitioners should refer asymptomatic children to a pediatric nephrologist before undertaking diagnostic investigations.

EVALUATION AND MANAGEMENT

In children with a single kidney, monitoring during childhood typically includes periodic ultrasound to assess for appropriate compensatory growth in the kidney, along with blood pressure measurement, urinalysis, and serum creatinine. In those with an MCDK, prior practice was to resect because of concerns for infection, pain, hypertension, and malignancy. Current data, however, suggest a conservative approach is best for most patients. MCDK generally involutes over time; periodic ultrasounds monitor for involution and compensatory growth in the contralateral kidney. Blood pressure screening is key because children with MCDK are at increased risk for hypertension. A recent systematic review estimates 3% will develop hypertension in childhood. Children with bilateral MCDK typically require chronic dialysis early in life.

Patients with isolated horseshoe kidney have an increased risk for developing Wilms tumor compared with the general population, but screening is not routine because the absolute risk remains low. Imaging for horseshoe kidney aims to identify VUR. Initial investigations include ultrasound to screen for hydronephrosis and VCUG to exclude VUR. A technetium 99m–labeled diethylenetriaminepentaacetic acid (DTPA) scan should be done if ultrasound shows obstruction. Most patients with horseshoe kidney need no specific treatment. If VUR or obstructive uropathy is identified, a pediatric urologist should follow the child. Antibiotic prophylaxis and corrective surgery may be necessary.

The diagnostic evaluation for double ureter includes renal ultrasound and VCUG. The goal of imaging is to identify VUR, ureteroceles, and obstructive uropathy. If found, surgical correction may be indicated. The standard evaluation of a newborn with prenatal ultrasound findings suggestive of UPJ obstruction includes a confirmatory postnatal ultrasound. If obstruction is persistent, a VCUG to assess for VUR should be considered. Urolithiasis and UTIs are possible complications of UPJ obstruction. If patients are symptomatic, surgical intervention frequently is indicated. The surgical options include reconstructive pyeloplasty or temporary nephrostomy tubes for more acute alleviation of pressure. If patients are managed by observation

alone, antibiotic prophylaxis usually is unnecessary unless there is evidence of VUR.

For patients with PUV, treatment first consists of ablation by a urologist. Children commonly develop postobstructive diuresis and should be monitored carefully for electrolyte and volume instabilities after ablation. The prognosis and treatment depends on the degree of preserved renal function after obstruction is relieved.

ARPKD treatment largely is supportive. The primary prognostic determinant in the newborn period is the degree of lung hypoplasia. Renal failure and portal hypertension are treated with medications, dialysis, or transplant depending on an individual patient's symptoms. In childhood, frequent features are chronic kidney disease, electrolyte abnormalities, and hypertension. The hypertension usually is responsive to angiotensin-converting enzyme inhibitors. Cholelithiasis is common, and ascending cholangitis is a potentially life-threatening concern.

The treatment of ADPKD in children is also largely supportive. Notably, UTIs are relatively common in patients with ADPKD, but may not show diagnostic pyuria or bacteriuria if infection is contained within a cyst. Conversely, a ruptured cyst may manifest as hematuria and pyuria in the absence of infection. Importantly, traditional first-line antibiotics for UTIs such as cephalosporins and aminoglycosides may not have adequate cyst penetration. A sulfonamide or quinolone usually is preferred. Screening for extrarenal manifestations, such as intracranial aneurysms, is not routinely recommended in children, with magnetic resonance angiography usually reserved for those with symptoms or a strong family history of cerebrovascular disease. Hypertension and proteinuria both can develop in ADPKD; appropriate medical management of these conditions is critical in preserving remaining kidney function. Tolvaptan, a vasopressin receptor antagonist, is approved for adults with ADPKD as the first drug treatment to slow kidney function decline in adults at risk for rapidly progressing ADPKD.

FUTURE DIRECTIONS

Advances in prenatal, neonatal, dialysis, and transplant care have improved outcomes and survival for children with the most severe forms of CAKUT. Knowledge continues to increase about the genetic causes of CAKUT (Table 106.2). As an early example, a frameshift mutation in *PAX2* was identified as causative for the constellation of optic nerve colobomas, renal hypoplasia, and VUR. At present, roughly 30% of CAKUT have a known monogenic cause. As whole exome data become available for more children, this proportion likely will continue to increase.

SUGGESTED READINGS

Available online.

107

Infections of the Urinary Tract

Selasie Q. Goka

 CLINICAL VIGNETTE

A 23-month-old girl presents to the emergency department (ED) with fever of 2 days, duration. The highest recorded temperature was 102.6°F (39.2°C). Her parents have been administering acetaminophen around the clock. She is fussier than usual and vomited once overnight but has normal oral intake and is making the same number of wet diapers. She has a history of intermittent constipation and her last stool was 3 days ago. She was born at full term, and there were no abnormal findings on prenatal ultrasound. She has no medical, surgical, or significant family history, and all her immunizations are up to date. Review of her vital signs shows a febrile and tachycardic toddler. After she is calmed, a blood pressure is obtained and is found to be normal for age. On physical examination, there is apparent lower abdominal discomfort and a mass suggestive of stool in the left lower quadrant. An external genitourinary examination shows no erythema or discharge. Dipstick testing of a catheterized urine sample shows leukocytes and nitrites. A urine sample is sent to the laboratory for culture, and she is started empirically on cephalexin pending the results of the culture. She tolerates the first dose by mouth and is discharged to follow-up with her pediatrician the next day with strict instructions to return to the ED for further vomiting or inability to take medications or maintain oral intake. The urine culture grows *Escherichia coli* that is susceptible to cephalexin, and she ultimately completes a 7-day course of antibiotics. The history of constipation is identified as a risk factor for urinary tract infection and she is started on a bowel regimen.

Urinary tract infections (UTIs) encompass infections of both the lower (bladder) and upper (kidneys) urinary tracts, also referred to as cystitis and pyelonephritis, respectively. A nonfebrile UTI is typically considered to be cystitis, whereas a febrile UTI is diagnosed as pyelonephritis. UTIs are very common in children and adolescents. Typically caused by bacteria, the incidence of UTIs varies based on different factors, including age and sex. They are diagnosed frequently in infants younger than 12 months of age, during which period uncircumcised males are at higher risk than females while the incidence in toddlers and older girls is about three times higher than that in boys. Recurrence is seen in up to 30% of patients and is more likely to occur in patients with bowel and bladder dysfunction or abnormalities of the kidneys and urinary tract, the most common being vesicoureteral reflux (VUR). The sequelae of an untreated UTI can include progression to sepsis in the immediate time period and/or renal scarring with resultant hypertension and chronic kidney disease.

By the end of this chapter, the reader should be able to describe the presentation of children with UTI as well as current recommendations on workup and management. Fig. 107.1 provides a broad overview of the material covered.

ETIOLOGY AND PATHOGENESIS

A UTI develops after introduction of the causative organism to the urinary tract and evasion or overpowering of the genitourinary (GU) defense mechanisms, which include urethral washout, epithelial shedding, and paraurethral glandular secretion. Bacteria are introduced to the urethra after crossing the perineum from the rectal region, then ascend into the bladder and, in some cases, the upper urinary tract. Less than 1% of UTIs are due to hematogenous seeding of the urinary tract. The patient's immune response to the bacteria ultimately determines the severity of the UTI.

The most common bacteria isolated in the urine of patients confirmed to have UTI come from the gram-negative Enterobacteriaceae family. *Escherichia coli* is by far the most likely etiologic agent; others include *Klebsiella*, *Proteus* species, *Enterobacter*, *Citrobacter* species, and *Pseudomonas*. Gram-positive bacteria causing UTI include *Enterococcus* species, *Staphylococcus saprophyticus*, and, less commonly, *Staphylococcus aureus* (in patients with hematogenous spread). Group B streptococci are seen in neonatal UTIs, and patients with abnormal urinary tracts or chronic need for urinary catheterization are more likely to grow *Pseudomonas* and *Enterococcus*. Some atypical pathogens may be found in special populations. For example, BK polyomavirus in immunocompromised patients, fungi such as *Candida* in patients with indwelling catheters on chronic antibiotic therapy, and *Schistosoma* in recent travelers from regions where it is endemic.

CLINICAL PRESENTATION

Presenting symptoms in pediatric UTI range from nonspecific, generalized symptoms in the very young to specific and localizing complaints in older children and adolescents. In neonates and young infants, the chief complaint may include fever, poor oral intake, vomiting, irritability, lethargy, failure to thrive, or jaundice. Parents may provide a history of foul-smelling urine or blood in the diaper. Older children can verbalize dysuria, urinary frequency, urgency or new incontinence, hematuria, abdominal pain (especially in the suprapubic region) and back or flank pain. There may be a subjective history of decreased urinary output in patients who are holding their urine as a result of dysuria. Fever and vomiting also may be present.

The medical history should include questions about urinary output and appearance. Additional history should assess for factors that may put patients at higher risk for UTI, such as recent toilet training, constipation, dysfunctional voiding, known genitourinary abnormalities, prior history of UTI, family history of UTI, and, in adolescents, recent sexual activity.

A complete physical examination should be performed in all pediatric patients presenting with history or symptoms concerning for UTI. Examinations may be more focused in older children who can give a clear and classic history and who are not ill appearing. Temperature should be taken to assess if the patient is febrile, a weight should be obtained because it may give an indication of failure to thrive or dehydration, especially in younger patients. A blood pressure should

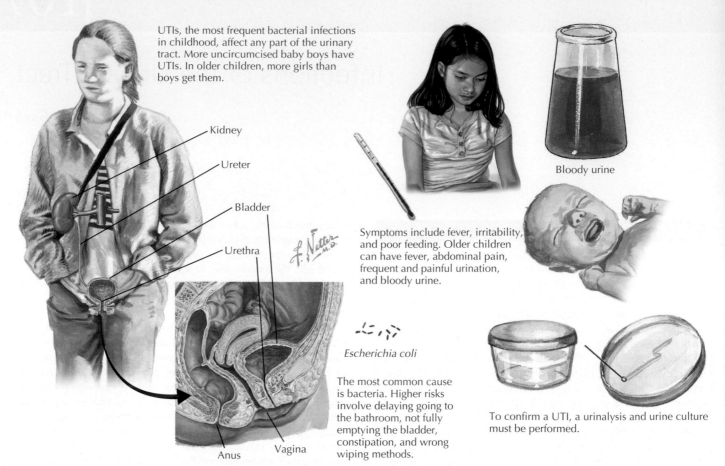

UTIs, the most frequent bacterial infections in childhood, affect any part of the urinary tract. More uncircumcised baby boys have UTIs. In older children, more girls than boys get them.

Kidney

Ureter

Bladder

Urethra

Anus

Vagina

Bloody urine

Symptoms include fever, irritability, and poor feeding. Older children can have fever, abdominal pain, frequent and painful urination, and bloody urine.

Escherichia coli

The most common cause is bacteria. Higher risks involve delaying going to the bathroom, not fully emptying the bladder, constipation, and wrong wiping methods.

To confirm a UTI, a urinalysis and urine culture must be performed.

Fig. 107.1 Urinary Tract Infection (UTI): An Overview.

be recorded to ensure there is no hypertension, because this may be evidence of underlying kidney disease. Abdominal examination may elicit pain, especially in the suprapubic region. Costovertebral angle tenderness is also suggestive of UTI. An external GU examination may be useful in certain age groups, such as female toddlers, to determine if symptoms may be due to vulvovaginitis or sexually active patients, in which case GU discharge might raise suspicion for a sexually transmitted infection (STI). An enlarged bladder should raise concern for abnormal anatomy (e.g., posterior urethral valves or neurogenic bladder as a risk factor for UTI).

Conditions such as sepsis, vulvovaginitis, vaginal foreign object, STI, pelvic inflammatory disease, gastroenteritis, and appendicitis, among others, can be considered in the differential diagnosis depending on the chief complaint, other risk factors, and age of the patient.

EVALUATION AND MANAGEMENT

The most crucial step in evaluation is a urine screen, either by point-of-care urinary dipstick testing or formal laboratory urinalysis and microscopy. If the screen is suggestive of a UTI, a urine sample should be sent for urine culture because this is the gold standard for diagnosis. The optimal way of obtaining a urine sample differs based on the age of the patient. In toilet-trained children and adolescents, a clean catch midstream specimen is adequate. In younger children, and those who are not toilet-trained, urine should ideally be obtained by bladder catheterization (Fig. 107.2). In some children 2 months of age and older, who are not high risk or ill enough to require immediate antibiotic treatment, a bagged urine specimen can be obtained for initial screen. However, any positive finding will require obtaining a new specimen

by catheterization, because of high rates of false positive results when using bagged specimens.

With urinalysis, the sample is examined for the presence of leukocyte esterase (LE) and/or nitrites, and microscopy provides information on the presence of bacteria and/or the number of white blood cells per high-power field (WBCs/hpf). A positive leukocyte esterase is reflective of the presence of WBCs and is considered highly sensitive for a diagnosis of UTI, especially in the correct clinical context. It is, however, not specific for UTI because other conditions can cause pyuria. The presence of nitrites is an indicator of enteric gram-negative bacteria in the urine that are able to convert dietary nitrates to nitrites. This has 98% specificity for UTI but is not highly sensitive, especially in infants, because a urine sample has to have been in the bladder for at least 4 hours in order for nitrites to be made. Of note, if the UTI is caused by a non–nitrite producing pathogen, the nitrite test will be negative.

On microscopy, the presence of bacteria and pyuria (>5 WBCs/hpf) makes UTI extremely likely. Bacteriuria alone does not usually indicate a true UTI but may be representative of asymptomatic bacteriuria, especially in older girls. Care should be taken in analyzing the urinary results of immunosuppressed patients because they might not mount a WBC response even in the context of a true UTI. Urinalysis may, in some cases of UTI, show red blood cells and/or protein; however, the clinician should be careful to think about the possibility of glomerulonephritis if the clinical presentation is not convincing for a UTI.

Guidelines from various regions specify different quantitative threshold criteria for diagnosis of UTI by culture. The thresholds also differ based on the method of sample collection. In general, a midstream sample is thought to have clinically significant bacteriuria if

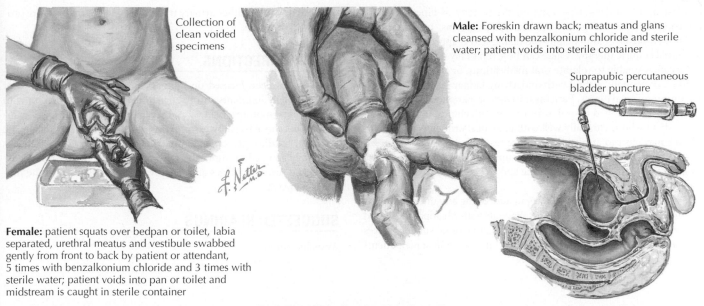

Male: Foreskin drawn back; meatus and glans cleansed with benzalkonium chloride and sterile water; patient voids into sterile container

Collection of clean voided specimens

Suprapubic percutaneous bladder puncture

Female: patient squats over bedpan or toilet, labia separated, urethral meatus and vestibule swabbed gently from front to back by patient or attendant, 5 times with benzalkonium chloride and 3 times with sterile water; patient voids into pan or toilet and midstream is caught in sterile container

Fig. 107.2 Urine Specimen Collection.

TABLE 107.1 Summary of Workup and Management of Patients at Risk for Urinary Tract Infection

At Risk for UTI?	Obtain Urine if Age 2–24 Months and Any of Risk Factors Below	Obtain Urine if Age >24 Months and Any of Risk Factors Below	Workup	Treatment
Uncircumcised male infant Dysfunctional voiding Recent potty training History of UTI VUR or abnormal anatomy Family history Sexual activity	History of UTI, VUR or abnormal anatomy Uncircumcised male Circumcised male with fever (>102.2°F [>39°C]) or lasting >24 hours or without a clear source Girls age <12 months, fever (≥102.2°F [≥39°C]) or lasting ≥48 hours or without a clear source Concerning findings on examination (suprapubic tenderness) Ill appearance	History of UTI, VUR or abnormal anatomy Urinary symptoms (dysuria, frequency, etc.) Concerning findings on examination (suprapubic tenderness, costovertebral angle tenderness) Ill appearance	UA, culture If UTI diagnosed, RBUS[a]: children <2 years with first febrile UTI, older children with recurrent UTI VCUG: if abnormality on RBUS or after second febrile UTI	Empiric antibiotics while awaiting results of urine culture and completion of 7–14-day course of organism-specific antibiotics after culture results available

[a]Does not need to be during acute illness if patient improves quickly
RBUS, Renal bladder ultrasound; *UA,* urinalysis; *UTI,* urinary tract infection; *VCUG,* voiding cystourethrography; *VUR,* vesicoureteral reflux.

there are more than 10^5 colony-forming units (CFU)/mL of a single uropathogenic organism. For samples obtained by bladder catheterization, significant growth is greater than 5×10^4 CFU/mL of a single organism, in addition to the presence of pyuria.

Workup such as blood work and imaging beyond urine testing is not necessary in many cases of UTI. Clinicians can decide on the need for broader workup based on other factors, including the age of the patient, how ill-appearing they are, associated risk factors for developing UTI (e.g., history of anatomic abnormalities), and any physical examination findings that might suggest the need for other testing. A febrile neonate or an ill-appearing child of any age should have bloodwork completed, including complete blood count, electrolytes, and serum creatinine. A blood culture should be considered.

Imaging recommendations have changed over the years to minimize unnecessary testing; however, a clear consensus is still lacking. A renal bladder ultrasound (RBUS) is a simple noninvasive test that is useful for identifying anatomic abnormalities of the urinary tract.

Voiding cystourethrograms are useful for identifying the presence and severity of VUR and, in some cases, urethral obstruction. A dimercaptosuccinic acid (DMSA) scintigraphy scan can be obtained in the acute phase of illness in the rare patient in whom definitive imaging diagnosis of pyelonephritis is warranted and can be used in select patients well after resolution of a UTI to assess for renal scarring. A summary of the suggested workup is included in Table 107.1.

Antibiotics are the mainstay of treatment for UTI. The timing and route of antibiotic administration as well as the choice of antibiotic depends on the clinical scenario, awareness of the most likely causative organisms, and local susceptibility patterns. Most patients should be started on an antibiotic to cover the most common uropathogens while awaiting results of the urine culture, after which a more targeted antibiotic can be used to complete the treatment course if needed. In those presenting with a recurrent UTI, review of organisms previously cultured can be helpful in ensuring that empiric therapy is adequately broad. Therapy should be given for a minimum of 7 days and can last up to 14 days depending on the severity of illness and risk for complications. All guidelines list cephalosporins, trimethoprim-sulfamethoxazole or amoxicillin-clavulanic acid as appropriate choices for initial empiric therapy. These can be given orally unless the patient is very ill, is unable to tolerate oral medications, or is at high risk; for example, a neonate, a child with underlying kidney disease, or immunocompromised patients. Patients initiated on parenteral medications should be transitioned to oral formulation with clinical improvement. In a patient who is clinically well with equivocal urinalysis results, clinicians may elect to await urine culture results before starting antibiotic therapy, as long as reliable follow-up with the patient is ensured. In general, repeat urine testing at the end of treatment to document a cure is not necessary

Prevention of recurrent UTI lies in addressing any underlying risk factors for the development of UTIs. Patients with constipation should be placed on a bowel regimen; those with dysfunctional voiding patters can be asked to void at regular, specified intervals; and some patients with severe VUR or other urinary tract abnormalities may require prophylactic antibiotics.

FUTURE DIRECTIONS

Research has been focused on biomarkers to aid in the diagnosis of UTI, especially in infants and young children, who often present with nonspecific symptoms. Urinary and serum neutrophil gelatinase–associated lipocalin have shown some promise for improving diagnostic accuracy. Studies into other biomarkers are ongoing. D-mannose is being studied in adult women as a means to reduce risk for UTI recurrence, and several vaccines are being researched in adults for the prevention of UTI.

SUGGESTED READINGS

Available online.

Neurology

Jennifer L. McGuire

108

Seizures

Jillian L. McKee and Sudha Kilaru Kessler

A seizure is caused by abnormal, excessive, synchronous electrical discharges from neurons. Clinically, this electrical disturbance can manifest as involuntary changes in movement, sensation, awareness, or behavior. Epilepsy is characterized by an enduring predisposition to generate seizures, but also by the neurobiologic, cognitive, psychological, and social consequence of the condition.

Epilepsy is a common neurologic condition affecting 50 million people worldwide with a prevalence around 1.2% in the United States. Incidence peaks during infancy and late adulthood. One-third of children with epilepsy may have pharmacoresistant seizures. Comorbid behavioral and cognitive difficulties are common.

ETIOLOGY AND PATHOGENESIS

Provoked seizures are caused by a transient factor acting on a normal brain to temporarily lower the seizure threshold. Common provocations include electrolyte derangements (hypoglycemia, hyponatremia or hypernatremia, hypocalcemia, hypomagnesemia), acute anoxia, drug intoxication or withdrawal, or systemic or intracranial infection. Epilepsy is diagnosed when a person has at least two unprovoked (or reflex) seizures occurring more than 24 hours apart, one unprovoked (or reflex) seizure and a probability of further seizures of at least 60% over the next 10 years, or an identified epilepsy syndrome. The many potential causes of epilepsy (Fig. 108.1) include structural lesions (tumor, infarct, vascular malformation, encephalomalacia, and developmental malformations), infections (such as cysticercosis), metabolic abnormalities, immunologic disorders, or genetic conditions. A cause is not always identified.

CLINICAL PRESENTATION

Seizure Classification

Classifying seizure type is important for diagnosis and treatment. In focal-onset seizures, abnormal electrical activity begins in one hemisphere; this activity may be localized to a discrete area or widely distributed. In contrast, generalized-onset seizures originate within bilaterally distributed neuronal networks. Unknown-onset seizures cannot be accurately classified as focal onset or generalized onset with the currently available clinical information.

Focal-onset seizures can be further classified by level of awareness, as either "aware" or "impaired awareness" (Fig. 108.2). Focal seizures that evolve to engage broad bilateral brain regions are now referred to as "focal to bilateral tonic-clonic" seizures, a term that replaces the old expression "secondarily generalized." Generalized seizures are usually associated with impaired awareness.

All types of seizures can be further classified as either motor or nonmotor onset, based on the clinical semiology. The motor component of seizures may include an atonic drop, tonic stiffening, clonic jerking, asynchronous hyperkinetic movements, myoclonic jerks, or automatisms. Features seen in nonmotor seizures include autonomic signs (diaphoresis, heart rate changes), behavioral arrest, perceptual impairments (visual hallucinations), and emotional or sensory phenomena. Examples of generalized motor seizures include tonic-clonic, clonic, tonic, myoclonic, myoclonic-tonic-clonic, myoclonic-atonic, atonic, and epileptic (including infantile) spasms. Generalized nonmotor–onset seizures, otherwise known as absence seizures, can be typical, atypical, myoclonic, or involve eyelid myoclonia. Obtaining a detailed description of seizures from the child's caregivers is more important than assigning terminology.

Febrile Seizures

Febrile seizures affect 2% to 5% of children between the ages of 6 months and 5 years, with peak incidence between 12 and 18 months. Seizures occur in the setting of a fever, but are sometimes the manifesting feature of a febrile illness. Simple febrile seizures occur in developmentally normal children, last less than 15 minutes, are generalized onset, and only occur once in a 24-hour period. Complex febrile seizures have a focal onset, are prolonged (>15 minutes), and/or recur within 24 hours. Simple febrile seizures do not confer an increased risk for future epilepsy. The risk for future epilepsy is increased in children with complex febrile seizures, an abnormal neurologic examination, developmental delay, or a family history of epilepsy. Febrile seizures are also a common manifesting sign of Dravet syndrome, a genetic epilepsy.

Common Epilepsy Syndromes

Common clinical presentations of epilepsy combined with specific electroencephalogram (EEG) patterns in children may be classified into syndromes (Fig. 108.3). Accurate diagnosis of syndromes can guide treatment choices and aid in predicting developmental outcomes.

West syndrome is the clinical triad of infantile spasms, a high-voltage and disorganized EEG pattern called hypsarrhythmia, and developmental delay or regression. Infantile spasms are sudden, brief

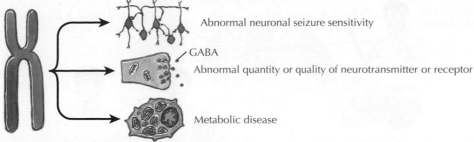

Genetic influences may predispose to seizure activity

Abnormal neuronal seizure sensitivity

GABA

Abnormal quantity or quality of neurotransmitter or receptor

Metabolic disease

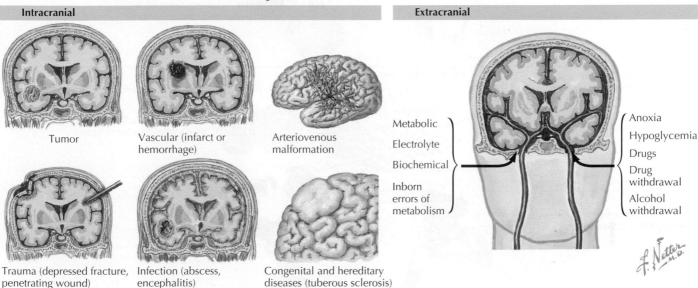

Intracranial

Tumor

Vascular (infarct or hemorrhage)

Arteriovenous malformation

Trauma (depressed fracture, penetrating wound)

Infection (abscess, encephalitis)

Congenital and hereditary diseases (tuberous sclerosis)

Extracranial

Metabolic
Electrolyte
Biochemical
Inborn errors of metabolism

Anoxia
Hypoglycemia
Drugs
Drug withdrawal
Alcohol withdrawal

Fig. 108.1 Causes of Seizures.

flexor or extensor jerks that often occur in clusters. Onset is typically in the first year of life, and the syndrome can occur in infants with known neurologic disorders or in previously healthy infants. The list of possible causes is broad, and it is not uncommon for the cause to remain unclear after a thorough diagnostic evaluation. Although spasms usually remit by 2 years of age, other seizure types may then emerge.

Lennox-Gastaut syndrome is a severe form of childhood-onset epilepsy characterized by multiple seizure types (including atonic, tonic, myoclonic, generalized tonic clonic, and atypical absence seizures), slow spike-and-wave pattern on EEG and intellectual disability. Seizures are often refractory to multiple therapies.

Childhood epilepsy with centro-temporal spikes, formerly known as benign epilepsy with centro-temporal spikes or benign rolandic epilepsy, is a common focal epilepsy occurring between the ages of 3 and 14 years in otherwise healthy children. Seizures occur out of sleep and involve unilateral facial motor or sensory symptoms, often with speech arrest, with or without impairment in consciousness. The EEG shows unilateral or bilateral central temporal epileptiform discharges that always occur more often in sleep. Seizures remit by adolescence.

Childhood absence epilepsy (CAE) is a common genetic generalized epilepsy syndrome affecting developmentally normal children between the ages of 4 and 10 years. Absence seizures are frequent brief behavioral pauses with staring and loss of awareness, and sometimes repetitive blinking and automatisms of the face or hands. The EEG shows generalized 3-Hz spike-and-wave discharges during a seizure, which can be provoked by hyperventilation. The majority of children respond to antiseizure medication. CAE remits in adolescence in most patients, but 15% may progress to juvenile myoclonic epilepsy (JME).

JME is another genetic generalized epilepsy syndrome that begins in adolescence. Patients with JME have myoclonic jerks (usually shortly after waking), bilateral tonic-clonic seizures, and occasionally absence seizures. The EEG shows 3- to 6-Hz generalized polyspike-and-wave discharges that are provoked by photic stimulation. Seizures typically respond to medication, but lifelong treatment may be needed.

Status Epilepticus

Status epilepticus (Chapter 117) describes abnormally prolonged seizures or repeated seizures with persistent mental status alteration in between. Prolonged seizures require urgent treatment. Treating a generalized tonic-clonic seizure lasting longer than 5 minutes with emergency medication is generally recommended, but the critical time point for treatment of other seizure types such as focal impaired awareness seizures or absence seizures is less clear.

DIFFERENTIAL DIAGNOSIS

Because the diagnosis of epilepsy is based on clinical history and the presentation may be varied, epilepsy is commonly misdiagnosed. Conditions frequently misdiagnosed as seizures in children include psychogenic nonepileptic events, syncope, gastroesophageal reflux (Sandifer syndrome), stroke, tics or other movement disorders, benign myoclonus of infancy, migraine, breath-holding or shuddering spells, and parasomnias. At times, normal childhood behaviors, including daydreaming, temper tantrums, self-stimulation, and inattention, can be misinterpreted as seizures.

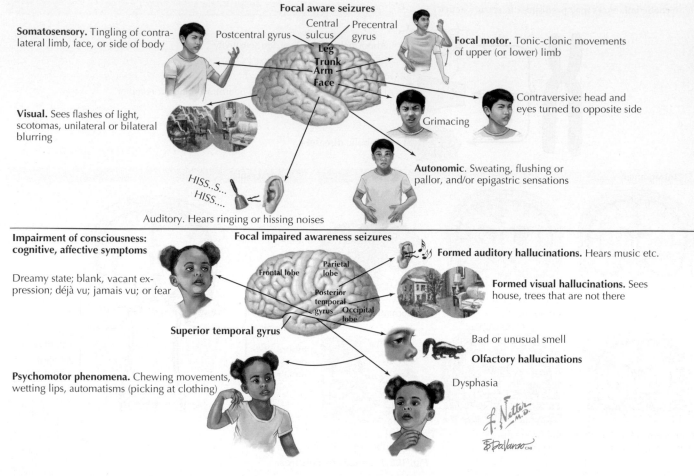

Focal aware seizures

Somatosensory. Tingling of contralateral limb, face, or side of body

Focal motor. Tonic-clonic movements of upper (or lower) limb

Central sulcus — Precentral gyrus

Postcentral gyrus

Leg
Trunk
Arm
Face

Contraversive: head and eyes turned to opposite side

Grimacing

Visual. Sees flashes of light, scotomas, unilateral or bilateral blurring

Autonomic. Sweating, flushing or pallor, and/or epigastric sensations

HISS..S...
HISS....

Auditory. Hears ringing or hissing noises

Focal impaired awareness seizures

Impairment of consciousness: cognitive, affective symptoms

Dreamy state; blank, vacant expression; déjà vu; jamais vu; or fear

Frontal lobe — Parietal lobe

Posterior temporal gyrus — Occipital lobe

Formed auditory hallucinations. Hears music etc.

Formed visual hallucinations. Sees house, trees that are not there

Superior temporal gyrus

Bad or unusual smell
Olfactory hallucinations

Psychomotor phenomena. Chewing movements, wetting lips, automatisms (picking at clothing)

Dysphasia

Fig. 108.2 Focal Seizures.

EVALUATION

Evaluation of a first seizure depends on the history and clinical manifestation, but should focus on whether the event was provoked by a transient or treatable abnormality (e.g., hypoglycemia), or signals an acute neurologic problem (e.g., intracerebral hemorrhage or meningitis).

EEG can support a clinical diagnosis of seizure and can help with the classification of seizure type. However, 50% of patients with epilepsy may have a normal interictal EEG. Certain techniques, such as hyperventilation and photic stimulation, may bring out abnormalities, particularly in certain epilepsy syndromes. Sometimes prolonged ambulatory or inpatient video EEG are required to capture an event and diagnose a seizure, differentiate from nonepileptic events, or clarify seizure type (Fig. 108.4).

Initial evaluation of epilepsy should focus on finding a cause and evaluating for psychosocial comorbidities that are common in children with epilepsy. Except in idiopathic epilepsy syndromes (such as CAE or JME), evaluation typically includes brain magnetic resonance imaging (MRI) to identify any structural abnormalities. Other diagnostic evaluation may include genetic testing to look for chromosomal copy number variants, or pathogenic variants in genes known to be associated with epilepsy. Advanced imaging techniques (e.g., magnetoencephalography, functional MRI, and positron emission tomography) are used to evaluate patients with pharmacoresistant epilepsy.

MANAGEMENT

Seizure First Aid

On encountering a seizing child, remain calm. Ensure that the child is safe from injury from surrounding objects and placed in a lateral decubitus position in the event of emesis. Avoid restraining the patient, and do not attempt to open a clenched jaw. Patients with epilepsy may carry a rescue medication such as rectal diazepam, orally disintegrating clonazepam, or nasal spray midazolam or diazepam, which can be administered to abort a prolonged seizure, often defined as 5 minutes or longer. Most seizures are self-limited and do not by themselves cause permanent brain injury. The patient may be sleepy, confused, or disorientated after a seizure.

Antiseizure Medications

Antiseizure medications are recommended when a child is diagnosed with epilepsy given the high risk for recurrent seizures. Key factors in choosing a medication include type of epilepsy (focal versus generalized onset, epilepsy syndromes; Table 108.1), comorbidities, and the side effect profile of a medication. For new-onset focal epilepsy in a child, the most common choices currently are oxcarbazepine or levetiracetam. Medications that treat a broad spectrum of seizure types are preferred when the mechanism of onset is unclear. Identification of a specific seizure syndrome may influence medication choice—for example, sodium channel blocking drugs such as oxcarbazepine

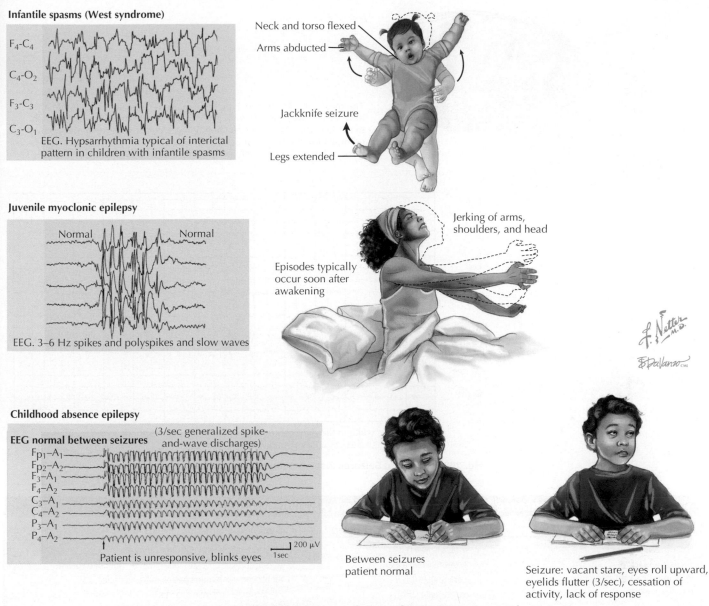

Infantile spasms (West syndrome)

F_4-C_4
C_4-O_2
F_3-C_3
C_3-O_1

EEG. Hypsarrhythmia typical of interictal pattern in children with infantile spasms

Neck and torso flexed
Arms abducted
Jackknife seizure
Legs extended

Juvenile myoclonic epilepsy

Normal   Normal

EEG. 3–6 Hz spikes and polyspikes and slow waves

Jerking of arms, shoulders, and head

Episodes typically occur soon after awakening

Childhood absence epilepsy

EEG normal between seizures
(3/sec generalized spike-and-wave discharges)
Fp_1-A_1
Fp_2-A_2
F_3-A_1
F_4-A_2
C_3-A_1
C_4-A_2
P_3-A_1
P_4-A_2

200 µV
1sec
Patient is unresponsive, blinks eyes

Between seizures patient normal

Seizure: vacant stare, eyes roll upward, eyelids flutter (3/sec), cessation of activity, lack of response

Fig. 108.3 Common Epilepsy Syndromes.

are contraindicated in Dravet syndrome, which is caused by a mutation in a sodium channel subunit gene. For new-onset CAE without generalized tonic-clonic seizures, ethosuximide is the first-line treatment. Comorbid conditions also affect the choice of medication. For example, levetiracetam may exacerbate mood or behavior disturbances and topiramate also can be used to treat migraine headaches. A medication's toxicities also affect its use—valproate may be teratogenic and is generally avoided in adolescent girls and women of childbearing age.

Other Therapies

Pharmacoresistance, or intractability, is defined as failure of two appropriately chosen and adequately dosed medications. Children with pharmacoresistant epilepsy should be evaluated by an epilepsy specialist for consideration of other treatment options, including the ketogenic diet and its variants, epilepsy surgery, and implantable devices such as a vagus nerve stimulator or responsive neurostimulator.

Management of Comorbidities

Learning disabilities, depression, anxiety, and attention deficit hyperactivity disorder (ADHD) are common in children with epilepsy. Screening for these conditions followed by appropriate referral to behavioral health professionals is critical. Identification of comorbid psychiatric or medical conditions may influence the choice of antiseizure medications or other treatment options.

FUTURE DIRECTIONS

Advances in identifying the genetic causes of epilepsy is fueling better understanding of the mechanisms underlying seizures and epilepsy comorbidities. Drug discovery continues to proceed rapidly. Disease modifying therapies, including gene therapies, are in development. Research to understand complex brain networks underlying epilepsy may lead to better approaches to epilepsy surgery and more effective implantable electrical stimulation devices.

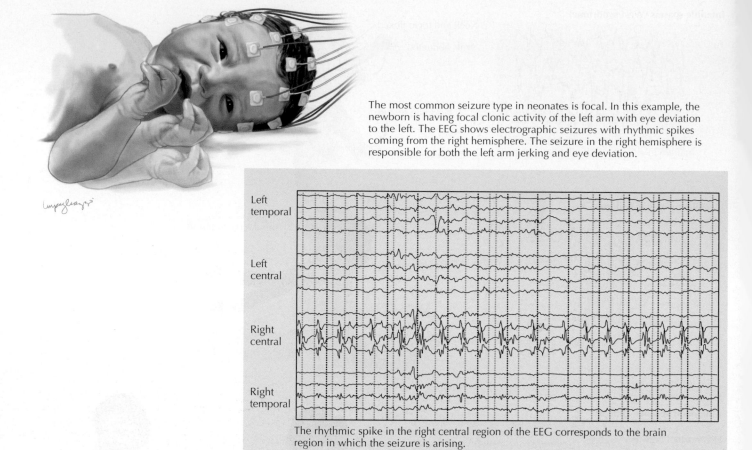

The most common seizure type in neonates is focal. In this example, the newborn is having focal clonic activity of the left arm with eye deviation to the left. The EEG shows electrographic seizures with rhythmic spikes coming from the right hemisphere. The seizure in the right hemisphere is responsible for both the left arm jerking and eye deviation.

Left temporal

Left central

Right central

Right temporal

The rhythmic spike in the right central region of the EEG corresponds to the brain region in which the seizure is arising.

Fig. 108.4 Neonatal Seizures Electroencephalogram.

TABLE 108.1 Antiseizure Medications: Choices by Seizure Type

Focal	Focal and/or Generalized	Syndrome-Specific
Oxcarbazepine (OXC)	Valproic acid (VPA)	Ethosuximide (ETX)—absence seizures
Lacosamide (LCM)	Levetiracetam (LEV)	Adrenocorticotropic hormone (ACTH)—infantile spasms
Eslicarbazepine (ESL)	Lamotrigine (LTG)	Vigabatrin—infantile spasms, tuberous sclerosis
Phenytoin (PHT)	Topiramate (TPM)	Prednisone—infantile spasms
Carbamazepine (CBZ)	Zonisamide (ZNS)	Stiripentol—Dravet syndrome
Vigabatrin (VGB)	Clobazam (CLB)	Fenfluramine—Dravet syndrome
Gabapentin (GBP)	Brivaracetam (BRV)	
Phenobarbital (PHB)	Rufinamide (RFM)	
Pregabalin (PGB)	Perampanel (PMP)	
	Felbamate (FBM)	
	Cannabidiol (CBD)	

SUGGESTED READINGS

Available online.

109

Headache

Christina Lynch Szperka, Marissa Anto, and Donna J. Stephenson

CLINICAL VIGNETTE

A 12-year-old girl presents to the neurology clinic with 7 months of headaches. She has no significant medical history and was born at full term with normal development and school performance. With menarche at age 11, she began to have intermittent throbbing headaches occurring four to six times per month accompanied by nausea, photophobia, and phonophobia. She denies visual aura. Her headaches improve if she is able to lie down in a dark room and sleep. In the past few months, she started to have headaches at school, which have caused her to miss class. She drinks about 30 oz of water a day, skips breakfast and lunch, exercises once a week, and sleeps on average 8 hours nightly. Relevant family history includes mother, father, and older brother with migraines. She was prescribed naproxen and metoclopramide as abortive therapy for severe headaches to be taken no more than twice a week. She was advised to start magnesium and riboflavin as daily preventive therapy. She was given a "Headache Action Plan" permitting her to carry a water bottle and to take naproxen and metoclopramide in school if needed. After 8 weeks, she returned for follow up and reported headaches only occur once a month and are responsive to abortive therapy. She is no longer missing class.

CLINICAL VIGNETTE

A 4-year-old boy with no significant medical history presents for evaluation of new-onset headache for the past month. Mom reports he complains of a headache on awakening in the morning and has woken in the middle of the night with a headache. Occasionally he has associated emesis. The child describes pain that is worse when he lies down. Additionally, he reports the headache is getting progressively worse. He denies photophobia and phonophobia. Mom has noted that his right eye has become slightly droopy in the past week. There is no family history of headache. After neurologic evaluation, brain magnetic resonance imaging is performed and reveals a posterior fossa mass. He is admitted to the hospital for further evaluation and treatment.

Headache is a very common symptom in children. Epidemiologic studies estimate that approximately 20% of children have experienced a headache by the age of 5 years, jumping to 60% to 80% by school age. Data are limited about the prevalence of headaches of a specific cause other than migraine. Overall, its prevalence is in the single digits for children ages 7 to 10 years and increases to about 20% in teens. Young children with migraines are more commonly boys, but this pattern switches at the time of preadolescence.

ETIOLOGY AND PATHOGENESIS

The pathophysiologic process of headache is not fully understood. The blood vessels and meninges sense pain but refer it to the anterior or posterior scalp, explaining why pain from multiple causes and locations can feel similar. The mechanism of migraine pain has been studied most extensively. Cortical spreading depression, which is associated with aura, is a rapid depolarization of neurons followed by prolonged hyperpolarization, which propagates as a wave through the brain. The initial phase of a migraine involves activation of the trigeminovascular reflex, which causes the release of vasoactive peptides (e.g., calcitonin gene-related peptide [CGRP], neurokinin A, and substance P) from trigeminal afferents supplying dural blood vessels. This leads to vasodilation and sterile inflammation in dural vessels, initiating the activation of first-order trigeminal afferents, which is called peripheral sensitization. Peripheral sensitization is manifested clinically by throbbing pain. As the migraine proceeds, activation of second- and third-order trigeminothalamic and thalamocortical neurons is mediated by nitric oxide and glutamate, which results in central sensitization. Central sensitization is manifested by cutaneous allodynia.

CLINICAL PRESENTATION

Headache syndromes vary widely in their presentation depending on cause. Relevant elements of the history are listed in Table 109.1. The physical examination must include vital signs, a general examination, and a neurologic examination, including funduscopic examination. The goal of initial evaluation is to differentiate primary from secondary headaches. Primary headaches, in which the headache itself is the disorder, include migraine, tension type headache, and others and often do not require further diagnostic testing. Secondary headaches are caused by an underlying medical condition, which must be identified; treatment of the underlying condition should then lead to improvement in headache. Table 109.2 outlines typical characteristics of primary and secondary headaches, the recommended evaluation, and treatment where applicable (Fig. 109.1).

EVALUATION AND MANAGEMENT

See Table 109.2 for recommended evaluation and management of headache based on cause. Overall indications for neuroimaging are summarized here:

- Acute-onset, severe headache should be imaged emergently. The American Academy of Neurology Practice Parameter recommends imaging for any headache of less than 1 month duration.
- Alteration of consciousness.
- Signs or symptoms that suggest a focal brain pathologic condition (consider structural and vascular imaging to rule out ischemia).
- Signs or symptoms that suggest increased intracranial pressure (ICP) (consider structural and vascular imaging to rule out mass lesions and cerebral sinus venous thrombosis).
- Comorbid seizures.

TABLE 109.1	**Headache History**
Description of the headache	Location and radiation
	Quality and severity of pain
	Frequency and duration of attacks
	Awaken from sleep?
	Pattern over time
	School absence
Triggers and exacerbating factors	Stress at home and school
	Food (monosodium glutamate [MSG], caffeine, alcohol)
	Sleep changes
	Valsalva maneuver, cough, sneeze
	Posture (supine, recumbent, upright)
Alleviating factors	Medication: clarify frequency and duration
	Sleep
Associated symptoms	Nausea or vomiting
	Photophobia or phonophobia
	Weakness—general or focal
	Sensory changes—positive (tingling) or negative (numbness)
	Visual symptoms—positive or negative
	Lacrimation or rhinorrhea
	Ptosis, pupillary changes
	Pulsatile tinnitus
Other	Allergic symptoms
	Snoring or teeth grinding
	Blurred vision
	Family history

- Change in headache quality, frequency, or severity.
- Consider for any recurrent headache in which there is *no* family history of headache.

Generally, magnetic resonance imaging (MRI) of the brain is the preferred neuroimaging modality for evaluation of headache because it provides excellent structural detail and resolution. Head computed tomography (CT) may be used in emergent situations when MRI is not available to look for intracranial hemorrhage, large mass lesion, hydrocephalus, cerebral edema, or bony changes. Vascular imaging, such as MR angiogram (MRA) and MR venogram (MRV), are suggested for evaluation of some secondary causes of headache (Table 109.2).

Screening neuroimaging is also sometimes necessary before lumbar puncture. Neuroimaging is indicated if a patient has an abnormal physical examination finding, to ensure that it is safe to perform the lumbar puncture (no signs of herniation nor significant edema). Indications for lumbar puncture (with opening pressure) in the evaluation of headache include:

- Acute-onset, severe headache (looking for subarachnoid hemorrhage; the first and last tubes should be collected for a cell count to aid interpretation)
- Alteration of consciousness
- Symptoms or examination findings that suggest increased ICP
- Consider for symptoms or examination findings that suggest a focal brain pathologic condition when the differential diagnosis includes ischemic, infectious or inflammatory pathologic findings.

Treatment

Treatment should be guided by the cause of the headache as outlined in Table 109.2.

Abortive Medications

These should be used at most two or three times per week to prevent medication overuse, which may transform headache from episodic to chronic. All abortive therapies should be given as soon as possible after symptom onset to maximize efficacy. Other than analgesics, studies of medication efficacy pertain to patients with migraine headache, and the intravenous therapies listed are generally for migraine except as noted.

Analgesics. Remind patients of side effects; many of these are available over the counter:

- Nonsteroidal antiinflammatory drugs (NSAIDs): contraindicated in renal disease or history of gastrointestinal (GI) bleeding.
  - Ibuprofen: The 2019 American Academy of Neurology–American Headache Society (AAN-AHS) Acute Treatment Guidelines recommend this as first line for children and adolescents with migraine.
  - Naproxen
  - Ketorolac (preferred NSAID for IV use)
- Acetaminophen: contraindicated in liver disease
- Opioids and preparations with butalbital or caffeine should be avoided because they can be detrimental long term.

Triptans. Triptans are contraindicated in cardiovascular and liver disease, pregnancy, hemiplegic migraine, and patients with hypertension. Studies of triptans in teens with migraine have been limited by their extremely high response to placebo, making it difficult to prove a statistically significant benefit. Side effects include taste disturbance (for nasal sprays), burning (for injections), drowsiness, nausea or vomiting, dizziness, tingling, flushing, and infrequent chest tightness. The strongest evidence of benefit is for the following triptans, though others may be used:

- Sumatriptan + naproxen (Treximet): US Food and Drug Administration (FDA) approved for adolescents 12 to 17
- Zolmitriptan (Zomig): nasal spray, FDA approved in adolescents 12 to 17
- Rizatriptan (Maxalt): FDA approved in children 6 to 17
- Almotriptan (Axert): FDA approved in adolescents 12 to 17

Antiemetics. The 2019 AAN-AHS Treatment Guidelines specifically recommend treatment of nausea with an antiemetic if NSAIDs and/or triptans are insufficient. Medications that block dopamine, such as prochlorperazine (Compazine) and metoclopramide (Reglan), can be effective for migraine even in the absence of significant nausea. Side effects include potential dystonic reaction, which usually responds to diphenhydramine. Data are limited in children. Medications such as ondansetron (Zofran) may treat nausea but may not stop headache pain.

Steroids. Data are limited, and a variety of doses are used. Use with caution in patients with hypertension, renal disease, diabetes, active infections, and history of GI bleeding. Short-term side effects include increased appetite, weight gain, irritability or mood changes, insomnia, or hyperglycemia. Though there are limited and mixed data, steroids are most commonly used orally or intravenously for prolonged headache that did not respond to usual acute treatments, or intravenously to prevent recurrence of headache after other intravenous therapies.

- Prednisone
- Dexamethasone
- Methylprednisolone

Nerve block. Abortive therapy for status migrainosus or any debilitating persistent headache. Consider if a procedural specialist is available and headache is refractory to other therapies. The mechanism of action of therapeutic effect is unclear because the duration of pain relief often lasts longer than the duration of numbness.

Typically, local anesthetics such as lidocaine and/or bupivacaine are injected over some combination of the following locations to target

TABLE 109.2	Differential Diagnosis and Evaluation and Treatment of Headaches by Cause		
Headache Syndrome or Cause	**Pertinent History**	**Pertinent Physical Examination Findings**	**Further Evaluation and Treatment**
Primary Headaches *Migraine*			
Migraine without aura	• Unilateral or bilateral frontotemporal throbbing • Moderate to severe intensity • Aggravated by physical activity • Accompanied by nausea, vomiting, photophobia, and/or phonophobia • 2–72 hours when untreated	Normal, may have photophobia or phonophobia	• Imaging is NOT needed if history consistent with migraine without any "red flags" and examination is normal • Emergent neuroimaging if focal symptoms or signs • Nonurgent MRI if:
Migraine with aura	• Above + aura symptom for 5–60 minutes • Headache begins during the aura or within 60 minutes • Aura is fully reversible • Aura includes visual, sensory symptoms (positive or negative), and/or speech disturbance (see Fig. 109.1)	Normal; may fit aura	• Concern for secondary headache • New onset, escalating, or changing quality • Does not respond to medical therapy • No family history • Treat with analgesic, triptan, and/or antiemetic, and avoidance of triggers • Consider prophylaxis if >3 headaches per month or disabling
Chronic migraine	• ≥15 or more days per month for longer than 3 months	Normal or may have photophobia or phonophobia	• Treat with prophylaxis
Status migrainosus	Debilitating migraine lasting ≥72 hours	Normal or may have photophobia or phonophobia	• Treat with analgesic, antiemetic, or triptan • Consider IV fluids, prochlorperazine, ketorolac, valproic acid, DHE • IV steroids anecdotally efficacious; in adults, dexamethasone shown to decrease rebound headache
Familial hemiplegic migraine	• Migraine with aura, including motor weakness • Attacks can be triggered by mild head trauma • Positive family history; sometimes family history of cerebellar ataxia (same gene)	• May include: • Focal weakness, sensory changes, or aphasia • Altered consciousness, fever, confusion	• MRI with diffusion weighted imaging to rule out focal ischemia or other lesion • Consider lumbar puncture (may have CSF pleocytosis during attack) • Consider genetic testing • Treat as above, avoid triptans and DHE (may increase risk for stroke) • Consider prophylaxis
Sporadic hemiplegic migraine	• As above, no family history		
Migraine with brainstem aura	• Migraine with aura symptoms from brainstem or both hemispheres (dysarthria, vertigo, tinnitus, hypacusis, diplopia, ataxia, altered consciousness)	May reflect aura symptoms	
Retinal migraine	• Monocular positive or negative visual phenomena	Visual field examination results may be abnormal	• Ophthalmologic examination to evaluate for optic neuropathy • MRI/MRA to evaluate for carotid plaque or dissection
Cyclic vomiting	• Intense nausea and vomiting lasting 1 hour to 5 days; symptom-free between attacks • No gastrointestinal/renal disease	Normal or may have findings of dehydration	• Rule out gastrointestinal and other causes • May treat with abortive and preventive medications used for migraine
Abdominal migraine	• Abdominal pain lasting 2–72 hours: • Midline, periumbilical, or poorly localized • Dull or sore • Moderate to severe • Accompanied by ≥2 of the following: anorexia, nausea, vomiting, pallor • No GI or renal disease		
Benign paroxysmal vertigo of childhood	• Episodes of severe vertigo lasting minutes to hours • May be associated with nystagmus, vomiting, headache	Normal or may have nystagmus	• Consider EEG to evaluate for seizure

Continued

TABLE 109.2 **Differential Diagnosis and Evaluation and Treatment of Headaches by Cause—cont'd**

Headache Syndrome or Cause	Pertinent History	Pertinent Physical Examination Findings	Further Evaluation and Treatment
Tension-Type Headache			
Episodic	• Bilateral • Pressing or squeezing • Mild to moderate intensity • Lasts minutes to days • May have photophobia or phonophobia • May coexist with migraine	Normal or scalp may be tender	• Neuroimaging if escalating or does not respond to long-term therapy • Adult studies support use of analgesics for acute management and amitriptyline for chronic headache • Other medications used for migraine, as well as psychological and complementary therapies may be helpful
Chronic	• As above but ≥15 days per month for ≥3 months		
Cluster Headache, Paroxysmal Hemicrania, Hemicrania Continua, Other Forms of Trigeminal Autonomic Cephalgia (Very Rare in Children)			
	All involve unilateral, side-locked intense pain in orbital, supraorbital, temporal distribution and should be accompanied by one or more ipsilateral autonomic symptoms including conjunctival injection, lacrimation, nasal congestion, rhinorrhea, forehead/facial sweating, miosis, ptosis, and/or eyelid edema.	Can have ptosis, miosis, eyelid edema of affected side.	• If paroxysmal hemicrania or hemicrania continua are on differential, consider an indomethacin trial; a positive response can be diagnostic. • As these headaches can be secondary to pituitary lesions, MRI brain with and without contrast with fine cuts through pituitary should be considered.
Secondary Headaches			
Headache Attributed to Non-Vascular Intracranial Disorder			
Posttraumatic headache	• No characteristic features • Severe head trauma with loss of consciousness more likely to cause demonstrable injury, but mild head trauma can cause headache as part of postconcussive syndrome	Look for signs of head trauma and focal neurologic findings	• Neuroimaging if examination results are abnormal or severity escalating • Treat as the primary headache it resembles (migraine, tension type) • Consider magnesium supplementation; case series found low ionized magnesium in patients with posttraumatic headache
Intracranial neoplasm	• Headache worse in the morning • Progressive • Aggravated by physical activity, Valsalva maneuver, cough, sneeze, bending forward • Associated with nausea or vomiting	May have focal abnormality, papilledema, sixth nerve palsy, depressed mental status, abnormal gait	• Neuroimaging
Hydrocephalus	• Headache worse in the morning • Aggravated by physical activity, Valsalva maneuver, cough, sneeze, bending forward • Associated with nausea or vomiting	May be associated with papilledema, sixth nerve palsy, depressed mental status, gait instability, increased head circumference	• Neuroimaging
Idiopathic intracranial hypertension (pseudotumor cerebri)	• No characteristic features • May be associated with tinnitus, transient visual obscurations, diplopia, constriction of visual field, enlarged blind spot • May be secondary to obesity, anemia, Lyme disease, lupus, medications (Retin A, tetracycline or minocycline, oral contraceptives)	• Papilledema; may have eye movement abnormalities • Lumbar puncture: increased opening pressure ≥280 mm H_2O in children (≥250 mm H_2O if non-obese, unsedated), all in lateral decubitus position • CSF studies normal; if elevated protein or WBCs, consider infectious or inflammatory causes (Lyme disease, lupus)	• MRI. Should include contrast or MRV to exclude sinus venous thrombosis • Ophthalmologic examination with visual fields • Abnormal vision necessitates emergent therapy (lumbar puncture to drain fluid, acetazolamide ± steroids); otherwise treat underlying cause and start acetazolamide

Chiari type 1 malformation (cerebellar tonsils extend below foramen magnum into the cervical spinal canal)	• Occipital or posterior pain
	• Lasts hours to days
	• Worsens with cough or Valsalva maneuver
	• May have:
	  • Transient visual symptoms
	  • Dizziness, change in hearing, vertigo, nystagmus
	  • Other symptoms of brainstem, cerebellar, or cervical cord dysfunction, including spells of loss of consciousness
		Normal or may have:
		• Signs related to cervical cord, brainstem, lower cranial nerves, or ataxia or dysmetria
		• Signs of syrinx: abnormalities of sensation, strength, tone, reflexes
			• MRI of the brain
			• If Chiari malformation is present, MRI of the spinal cord to look for syrinx
			• Refer to neurosurgeon if syrinx present or if headache consistent with Chiari-type headache
			• Chiari is a common incidental finding, and decompression is not indicated in most cases

TABLE 109.2 Differential Diagnosis and Evaluation and Treatment of Headaches by Cause—cont'd

Headache Syndrome or Cause	Pertinent History	Pertinent Physical Examination Findings	Further Evaluation and Treatment
Intracranial hemorrhage (intraparenchymal, epidural, subdural)	• Acute onset; may be thunderclap headache • History of trauma suggests epidural or subdural • No history of trauma suggests intraparenchymal	Usually abnormal examination results, often with altered consciousness	• Head CT; may require emergent surgery
Vascular malformation (aneurysm, AVM, cavernous angioma)	• New headache; may be thunderclap (suggests hemorrhage) • AVM can mimic migraine, but it is uncommon	May have pupil-involving third nerve palsy (points to posterior communicating artery aneurysm)	• MRI brain and MRA or CTA head/neck
Sickle cell disease	• Increased incidence of migraine and tension-type headache in patients with sickle cell disease and possible association with pseudotumor cerebri • Headache can represent a pain crisis in scalp or face or symptom of stroke or moyamoya disease	Normal or may show focal signs of ischemia	• Neuroimaging and vascular imaging; urgent if focal symptoms or signs • Treat as for primary headache, with precautions (e.g., acetazolamide can precipitate sickling)
Headache Attributed to Infection			
Systemic infection	• Diffuse pain with symptoms of infection	Fever, signs of infection	• Guided by other symptoms or signs • Treat with analgesics
Intracranial infection	• Diffuse pain with nausea, photophobia, phonophobia • May develop chronic postmeningitis headache	May have focal findings, fever, meningismus, or altered mental status	• Head imaging if focal findings • CSF examination • Treat with antibiotics, analgesics
Headache Attributed to a Substance or Its Withdrawal			
Medication side effect	• Associated with many medications, especially hormonal contraceptives • Look for recent change in formulation (brand or generic) • Aseptic meningitis associated with ibuprofen, IVIG, penicillin, trimethoprim, and intrathecal injections	Normal, may have meningismus	• Consider changing medication or formulation • If meningismus, consider lumbar puncture
Medication overuse headache	• Near-daily headache after overusing headache treatment (analgesic, ergot, triptan, opioid) for at least 3 months	Normal	• Withdraw agent • Adult data show decreased withdrawal symptoms, less use of rescue medications when 6-day oral prednisone taper was used during withdrawal
Headache Attributed to Disorder of Homeostasis			
Hypoxia or hypercapnia related to sleep apnea	• Bilateral headache almost daily on awakening; resolves within 30 minutes • History of snoring	Enlarged tonsils, obese habitus may be present	• Evaluate with overnight polysomnography
Psychiatric disease	• Rarely the direct cause • Comorbid anxiety and depression lead to increased rates of school absenteeism and lower rates of remission of chronic headaches	May have altered affect	• Ask about mood and coping; refer for psychotherapy, biofeedback, psychiatry
Facial Pain			
Refractive error or eye misalignment	• Frontal or diffuse • Worse in afternoon or evening • History of blurred vision, eye strain, squinting	Decreased visual acuity, abnormal eye movements or alignment	• Refer to optometrist or ophthalmologist

Continued

TABLE 109.2 Differential Diagnosis and Evaluation and Treatment of Headaches by Cause—cont'd

Headache Syndrome or Cause	Pertinent History	Pertinent Physical Examination Findings	Further Evaluation and Treatment
Rhinosinusitis	• Frontal headache accompanied by pain in face, ears, or teeth • May have halitosis, fatigue, cough, hyposmia or anosmia • Should remit within 7 days of treatment	Purulent nasal discharge, fever, tenderness to palpation of sinuses may be present	• Neuroimaging if diagnosis unclear • Treat with antibiotics, decongestants, nasal steroids • May be confused with tension, migraine, or medication overuse headache
Teeth or jaw abnormalities	• Frontal or diffuse headache • History of bruxism or pain precipitated by chewing or jaw movement	Noise or tenderness at TMJ with jaw movement, dental caries	• Refer to dentist or oral surgeon • Consider mouth guard, tricyclic antidepressant (TCA), relaxation techniques for bruxism
Cervicogenic headache	• Pain referred from neck, perceived in head or face	Tense or sore neck or back muscles	• Consider MRI of brain and cervical spine to rule out posterior fossa lesion, C2 spinal nerve or joint problem, vascular imaging to rule out aneurysm • Treat cervicogenic with physical therapy • Treat with occipital nerve block; consider antiinflammatory or anticonvulsant medications
Occipital neuralgia	• Paroxysmal jabbing pain on the posterior scalp in the distribution of the occipital nerve • Primary headache syndromes (especially migraine) can also cause pain in a similar distribution	Tenderness of posterior scalp	

AVM, Arteriovenous malformation; *CSF,* cerebrospinal fluid; *CT,* computed tomography; *CTA,* computed tomography angiography; *DHE,* dihydroergotamine; *EEG,* electroencephalography; *GI,* gastrointestinal; *IV,* intravenous; *IVIG,* intravenous immunoglobulin; *MRA,* magnetic resonance angiography; *MRI,* magnetic resonance imaging; *MRV,* magnetic resonance venography; *TCA,* tricyclic antidepressant; *TMJ,* temporomandibular joint; *WBC,* white blood cell.

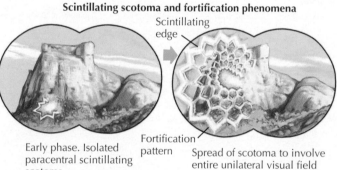

Scintillating scotoma and fortification phenomena

Scintillating edge

Early phase. Isolated paracentral scintillating scotoma

Fortification pattern

Spread of scotoma to involve entire unilateral visual field

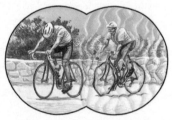

Wavy lines (heat shimmers)

Wavy line distortions in part of visual field similar to shimmers above hot pavement

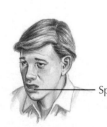

Vertigo

Speech disturbances

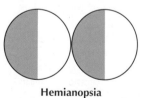

Focal neurologic phenomena

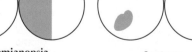

Hemianopsia

Scotoma

JOHN A. CRAIG—MD

C. Machado—M.D.

Fig. 109.1 Migraine Prodromes.

the areas of pain: greater occipital nerve, lesser occipital nerve, auriculotemporal nerve, supratrochlear nerve and supraorbital nerve. In some cases, a steroid may be added, although studies in adults did not demonstrate added benefit in patients with migraine.

Anticonvulsants. See discussion of valproic acid, later.

Dihydroergotamine. Contraindicated in cardiovascular, renal, and liver disease; pregnancy; hemiplegic migraine; and patients with hypertension or recent triptan use. Open-label case series of intravenous dihydroergotamine in children have shown that it is effective for the treatment of status migrainosus in children.

- Intranasal (migranal), intravenous
- Side effects include nausea or vomiting (can be improved by premedication with an antiemetic), vasoconstriction.

Preventive Medications

The 2019 AAN-AHS Guideline "Pharmacologic Treatment for Pediatric Migraine Prevention" highlights that high placebo response has limited the ability of randomized controlled trials (RCTs) to demonstrate efficacy of most preventive treatments for migraine in youth. Sometimes this is interpreted to mean that nothing works; on the contrary, approximately 60% of patients receiving amitriptyline, topiramate, or placebo had improvement in the CHAMP trial. Guideline recommendations include examination of lifestyle factors that influence headache, and management of comorbid conditions that can exacerbate headache. Clinicians should "engage in shared decision-making with patients and caregivers regarding the use of preventive treatments for migraine, including discussion of the limitations in the evidence to support pharmacologic treatments." The strongest evidence of benefit is for propranolol, topiramate, cinnarizine, and amitriptyline coupled with cognitive behavioral therapy (see Hershey et al., 2013, in Suggested Readings). Specific medication classes are reviewed below:

Antidepressants
- Amitriptyline
  - Side effects: sedation (advise taking 2 to 3 hours before bed), dry eyes, dry mouth, urinary retention, constipation (patients should drink plenty of water), worsening of underlying prolonged QT (check electrocardiogram [ECG] before starting), weight gain, risk for increased thoughts about suicide.
  - Other tricyclic antidepressants may have fewer side effects; these have not been studied in children.

Antiepileptics
- Topiramate
  - Side effects: metabolic acidosis causing tingling (can treat with vitamin C or sodium bicarbonate supplementation), oligohidrosis or hyperthermia, weight loss, cognitive dulling and word-finding problems; uncommon side effects are kidney stones, blurred vision, and decreased effectiveness of hormonal contraception (especially at doses ≥200 mg/day); it is teratogenic, so counsel adolescent girls to take daily folate.
- Valproic acid
  - Oral for prophylaxis; can use intravenously to treat status migrainosus.
  - Side effects: hepatic and pancreatic dysfunction, anorexia or weight gain, teratogenic (so should not be used long term in girls of child-bearing age; prescribe folate if used), tremor, and hair loss; it may be linked with polycystic ovarian syndrome.
- Gabapentin, zonisamide and levetiracetam, are also used.

NSAIDs
- Contraindicated in renal disease or history of GI bleeding
  - Naproxen: see earlier; prophylactic use in menstrual or other predictable headache
  - Indomethacin: for hemicrania continua and paroxysmal hemicrania

Antiserotonergic
- Cyproheptadine (may also work as calcium channel blocker and is an antihistamine)
  - Side effects: sedation, appetite stimulation, weight gain

Antihypertensive
- Calcium channel blockers
  - Cinnarizine has good evidence but is not available in the United States (it is also an antihistamine); verapamil is sometimes used.
  - Side effects: sedation, weight gain, depression, constipation, arrhythmia (check ECG); contraindicated in patients with heart failure
- β-Blockers: best evidence for propranolol, though other medications in the class, such as metoprolol, also may be used.
  - Side effects: decreased exercise tolerance, hypotension or orthostasis, low energy, depression, vivid dreams, contraindicated in patients with asthma or existing depression

Novel preventive therapies
- CGRP inhibitors (erenumab, galcanezumab, fremanezumab, eptinezumab) are monoclonal antibodies that have been FDA approved in adults older than 18 years or the preventive treatment of migraines. Pediatric studies are in progress. CGRP is a multifunctional neuropeptide involved in vasodilation, nociception, and neurogenic inflammation. CGRP levels have been found to be elevated in patients with migraine during an attack. Erenumab targets the CGRP receptor and the others target the CGRP molecule. Eptinezumab is administered intravenously, whereas the others are self-administered monthly injections.
  - Side effects include injection site discomfort and constipation.
- Botox: Botulinum toxin has been approved by the FDA for chronic migraine in people 18 years and older, although some insurances will approve for people younger than 18 years if they are refractory to multiple therapies. The treatment is administered every 3 months by 31 injection sites around the head. The proposed mechanism of action is through blocking neurotransmitter release from primary afferents, decreasing nociception in migraine.

Nonpharmaceutical
- Riboflavin (vitamin B_2): limited pediatric data; adult studies have been mixed
  - Side effects: turns urine bright yellow, diarrhea, polyuria
- Magnesium: uncontrolled pediatric studies have been positive; one RCT was equivocal
  - Side effects: diarrhea, GI upset
- CoQ10: no RCT, an open-label pediatric study in patients found to be deficient in CoQ10, showed improvement in headache frequency and disability as level normalized
  - Side effects: stomach upset, procoagulant (may decrease efficacy of Coumadin)

Nonpharmacologic Therapies

Nonpharmacologic therapies can be the mainstay of therapy or can complement medications.

Lifestyle changes and avoidance of triggers. Although these efforts are time consuming, they are very safe and can be quite effective. If patients find a lifestyle trigger, they often benefit from recognizing its predictability (Fig. 109.2). In reviewing these factors, avoid blaming the patient and think broadly about how to troubleshoot solutions with them. For example, high school students may sleep few hours because of demanding work and homework schedules with an early school start time. Food insecurity may contribute to missed meals.

- Sleep hygiene: sufficient sleep, consistent bedtime and wake-up time.
- Diet: avoid fasting; eat regularly; avoid dehydration; drink at least 72 oz daily of noncaffeinated fluids; there is poor evidence for some things

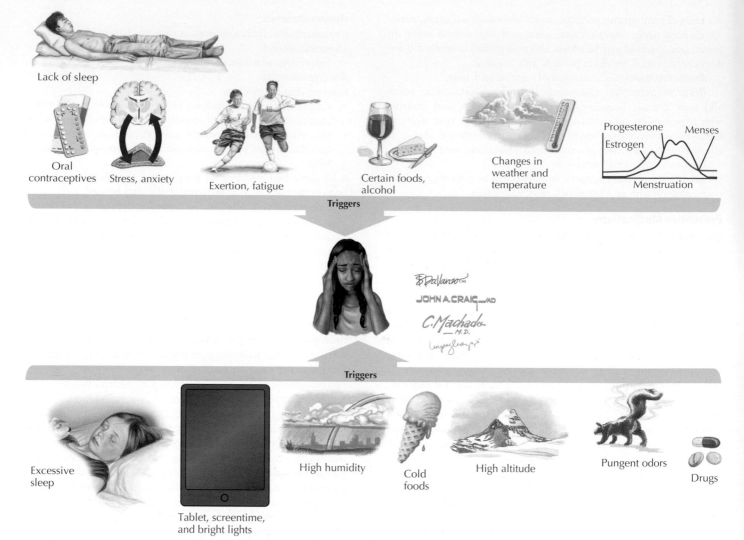

Lack of sleep

Oral contraceptives   Stress, anxiety   Exertion, fatigue   Certain foods, alcohol   Changes in weather and temperature   Progesterone   Menses   Estrogen   Menstruation

Triggers

Triggers

Excessive sleep   Tablet, screentime, and bright lights   High humidity   Cold foods   High altitude   Pungent odors   Drugs

Fig. 109.2 Triggers of Migraine.

thought of as common dietary triggers, such as chocolate; the best evidence is for caffeine, alcohol or wine, and monosodium glutamate.
- Exercise: thought to be preventive (evidence in adults shows benefit, but it has not been tested in children/adolescents)
- Stress: recognition of stressful life events at home and school, improvement of situation where possible, learning coping mechanisms (see later); stress letdown can also trigger headaches
- Hormonal fluctuations: can be anticipated; may be appropriate to use prophylaxis for a few days around the time a headache is predicted
- Weather: can be anticipated; barometric changes are usually too frequent to use intermittent prophylaxis
- Odors: avoidance of smoke and perfumes
  Psychological therapies
- Individual cognitive behavioral therapy with a psychologist is more beneficial than headache education when added to amitriptyline for children who have not had sufficient benefit from amitriptyline alone.
- Biofeedback has been shown to be effective in children as young as 9 years of age.

- A list of certified biofeedback practitioners is available at http://www.bcia.org.
  Acupuncture
- Small pediatric trials, some uncontrolled, have shown a trend in reduction of headache frequency and severity for both migraine and tension-type headache.

FUTURE DIRECTIONS

Most of the therapies used to treat pediatric headache are used off label, and there are limited supportive data. Moving forward, additional research should help characterize the efficacy of current therapies and shed light on newer treatments such as nerve blocks, botulinum toxin, and CGRP inhibitors that are increasingly being used in adolescents.

SUGGESTED READINGS

Available online.

110

Stroke

Maya R. Silver and Lauren A. Beslow

✳ CLINICAL VIGNETTE

A previously healthy 4-year-old boy presented to the emergency department with 1 day of irritability, difficulty speaking, and right-sided weakness. His parents noticed that he was not using his right arm and was walking with an uneven gait (dragging right leg). Physical examination revealed an alert, irritable child with a right lower facial palsy, right hemiparesis, and dysarthria. Deep tendon reflexes were 2+ on the left and 3+ on the right.

Head computed tomography was normal. Brain magnetic resonance imaging demonstrated an acute infarct in the left basal ganglia. Magnetic resonance angiography showed narrowing of the distal M1 segment of the left middle cerebral artery (MCA). He was started on a low molecular weight heparin and eventually transitioned to aspirin. Workup for coagulopathy was unrevealing. An echocardiogram was normal. On further history, his parents recall he had "the chickenpox" a month ago. He was diagnosed with a focal cerebral arteriopathy (FCA) secondary to varicella and experienced a stuttering course over the next few months with recurrence of stroke in a similar distribution. He ultimately stabilized. He participated in physical, occupational, and speech therapies, with significant improvement in his deficits.

Focal neurologic deficits should raise concern for acute stroke and prompt emergent brain imaging. A common cause of arterial ischemic stroke in childhood, FCA, is a focal unilateral stenosis of a cerebral artery causing ischemia. Involvement of the proximal branches of the MCA is classic. FCA is often postinfectious, as in this case. Treatment includes antithrombotic medications and intensive therapies to maximize recovery.

Stroke refers to acute vascular events involving the brain or brainstem. Childhood stroke occurs at a rate approximating that of childhood brain tumors. Stroke is among the top 10 causes of death in children and is a significant cause of morbidity among survivors. Pediatric stroke can be subdivided into categories of perinatal stroke, occurring from 20 weeks' gestation to 28 days of life, and childhood stroke, occurring 29 days of life to 18 years. Important subtypes of stroke include arterial ischemic stroke (AIS), watershed infarction, hemorrhagic stroke, and cerebral sinovenous thrombosis (CSVT). AIS is defined as an acute neurologic deficit of any duration corresponding to an infarction in an arterial territory on brain imaging. AIS can be due to thrombosis, embolism, hypoperfusion, and, in rare circumstances, arterial compression or vasospasm. Unlike AIS, "metabolic strokes" are caused by inherited defects in metabolic pathways that lead to an inability to compensate for metabolic stresses and ultimately cell death. They do not follow a vascular distribution and are not true strokes. Transient ischemic attacks (TIAs) are defined as focal deficits in a vascular territory lasting less than 24 hours, with some authors including the caveat that there must be no magnetic resonance imaging (MRI) evidence of infarction (Fig. 110.1).

The incidence of stroke in children is approximately 1 to 2 per 100,000 children per year. As opposed to adults, in whom intracerebral hemorrhage (ICH) accounts for about 15% of stroke, ICH accounts for about half of pediatric stroke. The incidence of perinatal stroke is approximately 1:1600 to 1:4200 live births, with 80% of these secondary to AIS. One-quarter of all strokes in children take place during the perinatal period. The incidence of CSVT is approximately 0.6 per 100,000 per year, with almost half of these occurring in the perinatal period. Strokes are more common in boys than in girls, with about 55% to 60% of all childhood strokes occurring in boys. In the United States, strokes are more common among African American children, even when controlling for the presence of sickle cell disease (SCD).

ETIOLOGY AND PATHOGENESIS

AIS occurs when occlusion of an artery with a thrombus or embolus decreases or prevents blood flow to the region supplied by that artery. In watershed infarctions, hypoperfusion preferentially damages areas on the border of two different vascular territories. In some circumstances, AIS can occur as a result of direct arterial compression (e.g., tumor) or vasospasm (e.g., after subarachnoid hemorrhage). The end result is a complex chain of events in cerebral neurons and support cells in which lack of oxygen and glucose leads to mitochondrial dysfunction, ion pump failure, calcium influx, and glutamate-induced neurotoxicity, eventually producing cell necrosis or apoptosis. The extent of ischemic damage to the region is determined by oxygen demand, collateral blood flow, and time to reperfusion. After an acute ischemic insult, there is a core area of infarction in which cells have sustained irreversible injury. This core is surrounded by an area with reversible ischemia known as the *ischemic penumbra*. If no further improvement of blood flow takes place or if additional insults occur, the tissue within the penumbra will eventually infarct, potentially causing additional neurologic impairment. In TIAs, perfusion is restored before infarction can take place, and neuronal dysfunction induced by ischemia is reversed.

Unlike adults, in whom hypertension, diabetes, and atherosclerosis predominate as risk factors for ischemic stroke, children presenting with AIS have much more varied causes. Approximately 50% of children presenting with stroke have a known risk factor at the time of presentation, including arteriopathy, congenital heart disease, sickle cell disease, inherited or acquired prothrombotic states, trauma, and/or infections (Box 110.1). However, after investigation, the cause remains unknown (cryptogenic) in at least 10% to 30% of childhood AIS. In older teenagers, traditional risk factors for adults, such as hypertension, diabetes, high cholesterol, and smoking, may also play a role. Cocaine or sympathomimetic medications are additional potential risk factors. Watershed strokes can be seen after cardiac arrest or other causes of shock, near drowning, and cardiac surgery.

In *hemorrhagic stroke,* blood extravasates into the brain parenchyma (ICH), into the ventricles (intraventricular hemorrhage), or

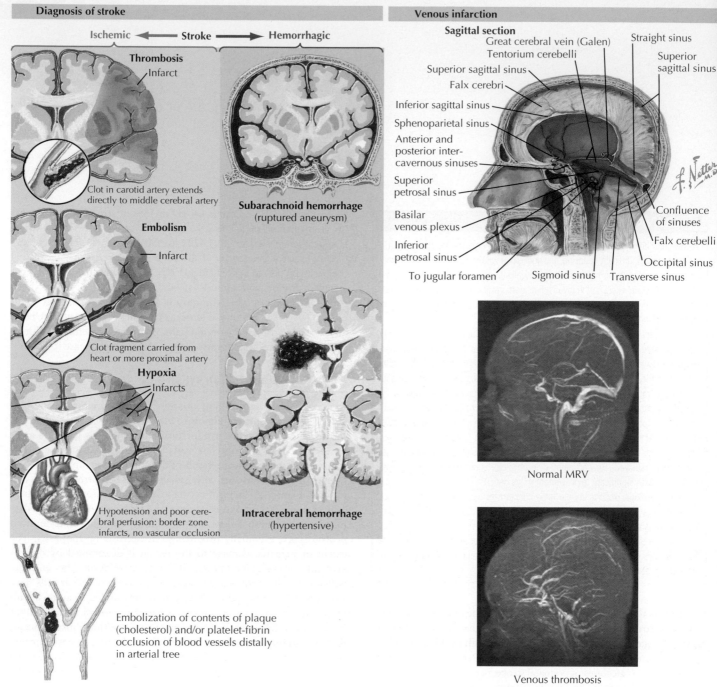

Fig. 110.1 Pathophysiology of Stroke. *MRV,* Magnetic resonance venography.

into the subarachnoid space (subarachnoid hemorrhage). ICH causes neuronal damage through a combination of mechanical damage and chemical irritation. Secondary ischemic stroke can occur as well because of mechanical deformation of cerebral vasculature by mass effect, vasospasm, or altered pressure dynamics, leading to decreased cerebral perfusion pressure. Intraventricular hemorrhage can lead to hydrocephalus.

ICH in children is also etiologically distinct from ICH in adults. Unlike adults, in whom hypertension and amyloid angiopathy are the most common causes, childhood ICH is most commonly caused by ruptured vascular malformations (e.g., arteriovenous malformations, cavernous malformations, and aneurysms), hematologic abnormalities, and brain tumors (Box 110.2 and Fig. 110.2).

In CSVT, obstruction of venous blood by clot formation alters blood flow dynamics and overall venous drainage is decreased. Increased cerebral venous pressure causes resistance to cerebral perfusion and can cause venous infarction or hemorrhage. The major risk factors for CSVT include dehydration, head and neck infections, hypercoagulable states, malignancies, congenital heart disease, inflammatory bowel disease, oral contraceptives, and the use of certain chemotherapeutics.

CLINICAL PRESENTATION

The clinical presentation of a child with stroke depends on the location, type, and size of the stroke and the age and developmental stage of

BOX 110.1 Etiologies of Pediatric Arterial Ischemic Stroke

Arteriopathy
- Focal cerebral arteriopathy of childhood
- Moyamoya disease and syndrome
- Cervicocephalic dissection of carotid or vertebral artery
- Fibromuscular dysplasia
- Congenital vascular anomalies
- Radiation-induced arteriopathy
- HIV-related arteriopathy
- Arteriopathy secondary to meningitis or encephalitis
- Primary or secondary CNS vasculitis

Hematologic
- Sickle cell disease
- Inherited or acquired prothrombotic disorders
- Disseminated intravascular coagulation
- Hemolytic-uremic syndrome
- Thrombotic thrombocytopenic purpura
- Hypercoagulable state caused by malignancy

Cardiac
- Congenital heart disease
- Valvular heart disease
- Intracardiac septal defect permitting passage of peripheral embolus
- Intracardiac tumors: atrial myxoma, fibroelastoma, or rhabdomyoma
- Cardiomyopathy
- Myocarditis
- Endocarditis
- Arrhythmia

- Cardiac surgery or cardiac catheterization
- Ventricular assist device related
- Extracorporeal membrane oxygenation related

Infectious
- Arteriopathy secondary to meningitis or encephalitis
- Post-varicella vasculopathy
- HIV-related arteriopathy
- Endocarditis
- Myocarditis
- Syphilis

Rheumatologic
- Primary or secondary CNS vasculitis
- Antiphospholipid syndrome

Metabolic
- Fabry disease
- Homocystinuria
- CADASIL
- Organic and amino acidurias

Other
- Traumatic vascular disorders
- Drug abuse, especially cocaine and amphetamines
- Inherited connective tissue disorders (e.g., Marfan syndrome, Ehlers-Danlos syndrome)
- Migrainous infarct

CADASIL, Cerebral autosomal dominant arteriopathy with subcortical infarcts and leukoencephalopathy; *CNS,* central nervous system; *HIV,* human immunodeficiency virus.

BOX 110.2 Etiologies of Pediatric Hemorrhagic Stroke

- Vascular malformations
- Coagulopathy
- Thrombocytopenia
- Hypertension
- Malignancy
- Mycotic aneurysms
- Hemorrhagic encephalitis or meningitis

the child. The diagnosis is often missed or delayed in children because of a low index of suspicion on the part of parents and care providers. In addition, children are much more likely than adults to present with headaches, seizures, or altered mental status as the first sign of stroke. Any child with acute onset of a focal neurologic deficit should be investigated for possible stroke. Additional situations that should be investigated for possible stroke include seizures in the newborn, seizures in a child of any age occurring after cardiac surgery, and changes in mental status associated with headache.

Approximately 75% of AISs in children occur in the anterior circulation (internal carotid arteries and their branches). Older children with ischemic strokes most commonly present with acute hemiparesis, hemisensory loss, or aphasia but may also present with isolated seizures or hemichorea. Children with posterior circulation strokes affecting the vertebrobasilar system may present with ataxia, vertigo,

visual field cut, or brainstem signs. Children with watershed strokes can present with proximal greater than distal weakness.

ICH classically presents with focal neurologic signs or seizures accompanied by severe headache, emesis, and altered mental status, but they may be difficult to distinguish from AIS based on clinical features alone because presentations vary and can also include hemiparesis and cortical signs (see Fig. 110.2). Children with subarachnoid hemorrhage often present with severe headache, neck pain, emesis, and altered mental status. Children with CSVT may present acutely with headaches, emesis, seizures, altered mental status, or focal neurologic signs but can also present more insidiously with symptoms of elevated intracranial pressure (ICP) such as headache, blurry vision, or diplopia secondary to sixth nerve palsies.

DIFFERENTIAL DIAGNOSIS

The most common mimics of stroke in children are complicated migraine, Bell's palsy, and postictal Todd's paralysis. Other considerations are hypoglycemia and other metabolic derangements, syncope, cerebral mass lesions such as brain tumor or abscess, demyelinating diseases, and functional disorders. Clues to the diagnosis of complicated migraine include a strong personal or family history of migraine, headache appearing after the onset of neurologic symptoms, and the presence of positive visual phenomena such as scintillating scotoma. Clues to the diagnosis of Todd's paralysis include a history of seizures. It is crucial to recognize that diagnoses such as complicated migraine are diagnoses of exclusion.

Pathology	CT scan	Pupils	Eye movements	Motor and sensory deficits	Other
Caudate nucleus (blood in ventricle)		Sometimes ipsilaterally constricted	Conjugate deviation to side of lesion; slight ptosis	Contralateral hemiparesis, often transient	Headache, confusion
Putamen (small hemorrhage)		Normal	Conjugate deviation to side of lesion	Contralateral hemiparesis and hemisensory loss	Aphasia (if lesion on left side)
Putamen (large hemorrhage)		In presence of herniation, pupil dilated on side of lesion	Conjugate deviation to side of lesion	Contralateral hemiparesis and hemisensory loss	Decreased consciousness
Thalamus		Constricted, poorly reactive to light bilaterally	Both lids retracted; eyes positioned downward and medially; cannot look upward	Slight contralateral hemiparesis, but greater hemisensory loss	Aphasia (if lesion on left side)
Occipital lobar white matter		Normal	Normal	Mild, transient hemiparesis	Contralateral hemianopsia
Pons		Constricted, reactive to light	No horizontal movements; vertical movements preserved	Quadriplegia	Coma
Cerebellum		Slight constriction on side of lesion	Slight deviation to opposite side; movements toward side of lesion impaired, or sixth cranial nerve palsy	Ipsilateral limb ataxia, no hemiparesis	Gait ataxia, vomiting

Fig. 110.2 Intracerebral Hemorrhage: Clinical Manifestations Related to Site.

EVALUATION

The initial evaluation of a child with suspected stroke should focus on confirming the diagnosis and ruling out common stroke mimics. The initial history and physical examination should assess the child's ability to maintain a natural airway and adequate perfusion. Brain imaging should be performed as soon as possible. Initial testing should include a complete blood count, electrolytes, blood glucose, prothrombin time, international normalized ratio, partial thromboplastin time, toxicology screen, and electrocardiography (ECG).

Initial diagnostic brain imaging is most often head computed tomography (CT) or MRI. CT of the head allows for the quick assessment of hemorrhage or large mass lesions. It is widely available, fast, and does not require sedation. In early AIS, a hyperdense MCA sign or blurring of the gray-white matter border can sometimes be seen, although the sensitivity of head CT for AIS is only 53%, and CT may miss many stroke mimics. The advent of rapid brain MRI protocols has allowed many centers to expedite diagnosis of stroke and evaluation for potential therapeutic intervention. These protocols, where available, generally last 15 to 20 minutes and include diffusion weighted imaging with apparent diffusion coefficient to detect ischemia, and susceptibility weighted imaging or gradient echo sequences to detect hemorrhage (Fig. 110.3). However, a complete MRI scan may need to be performed in patients in whom a full study is not obtained in the acute setting.

Initial imaging should also include imaging of the vessels of the head and neck with computed tomography angiography (CTA) or magnetic resonance angiography (MRA). MRA is often preferred because it avoids radiation. In AIS, arterial imaging may show arterial thrombus,

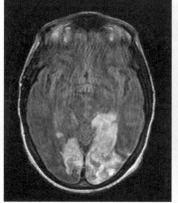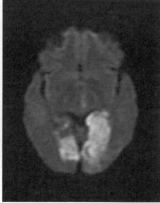

Cerebral infarction: Bilateral posterior cerebral artery infarction affecting both occipital lobes. Left panel shows the FLAIR image, which is most sensitive for pathology. Right panel shows the diffusion weighted imaging (DWI) which is sensitive for acute or subacute infarction.

Fig. 110.3 Arterial Ischemic Stroke on Magnetic Resonance Imaging. *FLAIR*, Fluid-attenuated inversion recovery.

arterial dissection (Fig. 110.4), or other arteriopathy. In some cases, dedicated vessel wall imaging also may be helpful because it can help identify inflammatory arteriopathies. In hemorrhagic stroke, MRA or CTA head may reveal an underlying vascular malformation. If no cause of hemorrhage is identified, conventional catheter angiography should be performed for a more sensitive assessment. Catheter angiogram is often required even if a vascular malformation is identified on noninvasive

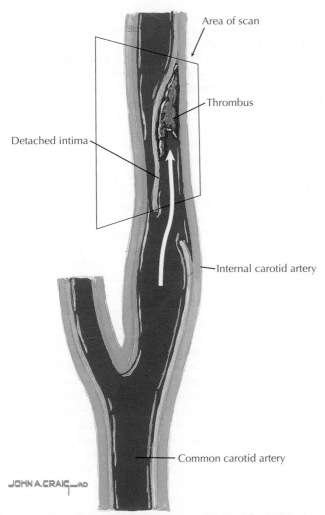

Intimal tear allows blood flow to dissect beneath intimal layer, detaching it from arterial wall. Large dissection may occlude vessel lumen.

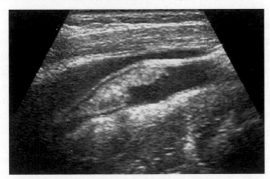

Carotid dissection: Ultrasound of the carotid artery with clot formed between layers of the artery.

Fig. 110.4 Arterial Dissection.

imaging to define the malformation better or for treatment. If a vascular lesion is suspected but is not found in the acute setting, arterial imaging should be repeated at later intervals because overlying hemorrhage may obscure the detection of vascular malformations. The interval for repeat vascular imaging is often case dependent but may be performed at about 3 months and 1 year after the initial hemorrhage. In children with suspected or confirmed CSVT, MRI brain with and without contrast and MR venography or CT venography are the modalities of choice to evaluate the dural sinuses for clot.

CT, Computed tomography; *CTA,* computed tomography angiography; *MRA,* magnetic resonance angiography; *MRI,* magnetic resonance imaging; *MRV,* magnetic resonance venography.

In children with either AIS or CSVT, an evaluation for prothrombotic states should be performed in most cases. Both inherited and acquired thrombophilias have been associated with pediatric AIS, often in concert with other predisposing conditions, such as cardiac disease or acute infection. Inherited thrombophilias include elevated lipoprotein(a), protein C and S deficiency, factor V Leiden mutation, prothrombin gene mutation, low antithrombin III level, elevated factor VIII level, and elevated homocysteine (e.g., due to methylene tetrahydrofolate reductase *[MTHFR]* mutation). Acquired thrombophilias include antiphospholipid antibodies (anticardiolipin antibodies, β2-glycoprotein antibodies, and lupus anticoagulant). It is important to consider that levels of many proteins involved in hemostasis vary with patient age and may also be affected by acute illness. If thrombophilia is suspected, a hematologist should be consulted to aid in the evaluation.

In the appropriate clinical setting, testing for infectious causes of arteriopathy including varicella, herpesviruses, and human immunodeficiency virus (HIV) should be considered. Evaluation of the heart for cardiac sources of thrombi should be performed in all children with AIS. Transthoracic echocardiography is usually the initial cardiac imaging modality, but if there is a strong suspicion for a cardiac source, transesophageal echocardiography should be considered, even when the transthoracic test results are normal. A "bubble study" (agitated saline contrast) during the echocardiogram is used to detect any abnormal arterial–venous connections. Delayed return of "bubbles" could be indicative of a pulmonary arteriovenous malformation. More extensive testing may be appropriate if the initial evaluation does not demonstrate a clear cause or if an underlying metabolic, infectious, or inflammatory disease is suspected (Box 110.3).

MANAGEMENT

The phrase "time is brain" has been used in adult stroke care to emphasize that a stroke is a "brain attack" that should be recognized and treated emergently. Unfortunately, treatment of childhood stroke is often delayed by more than 24 hours because parents and physicians do not recognize childhood stroke immediately. The goal of therapy in acute ischemic stroke is to save as much of the penumbra, or marginally perfused brain tissue, as possible by restoring perfusion. Other acute goals are minimizing metabolic demand (e.g., euthermia, seizure control) and avoiding additional insults such as hyperglycemia.

Each patient should be rapidly assessed for potential candidacy for hyperacute therapies such as intravenous alteplase (tPA) or endovascular therapy. Studies in adults have shown that intravenous tPA and endovascular mechanical thrombectomy for large vessel occlusion improves outcomes in select populations when performed within specific time windows (e.g., within 4.5 hours of last seen normal for tPA and within 6 hours of last seen normal for endovascular therapy [within 24 hours with perfusion imaging in certain populations]). Application of these "hyperacute" therapies in the setting of childhood stroke remains controversial. Hyperacute therapies may be considered on a case-by-case basis in pediatric stroke centers with the requisite specialists and technology, and complication rates have been low in retrospective analyses.

In the acute setting, if AIS is suspected, the child should lie supine with the head of the bed flat and isotonic intravenous fluids given to maximize perfusion. Hypertension is an adaptive response to ischemia, and thus outside of extreme hypertension, blood pressure should not be aggressively reduced. In most cases, aspirin should be given after hemorrhage has been excluded with neuroimaging. In certain cases of AIS such as cardioembolism or a known prothrombotic disorder, anticoagulation should strongly be considered. Fever and seizures should be treated to minimize additional metabolic demands, and normoglycemia should be maintained. After the neonatal period, dextrose-free fluids are preferred to minimize the risk of hyperglycemia.

After the child has been stabilized, attention should be directed at identifying the cause of the stroke and minimizing risk factors for recurrence. Speech, physical, and occupational therapies and other rehabilitation services should be involved early in the child's hospitalization course so a recovery plan can be initiated in a timely manner.

In the acute management of patients with hemorrhagic stroke and CSVT, the head of the bed should be elevated to at least 30 degrees to promote venous drainage and thereby lower ICP. The management of hemorrhagic stroke is sometimes endovascular and/or surgical, and prompt consultation with a neurosurgeon is advised. The need for acute lowering of ICP should be continuously reassessed. In CSVT, anticoagulation should be strongly considered, even in the presence of associated hemorrhage. In neonatal CSVT, anticoagulation is generally considered safe and beneficial, although the use of anticoagulation in the setting of neonatal CSVT with hemorrhage is an area of debate. Endovascular thrombolysis or thrombectomy may be considered in certain cases of CSVT.

SPECIAL CONSIDERATIONS

Perinatal Arterial Ischemic Stroke

The perinatal period is the most common period in childhood for ischemic stroke. The most common manifestation of perinatal AIS is seizure during the first few days of life, but it may also manifest only with lethargy or irritability, poor feeding, or alterations in tone. Many infants who have perinatal AIS are initially asymptomatic and are only diagnosed later upon detection of early hand preference, developmental delay, emerging hemiparesis, or seizures.

The pathophysiology of perinatal AIS is incompletely understood but is thought to be secondary to intrinsic hypercoagulability, dehydration, and shifts from the fetal to the mature circulation that lead to clot formation. A leading hypothesis is that emboli arise in the placenta, move into the fetal circulation and then across the foramen ovale, and ultimately enter the cerebral vasculature. The majority of perinatal AIS cases are in the anterior circulation, and there is a predilection for the MCA territory. There is a moderate preponderance of left-sided AIS in the perinatal period, presumably secondary to the anatomy of the carotid arteries as they arise from the aortic arch. Watershed infarcts

can occur, both in the classic distribution between the MCA and anterior cerebral artery territories and in a watershed area unique to the perinatal period between the territory of the long circumferential and paramedian penetrating branches of the basilar artery. This leads to a linear-shaped infarction affecting structures in the brainstem governing feeding and respiratory drive and thus can manifest solely with unexplained apnea or poor feeding.

Risk factors for perinatal AIS include complications during pregnancy or delivery, congenital heart disease, infection, and thrombophilias in both the infant and the mother. However, in about 50% of cases of perinatal AIS, no specific cause can be identified. Evaluation of the neonate with suspected AIS should include the same elements as that of the older child, although infectious causes and maternal prothrombotic states should also be investigated. There is low utility for routine thrombophilia testing of the neonate, although it should be investigated if there is a family history suggestive of thrombophilia, in neonates with congenital heart disease, or in neonates with systemic clots. The standard for diagnosis of perinatal AIS is MRI, often with MRA and MRV. Other studies, including echocardiogram, can be considered. The placenta should be evaluated for pathologic conditions when possible.

Similar to management of AIS in older children, management of a neonate with suspected AIS should include control of seizures, optimization of oxygenation, and correction of dehydration. Unlike in older children, intravenous thrombolysis and mechanical thrombectomy are not typically offered. Likewise, antiplatelet therapy or anticoagulation is rarely used unless there is high risk of recurrence as a result of a complex congenital heart disease or a known thrombophilia.

The prognosis depends on the extent and location of the injury, with complete MCA territory infarction and basal ganglia infarction portending a poor prognosis in almost all cases. Cerebral palsy is a common sequela, occurring in 30% to 60% of survivors of perinatal AIS. Because most perinatal AIS is secondary to factors unique to the perinatal period, recurrence is rare.

Sickle Cell Disease

Children with SCD, particularly those with hemoglobin SS and Sβ^0 thalassemia, are at increased risk for stroke both secondary to sludging from sickling and from arteriopathy (see Chapter 80). Stroke is an important cause of morbidity and mortality among patients with SCD; in one study stroke accounted for 12% of all SCD-related deaths. The cumulative risk of stroke in children with SCD increases with age, with up to 37% showing MRI evidence of stroke by age 14 years. Even in children with so-called "silent" infarctions, MRI evidence of ischemia is associated with cognitive deficits and learning and behavior problems. Stroke risk for children with SCD can be predicted by increased blood flow velocity on transcranial Doppler (TCD) ultrasonography, with high-risk children having an annual stroke risk of up to 10% per year if untreated. Thus, children with SCD should be followed with annual TCD. For children with elevated TCD, an MRI and MRA can be obtained to evaluate for intracranial stenosis. Children with elevated TCDs are placed on at least 1 year of chronic transfusions and then may be transitioned to hydroxyurea if there is no stenosis. For secondary stroke prevention, data support chronic transfusions. In the setting of acute stroke, aspirin may be less helpful than in other causes of stroke, and exchange transfusion (or simple transfusion to increase total hemoglobin but not to exceed 10 g/dL followed by exchange transfusion to reduce hemoglobin S) should be considered. Emerging therapies under investigation include hematopoietic stem cell transplantation and surgical revascularization for children with SCD and moyamoya arteriopathy.

Focal Cerebral Arteriopathy of Childhood

FCA is a term that describes a focal unilateral stenosis in a cerebral artery, usually of the anterior circulation. FCA can lead to AIS or TIA. Lenticulostriate branches of the MCA are preferentially affected, often leading to strokes in the basal ganglia. The inflammatory subtype of FCA (FCA-i) includes infectious and postinfectious arteriopathies—for example, from varicella or herpesvirus. The dissection subtype (FCA-d) refers to dissection of an intracranial vessel. There is a high recurrence rate in stroke because of FCA, between 19% and 25%. Therapy depends on cause, and steroids may be considered in some cases, although this treatment has not yet been tested in the setting of a clinical trial.

Moyamoya Disease and Syndrome

Moyamoya disease is a noninflammatory vasculopathy in which gradual occlusion of one or both internal carotid arteries leads to the formation of fragile collaterals that give a characteristic "puff of smoke" appearance on angiography. Idiopathic moyamoya disease is more common among children of Japanese descent and classically manifests with ischemic strokes in the first decade of life and intracranial hemorrhages thereafter. However, multiple other syndromes also can be associated with moyamoya vessels, including SCD, trisomy 21, Williams syndrome, neurofibromatosis type 1, and Alagille syndrome. In most patients, a revascularization procedure should be considered; however, the benefit of revascularization procedures is less clear in patients with SCD. Revascularization should not be performed in the immediate poststroke setting in most cases. Most pediatric patients with moyamoya are treated with aspirin unless the manifestation is hemorrhagic stroke.

Arterial Dissection

Arterial dissection is a common cause of arteriopathy in children and can affect the carotid or vertebral arteries in the neck and the intracranial vessels. Arterial dissection is caused by a tear along the inner wall of an artery. A small pouch called a "false lumen" can form, in which blood can pool (see Fig. 110.4). Strokes can occur if a pseudoaneurysm impedes blood flow or even ruptures, or if clot forms in the false lumen and then embolizes distally. Dissection can occur after minor or major trauma but can sometimes occur spontaneously, especially in patients with connective tissue disorders. Dedicated arterial imaging of the head and neck is required to make a diagnosis of dissection.

Vasculitis

Central nervous system (CNS) vasculitis is an inflammatory arteriopathy of the brain and meninges and is a rare cause of childhood stroke. It is primary when the process is isolated to the CNS (primary angiitis of the CNS) and is not explained by another condition. Vasculitis is secondary when it is the result of another process, including rheumatologic diseases such as lupus, infection such as meningitis, or drugs such as amphetamines. Large-, medium-, or small-caliber vessels can be affected. Conventional catheter angiography and sometimes brain and meningeal biopsy are required to confirm the diagnosis. Treatment depends on the underlying cause, but systemic immunosuppression may be necessary.

SUMMARY AND FUTURE DIRECTIONS

Stroke is a common cause of morbidity and mortality in children. Childhood stroke includes AIS, hemorrhagic stroke, and CSVT. The outcome of stroke in children varies from severe deficits to complete recovery and may depend in part on timely recognition and treatment. Efforts to reduce the delay of diagnosis in pediatric stroke include education of the community, pediatricians, emergency medical personnel, and specialists who care for high-risk patients such as those with SCD or congenital heart disease. Also, development of comprehensive pediatric stroke centers and protocols for rapid identification and treatment of pediatric stroke are necessary. Further studies are required to determine the risk-to-benefit ratio of hyperacute stroke therapies in children and optimal prevention strategies and treatment of stroke in specific high-risk populations.

SUGGESTED READINGS

Available online.

111

Neurocutaneous Disorders

Stephanie N. Brosius and Katherine S. Taub

CLINICAL VIGNETTE

A 7-year-old previously healthy boy presents to the neurology clinic with concerns regarding attention and learning. His teachers first noticed differences in kindergarten as he became bored easily and wandered off in the middle of activities. Since starting first grade, he frequently forgets assignments and leaves projects unfinished. His teacher often finds him staring out the window and taps him to regain attention. He has similar staring episodes at home and his parents state he races through activities, making careless mistakes or requiring frequent redirection in order to complete most tasks. He was born at term after an uncomplicated pregnancy. He reached all of his developmental milestones on time. There is no family history of any neurologic disease, genetic disorder, or developmental delay. His examination is notable for macrocephaly, Lisch nodules in bilateral eyes, 8 café-au-lait macules up to 9 mm in diameter and freckling in the axillary and inguinal regions. Vanderbilt screening surveys were positive for attention-deficit hyperactivity disorder with mixed inattentive and hyperactive symptoms. Genetic testing reveals a loss of function mutation in neurofibromin, consistent with a diagnosis of NF1. He is treated with a stimulant with improvement in symptoms.

Neurocutaneous diseases, or phakomatoses, encompass a diverse group of diseases affecting the nervous system and skin as a result of embryologic defects involving the ectoderm. Over 40 such diseases have been described, the majority of which have known causative genetic mutations. This chapter describes the most common neurocutaneous disorders.

TUBEROUS SCLEROSIS COMPLEX

Tuberous sclerosis complex (TSC) is a multisystem disorder affecting the eyes, heart, lung, kidney, brain, and skin (Fig. 111.1) occurring in 1:6000 to 1:10,000 live births. Symptoms are caused by autosomal dominant mutations in *TSC1* on chromosome 9q34 or *TSC2* on chromosome 16p13, which encode for hamartin and tuberin, respectively. Hamartin and tuberin form a protein complex involved in the negative regulation of cell growth by mammalian target of rapamycin complex 1 (mTOR1), and loss of function results in uncontrolled cell growth. TSC is diagnosed genetically with identification of a pathogenic mutation in *TSC1* or *TSC2*, or clinically based on the TSC diagnostic criteria from the Consensus Conference of 2012 (Box 111.1). Patients require two major features or one major and two minor features to establish a definitive TSC diagnosis. Patients with one major and one minor feature are diagnosed with probable TSC. Given the variable expressivity of the disease, surveillance for the multisystemic manifestations of TSC is crucial (Table 111.1).

Cutaneous stigmata of TSC arise throughout the lifetime of patients. Ash leaf spots are hypopigmented macules occurring in 90% of patients and emerging during infancy; they are best visualized using a Wood's lamp. Facial angiofibromas (adenoma sebaceum) commonly manifest on the nose and cheeks in preschoolers and become more prominent in adolescents. Treatment is with laser therapy or topical rapamycin. Shagreen patches are fleshy, raised lesions often located on the lower back in teenagers. Ungual fibromas, nodular lesions underneath the nail at the cuticle, also appear in teenagers and adults.

The neurologic hallmarks of TSC include tubers, subependymal nodules, and giant cell tumors. Tubers are dysplastic, cortical lesions resulting from disrupted neuronal proliferation, migration, and differentiation in early fetal life. Clinically, tubers are associated with the triad of seizures, intellectual disability, and tuberous sclerosis–associated neuropsychiatric disorders (TAND). Epilepsy occurs in 80% to 90% of patients with TSC and can begin as early as infancy with focal seizures or infantile spasms. Vigabatrin is the gold standard treatment for infantile spasms caused by TSC. Medically refractory focal seizures can be treated with an mTOR inhibitor, such as everolimus. Seizure control has been linked with cognitive outcomes. About 50% of children with TSC have intellectual disability ranging from mild to severe. Many are affected by TAND, which include autism spectrum disorder, aggressive behaviors, attention-deficit hyperactivity disorder (ADHD), mood disorders, and learning differences.

Subependymal nodules are hamartomas protruding from the ventricle walls that are seen in more than 90% of TSC patients. Subependymal giant cell tumors are benign glioneuronal tumors measuring more than 1 cm that can obstruct the foramen of Monro causing hydrocephalus, which can manifest as lethargy, change in behavior, emesis, limited upgaze, headaches, and increased seizure frequency. Tumors causing hydrocephalus are surgically resected, whereas asymptomatic patients with growing tumors are managed medically with mTOR inhibitors.

Cardiac rhabdomyomas occur in 50% to 70% of infants with TSC and are often detected on fetal ultrasound. Although these benign tumors frequently regress spontaneously, they can cause dysrhythmias, including Wolff-Parkinson-White syndrome, and are treated with medical management. They can also cause cardiac outlet obstruction and are treated either surgically or with mTOR inhibitors.

TSC-associated renal abnormalities increase in prevalence with patient age and are a significant source of morbidity and mortality. Renal cysts are often detected in infants and children. Although frequently asymptomatic, they can cause hypertension or renal failure, particularly in patients with TSC and polycystic kidney disease. Angiomyolipomas occur in approximately 50% to 75% of patients with TSC who are older than 10 years of age. They have abnormal vasculature with increased bleeding risk, especially if larger than 3 to 4 cm.

Retinal hamartomas may be asymptomatic or cause visual impairments, retinal detachment, or vitreous hemorrhage. Adult-aged women may have lung involvement with lymphangiomyomatosis, causing shortness of breath, hemoptysis, or a pneumothorax. These are also treated with mTOR inhibitors.

Tuberous Sclerosis Complex

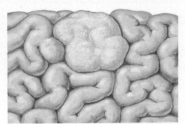

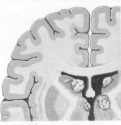

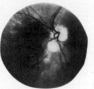

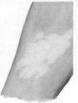

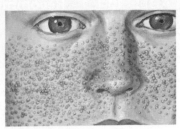

Tuber of cerebral cortex. Consisting of many astrocytes, scanty nerve cells, some abnormal sites

Multiple small tumors. Caudate nucleus and thalamus projecting into ventricles

Tuber of ocular fundus

Depigmented skin area

Adenoma sebaceum. Over both cheeks and bridge of nose

Tuberous Sclerosis Complex

Sturge–Weber Syndrome

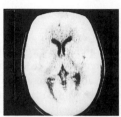

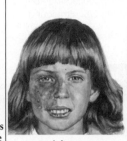

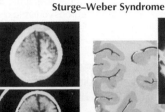

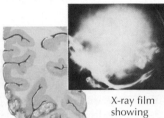

CT scan. Showing one of many calcified lesions in periventricular area

Multiple small angiomyolipomas or hamartomas in kidney

Rhabdomyomas of heart muscle

Facial nevus

CT scan. Showing calcifications and atrophy in temporoparietal area

Calcific deposits and hypervascularity. In leptomeninges and gray matter of brain

X-ray film showing "railroad" calcification

Fig. 111.1 Tuberous Sclerosis Complex and Sturge-Weber Syndrome.

BOX 111.1 Tuberous Sclerosis Complex Diagnostic Criteria

Major Criteria

- Angiofibromas (≥3) or fibrous cephalic plaque
- Nontraumatic ungual or periungual fibroma (≥2)
- Hypomelanotic macules (≥3 lesions, each ≥ 5 mm in diameter)
- Shagreen patch
- Cortical dysplasias (tubers, cerebral white matter radial migration lines)
- Subependymal nodules
- Subependymal giant cell tumor
- Multiple retinal nodular hamartomas
- Cardiac rhabdomyoma
- Lymphangiomyomatosis
- Renal angiomyolipomas (≥2)

Minor Criteria

- Dental enamel pits (>3)
- Bone cysts
- "Confetti" skin lesions
- Gingival fibromas (≥2)
- Retinal achromic patch
- Nonrenal hamartoma
- Multiple renal cysts

VON HIPPEL–LINDAU DISEASE

Von Hippel–Lindau (VHL) disease is a neurocutaneous disorder characterized by benign and malignant tumors of the central nervous system (CNS), retina, ear, and pancreas. It occurs in 1:30,000 live births

as a result of mutations in *VHL* on chromosome 3p25, which encodes a tumor suppressor. About 80% of cases are inherited in an autosomal dominant manner. According to the Massachusetts General Hospital Center for Cancer Risk Analysis and VHL Center, patients should be screened for VHL disease if they meet the criteria listed in Box 111.2. VHL disease–associated lesions are summarized in Fig. 111.2.

Hemangioblastomas of the CNS are benign tumors with a rich capillary blood supply arising in the second decade of life. They are the most prevalent lesions associated with VHL, occurring in approximately 70% of all patients. Hemangioblastomas are located most commonly in the cerebellum, spinal cord, and brainstem and can compress adjacent structures or bleed. Surgical resection is indicated with accelerated growth or symptomatic lesions.

Retinal angiomas are hemangioblastomas of the retina or optic nerve that develop during childhood and may be asymptomatic early in the disease course. Complications include hemorrhage leading to glaucoma, vision loss, or retinal detachment. Ophthalmic treatment for retinal lesions includes laser photocoagulation and cryotherapy.

Table 111.2 shows tests and screening recommended for VHL disease. Renal cell carcinoma is the most common malignancy in VHL disease, though it rarely develops before 20 years of age. Patients present with hematuria, flank pain, or a palpable mass. Tumors larger than 3 cm are surgically excised because of the risk for metastasis. Pheochromocytomas present in childhood and are often asymptomatic. Endolymphatic sac tumors are papillary cystadenomas located within the posterior temporal bone that present with hearing loss, vertigo, nystagmus, and facial muscle weakness. Treatment is surgical. Pancreatic lesions include cysts and serous cystadenomas, which are surgically excised when larger than 3 cm. VHL disease is also associated with asymptomatic papillary cystadenomas of the epididymis and broad ligament.

TABLE 111.1   Recommended Tests and Surveillance for Tuberous Sclerosis Complex

Assessment	Initial Testing	Frequency
MRI brain with and without contrast	At diagnosis	Every 1–3 years until age 25 years
Renal US or MRI	At diagnosis	Every 1–3 years
Creatinine clearance	At diagnosis	Annually
Ophthalmic examination	At diagnosis	Annually
Neurodevelopmental testing	At diagnosis	Annually by TAND checklist
ECG	At diagnosis	Every 3–5 years
ECHO	At diagnosis	Every 1–3 years until rhabdomyoma regression
EEG	Routine EEG at diagnosis, if abnormal and no clinical seizures, 24-hour video EEG recommended	As indicated
Chest CT	Adult women	As indicated

CT, Computed tomography; *ECG*, electrocardiography; *ECHO*, echocardiography; *EEG*, electroencephalogram; *MRI*, magnetic resonance imaging; *TAND*, tuberous sclerosis-associated neuropsychiatric disorders; *US*, ultrasound.

BOX 111.2   Screening for von Hippel–Lindau Disease

- Blood relative with VHL disease
- Hemangioblastomas diagnosed before 30 years old
- More than two CNS hemangioblastomas
- Clear cell renal carcinoma diagnosed before 40 years old
- Bilateral or multiple pheochromocytomas
- Family history of pheochromocytomas
- More than one pancreatic serous cystadenoma or neuroendocrine tumor
- Multiple pancreatic cysts and any VHL disease–associated lesion
- Middle ear endolymphatic sac tumor
- Epididymal papillary cystadenoma
- Bilateral epididymal cysts

CNS, Central nervous system; *VHL*, von Hippel–Lindau.

NEUROFIBROMATOSIS TYPE 1

Neurofibromatosis type 1 (NF1) is an autosomal dominant tumor susceptibility disorder caused by loss of function mutations in the tumor suppressor neurofibromin, encoded by *NF1* on chromosome 17. With an incidence of 1:3000 individuals, it is the most common genetic disorder affecting the nervous system. About 50% of cases are secondary to de novo mutations. To diagnose NF1, the patient must have two or more of the criteria in Table 111.3. The differential diagnosis for NF1 also includes Legius syndrome, caused by mutations in the *SPRED1* gene, which manifests with similar neurocutaneous findings but does not carry a risk for tumor development.

Neurofibromas are the hallmark lesions of NF1 and are benign Schwann cell tumors of the peripheral nervous system arising either from the cutaneous nerves (dermal neurofibromas), or from multiple nerve fascicles (plexiform neurofibromas). Dermal neurofibromas typically emerge in teenage years and may be asymptomatic or cause cosmetic deformity, pruritus, or pain (Fig. 111.3). Plexiform neurofibromas are congenital lesions that grow along the length of the nerve and may invade the surrounding tissues with the potential to cause deformity, neuropathy, and weakness. These lesions can appear anywhere along the neuro-axis and are treated with mitogen-activated protein kinase (MEK) kinase inhibitors, if symptomatic and inoperable. Plexiform neurofibromas may spontaneously transform into malignant peripheral nerve sheath tumors, which carry a poor prognosis and

manifest by rapid growth, severe pain, and focal neurologic deficits. Diagnosis is made with positron emission tomography (PET)/computed tomography (CT), and the mainstay of treatment is resection.

Optic gliomas occur in 15% to 25% of children with NF1. Patients may be asymptomatic or present with diminished visual acuity, visual field deficits, optic disc edema, strabismus, or precocious puberty. Annual vision screening is recommended until at least age 10 years, after which tumors are unlikely to become vision threatening. Lesions causing progressive vision impairment are treated with chemotherapy.

Children with NF1 also have increased risk for other malignancies, including leukemia and pheochromocytoma. Gliomas tend to be low grade with an indolent course, though brainstem gliomas require close observation for hydrocephalus and cranial nerve deficits. Additional common neurologic manifestations of NF1 include headaches, seizures, learning disabilities, and ADHD.

Children can also present with moyamoya syndrome, a type of noninflammatory vasculopathy that may result in stroke. It may be treated with surgical revascularization and/or aspirin (Chapter 110). Other systemic vasculopathies include renal artery stenosis, coarctation of the aorta, and aortic stenosis. Teenagers may present with essential hypertension.

Multiple bony abnormalities are observed in patients with NF1, including short stature, osteopenia and vitamin D deficiency, sphenoid wing dysplasia (often associated with underlying intracranial neurofibroma), and long-bone dysplasia, especially tibial pseudoarthrosis.

NEUROFIBROMATOSIS TYPE 2

Neurofibromatosis type 2 (NF2) is an autosomal dominant tumor susceptibility disorder caused by mutations in *NF2* on chromosome 22, which encode the tumor suppressor merlin. NF2 occurs in approximately 1:33,000 patients and is diagnosed based on the Manchester criteria if one of the four conditions is met:

1. Bilateral vestibular schwannomas (VS)
2. Unilateral VS *and* first-degree relative with NF2
3. First-degree relative with NF2 *or* unilateral VS, and two of the following:
   - Meningioma, juvenile cataracts, glioma (classically ependymoma), neurofibroma, schwannoma
4. Multiple meningiomas *and* unilateral VS *or* two of the following:
   - Juvenile cataracts, glioma, neurofibroma, schwannoma

Any child who meets these criteria or presents with an NF2-associated tumor should undergo genetic testing to confirm the

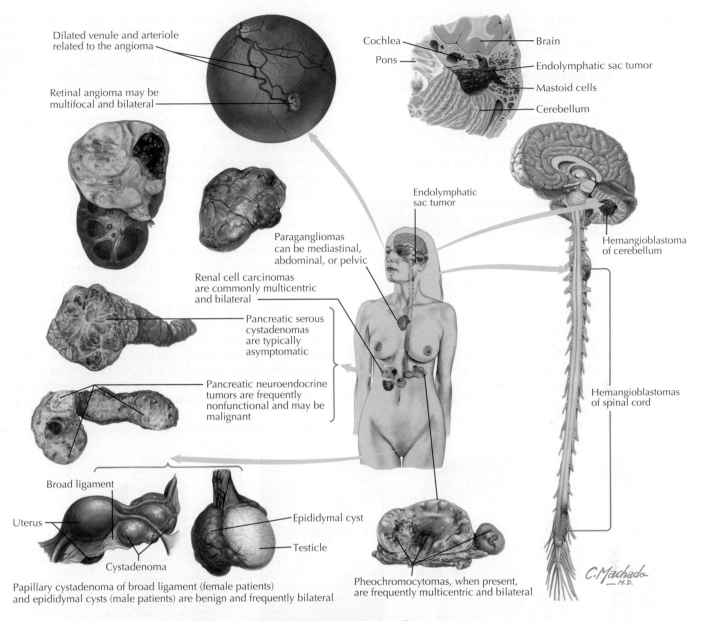

Fig. 111.2 von Hippel–Lindau Disease.

Within the figure, the following labels appear:

Dilated venule and arteriole related to the angioma

Retinal angioma may be multifocal and bilateral

Cochlea

Pons

Brain

Endolymphatic sac tumor

Mastoid cells

Cerebellum

Endolymphatic sac tumor

Paragangliomas can be mediastinal, abdominal, or pelvic

Renal cell carcinomas are commonly multicentric and bilateral

Pancreatic serous cystadenomas are typically asymptomatic

Pancreatic neuroendocrine tumors are frequently nonfunctional and may be malignant

Hemangioblastoma of cerebellum

Hemangioblastomas of spinal cord

Broad ligament

Uterus

Cystadenoma

Epididymal cyst

Testicle

Papillary cystadenoma of broad ligament (female patients) and epididymal cysts (male patients) are benign and frequently bilateral

Pheochromocytomas, when present, are frequently multicentric and bilateral

C. Machado —M.D.

TABLE 111.2 Recommended Tests and Screening in von Hippel–Lindau

VHL-Associated Tumor	Screening Exam	Frequency	Screening onset
Retinal hemangiomas	Eye examination	Every 6–12 months	Infancy
Pheochromocytomas	Plasma metanephrines	Annually	5 years
Hemangioblastomas	MRI brain and spinal cord with and without contrast	Every 2 years	>11 years
Renal tumors and pancreatic tumors	Abdominal MRI	Every 2 years	>15 years
Endolymphatic sac tumors	MRI internal auditory canal	Once	15 years

MRI, Magnetic resonance imaging; *VHL,* von Hippel Lindau.

diagnosis given the overlap with the diagnostic criteria for familial schwannomatosis.

Symptoms begin in the second decade with progressive hearing loss, tinnitus, ataxia, vertigo, or facial nerve palsy. Cutaneous manifestations include plaque-like lesions, subcutaneous nodules, and cutaneous schwannomas. Peripheral neuropathy can manifest with sensory or motor deficits as well as muscle wasting and is typically caused by neurofibromatous changes to the nerve versus underlying schwannoma. Once diagnosed, screening with contrast-enhanced magnetic resonance imaging (MRI) of the brain and internal auditory canal is recommended annually beginning at age 10 years. MRI of the spine should be obtained at baseline and every 2 to 3 years afterward. Hearing screening should be performed, and annual vision examinations are important given the risk for ophthalmic manifestations. Surgical resection remains the mainstay of tumor management.

STURGE-WEBER SYNDROME

Sturge-Weber syndrome (SWS) is a congenital disorder caused by somatic mutations in *GNAQ*, which is required for vascular development. Its incidence is between 1:20,000 and 1:50,000 births. Manifestations of SWS include cutaneous angiomas known as port-wine stains, leptomeningeal angiomas, and glaucoma. Most children

with port-wine stains do not have SWS, especially if limited to the midline of the forehead (nevus simplex). Port-wine stains in SWS typically involve the V1 and V2 distribution of the trigeminal nerve. Involvement of both the upper and lower eyelid has a greater association with ipsilateral leptomeningeal angiomas than isolated upper lid involvement, as do bilateral lesions. Port-wine stains may also involve the trunk or extremities and evolve with age, becoming larger with hypertrophy of the surrounding soft tissues and increasing hyperpigmentation. Venous angiomas form in the parietal-occipital region of the ipsilateral pia mater and cause venous congestion leading to parenchymal hypoxia, hemispheric atrophy, and parenchymal calcifications. Contrast-enhanced MRI of the brain is the study of choice to diagnose leptomeningeal angiomas, although classic MRI findings may not be apparent at birth. Therefore MRI should be performed after 1 year of age unless the infant presents with seizures, ocular findings, or hemiparesis.

Nervous system manifestations of SWS include epilepsy, stroke-like episodes, migraine with aura, and intellectual disability. Epilepsy occurs in approximately 80% of SWS patients, typically presenting by age 2 years. Hemiparesis and limb atrophy on the contralateral side of the leptomeningeal angioma often develop with seizure onset. Neurocognitive outcomes range from mild to severe. More severe outcomes have been linked to young age of epilepsy onset and to greater overall seizure burden. Stroke-like episodes manifest as transient hemiparesis or visual field deficits and can be challenging to differentiate from a postictal Todd's paralysis. These are postulated to be due to transient cortical ischemia related to venous congestion and thrombosis within leptomeningeal angiomas and may benefit from prophylactic low-dose aspirin, though no prospective trials evaluating

TABLE 111.3 **Neurofibromatosis Type 1 Diagnostic Criteria**	
Café-au-lait spots	≥6 lesions (>5 mm if prepubertal and >15 mm if postpubertal)
Neurofibromas	≥2 neurofibromas of any type or 1 plexiform neurofibroma
Freckling	Axillary or inguinal region
Lisch nodules	≥2
Optic glioma	
Bony lesion	Sphenoid dysplasia, thinning of long-bone cortex, scoliosis
First-degree relative with NF1	

NF1, Neurofibromatosis type 1.

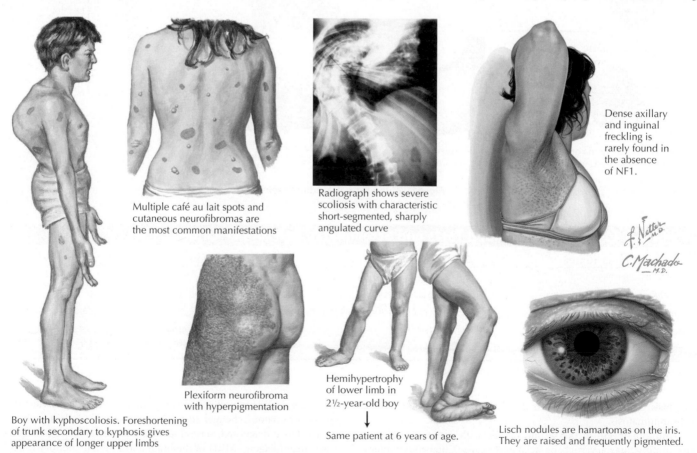

Boy with kyphoscoliosis. Foreshortening of trunk secondary to kyphosis gives appearance of longer upper limbs

Multiple café au lait spots and cutaneous neurofibromas are the most common manifestations

Plexiform neurofibroma with hyperpigmentation

Radiograph shows severe scoliosis with characteristic short-segmented, sharply angulated curve

Hemihypertrophy of lower limb in 2½-year-old boy
↓
Same patient at 6 years of age.

Dense axillary and inguinal freckling is rarely found in the absence of NF1.

Lisch nodules are hamartomas on the iris. They are raised and frequently pigmented.

Fig. 111.3 Neurofibromatosis Type 1.

its efficacy exist. Comorbid ADHD occurs in 40% of children with SWS. Screening for ADHD should begin at age 4 years.

Patients with SWS have elevated risk for vision loss caused by glaucoma or other vascular abnormalities of the eye. Glaucoma occurs in 30% to 70% of children with SWS, with 60% of cases presenting in infancy. Although frequent screening can capture symptoms before becoming vision-threatening, glaucoma in SWS is often refractory to medical therapy and requires surgical management.

FUTURE DIRECTIONS

Advances in our understanding of the genetic and molecular underpinnings of individual neurocutaneous disorders are leading to promising targeted therapeutic trials. Ongoing studies include the use of MEK inhibitors or mTOR inhibitors to abrogate cognitive impairment in children with NF1 and Sturge-Weber syndrome, respectively. Investigation of biomarkers for disease is underway for both tuberous sclerosis and SWS to aid in earlier diagnosis to prevent infantile complications. Finally, there are active trials for vestibular schwannoma, ependymoma, and inoperable meningiomas in patients with NF2 targeting several tyrosine-kinase signaling cascades.

SUGGESTED READINGS

Available online.

112

Movement Disorders

Jaclyn Tencer and Andres Deik

CLINICAL VIGNETTE

A 7-year-old boy presents to neurology clinic with reduced school performance and involuntary movements. His teachers have noticed that he seems to have difficulty paying attention and remaining seated while in class. Over the last 6 months he has also developed frequent sniffing and shoulder shrugging. He is not on any medications. In the neurologist's office he has a normal neurologic examination but exhibits fast, stereotyped, suppressible movements. The movements are most consistent with tics; no further diagnostic testing is pursued. Over the following months, his family works with his school to initiate an individualized education plan and his school performance improves. At his most recent follow-up, he still has intermittent tics, but they do not seem to bother him and medication is not recommended.

Tics are the most common movement disorder in children. With a normal neurologic examination and a typical time course, often no further diagnostic testing is needed. Tics can be associated with attention-deficit/hyperactivity disorder (ADHD) and obsessive-compulsive disorder (OCD). Treatment of tics depends on severity, with options including clinical monitoring with no active treatment, cognitive-behavioral therapy, or medical management. Often the most important treatment is to address any comorbid ADHD and OCD symptoms. This patient does not meet criteria for Tourette syndrome at this time given symptom duration less than 1 year; however, he should be followed over time.

Movement disorders are neurologic conditions featuring abnormal involuntary movements, abnormal quality of voluntary movements, or decreased movements. In children, causes of these disorders range from common conditions (e.g., tics) to rare genetic syndromes.

ETIOLOGIES AND PATHOPHYSIOLOGY

The basal ganglia (BG) are deep brain nuclei, including the caudate, putamen, globus pallidus, subthalamic nucleus, and substantia nigra (Fig. 112.1), that regulate initiation, scaling, control, and direction of movement. Most movement disorders arise from the disruption of the circuitry connecting the BG to the cerebral cortex, thalamus, and cerebellum. A simplified view of this circuitry is as follows: the BG receive input from the cerebral cortex (and, sometimes, the cerebellum) and generate output signals that mainly relay back to the cortex by way of the thalamus. From there, the signals are transmitted to the brainstem and spinal cord and eventually translated into muscle contractions (Fig. 112.2). The balance of excitatory and inhibitory signals within this system determines the speed and amplitude with which individuals move. Disruptions in the system can lead to excessive (hyperkinetic) or reduced (hypokinetic or parkinsonian) movements. Although not considered part of the basal ganglia, recent research has also recognized the role of the cerebellum in the genesis of some movement disorders, though primary cerebellar dysfunction causes ataxia.

CLINICAL PRESENTATION

Movement disorders have distinct features and patterns (phenomenologies) that distinguish them from each other. Hyperkinetic movement disorders (most common in children) include tics, tremor, chorea, ballism, athetosis, dystonia and myoclonus (Table 112.1). Hypokinetic movement disorders include Parkinson disease, the atypical parkinsonian syndromes and secondary parkinsonism (result of medications or structural brain abnormalities).

Tic Disorders and Tourette Syndrome

Tics are the most common movement disorder in children. They are involuntary or semi-voluntary, intermittent, repetitive movements (motor tics) or sounds (vocal or phonic tics, includes sounds not generated at the larynx, such as sniffing) (Fig. 112.3). They can be classified as simple (coughing, grunting, sniffing, blinking, shoulder shrugging, etc.) or complex (stereotyped sequence of movements or sounds). Tics are typically temporarily suppressible, do not occur during sleep, and are often associated with a "premonitory urge" and a sense of relief when performing them.

The typical age of onset is 3 to 8 years old with a peak in symptom severity between the ages of 10 and 12. Tics often change in frequency, character, or intensity over time and usually have a waxing and waning course. Most children experience improvement or resolution over time, usually by adolescence. When tics resolve within 1 year of onset, they are classified as transient. However for some patients, tics may persist into adulthood.

Tourette syndrome is a diagnosis that applies to a subset of children with persistent motor and vocal tics (Box 112.1); these patients frequently also experience comorbid ADHD, OCD, and/or anxiety.

Tremor

A tremor is an abnormal, rhythmic, oscillatory movement resulting from alternating contractions of opposing muscles. Tremor most often involves the hands, but can also affect the legs, trunk, head, and voice. Tremors can vary in frequency and amplitude, and the recognition of these features can aide in their classification. Types of tremor include:

- *Rest tremor*: Occurs when skeletal muscles are fully at rest (i.e., arms on lap). On examination, these can be enhanced by distraction (i.e., performing a mental task). In adults, this is a hallmark of Parkinson disease. In children, this can be seen with parkinsonism, as well as some of the dystonias (see later), in which a coarse, jerky rest tremor may be observed. A rest tremor is always pathologic.
- *Action tremor*: Emerges with activity. Types of action tremor include kinetic, posture, and intention. *Kinetic tremor* is one that emerges

Horizontal sections through cerebrum

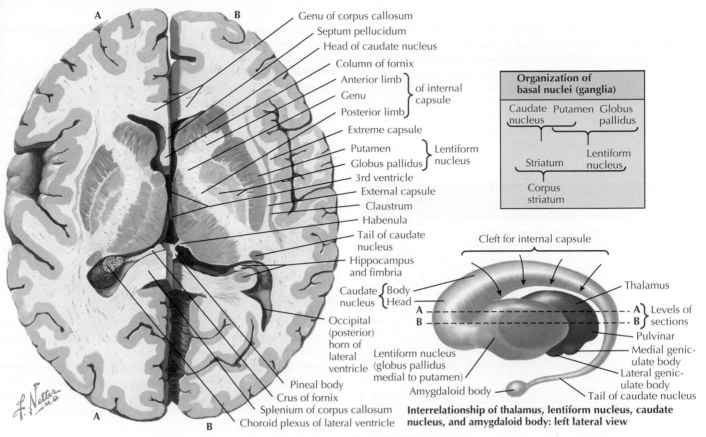

A   B   Genu of corpus callosum
Septum pellucidum
Head of caudate nucleus
Column of fornix
Anterior limb ⎫
Genu   ⎬ of internal capsule
Posterior limb ⎭
Extreme capsule
Putamen ⎫
Globus pallidus ⎬ Lentiform nucleus
3rd ventricle
External capsule
Claustrum
Habenula
Tail of caudate nucleus
Hippocampus and fimbria

Organization of basal nuclei (ganglia)

Caudate nucleus	Putamen	Globus pallidus
	Lentiform nucleus	
Striatum		
Corpus striatum		

Cleft for internal capsule
Thalamus
Caudate nucleus { Body, Head }
A ⎫ Levels of
B ⎬ sections
Pulvinar
Medial geniculate body
Lentiform nucleus (globus pallidus medial to putamen)
Lateral geniculate body
Amygdaloid body
Tail of caudate nucleus

Occipital (posterior) horn of lateral ventricle

Pineal body
Crus of fornix
Splenium of corpus callosum
Choroid plexus of lateral ventricle

Interrelationship of thalamus, lentiform nucleus, caudate nucleus, and amygdaloid body: left lateral view

Fig. 112.1 Anatomy of the Basal Ganglia.

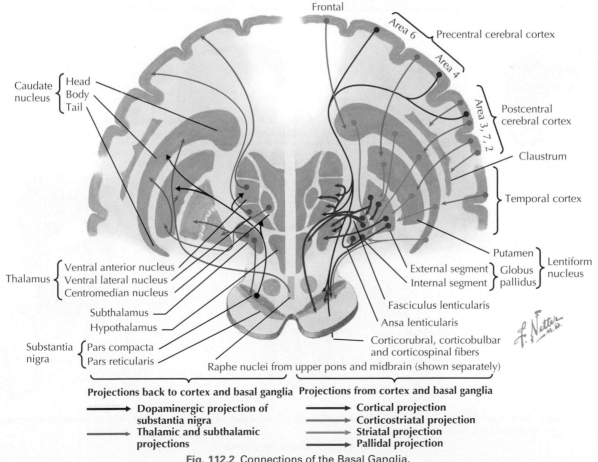

Frontal
Area 6
Precentral cerebral cortex
Area 4
Caudate nucleus { Head, Body, Tail }
Area 3, 7, 2
Postcentral cerebral cortex
Claustrum
Temporal cortex
Putamen ⎫
External segment ⎫ Globus
Internal segment ⎬ pallidus
⎬ Lentiform nucleus
Thalamus { Ventral anterior nucleus, Ventral lateral nucleus, Centromedian nucleus }
Subthalamus
Hypothalamus
Fasciculus lenticularis
Ansa lenticularis
Substantia nigra { Pars compacta, Pars reticularis }
Corticorubral, corticobulbar and corticospinal fibers
Raphe nuclei from upper pons and midbrain (shown separately)

Projections back to cortex and basal ganglia

→ Dopaminergic projection of substantia nigra
→ Thalamic and subthalamic projections

Projections from cortex and basal ganglia

→ Cortical projection
→ Corticostriatal projection
→ Striatal projection
→ Pallidal projection

Fig. 112.2 Connections of the Basal Ganglia.

during the execution of a motor task, like picking up a cup. *Postural tremor* emerges when attempting to maintain a specific posture against gravity (i.e., holding out arms) and is the most common type of tremor. Some postural tremor is normal (this is known as a physiologic tremor), but, when pronounced, it may indicate the presence of a metabolic derangement (like hyperthyroidism). *Intention tremor* arises (or increases in amplitude) as a limb approaches a target. This can be elicited by simple tasks such as performing the finger-to-nose maneuver. *Essential tremor*, a familial condition featuring progressive

tremor in otherwise normal individuals, often exhibits tremor that is more pronounced with intention than posture.

Chorea, Ballism, and Athetosis

Chorea, ballism (or ballismus), and athetosis are movement disorders within a spectrum of hyperkinesis. Chorea is a dance-like, involuntary movement that flows through contiguous body regions. Patients with chorea may exhibit parakinesia, in which the patient blends the involuntary movement into a volitional one (e.g., their arm flails over their head and they stroke their hair at the end). They may also experience motor impersistence, defined as the inability to sustain an ongoing movement. Common examples include the inability to maintain tongue protrusion (darting tongue) or a hand grip (milkmaid sign).

Ballism is similar to chorea, but more affects proximal limb musculature, resulting in violent, jerky, large-amplitude movements. When ballism affects one side of the body, it is termed hemiballism. Athetosis, in turn, consists of slower writhing movements that primarily affect distal locations.

Dystonia

Dystonia is defined as sustained or intermittent muscle contractions that lead to abnormal movements or postures. Dystonia is classified according to age at onset (childhood versus adulthood), body distribution (focal, segmental, multifocal or generalized), temporal pattern (paroxysmal versus sustained symptoms), associated features (either other movement disorders or other neurologic abnormalities), and cause (presence/absence of structural brain abnormalities, and inherited, acquired or sporadic).

Myoclonus

Myoclonus is a brief, shock-like, involuntary movement caused by muscular contraction or inhibition. It can be central or peripheral in

TABLE 112.1	**Hyperkinetic Movement Disorders**
Movement Disorder	**Phenomenology**
Tics	Intermittent, repetitive, and stereotyped movements or sounds under semi-voluntary control
Tremor	Rhythmic oscillatory movements from alternate contraction of opposing muscles
Chorea	Dance-like, irregular rapid and random movements that flow from one body part to another
Ballism	A form of chorea with large-amplitude jerking or flinging movements, usually of proximal extremities
Athetosis	Writhing movement of flexion, extension, pronation, supination of fingers, hands and sometimes toes and feet
Dystonia	Sustained muscle contraction, usually producing twisting movements or abnormal postures
Myoclonus	Shock-like or lightning-like contraction or jerk

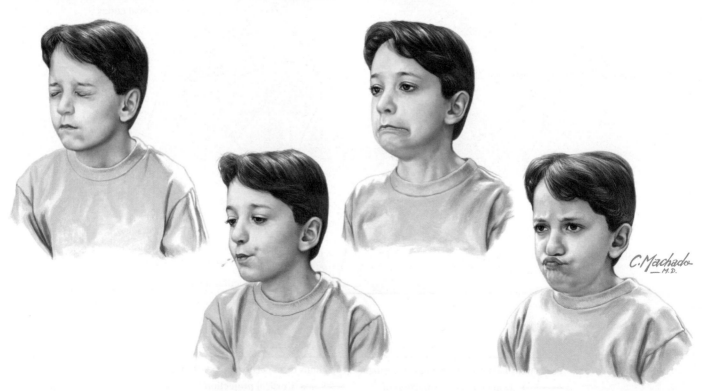

Tics involving the eyes, such as eye-blinking, are the most common tic in childhood-onset tic disorders. Patients with tic disorders frequently develop other motor tics of the head and neck, including grimacing and frowning.

Fig. 112.3 Tourette Syndrome.

origin and may arise in isolation, or as part of other neurologic conditions (e.g., epilepsy). Myoclonus is characterized by distribution (focal versus generalized), relation to activity (spontaneous or activity-induced), and pattern (rhythmic or irregular).

Functional Movement Disorders

Patients with functional movement disorders can exhibit movements that mimic organic disease (i.e., tremor, myoclonus, or dystonia). These are thought to be the somatic manifestation of a psychiatric stressor, but identification of such a trigger is not necessary for the diagnosis. Examination features that suggest functional disease include:

- Variability: movements change in phenomenology, amplitude, and frequency throughout the examination.
- Suggestibility: movements can be triggered during the examination.
- Distractibility: movements disappear or improve when the patient is distracted.

- Entrainment: for functional movements mimicking tremor, the affected limb can adopt the frequency of a movement that is performed volitionally on the opposite extremity.

Bradykinesia and Parkinsonism

Bradykinesia is the decrement in speed and amplitude that ensues while performing a repetitive movement (i.e., tapping the index and thumb, flexing and extending the fingers, pronating and supinating, toe and heel tapping).

DIFFERENTIAL DIAGNOSIS AND EVALUATION

Defining the phenomenology of an abnormal movement is the first step in formulating a differential diagnosis for the potential causes (Box 112.2).

Tics

The most common cause of tics in children is a primary tic disorder. However, secondary causes of tics include drug effects (central nervous system [CNS] stimulants, cocaine), genetic causes (Huntington disease, Wilson disease, neuroacanthocytosis), neurodevelopmental disorders (autism spectrum disorders), brain injury sequela (stroke, trauma, hypoxic injury), toxins (carbon monoxide poisoning), or infectious causes (Sydenham, human immunodeficiency virus [HIV]). Children with an abnormal neurologic examination or with clinical suspicion for a CNS pathologic condition should undergo brain imaging with magnetic resonance imaging (MRI).

BOX 112.1 Diagnostic Criteria of Tourette Syndrome

- Exhibit two or more motor tics and at least one vocal tic (may not happen at same time)
- Exhibit tics for at least 1 year
- Have tic onset before the age of 18 years
- Symptoms are not due to medications/drugs or another medical condition

---

BOX 112.2 Differential Diagnosis of Pediatric Movement Disorders

- Vascular causes
  - Basal ganglia, thalamic, or cerebellar infarct, injury, or hemorrhage
- Infectious causes
  - Human immunodeficiency virus
  - Poststreptococcal Sydenham chorea
- Toxins/substances
  - Alcohol
  - Amphetamines
  - Caffeine
  - Carbon monoxide
  - Cocaine
  - Heavy metals: manganese, lead, mercury, thallium, toluene
- Medications (selected)
  - Antidepressants
  - Antiemetics
  - Antiepileptics
  - Antipsychotics
  - β-Agonists
  - Corticosteroids
  - Dopamine blockers and agonists
  - Lithium
  - Stimulants
  - Thyroxine
- Nutritional disorders
  - Vitamin B_{12} deficiency
  - Beriberi (vitamin B_1, or thiamine, deficiency)
  - Pellagra (vitamn B_3, or niacin, deficiency)
- Metabolic derangements
  - Hypoglycemia or hyperglycemia
  - Hypomagnesemia and hypocalcemia
- Hyponatremia or hypernatremia
- Kernicterus
- Liver disease
- Inborn errors of metabolism/storage diseases
- Mitochondrial disease
- Neoplastic causes
  - Mass in basal ganglia
  - Pheochromocytoma
- Neuroautoimmune
  - Multiple sclerosis and other neuroinflammatory diseases
  - NMDA-R encephalitis
  - Opsoclonus-myoclonus ataxia syndrome (neuroblastoma)
  - Paraneoplastic disease
- Systemic autoimmune conditions
  - Antiphospholipid syndrome
  - Diabetes mellitus
  - Hyperthyroidism
  - Hypoparathyroidism
  - Lupus
- Genetic causes
  - Fahr syndrome
  - Huntington disease
  - Juvenile Parkinson disease
  - Neurodegeneration with brain iron accumulation (NBIA) disorders
  - Neuroferritinopathy
  - Wilson disease
  - Genetic dystonias
- Psychogenic movement disorder
- Physiologic movements

NMDA-R encephalitis, N-methyl-D-aspartate receptor encephalitis.

It can be difficult to distinguish tics from stereotypies. The latter are repetitive, purposeless movements that can overlap with certain habits. They are more common in children with autism and other intellectual disabilities, but occur in typically developing children as well. They can often be interrupted by distraction and are not associated with a premonitory urge. Examples include nail biting, hair twirling, thumb sucking, head nodding, body rocking or arm flapping. Isolated stereotypies do not indicate CNS pathology. Although these can have a younger age of onset than tics, they can persist through adulthood.

Tremor

Tremor in children should be investigated for a secondary cause. Although essential tremor can start in childhood, this benign diagnosis is typically one of exclusion. Hyperthyroidism, anxiety, and the use of medications that cause tremor (e.g., beta-agonists) are common and reversible causes of tremor. Other tremor-causing drugs include valproate, lithium, tricyclic antidepressants, cyclosporine, and stimulants such as cocaine, amphetamine, or caffeine. Toxic causes of tremor can include heavy metal poisoning with mercury, lead or manganese, to name a few. Metabolic causes of tremor are also important to consider and include hyperthyroidism, pheochromocytoma, hypomagnesemia, hypocalcemia, hypoglycemia, or hepatic encephalopathy. MRI of the brain should be considered for all children with tremor to exclude structural causes.

Chorea, Ballism, and Athetosis

Chorea can be hereditary or acquired, but most pediatric chorea is acquired. The most common cause of acquired chorea in children is Sydenham chorea. Sydenham chorea is an immune-mediated disorder that develops after a streptococcal infection. Other immune-mediated causes of chorea include N-methyl-D-aspartate (NMDA)-receptor antibody encephalitis (predominantly oro-bucco-lingual dyskinesias), and other autoimmune conditions (e.g., lupus or antiphospholipid syndrome). Metabolic derangements such as hyperglycemia, hyperthyroidism, hyponatremia, and liver failure can also lead to chorea, as can stroke. Finally, chorea and athetosis can be major features of cerebral palsy in children.

Hereditary forms of chorea are less common than acquired causes. These include Huntington disease, Fahr syndrome, neuroferritinopathy, neurodegeneration with brain iron accumulation (NBIA) disorders, and Wilson disease, among others.

Children with chorea, ballism, or athetosis should always undergo MRI of the brain, unless a secondary cause is readily identifiable. If a hereditary cause is suspected, targeted genetic evaluation may be warranted.

Dystonia

Dystonia may be caused by a primary genetic condition (including neurodegenerative diseases), an acquired disorder, or may be idiopathic. A genetic cause should be suspected for all children with isolated dystonia who are otherwise neurologically intact, even in the absence of a family history. Common forms of genetic dystonia include DYT-TOR1A dystonia (previously known as *DYT1*, most common in the Ashkenazi Jewish population), DYT-SGCE dystonia (previously known as *DYT11*, in children with both dystonia and myoclonus), and dopa-responsive dystonia/parkinsonism or Segawa disease (previously known as *DYT5*, in children with lower limb dystonia that worsens throughout the day but dramatically improves with levodopa). Of note, children with Segawa disease are often misdiagnosed as having dystonic cerebral palsy. Dystonia also can be seen in the setting of neurodegenerative conditions such as Wilson disease or NBIA disorders.

Juvenile Parkinson disease can debut with prominent dystonia, but this is exceedingly rare in children.

Acquired causes of dystonia are often acute or subacute in onset and include acute drug reactions to dopamine-blocking agents or delayed reactions after cerebrovascular conditions.

A basic dystonia workup includes complete blood count, comprehensive metabolic panel, antinuclear antibody, copper/ceruloplasmin, and MRI of the brain. Genetic testing and screening for inborn errors of metabolism also can be pursued if clinically indicated.

Myoclonus

Most pediatric myoclonus is acquired. Medications known to cause myoclonus include antidepressants (e.g., amitriptyline, nortriptyline, desipramine, fluoxetine, sertraline, lithium), stimulants (e.g., amphetamine, dextroamphetamine, methylphenidate, some asthma inhalers, caffeine), hepatotoxic medications, respiratory depressants, corticosteroids, amiodarone, acyclovir, bismuth, thallium, levodopa, and gabapentin. Metabolic abnormalities known to cause myoclonus include hyperthyroidism, hyponatremia, hypoglycemia and renal and liver failure. Patients with liver disease may exhibit negative myoclonus (i.e., asterixis). Myoclonus may also be present in some encephalopathies (including hypoxia), and with many pediatric epilepsy syndromes (see Chapter 108).

A rare, but important, cause of myoclonus is opsoclonus-myoclonus-ataxia (OMA) syndrome. Opsoclonus refers to conjugate, unpredictable, erratic eye movements. OMA is typically a paraneoplastic syndrome and children with this phenotype should be screened for neuroblastoma.

Whenever an acquired cause cannot be identified, a genetic cause should be suspected. The most common inherited forms of myoclonus are myoclonus-dystonia (DYT-SGCE dystonia, see previous section) and familial essential myoclonus.

Because most causes of myoclonus are acquired, a complete medical history should be obtained and children should be screened for medication exposures and metabolic abnormalities. Further testing to consider depending on clinical history includes MRI of the brain, electroencephalography, and cerebrospinal fluid sampling.

Bradykinesia and Parkinsonism

Parkinsonism is rare in children. Children with behavioral problems or tics who are exposed to neuroleptics or antiemetics (among other agents) can develop drug-induced parkinsonism, which, by definition, is reversible. Primary causes of parkinsonism in this population include dopa-responsive dystonia/parkinsonism or Segawa disease (see earlier), Wilson disease, Fahr disease and neurodegenerative conditions such as juvenile Parkinson disease, juvenile Huntington disease, and NBIA disorders. Of note, psychomotor retardation from severe depression can mimic bradykinesia in Parkinson disease.

MANAGEMENT

When movement disorders occur secondary to an acquired pathologic condition, treatment of the underlying condition can improve (or even fully reverse) symptoms. However, in children with primary movement disorders, treatment is targeted at symptom management.

Tics and Tourette Syndrome

Medical treatment of tics does not change the overall course or chance that the patient will outgrow the condition but can provide some symptomatic relief. Tics can be treated with cognitive-behavioral therapy (CBT) and/or pharmacologically. Common medications used include α-adrenergic agonists (guanfacine and clonidine), topiramate, or antidopaminergic drugs (risperidone, aripiprazole, fluphenazine, haloperidol).

Tremor

Action tremor can be treated with β blockers (propranolol is most common), benzodiazepines, topiramate or gabapentin. Deep brain stimulation (DBS) can be effective for refractory cases.

Chorea, Ballism, and Athetosis

Chorea can be treated with benzodiazepines, neuroleptics, or vesicular monoamine transporter 2 (VMAT2) inhibitors (tetrabenazine, deutetrabenazine, valbenazine). For patients with Sydenham chorea, treatment with penicillin is critical (with lifelong prophylaxis if there is cardiac involvement). In refractory cases of Sydenham chorea (as well as in other immune-mediated processes), immunosuppressive therapies such as steroids, intravenous immunoglobulin and plasmapheresis have been used.

Dystonia

Acute dystonic reactions are treated with diphenhydramine. However, subacute dystonia that is thought to be primary should always be treated with levodopa to exclude dopa-responsive dystonia. If no significant change with levodopa, anticholinergics (i.e., trihexyphenidyl), benzodiazepines (i.e., clonazepam or diazepam), or VMAT2 inhibitors can be considered. Focal dystonias can be treated with botulinum toxin injections, and cases of generalized dystonia should be evaluated for DBS.

Myoclonus

Treatment with valproate, levetiracetam, and/or clonazepam is the mainstay of myoclonus treatment for both epileptic and nonepileptic causes.

FUTURE DIRECTIONS

Advances in next-generation sequencing have allowed a substantial increase in the diagnostic yield of previously undiagnosed movement disorders. Unfortunately, this increase has not translated into a significant rise in disease-modifying treatments. Until we can have true personalized medicine, the treatment of movement disorders will remain largely symptomatic. Thus the correct identification of the abnormal movement a child experiences continues to be the first and most important step in the management of these patients. Until personalized medicine approaches become widely available, DBS and neuromodulation remain an exciting symptomatic therapy.

SUGGESTED READINGS

Available online.

113

Encephalopathies

Laura M. McGarry and Marissa DiGiovine

A 12-year-old girl with no chronic medical history was brought to the emergency department (ED) after an episode of incoherent speech and agitation. Her parents have noticed 2 days of behavioral changes with marked restlessness and anxiety. She has had difficulty sleeping and refused to sleep alone in her room. The day before presentation she had a transient hallucination in which she saw a deceased grandparent. One week before presentation she had rhinorrhea, dry cough, and fatigue. She has not had any fevers. In the ED, her initial examination was notable for speech changes with sometimes incoherent responses and delayed response time. While in the ED she has an episode of tachycardia, tachypnea, sweating, and tremulous movements consistent with panic. She was treated with lorazepam and discharged with referral to an outpatient psychiatry specialist. After discharge she continued to have episodes of agitation accompanied by hallucinations and developed choreoathetoid and dystonic movements of her extremities. She returned to the ED, where examination was notable for incoherent speech and motor agitation with periods of dystonia. Head computed tomography was normal. Lumbar puncture performed with basic studies was notable for a lymphocytic predominant pleocytosis. Further cerebrospinal fluid (CSF) studies, including anti–N-methyl-D-aspartate (NMDA) receptor antibodies were collected. She was admitted with a presumed diagnosis of autoimmune encephalitis. Treatment was initiated with intravenous methylprednisolone 20 mg/kg daily and intravenous immunoglobulin, as well as lorazepam and risperidone for agitation. A pelvic ultrasound performed to screen for ovarian teratoma was normal. Magnetic resonance imaging of the brain was normal. Several days later she had frequent brief episodes of arm stiffening and eye deviation, confirmed on electroencephalogram to be seizures. She was started on levetiracetam. Anti-NMDA receptor antibodies in serum and CSF were positive 1 week after admission. She began to have brief apneic episodes with decreased responsiveness prompting transfer to the pediatric intensive care unit. She received additional immunosuppressive therapy of plasmapheresis and rituximab with gradual improvement after multiple treatment rounds. One month after her initial presentation she was discharged to a rehabilitation program. At the time of discharge her hallucinations and dystonia were resolved, but she still had difficulty with speech articulation, emotional lability, insomnia and difficulty concentrating.

The term encephalopathy refers broadly to altered mental status caused by impaired brain function. Encephalopathy can be acute or chronic and can vary in severity, ranging from mild confusion to coma (Table 113.1). There are many possible causes of encephalopathy, some of which are static, some reversible, and others progressive. Prompt diagnosis and intervention are necessary, but given the diagnostic complexity of this diagnosis, a systematic approach to evaluation is important.

ETIOLOGY

Level of consciousness is regulated by the brain's ascending reticular activating system, a complex, highly interconnected network of nuclei in the brainstem, midbrain, hypothalamus, and the thalamus (Fig. 113.1) that sends extensive projections throughout the cortex using multiple different neurotransmitter systems. Consciousness requires an intact reticular activating system and at least one cortical hemisphere. Any process that diffusely impairs neuronal function or focally affects an area of the brain needed for arousal can result in altered mental status. Table 113.2 lists a broad differential diagnosis for encephalopathy. Seizures, particularly subclinical seizures, can mimic encephalopathy but are a distinct cause of altered mental status.

CLINICAL PRESENTATION

The presentation of encephalopathy can vary in severity, ranging from subtle (e.g., confusion) to severe (e.g., coma) (Table 113.1). A child can also fluctuate rapidly between various levels of consciousness. There are several standard scoring systems used to describe severity of encephalopathy. The AVPU scale categorizes the patient as **A**lert, response to voice (**V**erbal), response to **P**ain, and **U**nresponsive; this scale is straightforward and commonly used. The Glasgow Coma Scale (GCS), designed for head trauma, provides a more detailed scale rating eye response, motor responses, and verbal responses (Chapter 117, Table 117.1). Some modifications to these scales may be required in the cases of nonverbal patients or infants.

Neurologic Examination: Noncomatose Child

The neurologic examination can be a challenge in the noncomatose encephalopathic child but can lend significant insight into the cause of encephalopathy. As with much of the neurologic examination in children, observation alone can be very revealing. Watching how alert the child is to environmental stimuli, how the child communicates with caregivers, if the child walks, or if the child makes other spontaneous movements, including abnormal movements, are all informative. Orientation, affect, attention, language, executive function, fund of knowledge, and memory can be assessed with simple age-appropriate questions, whether asked by examiner or caregiver.

Changes in personality, erratic behavior, and psychiatric changes resembling psychosis can be seen with encephalopathies caused by frontal and temporal cortex dysfunction. These encephalopathies may also include movement disorders with involvement of the frontostriatal pathways (Chapter 112). The presence of certain movement disorders may suggest a specific underlying encephalopathic cause, such as opsoclonus-myoclonus-ataxia syndrome, which suggests neuroblastoma, or asterixis (flapping tremor) and bradykinesia which suggest hepatic encephalopathy. Impaired language may occur because of aphasia (frontal and/or temporal cortex dysfunction) or motor dysfunction (dysarthria; upper motor neuron, lower motor neuron, cerebellum, and/or extrapyramidal system dysfunction). Encephalopathy with associated vision deficits may be caused by posterior cortex

TABLE 113.1 States of Impaired Consciousness

State of Impaired Consciousness	Definition	Key Examination Findings
Confusion	Minimal reduction in alertness. Specific to global cognitive deficits	Unable to follow commands or complete age-appropriate cognitive tasks (serial 7s, counting backward), poor recall of events
Delirium	Minimal reduction in alertness, often agitated. Disorientation to environment	Disoriented to time, place and/or self. May have delusions or hallucinations.
Obtunded	Moderately depressed alertness and responsiveness to external stimuli	Lethargic, responds to auditory or vigorous tactile stimuli, spontaneous eye opening.
Stupor	Severely depressed awareness resembling sleep from which can briefly be aroused	Responds briefly and minimally to painful stimuli
Coma	Severely depressed awareness, unarousable state	No response to painful stimuli

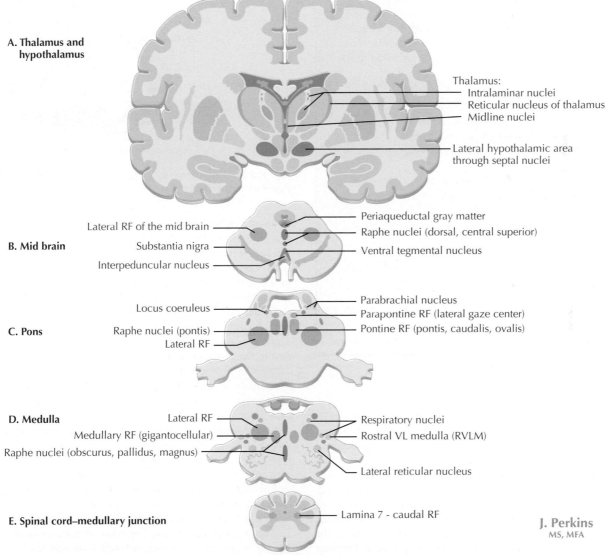

A. Thalamus and hypothalamus

Thalamus:
Intralaminar nuclei
Reticular nucleus of thalamus
Midline nuclei

Lateral hypothalamic area through septal nuclei

B. Mid brain

Lateral RF of the mid brain
Substantia nigra
Interpeduncular nucleus

Periaqueductal gray matter
Raphe nuclei (dorsal, central superior)
Ventral tegmental nucleus

C. Pons

Locus coeruleus
Raphe nuclei (pontis)
Lateral RF

Parabrachial nucleus
Parapontine RF (lateral gaze center)
Pontine RF (pontis, caudalis, ovalis)

D. Medulla

Lateral RF
Medullary RF (gigantocellular)
Raphe nuclei (obscurus, pallidus, magnus)

Respiratory nuclei
Rostral VL medulla (RVLM)

Lateral reticular nucleus

E. Spinal cord–medullary junction

Lamina 7 - caudal RF

J. Perkins
MS, MFA

Fig. 113.1 Brainstem and Diencephalon Nuclei That Compose the Reticular Activating System. *RF,* Reticular formation.

dysfunction, as can be seen in disorders such as posterior reversible encephalopathy syndrome.

Neurologic Examination: Comatose Child

The neurologic examination of the comatose patient focuses on cranial nerve (CN) examination, tone, and motor responses, which can provide clues about the cause of encephalopathy. First assess for pupil size and pupillary light response. Examine the pupil size in both normal and dim lights to help highlight any differences in size. Shining a bright light at each individual pupil should result in brisk and equal constriction of both pupils. This reflex depends on the parasympathetic pupilloconstriction pathway (Fig. 113.2), which includes the optic nerve,

TABLE 113.2 Differential Diagnosis of Encephalopathy VITAMINS, Please Guys!

Etiologies	Differential Diagnosis
Vascular	Global hypoxic-ischemic injury (typically secondary to asphyxiation, cardiorespiratory arrest or profound hypotension)
	Arterial ischemic stroke
	Cerebral sinus venous thrombosis
	Hemorrhagic stroke
	Hypertensive encephalopathy
	Vasculitis
Infectious/Inflammatory	Sepsis
	Meningitis
	Encephalitis
Trauma/toxins	Traumatic brain injury
	Toxins: opiates, anticholinergics, tricyclic antidepressants, salicylates, antiseizure medications, carbon monoxide, sedatives, others
Autoimmune	Acute demyelinating encephalomyelitis (ADEM)
	Lupus cerebritis
	Autoimmune encephalitides (e.g., anti–NMDA-receptor antibody encephalitis)
Metabolic/endocrine	Derangements in glucose, ammonia, urea, sodium, calcium, or magnesium, others
	Metabolic/respiratory acidosis
	Thyrotoxicosis
	Inborn errors of metabolism
Increased intracranial pressure	See Chapter 117, Table 117.4
Neoplastic	Neoplasm or paraneoplastic syndrome
Seizure	Seizures, status epilepticus, post-ictal state
PRES/Psych	Posterior reversible encephalopathy syndrome (PRES)
	Psychiatric disorders
Genetic/general	Genetic epileptic encephalopathies
	Systemic illnesses: intussusception, shock, hypoxemia

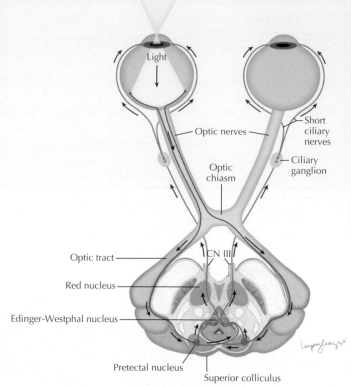

Fig 113.2 Parasympathetic Pupilloconstriction Pathway for the Pupillary Light Reflex.

pretectal and oculomotor nuclei in the upper midbrain, and the CN III fibers that innervate the parasympathetic ciliary ganglion. Dilated and poorly reactive bilateral pupils are seen during hypoxia or ischemia of the brain and also anticholinergic toxicity. A unilateral unreactive and dilated pupil is most often caused by external compression of cranial nerve III, such as with a compressive aneurysm, uncal herniation, other mass effect, or increased intracranial pressure. Injury to the nuclei of this pathway in the midbrain can cause bilateral midsized to dilated fixed pupils. Small but reactive pupils can be seen in injury above the midbrain, in metabolic causes, or with Horner syndrome. Pinpoint fixed pupils can be seen with injury to the pons or certain intoxications such as opioids. Seizures mimicking encephalopathy may cause transient bilateral or unilateral changes in pupil size and reactivity.

Eye movements are controlled by CN III, IV, and VI, which arise from midbrain and pontine nuclei and are influenced by many inputs from the cortex, other brainstem nuclei including the vestibular system, and sympathetic/parasympathetic systems (Fig. 113.3). The oculocephalic reflex is assessed by turning the patient's head briskly to one side while observing for eye movement in the opposite direction (toward midline), the so-called "doll's eye" response. This reflex will not be present in awake and alert patients because voluntary gaze control overrides this reflex. If the oculocephalic reflex is not present in a comatose patient (or unable to be assessed because of cervical spine immobilization or injury), eye movements can be assessed with vestibular caloric stimulation of the vestibulo-ocular reflex. Here, ice water is instilled by syringe in the ear canal with the head elevated 30 degrees, to cool the tympanic membrane, creating a convective current in the endolymph of the adjacent semicircular canal, and thus a decrease in basal activity of ipsilateral vestibular neurons. This change in vestibular neuron activity mimics head turning to the opposite side and should result in conjugate eye movement toward the side of the cold-water stimulus with corrective saccades back to midline, causing a horizontal jerk nystagmus toward the opposite side. This is very uncomfortable (often causes vertigo, nausea, and/or emesis) and thus is only very rarely performed on an awake child. In comatose patients with an intact brainstem, conjugate eye movement occurs toward the side of cold-water stimulation, but without associated nystagmus. In a child with a brainstem dysfunction at the level of these pathways, the eyes will remain fixed at midline.

Motor examination tests whether stimulation can provoke a specific motor response such as single limb withdrawal or pushing away the examiner. Often painful stimuli such as nail bed pressure or sternal rub must be used to produce a response. The presence of a purposeful response indicates an intact spinal cord and brainstem. Patients who do not demonstrate a specific motor response to stimuli may respond with nonspecific posturing. Decorticate posturing describes a reflexive posture with upper extremity flexion and lower extremity extension and inward rotation. It indicates significant injury of the cerebral hemispheres, internal capsule, thalamus,

Doll's eye phenomenon

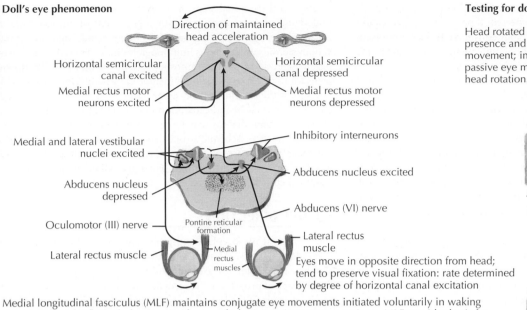

Direction of maintained head acceleration

Horizontal semicircular canal excited

Horizontal semicircular canal depressed

Medial rectus motor neurons excited

Medial rectus motor neurons depressed

Inhibitory interneurons

Medial and lateral vestibular nuclei excited

Abducens nucleus excited

Abducens nucleus depressed

Abducens (VI) nerve

Oculomotor (III) nerve

Pontine reticular formation

Lateral rectus muscle

Medial rectus muscles

Lateral rectus muscle

Eyes move in opposite direction from head; tend to preserve visual fixation: rate determined by degree of horizontal canal excitation

Medial longitudinal fasciculus (MLF) maintains conjugate eye movements initiated voluntarily in waking state or induced reflexively from cervical or vestibular inputs in comatose patients. MLF provides basis for doll's eye testing and caloric stimulation of semicircular canals.

Ice water caloric testing of the semicircular canals in the comatose patient

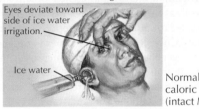

Eyes deviate toward side of ice water irrigation.

Ice water

Normal caloric test (intact MLF)

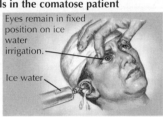

Eyes remain in fixed position on ice water irrigation.

Ice water

Abnormal caloric test (disrupted MLF)

JOHN A. CRAIG—MD

Testing for doll's head conjugate eye movement

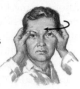

Head rotated and observed for presence and direction of eye movement; intact MLF prevents passive eye movement; with head rotation.

Normal doll's head (intact MLF)
← Direction of head rotation

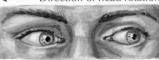

Apparent eye movement →
Eyes remain in primary position in relation to examiner or appear to "move opposite" to direction of head rotation.

Abnormal doll's head (disrupted MLF)
← Direction of head rotation

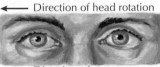

← Direction of eye movement
Eyes remain centered following same direction as rotation of head.

One ear irrigated with ice water solution and patient observed for presence and direction of eye movement relative to side of irrigation

Fig. 113.3 Brainstem Pathways and Testing of Vestibulo-ocular Reflexes.

and/or midbrain. Decerebrate posturing describes reflexive extension and internal rotation of upper and lower extremities with arching of the spine. It indicates extensive injury involving the midbrain, pons, and sometimes cerebellum. Progression from decorticate to decerebrate posturing suggests uncal or tonsillar brain herniation. Flaccid lower extremities can be seen with injury to the lower brainstem or spinal cord.

EVALUATION

After attending first to basic emergency care, including vital signs, airway, breathing, and circulation (ABCs), a pertinent history and neurologic examination must be performed. This history is often obtained from the parent or other caregiver when the child is encephalopathic. Relevant past history includes the child's baseline neurologic status, known medical conditions, and developmental and birth history. The timing and progression of the current presentation should be elicited, as well as any preceding events such as febrile illness, seizures, vomiting, possibility of drug or toxin ingestion, travel, and trauma. Family history of metabolic, mitochondrial, neurologic, or vascular disease is especially pertinent.

Beyond the history and examination, the laboratory and imaging studies needed are determined based on differential diagnosis (Table 113.2). In almost all cases, basic laboratories to be sent include a toxicology screen (urine and/or serum, and drug levels of any medications in the home), an arterial blood gas, electrolytes, glucose, liver function tests, ammonia level, complete blood count, blood cultures and urine analysis. Consultation with a pediatric neurologist can help guide further workup, including the need for neuroimaging (computed tomography [CT] and/or magnetic resonance imaging [MRI] of the brain),

lumbar puncture (LP) for cerebrospinal fluid (CSF) analysis, and/or electroencephalogram (EEG).

If an infection or parainfectious process is suspected, LP for CSF studies is essential (Chapter 118). Head CT before LP should be considered if there is concern for increased intracranial pressure (Chapter 117) or mass lesion. MRI of the brain is more sensitive than head CT for vasculitis, inflammation related to encephalitis, postinfectious or neuroinflammatory disorders such as acute disseminated encephalomyelitis, and posterior fossa pathologic conditions, such as cerebellitis. EEG in encephalitis may show slowing, epileptiform discharges, triphasic waves, or seizures. Focal, especially temporal, or lateralized findings are suspicious for herpes simplex virus.

If an autoimmune or paraneoplastic cause is suspected, blood and CSF testing for causative antibodies can ultimately provide a definitive diagnosis but results often take days to weeks to return. Blood and CSF samples are often collected to examine for oligoclonal bands and intrathecal antibody production. MRI of the brain should be performed. Evaluation for a primary tumor causing a paraneoplastic process is important.

In a child with known or suspected metabolic disease, relevant laboratory tests to perform include plasma amino acids, urine organic acids, lactate, pyruvate, and acylcarnitine profile. Consultation with specialists in pediatric metabolic disorders or neurology will help direct further studies. MRI and magnetic resonance spectroscopy (MRS) are important imaging studies in evaluating for metabolic disease. Endocrine causes of metabolic disturbances such as diabetic ketoacidosis will be identified on electrolyte and glucose laboratory tests. Thyroid function tests should be sent if the cause remains unknown.

When drug or toxin ingestion is possible, serum and urine toxin and drug screening should be ordered, including for salicylates and heavy metals. Sometimes children may ingest adult prescription medications in the house. If this is suspected, a prescription medication screen should be ordered and toxicology consulted. If the patient is on antiseizure medications (or if another family member has these in the house), levels should be obtained to rule out toxicity.

In a child with a history of trauma or suspected nonaccidental trauma, head CT is the first imaging study to evaluate for intracranial hemorrhage and/or skull fractures. If hypoxic-ischemic injury is suspected, head CT may show early signs, but MRI is more sensitive to subtle parenchymal injury. If a child presents with a focal neurologic deficit or stroke syndrome, neuroimaging (including vascular imaging) should be performed (Chapter 110). If an intracranial neoplasm is suspected, head CT is often the first-line imaging study. Head CT may miss posterior fossa tumors or small tumors. MRI of the brain will almost always be needed for further characterization and for surgical planning.

Seizures can mimic encephalopathy, in both the ictal and postictal phases. This may occur in children with epilepsy, or in children with new-onset seizures. EEG can identify nonconvulsive seizures and/or background abnormalities associated with specific epileptic encephalopathies (beyond the scope of this chapter).

MANAGEMENT

Initial management of the encephalopathic child includes emergency care (ABCs) and attention to reversible causes. Children presenting with obtundation, stupor, or coma require urgent intubation for airway protection and control of ventilation and oxygenation, in which case admission to the pediatric intensive care unit (PICU) will be necessary. Elevated intracranial pressure should be managed aggressively (Chapter 117). Hypoglycemia and electrolyte disturbances should be corrected appropriately. If a central nervous system infection is suspected, broad-spectrum intravenous antibiotics and acyclovir should be promptly initiated (Chapter 118). If metabolic disease is suspected, feeds should be withheld, dextrose containing intravenous fluids started, and metabolism consulted.

Beyond these initial steps, management should be directed at the underlying cause of encephalopathy. Treatment of autoimmune or inflammatory causes of encephalopathy often include high-dose intravenous steroids, intravenous immunoglobulin, and in refractory cases, plasmapheresis and/or immunosuppressant medications. Treatment plans for toxic exposures should include early involvement of toxicology and/or the poison control center. Depending on the toxin, a specific antidote may be indicated, or removal of the toxin with activated charcoal or hemodialysis may be recommended. Treatment of vascular causes such as ischemic stroke or venous thrombosis may require anticoagulation or aspirin (Chapter 110). Treatment of seizures is with standard anti-seizure medications. For a discussion on management of status epilepticus, see Chapter 117.

FUTURE DIRECTIONS

The treatment of encephalopathy ultimately depends on identifying the underlying cause. Many recent advances have been made in understanding neurologic disease mechanisms and improving testing. For example, great progress in the recognition of autoimmune encephalitis has been made in the last 15 years driven by the discovery of antineuronal antibodies. NMDA-receptor antibody encephalitis, which is now the most commonly identified autoimmune encephalitis, was not recognized until 2007. This recognition increased awareness of autoimmune encephalitis more broadly as a result, and with newer availability of antibody-based testing, has led to earlier immunosuppressive treatment and improved outcomes. Current research continues to expand the understanding of the heterogeneous mechanisms of neuroinflammation and the role of different immune modulators in CNS disease, such as monoclonal antibodies. Advances in genetic testing have led to increased identification of metabolic and mitochondrial disorders that can cause both acute and progressive encephalopathy.

SUGGESTED READINGS

Available online.

114

Demyelinating Diseases

Whitney Fitts and Amy T. Waldman

 CLINICAL VIGNETTE

A 13-year-old girl presented to her ophthalmologist complaining of "blurry vision" and eye pain. The blurry vision began a week before her presentation, and she noted pain with eye movements. Her examination was notable for 20/80 vision in the left eye, 20/20 vision in the right eye using a Snellen wall chart, and a left relative afferent pupillary defect. Her neurologic examination was otherwise unremarkable. Magnetic resonance imaging (MRI) demonstrated T2 signal abnormality and enhancement of the left optic nerve using fat-saturated imaging techniques but no other lesions outside the optic nerves. She was diagnosed with optic neuritis. She was treated with pulse methylprednisolone, after which her eye pain resolved. Antibodies to myelin oligodendrocyte glycoprotein and aquaporin-4 were negative. Her visual acuity improved over time. She was followed prospectively with serial MRI scans to screen for multiple sclerosis.

Optic neuritis (ON) may be an initial manifestation of multiple demyelinating conditions, and a thorough history and examination are necessary to look for other neurologic abnormalities. The overall prognosis for visual recovery depends on the presence of coexisting neurologic syndromes.

Demyelinating diseases are acquired autoimmune disorders affecting the central nervous system (CNS) of children and adolescents. The initial clinical presentations are often similar across various demyelinating diseases; however, differentiating between each specific disease is important for treatment and prognostication. Some demyelinating diseases, such as acute disseminated encephalomyelitis (ADEM), can be self-limited with a generally favorable prognosis, whereas others, such as multiple sclerosis (MS) and neuromyelitis optica–spectrum disorders (NMOSDs), are chronic relapsing conditions that are potentially disabling.

ETIOLOGY AND PATHOGENESIS

The pathogenesis of demyelinating diseases is complex, incompletely understood, and varies by specific disease. Autoimmune mechanisms have a fundamental role in the pathogenesis of MS, possibly initiated by an environmental trigger in a genetically susceptible individual. Previously, MS was thought to be primarily driven by a T cell–mediated process; however, B cells, macrophages, and microglia have now also been identified to have a role. Environmental factors, including Epstein-Barr virus (EBV) and human herpes virus-6 (HHV-6), have been implicated in the pathogenesis of MS. Twin studies of adults with MS have revealed a 30% concordance rate among identical twins; multiple genes are probably involved. Although demyelination is a key feature of these disorders, there is also axonal injury and neuronal loss, particularly in MS and relapsing disease, which may be the primary cause of chronic morbidity. In NMOSD and myelin oligodendrocyte glycoprotein (MOG)-antibody associated disorders, immunoglobulins play a direct role in the pathogenesis.

CLINICAL PRESENTATION AND DIFFERENTIAL DIAGNOSIS

Acute Disseminated Encephalomyelitis

Historically, ADEM was defined by the development of neurologic symptoms after a vaccination or a viral or bacterial infection. However, the most recent consensus definition of the International Pediatric MS Study Group (IPMSSG) now describes ADEM as a first demyelinating or inflammatory event in which the child has a polyfocal CNS event with concurrent encephalopathy. Encephalopathy can be mild (e.g., confusion or irritability) but must be present and should not be explained by fever, infection, or a postictal state. Although a preceding illness or infection is identifiable in approximately 75% of children (with an average latency between the illness and symptoms of 7 to 14 days), such an event is not required for the diagnosis. Magnetic resonance imaging (MRI) of the brain typically reveals multiple large (>1 to 2 cm) asymmetric lesions affecting the supratentorial and infratentorial white matter that are visualized using T2-weighted and fluid-attenuated inversion recovery (FLAIR) sequences. Symmetric gray matter involvement of the thalami and basal ganglia and confluent spinal cord lesions have also been described in ADEM. MRI findings must be present for the diagnosis. Cerebrospinal fluid (CSF) analysis may demonstrate an elevated white blood cell (WBC) count with a lymphocytic or monocytic predominance or elevated protein. CSF-specific oligoclonal bands are rare in ADEM. Patients with these clinical and radiographic findings should be tested for the presence of antibodies to MOG (see below).

Clinically Isolated Syndrome

The IPMSSG defines a clinically isolated syndrome as a first demyelinating event that may be monofocal or multifocal in the absence of encephalopathy (with the exception of a brainstem lesion, which may result in altered mental status or coma). These disorders may be isolated or may herald the initial presentation of MS. Transverse myelitis (TM) and optic neuritis (ON) are two common subtypes of clinically isolated syndrome.

Transverse Myelitis

TM is characterized by acute bilateral sensory, motor, or autonomic dysfunction localizable to the spinal cord. Neurologic symptoms manifest rapidly, within hours to days, often beginning with sensory symptoms. Weakness, urinary dysfunction, and pain frequently occur depending on the extent and location of disease. According to guidelines proposed by the Transverse Myelitis Consortium working

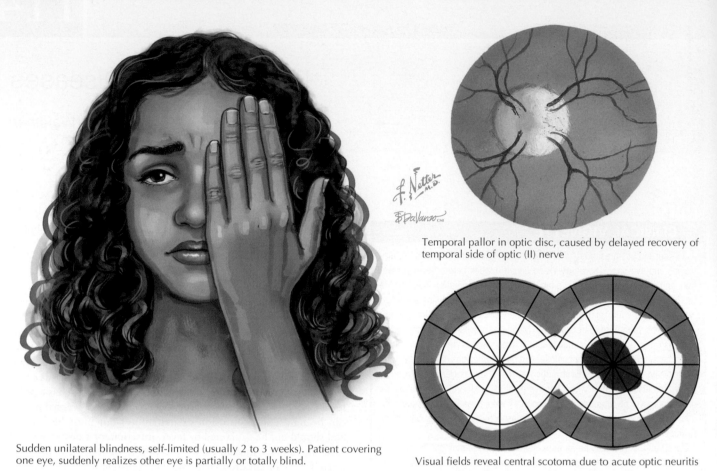

Temporal pallor in optic disc, caused by delayed recovery of temporal side of optic (II) nerve

Sudden unilateral blindness, self-limited (usually 2 to 3 weeks). Patient covering one eye, suddenly realizes other eye is partially or totally blind.

Visual fields reveal central scotoma due to acute optic neuritis

Fig. 114.1 Ocular Manifestations of Multiple Sclerosis.

group in 2002, inflammation in the spinal cord must be demonstrated by CSF analysis (pleocytosis or elevated immunoglobulin G [IgG] index) or MRI (gadolinium enhancement), which helps differentiate noninflammatory causes of spinal cord disease (e.g., fibrocartilaginous emboli, anterior spinal artery infarction) from TM. These criteria have not been validated in children, and normal CSF profiles have been reported. If inflammation is not detected in the CSF or on MRI, a repeat spinal tap or MRI 2 to 7 days after symptom onset should be performed to further look for signs of inflammation. There are no criteria for the size or extent of the lesion upon neuroimaging of the spine. TM is often associated with longitudinally extensive lesions (greater than three or more vertebral segments). Discrete lesions are more common in the initial presentation of MS. The prognosis for full recovery is less favorable than for the other demyelinating diseases because of residual disability in ambulation, sensation, or bladder function. Additional information on TM is found in Chapter 115.

Optic Neuritis

ON is characterized by acute or subacute visual loss, altered color vision, periorbital pain that is exacerbated by eye movements, and visual field defects. The neuro-ophthalmologic examination may reveal a relative afferent pupillary defect (if unilateral) or optic disc edema (Fig. 114.1). MRI of the orbits using fat-saturated images often reveals T2/FLAIR abnormality in the optic nerve or chiasm with or without enhancement using gadolinium. Visual recovery from idiopathic ON is excellent for most children, especially in the absence of alternative diagnoses such as NMOSD or MS.

Acute Flaccid Myelitis

Acute flaccid myelitis (AFM) occurs as a result of dysfunction or death of the anterior horn cells in the gray matter of the spinal cord. Children typically present with acute-onset flaccid limb weakness in the setting of a recent febrile illness. AFM most often occurs in the setting of viral infection, particularly enterovirus D68 and enterovirus A71 in recent outbreaks. MRI is helpful in distinguishing AFM from TM based on the location of signal abnormality (anterior horn cells in AFM, transverse cord in TM). Outcomes vary widely depending on the location and extent of spinal cord involvement. For further information on AFM, see Chapter 116.

Multiple Sclerosis

MS is a chronic demyelinating inflammatory disorder characterized by the dissemination of neurologic signs and symptoms in time and space in both children and adults. The development of a neurologic symptom lasting more than 24 hours is referred to as an "attack" or "flare." Children most often present with paresthesias or ON. Motor dysfunction, ataxia, cranial nerve palsies, vestibular symptoms, and other neurologic symptoms also may occur. Compared with clinically isolated syndrome, patients with MS meet the criteria of both dissemination in space and dissemination in time. Using the 2017 Revisions to the McDonald Criteria established for adults, dissemination in time is defined by two or more clinical attacks, the appearance of a new T2 or FLAIR lesion (compared with a reference scan) in the brain or spinal cord, the simultaneous presence of both gadolinium enhancing and nonenhancing lesions, or by CSF-specific oligoclonal bands. Dissemination in space is defined by objective clinical evidence of

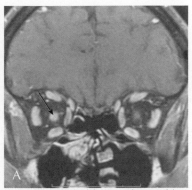

(A) Coronal T1-weighted, fat-saturated, post–gadolinium-enhanced image shows enhancement and enlargement of the right optic nerve (arrow).

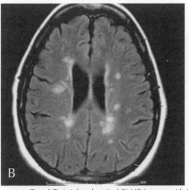

(B and C) Axial and sagittal FLAIR images with increased T2 signal within the corpus callosum and paraventricular white matter with extension into central white matter along vascular pathways

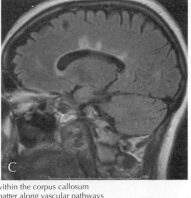

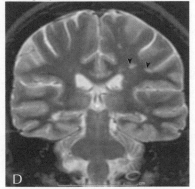

Also illustrated in D, coronal T2, where the typical oval lesions are oriented along vascular pathways, typical of "Dawson fingers" (arrowheads).

Reprint with permission from Misulis K, Heat T. Netter's Concise Neurology, page 303. Saunders, Elseiver 2007.

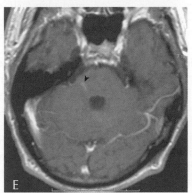

(E) Axial T1-weighted post–gadolinium-enhanced image shows enhancement of T2 bright lesion shown in other sequences in the right cerebellar peduncle. The enhancement suggests disease activity.

(F) Sagittal T2-weighted image shows T2 bright lesion in posterior cord at C2-3.

Fig. 114.2 Imaging of Multiple Sclerosis.

two or more lesions or an MRI with a T2 hyperintense lesion in at least two of the following four characteristic locations: periventricular, cortical/juxtacortical, infratentorial, and spinal cord (Fig. 114.2). The McDonald Criteria are overall applicable to children, with sensitivity estimated greater than 70%, specificity of greater than 95%. However, greater caution should be used in children, because of the higher rates of MOG-associated demyelination, NMOSD, and other demyelinating disorders, especially under the age of 11 years. Most children have relapsing-remitting MS; primary progressive MS and progressive relapsing MS are rare. Although there are limited data, the natural history of pediatric MS suggests a slower progression of disease than in adults. However, children develop secondary progressive MS at younger ages than adults and cognitive changes can be seen soon after diagnosis.

Neuromyelitis Optica Spectrum Disorder

NMOSD is a chronic, relapsing demyelinating disease affecting the optic nerves and spinal cord either concurrently or sequentially (with attacks separated by months). The symptoms can be significant with complete vision loss and quadriplegia or paraplegia depending on the location and extent of spinal cord involvement. Clinical criteria for the diagnosis differ depending on whether the individual has a positive NMO-IgG antibody. This autoantibody binds selectively to the aquaporin-4 water channel, a component of a protein complex found in astrocytes at the blood-brain barrier, causing complement activation and disrupting glutamate transport. The 2015 consensus guidelines defined six core characteristics of NMOSD: ON, acute myelitis, area postrema syndrome, acute brainstem syndrome, symptomatic narcolepsy or diencephalic syndrome with characteristic MRI lesions, and symptomatic cerebral syndrome with typical brain lesions. With positive NMO-immunoglobulin (Ig) G antibodies, a single core characteristic is necessary. Without NMO-IgG antibodies, two core clinical characteristics are required, of which one must be ON, area postrema syndrome, or acute myelitis with an MRI lesion extending at least three segments (longitudinally extensive). In children, the finding of a longitudinally extensive lesion is less specific to NMOSD than in adults and may be found in other demyelinating disorders as well. CSF analysis, although not required for the diagnosis, may reveal a pleocytosis (≥50 WBCs) or positive CSF NMO-IgG, although serum is preferred for the detection of the autoantibody. Patients with antibodies to NMO-IgG may have additional antibodies to other targets or have comorbid autoimmune conditions, including Sjögren disease, lupus, sarcoidosis, or antiphospholipid antibody syndrome, or antibodies to N-methyl-D-aspartate-type (NMDA-type) glutamate or other receptors. NMDSD has an overall poorer recovery from attacks compared with MS relapses.

Myelin Oligodendrocyte Glycoprotein (MOG) Antibody–Associated Demyelinating Disorders

MOG is a component of the myelin sheath. Approximately one-third of pediatric patients with demyelinating disease will have positive anti-MOG antibodies. In younger children, MOG is likely to present as ADEM while in older children it is more likely to present as ON and TM. CSF findings include a pleocytosis, elevated protein, and absence of oligoclonal bands. Approximately 40% of patients with positive MOG antibodies will have recurrent disease. Patients with persistently high anti-MOG antibody titers are more likely to have recurrent disease and poorer outcomes.

EVALUATION AND MANAGEMENT

The evaluation of a child with suspected demyelinating disease varies slightly based on the suspected disorder. Neuroimaging (MRI of the brain and cervical or thoracic spine), a lumbar puncture, neurophysiologic testing (visual evoked potentials, somatosensory evoked potentials, and brainstem auditory evoked potentials) aid in the detection of diffuse inflammation; blood work may be performed to exclude other nutritional, metabolic, and inflammatory conditions. A referral to a pediatric neuro-ophthalmologist may be helpful to characterize the extent of disease, including subclinical involvement of a seemingly unaffected eye. Further genetic, infectious, inflammatory, or metabolic tests depend on the clinical presentation.

Acute Therapy

Corticosteroids are used to decrease inflammation associated with demyelinating attacks. Methylprednisolone (20 to 30 mg/kg/day IV; maximum, 1 g) is given for 3 to 5 days depending on the clinical presentation and physician judgment. Oral corticosteroid tapers are not always necessary after an intravenous course. In general, intravenous corticosteroids do not alter the long-term prognosis but may hasten recovery compared with oral steroids. One trial found decreased recurrence using intravenous versus oral steroids in optic neuritis, though others have found no difference in treatment of multiple sclerosis flares. Second-line therapies include intravenous immunoglobulin (IVIG) and plasma exchange. There have been no clinical trials performed in children to evaluate the efficacy of corticosteroids, IVIG, plasma exchange, or any other therapy in acute demyelinating attacks.

Special Considerations
Multiple Sclerosis

Disease-modifying therapies (DMTs) are used in MS to alter the course of disease by decreasing the severity and number of relapses and reducing the number of new lesions on MRI. Cohort studies have reported safety and efficacy data for the use of DMTs in children, including intramuscular or subcutaneous interferon β-1a, subcutaneous interferon β-1b, and glatiramer acetate. Side effects of DMTs are common. Flu-like symptoms may occur with the interferons, which may be reduced with acetaminophen or ibuprofen before the injection. Subcutaneous injections may cause local irritation. There has been only one published randomized controlled trial (RCT) examining DMTs in pediatric MS. The PARADIGMS trial compared the efficacy of fingolimod to interferon β-1a and found that fingolimod was associated with a lower rate of relapse and fewer MRI lesions, but greater rates of adverse events. Fingolimod is the only DMT with US Food and Drug Administration (FDA) approval for pediatric MS; however, other therapies are frequently used given their safety and tolerability profile. Fingolimod is associated with cardiac rhythm abnormalities and macular edema. Natalizumab is also commonly used for pediatric patients with relapsing MS and requires periodic monitoring because of the association with progressive multifocal leukoencephalopathy and leukopenia.

Neuromyelitis Optica Spectrum Disorders

NMOSD attacks are more debilitating than other demyelinating diseases and do not respond to the immunomodulatory medications used to treat MS, making the distinction between the two important for therapeutic considerations. No RCTs have been completed in children, although small cohort studies have proposed immunosuppressive agents, such as rituximab, azathioprine, or mycophenolate mofetil, may be effective. There are a few FDA-approved treatments for NMDSD in adults. These include eculizumab, an antibody that inhibits the formation of the membrane attack complex; satralizumab, an interleukin-6 (IL-6) receptor antagonist; and inebilizumab, a monoclonal antibody against CD19 cells. Clinical trials of these medications are being performed in children.

Myelin Oligodendrocyte Glycoprotein (MOG) Antibody–Associated Demyelinating Disorders

There are no RCTs examining treatment in MOG antibody–associated disorders. Observational studies have shown that DMTs typically used in MS are ineffective, whereas other immunosuppressants, including IVIG, may have benefit in a single course or monthly regimen. Rituximab, azathioprine, or mycophenolate mofetil also may be used for relapsing patients; however, some patients have had clinical relapses despite B-cell depletion from rituximab.

Transverse Myelitis

Prompt evaluation and treatment with intravenous methylprednisolone and plasmapheresis may result in greater recovery. Supportive care, such as mechanical ventilation, may be required for cervical involvement. Relapses can occur, raising clinical suspicion for MS or NMOSD.

FUTURE DIRECTIONS

Greater recognition of pediatric demyelinating disorders moving forward is critical. Validation of the definitions set forth by the IPMSSG and others will allow for better understanding of the spectrum of these disorders in children. Additional clinical trial data about the safety and efficacy of the immunomodulatory and immunosuppressive medications in children are needed to decrease disability, especially in relapsing diseases such as MS and NMOSD.

SUGGESTED READINGS

Available online.

115

Spinal Cord Disorders

Alexis R. Karlin and Sona Narula

 CLINICAL VIGNETTE

An 8-year-old girl with asthma presented with a right wrist fracture and weakness after falling while doing cartwheels. On initial evaluation, her arm weakness was out of proportion to that expected with just a wrist fracture. Imaging of the brachial plexus was obtained to rule out proximal nerve/plexus injury. Magnetic resonance imaging (MRI) revealed normal brachial plexus, but there was signal abnormality in the cervical spine. She subsequently had complete spine and brain imaging, which revealed abnormalities in the bilateral midbrain and cervical spinal cord from C2 through C7. She was started on methylprednisolone and intravenous immuno-globulin (IVIG) for treatment of myelitis. In the next few hours, measurements of her negative inspiratory force decreased, from normal range of −40 to −20. On reassessment, she had suprasternal retractions and a weak cough, and could only speak in one- or two-word sentences. Mental status and cranial nerves were normal. On motor examination, she was no longer able to lift her right arm against gravity. She had some strength against resistance in the left arm but was weaker than the day prior. She had full strength in her legs and normal sensation throughout. She was transferred urgently to the intensive care unit. She was intubated and underwent plasmapheresis. Despite treatment, she became progressively weaker over the following days. Because of inability to wean off the ventilator, she underwent tracheostomy. On discharge to rehabilitation, motor function was limited to antigravity left arm movement and some leg movement. Two years later she can write and ambulate with assistance. She requires mechanical ventilation overnight and has required bilateral rod placement for progressive neuromuscular scoliosis.

Spinal cord disorders, termed myelopathies, typically conform to neuroanatomic pathways and vascular territories, which can result in a number of classic neurologic syndromes. These syndromes involve motor, sensory, and autonomic pathways. Causes of spinal cord disorders are diverse, including traumatic, vascular, inflammatory/autoimmune, toxin-mediated, metabolic, infectious, neoplastic, or congenital causes. We will focus our discussion on transverse myelitis (TM), which affects about 2 million children per year, and is preceded by mild illness in approximately two-thirds of cases. Acute flaccid myelitis (AFM) is a subset of TM associated with enterovirus D68 and A71 (Chapter 116). Pediatric spinal cord injury is rare, with about 2 to 4 cases per million per year, most occurring in children (majority over 15 years of age).

ANATOMY OF THE SPINAL CORD

The spinal cord is divided into four sections: cervical, thoracic, lumbar, and sacral. The termination of the spinal cord, conus medullaris, lies at vertebral body level L2-L3 in infants or level L1–L2 in older children and adults. The cauda equina is a collection of intradural lumbar, sacral, and coccygeal nerve roots that descend from the conus medullaris and exit by each root's respective foramen. The filum terminale is non-neural fibrous tissue that extends from the conus medullaris to the coccyx, anchoring the cord to the vertebral column.

The cervical cord innervates the upper body and the diaphragm. The thoracic cord innervates the muscles of expiration and contains preganglionic sympathetic fibers to the face, heart, and abdominal organs. The lumbosacral nerve roots innervate the lower extremities. The sacral cord provides parasympathetic innervation to pelvic and abdominal organs.

The spinal cord is composed of a central butterfly-shaped region of gray matter, containing neuron cell bodies. The gray matter is surrounded by white matter, which contains myelinated axons carrying signals between the brain and body (Fig. 115.1).

The major *descending* white matter tract is the lateral corticospinal tract located posterolaterally within the cord. The upper motor neurons contained within this tract originate in the primary motor cortex and decussate in the medulla before descending down the spinal cord. Exiting fibers travel medially to the anterior horns, where they synapse with the lower motor neurons. Axons of the lower motor neurons then exit by the ventral root to synapse at the neuromuscular junction.

There are two major *ascending* tracts carrying sensory information from the body to the cortex. The dorsal columns contain proprioceptive and vibratory information. These fibers enter the spinal cord by the dorsal horn, ascend medially and decussate in the medulla before traveling to the sensory cortex. The spinothalamic tract is located anterolaterally and carries pain, temperature, and crude touch sensory information. These sensory fibers enter the spinal cord, ascend ipsilaterally for 2 to 3 levels, then decussate across the anterior commissure.

The vascular anatomy of the spinal cord is composed of one anterior spinal artery, which supplies the anterior two-thirds of the spinal cord, and two posterior spinal arteries, which primarily supply the dorsal columns. Both anterior and posterior spinal arteries receive their vascular supply from the vertebral arteries. In the thoracic and lumbar spine, radicular arteries branch off the aorta to provide additional perfusion. Venous drainage of the cord consists of two major spinal veins. Spinal veins do not have valves; therefore significant increase in intraabdominal pressure may result in venous congestion and decreased cord perfusion.

CLINICAL PRESENTATION AND DIFFERENTIAL DIAGNOSIS

The clinician should suspect a spinal cord pathologic condition when a patient reports bilateral (sometimes asymmetric) or segmental sensorimotor signs and symptoms. Patients may have bladder or bowel dysfunction and/or back pain. The history should address preceding illnesses, immunocompromised status, trauma, pain, and time-course of symptoms. If there is a history of trisomy 21 or rheumatoid arthritis, consider cervical spine pathologic processes because these patients

Sections through spinal cord at various levels

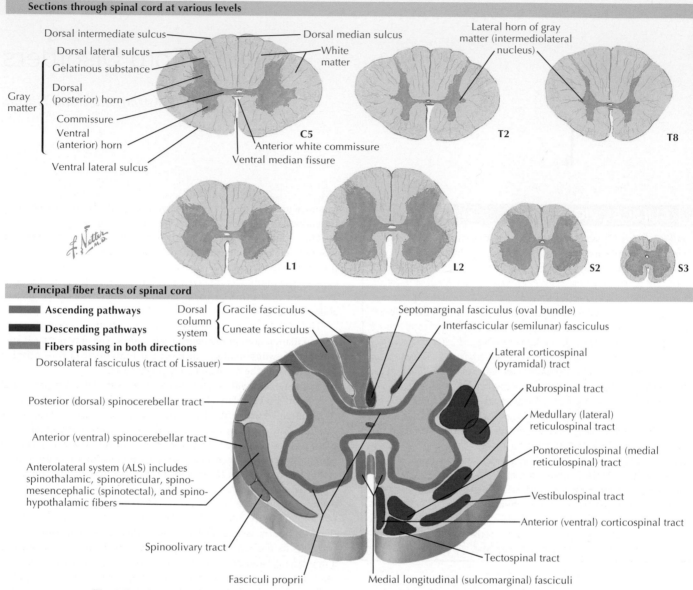

Fig. 115.1 Cross Section Through the Spinal Cord. Gray and white matter with ascending and descending pathways. Variable anatomy in cervical, thoracic, and lumbar regions. Note increased size of anterior gray matter in cervical and lumbar spine, reflecting anterior horn cells innervating upper and lower extremities, respectively.

may be at higher risk for atlantoaxial instability leading to cervical spine injury. The examination is key to localizing symptoms and guiding evaluation.

Assessment first addresses airway, breathing, circulation (ABCs), and vitals. General examination should include close attention to respiratory effort. The single-breath test is a simple bedside test that estimates a patient's vital capacity by asking the patient to take a deep breath and count aloud as high as they can in a single breath. (Normal range depends on age and gender. For example, for patients older than 11 years, normal is >30.) Respiratory function should be formally evaluated by a respiratory therapist. Spinous processes and paraspinal tissues should be palpated to assess for tenderness, swelling, or fractures.

On neurologic examination, it is important to assess mental status and cranial nerves to rule out signs or symptoms concerning for brainstem or supratentorial involvement. Examination should be as detailed as possible, including motor (bulk, tone, and strength), sensory, reflex, and gait assessments to determine patterns of weakness and elicit upper versus lower motor neuron signs. Upper motor neuron (UMN)

signs, including spasticity, hyperreflexia, clonus, or upgoing toes, indicate central nervous system (brain or spinal cord above the level of the affected anterior horn cell) involvement. Lower motor neuron (LMN) signs, including flaccid weakness, atrophy, fasciculations, and hypore-flexia/areflexia, indicate involvement of the peripheral nervous system and/or anterior horn cells. Involvement of specific muscle groups may help to localize the lesion in the spinal cord (Fig. 115.2), though it is important to note that a lesion anywhere in the spine may affect the lower extremities as well as bladder/bowel function, whereas only cervical spine lesions and above will affect the upper extremities.

Sensory examination should elicit the pattern of reported sensory loss and include a sensory level, defined by sensation to pin. Perineal sensation, rectal tone, and bowel and bladder function (typically with bladder scan) should be assessed. Lhermitte sign, indicative of a cervical spine pathologic condition, may be elicited by having the patient flex her neck forward; if the patient reports a sensation of electrical shock or vibration radiating downward, this is a positive sign TO Lhermitte sign may be elicited by having the patient flex her neck forward. If the

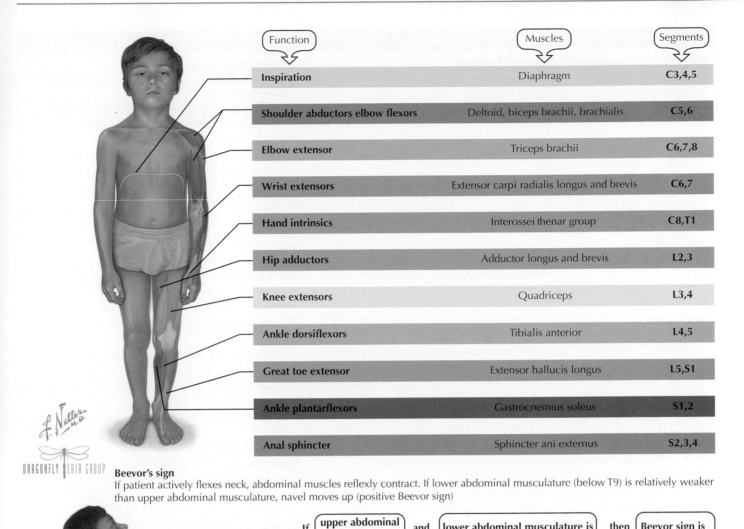

Function	Muscles	Segments
Inspiration	Diaphragm	C3,4,5
Shoulder abductors elbow flexors	Deltoid, biceps brachii, brachialis	C5,6
Elbow extensor	Triceps brachii	C6,7,8
Wrist extensors	Extensor carpi radialis longus and brevis	C6,7
Hand intrinsics	Interossei thenar group	C8,T1
Hip adductors	Adductor longus and brevis	L2,3
Knee extensors	Quadriceps	L3,4
Ankle dorsiflexors	Tibialis anterior	L4,5
Great toe extensor	Extensor hallucis longus	L5,S1
Ankle plantarflexors	Gastrocnemius soleus	S1,2
Anal sphincter	Sphincter ani externus	S2,3,4

Beevor's sign
If patient actively flexes neck, abdominal muscles reflexly contract. If lower abdominal musculature (below T9) is relatively weaker than upper abdominal musculature, navel moves up (positive Beevor sign)

If	upper abdominal musculature is	and	lower abdominal musculature is	then	Beevor sign is
	Normal		Normal		Negative
	Normal		Weak or nonfunctioning		Positive
	Weak		Nonfunctioning		Positive
	Nonfunctioning		Nonfunctioning		Negative

Fig. 115.2 Myotomes. Myotomes relating spinal level to muscle innervation. The Beevor sign may help to localize to the thoracic spine.

patient reports a sensation of electrical shock or vibration radiating downward, this is a positive sign and indicative of a pathological cervical spine condition. An acute spinal cord lesion can present with signs of spinal shock with LMN signs. UMN signs evolve later.

Spinal Cord Syndromes

There are common patterns of motor and sensory involvement depending on the localization of disease within the spinal cord. Table 115.1 and Fig. 115.3 describe the features of typical patterns of spinal cord disease, their common causes, and the expected time-course.

EVALUATION AND MANAGEMENT

In the acute setting, initial management of a spinal cord disorder involves hemodynamic and cardiorespiratory stabilization. If there is suspicion of an acute spinal cord lesion, clinicians should an order urgent MRI of the spine with and without contrast, including diffusion weighted imaging.

Transverse Myelitis

TM typically affects segments of the spinal cord and can result in weakness and/or sensory changes below the lesion, sometimes with bladder or bowel dysfunction. As the cause of TM is so diverse, ranging from demyelinating, infectious/postinfectious, and rheumatologic, these patients typically require extensive workup. MRI of the brain should be performed to look for lesions above the foramen magnum that may suggest a demyelinating process such as multiple sclerosis, myelin oligodendrocyte glycoprotein (MOG)-associated demyelination, neuromyelitis optica spectrum disorder (NMOSD), or acute disseminated encephalomyelitis (ADEM; if encephalopathy is also present) (Chapter 114). Serum tests should include aquaporin-4 antibody testing, MOG antibody testing, and inflammatory markers. If there is concern for systemic features, consider rheumatologic evaluation. If infectious causes are being considered, evaluation for West Nile virus, varicella-zoster, herpes simplex virus, human lymphotropic virus, human immunodeficiency virus (HIV), and Zika virus may be pursued in

TABLE 115.1   Spinal Cord Syndromes

Spinal Cord Syndromes	Clinical Features	Differential Diagnosis
Segmental (transection) syndrome	Loss of all sensory modalities, weakness below affected level, bladder dysfunction At risk for autonomic instability	**Hyperacute/acute:** atlantoaxial instability, trauma (blunt or penetrating wounds) **Acute/subacute:** transverse myelitis, extrinsic cord compression secondary to epidural abscess, epidural hematoma
Anterior cord	LMN at level of the lesion + UMN signs below the lesion Preserved vibration and proprioception sensation	**Hyperacute/acute:** • Vascular: arteriovenous malformation, ischemic infarct, profound hypotension (typically affects thoracic cord) • Trauma • Cerebellar herniation • Radiation • Myelitis
Dorsal cord	Decreased proprioception and vibration ± gait ataxia ± UMN signs Preserved pinprick and light touch sensation	**Acute:** vascular (rare) **Acute/subacute:** myelitis **Slowly progressive:** toxic/metabolic—subacute combined degeneration syndrome, vitamin E deficiency, copper deficiency; Infectious—HIV/AIDS myelopathy, tabes dorsalis
Central cord	Arm > leg weakness "Suspended sensory level" (loss of pain and temperature sensation at level of lesion because of interruption of anterior commissure) +/- urinary retention	**Subacute to slowly progressive:** • Syringomyelia • Neoplastic or infiltrative: intramedullary tumor, drop metastases
Brown-Séquard (hemicord)	Ipsilateral UMN and impaired vibration/proprioception Contralateral loss of pain/temperature Spared bladder and bowel function	**Acute:** trauma **Acute to subacute:** transverse myelitis
Pure motor syndrome	Weakness without sensory loss or bladder involvement. May involve upper and lower motor neurons	**Acute to subacute:** acute flaccid myelitis **Progressive:** spinal muscular atrophy
Cauda equina	Low back pain and asymmetric radicular pain Asymmetric LMN signs in lower extremities ± bladder/rectal dysfunction	**Variable:** cord compression
Conus medullaris	Sphincter dysfunction with flaccid paralysis of bladder and rectum, saddle anesthesia ± UMN signs in lower extremities	**Variable:** cord compression, myelitis
Variable	Variable features	**Slowly progressive:** • Structural or congenital: spina bifida, tethered cord, myelomeningocele, hereditary spastic paraplegia, Friedreich ataxia • Neoplastic: extradural tumor • Vascular: intramedullary spinal arteriovenous malformation

AIDS, Acquired immune deficiency syndrome; *HIV,* human immunodeficiency virus; *LMN,* lower motor neuron; *UMN,* upper motor neuron.

the appropriate clinical context. Enterovirus species D68 and A71 have been implicated in causing AFM, a subset of TM. Enterovirus polymerase chain reaction (PCR) should be sent from rectal and nasopharyngeal swabs as well as urine, serum, and cerebrospinal fluid (CSF) if possible. Bacteria that have been implicated in TM include *Mycoplasma, Borrelia, Listeria,* and *Treponema pallidum.* Consider evaluation for tuberculosis in the setting of pertinent risk factors. CSF analysis includes cell counts, glucose, protein, culture, cytology, oligoclonal bands, and viral studies as indicated. For children with gastrointestinal or metabolic disorders, vitamin levels, including B_{12}, B_9 (folate), and vitamin E, and copper should be ordered. Treatment for AFM and virally mediated transverse myelitis is typically supportive. Inflammatory myelitis may be treated with immunomodulatory therapies such as methylprednisolone, IVIG, or plasmapheresis depending on the severity of symptoms.

Cord Compression

If there is concern for cord compression on initial neuroimaging, a pediatric neurosurgeon should be urgently consulted to determine if a surgical intervention is warranted. Use of steroids may be considered. Epidural abscesses may be drained and treated with broad-spectrum antibiotics. Other lesions are treated according to cause. For traumatic spinal cord injuries, steroid administration is controversial; recent studies have shown that risks likely outweigh the benefits of steroid treatment in pediatric traumatic spinal cord injury.

Spinal Cord Ischemia

Spinal cord ischemia may preferentially affect the gray matter because of higher metabolic demand in this region. In addition to acute supportive management, the aim is to increase cord perfusion with intravenous fluids and vasopressors if needed.

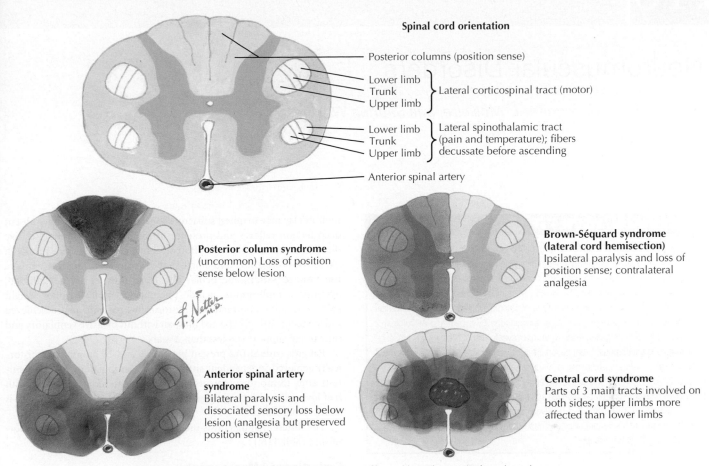

Spinal cord orientation

Posterior columns (position sense)

Lower limb
Trunk
Upper limb } Lateral corticospinal tract (motor)

Lower limb
Trunk
Upper limb } Lateral spinothalamic tract (pain and temperature); fibers decussate before ascending

Anterior spinal artery

Posterior column syndrome
(uncommon) Loss of position sense below lesion

Brown-Séquard syndrome (lateral cord hemisection)
Ipsilateral paralysis and loss of position sense; contralateral analgesia

Anterior spinal artery syndrome
Bilateral paralysis and dissociated sensory loss below lesion (analgesia but preserved position sense)

Central cord syndrome
Parts of 3 main tracts involved on both sides; upper limbs more affected than lower limbs

Fig. 115.3 Spinal Cord Syndromes. Regions affected in various spinal cord syndromes.

Other Causes

If physical examination or imaging suggests a congenital spinal cord or vertebral anomaly the child should be assessed for other structural anomalies including cardiac, renal, and tracheoesophageal differences (VACTERL). For neoplasms, treatment depends on grade and subtype of tumor. For all other causes of spinal cord dysfunction, treatment should address the underlying disorder and may include antibiotics, dietary supplementation, supportive management, and neurosurgical intervention.

FUTURE DIRECTIONS

Future steps include further investigation into the molecular mechanisms of inflammation within the spinal cord to better develop directed therapies and improve outcomes. Improved imaging techniques will allow for greater diagnostic accuracy. Vaccine development for enterovirus subtypes that are associated with AFM is being considered.

SUGGESTED READINGS

Available online.

116

Neuromuscular Disorders

Giulia S. Porcari, Jennifer L. McGuire, and Sabrina W. Yum

CLINICAL VIGNETTE

A 2-month-old infant is seen at his well-child check. He was delivered vaginally at term following an uncomplicated pregnancy with uneventful perinatal course. He is smiling, cooing, and responding to sound, but is unable to lift his head during tummy time. On assessment, he is well appearing, without signs of infection, and nondysmorphic, but has generalized hypotonia with slip-through on vertical suspension and a positive scarf sign. Examination by a pediatric neurologist 2 weeks later confirms generalized hypotonia, reveals absent reflexes and presence of tongue fasciculations. Creatine kinase (CK) is normal. *SMN1* testing shows a homozygous deletion, indicating a diagnosis of spinal muscular atrophy (SMA) type 1. After careful discussion, parents choose to pursue gene therapy. He receives onasemnogene abeparvovec at 3 months. Treatment is complicated by an asymptomatic transaminitis that resolves on prednisolone, which is discontinued after a month. At his 6-month visit, his head control is remarkably improved and he is beginning to sit with support.

Neuromuscular disorders are a variable group of diseases of the peripheral nervous system (Fig. 116.1). In this chapter, several of the more common pediatric disorders are reviewed and classified based on their level of neuroaxis involvement.

ANTERIOR HORN CELL

Spinal Muscular Atrophy

Spinal muscular atrophy (SMA) is a genetic disorder characterized by progressive degeneration of anterior horn cells in the spinal cord and motor nuclei in the lower brainstem. The term SMA commonly refers to the autosomal recessive disorder arising from mutations in the survival motor neuron 1 (*SMN1*) gene on chromosome 5q13, which accounts for approximately 95% of cases. Other "non-5q" forms exist. Altogether, SMA occurs in about 1 in 10,000 live births.

Etiology and Pathogenesis

SMN protein is involved in ribonucleic acid (RNA) processing and is ubiquitously expressed but particularly important in motor neurons. Humans have a near-identical homocopy, *SMN2*, but approximately 90% of these transcripts are degraded as a result of exclusion of exon 7 during alternative splicing (Fig. 116.2). *SMN2* copy number is inversely related to disease severity.

Clinical Presentation

SMA is subclassified based on age of onset and maximal motor skills achieved. SMA type 1 (SMA1) is the most common and severe, accounting for approximately 60% of cases. It manifests between birth and 6 months with generalized hypotonia, symmetric flaccid weakness (proximal greater than distal), and frequently feeding difficulty. Gross motor delay may manifest subacutely or indolently. Infants have absent deep tendon reflexes and presence of tongue fasciculations. Relative diaphragmatic sparing with intercostal muscle involvement results in paradoxical breathing and a bell-shaped torso (Fig. 116.3). Cognitive function, sensation, and ocular and facial muscles are not affected. Systemic complications include pneumonia, scoliosis, poor weight gain, and joint contractures. Historically, patients never achieved independent sitting; expected lifespan without invasive ventilatory and nutritional support was less than 2 years.

Patients with SMA2 present between 6 and 18 months and historically achieved independent sitting but not ambulation. SMA3 manifests after 18 months; patients historically achieved ambulation, with half losing this ability by age 10. SMA4 manifests in adulthood and is slowly progressive.

The differential diagnosis includes poliomyelitis and infantile botulism (Table 116.1).

Evaluation and Management

SMA diagnosis is confirmed with testing for biallelic mutations of *SMN1*, typically homozygous deletions. Given treatment advances, early diagnosis is of the essence. In the United States, SMA is gradually being included in state newborn screens to enable presymptomatic diagnosis, but it may be missed in rare cases.

Three US Food and Drug Administration (FDA)-approved disease-modifying therapies are available. Nusinersen (Spinraza) is an antisense oligonucleotide that modulates *SMN2* alternative splicing to promote inclusion of exon 7, thereby increasing translation of functional protein. It has been shown to benefit symptomatic patients with SMA 1 to 4, as well as presymptomatic infants expected to have SMA 1 or 2 based on genetic testing. Benefits include improved survival, decreased need for permanent respiratory support, and, among younger children, remarkable acquisition of motor milestones. It is administered intrathecally every 4 months after loading doses. Adverse effects include respiratory tract infection and constipation; patients should be monitored for coagulation abnormalities, thrombocytopenia, and renal toxicity.

Onasemnogene abeparvovec (Zolgensma), a one-time gene replacement therapy consisting of an adenovirus-associated viral vector (AAV-9) for delivery of the human *SMN1* gene, is approved in patients younger than 2 years. Clinical trials in children younger than 6 months and expected to have SMA 1 or 2 demonstrated improved survival and decreased need for permanent ventilation at 2 years, with nearly all able to sit unsupported and some even able to pull to stand and walk. Dosing is intravenous and well tolerated. Typical side effects include vomiting and asymptomatic transaminitis responsive to steroids. Severe liver injury and thrombotic microangiography have also been reported.

Risdiplam (Evrysdi) is approved for patients older than 2 months. It also targets *SMN2* alternative splicing but is administered orally.

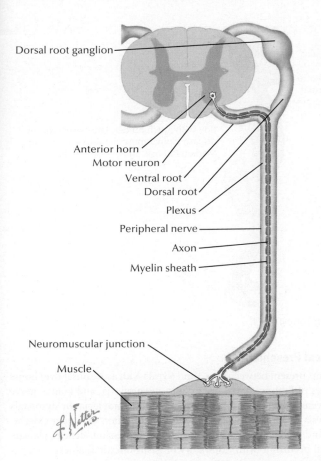

Motor neuron
Primary motor neuron diseases
  Amyotrophic lateral sclerosis
  Spinal muscular atrophy
    Type 1: Werdnig-Hoffmann disease
    Type 2: Intermediate form
    Type 3: Kugelberg-Welander
  Progressive muscular atrophy
  Poliomyelitis
  Acute flaccid myelitis

Dorsal root ganglion
  Herpes zoster
  Friedreich ataxia
  Hereditary sensory neuropathy

Spinal nerve (dorsal and ventral roots)
  Disk extrusion or herniation
  Tumor

Plexus
  Erb palsy
  Tumor
  Trauma
  Idiopathic plexopathy
  Diabetic plexopathy

Peripheral nerve
  Metabolic, toxic, nutritional, idiopathic neuropathies
  Arteritis
  Hereditary neuropathies (e.g., Charcot-Marie-Tooth disease)
  Infectious, postinfectious, inflammatory neuropathies (Guillain-Barré syndrome)
  Entrapment and compression syndromes
  Trauma

Neuromuscular junction
  Myasthenia gravis
  Lambert-Eaton syndrome
  Botulism
  Congenital myasthenic syndrome

Muscle
  Duchenne muscular dystrophy
  Myotonic dystrophy
  Limb-girdle muscular dystrophy
  Congenital muscular dystrophy
  Congenital myopathies
  Polymyositis/dermatomyositis
  Potassium-related myopathies
  Endocrine dysfunction myopathies
  Metabolic myopathies
  Rhabdomyolysis

Labels on figure: Dorsal root ganglion, Anterior horn, Motor neuron, Ventral root, Dorsal root, Plexus, Peripheral nerve, Axon, Myelin sheath, Neuromuscular junction, Muscle

Fig. 116.1 Classification of Neuromuscular Disorders by Level in the Neuroaxis.

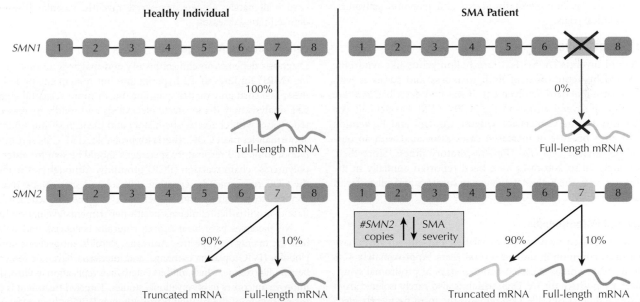

Fig. 116.2 Contribution of *SMN1* and *SMN2* to Survival Motor Neuron Protein Translation. *SMA*, Spinal muscular atrophy

Early clinical trial data suggest benefit in patients with SMA 1 to 3. Common adverse reactions are fever, diarrhea, and rash.

For approved therapies, younger age and higher baseline motor function are associated with greatest benefit. There are no head-to-head comparisons to date of the approved therapies; choice of agent should be guided by patient preference and risk-benefit analysis. Patients with AAV-9 antibodies are not candidates for onasemnogene abeparvovec.

Multidisciplinary supportive care remains essential, including neuromuscular, pulmonary, gastrointestinal/nutrition, genetics, orthopedic, rehabilitation, and palliative care specialists. Need for bilevel positive airway pressure (BLPAP), cough assist, and secretion management should be followed closely. Respiratory infections should be addressed promptly. Poor growth and dysphagia with risk for aspiration are historically common in SMA1, necessitating gastrostomy tube

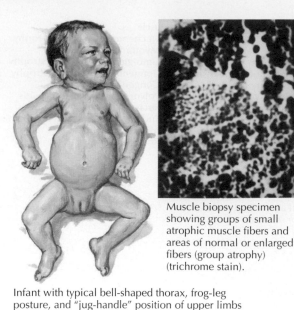

Baseline tremor in otherwise normal electrocardiogram

Boy with much milder, late-onset form of disease (Spinal muscular atrophy type III). Marked lordosis and eversion of feet

Muscle biopsy specimen showing groups of small atrophic muscle fibers and areas of normal or enlarged fibers (group atrophy) (trichrome stain).

Infant with typical bell-shaped thorax, frog-leg posture, and "jug-handle" position of upper limbs

Fig. 116.3 Spinal Muscular Atrophy Type I.

placement. Gastrointestinal reflux, delayed gastric emptying, and constipation are common in nonambulating patients. Orthopedic intervention may be required to address scoliosis and contractures. Genetic counseling and carrier testing should be pursued.

Future Directions

Active lines of research in SMA include gene therapy in older patients, and long-term safety and efficacy of approved therapies. Another *SMN2* splicing agent, branaplam, and agents targeting downstream muscle homeostasis (antimyostatin agents and troponin activators) are also in clinical trials.

Acute Flaccid Myelitis

Acute flaccid myelitis (AFM) is a rare poliomyelitis-like syndrome characterized by acute onset of limb weakness and paralysis with anterior horn spinal cord involvement. It was first described as a rare complication of several viruses in the 2000s. AFM was defined as a distinct entity by the Centers for Disease Control and Prevention (CDC) in 2014 because of increased cases associated with an outbreak of enterovirus D68 (EV-D68) respiratory illness. Since then, approximately 50 to 200 cases have been reported annually in the United States, with the highest incidence in summer and fall and with biennial periodicity.

Etiology and Pathogenesis

AFM is likely caused by a variety of viruses, but enteroviruses have been the most common in the last several years. Approximately 47% of respiratory specimens collected within 7 days of prodromal symptom onset are positive for EV-D68, which is also rarely isolated from cerebrospinal fluid (CSF). EV-D68 remains the most frequently identified pathogen despite extensive clinical and research testing, although other nonpolio enteroviruses have been detected (coxsackieviruses, other enterovirus serotypes, and rhinovirus). Test positivity decreases with time from symptom onset, suggesting testing latency may limit pathogen detection.

Pathogenesis is not well understood. Given the neurotropic nature of enteroviruses, similarity of lesions with poliovirus, and short interval between viral prodrome and neurologic symptoms, direct tissue invasion is suspected, but a postinfectious process remains possible.

Clinical Presentation

Patients present between ages 3 and 6 years with acute onset over hours to days of limb weakness, hypotonia, hyporeflexia, and cranial nerve involvement, leading to facial droop, ophthalmoplegia, or dysphagia Paralysis is typically asymmetric, with predilection for upper extremities and proximal muscles. After initial progression, deficits plateau. A viral prodrome with respiratory or gastrointestinal illness is recognized in approximately 80% of cases, typically occurring about 5 days before neurologic symptoms. Differential diagnosis includes spinal cord malignancy, abscess, transverse myelitis, vascular disease, and demyelinating diseases.

Evaluation and Management

Diagnosis depends on clinical history and magnetic resonance imaging (MRI) findings of T2 hyperintense but nonenhancing lesions in the spinal cord gray matter spanning one or more vertebral segments. CSF analysis may demonstrate pleocytosis and mildly increased protein. Cases with characteristic history and pleocytosis but no imaging abnormalities meet CDC criteria for probable AFM. CSF, serum/whole blood, stool, and respiratory specimens should be sent for enterovirus polymerase chain reaction (PCR) promptly. Although not mandated, the CDC recommends reporting all cases and sharing specimens for confirmatory testing and surveillance (https://www.cdc.gov/acute-flaccid-myelitis/hcp/clinicians-health-departments/evaluation.html).

No therapies have been proven clinically beneficial, and published data are mainly retrospective. Antivirals, steroids, intravenous immunoglobulin (IVIG), plasma exchange, and interferon have not shown clear benefit. Fluoxetine, which inhibits enterovirus replication in vitro, did not improve outcomes in observational studies. Targeted treatment is thus at the discretion of the treating team, although IVIG is frequently used in clinical practice. Care is otherwise supportive; intensive care monitoring should be considered, particularly in children with cervical spinal lesions who are at increased risk for respiratory failure and autonomic instability. Management should include early, intensive rehabilitation. Most patients have residual deficits and complete recovery is uncommon. Nerve transfer procedures have been used with some success.

A network of providers experienced with AFM is available around the clock for consultation (https://wearesrna.org/living-with-myelitis/resources/afm-physician-support-portal/).

TABLE 116.1 Differential Diagnosis of the Floppy Baby, Infant, and Child

Localization	Diagnoses (Examples)
Brain/systemic	Hypoxemic-ischemic encephalopathy
	Chromosomal (Turner syndrome, trisomy 21, Prader-Willi syndrome)
	Brain malformations
	Infection (sepsis, meningitis, encephalitis, TORCH infections, tick paralysis)
	Metabolic (electrolyte abnormalities, hypothyroidism, hepatic encephalopathy, mitochondrial and peroxisomal disorders, amino and organic acidemias)
	Toxins (alcohol, narcotics, heavy metal poisoning, organophosphates, anticholinergics)
	Trauma
	Benign congenital hypotonia
Spinal cord	Hypoxic-ischemic myelopathy
	Compression
	Syringomyelia
Anterior horn cell	Spinal muscular atrophy, infantile neuroaxonal dystrophy
	Acute flaccid myelitis (associated with poliovirus, coxsackie viruses, enteroviruses, and others)
	Cytochrome C oxidase deficiency
Peripheral nerve	Demyelinating (Guillain-Barré syndrome, Charcot-Marie-Tooth disease, congenital hypomyelinating neuropathy, tick paralysis)
	Axonal (familial dysautonomia, Charcot-Marie-Tooth disease, tick paralysis)
Neuromuscular junction	Infection (infantile botulism, tick paralysis)
	Juvenile myasthenia gravis, transient neonatal myasthenia gravis, congenital myasthenic syndrome
Muscle	Congenital myopathies, congenital muscular dystrophies, congenital myotonic dystrophy
	Metabolic (acid maltase deficiency, hypothyroid or hyperthyroid myopathy, carnitine deficiency)
	Inflammatory (dermatomyositis, polymyositis)
	Mitochondrial myopathies

Future Directions

Mouse models are allowing for the study of EV-D68 neutralizing antibodies for potential early treatment. Additional research areas include vaccine development and identification of host risk factors, given that, similar to poliomyelitis, less than 1% of patients with EV-D68 respiratory illness develop AFM. Widespread systems of surveillance, which would aid epidemiologic studies and clinical trial recruitment, are under development.

PERIPHERAL NERVE

Charcot-Marie-Tooth Disease

Charcot-Marie-Tooth disease (CMT), also known as hereditary motor and sensory neuropathy, encompasses a group of peripheral nerve disorders first described in 1886. They are the most common inherited neuromuscular disorders, with estimated prevalence of 10 to 28 in 100,000 individuals.

Etiology and Pathogenesis

CMT diseases are associated with mutations in more than 100 different genes, although approximately 90% of patients with positive genetic testing have mutations in one of four genes: *PMP22*, *GJB1*, *MPZ*, and *MFN2*. Pathophysiology is complex and poorly understood, with defects in myelin proteins, protein degradation, axonal transport, trophic support, and energy production leading to nerve demyelination or axonal degeneration, and resulting in slowly progressive, typically length-dependent weakness and sensory impairment. Based on nerve conduction studies (NCS)/electromyography (EMG), CMT is classified into two broad groups, CMT1 and CMT2, in which pathologic processes are primarily demyelinating and axonal, respectively. Further subclassification is based on genetics and inheritance pattern.

Clinical Presentation

Children with CMT typically have normal early motor milestone acquisition followed by a slowly progressive gait disorder with clumsiness, frequent falling, toe walking, foot drop, and progressive foot deformity with pes cavus and hammertoes. Loss of proprioception and vibration sense contributes to unsteady gait. Hand weakness may cause fine motor difficulties. Less commonly, children present with earlier onset and delayed walking. Most children remain ambulatory with or without orthotics, but some patients with certain types (such as CMT2A) have a more rapidly progressive course with early loss of ambulation. Hearing impairment, scoliosis, and musculoskeletal pain may occur. Classic findings include distal muscle weakness and atrophy, absent to diminished ankle reflexes, and high steppage gait. A rare severe type of CMT (CMT3) manifests with infantile onset of generalized hypotonia, feeding difficulties, hip dysplasia, and respiratory involvement. Differential diagnosis for childhood CMTs is broad, including other inherited conditions such as distal myopathy, Friedreich ataxia, leukodystrophies, mitochondrial diseases with sensorimotor neuropathy, and acquired peripheral neuropathies associated with systemic diseases, nutritional/vitamin deficiency, immune-mediated disorders, and toxin exposure.

Evaluation and Management

NCS/EMG distinguishes CMT from other diagnoses, determines type, and guides genetic testing. Uniform slowing on NCS suggests demyelinating CMT subtypes, while decreased amplitude of sensory and motor responses points to axonal subtypes. Testing for *PMP22* del/dup should be considered first in those with demyelinating disease as CMT1A. Duplication of *PMP22* accounts for 60% of CMT. Increasingly, next-generation sequencing strategies are used.

There are no disease-modifying agents for CMT. Treatment is largely supportive, aimed at maximizing strength and balance and addressing contractures and scoliosis. A multidisciplinary approach is key, involving neurologists, genetic counselors, rehabilitation specialists, occupational and physical therapists, and orthotists. Proper footwear and bracing, along with home stretching and strengthening, are essential. Orthopedic surgery for scoliosis and severe pes cavus/foot drop may benefit select cases.

Agents known to cause peripheral neuropathy should be avoided if possible, namely chemotherapy agents (vincristine, cisplatin), nitrofurantoin, metronidazole, isoniazid, and pyridoxine.

Future Directions

A phase III trial is evaluating PXT3003, a combination of sorbitol, naltrexone, and baclofen shown in preclinical studies to lower *PMP22* expression. Alternative approaches to down-regulate *PMP22*, such as progesterone antagonists or gene silencing, are in preclinical studies. Other areas of preclinical research include gene therapy, ion channel modulation (e.g., sodium channel blockers), and axonal transport optimization (e.g., histone deacetylase [HDAC] inhibitors).

Guillain-Barré Syndrome

Guillain-Barré syndrome (GBS) encompasses a variety of acute immune-mediated polyneuropathies. It is the most common cause of acute flaccid paralysis in children in the postpolio era, with annual incidence of 0.38 to 0.91 cases per 100,000 children. Between 50% and 82% of pediatric cases have antecedent respiratory or gastrointestinal infections associated with various organisms, most commonly *Campylobacter jejuni*. Occasionally, GBS is reported days to weeks after the influenza vaccine, but this association is not well established. Here we discuss acute inflammatory demyelinating polyradiculoneuropathy (AIDP), which accounts for 85% to 90% of cases. A chronic form, known as chronic inflammatory demyelinating polyneuropathy (CIDP), also exists but is rare in childhood.

Etiology and Pathogenesis

GBS is an autoimmune disorder thought to be mediated by antibodies cross-reacting to gangliosides expressed in peripheral and cranial nerves, resulting in demyelination or axonal degeneration. *Campylobacter* infections are known to result in molecular mimicry with the GM1 ganglioside. The relative contribution of T cells and macrophages remains unclear.

Clinical Presentation

AIDP manifests 2 to 4 weeks after a respiratory or gastrointestinal illness with extremity paresthesias, pain, and symmetric, ascending weakness with areflexia over hours to days. About 50% of cases also exhibit autonomic dysfunction, including arrhythmias, blood pressure fluctuations, and bladder dysfunction.

Differential diagnosis includes other causes of peripheral neuropathy (toxic neuropathy, critical care neuropathy, and tick paralysis), neuromuscular junction (NMJ) disease, and spinal cord pathologic conditions.

Evaluation and Management

Patients should be evaluated with a lumbar puncture, which classically shows albuminocytologic dissociation. CSF may be normal within the first week, and in a child with clinical GBS and normal CSF, treatment should still be initiated. EMG/NCS demonstrate multifocal demyelination or axonal degeneration. Spine MRI with contrast should be considered with atypical presentation and often demonstrates enhancing nerve roots.

Forced vital capacity (FVC) and negative inspiratory force (NIF) should be followed regularly, and cardiorespiratory status monitored closely. Hypertension may require intervention. About 15% to 20% of children develop respiratory failure requiring assisted ventilation, particularly in the presence of facial or bulbar weakness, dysautonomia, or axonal disease. In children with stable or improving weakness without respiratory distress, supportive care may be sufficient. Rapidly worsening weakness or respiratory status, bulbar involvement, or inability to walk are indications for more aggressive therapy with IVIG or plasmapheresis. Corticosteroids are not effective.

Children typically have a shorter course with more complete recovery (~85%) compared with adults. Recurrence is uncommon.

NEUROMUSCULAR JUNCTION

Myasthenia Gravis

Childhood neuromuscular transmission disorders include congenital myasthenic syndromes (CMSs), transient neonatal myasthenia gravis (MG), and juvenile MG (JMG).

CMSs are caused by genetic defects in presynaptic, synaptic basal lamina, and postsynaptic components of the NMJ with over 20 genes leading to defects in the acetylcholine receptor (AChR) and endplate development and maintenance. These often manifest with ptosis, fluctuating hypotonia, and life-threatening episodes of apnea in early infancy. Symptoms may improve with age; however, patients remain at risk for severe decompensations with illness. Treatment is disease-specific, using cholinesterase inhibitors such as pyridostigmine, adrenergic agonists, and ion channel blockers.

Transient neonatal MG occurs in 10% to 20% of infants born to myasthenic mothers, mediated by transplacental maternal antibody transfer. It typically self-resolves by 2 months of age as maternal antibodies are cleared.

MG is the most common disorder of neuromuscular transmission in the United States with a prevalence of about 12.5 cases per 100,000 people. Approximately 11% to 24% of patients have symptom onset in childhood or adolescence, referred to as JMG, which we review here.

Etiology and Pathogenesis

MG is caused by antibody-mediated attack of the nicotinic acetylcholine receptor on the postsynaptic motor endplate (Fig. 116.4). Two specific antibodies account for most cases. Antibodies directed against the acetylcholine receptor (anti-AChR antibodies) are positive in 50% to 80% of JMG, more likely in generalized MG and less likely in ocular or prepubertal cases. Antibodies against muscle specific kinase (anti-MuSK antibodies) are found in 5% to 8% of all MG cases. Antibodies against low-density lipoprotein receptor-related protein 4 (LRP4) are reported in 3% to 18% of so-termed double-seronegative adults. The mechanism by which anti-MuSK and anti-LRP4 antibodies lead to disease is poorly understood, however, these proteins are known to interact at the postsynaptic NMJ, where they play a key role in clustering AChRs during NMJ formation.

Patients with MG are particularly sensitive to nondepolarizing neuromuscular blocking drugs, aminoglycoside antibiotics, phenytoin, magnesium, and β blockers. If a patient presents with a sudden flare of uncertain cause, their medications should be closely reviewed.

Clinical Presentation

JMG typically manifests after 10 years of age but can manifest under a year old. The clinical hallmark of MG is fatigable weakness, which can be limited to ocular muscles (ocular MG) or more generalized (generalized MG). Most patients present with fatigable ptosis and variable ophthalmoparesis; however, some may present with generalized fatigue/weakness, swallowing/chewing dysfunction, slurred/nasal speech, or acute respiratory failure. Patients with anti-MuSK antibodies frequently have early facial, bulbar, and respiratory weakness, whereas disease is typically milder in patients with anti-LRP4 antibodies. Of note, about 15% of all patients have a second autoimmune condition.

Evaluation and Management

Eliciting fatigability with sustained or repetitive muscle activation (e.g., eyelid droop with sustained upward gaze) is helpful. Neck flexion and extension strength may correlate with respiratory muscle strength.

The edrophonium (Tensilon) test is useful when there is weakness that can be objectively assessed for change. It should be conducted in a controlled setting with cardiac monitoring and atropine available, as bradycardia may develop. Positive anti-AChR or anti-MuSK antibodies confirm the diagnosis. More than a 10% decrement of the compound muscle action potential on repetitive stimulation test supports the diagnosis. Single-fiber EMG is most sensitive but requires significant cooperation. Thymic imaging (mediastinal computed tomography [CT] or MRI) should assess for a thymoma, which, despite being rare in children, is an indication for thymectomy.

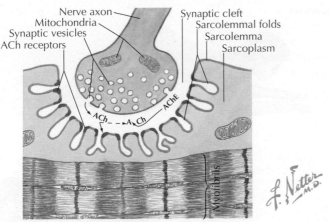

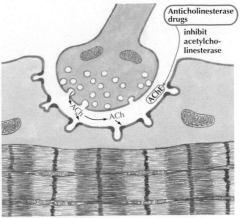

Normal neuromuscular junction
Synaptic vesicles containing acetylcholine (ACh) form in nerve terminal. In response to nerve impulse, vesicles discharge ACh into synaptic cleft. ACh binds to receptor sites on muscle sarcolemma to initiate muscle contraction. Acetylcholinesterase (AChE) hydrolyzes ACh, thus limiting effect and duration of its action.

Myasthenia gravis
Marked reduction in number and length of subneural sarcolemmal folds indicates that underlying defect lies in neuromuscular junction. Anticholinesterase drugs increase effectiveness and duration of ACh action by slowing its destruction by AChE.

Fig. 116.4 Myasthenia Gravis Pathophysiology.

Most children who require maintenance therapy are treated with anticholinesterase agents (e.g., pyridostigmine), with or without other immunosuppressants. Oral corticosteroids may help and reduce incidence of disease generalization in patients with ocular MG. Steroid-sparing immunosuppressants include azathioprine, cyclosporine, mycophenolate, cyclophosphamide, and rituximab. Plasmapheresis or IVIG may be used in refractory cases. IVIG is also sometimes the preferred first-line chronic therapy over corticosteroids in growing children. Eculizumab, a C5-specific monoclonal antibody, received FDA approval for adults with anti-AChR antibody generalized MG, but experience in JMG is minimal. In anti-AChR antibody positive children with refractory disease, thymectomy is associated with better outcomes in case series.

For myasthenic crisis, FVC, NIF, and examination should be followed closely. Plasmapheresis and IVIG are frequently used. For a patient on pyridostigmine in crisis, differential should include anticholinergic medication overuse.

Future Directions

Research areas in MG include triggers of autoimmunity, pathophysiology of recently described autoantibodies, and targets of autoimmunity in seronegative patients. Therapeutic strategies under investigation include modulating NMJ electrophysiology to augment ACh release by 3,4-diaminopyridine, a voltage-dependent potassium channel.

Infantile Botulism

Infantile botulism is a rare, potentially life-threatening toxin-mediated neuroparalytic disorder. The toxins are produced by *Clostridium botulinum,* a gram-positive, spore-forming, anaerobic organism found in soil, marine animals, and bird intestines. These toxins irreversibly block presynaptic cholinergic transmission, resulting in smooth and skeletal muscle weakness and autonomic dysfunction. Approximately 70 to 100 cases occur annually throughout the United States, affecting infants younger than 12 months, with greatest prevalence in California, Pennsylvania, and Utah.

Etiology and Pathogenesis

Botulinum spores reside in soil and are disrupted by construction or agricultural cultivation. Less commonly, they may be found in honey or home-canned foods. Infection occurs when ingested spores germinate in the intestines, leading to bacterial colonization and toxin

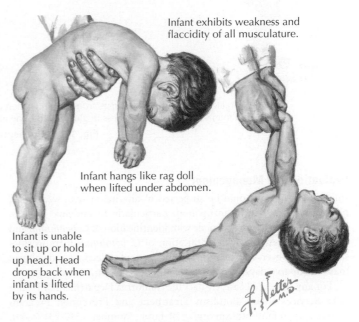

Infant exhibits weakness and flaccidity of all musculature.

Infant hangs like rag doll when lifted under abdomen.

Infant is unable to sit up or hold up head. Head drops back when infant is lifted by its hands.

Fig. 116.5 The Floppy Baby.

release. Infants may be more susceptible because of age-related changes in competitive intestinal flora.

Clinical Presentation

Infants incubate botulinum spores for 3 to 30 days, after which they present with progressive neuromuscular blockade, with nadir at 1 to 2 weeks. Poor feeding and constipation are followed by subacute descending bulbar and extremity hypotonia and weakness (Fig. 116.5). Cranial nerve dysfunction manifests early as pupillary paralysis, ptosis, ophthalmoparesis, facial diplegia, and weak suck and gag. Autonomic dysfunction manifests with decreased salivation and tearing, cardiovascular instability, and flushed skin. Decreased extremity movement and areflexia are later signs, followed by flaccid paralysis and respiratory failure in 50% to 70%.

Differential diagnosis includes other neurologic causes of hypotonia in the infant (Table 116.1), with SMA type 1 and metabolic disorders, the most frequent neurologic mimics, as well as sepsis and meningitis.

Gower maneuver

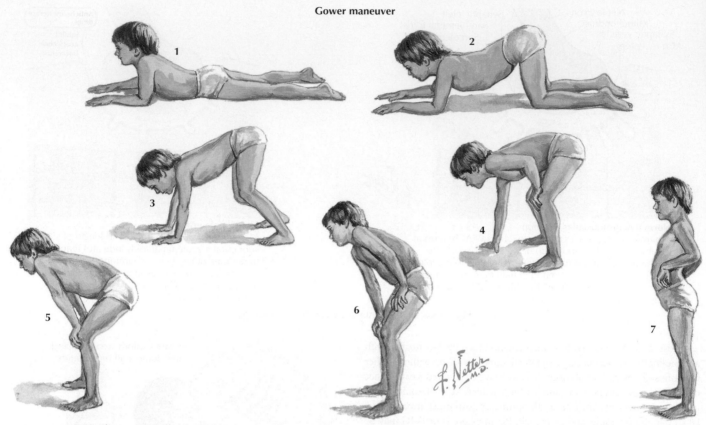

Characteristically, the child arises from prone position by pushing himself up with hands successively on floor, knees, and thighs, because of weakness in gluteal and spine muscles. He stands in lordotic posture.

Fig. 116.6 Duchenne Muscular Dystrophy.

Evaluation and Management

Infantile botulism should be suspected in any infant with weak suck, ptosis, inactivity, and constipation, particularly in endemic regions. Definitive diagnosis can be made with identification of *C. botulinum* and toxin in stool samples. is identification of *C. botulinum* toxin in stool samples. However, constipation may delay stool collection, and cultures may take up to 6 days, so empiric treatment is recommended.

For any suspected case, contact the California Department of Health Care Services Infant Botulism Treatment and Prevention Program (http://www.infantbotulism.org/, 24-hour number 510-231-7600), and immediately treat with intravenous botulism immune globulin (BabyBIG). Prompt therapy significantly decreases both mean hospital stay and duration of mechanical ventilation. Aminoglycoside antibiotics should be avoided because they can potentiate toxin effects. Supportive therapy and close monitoring are essential. With appropriate treatment, case fatality rate is under 2%, and full recovery is expected.

Future Directions

Botulism vaccines are currently in clinical trials for the general population, with some vaccines already available to at-risk adults, particularly military (bioterrorism risk).

MUSCLE

Duchenne Muscular Dystrophy

Muscular dystrophies (MDs) are a heterogeneous group of genetic disorders characterized by progressive muscle weakness and degeneration. Dystrophinopathies are the most common, characterized by variable skeletal and cardiac muscles involvement as a result of mutations of the *DMD* gene encoding dystrophin. Here we discuss the most severe and common, Duchenne muscular dystrophy (DMD), and its less severe allelic form, Becker muscular dystrophy (BMD).

Etiology and Pathogenesis

DMD occurs in about 1 in 3500 live male births, and is transmitted in an X-linked recessive pattern; however, approximately 30% of cases are sporadic. *DMD* is the largest known human gene, spanning 2.4 million base pairs and 79 exons. Exon deletion accounts for 60% to 65% cases of BMD and DMD, duplication accounts for approximately 10% to 15%, and the remainder are due to point mutations. The reading-frame rule holds true for about 90% of cases: out-of-frame deletions usually cause DMD, with absent or very low dystrophin expression, while in-frame deletions lead to semi-functional dystrophin expression, causing BMD. Identifying the specific mutation is important for targeted treatment.

Clinical Presentation

Patients with DMD classically present around 3 years of age with gross motor delay, excessive falling, difficulty running, climbing stairs, and gait abnormalities. Calf hypertrophy and neck flexion weakness are evident by age 3 or 4 years. Hip girdle muscles are typically affected before shoulder girdle muscles, causing classic Trendelenburg gait and Gowers sign (Fig. 116.6). Weakness spreads distally, and joint contractures may develop. Untreated, DMD always leads to loss of walking by age 13, kyphoscoliosis, and finally cardiac and respiratory failure in the second decade.

Rarely, female carriers may be symptomatic because of uneven lyonization or coexisting Turner syndrome; they are also at increased risk of cardiomyopathy, requiring monitoring.

Differential diagnosis includes other MDs, myopathies (Table 116.1), inflammatory myositis, and SM3.

Evaluation and Management

Creatine kinase (CK) is elevated, typically 10,000 to 30,000 IU (reference <250 IU). EMG and muscle ultrasound may help distinguish myopathic from neurogenic processes, if in question. Definitive confirmation of dystrophinopathy is with molecular testing; diagnosis of DMD versus BMD remains clinical. Muscle biopsy is infrequently needed.

Glucocorticosteroids are standard of care. Long-term therapy has been shown to prolong ambulatory status, preserve upper limb and respiratory function, and decrease need for scoliosis surgery. The significant side-effects, however, require close monitoring. Deflazacort (Emflaza) is a long half-life steroid specifically approved for DMD.

Approved targeted therapies fall into two categories: exon skipping and ribosomal read-through of premature stop codons. Exon skipping strategies rely on antisense oligonucleotides that modulate alternative splicing of *DMD* transcripts. These skipping strategies result in shorter transcripts that preserve the *DMD* reading frame, enabling translation of semi-functional dystrophin as in BMD. Four exon-skipping agents, eteplirsen (targeting exon 51, applicable to 13% to 14% of patients), casimersen (targeting exon 45, applicable to approximately 8% of patients), golodirsen, and viltolarsen (both targeting exon 53, applicable to approximately 8% of patients), were granted accelerated FDA approval based on increased dystrophin levels in muscle biopsies. Motor improvement, however, remains unproven. Ataluren is a small molecule that suppresses nonsense mutations, so full-length dystrophin can be translated. Ataluren is a small molecule that promotes ribosomal read-through of nonsense mutations allowing translation of full-length dystrophin. It is applicable to 10% to 15% of DMD patients. It is not FDA-approved, given unclear clinical efficacy in studies to date, but is licensed for use in the European Union and the United Kingdom.

Care guidelines for DMD are published (see Suggested Readings), and multidisciplinary care is essential. Pulmonary manifestations result from weak intercostal and diaphragmatic muscles, and are complicated by scoliosis. Pulmonary function should be monitored regularly starting in early teen years, because deterioration of FVC can occur in the absence of dyspnea. A sleep study should be performed if there is concern for nocturnal hypoventilation. Treatment includes implementing a cough assist device and BLPAP, regular immunizations, and prompt attention to respiratory infections. Cardiac manifestations include dilated cardiomyopathy, regional wall motion abnormalities, arrhythmias, and chronic heart failure. Electrocardiography and echocardiography are recommended every 2 years up to age 10, then annually. Echocardiographic abnormalities are seen in all patients by their late teens. Angiotensin-converting enzyme inhibitors, such as lisinopril, are the mainstay of heart failure treatment; β blockers may be added. Patients with progressive scoliosis may require spinal fusion. With improved supportive care, mean age of mortality is now in the mid-twenties and some patients survive into their forties. Death is usually from cardiomyopathy.

Boys with DMD overall have an intelligence quotient (IQ) curve shifted to the left. They are also more prone to behavioral issues, attention-deficit hyperactivity disorder (ADHD), and major depressive disorder.

There are several drug considerations when caring for DMD patients. They should not receive anticholinergic drugs, ganglionic blocking, or cardiotoxic agents. They may also be more susceptible to malignant hyperthermia.

Future Directions

Gene therapy approaches are currently under study. Given viral vector size constraints, as well as knowledge that shorter, but semi-functional dystrophins result in milder phenotypes, these approaches have used minidystrophins and microdystrophins, engineered dystrophin variants with deletions in non-key domains. Early data are encouraging. There are, however, concerns about efficacy of this strategy given some evidence of pre-existing T-cell immunity to dystrophin as well as instability of the dystrophin transgenes during muscle cell turnover. Gene editing via (CRISPR)-Cas9 is also being studied in the preclinical setting. Pharmacologic therapies are also targeting modulation of muscle growth, skeletal muscle progenitors, fibrosis, and inflammation.

Congenital Myopathies

Congenital myopathies are rare nondystrophic muscle diseases characterized by early-onset stable or slowly progressive muscle weakness, with variable severity and distinctive muscle biopsy findings. They are genetically heterogeneous, with over 20 genes implicated, encoding proteins involved in skeletal muscle calcium homeostasis, excitation-contraction coupling, and sarcomeric filament function. They are classified into four main diseases based on histology: central core disease, multi-minicore disease, centronuclear myopathy, and nemaline myopathy. Patients present with marked proximal and axial weakness with variable involvement of extraocular, bulbar, cardiac, respiratory, and distal muscles. *RYR1* mutations are most common; these patients are susceptible to malignant hyperthermia. Treatment is largely supportive, although targeted therapeutics are under investigation ranging from calcium modulation and muscle homeostasis to gene therapy.

SUGGESTED READINGS

Available online.

117

Neurologic Emergencies

Alexis R. Karlin and Rebecca N. Ichord

Pediatricians frequently encounter neurologic emergencies caused by primary nervous system dysfunction or related to systemic illness with secondary neurologic disease. This chapter aims to provide an overview of neurologic emergencies for the general pediatrician.

BASIC PRINCIPLES OF EMERGENT NEUROLOGIC EVALUATION

As with any critical illness, initial evaluation includes vital signs and assessment of airway, breathing, and circulation (ABCs). The Glasgow Coma Scale (GCS, Table 117.1) is calculated on presentation. Pupils are assessed for size, symmetry, and reactivity. History addresses present illness, past medical history, recent trauma, and ingestions. In the emergent setting, general examination prioritizes cardiorespiratory evaluation, abdominal examination to assess for organomegaly, assessment of nuchal rigidity, and skin examination to look for rashes, bruises/lacerations, and neurocutaneous lesions. Targeted neurologic examination should include assessment of mental status, pupils, eye movements, and basic sensorimotor examination, including sensory level and assessment of bladder/bowel function. Fundoscopic examination is performed to look for signs of retinal hemorrhage or papilledema.

Neurodiagnostic tools include neuroimaging (head computed tomography [CT] often the most rapid), lumbar puncture (LP), and electroencephalogram (EEG). The basic serum and cerebrospinal fluid (CSF) studies recommended for neurologic emergencies are listed in Table 117.2. LP should include an opening pressure when possible. Neuroimaging is often required before performing an LP, particularly in cases of suspected increased intracranial pressure (ICP) in which there may be risk for herniation.

ALTERED MENTAL STATUS

Etiology and Pathogenesis

Altered mental status (AMS) is a broad term used to characterize a wide spectrum of clinical presentations, from subtle alterations in responsiveness and attention to deep coma. Along the neuroaxis, AMS may localize to global cerebral dysfunction, dysfunction of bilateral thalami, or dysfunction in the brainstem reticular activating system.

Differential Diagnosis

The mnemonic *VITAMINS, Please Guys!* helps to guide the differential for AMS (Table 117.3).

Evaluation and Management

Although the differential diagnoses list is broad, diagnostic evaluation should be prioritized according to history and clinical examination. Typically, workup will include urgent neuroimaging with or without LP. Patients may require continuous video EEG monitoring to assess for and manage nonconvulsive status epilepticus (SE). In cases of metabolic derangements or toxin exposures, testing should include electrocardiogram (ECG) to assess for potentially fatal arrhythmias.

Patients presenting with obtundation, stupor, or coma require urgent intubation to protect the airway and control ventilation and oxygenation. Patients may require fluid resuscitation. Other interventions that should be considered early on include empiric antimicrobials for infection, naloxone for suspected opiate overdose, and benzodiazepine for suspected seizure.

STATUS EPILEPTICUS

Etiology and Pathogenesis

According to the 2015 guidelines by the International League Against Epilepsy (ILAE), SE is defined as seizure activity longer than 5 minutes, or as repeated seizures with persistent mental

TABLE 117.1 Glasgow Coma Scale

Behavior	Adults and Children 2 Years and Older	Modified for Children Younger Than 2 Years
Eye opening response	4: Spontaneous eye opening 3: To verbal stimuli 2: To painful stimuli 1: No eye opening	4: Spontaneous eye opening 3: To speech 2: To painful stimuli 1: No eye opening
Best verbal response	5: Oriented to time, place, and person 4: Confused 3: Inappropriate speech 2: Incomprehensible speech 1: No verbal response	5: Coos or babbles 4: Irritable and continually cries 3: Cries to pain 2: Moans to pain 1: No verbal response
Best motor response	6: Follows commands 5: Localizes to painful stimuli 4: Flexion withdrawal from pain 3: Abnormal flexion (decorticate) 2: Abnormal extension (decerebrate) 1: No motor response	6: Moves spontaneously or purposefully 5: Withdraws from touch 4: Withdraws from pain 3: Abnormal flexion to pain 2: Extension to pain 1: No motor response

status alteration in between. Although strict definitions of SE vary between seizure types, for the purposes of the general pediatrician, if seizure activity persists for longer than 5 minutes, it is unlikely to self-resolve and therefore requires pharmacologic rescue. SE may ultimately lead to neuronal death, injury, and alteration of neuronal networks. In the case of generalized tonic-clonic seizures, irreversible damage may occur by 30 minutes; for focal seizures with impaired consciousness, irreversible damage may occur at 60 minutes. Nonconvulsive seizures may manifest clinically as AMS, even coma, with or without subtle motor phenomena; for nonconvulsive SE, the time-course within which irreversible damage occurs is unknown.

Differential Diagnosis

The differential diagnosis for SE may be divided into three general causes: (1) acute symptomatic seizures secondary to an underlying central nervous system (CNS) process, (2) explosive onset of new epilepsy, or breakthrough SE in a child with a seizure disorder, and (3) idiopathic (rare).

In a child with *or* without known epilepsy, the differential diagnosis for acute symptomatic seizures is similar to that of AMS, including vascular events, head trauma, metabolic derangement, toxins, and infection. Other considerations include febrile SE, posterior reversible encephalopathy syndrome (PRES), or autoimmune or inflammatory conditions such as anti–N-methyl-D-aspartate (NMDA) receptor encephalitis. Structural abnormalities such as focal cortical dysplasia, or genetic syndromes, including neurocutaneous disorders, may first manifest with explosive-onset epilepsy and SE. Common causes of acute symptomatic seizures in neonates include hypoxic-ischemic injury (most common by far), followed by perinatal stroke or hemorrhage, infection (e.g., sepsis/meningitis or congenital infections [e.g., toxoplasmosis, syphilis, cytomegalovirus, and herpes viruses]), or genetic/metabolic disorder.

In a child with known epilepsy, SE may occur secondary to concomitant illness resulting in lowered seizure threshold, missed medications or change in medication, or evolution of existing seizure disorder. Idiopathic SE includes new-onset refractory SE (NORSE) and febrile infection-related epilepsy syndrome (FIRES). Both of these entities may be refractory to anti-seizure medications (ASMs) (failure to

TABLE 117.2 Basic Serum and Cerebrospinal Studies in Neurologic Emergencies

Serum	Cerebrospinal Fluid Studies[a]
Point-of-care glucose, venous or arterial blood gas, basic metabolic panel, magnesium, phosphorus, ± liver function tests, ammonia	Opening pressure, cell counts (tubes 1 and 4)
Complete blood count, ± C-reactive protein and erythrocyte sedimentation rate	Glucose, protein
Blood culture	Gram stain, culture
Toxicology screen: salicylates, acetaminophen, ethanol (and urine drug screen)	± Viral studies
± Creatine kinase, thyroid studies	± Oligoclonal bands

[a]Consider additional CSF for "save our specimen" to access later if further testing is indicated.

TABLE 117.3 Altered Mental Status Differential Diagnosis: VITAMINS, Please Guys!

Etiologies	Differential Diagnosis
Vascular	Global hypoxic-ischemic injury (typically secondary to asphyxiation, cardiorespiratory arrest or profound hypotension) Arterial ischemic stroke Cerebral sinus venous thrombosis Hemorrhagic stroke Hypertensive encephalopathy Vasculitis
Infectious/inflammatory	Sepsis Meningitis Encephalitis
Trauma/toxins	Traumatic brain injury Toxins: opiates, anticholinergics, tricyclic antidepressants, salicylates, antiseizure medications, carbon monoxide, sedatives
Autoimmune	Acute demyelinating encephalomyelitis (ADEM) Lupus cerebritis Autoimmune encephalitides (e.g., anti-NMDA-receptor antibody encephalitis)
Metabolic/endocrine	Derangements in glucose, ammonia, urea, sodium, calcium, or magnesium, etc. Metabolic/respiratory acidosis Thyrotoxicosis Inborn errors of metabolism
Increased intracranial pressure	See Table 117.4
Neoplastic	Neoplasm or paraneoplastic syndrome
Seizure	Status epilepticus
PRES/Psych	Posterior reversible encephalopathy syndrome (PRES) Psychiatric Disorders
Genetic/general	Genetic epileptic encephalopathies Systemic illnesses: intussusception, shock, hypoxemia

respond to at least two different ASMs, including one benzodiazepine) or even super-refractory (failure to respond to anesthetic infusions).

Evaluation and Management

Most patients with SE require urgent head CT and may require LP. Neuroimaging may be deferred, however, if the patient has known epilepsy with clear provoking features suggestive of breakthrough seizures. Consideration must be given to continuous EEG monitoring to assess for and manage nonconvulsive SE.

Management of SE aims to stop seizure activity as quickly as possible and to address underlying causes. The goal of treatment for overt convulsive SE is seizure cessation by administering ASM within 5 minutes and repeating at 5-minute intervals as needed either until seizures have ceased, or until the threshold for starting continuous anesthetic infusion has been reached (see example of protocol listed in references). Metabolic derangements should be corrected accordingly. Benzodiazepines are first-line ASMs. Intravenous lorazepam should be administered at 0.1 mg/kg/dose. If there is no intravenous access, buccal, intranasal, or rectal forms of benzodiazepines should be given. Treatment should not be delayed to attain intravenous access. Benzodiazepines may be administered a second time if seizure persists. Next-line agents include levetiracetam, fosphenytoin, and phenobarbital. For refractory status epilepticus, clinicians should prepare to transfer the child to the intensive care unit (ICU) with consideration of a next-line agent versus pharmacologic coma with midazolam, pentobarbital, or ketamine infusions. Each of these agents can have an impact on the hemodynamic status of the patient and should be carefully considered in light of a given patient's comorbidities.

For suspected infection, broad-spectrum antimicrobials should be started immediately, including a third-generation cephalosporin for empiric treatment of bacterial meningitis, and acyclovir for empiric treatment of herpes simplex virus meningoencephalitis. Steroids and intravenous immunoglobulin (IVIG) may be considered for suspected autoimmune or inflammatory process.

INCREASED INTRACRANIAL PRESSURE

Etiology and Pathogenesis

To understand the pathogenesis of increased ICP, we must review the Monro-Kellie doctrine: the sum of the volumes of intracranial blood (~10%), CSF (~10%), and brain parenchyma (~80%) is constant given the fixed volume of the cranium (with exception of infants with open fontanelles). If there is an increase in any of these components, or if there is a component (e.g., a mass lesion) *added* to this system, the volumes of the others must decrease in order to compensate. Multiple interrelated regulatory systems subsequently interact to maintain adequate cerebral oxygen delivery in the face of fluctuations in ICP, cerebral metabolic rate, and systemic physiologic variables, including blood pressure, SaO_2, and CO_2. These mechanisms serve to maintain a normal ICP with small fluctuations in intracerebral volume. With severe pathologic conditions, these regulatory mechanisms fail, resulting in increased ICP and, in the most severe cases, in herniation and death. Figure 117.1 reviews herniation syndromes.

Cerebral perfusion pressure (CPP) is maintained via regulatory mechanisms that increase systemic blood pressure in response to an increase in ICP:

$$CPP = Mean\ arterial\ pressure\ (MAP) - ICP$$

As ICP increases, changes in the patient's vital signs may alert the clinician of impending herniation. These changes, known as Cushing's triad, occur sequentially as the patient's condition worsens without intervention: (1) increase in MAP to maintain CPP, (2) reflex bradycardia, and (3) abnormal respirations resulting from brainstem compression.

Children with increased ICP may present with headache, AMS, or vomiting. Primary CNS processes such as meningitis, neoplasm, hemorrhage, or focal/generalized edema may cause both elevated ICP and acute symptomatic seizures, in which seizures in turn exacerbate the elevation in ICP. "Red flag" headache features that raise suspicion for elevated ICP include progressive worsening, headache worse in the morning or with lying flat, nocturnal awakening, and worsening with Valsalva maneuvers (cough, defecation, micturition). Infants may have a bulging fontanelle, poor feeding, lethargy, and "sun-setting" of the eyes (eyes driven downward bilaterally). Fundoscopic examination may reveal papilledema, but the absence of this finding does not rule out increased ICP, especially in acute cases. Dilated pupils (unilateral or bilateral) may occur along with cranial nerve palsies (most commonly third and sixth nerves).

Differential Diagnosis

Causes of increased ICP are outlined in Table 117.4. Broad categories include:

1. Obstruction to CSF flow or absorption causing hydrocephalus (Fig. 117.2)
2. Increased CSF production
3. Venous congestion or venous outflow obstruction
4. Space-occupying lesion
5. Cerebral edema

Evaluation and Management

Evaluation includes urgent neuroimaging and other studies noted previously. Medical management aims to immediately stabilize ABCs, address metabolic derangements including glucose, and to optimize cerebral perfusion pressure via the following mechanisms:

1. *Raise the head of the bed to 30 degrees and maintain head midline.* This optimizes venous drainage, thereby lowering ICP.
2. *Intubate to protect airway and control oxygenation and ventilation, with normocarbia and normoxia goals.* For suspected active or impending herniation, hyperventilation is used as an acute rescue intervention, with goal $PaCO_2$ 30 to 35 mm Hg. Lowering cerebral arterial CO_2 causes arterial vasoconstriction and therefore lowers ICP. However, this is not a long-term strategy, particularly as vasoconstriction will ultimately result in decreased cerebral perfusion.
3. *Obtain venous access* to manage fluids and support blood pressures with a goal of normal blood pressures per age and normoglycemia.
4. *ASM as needed.* Consider continuous EEG monitoring. Consider prophylactic ASM for those at increased risk. Be wary to use ASM that may lower blood pressure and interfere with the body's physiologic compensatory mechanism to maintain CPP.
5. *Targeted temperature control with antipyretics and cooling blankets as needed to maintain normothermia.* This lowers cerebral metabolism and oxygen extraction.
6. *ICP monitoring.* Consider invasive and noninvasive multimodal neuromonitoring tools in order to guide titration of pharmacologic therapies.
7. *Pharmacologic therapies*
   a. Osmotic therapies: Hypertonic saline with goal sodium no higher than 160 mEq/L. This establishes an osmotic gradient between plasma and brain parenchyma, lowering brain water content. Mannitol may be considered. However, because mannitol is an osmotic diuretic, there is risk for hypovolemia and subsequent hypotension, leading to a decrease in CPP despite improving ICP.

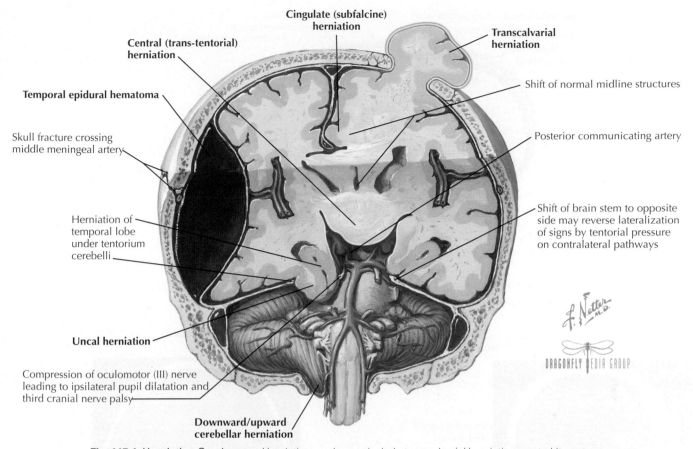

Fig. 117.1 Herniation Syndromes. Herniation syndromes include transcalvarial herniation, central (transtentorial), cingulate (subfalcine), uncal, and downward/upward cerebellar herniation. Cerebral herniation syndromes may occur as a result of mass effect (including epidural, subdural, or intraparenchymal bleed or mass lesion) or other syndromes of increased ICP. Clinical manifestations are variable and include altered mental status and coma, focal neurologic deficits, pupillary changes, and coma/death.

Labels in figure:
- Cingulate (subfalcine) herniation
- Central (trans-tentorial) herniation
- Temporal epidural hematoma
- Skull fracture crossing middle meningeal artery
- Herniation of temporal lobe under tentorium cerebelli
- Uncal herniation
- Compression of oculomotor (III) nerve leading to ipsilateral pupil dilatation and third cranial nerve palsy
- Downward/upward cerebellar herniation
- Transcalvarial herniation
- Shift of normal midline structures
- Posterior communicating artery
- Shift of brain stem to opposite side may reverse lateralization of signs by tentorial pressure on contralateral pathways

TABLE 117.4	Differential Diagnosis by Category of Increased Intracranial Pressure
Causes	**Differential Diagnosis**
Decreased CSF absorption	• Outflow obstruction (aqueductal stenosis, colloid cyst, mass) • Infiltrative meningeal process (leukemic infiltration or carcinomatosis, severe bacterial meningitis, subarachnoid hemorrhage)
Increased CSF production (rare)	• Choroid plexus tumor
Venous congestion/outflow obstruction	• Sinus venous thrombosis
Space-occupying lesion or focal edema	• Intracranial hemorrhage • Tumor • Abscess • Ischemic infarct with surrounding edema • Posterior reversible encephalopathy syndrome (PRES)
Generalized cerebral edema	• Liver failure, hyperammonemia • Hypercarbia • Hypertension • Diabetic ketoacidosis • Head trauma (peak swelling 3–5 days) • Malignant edema following large ischemic stroke, watershed injury, or hypoxic ischemic injury
Idiopathic	• Idiopathic intracranial hypertension
Closed sutures	• Craniosynostosis

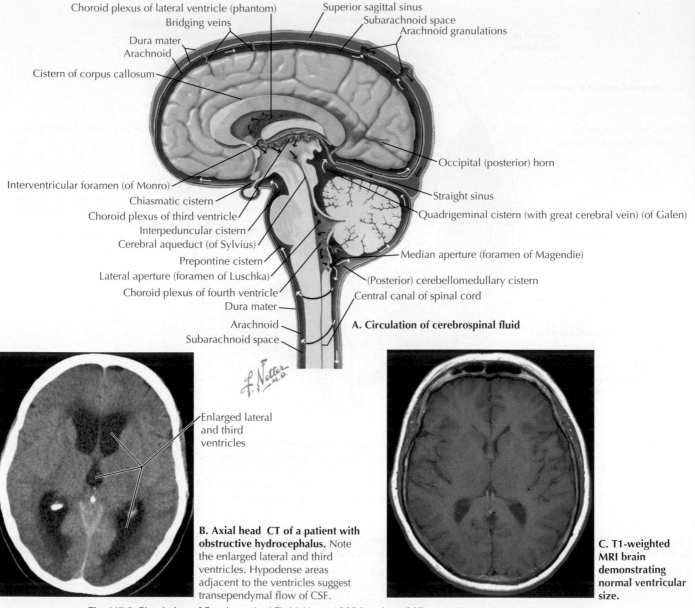

Choroid plexus of lateral ventricle (phantom)
Bridging veins
Dura mater
Arachnoid
Cistern of corpus callosum
Superior sagittal sinus
Subarachnoid space
Arachnoid granulations
Occipital (posterior) horn
Interventricular foramen (of Monro)
Chiasmatic cistern
Choroid plexus of third ventricle
Interpeduncular cistern
Cerebral aqueduct (of Sylvius)
Prepontine cistern
Lateral aperture (foramen of Luschka)
Choroid plexus of fourth ventricle
Dura mater
Arachnoid
Subarachnoid space
Straight sinus
Quadrigeminal cistern (with great cerebral vein) (of Galen)
Median aperture (foramen of Magendie)
(Posterior) cerebellomedullary cistern
Central canal of spinal cord

A. Circulation of cerebrospinal fluid

Enlarged lateral and third ventricles

B. Axial head CT of a patient with obstructive hydrocephalus. Note the enlarged lateral and third ventricles. Hypodense areas adjacent to the ventricles suggest transependymal flow of CSF.

C. T1-weighted MRI brain demonstrating normal ventricular size.

Fig. 117.2 Circulation of Cerebrospinal Fluid. Normal CSF flow from CSF production at choroid plexus to resorption at arachnoid granulations. Images demonstrate obstructive hydrocephalus (B) and normal ventricular size (C).

b. **Sedation ± pharmacologic paralysis.** Goal is to decrease cerebral metabolism and oxygen extraction, as well as optimize airway management and prevent triggers of ICP elevation such as cough and Valsalva.

c. **Consider steroids** to reduce vasogenic edema.

8. *Consider neurosurgical management*: includes ventriculostomy or external ventricular drain placement for acute hydrocephalus, evacuation or resection of a space-occupying lesion, or decompressive hemicraniectomy (allows space for swelling).

NEUROLOGIC CAUSES OF RESPIRATORY FAILURE

Etiology and Pathogenesis

It is critical to consider neurologic or neuromuscular causes for patients presenting with weakness and difficulty breathing or with hypercapnic respiratory failure of unclear origin. Unlike primary

pulmonary disorders, there may be no change in oxygen saturation preceding acute decompensation.

Respiratory failure of neurologic or neuromuscular origin may localize to any component of the nervous system. Any process contributing to AMS may lead to decreased respiratory drive. Disruption of the respiratory centers in the pons and medulla (receiving input from chemoreceptors, stretch receptors, and irritant receptors) may result in abnormal breathing patterns or altered respiratory drive. Spinal cord disease above the level of C5 can cause abrupt cessation of respiration as a result of autonomic dysfunction or diaphragmatic weakness (phrenic nerve supplied by C3–C5). Injury at the thoracic level up to C5 may result in weakness of accessory respiratory muscles. Similarly, pathologic conditions affecting the anterior horn cell, nerve roots, peripheral nerves, neuromuscular junction, or muscles may also lead to respiratory failure.

Differential Diagnosis

If a lesion is localized to the brainstem, consider demyelinating lesion, hemorrhagic or ischemic stroke, tumor, or genetic disorder. If there are both sensory and motor symptoms, lesion may localize to the spinal cord, nerve roots, or peripheral nerves. For spinal cord, consider transverse myelitis and cord transection (Chapter 115). For nerve roots or peripheral nerves, consider Guillain-Barré syndrome (GBS), particularly if the patient has ascending weakness. GBS also affects the peripheral cranial nerves and may disrupt the gag reflex, contributing to loss of the patient's ability to protect the airway. GBS variants include Bickerstaff encephalitis and Miller-Fisher syndrome.

Anterior horn cell, neuromuscular junction (NMJ), and muscular disorders should be considered in cases of pure motor symptoms (Chapter 116). Anterior horn cell disorders include acute flaccid myelitis (AFM) or spinal muscular atrophy (SMA). NMJ disorders include myasthenia gravis/myasthenic crisis, infant botulism, *Clostridium* tetany, and, more rarely, tick paralysis and other toxins that inhibit transmission at the NMJ. Infant botulism is often preceded by constipation and poor feeding because of poor intestinal motility and classically manifests with descending weakness and dilated pupils as a result of disruption of parasympathetic innervation.

Evaluation and Management

Initial evaluation should include evaluation of respiratory status (with formal evaluation of negative inspiratory force by a respiratory therapist) and assessment of cough/gag. Complete neurologic examination should be performed to localize weakness and investigate other diagnostic clues. The patient should be placed on a continuous cardiorespiratory monitor, and a bladder scan should be performed to assess the need for catheterization. Evaluation should be based on clinical examination and may include magnetic resonance imaging of the brain and/or spine and LP. Additional serum studies may include antiganglioside antibodies (for GBS variants), anti–aquaporin-4 antibodies (for neuromyelitis optica spectrum disorders [NMOSDs]) and anti–myelin oligodendrocyte glycoprotein (MOG) antibody testing. Finally, electromyography may play a role in the acute setting to differentiate NMJ and neuropathic disorders, though a normal study does not rule out pathologic conditions. For suspected infant botulism, a stool sample should be sent for botulism testing (this may not be feasible in the acute period given constipation). Thus for cases of suspected botulism, babies should be treated empirically with botulism immunoglobulin therapy. Further management for other causes may include IVIG, plasmapheresis, and other immunomodulatory therapies, along with supportive management.

FUTURE DIRECTIONS

Pediatric neurocritical care is an emerging field, with ongoing studies on neuromonitoring in the ICU, including both invasive (ICP monitoring with bolt or external ventricular drain, or CSF diversion) and noninvasive (long-term EEG monitoring, near-infrared spectroscopy, and pupillometry) tools.

SUGGESTED READINGS

Available online.

118

Infectious Diseases of the Central Nervous System

Allison M. Blatz and Sanjeev Swami

CLINICAL VIGNETTE

A previously healthy 10-year-old boy presents with 1 day of fever, headache, and rash. His vital signs include a temperature of 103.6°F (39.8°C), heart rate of 122 beats/min, respiratory rate 16 breaths/min, SpO₂ 98%, blood pressure 118/78 mm Hg. He is somnolent and intermittently follows commands. He has meningismus and groans when you extend his legs. Other pertinent findings include a nonblanching, purpuric rash on his arms and legs. A lumbar puncture is performed that shows an elevated opening pressure of 34 cm H₂O. Cerebrospinal fluid (CSF) is obtained and shows 462 white bloods cells (WBCs)/mm³, 0 red blood cells (RBCs)/mm³, glucose of 18 mg/dL, and protein of 82 mg/dL. Gram stain shows many white blood cells and gram-negative rods. He is diagnosed with bacterial meningitis, given meropenem, and admitted to the intensive care unit for close monitoring. Eighteen hours later, his CSF culture grows *Neisseria meningitidis*. Over the next 2 days, his mental status returns to normal. He completes a 7-day course of therapy with ceftriaxone and is discharged home.

MENINGITIS AND MENINGOENCEPHALITIS

Meningitis is defined as inflammation of the leptomeninges. Meningoencephalitis is inflammation of the meninges and brain parenchyma.

Etiology, Epidemiology, and Pathogenesis

Meningitis is usually an acute process caused by either bacteria or viruses. Meningoencephalitis is predominantly caused by viruses. Enteroviruses are the most common cause of viral meningitis and meningoencephalitis; the incidence of these infections peaks in summer and fall and wanes in winter. Parechovirus is another common cause of viral meningitis in infants and toddlers with the same seasonal pattern. Herpes family viruses, such as herpes simplex virus (HSV) and varicella zoster (VZV), also cause meningoencephalitis, as can numerous other pathogens (Box 118.1).

Historically, the most common causes of bacterial meningitis beyond the neonatal period were *Streptococcus pneumoniae*, *Neisseria meningitidis*, and *Haemophilus influenzae* type b (Hib). Fortunately, there has been a dramatic reduction in the incidence of Hib infections after the introduction of the conjugate Hib vaccine in 1987. Additionally, there has been a reduction in the incidence of meningitis caused by *S. pneumoniae* since the introduction of the pneumococcal conjugate vaccine. However, some serotypes not contained in this vaccine do have the ability to cause disease in humans, so this vaccine's effect has not been as dramatic as the Hib vaccine. There are currently two licensed vaccine types for *N. meningitidis*: one covers serogroups A, C, W135, and Y, and the second covers serogroup B.

These bacteria colonize the upper respiratory tract. They invade through the mucosal epithelium, usually when it is inflamed due to a viral infection, and enter the bloodstream. The bacteria circulate in the bloodstream and gain access to the central nervous system (CNS) via the choroid plexus. The bacteria readily replicate in the subarachnoid space within the cerebrospinal fluid (CSF) because this area is normally sequestered from the immune system. In response to bacterial replication, white blood cells (WBCs) migrate to the CSF, and the ensuing inflammatory response leads to the signs and symptoms of meningitis.

In addition to this hematogenous seeding of the CSF, bacteria can also gain access to the CNS by direct extension. Congenital malformations, such as dermoid sinuses, or traumatic injuries, including basilar skull fractures and penetrating trauma, can allow bacteria to enter the CSF. Infections of the sinuses, mastoid air cells, or middle ear can also act as portals of entry (Fig. 118.1).

In neonates, the three most common causes of bacterial meningitis are *Streptococcus agalactiae* (group B streptococcus [GBS]), *Escherichia coli*, and *Listeria monocytogenes*. GBS and *E. coli* are acquired perinatally through the maternal genitourinary tract during delivery, whereas *L. monocytogenes* is usually acquired transplacentally after a mother is exposed to unpasteurized dairy or lunch meat. Rarer causes of meningitis in older children include *Borrelia burgdorferi*, which causes Lyme disease, gram-negative bacilli besides *E. coli*, fungal, and parasitic pathogens.

Clinical Presentation

Neonates and infants with meningitis often present with nonspecific symptoms. The most common parental complaint is fever, often associated with irritability and poor feeding. Infants also may be hypothermic and can develop vomiting and a bulging fontanelle. In severe cases, infants may present with lethargy or seizure and have focal neurologic deficits on examination. Although neonates and infants with meningitis can present in many ways, toddlers and school-aged children are more likely to present with "classic" signs and symptoms. These include high fever, photophobia, headache, neck stiffness, vomiting, and altered consciousness. Of these, fever and headache are most common. On physical examination, these patients may have nuchal rigidity as well as Kernig and/or Brudzinski signs (Fig. 118.2). Children with disseminated *N. meningitidis* infections may have a petechial or purpuric rash. Infants with enteroviral meningitis often have an erythematous, macular rash. Papilledema may be found in children with acute bacterial meningitis, though sometimes it may lag behind other symptoms.

Differential Diagnosis

The patient's presenting signs and symptoms, along with age, exposures, and vaccination status narrow the differential diagnosis of meningitis and meningoencephalitis.

The combination of fever and irritability in an infant or toddler has a broad differential diagnosis, including infectious and noninfectious

BOX 118.1 Microbiologic Causes of Meningitis

Common
- *Neisseria meningitidis*
- *Streptococcus pneumoniae*
- *Borrelia burgdorferi*
- Enteroviruses

Uncommon
- West Nile virus
- Herpes simplex virus
- Parechovirus

Special Circumstances
- Neonates
  - Group B streptococcus
  - *Escherichia coli*
  - *Listeria monocytogenes*
  - *Citrobacter* species
- Immunocompromised
  - *Listeria monocytogenes*
  - *Candida* species
  - Cryptococcus (HIV-positive patients)
  - Lymphocytic choriomeningitis virus
  - Cytomegalovirus
  - Epstein-Barr virus
  - Human herpes virus-6
- Unimmunized
  - *Haemophilus influenzae* type b
  - *Streptococcus pneumoniae*
  - Measles virus
  - Mumps virus
  - Poliovirus
  - Varicella-zoster virus
- Other rare circumstances
  - *Staphylococcus aureus*: postoperative wound infection, ventriculoperitoneal shunt
  - Gram-negative bacilli: nosocomial infection, postoperative wound infection
  - Arboviral infections: Eastern equine encephalitis virus, Western equine encephalitis virus, West Nile virus, St. Louis encephalitis virus, La Crosse virus
  - Tick-borne infections: Rocky Mountain spotted fever, *Ehrlichia*, Powassan virus, tick-borne encephalitis virus
  - HIV

HIV, Human immunodeficiency virus.

causes. A detailed history and thorough physical examination are critical in narrowing the differential diagnosis. There will almost always be additional information that helps to focus the differential. A history of vomiting or diarrhea points toward gastroenteritis. Tachypnea or focal findings on lung auscultation are a sign of pneumonia, either viral or bacterial. Torticollis or other unusual positioning of the head and neck or a history of drooling suggest a focal infection in the neck or upper thorax, such as a retropharyngeal abscess. Another consideration in this scenario, especially for toddlers with low-grade fevers rather than high fevers, is a foreign body in the upper airway, esophagus, or trachea. Cardiac and metabolic abnormalities are also important considerations in neonates and infants who present with fever, irritability, poor feeding, and vomiting.

Neck stiffness or pain on neck flexion also may be caused by a number of processes. These include peritonsillar or retropharyngeal abscesses, cervical lymphadenitis, muscle strain or spasms, cervical epidural infections, and upper lobe pneumonia.

Seizures as an isolated symptom have many possible causes (Chapter 108). These include epilepsy, brain tumors, CNS infections, metabolic abnormalities (especially hypoglycemia), and secondary to trauma.

As patient age increases and children are better able to verbalize symptoms, the differential diagnosis becomes more focused. However, children and adolescents who present with fever and altered mental status may not be able to communicate to describe their symptoms. The differential diagnosis of fever and altered mental status in an older child includes CNS infections, ingestions or drug use, and metabolic abnormalities (such as diabetic ketoacidosis).

Evaluation

The most important diagnostic procedure in the evaluation of a child with suspected bacterial meningitis is an LP (Fig. 118.1). An opening pressure should be measured at the time of the LP, and fluid should be sent for cell count with differential, Gram stain and culture, protein, and glucose. If viral meningitis or meningoencephalitis is suspected, polymerase chain reaction (PCR) tests for enteroviruses and HSV are useful. Various CNS infections have typical CSF parameters that can aid the clinician while cultures and PCRs are pending (Table 118.1). If examination is concerning for elevated intracranial pressure (ICP) with clinical signs such as papilledema or focal neurologic findings, a head computed tomography (CT) scan or magnetic resonance imaging (MRI) of the brain should be performed before proceeding with LP. These studies allow the clinician to determine whether there is a space-occupying lesion, such as an abscess or tumor, significant cerebral edema, or ventricular dilation. These critical findings indicate risk for brain herniation if a lumbar puncture were performed, so clinicians should proceed with caution and discuss with subspecialists if this situation arises.

Blood tests can be helpful in children with meningitis but are rarely diagnostic in isolation. Although blood cultures are seldom positive, it is useful to obtain samples before the administration of antibiotics, especially if there may be a delay in performing the LP. A complete blood count (CBC) occasionally has an elevated WBC count, which is a nonspecific finding. The remainder of the CBC is usually normal, but platelets may be elevated as a sign of diffuse inflammation. The results of a basic metabolic panel are rarely abnormal, although some patients develop syndrome of inappropriate antidiuretic hormone secretion with subsequent hyponatremia. Inflammatory markers such as an erythrocyte sedimentation rate and C-reactive protein are rarely helpful and do not reliably differentiate between bacterial meningitis and other causes of meningitis. If Lyme meningitis is suspected, tests for serologic evidence of Lyme exposure are useful.

Management

Patients with bacterial meningitis may be critically ill and require admission to an intensive care unit. In addition to respiratory and cardiovascular support, antibiotics are the most important intervention for patients with bacterial meningitis. In patients in whom the risk for bacterial meningitis is high, antibiotics should not be withheld pending the results of diagnostic procedures or radiographic scans. Empiric antibiotic selection should be made based on local resistance patterns, risk factors, and the child's age. The final treatment decision should be made based on the CSF culture and sensitivity reports. In general, the combination of an intravenous third-generation cephalosporin, such as ceftriaxone or cefotaxime, plus vancomycin offers excellent activity against most common pathogens. If gram-negative

Sources of infection

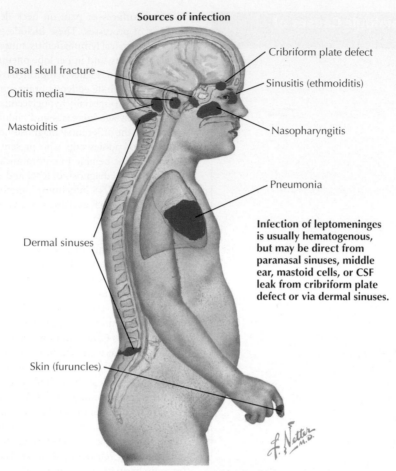

Basal skull fracture

Otitis media

Mastoiditis

Dermal sinuses

Skin (furuncles)

Cribriform plate defect

Sinusitis (ethmoiditis)

Nasopharyngitis

Pneumonia

Infection of leptomeninges is usually hematogenous, but may be direct from paranasal sinuses, middle ear, mastoid cells, or CSF leak from cribriform plate defect or via dermal sinuses.

Fig. 118.1 Bacterial Meningitis.

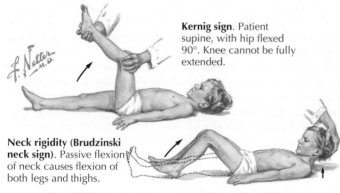

Kernig sign. Patient supine, with hip flexed 90°. Knee cannot be fully extended.

Neck rigidity (Brudzinski neck sign). Passive flexion of neck causes flexion of both legs and thighs.

Fig. 118.2 Kernig Sign and Brudzinski Neck Sign.

bacilli are seen on the CSF Gram stain, some experts recommend broader gram-negative coverage with meropenem and consideration of adding an aminoglycoside while awaiting results of the CSF culture. The recommended duration of therapy varies according to the causative pathogen. In general, *N. meningitidis* meningitis is treated for 7 days, Hib meningitis for 7 to 10 days, and pneumococcal meningitis for 14 days.

The treatment of most viral causes of meningitis consists of supportive care of the patient. If HSV disease is suspected, intravenous acyclovir should be administered before the return of results, given the mortality and morbidity associated with this infection. For Lyme meningitis, treatment is intravenous ceftriaxone or oral doxycycline for 14 days.

The role of dexamethasone in the treatment of children with bacterial meningitis remains controversial. Studies of patients with Hib meningitis found that children treated with dexamethasone had decreased morbidity and mortality. Studies in adults with pneumococcal meningitis treated with steroids have shown a mortality benefit, but these findings have not been reproduced in children.

The most common sequela of bacterial meningitis is sensorineural hearing loss, and all children with meningitis should have a hearing test after completion of therapy. Nonobstructive hydrocephalus may also develop either acutely or in the ensuing weeks to months. Most patients with enteroviral meningitis recover with no long-term sequelae. Neonates with HSV meningoencephalitis have a high rate of morbidity and mortality, and older children with HSV meningitis often have long-term neurologic deficits.

FOCAL SUPPURATIVE INFECTIONS

Brain Abscess

Brain abscesses are focal infections of the cerebrum or cerebellum.

Etiology and Pathogenesis

Many microbes can form a focal suppurative infection of the CNS, including fungi, parasites, and bacteria, with bacteria being most common. Bacterial brain abscesses are often polymicrobial, and the causative organisms vary by age and pathogenesis. Overall, streptococci are most common, followed by staphylococci and then gram-negative organisms. Organisms gain access to the brain parenchyma by a number of different mechanisms. These include hematogenous seeding,

TABLE 118.1	Typical Cerebrospinal Fluid Parameters				
	Bacterial	**Viral**	**Tuberculosis**	**Lyme Disease**	**Epidural Abscess**
Opening pressure	Elevated	Normal or mildly elevated	Elevated	Normal or elevated	Normal
Gram stain	Occasionally positive	Negative	Negative	Negative	Rarely positive
WBC count	Elevated	Mildly elevated	Very elevated	Mildly elevated	Normal or mildly elevated
WBC differential	Neutrophil predominance	*Early:* neutrophil predominance *Late:* lymphocyte and monocyte predominance	Lymphocyte predominance	Lymphocyte and monocyte predominance	Neutrophil predominance
Glucose	Low	Low or normal	Very low	Low or normal	Normal
Protein	High	Normal or mildly elevated	Very high	Normal or mildly elevated	Normal

direct extension from infections of the middle ear or sinuses, or by inoculation after a surgical procedure or penetrating trauma.

Neonates with no predisposing factors can develop brain abscesses after an episode of bacteremia. These infections are usually caused by Enterobacteriaceae such as *E. coli* or *Citrobacter* species. Infants with cyanotic congenital heart disease are at especially high risk for developing brain abscesses because part of their venous blood flow bypasses the lungs. Infected emboli in the venous system therefore have direct entry into the arterial circulation and from there can travel to the brain. One large case series of children with brain abscesses found that 25% of the patients had congenital heart disease as a risk factor. Another study estimated that up to 6% of people with cyanotic congenital heart disease develop a brain abscess over the course of their lives.

Older children are at risk for brain abscesses from direct extension of other infections, particularly sinusitis or otitis media with mastoiditis. Brain abscesses that arise secondary to these infections are often polymicrobial and may include both aerobic and anaerobic organisms. The most commonly isolated organism from these infections is *Staphylococcus intermedius*, which is part of the *Streptococcus milleri* group. Other commonly isolated organisms include viridans streptococci and *Staphylococcus aureus*. Many additional pathogens have been reported as causative agents of brain abscesses (Box 118.2).

Recently, fungal brain infections have become more common in a subset of pediatric patients with immune dysfunction. Many of these children are on immunosuppressive medications in the setting of solid organ transplant or malignancy and have had long periods of neutropenia before development of the fungal infection. Primary immunodeficiencies and human immunodeficiency virus (HIV) have not been reported as common risk factors for fungal brain abscesses in children.

Clinical Presentation

Children with brain abscesses often have a clinical presentation similar to that of meningitis. They present with fever and headache and may have nausea or vomiting. Sometimes, they present to medical attention after a seizure or with focal neurologic abnormalities. If the abscess is in a location that affects CSF flow leading to obstructive hydrocephalus, patients can present with signs of increased ICP—vital sign abnormalities (bradycardia, hypertension, and abnormal respirations) altered mental status, and/or papilledema. The examination for patients with brain abscess usually lacks nuchal rigidity and Kernig and Brudzinski signs, in contrast to meningitis.

Evaluation

The most important diagnostic procedure is neuroimaging with contrast, either head CT scan or MRI of the brain (Fig. 118.3). Head CT scans are fast, effective at identifying acute problems that require intervention (e.g., hemorrhage, large mass, obstructive hydrocephalus, or large vascular territory infarction), and usually do not require

BOX 118.2 Risk Factors and Organisms Associated With Brain Abscesses

Common Organisms
- *Streptococcus milleri*
- *Streptococcus pyogenes*
- *Staphylococcus aureus*
- Anaerobic streptococci
- *Peptostreptococcus*

Rare Organisms
- *Streptococcus agalactiae*
- Coagulase-negative staphylococci
- *Pseudomonas* species
- *Klebsiella* species
- *Haemophilus influenzae*
- *Nocardia* species
- *Citrobacter* species
- *Escherichia coli*
- *Enterobacter* species
- *Aspergillus* species
- *Candida* species

Common Risk Factors
- Cyanotic congenital heart disease
- Sinus or otic infection
- Immunosuppression (solid organ transplant, malignancy)

Rare Risk Factors
- Ventriculoperitoneal shunt
- Trauma
- Dental procedure
- Neurosurgical procedure

sedation. Although MRI is a longer study and may require sedation, it is much more sensitive for small structural lesions, inflammation (including meningeal enhancement), and ischemia. Abscesses found on either modality appear as rim-enhancing, space-occupying lesions, often with surrounding cerebral edema. After an abscess is identified, the patient should be promptly evaluated by a neurosurgeon for possible drainage. Surgical samples should be sent for Gram stain and aerobic and anaerobic culture.

Management

Surgery and antibiotics are the mainstays of therapy for brain abscesses. If a neurosurgeon is not immediately available, antibiotics should not be held awaiting surgery for clinical specimens to be sent for culture.

Brain abscess

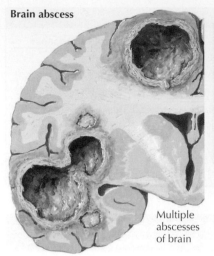

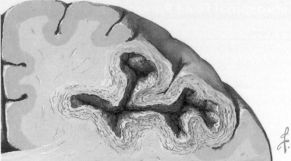

Scar of healed brain abscess, with collapse of brain tissue into cavity

Multiple abscesses of brain

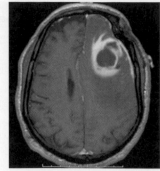

Axial T1-weighted gadolinium enhancing left frontal mass with central hypointensity

Epidural abscess

Fat in epidural space

Anterior spinal artery

Dura

Arachnoid

Venous plexus

Dura

Posterior spinal arteries

Abscess in epidural space compressing spinal cord and its blood supply

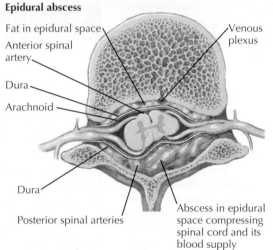

Subdural abscess

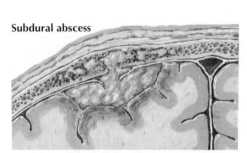

Osteomyelitis of skull, with penetration of dura to form subdural "collar button" abscess

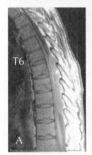

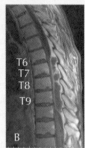

Epidural abscess. Sagittal T1-weighted images without (**A**) and with (**B**) gadolinium enhancement demonstrate an extensive posterior epidural process from T6 to T11. Enhancement of the granulation tissue allows appreciation of nonenhancing focal pus collections.

Fig. 118.3 Parameningeal Infections.

Empiric antibiotic therapy should be broad and include activity against anaerobes, streptococci, *S. aureus*, and gram-negative organisms. A commonly used regimen is intravenous vancomycin, a third-generation cephalosporin, and metronidazole. β-Lactam and β-lactamase inhibitor combinations or clindamycin should not be used because the β-lactamase inhibitors and clindamycin do not achieve adequate concentrations in the CNS. For a broader spectrum of gram-negative activity, carbapenems can be used to replace the third-generation cephalosporin and metronidazole. If the patient shows signs of increased ICP, therapy to reduce pressure may be necessary before abscess drainage (Chapter 117).

Culture samples sent from abscess drainage typically reveal the causative organisms, but antibiotics given before drainage can affect culture results. These infections require a prolonged course of intravenous antibiotics. The decision to stop antibiotics is guided by the patient's clinical response in addition to follow-up imaging. Long-term sequelae are difficult to predict and depend on many factors, including patient comorbidities, location of the abscess, presence of increased ICP and related complications, seizures, and number of neurosurgical procedures.

Subdural Empyema

Subdural empyema is an infection of the potential space between the dura mater and arachnoid membrane that can spread over the surface of the cerebral cortex.

Etiology, Epidemiology, and Pathogenesis

Subdural empyema is most commonly associated with infection of the paranasal sinuses, and mostly affects children in their second decade of life. It is the most common suppurative complication of sinusitis and affects boys more than girls (the male-to-female ratio ranges from 1.3:1 to 4.5:1). It can occur by one of two mechanisms: direct extension of the infection, usually from the frontal sinus that passes through the dura into the subdural space, or by thrombophlebitis of the valveless diploic veins. Subdural empyema can also occur after penetrating trauma or neurosurgery, or as a superinfection of subdural effusions as a result of neonatal meningitis.

The microbiology of subdural empyema is determined by the mechanism of the infection. *S. intermedius* is the most common pathogen in subdural empyema that arises as a complication of sinusitis. These infections are often polymicrobial and include anaerobes such as *Fusobacterium* or *Prevotella* species. Some data suggest these anaerobes increase the virulence of *S. intermedius*, which may explain the frequent polymicrobial nature of these infections. Other flora that commonly cause bacterial sinusitis, including *S. pneumoniae*, *Moraxella catarrhalis*, and nontypable *H. influenzae*, do not commonly lead to subdural empyema. *S. aureus* is a common cause of subdural empyema after penetrating trauma or neurosurgery. Historically, Hib was a common cause of subdural empyema infecting subdural effusions complicating Hib meningitis, but since the introduction of the Hib vaccine this is now extremely rare.

Clinical Presentation

The clinical presentation for pediatric subdural empyema is broad. The most frequently associated symptoms are fever, headache, and vomiting. Because vomiting is an uncommon feature of sinusitis, the combination of sinusitis, fever, and vomiting is concerning for intracranial extension of infection. Other presenting signs include focal neurologic deficits, seizures, and decreased sensorium. The severity of presentation is usually related to the extent of the infection and the degree of elevated ICP. Patients also may be asymptomatic, or a subdural empyema can be an incidental finding in patients with bacterial sinusitis.

Evaluation

When subdural empyema is suspected, the most important diagnostic procedure is neuroimaging, preferably with an MRI with contrast; a head CT scan with contrast may miss a small collection or may underestimate the extent of infection. An MRI with contrast offers excellent visualization of the subdural space and allows for differentiation between blood and purulent fluid. It often is sufficient for localization and assessing the presence or absence of loculations for neurosurgeons to determine whether surgical approach with a burr hole is adequate or whether a craniotomy is needed for drainage.

Routine blood work does not give significant information to aid in the diagnosis of subdural empyema but may be important for overall management of the patient. If antibiotics have not been administered, it is useful to obtain a blood culture. Although bacteremia is uncommon in patients with subdural empyema, it occurs in some of the other processes that are part of the differential diagnosis. An LP is not diagnostic of subdural empyema because the infection is sequestered within the subdural space and may be contraindicated in the setting of increased ICP. Unlike meningitis, the pathogen does not freely circulate throughout the CSF. If an LP is performed, the CSF often has a mild pleocytosis, but the CSF culture rarely grows an organism.

Management

When a subdural empyema is diagnosed, the most important step is neurosurgical consultation. Most patients require surgical source control, although there are reports of some patients with small subdural empyemas being managed with medical therapy alone. The drained fluid should be sent for Gram stain and aerobic and anaerobic culture.

Empiric antibiotic regimens for subdural empyema are the same as regimens for brain abscesses and should include broad coverage of aerobic and anaerobic streptococci, oropharyngeal anaerobes, and gram-negative organisms. Antibiotics should be given immediately and should not be delayed while awaiting surgical intervention. Patients with subdural empyema require intensive care management even if they do not require surgery. Before surgery, they can have vital sign instability if there is significant elevation of ICP, and they can develop rapid changes in their neurologic function. Postoperatively, they require close monitoring of their cardiorespiratory and neurologic status. The duration of antibiotics depends on clinical course but is usually 4 to 6 weeks. Many patients experience some long-term sequelae from these infections, but death is rare.

Epidural Abscess

Epidural abscesses are collections of infected fluid that are located between the outermost layer of the meninges (the dura) and the bony structures protecting the CNS (the skull or vertebrae).

Etiology and Pathogenesis

Epidural abscesses can occur within the cranium or within the spinal canal (Fig. 118.3). Overall, epidural abscesses are quite rare in pediatrics. The pathogenesis and infectious organisms associated with these infections vary according to the site of infection. Most intracranial epidural abscesses occur as a complication of sinusitis. Multiple case series have found an increased incidence during adolescence, which is thought to be attributable to the rapid growth of the sinuses during that time, along with increased vascularity of the diploic veins. These

case series have also described male predominance, although the cause is unclear. The frontal sinuses are usually the primary site of infection. It has been hypothesized that epidural abscesses are seen more often in conjunction with frontal sinusitis because of a larger potential space between the frontal sinuses and the cranial vault compared with other locations, where the dura is more adherent to the cranium. Less commonly, epidural abscesses can occur as a complication of otitis media and mastoiditis.

The microbiology of intracranial epidural abscesses resulting from sinusitis is similar to the microbiology of subdural empyema because they have the same primary source of infection. Organisms of the *S. milleri* group are the most commonly identified. These infections also can be polymicrobial and include anaerobic bacteria.

Spinal epidural abscesses are rarer than intracranial epidural abscesses. In pediatric patients, the pathophysiology is usually hematogenous seeding of the epidural space with subsequent response by the immune system leading to abscess formation. These abscesses can occur anywhere from the cervical spine to the sacrum. Whereas most pediatric patients with spinal epidural abscesses do not have any comorbidities, the majority of adults who develop these infections have underlying risk factors (e.g., diabetes mellitus, spinal cord injury, immunocompromised condition).

S. aureus is the most common pathogen associated with pediatric spinal epidural abscesses. Often, there is also evidence of osteomyelitis, discitis, or paraspinal pyomyositis. These infections are very rarely polymicrobial, and anaerobes have not been described as part of this syndrome. Other pathogens that have been reported to cause spinal epidural abscesses include *Pseudomonas aeruginosa*, *S. pneumoniae*, *Salmonella* species (in children with sickle cell disease), *E. coli*, *Fusobacterium* species, and viridans streptococci. Children receiving chemotherapy for malignancies or with primary immunodeficiencies have been reported to have infections caused by unusual pathogens, including *Aspergillus*, *Mycobacterium*, and *Candida* species.

Clinical Presentation

The clinical presentation of patients with epidural abscesses depends on the anatomic location of the infection. Patients with intracranial epidural abscesses arising from the frontal sinuses typically present with intermittent headaches, for a few days to a few weeks. They also may have fever, nausea, and vomiting. Occasionally, patients with these infections develop cerebritis and may develop personality changes or other focal neurologic symptoms. Epidural abscesses can also result as a complication of mastoiditis. In these situations, patients may present with headache, nausea, and vomiting in addition to the signs and symptoms of mastoiditis. The symptoms seen in spinal epidural abscesses are attributable to inflammation of or mass effect on the spinal nerve roots arising in the affected area. Patients with cervical epidural abscesses may present with neck stiffness or focal arm pain or weakness. Patients with epidural abscesses in the lumbosacral region may present with back pain, gait abnormalities, changes in bowel or bladder function, weakness or pain of the lower extremities.

Evaluation

If an intracranial epidural abscess is suspected, the first diagnostic step is MRI of the brain with contrast or head CT with contrast. Noncontrast studies are less useful because contrast improves the sensitivity and displays a better outline of the abscess. For spinal lesions, MRI is the preferred modality because of its superiority in identifying bone and soft tissue inflammation compared with CT. After an abscess has been identified, a neurosurgeon should be consulted to discuss drainage of the lesion. If sinusitis is also identified on imaging, an otolaryngologist

TB with involvement of basal cistern with vasculitis and ischemia

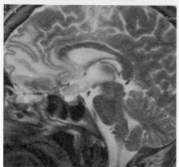

Midsagittal T2-weighted image shows increased T2 signal within ischemic frontal lobe.

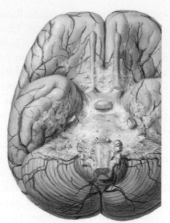

Tuberculous basilar meningitis

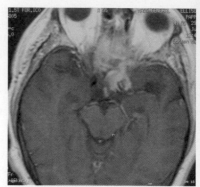

Axial T1-weighted gadolinium-enhanced image with enhancing mass at left basal cisterns and subfrontal region.

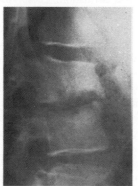

X-ray film: destruction of disk space and adjacent end plates of vertebrae

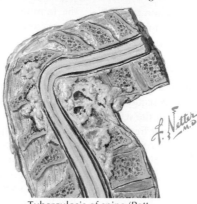

Tuberculosis of spine (Pott disease) with marked kyphosis

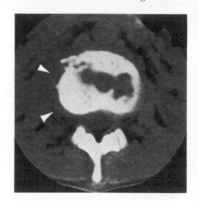

CT scan: paraspinous abscess in addition to bony destruction

Fig. 118.4 Tuberculosis of the Brain and Spine.

should be consulted to discuss possible sinus drainage. Some spinal epidural abscesses may be drained by an interventional radiologist under ultrasound or CT guidance. Occasionally, small abscesses do not require drainage and can be treated with antibiotics alone. If an abscess is drained, samples should be sent for Gram stain and aerobic and anaerobic culture.

Management

For small intracranial epidural abscesses or those that are difficult to approach surgically, medical therapy with antibiotics is the initial step in management. The location of the infection guides empiric antibiotic therapy. The microbiology of intracranial epidural abscesses arising from sinusitis or mastoiditis is similar to the microbiology of subdural empyemas and brain abscesses. The combination of an intravenous third-generation cephalosporin, vancomycin, and metronidazole offers broad activity with good CNS penetration (in case there is a subdural component of the infection). Antibiotic therapy can be narrowed based on culture results from drainage. These infections are usually treated for a minimum of 3 weeks, but total duration depends on the size of the abscess, whether it was drained, and the patient's clinical response. In most cases, there are no long-term sequelae, but the risk for morbidity is increased if there is associated subdural empyema or if the patient presented with focal neurologic signs suggesting injury of the subjacent brain parenchyma.

Empiric antibiotic selection for patients with spinal epidural abscesses without any underlying conditions should focus on *S. aureus*. Recently, community-acquired methicillin-resistant *S. aureus* (CA-MRSA) has become a common pediatric pathogen, so this should be considered. Clindamycin has good activity against most CA-MRSA isolates and is a good empiric choice, though vancomycin should be considered if community resistance is high to clindamycin. In patients with predisposing conditions (e.g., malignancy or sickle cell disease), empiric coverage should be broader and include gram-negative organisms, and treatment will likely be longer. Factors to take into consideration include size of the abscess, whether it was drained, whether the patient has a predisposing medical condition, and patient's response to therapy. Most patients recover fully unless focal neurologic findings were present at time of presentation, again suggesting injury of the subjacent spinal cord parenchyma.

OTHER INFECTIONS

Tuberculosis Meningitis

Meningitis caused by *Mycobacterium tuberculosis* is very rare in the developed world, but has become more common in areas with a high prevalence of HIV infection (Fig. 118.4). It usually occurs in children younger than 2 years of age with tuberculosis (TB) because they are at higher risk for developing extrapulmonary disease. In most cases, the child has a household contact or a caregiver with active pulmonary TB, which is often undiagnosed.

Unlike typical bacterial meningitis, TB meningitis (TBM) is often indolent in nature, and most children present with advanced disease. TBM is classified in three stages. Stage 1 includes irritability, anorexia, fever, personality changes, and listlessness. Stage 2 is characterized by signs of increased ICP and cerebral damage. Stage 3 disease manifests as coma, irregular pulse and respirations, and rising fever.

Children with suspected TBM should be tested for HIV if their status is unknown. In addition, they should be tested with a tuberculin skin test or interferon-γ release assay, depending on age, and a chest radiograph. The interpretation of the skin test will depend on the HIV status, age, and nutritional status of the patient. In general, 50% of patients who are HIV positive and have TBM will have a positive skin test result. Chest radiographs are helpful if the results are abnormal, but a normal result does not exclude extrapulmonary TB disease.

If the patient is clinically stable, an LP should be performed. CSF should be sent for routine testing, acid-fast bacillus (AFB) smear and culture, and TB PCR. The sensitivity of the AFB smear can be increased by sending a large volume of CSF (5 to 10 mL) and centrifuging the sample before examination. The AFB smear result is often negative, and culture can take weeks to grow, even in the presence of true disease.

Management of patients with TBM is outside of the scope of this chapter. See Chapter 87 for more information on TB infection. TBM is frequently associated with vasculitis, which can lead to strokes. Therefore many children have permanent disabilities as a consequence of this infection.

Acute Flaccid Myelitis

Acute flaccid myelitis (AFM) is a rare condition in children that has come to national attention in the past decade in the context of case clusters occurring in 2014, 2016, and 2018. AFM is further discussed in Chapter 116.

SUGGESTED READINGS

Available online.

Nutrition

Jennifer Robbins

119

Nutritional Requirements and Growth

Yoshi M. Rothman

✳ CLINICAL VIGNETTE

A 4-month-old girl born at 39 weeks and her 4-year-old brother present to their pediatrician for their well-child visits. The mother reports she is breastfeeding her baby and continues to supplement 400 IU of vitamin D daily, but she does not always recognize when her baby is hungry. She is not yet eating solid foods. The 4-year-old eats cereal with milk for breakfast, a sandwich with deli meat on white bread with potato chips for lunch, and usually eats chicken or meat with rice, potatoes, or pasta for dinner. He will occasionally snack on apple slices with peanut butter, but he mostly snacks on crackers or cookies. The mother states she has not really offered him many vegetables. He does drink two or three glasses of whole milk daily and drinks water throughout the day. He gets juice at most once per week.

The mother is counseled on distinguishing the signs of hunger and satiety in infants. Moving lips, sucking on hands, and rooting are some signs of hunger that precede fussing or crying. Releasing the nipple, biting the nipple, pulling head away, and shaking the head are some signs of satiety. Responding to the baby's cues rather than adhering to a feeding schedule will encourage appropriate eating habits. In addition, confirming that the baby is adequately gaining weight can be reassuring. The mother is counseled to continue breastfeeding exclusively for the first 6 months (see Fig. 119.2). Breastfeeding should continue through at least the first year of life; however, at 6 months solid foods should be introduced. Initially, iron-rich, high-protein foods, iron-fortified cereals, and pureed fruits, vegetables, and meats should be given to the infant. Over time more complex textures can be introduced as tolerated, always avoiding foods that could cause choking.

The mother is also encouraged to optimize her son's diet by following a healthy eating pattern that includes the following six categories: fruits, vegetables, protein, dairy, grains, and oil (see Fig. 119.1). In addition, limiting saturated and trans fats, added sugars, and sodium are important steps. These are changes that can occur gradually, and should take into account cultural and personal preferences. The mother agrees that she can work toward incorporating vegetables into meals, substitute fresh, lean meat for deli meat, and offer fruits and mixed nuts for snacking. The mother plans to follow up in 2 months for her daughter's 6-month visit and to check in on how her son's dietary changes are going.

NUTRITIONAL REQUIREMENTS

Energy

Estimated energy requirement (EER) is the predicted average caloric intake required to maintain energy balance in healthy individuals. EER, in kilocalories (kcal) per day, is calculated by adding total energy expenditure to energy deposition, which is the energy required for new tissue production. Energy requirements are often expressed in kcal/kg/day in infants and toddlers, and in kcal/day as children reach school age and adolescence.

Caloric requirements are highest in infancy and steadily decrease over time. Neonates require approximately 110 to 120 kcal/kg/day to achieve adequate growth, whereas toddlers' needs decrease to around 90 kcal/kg/day. At age 3 years, EER varies based on age, sex, weight, height, and amount of physical activity. When offered but not forced to take food, most infants and children are able to self-regulate their energy intake. Children are generally able to increase their calories when needed, such as during brief periods of rapid growth in infancy and puberty, and then decrease their intake back to appropriate levels for typical growth. However, children with chronic medical problems may be unable to self-regulate energy intake, and thus frequent assessment of nutritional status may be warranted.

Energy sources in children come from the following macronutrients: fat (~9 kcal/g), protein (4 kcal/g), and carbohydrates (4 kcal/g) (Fig. 119.1). The EER does not specify a proportional contribution of each macronutrient. Acceptable macronutrient distribution ranges have been devised and are expressed as a percentage of total energy intake.

Fat

Fat is an important nutrient that contributes to nervous system myelination, hormone production, and cell membrane structure and function. For infants, human milk and formula are the primary sources of dietary fat intake. Children and adolescents often get their fat from animal products, vegetable oils, nuts, and seeds. Children between the ages of 1 and 3 should get approximately 30% to 40% of calories from fat, whereas children between the ages of 4 and 18 should get 25% to 35% of calories from fat.

Protein

Protein has a wide variety of roles in the body, ranging from enzymatic function within each cell to coordination of large skeletal muscle contraction (Fig. 119.1). Protein is made up of amino acids, some of which can be synthesized by humans; others, however, are essential amino acids and must be obtained through diet. Human milk and animal protein provide adequate levels of all essential amino acids. Plant sources of protein, such as legumes, nuts, seeds, and grains, individually do not contain adequate levels of all essential amino acids. However, when a variety of plant sources are consumed, adequate intake of essential amino acids can be achieved.

Similar to fat, infants receive the majority of their dietary protein from human milk and formula. Older children get their protein from animal products, legumes, grains, nuts, and seeds. Protein requirements start at approximately 1.5 g/kg/day for infants and steadily decrease to 0.85 g/kg/day for adolescents. This amounts to 5% to 20% of calories from protein between the ages of 1 and 3, and 10% to 30% of calories from protein between the ages of 4 and 18.

1. Follow a healthy eating pattern across the lifespan. All food and beverage choices matter. Choose a healthy eating pattern at an appropriate calorie level to help achieve and maintain a healthy body weight, support nutrient adequacy, and reduce the risk of chronic disease.

Follow a healthy eating pattern over time to help support a healthy body weight and reduce the risk of chronic disease.

A Healthy Eating Pattern Includes:

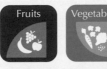 Fruits
 Vegetables
 Protein

 Dairy
 Grains
 Oils

A Healthy Eating Pattern Limits:

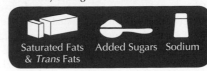 Saturated Fats & *Trans* Fats   Added Sugars   Sodium

---

2. Focus on variety, nutrient density, and amount. To meet nutrient needs within calorie limits, choose a variety of nutrient-dense foods across and within all food groups in recommended amounts.

Choose a variety of nutrient-dense foods from each food group in recommended amounts.

Example Meal:

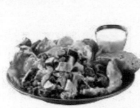

 Fruits — Apples & Grapes
 Vegetables — Lettuce & Celery
 Protein — Chicken Breast & Unsalted Walnuts

Dairy — Fat-Free Milk
Grains — Whole-Grain Bread
Oils — Mayonnaise

---

3. Limit calories from added sugars and saturated fats and reduce sodium intake. Consume an eating pattern low in added sugars, saturated fats, and sodium. Cut back on foods and beverages higher in these components to amounts that fit within healthy eating patterns.

Consume an eating pattern low in added sugars, saturated fats, and sodium.

Example Sources of:

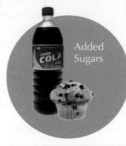 Added Sugars
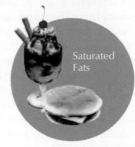 Saturated Fats
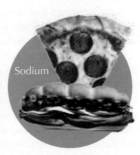 Sodium

---

4. Shift to healthier food and beverage choices. Choose nutrient-dense foods and beverages across and within all food groups in place of less healthy choices. Consider cultural and personal preferences to make these shifts easier to accomplish and maintain.

Replace typical food and beverage choices with more nutrient-dense options. Be sure to consider personal preferences to maintain shifts over time.

Example:

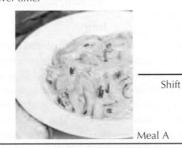 Meal A   Shift →   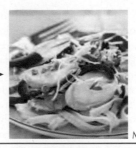 Meal B

---

5. Support healthy eating patterns for all. Everyone has a role in helping to create and support healthy eating patterns in multiple settings nationwide, from home to school to work to communities.

Everyone has a role in helping to create and support healthy eating patterns in places where we learn, work, live, and play.

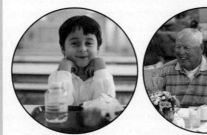 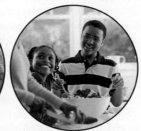 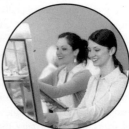

Fig. 119.1 Dietary Guidelines for Americans 2015–2020: 5 Guidelines That Encourage Healthy Eating Patterns. The 2015–2020 Dietary Guidelines focuses on the big picture with recommendations to help Americans make choices that add up to an overall healthy eating pattern. To build a healthy eating pattern, combine healthy choices from across all food groups—while paying attention to calorie limits, too. (Reused from U.S. Department of Health and Human Services and U.S. Department of Agriculture. 2015–2020 Dietary Guidelines for Americans. 8th ed. December 2015. Retrieved from http://health.gov/dietaryguidelines/2015/guidelines/.)

Carbohydrates

Carbohydrates are the primary source of energy in the human body. Most carbohydrate intake should come from complex carbohydrates rather than simple sugars, which contribute to dental caries and obesity. Fruits have significant amounts of sugar but also supply vitamins and fiber and are part of a healthy diet for children (Fig. 119.1). Most other sources of sugar, such as sugar-sweetened beverages, including fruit juice, candy, cookies, and other processed foods do not contain significant sources of other nutrients and should be limited.

Juice that is 100% fruit contains vitamins but lacks fiber and provides more concentrated sugar than whole fruit. Therefore the American Academy of Pediatrics (AAP) recommends no juice before 1 year of age, no more than 4 oz per day of 100% fruit juice between 1 and 3 years of age, no more than 4 to 6 oz per day of 100% fruit juice between 4 and 6 years of age, and no more than 8 oz per day of 100% fruit juice between age 7 and 18 years. Excess juice contributes to obesity by increasing caloric intake and can contribute to failure to thrive in children who drink juice in place of eating more nutritious food.

Children of all ages should get 45% to 65% of calories from carbohydrates. Low-carbohydrate diets are not generally recommended for children and should never be followed without the supervision of a dietitian or physician.

Fiber

Fiber is an important nutrient that does not contribute to energy intake, because it consists of nondigestible carbohydrates. Dietary fiber is processed by colonic bacteria, producing metabolites such as short-chain fatty acids that serve as a fuel source for colonic cells, and help regulate colonic function. Adequate fiber intake is important for the prevention of constipation. Fiber may have additional beneficial effects, and low dietary consumption has been associated with an increased risk for cardiovascular disease, diabetes, colon cancer, and other diseases. Dietary sources of fiber generally come from plants such as fruits, vegetables, and whole grains. Recommended intake of fiber for children over age 2 is the child's age in years plus 5 g/day and increases to 26 g/day in girls and 38 g/day in boys by adolescence.

Fluid and Electrolytes

Adequate fluid and electrolyte balance is important for many bodily processes, including thermoregulation, hemodynamics, and cardiac and neurologic functioning. In general, infants who are voiding six or more times in 24 hours are getting adequate fluids. Infants' immature kidneys are not capable of producing either very concentrated or very dilute urine; therefore it is essential that the fluid and electrolytes consumed be balanced. Breast milk and properly prepared commercial infant formula contain appropriate amounts of electrolytes for infants. Free water should not be given to infants younger than 6 months of age, and intake should be limited until 1 year of age. The electrolyte composition of cow's milk is not appropriate until 1 year of age.

Healthy children are generally able to regulate their own fluid intake when it is provided, and many children get a substantial amount of fluid through the high water content of most foods. Beverages can be rich in nutrients or a source of empty calories. Recommended beverages change with age, but avoiding high-calorie, sugar-rich beverages is consistently recommended throughout childhood (Table 119.1). Electrolytes such as sodium and chloride are found in table salt and are added to many foods during processing. Potassium is another important electrolyte that is obtained through fruits, vegetables, dairy, meat, and nuts. Urine output and signs and symptoms of dehydration can be used to assess fluid status in older children.

In situations in which children are unable to regulate fluid intake, weight-based recommendations for adequate fluids in children have been made based on metabolic rates. The Holliday-Segar method recommends 100 mL/kg/day for the first 10 kg of weight, 50 mL/kg/day

TABLE 119.1 Recommended Fluids by Age for Healthy, Typically Growing Children

Age	Fluid Recommendations
0–6 months	• Breast milk • Properly prepared commercial infant formula
6–12 months	• Breast milk • Properly prepared commercial infant formula • Water: no more than 8 oz/day • 0–4 oz/day of 100% fruit juice
12–24 months	• Breast milk if desired • Whole milk: 16–24 ounces/day • Water • 0–4 oz/day of 100% fruit juice
2–6 years	• Water • Low-fat milk (skim or 1% milk) • 0–4 oz/day of 100% fruit juice
6–18 years	• Water • Low-fat milk (skim or 1% milk) • 0–8 oz/day of 100% fruit juice

for the next 10 kg of weight, and then 20 mL/kg/day for each kilogram above 20 kg. This method has two notable limitations. First, this estimate does not account for excess losses; children with diarrhea, vomiting, severe burns, and other sources of fluid loss may require more fluids. Second, these estimates have not been tested in children, and may overestimate fluid requirements. The Holliday-Segar method ends up with similar values to the adequate intake of fluids, which starts at 0.7 to 0.8 L/day in the first year of life, and then increases to 2.7 L/day in girls and 3.7 L/day in boys by adolescence.

Micronutrients

This section briefly discusses three of the most important micronutrients and the problems that can arise when they are deficient. Chapter 122 addresses these and other deficiencies in more detail.

Iron

Iron contributes to red blood cell production and neurocognitive development. Iron deficiency is the most common micronutrient deficiency worldwide, putting children at risk for iron deficiency anemia and irreversible neurologic impairment. Between birth and 6 months of age breastmilk provides an adequate supply of highly bioavailable iron so long as the mother has accrued adequate iron stores through dietary or supplemental sources (Fig. 119.2). Commercial infant formulas that are fortified with iron are acceptable alternatives. Preterm infants require additional iron, which can be given as a multivitamin with iron. After 6 months of age, iron-rich foods should be introduced to provide adequate iron intake. Animal products such as meat and eggs and iron-fortified cereals are good sources of highly bioavailable iron. Iron is also found in many fruits and vegetables, but these sources contain iron in a less bioavailable form. The iron in cow's milk is not very bioavailable; cow's milk should not be given to any child younger than 1 year of age. In addition, cow's milk intake should be limited to 24 oz daily to reduce the risk for developing iron deficiency.

Vitamin D

Adequate vitamin D intake is important for long-term bone health, and recent research has shown its importance in a wide variety of other functions (Fig. 119.3). Vitamin D can be ingested or synthesized when the skin is exposed to ultraviolet light. Dietary sources of vitamin D include fatty fish, liver, and fortified products such as eggs, milk, and cereals. Vitamin D deficiency in infants causes rickets and when severe can lead to hypocalcemic seizures. Vitamin D deficiency is relatively common in the United States. Risk factors include breastfeeding, darker skin, limited sun exposure, and fat malabsorption. Infant formula is supplemented with vitamin D, but breastfed infants are at risk for rickets without supplementation. Infants who are breastfed should receive a vitamin D supplement with 400 IU of vitamin D per day to prevent rickets. Children between 1 and 18 years of age require 600 IU of vitamin D daily, and those who do not receive that amount in their diets also should receive supplementation.

Calcium

Adequate calcium intake during childhood is critical for long-term bone health, contributes to nervous system function, muscle contraction, and various other physiologic processes. Breast milk and infant formula provide the recommended calcium intake for infants (210 to 270 mg/day). Preterm infants who are formula fed should receive preterm formula with increased calcium. Dairy products are the most well-known source of calcium and can provide daily requirements at all age groups. Fortified plant-based milks such as soy milk serve as an acceptable alternative to obtain daily calcium requirements. However, not all plant-based milks are equal, and attention must be paid to nutrition facts to ensure adequate fortification. Alternative sources include leafy green vegetables, tofu, and fortified products such as orange juice. Children who are 1 to 3 years of age should receive 700 mg/day of calcium, children between 4 and 8 years of age need 1000 mg/day of calcium, and children older than 9 years of age need 1300 mg/day of calcium.

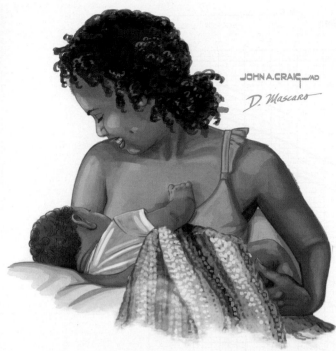

The AAP recommends breastfeeding for at least the first year of life, with exclusive breastfeeding for the first six months.

Fig. 119.2 Breastfeeding.

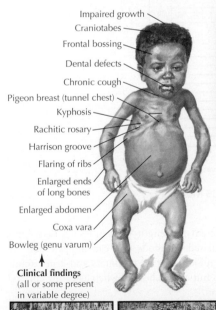

Clinical findings (all or some present in variable degree)

- Impaired growth
- Craniotabes
- Frontal bossing
- Dental defects
- Chronic cough
- Pigeon breast (tunnel chest)
- Kyphosis
- Rachitic rosary
- Harrison groove
- Flaring of ribs
- Enlarged ends of long bones
- Enlarged abdomen
- Coxa vara
- Bowleg (genu varum)

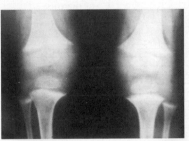

◄ Flaring of metaphyseal ends of tibia and femur. Growth plates thickened, irregular, cupped, and axially widened. Zones of provisional calcification fuzzy and indistinct. Bone cortices thinned and medullae rarefied

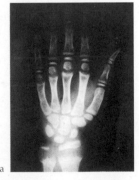

► Radiograph of rachitic hand shows decreased bone density, irregular trabeculation, and thin cortices of metacarpals and proximal phalanges. Note increased axial width of epiphyseal line, especially in radius and ulna

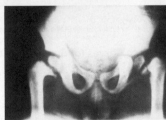

▲ Coxa vara and slipped capital femoral epiphysis. Mottled areas of lucency and density in pelvic bones

Radiographic findings

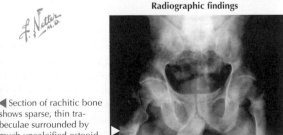

▲ Radiograph shows variegated rarefaction of pelvic bones, coxa vara, deepened acetabula, and subtrochanteric pseudofracture of right femur

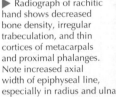

◄ Section of rachitic bone shows sparse, thin trabeculae surrounded by much uncalcified osteoid (osteoid seams) and cavities caused by increased resorption

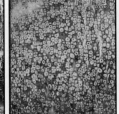

◄ (Left) Cartilage of epiphyseal plate in immature normal rat. Cells of middle (maturation) zone in orderly columns, with calcified cartilage between columns
◄ (Right) After 6 weeks of vitamin D- and phosphate-deficient diet. Large increase in axial height of maturation zone, with cells closely packed and irregularly arranged

Fig. 119.3 Bone Health.

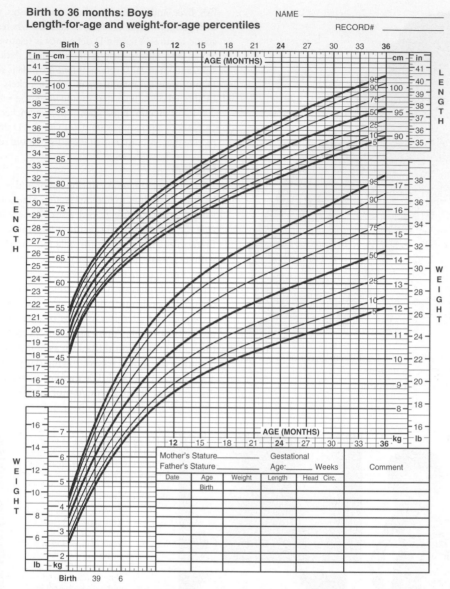

Birth to 36 months: Boys
Length-for-age and weight-for-age percentiles

NAME _____

RECORD# _____

Centers for Disease Control and Prevention, A National Center for Health Statistics. CDC growth charts: United States. http://www.cdc.gov/growthcharts/. May 30, 2000.

Fig. 119.4 Weight and Height Growth Curves for Boys Ages 0 to 36 Months.

GROWTH

During well-child visits, assessment of growth serves as a screening tool for a wide variety of medical problems. In children presenting with an illness, assessment of growth can provide clues about the nature and time course of the illness. Because there is such wide variation in the distribution of normal growth, the challenge for clinicians is to determine whether children with unusual growth patterns are unhealthy or if they are healthy patients with a less common growth pattern. This segment focuses on how to assess growth and growth patterns seen in healthy patients. Further information on disorders of growth can be found in this section, as well as the chapter on disorders of growth in the endocrinology section (Chapter 52).

Types of Measurements

Weight is the most important and most commonly used measure of growth in children. Length (in children younger than 2 years), height (in children 2 years or older), and head circumference are also useful.

From these measures, weight-for-length percentiles or body mass index (BMI) can be calculated. Methods that can indicate body fat percentage, such as subscapular skinfold thickness and arm circumference, are used less often but can be helpful when assessing children with suspected malnutrition.

Measurement Methods

It is crucial that all measurements are accurately assessed. Infants should be weighed without clothing or a diaper, and older children should be weighed with very light clothing because apparent weight loss or weight gain may be an artifact of differences in clothing. All staff taking measurements should be properly trained, and equipment should be calibrated to ensure proper measurements. A stadiometer should be used for measuring height.

Use of Growth Curves

Growth in children is typically assessed by plotting a child's measurement and age on a sex-specific growth curve (Fig. 119.4). Growth curves allow clinicians to compare a child's measurements with those of other children of the same age and to evaluate patterns in an individual child's growth if measurements from multiple points in time are plotted on the same curve. On weight and BMI charts, the upper lines are not true percentiles; they have been adjusted so that the increasing prevalence of obesity does not lead to the classification of overweight children as having a healthy weight.

Two standard forms are commonly used in the United States: the Centers for Disease Control and Prevention (CDC) charts published in 2000 based on data from multiple national cross-sectional studies including both healthy children and those with medical problems, and the World Health Organization (WHO) charts published in 2006 based on a prospective longitudinal study of healthy, breastfed children on six continents. The CDC and WHO's length curves are similar. The WHO curves classify more children as being overweight and fewer children as underweight than the CDC curves. The WHO curves also classify more children as being macrocephalic than the CDC curves.

Assessing a Child's Growth

Growth is usually assessed in two ways: (1) current, attained growth relative to same-age peers and (2) growth velocity relative to peers. Using the 5th and 95th percentile parameters as cutoffs for normal growth is sensitive but not specific. It is important to remember that in using these cutoffs, approximately 10% of all children will be labeled as outside the normal range, including many healthy children. A child's growth velocity can be estimated by determining if a child is following a certain percentile line or is crossing percentile lines. Crossing two or more major percentile lines can be indicative of a problem and may warrant further assessment. However, a shift in percentiles in the first year of life may merely reflect a child's transition to his or her genetic potential.

Weight

Neonates can lose up to 10% of their birth weight and should be at or above their birth weight by 10 to 14 days after birth. Expected weight gain early in infancy is approximately 30 g/day in the first 3 months, 20 g/day from 3 months to 6 months of age, and 10 g/day from 6 months to 12 months of age. Breastfed infants typically gain weight more quickly than formula-fed infants between 4 and 6 months but then gain weight more slowly and are ultimately slightly leaner, on average, than formula-fed infants. Children do not always gain weight steadily and may have periods of relatively little weight gain followed by periods of more rapid weight gain. If an infant or child loses weight or has not been gaining adequate weight, a careful history, physical examination, and focused workup should be initiated.

Height and Length

As with weight, periods of slower gain in height may be followed by more rapid gains. A significant change in height percentile is less common than for weight percentile, particularly after the first year of life.

The velocity of height change generally decreases slowly from infancy until puberty. The average gain in length is 4 cm/month in the neonatal period, decreasing to 0.8 cm/month at 2 years of age. By 12 months of age, infants usually increase in length by 50% of their birth length. At puberty, children have a growth spurt, gaining several inches in height, and have minimal gain in height after puberty. The pubertal growth spurt starts later and lasts longer in boys, which accounts for much of their increased average height.

Weight for Height and Body Mass Index

For infants and young children, weight relative to length can be evaluated with weight-for-length percentiles on the CDC 2000 or WHO growth curves or with the WHO curves for BMI. For older children, weight relative to height should be evaluated using BMI. These charts are helpful when evaluating children who have familial short or tall stature. If these children are out of the normal range on the weight growth curve but have a normal weight for height, one can be reassured that their abnormal weight is likely proportional to their height. Overweight and obesity are discussed further in Chapter 121.

Head Circumference

Head circumference should be measured by placing a tape measure around the head parallel to the floor with the tape just above the eyebrows in front and around the most prominent part of the occiput. In infants, a head circumference that is rapidly crossing increasing percentiles is concerning for hydrocephalus. A head circumference that is not increasing or is crossing decreasing percentile lines is concerning for failure of brain growth.

FUTURE DIRECTIONS

Obesity and starvation affect large populations of children around the world. Researchers are working on combating hunger through agricultural sustainability, government-sponsored micronutrient food fortification, and programs supporting maternal health and community nutrition education. Meanwhile, obesity prevention and treatment strategies are being investigated, including increasing rates of exclusive breastfeeding, establishing early weight monitoring and home intervention programs for high-risk infants, government initiatives to reduce added sugar consumption such as the sugar-sweetened beverage taxes, and identification and reduction in exposure to environmental obesogens. Research continues to evaluate timing of introduction of solid foods, particularly in relation to food allergies. Further research is ongoing regarding prevention of nutrient deficiencies.

SUGGESTED READINGS

Available online.

120

Acute and Chronic Malnutrition

Stanislaw J. Gabryszewski and Bridget D. Kiernan

CLINICAL VIGNETTE

A 2-month-old, 38-weeks gestation male infant was brought to the emergency department by his mother with complaint of occasional postprandial vomiting. The vomiting was not bilious, bloody, or projectile. It was characterized as small-volume and occurred infrequently, within 30 minutes of feeding. The infant was otherwise tolerating standard cow's milk formula. There was no associated lethargy, diarrhea, poor suck, respiratory distress, cyanosis, hypotonia, or back arching. The infant had regular, nonbloody bowel movements that were reportedly hard. Urine output was below average. The remainder of review of systems, medical history, pregnancy history, and birth history were unremarkable. Birth weight was 3.2 kg. The infant was not on any medications. Family history was notable for depression in the mother. Citing lack of additional caregivers to take care of her two older children, the mother confided that she was unable to arrange primary care visits beyond the infant's initial visit. Review of diet revealed transition from exclusive breastmilk to exclusive formula by 1 month of age. Most recently, the infant was taking in 60 to 90 mL of formula six times per day, although not consistently. On review of formula preparation, the mother revealed that she sometimes added extra water to make the formula last longer. She expressed concern about having enough food for the entire household.

The patient's vital signs were notable for mild tachycardia. His weight, length, and head circumference were 4.6 kg (7th percentile), 59 cm (61st percentile), and 39 cm (46th percentile), respectively. Weight-for-length *z* score was −2.7. On physical examination, the infant was active and not toxic-appearing. There were no visible signs of trauma. He had sunken eyes and produced few tears when crying. His extremities were well-perfused. The remainder of the physical examination was unremarkable. The patient received a bolus of 10 mL/kg normal saline. A limited laboratory workup was performed; complete blood count and liver function panel were grossly normal. The chemistry panel was notable for mild hyponatremia. His blood glucose level was normal. The patient was admitted to the hospital with a working diagnosis of malnutrition as a result of a nonorganic cause, with possible contribution from gastroesophageal reflux.

Upon admission, a clinical dietician and a social worker were consulted. The patient was initiated on a supervised schedule of frequent, small-volume feeds, after which he was burped and held upright for 30 minutes. Aside from infrequent, small-volume spit-ups, there was no vomiting. Pharmacologic acid suppression was not deemed necessary. After several days, the infant exhibited sustained weight gain and bowel movements and urine output normalized. The mother enlisted the help of her older sister, who expressed commitment to assist. Both the mother and her sister received education about formula preparation, feeding frequency, and reflux precautions. Relevant community resources were identified. The mother expressed interest in joining a support group for mothers. An authorization form was provided for the Women, Infants, and Children (WIC) Nutrition Program. The infant was discharged with a plan for serial weight checks with his pediatrician, including follow-up within 48 hours of discharge.

Malnutrition occurs as a result of inadequate bioavailability of macronutrients, vitamins, and minerals and is associated with negative effects on growth and health. Although malnutrition is often equated with underweight, overweight and obesity (discussed in Chapter 121) are also forms of malnutrition. Although the prevalence of malnutrition has gradually declined in developed countries, it remains a major global burden and is implicated in nearly half of deaths in children younger than five years. Because of the variability in defining malnutrition historically, standardized anthropometric criteria have been proposed to classify mild, moderate, or severe malnutrition. Malnutrition is also categorized as acute or chronic. Wasting (low weight and normal linear growth) and stunting (low weight and low linear growth) are characteristics that help distinguish between acute and chronic malnutrition, respectively.

Because of the significant growth and physiologic changes occurring in childhood, children are uniquely susceptible to effects of malnutrition. Failure to treat malnutrition may cause long-term neurocognitive sequalae, especially in the youngest patients. Among the goals of frequent health visits after birth is screening for irregularities of growth. Both failure to thrive and excessive growth warrant nutritional evaluation. Undernutrition is most commonly caused by inadequate nutrient provision due to limited availability, such that assessment of barriers to food access is an important component of a comprehensive malnutrition evaluation.

ETIOLOGY AND PATHOGENESIS

The differential diagnosis of malnutrition is extensive (Table 120.1). The most common causes for malnutrition are nonorganic. These include psychosocial causes, such as inadequate food availability, inappropriate food intake, feeding aversions, inconsistent feeding patterns and inappropriate food preparation (i.e., incorrect formula preparation). A complex interplay between psychosocial and organic factors further exacerbates malnutrition.

Organic causes of malnutrition are classified by the predominant mechanism. The three main mechanisms are (1) inadequate intake, (2) increased metabolic demand, and (3) malabsorption. The age of the child helps establish a differential diagnosis. In premature infants, metabolic demand is increased because of incomplete organ maturation and may be further increased by complications of prematurity, such as necrotizing enterocolitis or chronic lung disease. In infants and toddlers, organic causes of malnutrition include gastroesophageal reflux, oromotor dysfunction, congenital heart disease, food allergies, and genetic syndromes. The differential diagnosis for older children and adolescents includes eating disorders, mood disorders, and inflammatory bowel disease. Avoidant-restrictive food intake disorder is an eating disorder that affects all pediatric age groups.

TABLE 120.1 Etiologies of Pediatric Malnutrition

Inadequate Intake	Increased Metabolic Demand	Malabsorption
Inadequate food availability (e.g., food insecurity, low breastmilk production, restricted diet)	Prematurity	Food allergy (e.g., cow's milk protein allergy, food protein-induced enterocolitis, IgE-mediated food allergy)
Inappropriate food preparation (e.g., formula overdilution)	Infection (e.g., HIV, tuberculosis, giardiasis)	Chronic diarrhea (e.g., chronic nonspecific diarrhea, fructose malabsorption)
Neglect, abuse	Immunodeficiency (e.g., severe combined immunodeficiency)	Anatomic abnormality (e.g., pyloric stenosis, malrotation, superior mesenteric artery syndrome)
Food aversion	Chronic lung disease	Inborn error of metabolism (e.g., galactosemia)
Gastroesophageal reflux	Congenital heart disease	Celiac disease
Mechanical feeding problem (e.g., ankyloglossia, cleft lip, cleft palate)	Oncologic disease (e.g., leukemia)	Inflammatory bowel disease
Oromotor dysfunction (e.g., spinal muscular atrophy, cerebral palsy)	Endocrinopathy (e.g., type 1 diabetes, thyroid disease, growth hormone deficiency)	Pancreatic insufficiency (e.g., cystic fibrosis)
Eating disorder (e.g., rumination, anorexia, bulimia, avoidant-restrictive food intake disorder)	Renal disease (e.g., renal tubular acidosis)	Short gut syndrome
Mood disorder (e.g., depression, anxiety, psychosis)	Genetic syndrome (e.g., Russell-Silver syndrome, Turner syndrome)	Autoimmune enteropathy
Irritable bowel syndrome	Rheumatologic disease (e.g., juvenile idiopathic arthritis)	

HIV, Human immunodeficiency syndrome; *IgE,* immunoglobulin E.

Acute malnutrition triggers metabolic and hormonal changes that cause a series of physiologic changes (Table 120.2), including reduced cardiac output, malabsorption, and coagulopathy. As cellular metabolism shifts from anabolism to catabolism, there is resultant loss of muscle and fat mass. In the absence of adequate glucose intake, glycogenolysis and gluconeogenesis are increased. The basal metabolic rate is initially increased and then decreases. Electrolyte shifts and low protein availability result in edema. Levels of thyroid hormones, insulin, and insulin-like growth factor-1 (IGF-1) decrease, whereas growth hormone and cortisol increase, contributing to wasting. It is now increasingly appreciated that active inflammation directly mediates physiologic changes related to malnutrition. In cancer and infection, proinflammatory mediators (e.g., tumor necrosis factor-α) contribute to anorexia and wasting, a syndrome referred to as cachexia.

Chronic malnutrition is typified by stunting, defined as a length (or height) z score 2 or more standard deviations (SDs) below the population mean for age. Previous studies have established an association between low length for age and poor neurodevelopmental outcomes. However, the role of stunted growth in chronic malnutrition pathogenesis remains poorly understood. In settings where poor hygiene and food quality are common, chronic malnutrition is driven by repeat exposures to pathogens, which can cause small intestinal inflammation, villous atrophy, and dysbiosis. Associated complications include small intestine bacterial overgrowth, fat malabsorption, vitamin deficiency, and impaired immune function.

Malnourished patients are at risk for micronutrient deficiencies. In low-income countries, deficiencies in iron, vitamin A, iodine, and zinc are common. Specific vitamin deficiencies may arise as a result of dietary limitations or malabsorption. For instance, vegan patients are at higher risk for vitamin B_{12} deficiency and patients with fat malabsorption are at risk for deficiencies in vitamins A, D, E, and K.

CLINICAL PRESENTATION

The clinical features of malnutrition are diverse (Table 120.2). Concomitant micronutrient deficiencies may be suggested by specific clinical findings, such as conjunctival buildup of keratin (Bitot spots) in vitamin A deficiency, perifollicular hemorrhages in vitamin C deficiency, and fractures in vitamin D deficiency. The hallmark characteristic of acute malnutrition is wasting, and patients with chronic malnutrition exhibit stunted linear growth. Chronically malnourished infants progress through a sequence of low weight, low height, and ultimately low head circumference.

Extreme physical manifestations of malnutrition are most commonly seen in resource-poor settings. Three distinct forms of extreme protein-energy malnutrition have been described (Fig. 120.1). The first, marasmus, is associated with caloric deficiency and manifests as profound wasting. Affected patients appear emaciated, with reduced subcutaneous fat and prominent bones. They may be lethargic, bradycardic, and hypotensive. The second form, kwashiorkor, reflects a relative deficiency in protein and occurs even in the setting of near-normal caloric intake. Patients exhibit fluid retention, with a protuberant abdomen and pitting edema. The third form, marasmic kwashiorkor, represents a hybrid syndrome featuring both wasting and fluid retention.

Malnutrition related to psychosocial factors, such as inadequate food availability, behavioral difficulties, and health literacy issues, may be corroborated by elements of the history or through direct clinical observation. Findings such as bruises, lacerations, and poor grooming raise suspicion for neglect. Malnutrition secondary to an underlying disease may be suggested by pathognomonic clinical features. For example, postprandial vomiting responsive to acid suppression therapy suggests gastroesophageal reflux disease, while cyanosis and respiratory distress with feedings suggests congenital heart disease. A history of meconium ileus in an infant with chronic cough and clubbing suggests cystic fibrosis, and tooth decay, halitosis, and parotitis raises suspicion for an eating disorder.

EVALUATION

Diagnosis of the underlying cause responsible for malnutrition is greatly informed by the patient's age, clinical history, and physical

TABLE 120.2   Physical Manifestations of Pediatric Malnutrition

Physiologic Changes	Physical Findings[a]
Cardiovascular changes (decreased cardiovascular output, decreased blood volume)	Bradycardia, hypotension, weak pulses, orthostasis, syncope, sunken fontanelle, absent tears, dry mucous membranes, xerosis, poor skin turgor
Altered metabolism (catabolism of host tissues, low protein availability, depletion of glucose stores)	Low subcutaneous fat, low muscle mass, low weight, edema, jitteriness, sweating, fatigue
Electrolyte derangements (increased intracellular sodium, hypokalemia, hypophosphatemia, hypomagnesemia, hypocalcemia)	Edema, arrhythmias, paresthesias, seizures, weakness, tetany, cramps, abnormal deep tendon reflexes, constipation
Decreased gastrointestinal absorption, decreased intestinal motility	Abdominal distension, diarrhea, constipation
Impaired immunity	Signs of concomitant infection
Impaired wound healing	Delayed wound healing, ulceration
Hormonal dysregulation (dysregulation of thyroid, growth hormone, cortisol, and sex hormones)	Low height, fatigue, brittle hair, delayed sexual maturation, cold extremities
Micronutrient deficiencies (deficiencies in vitamin A, vitamin B$_{12}$, vitamin C, vitamin D, folate, iron, thiamine, zinc, and essential fatty acids)	Fatigue, pallor, corneal and conjunctival lesions (e.g., Bitot spots, keratomalacia), stomatitis, cheilosis, gingivitis, defective enamel, delayed suture fusion, prominent forehead, depressed ribs, bowlegs, petechiae, perifollicular hemorrhages, bruising, hemarthrosis, xerosis, skin peeling, hyperpigmentation, spoon-shaped nails, hair loss, flat affect, confusion

[a]Additional, cause-specific physical findings may be observed. Examples include fractures and burns in child abuse, cyanosis in congenital heart disease, bloody stools and perirectal fistulae in inflammatory bowel disease, and halitosis and dorsal hand calluses in bulimia.

examination. The history should include maternal pregnancy history, including relevant diagnostics, medications, and exposures. Maternal testing against human immunodeficiency virus (HIV), hepatitis, and syphilis should be reviewed. Birth history should include gestational age, medical complications, and review of passage of meconium and infant diet.

A review of feeding habits should be performed. The quantity and quality of intake over a 24-to 72-hour period should be documented and compared against estimated energy requirements (Chapter 119). The number of daily meals, intervals between meals, and, in older children, the setting of meals should be discussed. For infants, issues with breastmilk supply, latching, and formula preparation should be identified. Family dietary restrictions and history of adverse reactions to specific foods should be documented.

The timeline of weight loss and intentionality should be clarified. Developmental assessments and growth charts should be reviewed and compared against parental growth. Significant associated events (e.g., family stressors, illness), behaviors (e.g., purging, excessive exercise), and symptoms (e.g., poor suck, lethargy, emesis, diarrhea, respiratory distress) should be elicited. Additionally, the clinician should screen for evidence of dehydration and hypoglycemia.

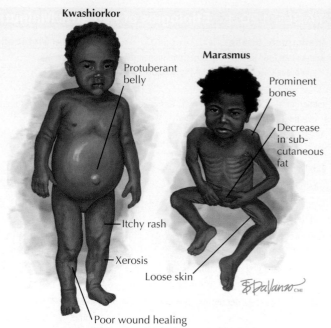

Fig. 120.1 Kwashiorkor and Marasmus.

Food insecurity is an established cause of malnutrition and should be explored. Eligibility for and access to community assistance programs, such as WIC, should be reviewed. The clinician should inquire about potential psychosocial stressors, such as significant changes in family structure (e.g., divorce, death, relocation). Risk factors for neglect should be explored. In select cases, involvement of child protective services may be warranted to assess the safety of the home environment.

Chronic morbidities should be identified during the initial assessment. A history of infections should be documented. A comprehensive review of systems should be performed, including a review of gastrointestinal symptoms (e.g., dysphagia, nausea, early satiety, abdominal pain, emesis, diarrhea, constipation, and bloody stools). The clinician should also inquire about fevers, malaise, neurologic changes, dyspnea, pain, joint swelling, dysuria, rashes, and bruising. Older children should be asked about hair loss, cold intolerance, mood changes, and delayed onset of puberty. As applicable, females should be asked about irregular or absent menses. Family history of early deaths, consanguinity, health issues in immediate family members, and conditions associated with malnutrition (e.g., inflammatory bowel disease, cystic fibrosis, immunodeficiency) should be documented. A careful review of medications may reveal agents that suppress appetite or cause gastrointestinal side effects, such as chemotherapies, antibiotics, stimulants, and anticonvulsants.

Vital signs, including orthostatic vital signs, should be reviewed to assess clinical stability and hydration status. Anthropometric measurements, including weight, recumbent length (age 0 to 2 years) or standing height (age older than 2 years), body mass index (BMI; weight in kilograms divided by height in meters squared), and head circumference (age 0 to 2 years) should be obtained and plotted on appropriate growth charts (Fig. 120.2). Determination of the mid-upper arm circumference (MUAC), a reflection of body composition, may be helpful. In the United States, growth is usually plotted on World Health Organization growth charts form birth until age 2 and on Centers for Disease Control and Prevention growth charts in subsequent years. As applicable, measurements may be plotted on growth charts tailored to specific patient populations. Examples include the Fenton and Olsen growth charts for preterm infants and disease-specific growth charts, such as those used for patients with cerebral palsy and Down syndrome.

Clinical indicators of mild, moderate, and severe malnutrition are based on deficits in growth and nutrient intake (Table 120.3). Agreed upon indicators include low z score for BMI (or weight-for-length), low height (or length), low MUAC, deceleration in z score for BMI or weight, significant weight loss, inadequate weight gain, and inadequate energy intake. Additional diagnostic criteria have been developed for preterm infants (gestational age <37 weeks) and neonates (gestational age ≥37 weeks and up to 28 days old) affected by malnutrition; these include failure to regain birth weight by 14 days, inability to gain about 20 to 30 g/kg/day and decline in weight-for-age z score greater than 0.8 SD below the mean.

A comprehensive physical examination should be performed. Often, the history and physical examination suffice in identifying the cause of malnutrition. Select laboratory studies may be considered to aid with diagnosis and help determine if acute medical intervention is warranted, as in cases of severe dehydration, hypoglycemia, infection, and electrolyte derangements. Diagnostic studies may include complete blood count, chemistry panel, liver function panel, inflammatory markers, Hemoccult testing, fecal elastase, fecal calprotectin, celiac serology, endocrine function testing, and vitamin deficiency screening. As applicable, additional studies such as feeding evaluation, imaging (e.g., video fluoroscopic swallow study, upper gastrointestinal series, or skeletal survey in the case of suspected abuse), and electrocardiography also may be performed. Specialists may be consulted to assist with workup and may include clinical dieticians, speech and language pathologists, gastroenterologists, and nutrition physician specialists.

MANAGEMENT

Management of malnutrition depends on the underlying cause and the severity of malnutrition. Treatment of the underlying cause is essential. Mild-to-moderate malnutrition may be managed in the outpatient setting with close follow-up. As applicable, the primary care provider may involve a lactation consultant, a clinical dietician, a social worker, a speech language pathologist, a behavioral specialist, and other relevant medical specialists. In some cases, patients may be enrolled in a multidisciplinary treatment program, such as family-based therapy, a mainstay of eating disorder treatment. Information about relevant resources, such as supplemental nutrition programs and community support groups, should be provided.

Patients with moderate-to-severe malnutrition may require hospitalization. Indications for hospitalization include clinical instability (e.g., syncope, seizures, severe dehydration), psychosocial emergency (e.g., acute food refusal, risk for neglect or abuse by caregiver), and

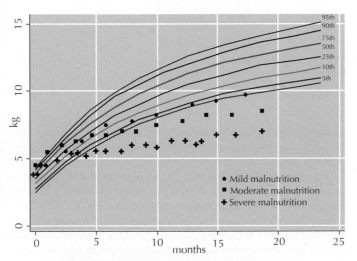

Fig. 120.2 Malnutrition Growth Trajectories.

TABLE 120.3	Criteria for Mild, Moderate, and Severe Pediatric Malnutrition		
Indicator	**Mild Malnutrition**	**Moderate Malnutrition**	**Severe Malnutrition**
Indicators of Neonatal Malnutrition[a]			
Nutrient intake	≤75% of estimated needs for 3–5 days	≤75% of estimated needs for 5–7 days	≤75% of estimated needs for >7 days
Decline in weight for age z score[b]	Decline of 0.8–1.2 SD	Decline of >1.2–2 SD	Decline of >2 SD
Weight gain velocity[b]	>50%–75% of norm	>25%–50% of norm	≤25% of norm
Days to regain birth weight[c]	15–18	19–21	≥22
Linear growth velocity[b,c]	>50%–75% of expected rate	>25%–50% of expected rate	≤25% of expected rate
Decline in length for age z score[b,c]	Decline of 0.8–1.2 SD	Decline of >1.2–2 SD	Decline of >2 SD
Indicators of Pediatric Malnutrition			
Nutrient intake	>50%–75% of estimated needs	>25%–50% of estimated needs	≤25% of estimated needs
Decline in weight for length (height) or body mass index for age	Decline across 1 z score line	Decline across 2 z score lines	Decline across 3 z score lines
Weight loss (age 2–18 years)	>5%–7.5% of usual body weight	>7.5–10% of usual body weight	>10% of usual body weight
Weight gain velocity (age ≤2 years)	>50%–75% of norm	>25%–50% of norm	≤25% of norm
Weight for length z score[c]	z >–2 to –1	z >–3 to –2	z ≤–3
Body mass index for age z score[c]	z >–2 to –1	z >–3 to –2	z ≤–3
Length (height) z score	NA	NA	z ≤–3
Mid-upper arm circumference (age <5 years)	z >–2 to –1	z >–3 to –2	z ≤–3

[a]Applicable for preterm infants and full-term neonates up to 28 days of life.
[b]Applicable only after first 2 weeks of life.
[c]More than one criterion required for malnutrition diagnosis.
NA, Not applicable; *SD,* standard deviations.

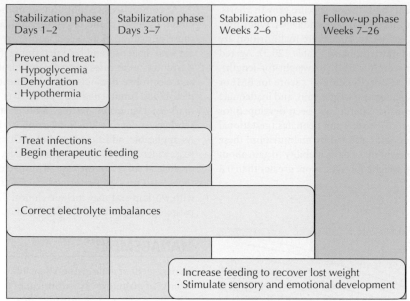

Stabilization phase Days 1–2	Stabilization phase Days 3–7	Stabilization phase Weeks 2–6	Follow-up phase Weeks 7–26

Prevent and treat:
· Hypoglycemia
· Dehydration
· Hypothermia

· Treat infections
· Begin therapeutic feeding

· Correct electrolyte imbalances

· Increase feeding to recover lost weight
· Stimulate sensory and emotional development

Fig. 120.3 Phases in Management of Severe Malnutrition.

failure of outpatient management. The stabilization phase of malnutrition treatment (Fig. 120.3) begins with acute stabilization, and correction of hypoglycemia and dehydration. Patients with severe dehydration should receive intravenous isotonic fluid. As workup for specific vitamin deficiencies is pursued, empiric treatment with multivitamins, including thiamine, iron, and zinc, is appropriate.

Once medical stability is achieved, therapeutic feeding should be initiated, preferably by the enteral route. Parenteral nutrition may be required in select instances (e.g., bowel obstruction, short gut syndrome). Oral rehydration solutions should be administered to correct dehydration, particularly in patients with diarrhea. In resource-poor settings, Rehydration Solution for Malnutrition (ReSoMal) is often used in conjunction with ready-to-use therapeutic food. Actual intake should be tracked and compared against requirements. Disease-specific considerations (e.g., volume limits in congenital heart disease) should be discussed. Caregivers should receive education about feeding cues and appropriate food preparation and administration. For breastfed infants, pre- and post-feed weights should be tracked. Input from a lactation consultant may be beneficial. To promote weight gain, breastmilk or formula may need to be fortified to increase caloric density. Extensively hydrolyzed or amino acid–based formula should be considered for patients with specific intolerances. Cases of oromotor dysfunction may require evaluation by a speech language pathologist, with possible initiation of nasogastric or orogastric feedings.

The nutritional rehabilitation plan should be individualized. Severely malnourished patients should be started at a fraction of goal feeds and closely monitored as feeds are increased, in part because of risk for refeeding syndrome. The clinical manifestations of refeeding syndrome are attributable to a transition from catabolic to anabolic cellular metabolism, which causes intracellular shifts of electrolytes, including potassium, phosphate, and magnesium. Patients may develop paresthesias, edema, or confusion. Further complications

include seizures, muscle paralysis, and heart failure. To reduce the risk for refeeding syndrome, daily electrolytes should be monitored, and deficient minerals should be supplemented.

Caregivers should learn how to create a consistent, supportive environment to facilitate continued recovery. Full recovery may not be achieved until weeks to months after initial diagnosis. Before discharge, patients should demonstrate sustained weight gain on a well-tolerated regimen. If there are concerns about the home environment, a home visit may be warranted. Families should commit to a follow-up plan that includes the primary care provider and relevant specialists.

FUTURE DIRECTIONS

Despite efforts to standardize the definition and categorization of malnutrition, multiple inconsistent definitions have been used, even in recent literature. There are ongoing discussions about the suitability of stunting as a marker for chronic malnutrition at the individual level as well as proposals to categorize malnutrition as illness-associated or non–illness-associated. Longitudinal studies examining clinical outcomes associated with specific subtypes of malnutrition will undoubtedly benefit from consensus definitions. The diagnosis and management of malnutrition-associated vitamin deficiencies as well as malnutrition-associated HIV infection represent additional areas of active interest. Because food insecurity accounts for a significant portion of malnutrition cases, collaboration among clinicians, public health advocates, and legislators will be needed to improve universal access to affordable, nutrient-dense foods to all children.

SUGGESTED READINGS

Available online.

121

Obesity

Zoe M. Bouchelle and Jennifer Robbins

✳ CLINICAL VIGNETTE

A 10-year-old boy presents for a well-child visit. His father reports that he has been well, without any acute illnesses in the past year. Birth and medical history are unremarkable. He has been developing appropriately. Family history is notable for parental obesity and type 2 diabetes. He takes no medications and has no allergies. Review of systems is negative. On examination, he is at the 51st percentile for height for age, 96th percentile for weight for age, and the 98th percentile for body mass index (BMI) for age. Vitals signs are normal. Examination is notable for an obese child with acanthosis nigricans affecting the neck folds. He has had gradual weight gain over the last several years with BMI at the 90th percentile at his visit at 9 years old.

With BMI at the 98th percentile, this child meets criteria for obesity. Obesity is multifactorial with environmental, genetic, and epigenetic influences. The family history of obesity and associated comorbidities suggest a genetic predisposition. Acanthosis nigricans is concerning for its association with the development of insulin resistance. The provider assesses for environmental factors by taking a dietary and activity history and finds that the patient eats 1 or 2 servings of fruits/vegetables daily, drinks juice with each meal, and has 3 to 4 hours of screen time daily. The provider explains the diagnosis of obesity and associated health risks and suggests screening laboratory tests including hemoglobin A1c, liver enzymes, and a lipid panel. Using motivational interviewing, the provider finds that the family is eager to make lifestyle changes, and they set a goal of reducing juice consumption to 6oz daily over the next month. A follow-up visit is scheduled in 4 weeks to review progress toward this goal.

Obesity is one of the most significant public health issues in the United States, and the prevalence is increasing worldwide. As the prevalence of obesity has increased, there has been a concomitant increase in the comorbid conditions associated with obesity, including diabetes, hypertension, dyslipidemia, nonalcoholic fatty liver disease, sleep apnea, early pubertal development, poor body image, and orthopedic problems.

Nearly one in five children and adolescents in the United States meet criteria for being obese, with notable disparities in prevalence among particular demographics. Rates of obesity are higher among American Indian, non-Hispanic black, and Hispanic youth compared with non-Hispanic white and Asian youth. The prevalence of obesity also decreases with increasing household educational attainment and income. There are significant direct and indirect costs associated with childhood obesity, with an even larger cost incurred when children with obesity develop into adults with obesity.

It is critical that health providers have the tools for prevention, diagnosis, and management of obesity in children and adolescents.

ETIOLOGY AND PATHOGENESIS

Obesity is caused by an imbalance between caloric intake and energy expenditure. Its development is often multifactorial with environmental, genetic, and epigenetic influences. Environmental factors, such as sedentary lifestyle, increased intake of calorie-dense foods with low nutritional value, and increased screen time, are implicated in nearly all cases of childhood obesity. Research suggests that obesity is also heritable; children with at least one biological parent with obesity have a 2-fold to 3-fold increased risk for developing obesity in their lifetime, and those with two biological parents with obesity have an up to 15-fold increased risk. Although rare, certain endocrine disorders, syndromes, and hypothalamic lesions are also associated with obesity. Finally, there is increasing evidence that environmental and nutritional status during gestation and infancy can predispose children to obesity through epigenetic mechanisms, termed "metabolic programming."

CLINICAL PRESENTATION

The standard measure of overweight and obesity for children 2 years of age and older is the body mass index (BMI) percentile. Before age 2 years, it is useful to rely on a patient's weight-to-height measurement. BMI percentiles are adjusted for age and sex and account for the typical pattern of increases in weight and height throughout childhood. Weight status definitions are as follows:
- *Underweight:* BMI <5th percentile
- *Normal weight:* BMI 5th to <85th percentile
- *Overweight:* BMI ≥85th to <95th percentile
- *Obese:* BMI ≥95th percentile
- *Severe obesity:* BMI ≥120% of the 95th percentile values or a BMI ≥35 kg/m² (whichever is lower)

BMI is calculated using the formula (weight (kg) ÷ [height (m)²]) and should be plotted on the appropriate standardized graph to ascertain the BMI percentile at every well-child visit.

The history and physical examination of a patient with obesity should focus on identifying treatable causes of obesity and comorbidities. The history should include a dietary assessment with focus on calorie-dense foods with low nutritional value (including sugar-sweetened beverages) and review physical activity and screen time. History should also include general eating behaviors, family dynamics around food, and assessment of food security. Medical history should assess for sleep problems, psychosocial concerns such as depression, and weight-promoting medications. Family history should include any siblings, parents, or grandparents with obesity, hypertension, cardiovascular disease, hyperlipidemia, or type 2 diabetes.

The differential diagnosis for obesity is broad. While the majority of obesity is caused by environmental factors, in rare cases there is an

TABLE 121.1   Evaluation for Comorbidities Associated With Obesity

Comorbidity	Relevant History	Physical Examination Findings	Laboratory and Radiologic Findings
Prediabetes	Family history	Acanthosis nigricans	Hemoglobin A1c, between 5.7% and 6.4% Fasting glucose, ≥100 mg/dL to 125 mg/dL
Diabetes	Family history, polyuria, polydipsia	Acanthosis nigricans	Hemoglobin A1c, ≥6.5% Fasting glucose ≥126 mg/dL
Hypertension	Family history		SBP or DBP≥95% on three separate encounters
Dyslipidemia	Family history	Central fat distribution	Fasting LDL ≥130 or fasting triglycerides ≥100 (age 0–9 years) or ≥130 (age 10–19 years) or fasting HDL <40 mg/dL
NAFLD	Asymptomatic/nonspecific complaints	RUQ pain, hepatomegaly	Elevated AST, ALT Diffusely hyperechogenic and enlarged liver on ultrasonography
Cholelithiasis	Abdominal pain, nausea, fatty food intolerance	RUQ pain, jaundice	Hyperechoic, shadowing, and mobile structures on ultrasonography
Metabolic syndrome	Family history	Waist circumference ≥90th percentile	See criteria for diabetes, hypertension and dyslipidemia
PCOS	Menstrual irregularity	Hirsutism, acne, acanthosis nigricans	Elevated total or free testosterone level Enlarged ovaries with numerous, small, peripheral follicles on ultrasonography
Idiopathic intracranial hypertension	Headache, vision abnormalities	Papilledema	Nonspecific imaging findings including flattening of the posterior sclera and partially empty sella turcica on brain MRI
Sleep apnea	Snoring, daytime sleepiness (may manifest as behavioral problems)	Enlarged tonsils/adenoids	Polysomnography meeting criteria for obstructive sleep apnea
SCFE	Hip, thigh, groin, or knee pain	Altered gait, limited internal rotation of the affected hip	Slipped capital femoral epiphysis on plain radiograph
Blount disease	Knee pain, instability	Altered gait, bowing of the knees	Varus bowing of the tibia on plain radiograph
Depression	Social history (specifically inquire about teasing and bullying)		

ALT, Alanine aminotransferase; *AST*, aspartate aminotransferase; *DBP*, diastolic blood pressure; *HDL*, high-density lipoprotein; *LDL*, low-density lipoprotein; *NAFLD*, nonalcoholic fatty liver disease; *PCOS*, polycystic ovarian syndrome; *RUQ*, right upper quadrant; *SCFE*, slipped capital femoral epiphysis; *SBP*, systolic blood pressure.

underlying genetic, endocrine, or hypothalamic cause (i.e., Prader-Willi syndrome, Beckwith-Wiedemann syndrome, hypothyroidism, high cortisol states, growth hormone deficiency, or hypothalamic lesions).

The physical examination should assess for signs of comorbidities (Table 121.1). It may also reveal evidence of an underlying cause (i.e., marked short stature, decreased linear growth, dysmorphic features, hypogonadism, or abnormal pubertal development) and may merit additional evaluation.

EVALUATION

Laboratory evaluation such as fasting glucose or hemoglobin A1c, liver enzymes, and fasting lipid panel are used to screen patients for common comorbidities. Some providers also screen for vitamin D deficiency (by measuring 25-hydroxyvitamin D) although the utility of routine screening is controversial. Screening may be repeated up to every 2 years or as indicated by risk factors and comorbidities. Further endocrine or genetic testing may be pursued based on history and examination.

MANAGEMENT

Prevention

All children and adolescents should receive family-centered counseling on healthful eating and activity regardless of BMI percentile at

each well-child visit. Simple messages should be repeated early and often. For example, "5210" recommendations may be reviewed at each visit—at least 5 servings of fruits/vegetables, 2 hours or less of recreational screen time, 1 hour or more of physical activity, and 0 sweetened drinks daily. Establishing these habits early can lead to a lifelong preventive approach.

Behavioral

Behavior change is the most useful modality in the treatment of pediatric obesity. Motivational interviewing can be used to assess the readiness of the patient and family to adopt lifestyle changes necessary for obesity management. Lifestyle interventions should focus on all areas of a child's life: home, school, and childcare settings (Fig. 121.1).

A staged approach to pediatric weight management is recommended. Initial management in the primary care setting can focus on positive behavior change and goal setting with visits every 1 to 2 months. Counseling should always use a sensitive, nonjudgmental approach. The provider must be cognizant of and attempt to minimize weight bias and provide information in a way that does not promote body dissatisfaction or disordered eating. The provider should also be aware of family and cultural food preferences and acceptability when making recommendations.

Children ages 2 to 5 with obesity should not lose more than 1 lb per month; older children and adolescents with obesity should not lose

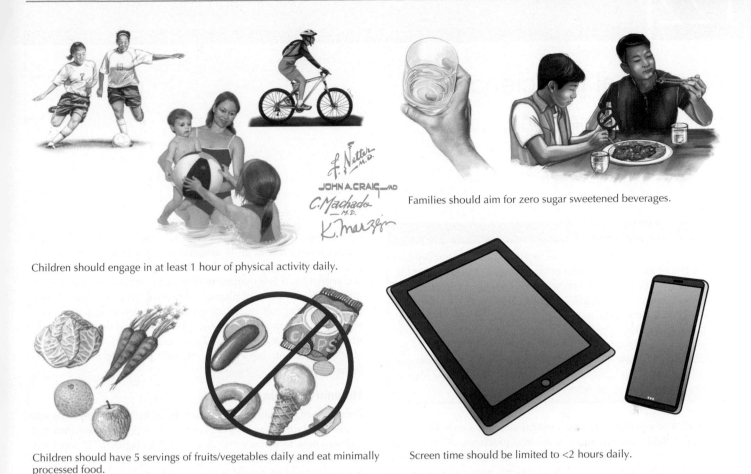

Children should engage in at least 1 hour of physical activity daily.

Families should aim for zero sugar sweetened beverages.

Children should have 5 servings of fruits/vegetables daily and eat minimally processed food.

Screen time should be limited to <2 hours daily.

Fig. 121.1 Lifestyle Interventions for Obesity Prevention and Treatment.

more than 2 lb per week. If after 6 months the BMI status has not stabilized or improved, providers may consider referral to a pediatric weight management clinic for a comprehensive multidisciplinary evaluation and more structured behavioral modification and consideration of pharmacotherapy and/or surgical intervention.

Pharmacotherapy

Pharmacologic treatment of obesity can be considered as an adjunct to dietary and behavioral modifications in adolescents. Orlistat is approved in the United States for weight loss in adolescents. Metformin is approved in the United States for adolescents with type 2 diabetes. Phentermine is approved in the United States for short-term use (12 weeks) in patients over 16 years of age. Many medications approved for weight loss in adults are being studied for efficacy and safety in adolescents. Such medications are considered under the surveillance of an experienced medical provider. Of note, liraglutide is one such medication that was recently approved for treatment of severe obesity in those 12 years of age and older.

Surgery

Surgical weight loss ("bariatric surgery") can be considered for adolescents with severe obesity and with medical comorbidities. The most widely performed procedures in adolescents are the sleeve gastrectomy and Roux-en-Y gastric bypass. These interventions should be performed in centers with experience in treating adolescents and require close follow-up to prevent associated nutrient deficiencies (e.g., iron, vitamin B_{12}, vitamin D, and thiamine) and address any complications. Centers caring for these adolescents should also provide psychological services, and mental health concerns should be addressed both before and after surgery.

FUTURE DIRECTIONS

Although there has been considerable progress in understanding the genetic, epigenetic, and environmental factors that contribute to pediatric obesity, greater investment is needed to identify preventive and treatment interventions that optimize child health into adulthood. Stemming the tide of childhood obesity will require a united and carefully calculated effort from local and federal governments, food manufacturers, health care providers and insurers, school systems, and communities.

SUGGESTED READINGS

Available online.

122

Nutritional Deficiencies

Yoshi M. Rothman and Bridget D. Kiernan

Assessment of a pediatric patient's nutritional status includes evaluation of the child's current and past medical problems, dietary intake, growth parameters, physical examination, and often laboratory tests. Establishing normal growth and development, prevention, and early identification of nutritional deficiencies is the goal in assessing a patient's nutritional status.

DEFICIENCIES

Vitamin A

Vitamin A is a fat-soluble micronutrient that has important roles in vision, immune system function, reproduction, and other metabolic functions. Vitamin A includes retinols, β-carotenes, and carotenoids. Retinols are the most bioactive form and are found in animal proteins. β-Carotenes are derived from plants, including leafy greens, carrots, sweet potatoes, and red and yellow peppers. Vitamin A deficiency, although uncommon in the United States, may be caused by increased requirements, decreased intake (often associated with food insecurity), or decreased intestinal absorption, including any process that decreases fat absorption.

Ocular manifestations are the most specific clinical findings for vitamin A deficiency. An early ophthalmologic consequence of vitamin A deficiency is delayed dark adaptation. As vitamin A deficiency progresses, a patient may develop Bitot spots caused by excessive keratin deposition in the superficial conjunctiva, xerophthalmia, keratomalacia, and ultimately irreversible blindness. However, before ocular findings, epithelial cell function may be altered, which can be illustrated by characteristic dermatologic manifestations, including dry skin, pruritus, dry hair, dry and cracked fingernails, and follicular hyperkeratosis. Deficiency is also associated with anemia, impaired osteoclast activity, and immune dysfunction (Fig. 122.1).

Vitamin B

The vitamin B complex includes eight water-soluble vitamins with distinct roles in cellular metabolism and is essential for neurologic, dermatologic, cardiac, hematologic, and musculoskeletal functioning. Nutritional sources of all B complex vitamins include animal products. Some B complex vitamins can be found in fortified cereals, fruits, and vegetables. It is important to note that vitamin B_{12} is not available through consumption of plants, and this should be considered when caring for vegan and vegetarian patients. Deficiency often arises from poor nutritional intake or malabsorptive states, and there are minimal stores of vitamin B in the body. Treatment with oral supplementation is often sufficient; however, occasionally injectable or intravenous therapy is required.

Thiamin (Vitamin B_1)

Deficiency of thiamin can cause "dry beriberi," with symptoms such as emotional disturbances, peripheral neuropathy, and extremity pain and weakness. Deficiency may also cause "wet beriberi," in which cardiac abnormalities are present (Fig. 122.2). Wernicke encephalopathy, the classic triad of mental status change, ataxia, and ocular symptoms, is rare in young children. Children with thiamine deficiency may instead present with failure to thrive, irritability, lethargy, ocular symptoms such as paralysis of eye movements, and gastrointestinal symptoms such as vomiting and diarrhea. There should be a high suspicion in breastfed infants of mothers with a history of alcoholism, or in adolescents or adults who have had bariatric surgery.

Riboflavin (Vitamin B_2)

Lack of riboflavin is associated with dermatologic findings such as cheilosis, angular cheilitis, glossitis, and seborrheic dermatitis. When maternal intake of riboflavin is low or if absorption is impaired because of birth control pills, congenital anomalies may result, such as cleft lip and palate, growth impairment, and congenital heart disease.

Niacin (Vitamin B_3)

Niacin deficiency initially manifests with nonspecific symptoms such as paresthesias and anorexia. Longer periods of deficiency may lead to pellagra, which is characterized by the classic triad of diarrhea, dermatitis, and dementia. Notably, the US food supply has been fortified with niacin because of high rates of deficiency in the 1930s and 1940s.

Pantothenic Acid (Vitamin B_5)

Pantothenic acid deficiency is quite rare; however, if present, symptoms may include emotional disturbances, fatigue, paresthesias, or muscle cramps.

Pyridoxine (Vitamin B_6)

Pyridoxine deficiency may manifest with failure to thrive, paresthesias, emotional disturbances, and seizures that are refractory to antiepileptic drugs. In infants with seizures resulting from vitamin B_6 deficiency, intramuscular or intravenous pyridoxine is the recommended treatment.

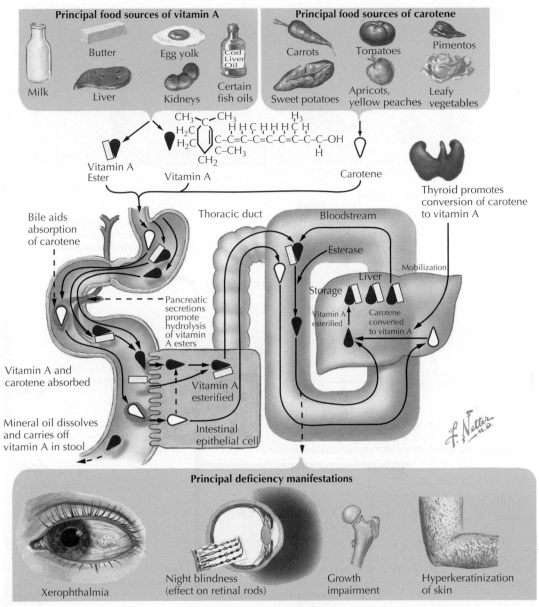

Principal food sources of vitamin A

Milk · Butter · Liver · Egg yolk · Kidneys · Cod Liver Oil · Certain fish oils

Principal food sources of carotene

Carrots · Tomatoes · Pimentos · Sweet potatoes · Apricots, yellow peaches · Leafy vegetables

Vitamin A Ester · Vitamin A · Carotene

Thyroid promotes conversion of carotene to vitamin A

Bile aids absorption of carotene

Thoracic duct · Bloodstream · Esterase

Pancreatic secretions promote hydrolysis of vitamin A esters

Mobilization · Liver · Storage

Vitamin A esterified · Carotene converted to vitamin A

Vitamin A and carotene absorbed

Vitamin A esterified

Mineral oil dissolves and carries off vitamin A in stool

Intestinal epithelial cell

Principal deficiency manifestations

Xerophthalmia · Night blindness (effect on retinal rods) · Growth impairment · Hyperkeratinization of skin

Fig. 122.1 Vitamin A Deficiency.

Biotin (Vitamin B₇)

Deficiency of biotin is rare, but has been linked to periorificial dermatitis, developmental delay, hypotonia, and paresthesias.

Folate (Vitamin B₉)

Folate deficiency in pregnancy may lead to neural tube defects; deficiency in children and adults may lead to macrocytic anemia. Dietary sources of folate include leafy greens, some fruits, and beans. Many breads, flours, and cereals are fortified with folate. Folate deficiency may occur with chronic diarrhea, congenital malabsorptive states, and drug interactions. Deficiency can be suggested by a peripheral blood smear demonstrating hypersegmented neutrophils and macrocytes, and confirmed by a serum folate level. Treatment may include increasing dietary intake, oral supplementation, or injection of folic acid.

Cobalamin (Vitamin B₁₂)

Cobalamin deficiency may lead to megaloblastic anemia, developmental delay, hypotonia, poor growth, and neurologic deficits. Deficiency

is rare in infants because of large vitamin B₁₂ stores but can be found in some inherited disorders of metabolism as well as in infants breastfed by mothers with vitamin B₁₂ deficiencies. More commonly, deficiency results from gastrointestinal malabsorption, or from strict vegan diets that fail to supplement with vitamin B₁₂. Diagnosis of deficiency is evident by a low vitamin B₁₂ level. Treatment of vitamin B₁₂ deficiency includes administration of oral supplementation or intramuscular injection.

Vitamin C (Ascorbic Acid)

Vitamin C plays an important role in collagen synthesis, and therefore skin integrity and wound healing. Citrus fruits are the most well-known source of vitamin C, but it is also present in many other fruits and vegetables. Vitamin deficiency manifests as scurvy with symptoms such as gingival hemorrhages, petechial rash, and ecchymosis caused by defective collagen synthesis of blood vessel walls. Children with vitamin C deficiency may also present with bone tenderness, pseudoparalysis, and poor wound healing. Vitamin C deficiency can be diagnosed

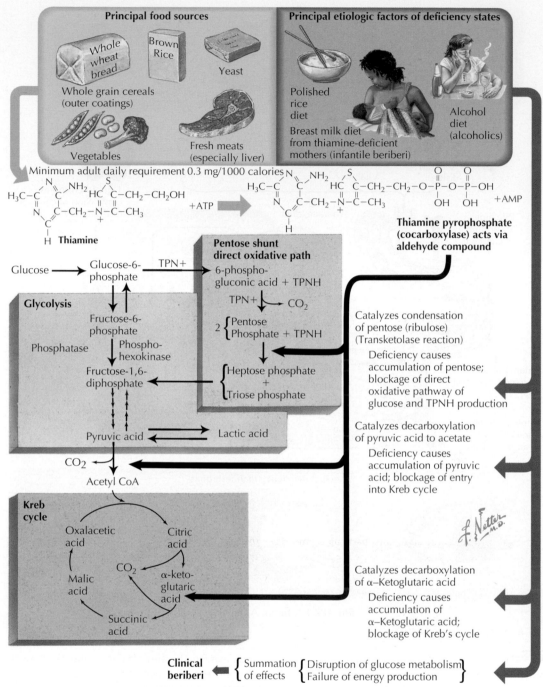

Fig. 122.2 Vitamin B$_1$ (Thiamine) Deficiency (Beriberi).

clinically by assessing physical signs and symptoms and characteristic radiologic findings, such as costochondral beading known as scorbutic rosary (Fig. 122.3).

Vitamin D

Vitamin D plays a major role in bone mineralization by regulating the levels of calcium and phosphorus in the body through absorption in the intestines and reabsorption in the kidney. Vitamin D has also more recently been shown to have roles in cellular growth, immune system and inflammatory response regulation, and neuromuscular function. Vitamin D$_2$ (ergocalciferol) is provided in the diet mostly from plants. Vitamin D$_3$ (cholecalciferol) is found in animal-derived foods such

as eggs and fatty fishes, and is produced in the skin from vitamin D$_2$ when it reacts with ultraviolet B (UVB) light. Many foods such as milk, cereal, and bread are fortified with vitamin D. Both vitamin D$_2$ and D$_3$ are prohormones and are subsequently hydroxylated in both the liver and kidney to become 1,25 dihydroxyvitamin D (1,25[OH]$_2$D), the physiologically active form of vitamin D known as calcitriol.

Vitamin D deficiency may result from a lack of exposure to UVB radiation, inadequate intake, fat malabsorption, or liver or kidney disease, which can impair its conversion to active metabolites, and rarely, genetic disorders. Deficiency is most commonly seen in breastfed infants with inadequate vitamin D supplementation. Dark-skinned children are at increased risk for vitamin D deficiency because

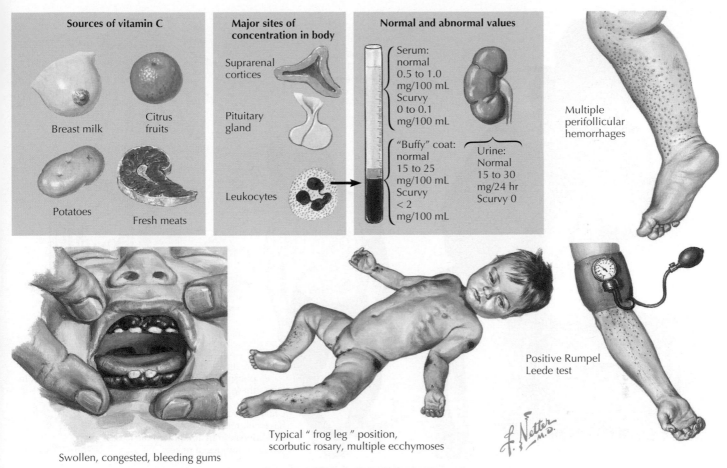

Fig. 122.3 Vitamin C Deficiency (Scurvy).

increased amounts of melanin reduce the production of endogenous vitamin D in response to sunlight exposure. American Academy of Pediatrics (AAP) guidelines, published in 2008, recommend supplementation of 400 IU/day vitamin D for all infants, particularly those who are exclusively or partially breastfed. The AAP also recommends that older children and adolescents who do not obtain 400 IU/day through diet should take a supplement daily.

Deficiency results in disorders of bone mineralization, leading to rickets in children (Fig. 122.4). Clinical presentation may include bone abnormalities such as genu valgus and varus, craniotabes, and costochondral deformities, which produce the classic "rachitic rosary" on chest radiography. Deficiency can also lead to hypophosphatemia or hypocalcemia, which can manifest with tetany or seizures.

Iron

Iron is important for red blood cell synthesis and neurocognitive development. Between birth and 6 months of age, breastmilk provides an adequate supply of highly bioavailable iron so long as the mother has accrued adequate iron stores. Commercial iron-fortified infant formulas are an acceptable alternative to breastmilk. Preterm infants require additional iron, which is usually supplied as an iron supplement or as a multivitamin with iron. At 6 months of age, infants begin to require additional iron that can be obtained from iron-rich foods such as animal products and iron-fortified cereals. Fruits and vegetables also contain iron but in a less bioavailable form. Iron in cow's milk is not very bioavailable and should not be given to any child less than 1 year of age. In children older than 1, no more than 16 to 24 oz of cow's milk should be consumed daily to prevent iron-deficiency.

Iron deficiency primarily manifests as anemia in infants, children, and adolescents. Iron deficiency anemia may lead to impaired neurocognitive development, decreased exercise capacity, pica, and thrombosis. The greatest risk factor for the development of iron-deficiency anemia in infants is introduction of cow's milk before 1 year of age. Additional risks include low iron stores in nursing mothers and cow's milk protein–induced colitis. In children and adolescents, iron deficiency anemia is often secondary to excessive ingestion of cow's milk (>24 oz daily), occult intestinal blood loss, gastrointestinal malabsorptive states such as inflammatory bowel disease, vegetarian or vegan diets, heavy menses in girls, and obesity.

Iron-deficiency anemia has decreased in the past 40 years as a direct result of universal screening guidelines as well as iron fortification of formulas and cereals. It is important for pediatricians to monitor their patients' iron intake because primary prevention is necessary to prevent irreversible mental, motor, and behavioral effects. The AAP recommends screening between 9 and 12 months of age, with additional screening between 1 and 5 years of age for patients at risk. Iron deficiency screening includes assessing dietary iron intake and laboratory testing with a complete blood count (CBC). Although a hemoglobin value determines anemia, a CBC with red blood cell indices helps to delineate iron deficiency from other anemias.

In most cases of iron deficiency anemia, counseling on dietary sources of iron is recommended and treatment with elemental iron is initiated. Repeat laboratory testing should be performed several weeks after treatment is initiated. Further iron therapy and laboratory

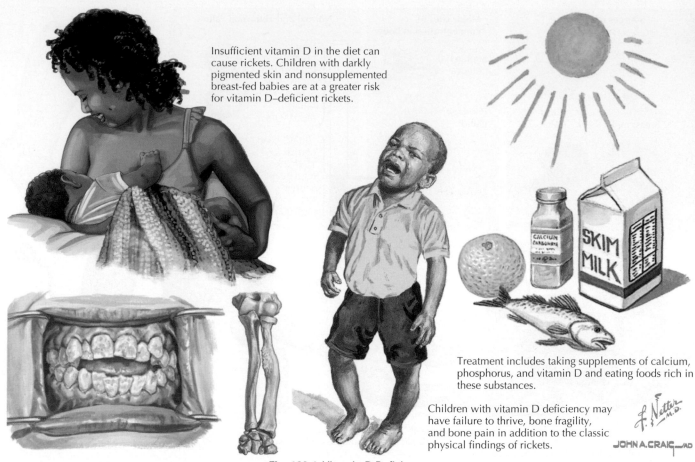

Insufficient vitamin D in the diet can cause rickets. Children with darkly pigmented skin and nonsupplemented breast-fed babies are at a greater risk for vitamin D–deficient rickets.

Treatment includes taking supplements of calcium, phosphorus, and vitamin D and eating foods rich in these substances.

Children with vitamin D deficiency may have failure to thrive, bone fragility, and bone pain in addition to the classic physical findings of rickets.

Fig. 122.4 Vitamin D Deficiency.

monitoring should be continued for at least several months after improvement.

Iodine

Iodine is an essential component of thyroid hormone that is crucial for growth and development. Iodine is absorbed through the intestines in the form of iodide and is then taken up by the thyroid gland for incorporation into thyroxine (T_4) and triiodothyronine (T_3). Before the iodization of salt in 1920, iodine deficiency was endemic in the United States, and it is among the most common preventable causes of intellectual disability worldwide. An iodine deficiency is the most common cause of goiter, an enlargement of the thyroid gland. Iodine deficiency and subsequent thyroid hormone deficiency can manifest with symptoms of hypothyroidism. The most severe consequence of iodine deficiency is congenital hypothyroidism, which manifests with intellectual disability, deaf-mutism, gait abnormalities, and short stature. This can be prevented by adequate iodine intake both during pregnancy and early infancy.

Zinc

Zinc is an essential cofactor necessary for growth and development. Full-term breastfed infants with mothers consuming adequate zinc and formula-fed infants typically have adequate zinc. Children and adolescents can obtain zinc from animal products, legumes, nuts, and fortified-cereals. Zinc deficiency is usually caused by intestinal loss from diarrhea or malabsorptive states but can also be associated with renal disease, malignancy, and skin conditions such as acrodermatitis enteropathica. The clinical diagnosis is supported by findings that include growth failure, an erythematous, scaly rash found on the face and perineal region, and impaired wound healing. Laboratory measurements of zinc are often unreliable because of fluctuations seen in various disease states, thus results must be correlated with the clinical presentation.

FUTURE DIRECTIONS

Research continues to evaluate the role of micronutrient supplementation for pregnant women to prevent congenital anomalies, as well as micronutrient fortification strategies to combat specific nutritional deficiencies globally. Current research is elucidating the more intricate functions of micronutrients in wound healing, metabolism, and immune regulation.

SUGGESTED READINGS

Available online.

Oncology

Lisa Wray

123

Leukemia

Rebecca Whitmire

✳ CLINICAL VIGNETTE

A 9-year-old previously healthy girl was in her usual state of health until 2 weeks before admission when she began to have decreased appetite with subjective weight loss. One week before admission, she developed a sore throat, diffuse myalgias, gum bleeding, and fatigue. On the evening of admission, she developed exertional dyspnea and so presented to the emergency department. On review of systems, the family noted easy bruising with only mild trauma over the past 1 to 2 months and, more recently, facial pallor. They denied fevers, night sweats, nausea, vomiting, abdominal pain, cough, upper respiratory tract infectious symptoms, rashes, bony pain, dysuria, hematuria, melena, hematochezia, or changes in urine output. In the emergency room, she was febrile to 100.8°F (38.2°C), tachycardic, tachypneic, and normotensive while maintaining an oxygen saturation of 100% on room air. On physical examination she was noted to be pale with petechiae on her buccal mucosa and ecchymoses on her shins and left lower quadrant of her abdomen. There was no increased work of breathing, and her lungs were clear to auscultation bilaterally; there were no murmurs appreciated. Her abdominal examination demonstrated both hepatomegaly and splenomegaly. Complete blood count with differential and peripheral smear, lactate dehydrogenase, uric acid, coagulation panel, type and screen, and comprehensive metabolic panel were obtained and notable for normocytic anemia, thrombocytopenia, and leukocytosis with 85% blasts and an absolute neutrophil count of 180 cells/μL, elevated uric acid, hyperkalemia, hyperphosphatemia, and hypocalcemia. A chest radiograph was obtained and did not demonstrate a mediastinal mass. Immediate management included transfusions with red blood cells and platelets, initiation of tumor lysis precautions with allopurinol and hyperhydration with alkalinized fluids, and starting empiric antibiotic therapy with cefepime after blood cultures were obtained. She was admitted to the oncology service. Bone marrow aspirate and biopsy confirmed a diagnosis of acute lymphoblastic leukemia (B-ALL) and lumbar puncture confirmed no central nervous system (CNS) disease. She began induction therapy with cytarabine, vincristine, dexamethasone, and pegaspargase. The patient's family met frequently with the oncology team, including the oncology social worker. They received oncology education, support to address the challenges surrounding a new cancer diagnosis, and resources to address their additional needs of food insecurity.

Leukemia is the most common childhood cancer, comprising 31% of pediatric malignancies with over 3100 new diagnoses annually in the United States in children younger than 15 years of age. Pediatric leukemia is a malignant clonal proliferation of mutated hematopoietic progenitor cells. Subtypes of leukemia are classified by cell lineage of origin, the most common of which is acute lymphoblastic leukemia (ALL). ALL accounts for 77% of all pediatric leukemia diagnoses. Acute myelogenous leukemia (AML) accounts for roughly 20% of all pediatric leukemias. Chronic myelogenous leukemia (CML) accounts for about 3% of pediatric leukemias (Fig. 123.1).

Survival rates continue to improve as genetic and molecular understanding of pediatric leukemias improve and are used to develop targeted therapies. Pediatric ALL has a survival rate of nearly 90%, and pediatric AML has a survival rate of approximately 70%.

EPIDEMIOLOGY AND PATHOGENESIS

Peak incidence of ALL occurs at 2 to 4 years old. AML has a bimodal distribution with peak incidence at 2 years of age or younger and between 13 and 20 years old. Pediatric CML peak incidence occurs in adolescence (Fig. 123.2).

Leukemia is caused by mutations affecting cell deoxyribonucleic acid (DNA) processes and death that permit the uncontrolled proliferation and impaired apoptosis of clones of mutated and dysfunctional hematopoietic blast cells. Although the cause of leukemia is almost always unknown, certain environmental exposures can increase the risk for leukemia, including exposure to ionizing radiation, alkylating agents (including chemotherapeutic agents), epipodophyllotoxins, and benzene.

Incidence of leukemia temporally correlates with age of initial infectious exposures for children in developed countries. Pediatric leukemia incidence is higher in developed nations than in developing nations. Additionally, studies assessing the odds for ALL diagnosis in children with and without daycare attendance and early childhood infections have demonstrated that children with early daycare attendance and earlier onset of exposure to childhood infections had decreased odds for developing ALL.

There are known racial and socioeconomic disparities in pediatric leukemia outcomes. Black children with AML are twice as likely to die during induction therapy as are White children. Publicly insured children also have significantly higher mortality rates during AML therapy than do privately insured children. Given that race is primarily a social construct rather than a biologic driver of disease, additional research is needed to better understand the factors contributing to both racial and socioeconomic disparities in leukemia outcomes in order to design interventions addressing these disparities.

Genetics

Fewer than 5% of all pediatric leukemia diagnoses can be explained by genetic syndromes (Box 123.1) or by prior chemotherapy or radiation exposure. Studies of twin concordance rates, neonatal blood spots (Guthrie cards), and cord blood demonstrate that mutations frequently seen in leukemic cells can be present at birth in both healthy patients and in patients later diagnosed with leukemia. For instance, a survey of several hundred umbilical cord blood samples demonstrated that 1% of newborns had a functional TEL-AML1, which is the most frequently identified chromosomal translocation in molecular analysis of patients with B-ALL. However, this rate is 100 times higher than the rate of childhood ALL in the general population, suggesting that these mutations are necessary but not sufficient to cause pediatric leukemia.

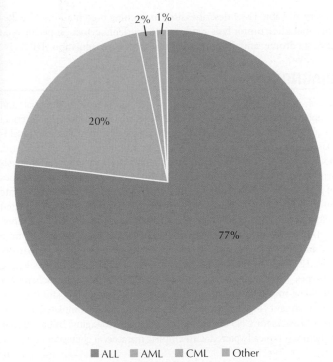

Fig. 123.1 Prevalence of Pediatric Leukemias. (Data from Raetz EA, Teachey DT. T-cell acute lymphoblastic leukemia. *Hematology Am Soc Hematol Educ Program.* 2016;2016(1):580-588. https://doi.org/10.1182/asheducation-2016.1.580; Elgarten CW, Aplenc R. Pediatric acute myeloid leukemia: updates on biology, risk stratification, and therapy. *Curr Opin Pediatr.* 2020;32(1):57-66. https://doi.org/10.1097/MOP.0000000000000855; Pui CH, Yang JJ, Hunger SP, et al. Childhood acute lymphoblastic leukemia: progress through collaboration. *J Clin Oncol.* 2015;33:2938-2948.)

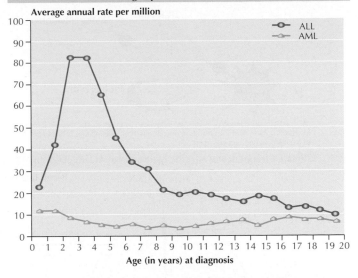

Race/Ethnicity	Male	Female
All races	1.9 per 100,000 men	1.4 per 100,000 women
White	2.0 per 100,000 men	1.5 per 100,000 women
Black	1.1 per 100,000 men	0.8 per 100,000 women
Asian/Pacific Islander	1.6 per 100,000 men	1.3 per 100,000 women
American Indian/Alaska Native	1.3 per 100,000 men	
Hispanic	2.4 per 100,000 men	2.1 per 100,000 women

*All statistics in this report are based on SEER incidence statistics. Most can be found within:

Altekruse SF, Kosary CL, Krapcho M, et al. *SEER Cancer Statistics Review, 1975-2007.* Bethesda, MD: National Cancer Institute. http://seer.cancer.gov/csr/1975_2007/, based on November 2009 SEER data submission, posted to the SEER web site, 2010.

Fig. 123.2 Incidence Rates of Acute Lymphoblastic Leukemia and Acute Myelogenous Leukemia.

BOX 123.1 Genetic Conditions Associated With Increased Risk of Leukemia

General Syndromes
- Trisomy 21
- Neurofibromatosis type 1
- Paroxysmal nocturnal hemoglobinuria
- Li-Fraumeni syndrome

Bone Marrow Failure Syndromes
- Fanconi anemia
- Schwachman-Diamond syndrome
- Kostmann syndrome
- Bloom syndrome

Primary immunodeficiencies
- Severe combined immunodeficiency
- Ataxia telangiectasia

Several genetic mutations have been identified as important prognostic factors in ALL and AML and are used to drive risk stratification and treatment protocols; evaluating cancer cell cytogenetics is thus a routine part of leukemia diagnosis (Fig. 123.3). Analysis of copy number variations across all ALL subtypes demonstrates that 40% of involved genes affect B cell differentiation and the rest affect cell cycle regulation, apoptotic pathway modifiers, and drug metabolism.

Genetic probes reflecting blast cell molecular biology profiles are used to detect small numbers of blast cells and have become essential to measuring disease activity throughout treatment. Use of this technology to measure blast cells at a threshold of 0.01% of marrow cells is defined as measurement of minimal residual disease (MRD). MRD measurement is used to guide therapy throughout treatment and serves as a strong prognostic factor.

Genetic polymorphism testing is also used to predict chemotherapy toxicity at the patient level. For instance, patients with leukemia frequently undergo pharmacogenetic testing for thiopurine-S-methyltransferase (*TPMT*) polymorphisms. This information allows for preemptive dose adjustments to chemotherapy while minimizing adverse effects.

CLINICAL PRESENTATION

Signs and symptoms of leukemia are consequences of bone marrow failure resulting from leukemic cell infiltrate (Fig. 123.4). These include signs and symptoms of anemia (pallor, shortness of breath, decreased exercise tolerance, lightheadedness/syncope, palpitations, tachycardia, dizziness, and orthostasis), thrombocytopenia (abnormal bleeding and bruising), and leukopenia (frequent infections). Signs and symptoms

of leukemic infiltrate of the marrow, lymph nodes, spleen, and mediastinum include bone pain (especially in long bones), hepatosplenomegaly, lymphadenopathy, and both symptomatic and asymptomatic anterior mediastinal masses. Constitutional symptoms such as fevers, malaise, decreased appetite, fatigue, and weight loss are frequently

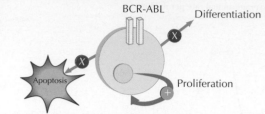

Pathways affected by BCR-ABL

Many signal transduction pathways are influenced by the BCR-ABL tyrosine kinase. Interrupting these pathways results in uncontrolled cell proliferation, a halt in cell differentiation, and reduced apoptosis.

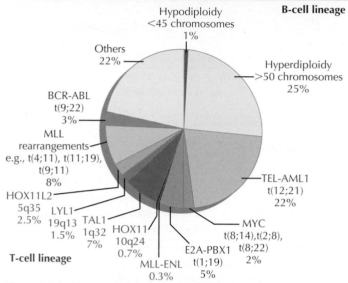

Estimated frequency of specific genotypes of ALL in children

The genetic lesions that are exclusively seen in cases of T-cell lineage leukemias are indicated in purple. All other genetic subtypes are either exclusively or primarily seen in cases of B-cell lineage ALL.

Reprinted with permission from Pui CH, Relling MV, Downing JR. Acute lymphoblastic leukemia. N Engl J Med. 2004;350:1535-1548.

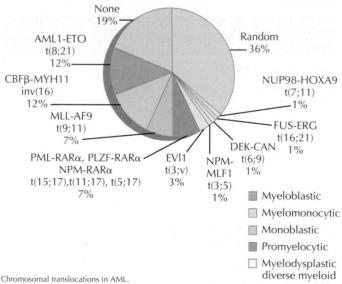

Estimated frequency of specific genotypes of AML in children

Chromosomal translocations in AML.

Reprinted with permission from Look AT. Oncogenic transcription factors in the Human Acute Leukemias. Science 1997;278:1059-1064.

Fig. 123.3 Genetics of Acute Lymphoblastic Leukemia and Acute Myelogenous Leukemia.

observed. Table 123.1 describes life-threatening presentations of leukemia, including tumor lysis syndrome, hyperleukocytosis, superior vena cava syndrome, and disseminated intravascular coagulation (DIC).

DIAGNOSIS

Initial workup includes complete blood count with differential and peripheral smear. Manual differential is essential as automated differential frequently misclassifies lymphoblasts as atypical lymphocytes and myeloblasts as monocytes; this can falsely suggest infectious diagnoses. Uric acid, potassium, calcium, and phosphorus are obtained to assess for tumor lysis syndrome. Coagulation studies should also be obtained as certain subtypes of AML often manifest as DIC. Chest radiograph is obtained to evaluate for mediastinal mass, which can be asymptomatic; this must be completed before diagnostic procedures requiring sedation to prevent airway collapse.

Definitive diagnosis of AML and ALL requires bone marrow aspirate and biopsy with identification of more than 25% blast cells in marrow (Fig. 123.5). Morphology of marrow cells is used to classify leukemic subtypes. Flow cytometry, cytogenetics, and immunohistochemistry provide a molecular profile of the cancer that guides risk stratification and treatment (Fig. 123.6). Lumbar puncture is also completed at diagnosis to assess for CNS disease, which is crucial to staging. Initial lumbar puncture is typically paired with empiric intrathecal chemotherapy.

DIFFERENTIAL DIAGNOSIS

Childhood leukemia can present similarly to more common childhood illnesses, including Epstein-Barr virus (EBV), cytomegalovirus (CMV), infectious lymphadenitis, coxsackievirus, parvovirus, postinfectious myelosuppression, idiopathic thrombocytopenic purpura, juvenile idiopathic arthritis, transient erythrocytopenia of childhood, and human immunodeficiency virus (HIV). Bone marrow analysis is required to confirm a diagnosis of leukemia.

Acute Lymphoblastic Leukemia
Classification
The World Health Organization (WHO) morphologic classification subdivides ALL into three categories: B lymphoblastic leukemia (85% of ALL diagnoses), T lymphoblastic leukemia (~15% of ALL diagnoses), and mature B-cell or Burkitt leukemia (<1% of ALL diagnoses).

Flow cytometry in patients with B-ALL demonstrates the presence of B cell surface markers (CD19, CD20, CD22, CD79a, CD10, and CD34) with absent T cell surface markers. Flow cytometry in patients with T-ALL demonstrates the presence of T cell surface markers (CD2, CD3, CD4, CD5, CD7, and CD8), the presence of terminal deoxynucleotidyl transferase, and the absence of B cell surface markers. Cytogenetic analysis provides important prognostic markers and guides risk stratification and treatment (Table 123.2).

Patients with B-ALL are stratified as standard or high risk at diagnosis. Standard risk criteria include age 1 to 10 years, white blood cell (WBC) count less than 50,000, absence of testicular disease, and CNS stage 1 or 2 disease. Patients younger than 1 year, leukemia with the Philadelphia chromosome, and patients with trisomy 21 have unique treatment plans. After induction therapy, patients are re-stratified based on day 29 bone marrow MRD.

Patients with T-ALL undergo risk stratification (standard risk, intermediate risk, and very high risk) based on steroid pretreatment, CNS and/or testicular disease, and MRD testing during therapy. Many cytogenetic abnormalities with prognostic implications in B-ALL are not frequently observed in T-ALL.

Mixed phenotypic acute leukemia (MPAL) accounts for 3% to 5% of all pediatric leukemias and is defined as poorly differentiated and

Acute lymphoblastic leukemia (ALL), acute myeloid leukemia (AML), and chronic myelogenous leukemia (CML)

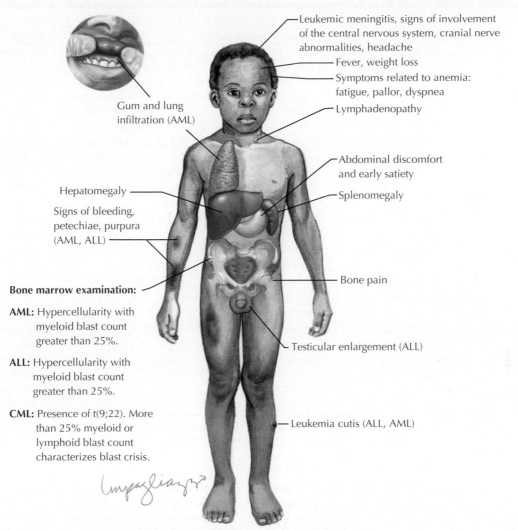

Leukemic meningitis, signs of involvement of the central nervous system, cranial nerve abnormalities, headache

Fever, weight loss

Symptoms related to anemia: fatigue, pallor, dyspnea

Lymphadenopathy

Gum and lung infiltration (AML)

Abdominal discomfort and early satiety

Splenomegaly

Hepatomegaly

Signs of bleeding, petechiae, purpura (AML, ALL)

Bone pain

Bone marrow examination:

AML: Hypercellularity with myeloid blast count greater than 25%.

ALL: Hypercellularity with myeloid blast count greater than 25%.

CML: Presence of t(9;22). More than 25% myeloid or lymphoid blast count characterizes blast crisis.

Testicular enlargement (ALL)

Leukemia cutis (ALL, AML)

Fig. 123.4 Clinical Presentation of Leukemia.

TABLE 123.1	**Life-Threatening Presentations and/or Complications of Leukemia**			
Life-Threatening Presentation	**Pathophysiology**	**Clinical Manifestations**	**Epidemiology**	**Treatment**
Febrile neutropenia, bacteremia, and sepsis	Organisms of concern: • **Gram negative: *Pseudomonas*,** *Escherichia coli, Klebsiella, Enterobacter* • **Gram positive:** *Staphylococcus aureus,* coagulase-negative staphylococci, *Streptococcus viridans* • **Viruses:** herpes simplex virus (HSV) and varicella zoster virus (VZV) • **Fungi** (less common): *Candida*	Symptoms can be mild, including isolated neutropenia, and can quickly progress to sepsis/septic shock	Patients at high risk of serious bacterial illness: • **Patient factors**: Ill-appearing, central access, age <6 months, implanted devices (shunts) • **Disease status:** relapsed leukemia with active disease, surgery in the past 2 weeks, bone marrow transplant within the past 12 months • **Laboratory test results:** ANC <200 or <500 and falling, prolonged neutropenia (>7 days)	**Initiate broad workup:** • Blood cultures, consider urine culture, CBC with differential (check ANC) • Promptly initiate broad-spectrum antibiotic therapy • Early sepsis recognition and management: fluids, electrolyte management, pressors

Continued

TABLE 123.1   Life-Threatening Presentations and/or Complications of Leukemia—cont'd

Life-Threatening Presentation	Pathophysiology	Clinical Manifestations	Epidemiology	Treatment
Tumor lysis syndrome	Rapid cell death/lysis leading to release of intracellular contents	Hyperuricemia, hyperkalemia, hyperphosphatemia, and hypocalcemia with increased risk of acute renal failure and arrhythmias	Increased risk in patients with ALL, elevated WBC count at presentation, anterior mediastinal mass (especially in patients with T-ALL), and Burkitt leukemia	Hyperhydration Reduce hyperuricemia: allopurinol or urate oxidase Frequent monitoring of electrolytes and renal function
Typhlitis	Necrotizing enterocolitis in the setting of neutropenia	Acute onset or severe abdominal pain ± signs of peritonitis on examination	Most frequently occurs in patients with profound neutropenia	Abdominal imaging, broad-spectrum antibiotics, bowel rest, pain control, and surgical management if perforation
Hyperleukocytosis	Increased WBC count resulting in increased blood viscosity and subsequent sludging	WBC >100,000/μL Hyperviscosity syndrome: stroke, renal insufficiency, pulmonary infarcts	AML > ALL	Hyperhydration Rapid initiation of chemotherapy Exchange transfusion or leukapheresis
Hemorrhage or DIC	Consumptive coagulopathy Thrombocytopenia	CNS hemorrhage Retinal hemorrhage Thrombosis	APL (M3 AML)	All-trans retinoic acid/chemotherapy Blood product support
Airway compression or SVC syndrome	Anterior mediastinal mass compression of the superior vena cava, airway, and other mediastinal structures	*Respiratory distress*, cough, orthopnea, changes in vocal quality *Headache, syncope* *Facial swelling/plethora* *Cardiogenic shock*	T-cell ALL	*Chest radiography* before sedation or anesthesia *Careful respiratory monitoring* in ICU *Treat leukemia rapidly* ± Steroids, radiation therapy

ALL, Acute lymphoblastic leukemia; *AML*, acute myelogenous leukemia; *ANC*, absolute neutrophil count; *APL*, acute promyelocytic leukemia; *CBC*, complete blood count; *CNS*, central nervous system; *DIC*, disseminated intravascular coagulopathy; *ICU*, intensive care unit; *SVC*, superior vena cava; *WBC*, white blood cell.

heterogeneous cancer cells with morphologic and immunologic properties of both myeloid and lymphoid blast cells. Research is ongoing to identify the most effective treatment regimens; currently, ALL therapy is considered the first-line chemotherapy regimen, with AML therapy and stem cell transplant used for patients with poorly responsive disease.

Nearly 80% of infants with ALL and about 50% of infants with AML have *KMT2A* mutations (previously called *mixed lineage leukemia [MLL]* gene mutation) resulting from translocation 11q23. These leukemias have aggressive clinical courses and are associated with poor outcomes of 40% to 50% 5-year survival, despite intensive chemotherapy and hematopoietic stem cell transplant.

Clinical Presentation

Pancytopenia is common at ALL diagnosis. Half of children will have hepatosplenomegaly and lymphadenopathy at diagnosis, and 50% to 60% of patients with T-ALL will have an anterior mediastinal mass. Few patients (2% to 3%) will have symptoms of CNS infiltration at diagnosis.

Treatment

Treatment of ALL is accomplished by multiagent chemotherapy with intensive therapy for 6 to 9 months, plus 2 to 3 years of maintenance therapy. Stages of therapy include induction (1 month of therapy with goal of inducing remission—includes a steroid, vincristine, pegaspargase, ± anthracycline, as well as intrathecal cytarabine and methotrexate), consolidation (1 to 2 months based on risk; includes prophylactic CNS treatment), interim maintenance (2 months relative respite from myelosuppressive chemotherapy with escalating doses of methotrexate), delayed intensification (2 months of reinduction and

reconsolidation), and maintenance therapy (lower dose, outpatient chemotherapy for 2 years for girls and 3 years for boys).

Patients with T-ALL have historically had poorer outcomes than patients with B-ALL; however, with more aggressive chemotherapy regimens for T-ALL, this gap is decreasing. Cranial radiation therapy was previously used for most patients with T-ALL and is now either eliminated from treatment regimens or reserved for patients with T-ALL with persistent positive MRD after consolidation or high CNS disease burden.

Approximately 3% to 4% of all childhood cancers are Philadelphia chromosome–positive (Ph[+]) leukemia (chromosome 9;22 translocation results in a BCR-ABL fusion protein). Targeted molecular therapy with imatinib, a receptor tyrosine kinase inhibitor, is added to intensive chemotherapy to treat patients with Ph(+) leukemia.

Adolescent and young adult patients with leukemia have been demonstrated to have improved outcomes using pediatric therapy protocols compared with adult protocols.

Relapse

Early relapse (within 18 months of diagnosis) has an extremely poor survival rate of less than 20%. Intermediate relapse (between 18 and 36 months from diagnosis) confers a survival rate of 18% to 36%. Late relapse (>36 months after diagnosis) has a survival rate of about 40%. Bone marrow transplant is the current standard relapse therapy; outcomes are best when remission is reinduced before transplant. Chimeric antigen receptor therapy (CART) is used in refractory or relapsed B-ALL; a patient's own T cells are isolated and transduced with a viral vector resulting in expression of receptors that bind CD19 on B cells. These engineered T cells are reintroduced into the patient, allowing the CART cells to bind to

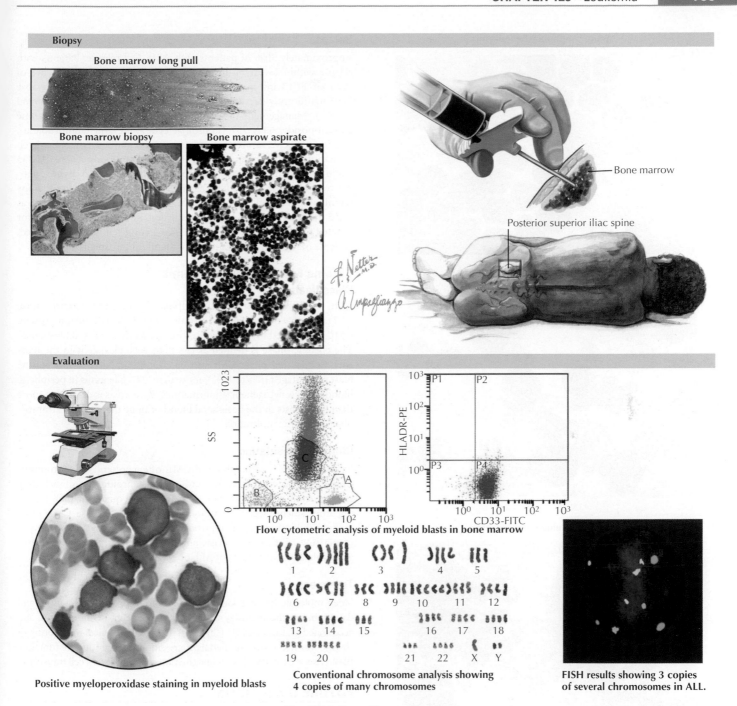

Biopsy

Bone marrow long pull

Bone marrow biopsy   **Bone marrow aspirate**

Bone marrow

Posterior superior iliac spine

Evaluation

Flow cytometric analysis of myeloid blasts in bone marrow

Positive myeloperoxidase staining in myeloid blasts

Conventional chromosome analysis showing 4 copies of many chromosomes

FISH results showing 3 copies of several chromosomes in ALL.

Fig. 123.5 Bone Marrow Biopsy

and kill malignant and healthy B cells expressing CD19. Additional immunotherapies used in relapsed ALL include blinatumomab, a bi-specific T cell engager that binds CD19(+) B cells as well CD3(+) T cells. This allows the body's T cells to be co-localized to and activated against leukemic B cells.

Acute Myelogenous Leukemia
Classification
The French-American-British (FAB) classification divides AML into subtypes M0 to M7 based on cell type and differentiation. The WHO classifies AML by morphology, flow cytometry, genetic mutations, and chromosomal abnormalities (Table 123.3). Staining for myeloperoxidase on bone marrow analysis helps confirm myelogenous cell origin. Cytogenetic analysis provides important prognostic markers (Table 123.2).

Clinical Presentation
Similar to ALL, patients with AML frequently present with signs and symptoms of bone marrow failure, constitutional symptoms, and symptoms of secondary organ infiltrate. In contrast to ALL, patients with AML may present with masses of tumor cells called chloromas; these may be found in the orbits or epidural space. Chloromas are frequently associated with AML t(8;21) and can rarely occur in the absence of bone marrow involvement. Leukemic infiltrate of the skin (leukemia cutis) occurs more frequently in patients with AML than in patients with ALL; lesions often appear violaceous and can be hemorrhagic.

Treatment
Treatment of AML begins with induction therapy (including intrathecal chemotherapy) with cytarabine and anthracycline-based myelosuppressive chemotherapy. Approximately 85% of patients achieve remission

Acute lymphoblastic leukemia

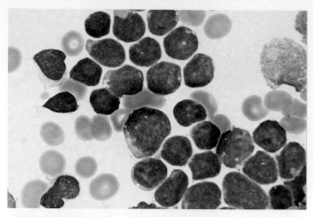

Acute myelogenous leukemia

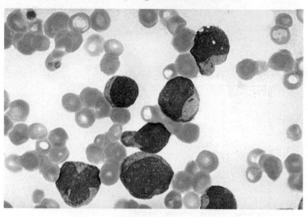

Chronic myelogenous leukemia

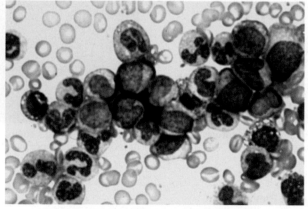

Fig. 123.6 Blood Smears of Leukemias.

after completion of induction therapy. Based on postinduction MRD and cancer cytogenetics, patients are risk stratified; patients at higher risk for poor outcomes progress to hematopoietic stem cell transplant after three total cycles of chemotherapy. Patients with no detectable MRD and more favorable cytogenetics such as t(8;21) and inv(16) complete consolidation with high-dose cytarabine for a total of four to five cycles of intensive chemotherapy. Children with trisomy 21 and AML have a unique classification of AML with almost uniformly *GATA1* mutation characterized disease; these children (especially those younger than 4 years old) generally have increased chemotherapy responsiveness and higher remission rates than other children with AML and therefore make up a subgroup for which dose reduction treatment protocols are ongoing.

Relapse

Approximately 30% of patients with AML will relapse. Patients with relapse within 1 year of diagnosis and patients with the presence of WT1 or FLT3 internal tandem duplications (ITDs) at first relapse have significantly decreased rates of second remission and of survival (~10%). Management of relapse may include high-dose cytarabine and etoposide, CPX-351 (liposomal cytarabine and daunorubicin), venetoclax (bcl-2 inhibitor), and conjugated antibody therapies such as gemtuzumab ozogamicin (a monoclonal antibody against CD33 conjugated to the antitumor antibiotic calicheamicin). Trials are ongoing to assess efficacy of these agents as part of initial chemotherapy regimens for AML. Use of additional small molecule inhibitors such as FLT3 inhibitors are also being investigated. Radiation may be used for isolated testicular or CNS relapse. Once second remission is achieved, patients may undergo hematopoietic stem cell transplant.

Chronic Myelogenous Leukemia
Classification

CML is characterized by Philadelphia chromosome (translocation 9;22) presence in leukemic cells resulting in BCR-ABL fusion protein. CML is described in three phases: chronic, accelerated, and blast crisis. The chronic phase is defined as less than 10% blast cells in the marrow. Accelerated phase CML can be established based on increasing blast percentage (10% to 19%), more than 20% basophils in peripheral blood, or new cytogenetic abnormalities. Blast crisis is defined as more than 20% blasts in the peripheral blood or bone marrow or extramedullary leukemic infiltration.

Clinical Presentation

Patients in the chronic phase of CML often present with symptoms caused by hyperleukocytosis and marrow proliferation, including respiratory distress, bone pain, and left upper quadrant pain resulting from splenomegaly. Symptoms of accelerated phase CML often include abdominal pain from worsening splenomegaly and symptoms of marrow failures. Blast crisis phase symptoms are largely indistinguishable from symptoms of ALL or AML.

Treatment

Small molecule tyrosine kinase inhibitors (TKIs), such as imatinib and dasatinib, are the mainstay of therapy for patients in the chronic and accelerated phases of CML. Chronic TKI therapy requires monitoring of thyroid, cardiac, growth/pubertal progression, and reproductive function. Blast crisis is treated with systemic chemotherapy and stem cell transplant.

FUTURE DIRECTIONS

As targeted therapies improve, studies are ongoing to incorporate these into upfront treatment rather than reserving them for relapsed and refractory disease. For instance, clinical trials are currently assessing blinatumomab's efficacy in initial consolidation therapy for specific subsets of patients with B-ALL. Additional research is needed to better understand molecular drivers of relapse, and targeted therapies are needed to address these pathogenic factors. Improved understanding of biologic drivers of clinical severity in leukemia will help refine risk stratification to provide effective chemotherapy regimens while minimizing toxicity. Finally, a deeper understanding of the ways in which social determinants of health contribute to racial and socioeconomic disparities in leukemia outcomes will provide opportunities for interventions to achieve equity in care for patients with leukemia.

SUGGESTED READINGS

Available online.

TABLE 123.2 Cytogenetics With Prognostic Significance

Cytogenetic Abnormality	Product/Function	Prognostic Significance
B-ALL		
Hyperdiploidy	>50 chromosomes	Favorable
t(12;21)	*ETV6-RUNX1* fusion gene	Favorable
Hypodiploidy	<45 chromosomes	Unfavorable
iAMP21	Internal duplication/amplification of chromosome 21 at the *RUNX1* gene	Unfavorable
Trisomy 4		Favorable
Trisomy 10		Favorable
Trisomy 17		Favorable
Phl chromosome t(9;22)	BCR-ABL fusion protein	Unfavorable
KMT2A (MLL) rearrangements, 11q23 abnormalities	KMT2A fusion proteins	Unfavorable
AML		
t(8;21)	*RUNX1-RUNX1T1* fusion	Favorable
CEPBA mutations	In-domain mutations and truncated protein product	Favorable
NPM1 mutations	Localization of NPM1 protein into the cytoplasm	Favorable
inv(16)(p13.1;q22) or t(16;16)(p13.1;q22)	CBFB-MYH11 fusion protein that sequesters CBFA2 in the cytoplasm, affecting differentiation of myeloid leukemia cells	Favorable
FMS-like tyrosine kinase (Flt3) internal tandem duplication (ITD)	Increased Flt3 activity	Unfavorable
Monosomy 5		Unfavorable
Monosomy 7		Unfavorable
KMT2A(MLL) rearrangements, 11q23 abnormalities	KMT2A fusion proteins	Unfavorable
t(6;9)	*DEK-NUP214* fusion	Unfavorable
t(7;12)	*MNX-ETV6* fusion	Unfavorable

TABLE 123.3 World Health Organization Classification of Acute Myeloid Leukemia

AML Classification Category	Specific Subtypes of AML
AML with recurrent genetic abnormalities	AML with t(8;21)(q22;q22), *RUNX1-RUNX1T1* AML with inv(16)(p13.1;q22) or t(16;16)(p13.1;q22), *CBFB-MYH11* APL with *PML-RARα* AML with t(9;11)(p21.3;q23.3), *MLLT3-KMT2A* AML with t(6;9)(p23;q34.1), *DEK-NUP214* AML with inv(3)(q21.3;q26.2) or t(3;3)(q21.3;q26.2), *GATA2, MECOM* AML (megakaryoblastic) with t(1;22)(p13.3;q13.3), *RBM15-MKL1* AML with *BCR-ABL1* (provisional entity) AML with mutated *NPM1* AML with biallelic mutations of *CEBPA* AML with mutated *RUNX1* (provisional entity)
AML with myelodysplasia-related features	
Therapy related myeloid neoplasms	
AML, not otherwise specified	AML with minimal differentiation AML without maturation AML with maturation Acute myelomonocytic leukemia Acute monoblastic/monocytic leukemia Pure erythroid leukemia Acute megakaryoblastic leukemia Acute basophilic leukemia Acute panmyelosis with myelofibrosis
Myeloid sarcomas	
Myeloid proliferations related to trisomy 21	Transient abnormal myelopoiesis (TAM) Myeloid leukemia associated with trisomy 21

AML, Acute myeloid leukemia.
Adapted from Arber DA, Orazi A, Hasserjian R, et al. The 2016 revision to the World Health Organization classification of myeloid neoplasms and acute leukemia. *Blood.* 2016;127:2391–2405.

124

Lymphomas

Kyle B. Lenz

CLINICAL VIGNETTE

A 15-year-old healthy girl is seen by her pediatrician for a painless bump on her left neck that she noticed after a necklace no longer fit. She notes that she has lost 12 lb in the past 2 months despite no changes to her routine. She applies daily acne medicine but otherwise has no medical issues.

Her examination showed a 3-cm left anterior cervical lymph node and a 1-cm left supraclavicular lymph node. Both were nontender, firm, and fixed. An initial chest radiograph showed an enlarged mediastinal silhouette concerning for malignancy. A computed tomography scan of the neck, chest, and abdomen was performed to assess disease burden. She underwent a lymph node biopsy that confirmed the diagnosis of Hodgkin lymphoma. Increased uptake was seen on a positron emission tomography scan, ultimately used for staging.

CLINICAL VIGNETTE

In the emergency room, a 5-year-old boy with asthma is seen for a palpable abdominal mass noted while his grandmother was bathing him. He has no associated symptoms. He has an inhaler that he uses intermittently for asthma flares.

His examination demonstrated a distended abdomen with a large, palpable mass in the left lower quadrant. He had no lymphadenopathy, skin breakdown, or other focal findings on examination. A chest radiograph showed clear lung fields whereas abdominal computed tomography demonstrated a 3- × 3.2- × 2.7-cm nonobstructing mass. Subsequent biopsy of the mass revealed non-Hodgkin lymphoma, Burkitt subtype.

It is important to note that a painless and enlarging mass with or without constitutional symptoms in a child or adolescent is highly suspicious for lymphoma, though other infectious or inflammatory causes also may be considered. Initial workup includes imaging to aid in diagnosis and acute management; patients also may present with a mediastinal mass that can occlude the airway or blood vessels, both of which are oncologic emergencies.

Lymphomas are defined as malignancies of the lymphatic system. They consist of two primary types, Hodgkin lymphoma (HL) and non-Hodgkin lymphoma (NHL). Together, they comprise 15% of pediatric cancers and are the third most common form of pediatric cancer. Between 1992 and 2017, there were 42,694 lymphoma diagnoses under the age of 20 in the United States. HL broadly occurs evenly in boys and girls, whereas NHL occurs more frequently in boys. This chapter focuses on pathogenesis, presentation, evaluation, management, and future treatments of these pediatric lymphomas.

HODGKIN LYMPHOMA

Etiology and Pathogenesis

HL is a neoplasm of B-lymphocytes and involves the lymphatic and reticuloendothelial systems. It can originate from lymphoid tissue, as shown in Fig. 124.1, such as the bone marrow or thymus, or it can develop from secondary organs such as the lungs, brain, skin, or liver. There are two variants of HL: classic HL (cHL) and nodular predominant HL (NPHL). CHL makes up 90% of HL cases and can be further divided into nodular sclerosis, mixed cellularity, lymphocyte-rich, and lymphocyte depleted subtypes, which offer prognostic ramifications. As a group, cHL is distinguished by its hallmark multinuclear cells called Reed-Sternberg cells. These cells express CD30 and CD15. NPHL instead have lymphocyte-predominant cells with folded, multilobulated nuclei. These cells express CD20 and not CD30 or CD15.

Epidemiologic studies show that HL is more common in school-age children in developing countries but is more common in adolescents in developed countries. The earlier onset pattern correlates with increased family size and decreased socioeconomic status. Other studies show increased risk for developing HL in monozygotic twins, suggesting a genetic component. The incidence of HL increases in both inherited and acquired immune deficiency syndromes. Epstein-Barr virus (EBV) infection has been connected to HL, particularly in the mixed cellularity cHL subtype. EBV-related HL also shows male predominance and is found more frequently in younger children.

Clinical Presentation

HL diagnosis requires a high index of suspicion because of a variety of nonspecific symptoms or asymptomatic manifestations. Patients typically have a painless, rubbery, enlarging mass in the cervical chain. However, enlarged lymph nodes also can be seen in infectious, autoimmune, or other self-limited causes, thereby making diagnosis challenging (Table 124.1). Lymphadenopathy in HL presents as a mediastinal mass in 60% of patients, which can provoke respiratory distress, orthopnea, cough, or chest pain. Such mass effect can also cause superior vena cava (SVC) syndrome with reduced circulatory blood flow. Hepatosplenomegaly is sometimes seen, which may help to further distinguish HL from other viral syndromes.

Patients may present with constitutional symptoms or "B symptoms," including fevers (temperature >100.4°F [38°C]) for 3 consecutive days, weight loss (>10% body weight over 6 months), and drenching night sweats. It is thought that cytokine production from Reed-Sternberg cells causes these systemic symptoms. Ultimately, B symptoms confer important staging information and therefore therapy decisions.

Evaluation and Staging

Patients should undergo a chest radiograph to assess for mediastinal disease burden. If without significant orthopnea, they should undergo computed tomography (CT) of the neck, chest, abdomen, and pelvis to determine extent of disease. An echocardiogram is necessary to evaluate baseline cardiac function and circulatory flow. Initial laboratory studies include complete blood cell count (CBC), erythrocyte sedimentation rate (ESR), ferritin, and electrolytes. Excisional biopsy of an involved lymph node informs the final diagnosis. After the initial

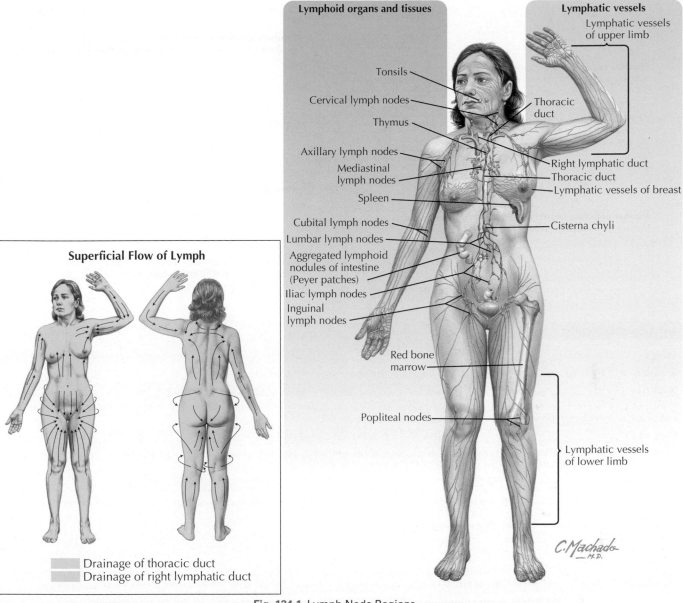

Lymphoid organs and tissues

- Tonsils
- Cervical lymph nodes
- Thymus
- Axillary lymph nodes
- Mediastinal lymph nodes
- Spleen
- Cubital lymph nodes
- Lumbar lymph nodes
- Aggregated lymphoid nodules of intestine (Peyer patches)
- Iliac lymph nodes
- Inguinal lymph nodes
- Red bone marrow
- Popliteal nodes

Lymphatic vessels

- Lymphatic vessels of upper limb
- Thoracic duct
- Right lymphatic duct
- Thoracic duct
- Lymphatic vessels of breast
- Cisterna chyli
- Lymphatic vessels of lower limb

C. Machado
M.D.

Superficial Flow of Lymph

☐ Drainage of thoracic duct
☐ Drainage of right lymphatic duct

Fig. 124.1 Lymph Node Regions.

TABLE 124.1	**Differential Diagnosis of Hodgkin and Non-Hodgkin Lymphomas**	
	Hodgkin Lymphoma	**Non-Hodgkin Lymphoma**
Infections	Lymphadenitis	Lymphadenitis
	Cat scratch disease	Cat scratch disease
	Mononucleosis (EBV, CMV)	Mononucleosis (EBV, CMV)
	Brucellosis	Tuberculosis
	Tuberculosis	Toxoplasmosis
	Toxoplasmosis	Atypical mycobacterial
	Atypical mycobacterial	infections
	infections	Appendicitis
Malignancies	ALL	ALL
	Rhabdomyosarcoma	AML
	Germ cell tumors	Neuroblastoma
	Lymphoproliferative disorders	Rhabdomyosarcoma
		Wilms tumor
		Lymphoproliferative disorders
Other	Bronchogenic cyst	Intussusception
	Lipoma	Sarcoidosis
	Teratoma	

ALL, Acute lymphoblastic leukemia; *AML,* acute myelogenous leukemia; *CMV,* cytomegalovirus; *EBV,* Epstein-Barr virus.

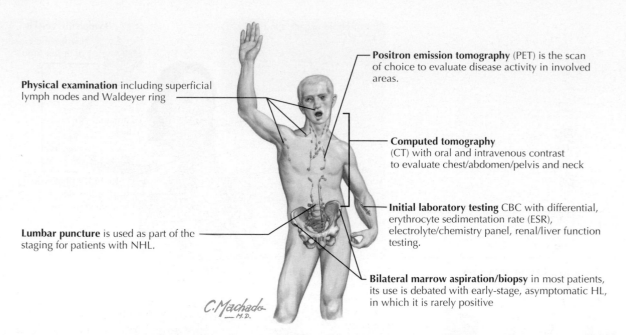

Physical examination including superficial lymph nodes and Waldeyer ring

Positron emission tomography (PET) is the scan of choice to evaluate disease activity in involved areas.

Computed tomography (CT) with oral and intravenous contrast to evaluate chest/abdomen/pelvis and neck

Initial laboratory testing CBC with differential, erythrocyte sedimentation rate (ESR), electrolyte/chemistry panel, renal/liver function testing.

Lumbar puncture is used as part of the staging for patients with NHL.

Bilateral marrow aspiration/biopsy in most patients, its use is debated with early-stage, asymptomatic HL, in which it is rarely positive

C. Machado
—M.D.

Ann Arbor Classification

Stage I

Involvement of a single lymph node region (I) or of a single extralymphatic organ or site (IE)

Stage II

Involvement of two or more lymph node regions on the same side of the diaphragm (II) or localized involvement of extralymphatic organ or site and of one or more lymph node regions on the same side of the diaphragm (IIE)

Stage III

Involvement of lymph node regions on both sides of the diaphragm (III), which may also be accompanied by localized involvement of extralymphatic organ or site (IIIE) or by involvement of the spleen (IIIS) or both (IIISE)

Stage IV

Diffuse or disseminated involvement of one or more extralymphatic organs or tissues with or without associated lymph node enlargement

Certain symptoms are commonly associated with lymphoma:
* Night sweats
* Temperature >38.5°C
* Weight loss >10%
These are called "B" symptoms and are included in the stage designated to a patient. For instance, a patient with involved lymph nodes in the neck and under the arms only, and without any of the "B" symptoms, has stage IIA disease. The same patient with night sweats has stage IIB disease.

Fig. 124.2 Malignant Lymphomas: Staging. *CBC,* Complete blood cell count; *HL,* Hodgkin lymphoma.

workup, a positron emission tomography scan assists in determining disseminated disease burden. A bone marrow aspirate and biopsy are performed under certain circumstances.

Staging for HL is based on the Ann Arbor Classification System, as illustrated in Fig. 124.2. B symptoms increase the stage and risk for disease.

Management

Treatment for HL is risk-adapted, multimodal, and based on risk stratification. Table 124.2 depicts the risk stratification of the Children's Oncology Group (COG). Standard treatment includes chemotherapy; some patients receive radiation. Also employed, though less commonly, are targeted therapy, immunotherapy, surgery, and stem cell transplant. Chemotherapy regimen selection depends on the initial risk stratification. The initial tumor response to therapy guides subsequent amounts and types of treatment. Different chemotherapy agents attack malignant cells by different mechanisms of action to reduce cancer cell resistance. Additionally, agents are preferentially partnered with others that have different side effects or toxicities.

TABLE 124.2 Risk Stratification of Patients With Hodgkin Lymphoma

Risk Category	Stages
Low risk	IA, IIA; no bulk disease[a]
Intermediate risk	IA and IIA with bulk disease[a]
	All IB and IIB
	All IIIA and IVA
High risk	All IIIB and IVB

[a]Bulk disease is defined as a mediastinal mass greater than 33% of the chest width or any nodal aggregate that is larger than 6 cm.

HL treatment commonly incorporates a combination of bleomycin, vinblastine/vincristine, etoposide, procarbazine, prednisone, methotrexate, doxorubicin, or cyclophosphamide. Each agent has a unique toxicity profile that requires careful monitoring (Table 124.3). Secondary malignancies are common in HL survivors, often because of accumulation of chemotherapy side effects and radiation exposure,

TABLE 124.3 Common Chemotherapy Side Effects

Agent	Side Effect(s)
Bleomycin	Pulmonary fibrosis
Vinblastine/vincristine	Peripheral neuropathy
Etoposide	Marrow suppression, secondary malignancy
Procarbazine	Marrow suppression
Prednisone	Appetite stimulation, irritability, hyperglycemia, adrenal suppression
Methotrexate	Mucositis, hepatotoxicity
Doxorubicin	Cardiac toxicity
Cyclophosphamide	Hemorrhagic cystitis

with up to 30% of survivors developing another malignancy within 30 years.

Despite potential side effects, HL has an overall excellent prognosis. Patients with early-stage disease have an overall 5-year survival (OS) of more than 95%. Patients with late-stage disease also fare well, with an event-free survival of 80% to 85% and OS of 90%. Prognosis remains good in the setting of relapse, but it varies based on time from completion of chemotherapy, relapsed disease burden, and quantity of initial chemotherapy administered. Patients that relapse more than 12 months from completion of therapy have the best prognosis. Relapses typically respond to standard chemotherapy regimens but sometimes require advanced approaches, such as stem cell transplant or immunotherapy.

Future Directions

In an effort to reduce the frequency of relapse and decrease the toxicity of treatment, studies are investigating radiation schedules and/or the implementation of targeted therapies. COG studies are investigating lessened radiation dose and frequency. Rituximab (anti-CD20) has shown encouraging evidence in treating NPHL. Brentuximab (anti-CD30) has demonstrated efficacy in treating cHL or refractory HL because it targets Reed-Sternberg cells. Another monoclonal antibody, nivolumab, prevents cancer cells from inactivating native immune system surveillance. It does this by binding to the PD-1 portion of T-cells and inhibiting the PD-L1 or PD-L2 on cancer cells from linking and thereby inactivating the T-cell.

NON-HODGKIN LYMPHOMA

Etiology and Pathogenesis

There are four separate subtypes of NHL: Burkitt (BL), diffuse large B cell (DLBC), lymphoblastic (LL), and anaplastic large cell (ALCL). In developed countries, most cases of NHL are idiopathic, but immunocompromised patients have an elevated risk for developing NHL. Countries in sub-Saharan Africa have shown a strong association with previous infections of malaria or EBV and subtypes of NHL. One of those subtypes, BL, is a mature B cell malignancy. Classically, it has a "starry-sky" appearance on histologic examination and expresses CD20 on cellular surfaces. Ninety percent of BL patients have a t(8;14) *c-myc* translocation with an immunoglobulin chain that drives the malignant process. DLBC lymphoma is also a mature B cell malignancy that expresses CD20 and CD22 and can be further divided into subtypes that dictate prognosis. The germinal center B cell–like type offers a favorable prognosis, whereas the activated B cell–like and primary

mediastinal B cell types have an unfavorable prognosis. LL has similar biological processes to leukemia and can be composed of precursor T or B cell lymphoblasts. ALCL consists of mature T cells, mature B cells, or null cells and expresses CD30 on the cellular surface. ALCL regularly has a driver t(2;5) translocation that constitutively activates anaplastic lymphoma kinase (ALK) and drives malignancy.

Clinical Presentation

HL presents gradually and indolently, whereas NHL develops more acutely. NHL also has distinct sites of primary malignancy and areas of metastasis based on its subtypes. For example, BL can masquerade as an abdominal mass that intermittently causes intussusception or small bowel obstruction. NHL can progress to a mediastinal mass, seen in 75% of LL. ALCL can manifest with lesions of skin or bone or systemically. NHL may disseminate to the central nervous system (CNS) or bone marrow, which is not commonly seen in HL.

The location of disease relates to symptoms at presentation. An enlarging lymph node may represent localized disease. Mediastinal masses may cause cough, chest pain, or orthopnea. Malignancy that obstructs venous return causes plethora and dyspnea seen in SVC syndrome. Bony pain can be seen in metastatic disease. Gonadal disease causes testicular enlargement and CNS involvement provokes encephalopathy or headache.

Evaluation and Staging

The workup for NHL is similar to the workup for HL. Chest radiograph, CT scan (neck, chest, abdomen, and pelvis), and echocardiogram are part of the initial workup. CBC and electrolytes should be ordered. BL has a high risk for tumor lysis syndrome, and therefore uric acid and lactate dehydrogenase also should be collected. NHL can metastasize to the CNS, and therefore a lumbar puncture should be performed.

There are multiple systems to stage and guide NHL treatment, including the International Pediatric Non-Hodgkin Lymphoma Staging System (IPNHLSS) or the more commonly used Murphy staging system (Table 124.4).

Management

NHL uses a combination of multimodal chemotherapy (including intrathecal treatment), radiation, and targeted therapy. Radiation is typically saved for oncologic emergencies, such as a mediastinal mass or CNS involvement. During initial diagnosis and in the first few days of treatment, NHL (especially BL and LL types), requires aggressive hydration and commonly a xanthine oxidase inhibitor to prevent tumor lysis syndrome. Fluids should be without potassium or phosphorus. For elevated potassium, patients may require diuretics, potassium binders, or dialysis. Other temporizing agents include albuterol, sodium bicarbonate, or insulin/glucose. Electrolyte levels can be checked up to every hour and intensive care unit stay may be necessary for serial monitoring. Elevated uric acid levels may require administration of a recombinant urate oxidase to prevent potential renal damage.

The specific treatment regimens for NHL vary based on the subtype and risk stratification. BL and DLBL have a similar treatment backbone. Localized disease commonly implements cyclophosphamide, vincristine, prednisone, and doxorubicin (COPAD) with high survival. Advanced disease requires chemotherapy, which is more intensive and of longer duration, resulting in disease-free survival (DFS) ranging from 45% to 70%. The addition of rituximab also has shown improved survival in advanced disease. Neither the stage nor phenotype of LL offers prognostic value. Treatment of CNS-positive disease incorporates intrathecal chemotherapy and may also include cranial radiation.

TABLE 124.4	**Murphy Staging System of Non-Hodgkin Lymphoma**
Stage	Definition
I	A single tumor (extranodal) or single anatomic area (nodal), excluding mediastinum or abdomen
II	A single tumor (extranodal) with regional node involvement, or a primary GI tract tumor with or without associated mesenteric node involvement, grossly completely resected; or, on the same side of the diaphragm, two or more nodal areas or two single (extranodal) tumors with or without regional node involvement
III	All primary intrathoracic tumors (mediastinal, pleural, thymic); or all extensive primary intraabdominal disease that is unresectable; or all primary paraspinal or epidural tumors regardless of other sites; or on both sides of the diaphragm, two single tumors (extranodal) or two or more nodal areas
IV	Any of the above with initial CNS or bone marrow involvement (<25%)

CNS, Central nervous system; *GI,* gastrointestinal.

ALCL can sometimes be treated with surgical resection alone if disease is localized; advanced disease requires chemotherapy. Recent studies with targeted therapies, brentuximab and crizotinib (ALK inhibitor), have shown promise in advanced and/or relapsed disease of various NHL forms.

Future Directions

The overall survival and prognosis of NHL is excellent, and current research aims to reduce long-term toxicity of therapy. Relapsed NHL is difficult to treat, and therapy sometimes results in future secondary malignancies. Ongoing investigations attempt to identify patients at high risk and reduce risk for relapse. Novel chimeric antigen receptor T cells (CART therapies) offer potential to target relapsed and refractory NHL.

SUGGESTED READINGS

Available online.

125

Brain Tumors

Stephanie N. Brosius, Kavita A. Desai, and Amish C. Shah

✳ CLINICAL VIGNETTE

An 8-year-old previously healthy boy presented to the emergency department for evaluation of new-onset headaches and emesis. Symptoms began 1 week before presentation with morning headaches described as pounding and associated with vomiting and photophobia. Headaches awakened him from sleep and improved throughout the day. He denied any vision changes, weakness, tingling, or gait abnormality.

Physical examination was notable for bilateral papilledema but otherwise intact cranial nerves, normal strength, reflexes, and gait. Head computed tomography (CT) revealed obstructive hydrocephalus and a hyperdense mass obstructing the fourth ventricle. He was started on dexamethasone because of mass effect. Magnetic resonance imaging of the brain and spine was notable for a 2- × 3-cm T2 hypointense lesion in the cerebellum with cystic nodules, avid enhancement, and heterogeneous diffusion restriction. Nodular enhancement was also seen along the spinal cord and brainstem consistent with leptomeningeal spread. He underwent gross total resection of the lesion with cerebrospinal fluid diversion. Pathology revealed non-WNT, non-SHH medulloblastoma; cytology on lumbar puncture was positive. He was subsequently treated with craniospinal irradiation and high-dose chemotherapy.

✳ CLINICAL VIGNETTE

A 5-year-old girl with no health problems presented to the emergency room with 3 weeks of persistent headache and gait disturbance. She awoke one morning with a diffuse headache that was unresponsive to over-the-counter medications. The headache subsequently worsened in severity and was associated with nausea and fatigue. Over the past 2 days she noted progressive difficulty with ambulation, prompting presentation. Physical examination was notable for papilledema but otherwise intact cranial nerves. Strength and reflexes were normal. She had dysmetria on finger-to-nose and heel-to-shin as well as a wide-based gait. Head computed tomography demonstrated a cystic mass in the cerebellar vermis with mural nodule. She was started on dexamethasone and acetazolamide for increased intracranial pressure. Magnetic resonance imaging of the brain showed a cystic lesion with an enhancing solid component as well as hydrocephalus with transependymal flow. She underwent gross total resection, and pathologic examination confirmed pilocytic astrocytoma with resolution of symptoms after rehabilitation hospitalization. She was followed with serial imaging longitudinally without evidence of recurrence.

Collectively, brain tumors are the most common solid tumor identified in children, accounting for 20% to 25% of all childhood cancers. The incidence ranges from 1 to 5 cases per 100,000 children annually, with variation dependent on country of origin. A slight male predominance is seen among children younger than 15 years of age, with a 1.3:1 male-to-female ratio. The cause for the vast majority of pediatric brain tumors is unknown, though several genetic syndromes have an increased risk and incidence of tumor development, including neurofibromatosis types 1 and 2, tuberous sclerosis complex, Li-Fraumeni syndrome, Turcot syndrome, and Gorlin syndrome. However, these syndromes account for less than 10% of all pediatric brain tumor diagnoses and the only clear environmental risk factor identified has been prior exposure to radiation. Despite improvement in imaging modalities, surgical techniques, and treatment protocols, brain tumors remain the greatest cause of mortality related to pediatric cancer.

Since 2010, there has been significant advancement in the understanding of the mutations and signaling cascades driving tumor pathogenesis, holding promise in the development of more targeted therapeutics for pediatric brain tumors. These advances are reflected in the 2021 World Health Organization (WHO) Classification of Pediatric Brain Tumors. This chapter will review the prevalence, pathogenesis, presentation, and management of the most common brain tumors impacting children.

CLINICAL PRESENTATION

The presenting symptoms of brain tumors in children are dependent on location, age, and rapidity of tumor growth (Fig. 125.1). Nearly half of all childhood brain tumors arise infratentorially in the brainstem, cerebellum, or fourth ventricle. Tumors in these locations, in addition to pineal, suprasellar, and tectal tumors, typically present manifest with symptoms of increased intracranial pressure secondary to obstructive hydrocephalus. In older children, hydrocephalus manifests as early morning headaches, ataxia, and emesis. Physical examination may reveal a sixth nerve palsy and papilledema. In contrast, infants frequently manifest with more nebulous signs and symptoms, including irritability, vomiting, increasing head circumference, developmental regression, failure to thrive, or a setting-sun phenomenon of the eyes because of upward-gaze paresis. Central nervous system (CNS) tumors can also manifest with focal deficits, which aid in localization of the lesion as summarized in Table 125.1.

DIFFERENTIAL DIAGNOSIS, EVALUATION, AND TREATMENT

After thorough neurologic examination, the first step in evaluation of a suspected brain tumor is obtaining neuroimaging. Initial imaging is frequently computed tomography (CT) because of the ease of obtaining images even in young children and ubiquity in most emergency departments. CT is most useful in evaluation of hydrocephalus or acute intracranial hemorrhage, and can detect 95% of CNS tumors. Once a patient is medically stabilized, higher resolution magnetic resonance imaging (MRI) with and without gadolinium contrast should be obtained. Though the differential diagnosis of a mass can be narrowed by anatomic location (Table 125.2), histologic confirmation is required in nearly all brain tumor cases with the exception of diffuse midline gliomas involving the pons, tectal gliomas, and optic pathway gliomas

Cystic astrocytoma of cerebellum

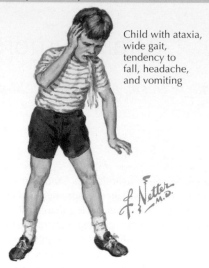

Child with ataxia, wide gait, tendency to fall, headache, and vomiting

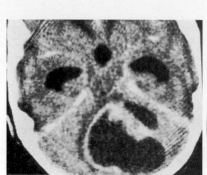

CT scan showing cystic tumor of cerebellum with nodule

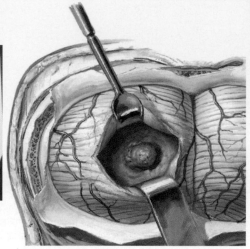

Cyst opened, revealing nodular tumor

Brain glioma

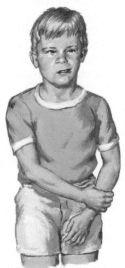

Child with sixth and seventh cranial nerve palsy on side of tumor and contralateral limb weakness

Glioma distorting brainstem and cranial nerves VI, VII, VIII

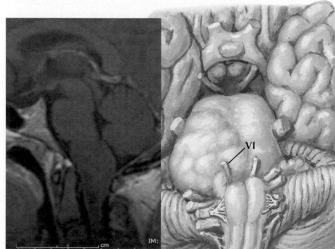

VI

Sagittal MR T1-weighted image shows expansion of medulla to the pons

Fig. 125.1 Clinical Manifestation of Brain Tumors.

in patients with neurofibromatosis type 1 (NF1). For these exceptions, neuroimaging may be sufficient for diagnosis. In other tumor types, operative management is required to obtain tissue for histologic diagnosis, which dictates management, and more recently, for genetic profiling, which confirms the diagnosis, clarifies prognosis, and guides therapy options. At the same time, maximal safe surgical debulking can be very useful. In the immediate 24 to 48 hours postoperatively, repeat brain MRI with and without contrast should be performed to better distinguish between postoperative inflammatory changes and residual tumor. Once a histologic diagnosis is established, staging of malignant tumors is completed. Unlike other malignancies, primary brain tumors rarely disseminate outside of the CNS but are capable of spreading into the subarachnoid space through cerebrospinal fluid (CSF) and distant seeding along the neuroaxis. As such, medulloblastoma, ependymoma, atypical teratoid rhabdoid tumors (ATRT), and germ cell tumors must be further evaluated with MRI of the spine with and without contrast and large volume lumbar puncture for cytologic examination (Fig. 125.2).

After surgical resection, the mainstays of brain tumor treatment can include radiation and/or chemotherapy. Craniospinal irradiation (CSI) plays a major role in the treatment of malignant brain tumors but is avoided in children younger than 3 years of age because of the devastating impact on brain development. Depending on tumor type, adjuvant chemotherapy is also used and is particularly intensified in younger children unable to receive radiotherapy. More detailed evaluation and management for the most common tumor types is outlined in the following section.

Embryonal Tumors
Medulloblastoma

Medulloblastoma is the most common malignant brain neoplasm, comprising about 20% of all pediatric brain tumors and can be seen in children with Gorlin syndrome. By definition, these tumors arise from the cerebellum. The 2021 WHO classification system utilizes molecular subgroupings of wingless (WNT), Sonic hedgehog (SHH), group 3, and group 4 with retention of the histologic and clinical subtypes as a

TABLE 125.1 Localizing Symptoms of Brain Tumors

Location	Tumor
Cerebral hemisphere	Seizures, hemiparesis, visual field deficits, and cognitive deficits
Brainstem	Weakness; cranial nerve deficits, including diplopia or dysphagia; and long tract signs (spasticity, hyperreflexia, clonus, and positive Babinski or Hoffmann reflexes)
Cerebellum	Ataxia, dysmetria, visual disturbances, and changes in speech
Pineal region	Parinaud syndrome (upward gaze palsy, convergence retraction nystagmus, bilateral eyelid retraction, and light-near dissociation)
Thalamus	Hemiparesis; prominent sensory symptoms, including paresthesias or pain; and psychomotor retardation
Neurohypophysis or suprasellar region	Bitemporal hemianopia, endocrine dysfunction, and changes in visual acuity
Spinal cord	Back pain, bowel or bladder dysfunction, and extremity weakness with sensory changes such as a sensory level

TABLE 125.2 Differential Diagnosis of Brain Tumors by Location

Location	Tumor
Cerebral hemisphere	Glioma Ependymoma
Pineal	Germ cell tumor Glioma (tectal glioma) Pineoblastoma Pineocytoma
Cerebellum	Pilocytic astrocytoma Medulloblastoma Ependymoma
Brainstem	Glioma Atypical teratoid rhabdoid tumor in children less than age 2
Suprasellar	Craniopharyngioma Optic pathway glioma Germ cell tumor Pituitary tumor
Spinal cord	Astrocytoma Ependymoma

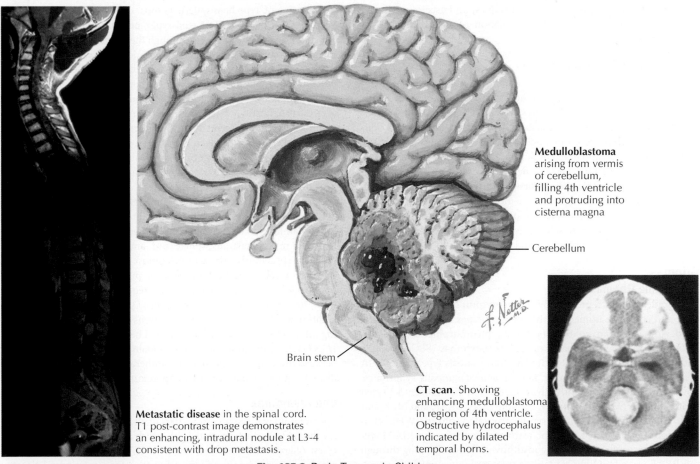

Medulloblastoma arising from vermis of cerebellum, filling 4th ventricle and protruding into cisterna magna

Cerebellum

Brain stem

Metastatic disease in the spinal cord. T1 post-contrast image demonstrates an enhancing, intradural nodule at L3-4 consistent with drop metastasis.

CT scan. Showing enhancing medulloblastoma in region of 4th ventricle. Obstructive hydrocephalus indicated by dilated temporal horns.

Fig. 125.2 Brain Tumors in Children.

TABLE 125.3	**Molecular Subgroups of Medulloblastoma and Their Key Features**			
	WNT	**SHH**	**Group 3**	**Group 4**
Prevalence	10%	30%	25%	30%
Age of onset	Older children and adults	Infants, children, adults	Infants and children	Older children and adults
Male-to-female	1:1	1:1	2:1	2:1
Histologic features	Classic	Diffuse/nodular, large-cell/anaplastic	Classic, large-cell/anaplastic	Classic, large-cell/anaplastic
Metastases	Rare	Uncommon	Very frequent	Frequent
Genetic alterations	*CTNNB1* Monosomy 6	*PTCH1/SUFU/SMO TP53* mutation *MYCN* amplification	*MYC* amplification	*CDK6* amplification Isochromosome 17q
Prognosis (5-year overall survival)	>95%	Infants (80%) With *TP53* mutation (30%) Adult (60%-70%)	50% If *MYC* amplified (30%)	75%

SHH, Sonic hedgehog; *WNT*, Wingless.
Adapted from Taylor MD, Northcott PA, Korshunov A, et al. Molecular subgroups of medulloblastoma: the current consensus. *Acta Neuropathol.* 2012;123:465-472.

second tier of classification. In addition to distinct molecular drivers of tumor pathogenesis, each subtype is unique in its demographics, metastatic potential, and prognosis as summarized in Table 125.3. Although all subtypes qualify as WHO grade IV tumors, prognostic stratification of risk is based on age, dissemination of disease, and extent of resection. Metastatic disease or residual tumor volume after resection of more than 1.5 cm³ qualifies as high-risk lesions, which are treated more aggressively with high-dose CSI followed by chemotherapy. Clinical trials are underway to confirm molecular stratification of medulloblastoma, assess targeted therapies, and ascertain whether lower-risk subtypes can tolerate deescalation of treatment intensity without affecting prognosis.

Atypical Teratoid Rhabdoid Tumor

Although ATRTs represent only 1% to 2% of all CNS tumors, they account for 10% to 20% of brain tumors identified in children younger than 3 years of age. They are aggressive (WHO grade IV) neoplasms derived from pluripotent fetal cells and characterized by poorly differentiated cells with eccentric nuclei, small nucleoli, an abundance of granular cytoplasm, and frequent mitotic figures. ATRTs are defined by mutations involving INI1 *(SMARCB1)* on chromosome 22. Treatment of ATRT has been notoriously challenging, with overall 5-year survival of less than 30% despite high-dose chemotherapy. Use of radiotherapy is often limited by the age of onset, though in older children with more localized disease, 5-year overall survival approaches 50% with combination of intensive chemotherapy and radiation.

Gliomas
Low-Grade Gliomas

Low-grade gliomas represent the most common brain tumor in children and comprise numerous histologic subtypes, including pilocytic astrocytomas, pilomyxoid astrocytomas, pleomorphic xanthoastrocytomas, and subependymal giant cell astrocytomas (SEGAs). Optic pathway gliomas in patients with neurofibromatosis type 1 and SEGA are detailed further in Chapter 111 on neurocutaneous syndromes. Low-grade gliomas frequently have mutations in the mitogen-activated protein kinase (MAPK) pathway, including Ras, BRAF, and MEK, but molecular subtypes have not been incorporated into the WHO classification. Over 70% of pilocytic astrocytomas carry the *KIAA1549-BRAF* fusion gene, resulting in constitutively active signaling through the BRAF cascade. Other mutations frequently encountered in low-grade gliomas include *BRAF V600E*, *NTRK1*, and *FGFR1*. After surgical resection, some low-grade gliomas require only serial imaging for

monitoring. Tumors unable to undergo gross total resection receive vincristine and carboplatin, though targeted molecular therapeutics are currently in late-stage trials. Five-year overall survival is 95% to 100% with complete resection in pilocytic astrocytoma and greater than 90% in other subtypes.

High-Grade Gliomas

High-grade gliomas encompass 10% of pediatric brain tumors and include anaplastic astrocytomas (WHO grade III), diffuse hemispheric gliomas, infant-type hemispheric glioma, diffuse pediatric high-grade glioma (H3 wild-type, IDH wild-type), and diffuse midline gliomas, which are all WHO grade IV. Although these tumors are histologically identical to adult tumors with high mitotic index, perivascular proliferation, and pseudopalisading necrosis, they are molecularly distinct entities. The molecular subtypes within pediatric high-grade gliomas segregate based on tumor location. Prognosis is overall poor, with the greatest prognostic indicator being extent of surgical resection. After surgical resection, patients typically undergo radiotherapy and high-intensity chemotherapy given the aggressive nature of disease, though no standard chemotherapeutic regimen exists. Five-year overall survival is approximately 30%, though children younger than 3 years of age have slightly better prognosis.

Diffuse midline gliomas are unique to the pediatric population and comprise 10% to 15% of childhood brain tumors. These lesions typically manifest in children between the ages of 4 and 9 years and can be found in the thalamus, spinal cord, and brainstem, particularly in the pons (previously referred to as diffuse intrinsic pontine gliomas). Biopsy is rarely required for diagnostic purposes but is increasing in frequency given ongoing clinical trials requiring molecular diagnosis. Over 70% of pontine tumors have an *H3.1 K27M* mutation, and an additional 20% carry activating mutations in *ACVR1*. Tumors involving other midline structures or cerebral hemispheres commonly have *H3.3 G34R/V* mutations. Radiation remains the mainstay of treatment, because there are no effective chemotherapeutic agents. Prognosis is dismal, with a median survival of approximately 10 months.

Ependymomas

Ependymomas make up 6% to 10% of all pediatric brain tumors and are thought to arise from radial glia, which are the progenitors of astrocytes, oligodendrocytes, and neurons. Histologically, ependymomas are characterized by round blue cells with perivascular pseudorosettes and true ependymal rosettes. The 2021 WHO criteria further classify ependymomas by location as well as histological and molecular features. Children typically present with WHO grade II or III tumors. Molecularly, the WHO also designates a subset of tumors with *ZFTA-RELA* fusion gene, which results in constitutive activation of the nuclear factor–kappa B (NF-κB) signaling cascade.

With regard to tumor location, 60% of ependymomas are found in the posterior fossa, 30% arise supratentorially, and 10% are of spinal origin. Of the supratentorial lesions, 70% will possess the *RELA* fusion gene. Staging of the tumor with spinal imaging and lumbar puncture with cytologic examination is imperative because approximately 10% of cases are disseminated at diagnosis.

Treatment involves surgical resection to achieve local control, followed by adjuvant radiation to the primary site. Myxopapillary subtypes are an exception and are followed by serial imaging after resection. In young children, chemotherapy can be used to delay radiation or improve surgical resection. Prognosis is most correlated with the extent of tumor resection. Five-year progression-free survival is 50% to 70% in the setting of gross total resection compared with less than 30% with subtotal resection. Other poor prognostic factors include age younger than 3 years at diagnosis, disseminated disease, and anaplastic features such as nuclear atypia, increased mitotic index, and vascularity, which suggest a more aggressive lesion. In contrast, supratentorial lesions have a more favorable prognosis. Recent studies have demonstrated that repeat irradiation is safe in patients with relapsed ependymoma, though no curative treatment exists.

Germ Cell Tumors

Germ cell tumors make up about 3% of childhood brain tumors. They typically arise in midline structures, including the pineal and suprasellar regions, though they also can be found in the basal ganglia, thalamus, and cerebellar hemispheres. Approximately 10% of tumors have dissemination with seeding along the ventricles at time of diagnosis. Teratomas are more prominent in the neonatal population, whereas malignant tumors typically present between the ages of 10 and 14 years. There is a male predominance with male-to-female ratio of 2 to 3:1. There are five subtypes of germ cell tumors: pure germinomas, teratomas, yolk sac tumors, embryonal carcinomas, and choriocarcinomas. Of these, germinomas have the highest prevalence. The others (the nongerminomatous germ cell tumors [NGGCTs]) provide an exception to the diagnostic steps discussed earlier. For NGGCTs, detection of germ cell markers and identification of the mass in characteristic locations can be sufficient for diagnosis—histologic confirmation may not be necessary.

Therefore all suspected germ cell neoplasms also require evaluation of tumor markers in the CSF and serum. Although pure germinomas may secrete low levels of beta human chorionic gonadotropin (β-hCG), high levels are characteristic of choriocarcinoma. Expression of α-fetoprotein (AFP) is observed in yolk sac tumors.

Prognosis varies based on the tumor subtype. Gross total resection is curative for mature teratomas, whereas immature teratomas require a mix of chemotherapy and radiation to achieve an overall survival of greater than 90% at 5 years. Pure germinomas, which are exquisitely sensitive to radiation, have greater than 90% 5-year overall survival. This contrasts starkly with NGGCTs, which have between 25% and 55% overall survival at 5 years when treated with surgical resection, chemotherapy, and CSI.

Craniopharyngiomas

Craniopharyngiomas account for 5% to 10% of all pediatric brain tumors and derive from remnants of the Rathke pouch in the suprasellar region or pituitary stalk. Although histologically classified as WHO grade I, craniopharyngiomas are often associated with significant morbidity because of their site of origin with associated symptoms of visual field deficits, endocrine abnormalities, headache, and growth failure. There are two subtypes of craniopharyngiomas: papillary tumors, which typically carry *BRAF* mutations, and adamantinomatous tumors, which are characterized by *CTNNB1* mutations and carry a higher risk for recurrence. Surgical resection is standard of care. However, there remains controversy on treatment modality and surgical approach as a result of the high morbidity associated with gross total resection as hypothalamic function is commonly disrupted. Radiotherapy is commonly used to treat residual disease or recurrent tumors but also portends the long-term risk for radiation side effects to the nearby circle of Willis, including cavernomas, moyamoya syndrome, or aneurysm development. Overall 5-year survival is 95%.

FUTURE DIRECTIONS

Although strides have been made in terms of long-term survival of children with brain tumors, there remains significant morbidity associated with therapies. Improved understanding of the molecular basis of pediatric brain tumors has allowed for greater stratification of the risk and prognosis of individual tumor subtypes with the hope of guiding more targeted treatment based on tumor biology. Furthermore, trials are under way that may decrease the long-term treatment toxicities by reduction of chemotherapy and radiation intensity in tumors with a favorable response profile. For many aggressive tumors, however, there remains a desperate need for effective chemotherapeutic agents in order to improve long-term survival. Ongoing areas of investigation include analysis of the contribution of tumor microenvironment to pathogenesis and the potential role of immunotherapy in treatment.

SUGGESTED READINGS

Available online.

126

Neuroblastoma

Haley Newman

✳ CLINICAL VIGNETTE

A 19-month-old boy presents to the pediatrician after his mother felt an abdominal mass while bathing him. He has not had vomiting, diarrhea, constipation, or changes in energy or activity level. On examination, the pediatrician palpates a left lower quadrant abdominal mass. She does not note lymphadenopathy, rashes, petechiae, or bruising. He has a normal neurologic examination. She orders an abdominal radiograph, which shows an intra-abdominal soft tissue mass displacing adjacent organs. Full body magnetic resonance imaging is performed. There is a large tumor within the left adrenal gland, as well as metastatic disease in the liver, spinal cord, and lungs. He undergoes metaiodobenzylguanidine scan, biopsy of the primary mass, and bilateral bone marrow aspirates and biopsies. Pathologic examination of the mass shows a small, round blue cell tumor, highly undifferentiated, and consistent with neuroblastoma. Molecular testing shows that the tumor is *MYCN* amplified. His tumor is categorized as high-risk, and treatment is initiated with chemotherapy with a plan for subsequent surgical resection of the primary tumor, myeloablative chemotherapy with autologous stem cell rescue, radiation, and maintenance immunotherapy/differentiation therapy.

Neuroblastoma is the most common extracranial solid tumor of childhood, accounting for 8% to 10% of all childhood cancers. It is also the most common malignancy diagnosed in the first year of life. Median age at diagnosis is 18 months and 90% of cases are diagnosed before age 10. The disease is quite rare in adolescents and adults, and when seen in this population it tends to be incurable.

Neuroblastoma is a unique childhood cancer in that its treatment and prognosis vary widely and depend on age, tumor biology, extent of disease, and tumor anatomy. Although some disseminated tumors in infants may spontaneously regress, metastatic tumors diagnosed in slightly older children carry a long-term survival rate of around 50%. Although many children with neuroblastoma require aggressive surgical resection and chemotherapy, some children can be safely observed over time. It is this dramatic heterogeneity of phenotypes that has prompted further evaluation of the implications of staging and treatment, as well as multimodal treatment for high-risk disease.

ETIOLOGY AND PATHOGENESIS

Neuroblastoma is characterized as a small, round blue cell tumor and arises from neural crest cells, which can lead to masses arising in the adrenal glands and/or anywhere along the sympathetic chain ganglia. The Shimada and Joshi staging system is based on the pathologic components of neuroblastoma. Important histologic components for classification include degree of neuroblast cell differentiation, mitosis-karyorrhexis index, and amount of stromal content. These components combined with age at diagnosis divide tumors into two categories: favorable and unfavorable histology.

A number of genetic aberrations have been observed in neuroblastoma, and some have recognized implications for classification and prognosis. Deoxyribonucleic acid (DNA) content of tumor cells is characterized as near-diploid or hyperdiploid, with hyperdiploid generally having a more favorable outcome. Other key genetic abnormalities include: *MYCN* amplification, deletion of the short arm of chromosome 1p, and deletion of chromosome 11q. *MYCN* amplification is seen in about 20% of patients and is associated with rapid tumor progression and poor prognosis. It is used as a biomarker for risk stratification. Anaplastic lymphoma kinase *(ALK)* amplification was identified as a predisposition gene for familial neuroblastoma; however, somatic mutations in *ALK* are also seen in about 14% of high-risk neuroblastoma and also portend poor prognosis. Loss of 1p occurs in about one-third of cases and correlates with *MYCN* amplification.

Neuroblastoma is most commonly an isolated diagnosis, but it has been associated with other neurocristopathies such as Hirschsprung disease, congenital central hypoventilation syndrome, and neurofibromatosis type 1. These syndromes are associated with germline loss-of-function mutation in the *PHOX2B* gene and can predispose to neuroblastoma. Additionally, a very small number of patients (1% to 2%) present as part of a familial neuroblastoma syndrome and should be tested for germline *ALK* mutations (Fig. 126.1).

CLINICAL PRESENTATION

Neuroblastoma can arise at any site along the sympathetic chain. Symptoms at diagnosis depend on the location and extent of disease. Primary tumors most commonly occur in the abdomen (65%) and typically present as a painless abdominal mass. These patients may also present with vomiting, constipation, or symptoms of intestinal obstruction. Other common sites of primary tumors include the neck, chest, and paraspinal region. Tumors arising from the chest may be found incidentally on chest radiography, and cervical tumors may present as Horner syndrome or more rarely with superior vena cava syndrome (Fig. 126.2).

Approximately half of patients have metastatic disease at the time of diagnosis. Infants with metastatic disease often present with massive hepatomegaly with or without respiratory compromise. Infants may also present with bluish, subcutaneous nodules, a hallmark of the disease in this population. Other symptoms of metastatic disease in any patient include anorexia, bone pain, irritability, fever, pallor, and hypertension (most often as a result of renal vascular compression). Periorbital ecchymosis and proptosis (from bony tumor infiltrate) are also characteristic of neuroblastoma. Rarely, children are symptomatic from tumor cell catecholamine release, resulting in flushing, sweating, headache, palpitations, and hypertension.

A small percentage of children (5%) present with symptoms of spinal cord compression. This oncologic emergency is associated with

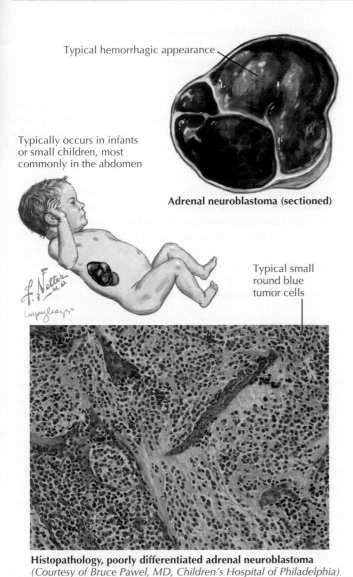

Typical hemorrhagic appearance

Typically occurs in infants or small children, most commonly in the abdomen

Adrenal neuroblastoma (sectioned)

Typical small round blue tumor cells

Histopathology, poorly differentiated adrenal neuroblastoma
(Courtesy of Bruce Pawel, MD, Children's Hospital of Philadelphia)

Fig. 126.1 Overview of Neuroblastoma.

paraspinal neuroblastomas, and associated findings include lower extremity weakness, bowel and bladder dysfunction, back pain, and sensory loss (Fig. 126.2). Neurologic function at the time of diagnosis has a strong association with long-term neurologic outcome.

In addition, there are distinct paraneoplastic syndromes associated with neuroblastoma. Secretion of vasoactive intestinal peptide by tumor cells results in intractable, watery diarrhea, hypokalemia, and poor growth. These tumors are often associated with favorable histologic findings and good prognosis. The syndrome of opsoclonus-myoclonus is characterized by rapid, involuntary eye movements in all directions; irregular, frequent muscle jerking; and ataxia, likely the result of autoimmune attack of the cerebellum. These children usually also have a low-stage tumor with favorable biologic features. The presenting neurologic symptoms of opsoclonus-myoclonus and ataxia typically resolve after treatment; however, the majority of children have residual developmental delay.

The previously described clinical symptoms should be carefully evaluated on physical examination. The abdominal examination should focus on the presence of a mass or hepatomegaly. Head and neck evaluation should include examination for proptosis, periorbital ecchymosis, and Horner syndrome (ptosis, miosis, anhidrosis, and ipsilateral facial flushing). One should perform an examination of the cervical, supraclavicular, axillary, and inguinal areas for lymphadenopathy. A careful neurologic examination is essential because subtle findings can indicate an evolving paraspinal mass. Key neurologic findings include lower extremity weakness, hyperreflexia or diminished reflexes, decreased rectal sphincter tone, bowel or bladder incontinence, and paraplegia.

DIFFERENTIAL DIAGNOSIS

Because of its varied presentation, the differential diagnosis of a patient with suspected neuroblastoma is broad and should be based on specific signs and symptoms. The clinical presentation can be divided into categories: an abdominal mass or symptoms, a mass in another location, spinal cord compression, and nonspecific neurologic symptoms. Table 126.1 summarizes the differential diagnosis of neuroblastoma using these categories of presenting symptoms.

An abdominal mass is the most common physical examination finding in a patient with neuroblastoma. When evaluating an

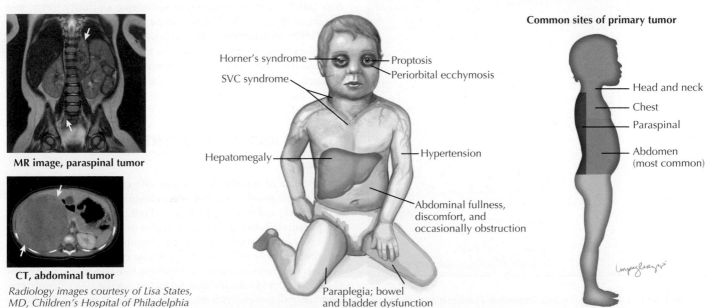

MR image, paraspinal tumor

CT, abdominal tumor

Radiology images courtesy of Lisa States, MD, Children's Hospital of Philadelphia

Horner's syndrome
SVC syndrome
Proptosis
Periorbital ecchymosis
Hepatomegaly
Hypertension
Abdominal fullness, discomfort, and occasionally obstruction
Paraplegia; bowel and bladder dysfunction

Common sites of primary tumor
Head and neck
Chest
Paraspinal
Abdomen (most common)

Fig. 126.2 Summary of Clinical Presentation of Neuroblastoma.

TABLE 126.1   Differential Diagnosis of Neuroblastoma

Presenting Symptom	Differential Diagnosis
Abdominal Mass	
Intra-abdominal mass	Neuroblastoma
	Wilms tumor
	Omphalocele
	Hernia
	Pheochromocytoma
	Adrenal hemorrhage
	Hemangioendothelioma
	Ovarian torsion
	Ovarian tumor
	Teratoma
	Lymphoma
	Hepatoblastoma
	Pancreatoblastoma
Intestinal mass	Bezoar
	Volvulus
	Megacolon
	Intussusception
	Abscess
Other intra-abdominal pathologic conditions	Pancreatic pseudocyst
	Choledochal cyst
	Hydrops of the gallbladder
	Enlarged uterus
	Constipation
	Cystic kidney disease
Thoracic Mass	
Oncologic	Neuroblastoma
	Lymphoma/leukemia
	Germ cell tumor
Non-oncologic	Congenital malformations
	• Bronchogenic cyst
	• Vascular malformations
	Tuberculosis
	Histoplasmosis
	Pneumonia
Spinal Cord Compression	
Oncologic	Sarcoma (most common)
	Neuroblastoma
	Leukemia
	Lymphoma
Non-oncologic	Trauma
	Infectious causes
	• Epidural abscess
	• Vertebral osteomyelitis
	• Tuberculosis
	Aortic dissection
	Thrombosis of the anterior spinal artery
	Arteriovenous malformation
	Transverse myelitis
	Vasculitis
	Guillain-Barré syndrome
	Acute demyelinating encephalomyelitis

abdominal mass, it is important to determine whether it is secondary to an enlarged organ (hepatomegaly or splenomegaly) or a discrete mass. Even though hepatomegaly may be mistaken for an abdominal mass,

an enlarged liver may be the result of an infection, storage disease, congenital hepatic fibrosis, or malignant infiltration. Splenomegaly may be attributable to leukemia or lymphoma, a hemolytic anemia, portal hypertension, or a storage disease.

There are many causes of spinal cord compression (Table 126.1) in addition to neuroblastoma. However, in the case of spinal cord compression, the cause may not be immediately known, and steroid treatment can be initiated before a definitive diagnosis is made in select cases. In cases in which neurologic symptoms are rapidly progressing, immediate treatment is warranted to increase the prospect for preservation of neurologic function.

Opsoclonus-myoclonus occurs in 2% to 4% of children with neuroblastoma. It represents a specific syndrome characterized by rapid, irregular eye movements, ataxia, and myoclonus. Approximately 50% of children with this syndrome are found to have a primary neuroblastoma, and diagnostic workup should be undertaken to identify a primary tumor in all children with these symptoms. The differential diagnosis is broad for any one of these symptoms; however, the constellation of symptoms significantly narrows the differential diagnosis.

EVALUATION

The initial workup for patients with suspected neuroblastoma includes laboratory and radiographic studies, and disease confirmation requires histologic assessment. Tumor stage and biology are determined at diagnosis as part of risk stratification and for guidance of treatment plan.

In a patient with suspected neuroblastoma, initial laboratory studies should include complete blood count, basic metabolic panel, hepatic function panel, lactate dehydrogenase, ferritin, and urine homovanillic acid (HVA) and vanillylmandelic acid (VMA). Elevated urine HVA and VMA are detected in 90% of all patients with neuroblastoma. Radiologic evaluation depends on primary tumor location. Computed tomography imaging is best for tumors of the mediastinum, abdomen, and pelvis, but magnetic resonance imaging is superior for evaluation of paraspinal lesions and potential spinal cord compression. Imaging is important to define the presence of image-defined risk factors that make complete or partial tumor resection more challenging at the time of diagnosis, for example, encasement of vasculature or intraspinal tumor extension.

If neuroblastoma is the likely diagnosis, a metaiodobenzylguanidine (MIBG) scan is important in identifying a primary tumor and metastatic disease. The MIBG isotope is concentrated in approximately 90% of neuroblastomas and is used in diagnosis and monitoring throughout therapy. Bilateral bone marrow aspirates and biopsies are necessary to evaluate for the presence of metastatic disease.

Tumor molecular biology is also assessed at diagnosis and includes testing for *MYCN* amplification, 11q aberration, and DNA index (ploidy).

STAGING AND MANAGEMENT

Staging

Classification of neuroblastoma is generally clear for patients at either end of the diagnostic spectrum: older children with metastatic disease are high risk, and infants with localized tumors are generally curable. The patients in between are more complex to categorize. Many staging systems have been used over time, but recently, efforts have been made to more uniformly define risk categories for cooperative group collaboration. The International Neuroblastoma Risk Group Staging System (Table 126.2) and Classification System was designed to identify *pretreatment* risk groups. With this system there are 16 distinct risk groups based on 13 potential prognostic factors; however, there are essentially four broad risk categories: very low risk, low risk, intermediate risk,

TABLE 126.2 International Neuroblastoma Risk Group Staging System (INRGSS)

L1	Localized tumor not involving vital structures (defined by list of image-defined risk factors) and confined to one body compartment
L2	Locoregional tumor with presence of one or more image-defined risk factors
M	Distant metastatic disease (except MS)
MS	Metastatic disease in children younger than 18 months with metastases confined to skin, liver, and/or bone marrow[a]

[a]MS treated like lower-risk disease.

and high risk. Five-year event-free survival rates for these groups are: greater than 85%, greater than 75% to less than 85%, greater than 50% to less than 75%, and less than 50%, respectively. Tumor risk assessment generally depends on stage at diagnosis (localized or metastatic), age at diagnosis, pathology, and genomic characterization (*MYCN* amplification, 11q status, and ploidy). Risk classification is essential in determining a treatment course and prognosis.

Risk Categories

Low risk. Infants less than 1 year with adrenal masses (<5 cm diameter) presumed to be neuroblastoma may be observed safely without tissue biopsy (unless tumors grow). For patients over 1 year with localized disease and absence of imaging defined risk factors, the tumor should be resected. In the absence of *MYCN*, no further treatment is necessary, and residual tumor after resection is not considered a risk factor for relapse.

Intermediate risk. Children with intermediate-risk neuroblastoma generally undergo two to eight cycles of moderate-intensity chemotherapy. When possible, surgery is performed for resection of residual primary tumor, but complete resection is not essential. Some children in this risk category have unresectable disease and unfavorable genomics and may also require radiotherapy.

High risk. Any child over 18 months with metastatic disease is classified as having high-risk disease. Unfavorable genomics may also place a child in this category. The current approach for high-risk neuroblastoma involves induction chemotherapy to reduce tumor burden, followed by surgery, as well as myeloablative chemotherapy followed by autologous hematopoietic stem cell rescue. Additionally, there is maintenance therapy with an anti-GD2 monoclonal antibody and a differentiating agent (isotretinoin).

Treatment Modalities
Surgery

Surgery is a mainstay of therapy and is important in confirming diagnosis as well as in disease treatment. Gross total resection is the goal, provided the tumor can be safely removed without damaging vital organs, but is not necessary in all cases. In patients with intermediate- and high-risk tumors, it may be necessary to attempt to reduce the tumor burden with chemotherapy before attempting resection. Surrounding lymph nodes are also sampled at the time of surgery.

Chemotherapy

A number of different chemotherapeutic regimens are used in patients with intermediate- and high-risk disease. The most common medications used for initial therapy include cisplatin, etoposide, doxorubicin, cyclophosphamide, topotecan, and vincristine.

Radiation

Radiation therapy is used in neonates with 4S disease (localized primary tumor with dissemination limited to skin, liver, or bone marrow) who develop respiratory distress as a result of hepatosplenomegaly and in whom chemotherapy alone is not effective in symptom resolution. Localized radiation therapy is also used for treatment of patients with high-risk disease after stem cell transplant. Additionally, radiation therapy can play an important role in palliation when required.

Relapsed Disease

The most effective treatments for relapsed neuroblastoma have included topotecan with cyclophosphamide, irinotecan with temozolomide, or topotecan with temozolomide. Iodine-131 MIBG therapy also has been used as a salvage treatment. Unfortunately, overall survival is only approximately 11 months for patients with relapsed disease.

FUTURE DIRECTIONS

Although patients with low-risk disease have a generally favorable outcome, those with high-risk disease experience significant morbidity. Even with aggressive treatment, approximately 50% of patients with high-risk neuroblastoma will experience disease relapse. Patients who survive may experience a number of long-term complications of treatment, including secondary malignancies later in life. As the specific molecular pathogenesis of neuroblastoma is more completely understood, the hope is to develop therapies that target these factors. Incorporation of anti-GD2 antibody in maintenance therapy has been a successful approach for some patients to prevent relapse. Future research may continue to explore antibody-mediated treatment and directed cell therapy in conjunction with, or perhaps someday in place of, cytotoxic treatment.

MIBG therapy has been used for several decades for relapsed/refractory neuroblastoma and has been shown to have some benefit in this patient population. Currently, there is research into use of MIBG up front for high-risk disease, with the aim of ultimately substituting this for other parts of treatment to reduce morbidity and long-term side effects.

The outlook for neuroblastoma depends on gaining a more detailed understanding of the genetic basis of disease initiation and progression in order to identify novel therapies offering decreased toxicity, improved outcomes, and enhanced quality of life.

ACKNOWLEDGMENT

The author would like to acknowledge Elizabeth M. Wallis, MD, and Nicholas Evageliou, MD, for their work on the previous edition chapter.

SUGGESTED READINGS

Available online.

127

Renal Neoplasms

Ajibike Lapite

✳ CLINICAL VIGNETTE

A 3-year-old boy is brought to clinic by his mother for evaluation of an abdominal mass. She noted the mass two nights before while bathing him. He has otherwise been well.

His vital signs are unremarkable. He is well appearing and interactive. He has a palpable, firm, nontender abdominal mass that does not cross the midline. There are no other notable findings on physical examination. His complete blood count and basic metabolic panel were within normal limits. Urinalysis demonstrated no hematuria or pyuria. He underwent abdominal ultrasound, which demonstrated a hyperechoic lesion of the left kidney with areas of heterogeneity. He subsequently underwent computed tomography of the chest, abdomen, and pelvis showing presumed Wilms tumor. No metastases were identified with imaging. He underwent nephrectomy. Subsequent pathologic examination confirmed favorable histology Wilms tumor. His disease was determined to be stage I and he received no chemotherapy or radiation.

Renal neoplasms account for 7% of pediatric cancers and can be divided into primary benign tumors, primary malignant tumors, and renal metastatic tumors. Outcomes for renal cancer are variable and depend on the cause, stage at presentation, and underlying histology. Survival rate for favorable histology Wilms tumor is estimated at more than 90%, with the survival rate for advanced rhabdoid tumor and renal medullary carcinoma estimated at less than 25%. Optimal therapy for renal tumors remains an active area of research.

ETIOLOGY AND PATHOGENESIS

Benign Renal Tumors
Angiomyolipoma

Angiomyolipomas are mesenchymal tumors characterized as neoplasms with perivascular epithelioid differentiation (PEComas). Epithelioid cells distributed around blood vessels serve as progenitors for these neoplasms. Tumors are composed of smooth muscle, fat, and abnormal blood vessels, which aid in imaging diagnosis. The majority of angiomyolipomas are sporadic with approximately 20% identified in patients with tuberous sclerosis (Chapter 111). Associations between angiomyolipoma and von Hippel–Lindau, Sturge-Weber, and autosomal dominant polycystic kidney disease have been described.

Congenital Mesoblastic Nephroma

Congenital mesoblastic nephroma is the most common and typically benign renal tumor of infancy and may be noted on prenatal ultrasound. Congenital mesoblastic nephromas have low malignant potential. The variants are classic, cellular (which is most common and resembles infantile fibrosarcoma), and mixed type (least common).

Metanephric Adenoma

Metanephric adenoma (also referred to as nephrogenic adenofibroma or embryonal adenoma) is an uncommon benign renal neoplasm of the renal cortex. Nearly all metanephric adenomas contain a *BRAF V600* mutation.

Multilocular Cystic Nephroma

Multilocular cystic nephromas appear cystic on ultrasound. These benign tumors cannot be distinguished from cystic Wilms tumor on imaging.

Ossifying Renal Tumor of Infancy

Ossifying renal tumor of infancy (ORTI) is a benign renal neoplasm arising from intralobar nephrogenic rests and demonstrating osteoid formation.

Malignant Renal Tumors
Wilms Tumor

Wilms tumor or nephroblastoma (Fig. 127.1) is the most common malignant pediatric renal tumor, accounting for 6% of all pediatric cancer and 90% of pediatric renal tumors. These tumors are embryonic, solid tumors often arising from the metanephros. Embryonic renal tissue (nephrogenic rests) is often noted at resection. The presence of multiple, diffuse nephrogenic rests is known as nephroblastomatosis, which can regress, differentiate into mature renal tissue, or transform into a Wilms tumor. Its presence warrants screening for malignant progression. Wilms tumor is frequently sporadic but can be associated with a number of genetic syndromes such as Denys-Drash, WAGR, Perlman, and Beckwith-Wiedemann. Approximately 5% of patients with Wilms tumor have a defect in Wilms tumor gene *(WT1)* located at 11p13. Deletions of this region are associated with WAGR syndrome and mutations are associated with Denys-Drash syndrome. When functional, *WT1* plays a role in DNA damage repair. Loss of heterozygosity (LOH) or loss of imprinting at the *WT2* gene located at 11p15 has been identified in patients with overgrowth syndromes such as Beckwith-Wiedemann and Perlman.

LOH of chromosomes 16q and 1p has been associated with a more aggressive form of Wilms tumor. Although 85% to 90% of Wilms tumor is deemed favorable histology, 5% to 10% is anaplastic. Anaplastic Wilms tumor is associated with alterations in the *TP53* gene. On histologic examination, these tumors have irregular mitoses and hyperchromatic cells with large nuclei throughout; the prognosis for anaplastic Wilms tumor is poor.

Clear Cell Sarcoma of the Kidney

Clear cell sarcoma of the kidney (CCSK) is the second most common pediatric renal cancer. This tumor is also called *bone metastasizing renal tumor of childhood* because of its proclivity for bone metastasis.

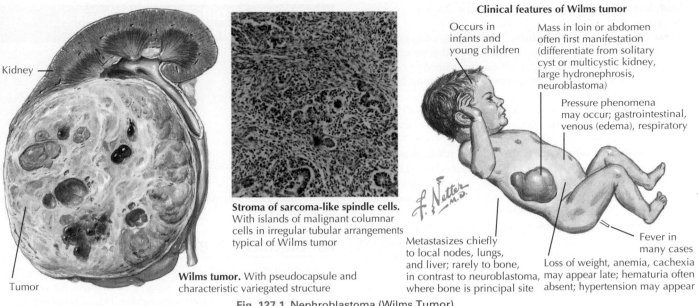

Kidney

Tumor

Stroma of sarcoma-like spindle cells. With islands of malignant columnar cells in irregular tubular arrangements typical of Wilms tumor

Wilms tumor. With pseudocapsule and characteristic variegated structure

Clinical features of Wilms tumor

Occurs in infants and young children

Mass in loin or abdomen often first manifestation (differentiate from solitary cyst or multicystic kidney, large hydronephrosis, neuroblastoma)

Pressure phenomena may occur; gastrointestinal, venous (edema), respiratory

Metastasizes chiefly to local nodes, lungs, and liver; rarely to bone, in contrast to neuroblastoma, where bone is principal site

Fever in many cases

Loss of weight, anemia, cachexia may appear late; hematuria often absent; hypertension may appear

Fig. 127.1 Nephroblastoma (Wilms Tumor).

Histologic examination typically reveals nests and cords of cell, but some histologic types may be difficult to differentiate from other renal cancers. Recent studies have demonstrated *BCOR* duplications as a genetic change that distinguishes CCSK among malignant renal tumors. Some tumors have been shown to have a balanced t(10;17) (q22;p13) chromosomal translocation with resultant *YWHAE-NUTM2* fusion and dysregulation of downstream signaling cascades.

Renal Cell Carcinoma

Renal cell carcinoma (RCC) is exceedingly rare in the pediatric population and has been identified as a distinct entity from adult RCC. Pediatric RCC is translocation-positive; translocations involve Xp11.2, the locus of the *TFE3* gene, which results in upregulation of met tyrosine kinase and downstream signaling. Bilateral RCC can be associated with von Hippel–Lindau syndrome (Chapter 111).

Renal Medullary Carcinoma

Renal medullary carcinoma (RMC) is another rare, aggressive pediatric cancer and is a subtype of RCC. RMC is found almost exclusively in patients with sickle cell trait/sickle hemoglobinopathy. Currently, the strong association is not well understood. All RMC tumors lack the INI1 protein, which is a tumor suppressor.

Rhabdoid Tumor of the Kidney

Rhabdoid tumor of the kidney (RTK) is one of the most aggressive pediatric cancers with peak incidence in infancy. RTK is characterized by defects in the *SMARCB1/INI1/hSNF5/BAF47* gene, which functions as a tumor suppressor.

CLINICAL MANIFESTATION

Clinical manifestation is variable; often, masses are asymptomatic and incidentally identified. Initial presentation depends on the pathologic processes and severity of the renal neoplasm. Common manifesting symptoms include a palpable abdominal mass that may or may not be painful, abdominal distension, and hematuria; some patients may present with constitutional symptoms, including fever, weight loss, and fatigue. Tumor-specific clinical manifestation is discussed in the following section.

Benign Renal Tumors

- **Angiomyolipoma:** The majority of angiomyolipomas are asymptomatic and are often incidentally noted on tuberous sclerosis screening. Larger angiomyolipomas are more likely to be symptomatic and may cause flank pain or hematuria. The abnormal vasculature component of this tumor can form aneurysms that may hemorrhage.
- **Congenital mesoblastic nephroma:** Of children with congenital mesoblastic nephroma, 90% present within the first year of life, with peak incidence at younger than 3 months of age. It can be identified on prenatal ultrasound; a palpable abdominal mass is the most common postnatal manifestation. Hematuria, proteinuria, acute kidney injury, and electrolyte disturbances secondary to the infiltrative nature of this neoplasm have been described.
- **Metanephric adenoma:** Metanephric adenomas are often incidentally noted; they are far more common in the adult population but have been diagnosed in the pediatric population. Incidence is greater in females than males. Symptomatic patients may present with flank pain in addition to dysuria and may exhibit hypertension, hypercalcemia, hematuria, and polycythemia.
- **Multilocular cystic nephroma:** Cystic nephromas have been identified in the pediatric population, although they are more common in the adult population. Cystic partially differentiated nephroblastoma is typically diagnosed in children 3 months to 4 years of age. The typical presentation includes a palpable abdominal mass.
- **Ossifying renal tumor of infancy:** ORTIs classically manifest with gross hematuria and less frequently with a palpable mass. Males are affected more often than females.

Malignant Renal Tumors

- **Wilms tumor:** Wilms tumor classically manifests as a palpable abdominal mass. Hypertension and hematuria may occur at presentation secondary to tumor mass effect on neighboring vasculature. The majority of patients are younger than 10 years, typically toddlers, at diagnosis. Patients with unilateral disease (95% of cases) present at 3 to 4 years of age, whereas patients with bilateral disease (5% of cases) present at 2 to 2.5 years of age. Metastasis at diagnosis is not uncommon. Approximately 85% of metastases are to the lungs. Other common sites are regional lymph nodes and liver. Metastases to the brain or bone are exceedingly rare but have been described.

- **Clear cell sarcoma of the kidney:** The majority of patients with CCSK present at 1 to 4 years of age. Patients often present with a palpable abdominal mass which can be accompanied by hematuria or flank pain. CCSK is known to metastasize to the lung, brain, soft tissues, and most often to bone.
- **Renal cell carcinoma:** Peak incidence occurs between 10 and 11 years of age. Patients present with a palpable abdominal mass, painless hematuria, and flank pain.
- **Renal medullary carcinoma:** Patients with RMC present with hematuria and flank pain; a palpable mass is less typical but when present is more likely to be right sided. Approximately 50% of patients will endorse constitutional symptoms such as weight loss, fever, and night sweats at presentation.
- **Rhabdoid tumor of the kidney:** RTK is identified in patients who are generally younger than 2 years of age. At presentation, fever and hematuria are common. Approximately 25% of patients have metastatic disease at diagnosis. Approximately 10% to 20% of patients have a concomitant brain tumor and exhibit neurologic symptoms at presentation.

EVALUATION AND MANAGEMENT

Along with a thorough history and physical examination, it is important to elucidate symptoms and duration thereof and to acquire a complete list of medical comorbidities that can guide diagnosis. A predisposition such as nephroblastomatosis is important to note. Although familial inheritance is uncommon, a complete family history should be acquired. The abdomen should be examined with care because an aggressive palpation can rupture a large tumor. A thorough assessment for lymphadenopathy is important. Anomalies can be detected that may suggest an underlying predisposition syndrome. Such features might include coarse facies (seen in patients with *WT1* mutations), aniridia or undescended testicles (seen in patients with WAGR), or hemihypertrophy, macroglossia, ear pits/tags/creases (seen in patients with Beckwith-Wiedemann). Identification of a predisposition syndrome will affect further diagnostics and management.

DIAGNOSTIC APPROACH

Initial laboratory evaluation can help differentiate a renal neoplasm from other renal lesions (Box 127.1). Initial studies should include a complete blood count (CBC), lactate dehydrogenase (LDH), uric acid, chemistries, and urinalysis. The CBC, LDH, and uric acid can help differentiate leukemic/lymphomatous infiltration of the kidney from other renal neoplasms. Chemistries are helpful to determine whether the patient has normal kidney function. Hypercalcemia has been identified in renal tumors secondary to paraneoplastic phenomenon. Urinalysis can be helpful to demonstrate hematuria, which can be present in neoplastic, infectious, or thrombotic causes or pyuria, which is more suggestive of an infectious process.

Abdominal ultrasound can identify the origin of the mass and determine whether the mass is cystic or solid. Computed tomography (CT) of the abdomen and pelvis is often performed to further characterize the lesion. Magnetic resonance imaging (MRI) or other imaging of the head and chest may be obtained to evaluate for metastatic disease (which is more likely for some neoplasms than others). Given that some renal tumors can extend into vasculature, including the inferior vena cava, and form tumor thrombi (Fig. 127.2), imaging of the renal/large vasculature is imperative. After radiographic evaluation, biopsy often follows; this is dependent on whether workup favors benign

---

> **BOX 127.1 Differential Diagnosis of Pediatric Renal Lesions**
>
> Abscess
> Cysts
> Hemorrhage
> Neoplasm (primary benign, primary malignant, or leukemic/lymphomatous infiltration)
> Pseudotumor
> Thrombus
> Vascular malformation

versus malignant cause and whether the mass is appropriate for surgical resection.

MANAGEMENT OF BENIGN RENAL TUMORS

- **Angiomyolipoma:** Identification of an angiomyolipoma (Fig. 127.3) should prompt brain imaging to evaluate for other syndromic features of tuberous sclerosis (Fig. 111.1). Imaging findings are usually characteristic such that biopsy is not necessary for diagnosis. Given the vascular element of the tumor, biopsy can carry a grave risk for hemorrhage. The risk for aneurysmal hemorrhage is increased for tumors greater than 4 cm. Catheter embolization is important for patients who have bleeds, and, if unsuccessful, partial nephrectomy is definitive. Routine renal surveillance is important for patients with tuberous sclerosis because of risk for angiomyolipoma.
- **Congenital mesoblastic nephroma:** Treatment for congenital mesoblastic nephroma is nephrectomy with wide surgical margins given the tumor's proclivity to infiltrate. Recurrence within the first year occurs in 5% to 10% of patients; serial surveillance ultrasounds are thus recommended. Patients who present with stage III disease, have the cellular subtype, or are older than 3 months at diagnosis are candidates for adjuvant chemotherapy.
- **Metanephric adenoma:** Metanephric adenoma is difficult to distinguish from malignant tumors on imaging. Partial nephrectomy is the treatment of choice.
- **Multilocular cystic nephroma:** Cystic renal lesions can be difficult to distinguish from cystic Wilms tumor upon imaging. Treatment of choice is nephrectomy or nephron-sparing surgery given the risk for carcinomatous degeneration.
- **Ossifying renal tumor of infancy:** ORTIs have characteristic imaging findings, appearing very similar to a staghorn calculus on CT. Partial nephrectomy is the treatment of choice.

MANAGEMENT OF MALIGNANT RENAL TUMORS

- **Wilms tumor:** Treatment of Wilms tumor depends on tumor stage and histology with less aggressive management for favorable histology Wilms tumor (Table 127.1) compared with anaplastic Wilms tumor (Table 127.2). Nephrectomy is followed by chemotherapy in the United States, given that the presence of tumor at time of chemotherapy up-stages the patient's disease; preoperative chemotherapy is indicated for patients with a large unresectable tumor or vascular extension. Preoperative chemotherapy is standard in Europe. Outcomes for subsequent and preoperative chemotherapy are similar. Patients with bilateral disease undergo nephron-sparing surgery so as to maintain renal function. Patients with predisposition for Wilms tumor undergo screening with renal ultrasound every 3 months until they are approximately 7 to 8 years of age.

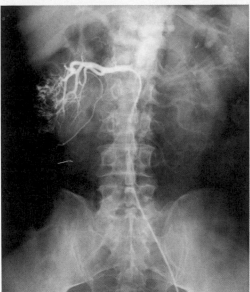

Renal cell carcinoma (hypernephroma). Selective right renal arteriogram showing typical tumor vessel pattern characteristic of a highly vascular renal neoplasm, such as renal cell carcinoma.

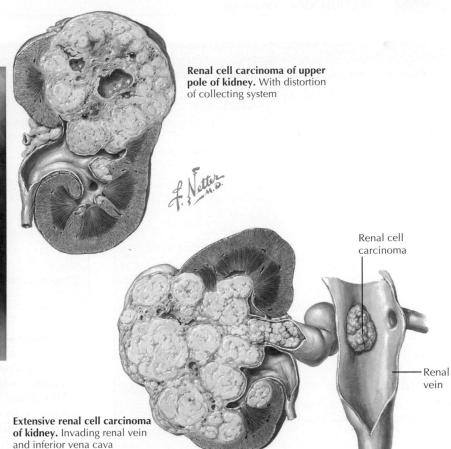

Renal cell carcinoma of upper pole of kidney. With distortion of collecting system

Renal cell carcinoma

Renal vein

Extensive renal cell carcinoma of kidney. Invading renal vein and inferior vena cava

Fig. 127.2 Malignant Tumors of the Kidney.

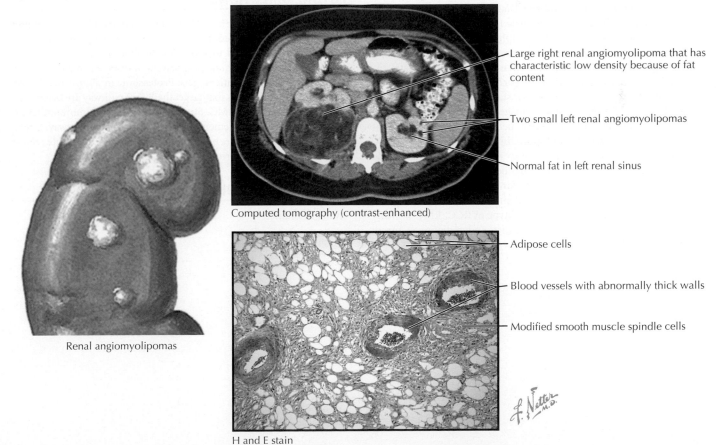

Large right renal angiomyolipoma that has characteristic low density because of fat content

Two small left renal angiomyolipomas

Normal fat in left renal sinus

Computed tomography (contrast-enhanced)

Adipose cells

Blood vessels with abnormally thick walls

Modified smooth muscle spindle cells

Renal angiomyolipomas

H and E stain

Fig. 127.3 Benign Renal Tumors: Angiomyolipoma.

TABLE 127.1   Current Management for Favorable Histology Wilms Tumor

Stage	Treatment
Stage I (favorable histology and patient younger than 2 years of age)	No chemotherapy or radiation
Stage I and II (favorable histology without LOH 1p and 16q)	Vincristine and actinomycin-D No radiation
Stage I and II (favorable histology with LOH 1p and 16q)	Vincristine, actinomycin-D, and doxorubicin No radiation
Stage III (favorable histology without LOH 1p and 16q)	Vincristine, actinomycin-D, and doxorubicin Radiation of flank or hemiabdomen
Stage III (favorable histology with LOH 1p and 16q)	Vincristine, actinomycin-D, doxorubicin, cyclophosphamide, etoposide Radiation of flank or hemiabdomen
Stage IV (favorable histology without LOH 1p and 16q)	Vincristine, actinomycin-D, and doxorubicin Radiation of flank or hemiabdomen
Stage IV (favorable histology with pulmonary metastasis ± other metastases, LOH 1p and 16q)	Vincristine, actinomycin-D, doxorubicin, cyclophosphamide, etoposide Radiation of the whole lung in addition to flank or hemiabdomen

LOH, Loss of heterozygosity.

TABLE 127.2   Current Management for Anaplastic Wilms Tumor

Stage	Treatment
Stage I (diffuse anaplastic)	Vincristine, actinomycin-D, and doxorubicin Radiation of flank or hemiabdomen
Stage I–III (focal anaplastic)	Vincristine, actinomycin-D, and doxorubicin Radiation of flank or hemiabdomen
Stage II and III (diffuse anaplastic)	Vincristine, actinomycin-D, doxorubicin, cyclophosphamide, etoposide, carboplatin Radiation of flank or hemiabdomen
Stage IV (focal anaplastic)	Vincristine, actinomycin-D, doxorubicin, cyclophosphamide, etoposide, carboplatin Radiation of flank or hemiabdomen
Stage IV (diffuse anaplastic)	Vincristine, actinomycin-D, doxorubicin, cyclophosphamide, etoposide, carboplatin, irinotecan Radiation of flank or hemiabdomen

- **Clear cell sarcoma of the kidney:** Diagnostic imaging for CCSK should include a bone scan to evaluate for metastases. Given nodal metastasis in one-third of cases, lymph node sampling is integral to staging. Treatment includes nephrectomy and chemotherapy. Radiation therapy is considered in circumstances of metastatic disease. The addition of doxorubicin for chemotherapy has increased survival rates to greater than 95% for stage I disease.
- **Renal cell carcinoma:** Initial management for suspected RCC should include imaging to assess for metastatic disease. Survival for stage I is greater than 90% and approximately 9% for stage IV. RCC is known to be poorly responsive to many chemotherapies and radiation. Current treatment includes nephrectomy. Immunotherapies for RCC have been approved for adult patients and remain under investigation for pediatric patients.
- **Renal medullary carcinoma:** As a subtype of RCC, RMC similarly is resistant to many chemotherapeutics and radiation. Current treatment of choice is nephrectomy.
- **Rhabdoid tumor of the kidney:** CT or MRI of the brain is recommended at diagnosis to evaluate for concurrent brain neoplasm. Prognosis is poor, with an overall survival rate of 25%. Treatment modalities include chemotherapy, radiation, and nephrectomy.

Chemotherapy regimens for malignant renal tumors often include vincristine, actinomycin-D, doxorubicin, cyclophosphamide, etoposide, and carboplatin. All patients treated for a malignant renal tumor warrant follow-up to evaluate for recurrence for a minimum of 5 years after diagnosis.

FUTURE DIRECTIONS

The significant difference in survival rates for favorable histology Wilms tumor compared with less common malignant renal tumors underlines the need for novel therapeutics for renal neoplasms. Ongoing research to identify the biological drivers of disease will aid efforts to identify unique therapeutic targets. Proteasome inhibitors in addition to pharmaceutical agents that target the EZH2 pathway are being evaluated for treatment of RMC. Studies to determine if immunotherapy is appropriate for management of pediatric RCC are underway. Efforts to identify tumor markers by urine continue and may indicate relapse sooner than current metrics.

SUGGESTED READINGS

Available online.

128

Bone Neoplasms

Timothy T. Spear and Jenna M. Gedminas

 CLINICAL VIGNETTE

A 16-year-old previously healthy boy presented with 3 months of dull, achy, right upper leg pain. He attributed this to overuse and denied recent injury. He denied fever or weight loss. Physical examination showed tenderness over the distal right femur with associated soft tissue mass. Plain radiograph of the right femur showed a "sunburst" lesion associated with periosteal elevation without fracture. Biopsy displayed osteoid-producing spindle cells, confirming a diagnosis of osteosarcoma. Computed tomography and positron emission tomography imaging showed no bony or pulmonary metastases. The patient underwent interdisciplinary orthopedic, surgical, and oncologic evaluation and received limb-sparing surgical resection with neoadjuvant and adjuvant chemotherapy.

Primary malignant bone tumors account for approximately 6% of all childhood cancers. Osteosarcoma (OS) and the Ewing sarcoma family of tumors (ESFTs) are the most common primary bone neoplasms and together have an annual incidence of 8.7 per million in patients younger than 20 years of age. Approximately 650 to 700 children, adolescents, and young adults are diagnosed with malignant bone tumors annually in the United States. Diagnosis is often delayed because many patients attribute pain to a nonspecific trauma or acute injury.

OSTEOSARCOMA

Epidemiology and Pathogenesis

OS is the most common primary malignant bone tumor in childhood, representing 15% of all primary bone tumors and 3% of childhood malignancies. There is a slightly higher incidence in African Americans than in Whites, with a male-to-female ratio of approximately 1.5:1. The incidence is highest in patients 10 to 20 years of age, coinciding with the adolescent growth spurt.

OS lacks characteristic translocations or other genetic molecular abnormalities. However, most OSs carry a complex unbalanced karyotype, and 3% patients with OS have a germline mutation in p53. Many such patients are affected by Li-Fraumeni syndrome, a familial cancer predisposition syndrome in which affected individuals may develop sarcomas, brain tumors, leukemia, breast cancer, and adrenal cortical carcinoma at young ages; this risk persists throughout patients' lifetimes. Patients with a history of hereditary retinoblastoma are at higher risk for OS, further implicating the p53 pathway in proposed pathogenesis. Secondary OS has been linked to prior exposure to ionizing radiation or previous chemotherapy.

Clinical Presentation

The most common clinical symptom at presentation is localized, dull, and aching pain, typically of several months' duration. Other complaints include a palpable mass with or without swelling. Systemic complaints are rare. Pathologic fracture can occur in 10% to 15% of cases. Eighty percent of OSs occur in the extremities and a mass (tender or nontender) may be noted on physical examination (Fig. 128.1). Examination may reveal decreased range of motion or muscle atrophy; regional lymphadenopathy is rare. The most common disease sites are the metaphyses of long bones, including the distal femur, proximal tibia, and proximal humerus, although OS may occur in any bone. Axial skeleton involvement is less common. Eighty percent of patients have localized disease at diagnosis. The lung is the most common site of detectable metastatic disease, although patients may present with multifocal bone disease without pulmonary involvement.

The differential diagnosis includes benign bone tumors, infections, and other malignancies. Benign tumors to be considered include unicameral bone cysts, osteoblastomas, giant cell tumors, eosinophilic granulomas, aneurysmal bone cysts, osteochondromas, and fibrous dysplasia. Infections to be considered include osteomyelitis and septic arthritis. Other malignancies to be considered include ESFT, chondrosarcoma, fibrosarcoma, leukemia, and metastases of other solid tumors.

Evaluation

Laboratory evaluation is usually normal, with some exceptions in fewer than half of patients, including elevated alkaline phosphatase, lactate dehydrogenase, and erythrocyte sedimentation rate; these abnormalities typically do not correlate with disease extent. Plain radiograph typically reveals a lytic or blastic lesion of the bone with poorly defined borders (Fig. 128.1). Other findings include periosteal elevation adjacent to the primary lesion, a "sunburst" appearance, or a pathologic fracture. If OS is suspected, chest computed tomography (CT) can be used to assess for pulmonary metastases, and positron emission tomography (PET) or bone scan can be used to detect bony metastases. Magnetic resonance imaging (MRI) should be performed to better characterize tumor extent and should include the joint above and below the involved area to assess for skip lesions and evaluate for impingement on critical neurovascular structures (Fig. 128.1).

The diagnosis of OS can only be made by biopsy. Biopsies should be performed by an experienced orthopedic oncologist. The surgical approach at the time of biopsy may have an impact on the feasibility of future limb-sparing surgeries, which are necessary for local control. Interventional radiologists may be able to obtain the necessary biopsies with active participation by orthopedic oncologists. Involvement of the surgeon who will later perform the definitive surgical resection is preferable.

Microscopically, OS cells are mesenchymal in origin, and classically appear to be composed of spindle cells associated with malignant osteoid (Fig. 128.1). The extent of osteoid production may vary among the osteoblastic, chondroblastic, fibroblastic, telangiectatic, and small cell subtypes; however, the presence of tumor osteoid is the key pathologic feature of this disease.

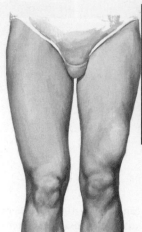

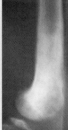

AP and lateral radiograph shows dense lesion and periosteal elevation

Mass on left distal femur palpable and tender but only slightly visible

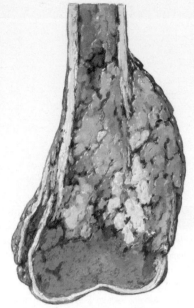

Tumor occupies entire metaphysis of distal femur and has extended into the soft tissues

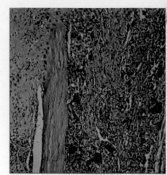

Highly malignant stroma with cartilaginous and osteoid components (H and E stain)

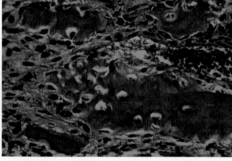

Masses of tumor cells with hyperchromatic nuclei interspersed with foci of malignant osteoid are typical histopathologic findings (H and E stain)

Osteosarcoma MRI of thigh showing pathologic fracture of distal femur and extensive soft tissue spread of osteogenic sarcoma into both anterior and posterior thigh compartments.

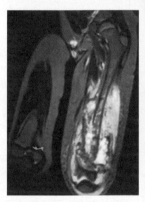

Fig. 128.1 Osteosarcoma.

Management

Advances in chemotherapy over the past 30 years have resulted in higher overall survival rates and improved rates of limb salvage for patients with OS. Chemotherapy is used initially both to decrease primary tumor size, facilitating surgical resection, and to treat pulmonary micrometastases. Current treatment protocols for OS include neoadjuvant and adjuvant chemotherapy. The total duration of treatment is 8 to 12 months and includes cisplatin, doxorubicin, and high-dose methotrexate.

Complete surgical resection with wide margins is necessary for cure. Modern approaches to limb salvage surgery have resulted in local recurrence rates similar to those achieved with amputation. Limb salvage has therefore become the standard of care except when limb preservation might compromise disease control. OS is not considered a radiosensitive tumor, although high-dose radiation may be considered for local control in rare cases in which tumor location precludes surgical resection. Surgery is employed for macroscopic pulmonary metastases.

Treatment of recurrent OS remains challenging given few effective therapeutic options. A small subset of patients are able to achieve subsequent surgical remission. More recently, ifosfamide alone or in combination with etoposide is being evaluated to treat recurrent disease. Other targets and agents under investigation include MTP-PE (an immune modulator that induces monocytes and macrophages to become tumoricidal), monoclonal antibodies directed against GD2 (a surface glycolipid expressed at high levels in OS), and targets involved in bone remodeling including RANK and RANKL.

Prognosis

Most patients with localized OS involving an extremity can be cured. The 5-year survival rate for nonmetastatic OS is approximately 60% to 70%. Patients with clinically detectable metastatic disease have a far worse prognosis; the overall survival rate is approximately 25% to 30% and is worse with bony compared with pulmonary metastasis. Factors that independently contribute to predicted worse outcomes include larger initial tumor burden, inadequate surgical margins, age less than 14, and male gender. Importantly, chemotherapy-induced degree of necrosis at surgical resection is an important prognostic factor for patients with localized disease. Relapse-free survival is higher in patients with near-complete eradication of viable tumor compared with patients who achieve a less extensive histologic response to therapy.

EWING SARCOMA FAMILY OF TUMORS

Epidemiology

ESFT is the second most common cancer of bone in children and adolescents, with an incidence of 2.1 per million children in the United States. Most patients are diagnosed during the second decade of life. ESFT includes Ewing sarcoma (ES) of bone, Askin tumor (ES of the chest wall), extraosseous ES (arising from soft tissue), and peripheral neuroectodermal tumor (PNET). ESFT is six times more common in Whites than African Americans and is slightly more common in males than females. The cause of ESFT remains largely obscure, though chromosomal translocations are the hallmark of ESFT and directly impact diagnostic and treatment approaches.

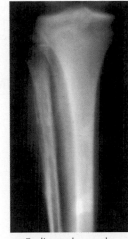

Tender bulge on proximal fibula with some inflammatory signs

Radiograph reveals mottled, destructive radiolucent lesion

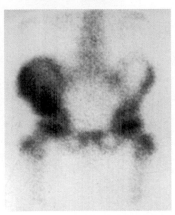

Bone scan shows lesion of mottled density involving anterior superior iliac spine

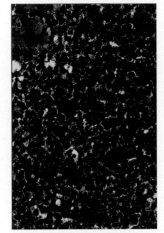

Section shows masses of small, round cells with uniformly sized hyperchromatic nuclei (H and E stain)

Fig. 128.2 Ewing Sarcoma.

Clinical Presentation

The most common presenting symptom of patients with ESFT of bone is pain; it is often more intermittent than in OS. Like OS, bone pain is often attributed to trauma, thereby delaying diagnosis. Patients may also present with swelling or a palpable, tender soft tissue mass (Fig. 128.2). Fever and weight loss are more common in the 25% of patients with metastatic disease at diagnosis but also may be seen in those with large, localized tumors. Patients with tumors of the axial skeleton may present with neurologic symptoms, including paraplegia or bowel or bladder dysfunction, secondary to spinal cord compression from paraspinal tumors.

The differential diagnosis in patients with ESFT and bony disease is similar to that of OS, including benign bone tumors, infections, and other malignancies. ESFT can be definitively distinguished from OS and other bony lesions only after a tumor biopsy. Other characteristics that differentiate ESFT from OS include more common involvement of the axial skeleton and localization within the diaphysis of long bones (as opposed to the metaphysis in OS).

Evaluation

Like OS, radiography is typically the first imaging modality used to evaluate disease (Fig. 128.2). "Onion skinning" of the periosteum

may be seen because of bony destruction. The Codman triangle may be seen resulting from tumor growth elevating the periosteum, forming a triangular interface between the tumor and normal bone. MRI of the primary site is critical in determining the extent and size of an ESFT involving bone, and the relevant bone or compartment should be imaged in its entirety.

Biopsies of suspected ESFT should be performed with the same care used for biopsies of other suspected bony malignancies. Because there may be extensive necrosis within an ESFT at presentation, frozen sections are often necessary to confirm presence of adequate diagnostic material within a biopsy. Importantly, biopsy samples should provide sufficient material for microscopy, immunohistochemical studies, and molecular diagnostic studies and should ideally be performed at a center with a pathologist experienced in their interpretation.

Microscopically, ESFTs are composed of sheets of small, round blue cells with scant cytoplasm (Fig. 128.2). The PNET variant of ESFT may appear to contain aggregates of cells known as Homer-Wright rosettes. ESFT cells are often positive for membranous CD99 (cluster of differentiation molecule) on immunohistochemistry. CD99 positivity also can be seen in other cells, including lymphoblasts. For this reason, molecular diagnostic studies are of critical importance. In 95% of cases, a rearrangement involving the *EWSR1* gene is detected. Most occur via a t(11;22) translocation, which results in production of the EWS-FLI1 fusion protein. In approximately 10% of cases, other members of the ETS transcription factor family, including *ERG*, *ETV1*, or *E1AF*, are involved in gene rearrangements, fusing with *EWSR1*.

After diagnosis of ESFT, staging evaluation is critical. The most common sites of metastases at diagnosis are lung, bone, and bone marrow. CT of the chest and fluorodeoxy-D-glucose (FDG) PET are used to detect pulmonary and skeletal metastases. Bilateral bone marrow aspirates and biopsies are performed to detect marrow involvement.

Management

Therapy for patients with ESFT involves multimodal treatment with chemotherapy, surgery, and radiation. Typically, treatment begins with neoadjuvant chemotherapy to decrease tumor burden before definitive local control. Treatment typically consists of vincristine, doxorubicin, and cyclophosphamide alternating with ifosfamide and etoposide on an every 2-week (interval compressed) schedule.

Local control for ESFT can be accomplished with surgery, radiation therapy, or a combination thereof. Complete surgical resection with margins clear of tumor is critical. In contrast with OS, ESFTs are radiosensitive; therefore radiation may serve as the primary therapeutic modality for local control in cases not amenable to surgical resection. Radiotherapy is also used postoperatively if tumor is detected at resection margins. Patients receive adjuvant systemic chemotherapy after local control. Total duration of ESFT therapy using modern intensive regimens is approximately 8 to 9 months.

The presence of unique fusion proteins in ESFT provide opportunities for the development of small molecule inhibitors as novel adjunctive therapeutic options, a number of which are currently being evaluated in clinical trials.

Prognosis

The most important prognostic factor in ESFT is disease extent at diagnosis. Despite aggressive treatment, the overall survival for patients with metastatic disease at diagnosis is approximately 25%. In patients with localized disease, 5-year event-free survival rates near 80% to 85% are recently reported. Age, site of disease, serum lactate dehydrogenase level, tumor size, and histologic response to chemotherapy have been identified as potential prognostic factors in newly diagnosed patients.

FUTURE DIRECTIONS

The successful treatment of patients with localized OS and ESFT is a result of integrated, intensive multimodality and interdisciplinary care. Dramatic improvements in outcome have been achieved in the past 30 years, although late effects of required therapies can be significant. The need to develop more targeted, less toxic therapies is therefore pressing to improve outcomes, reduce adverse events, and provide options for metastatic or relapsed disease. Enhanced understanding of the basic biology of sarcomas may improve the ability to develop rationally designed immunotherapeutic or fusion-targeted approaches for patients with bone tumors.

SUGGESTED READINGS

Available online.

129

Rhabdomyosarcoma

Jeremy M. Grenier and Jenna M. Gedminas

 CLINICAL VIGNETTE

A 10-year-old girl presents with an enlarging left periorbital mass. On history, parents report noticing mild unilateral eyelid swelling several months earlier that has slowly grown in size and now completely surrounds her eye. The patient has had some intermittent double vision but denies fever or pain. On examination, there is a 3-cm firm, immobile, nontender mass along the temporal border of the left orbit and intermittent left cranial nerve VI palsy. There is no overlying erythema, fluctuance, or lymphadenopathy. Head magnetic resonance imaging confirms your suspicion, showing a heterogeneous solid lesion infiltrating the lateral border of the left orbit, concerning for sarcoma (Fig. 129.2). Biopsy confirms rhabdomyosarcoma. She is referred to a pediatric oncologist and undergoes imaging for staging, which confirms localized disease. She undergoes systemic chemotherapy and radiation for local control with complete resolution of her primary tumor.

Rhabdomyosarcoma (RMS) is a soft tissue tumor consisting of partially differentiated mesenchymal cells with skeletal muscle characteristics. It is the third most common extracranial solid tumor in children, representing 3% of childhood cancers and 50% of soft tissue sarcomas in children, with an annual incidence of 400 new cases throughout the United States.

ETIOLOGY AND GENETICS

The majority of cases of RMS are sporadic; however, several inherited conditions have been associated with increased incidence of RMS, including Li-Fraumeni syndrome, Noonan syndrome, Costello syndrome, neurofibromatosis I, and Beckwith-Wiedemann syndrome, particularly in patients who are younger than 3 years of age. Alveolar RMS (ARMS) tumors frequently contain a characteristic fusion protein with *FOXO1* paired with either *PAX3* or *PAX7*. These fusion products are more transcriptionally active than their normal counterparts and are thought to contribute to decreased apoptosis, disruption of typical skeletal muscle differentiation, and tumorigenesis. Embryonal RMS (ERMS) tumors frequently exhibit loss of heterozygosity at the 11p15 locus, leading to duplication of the paternal copies and silencing of maternal copies of genes within this locus. ERMS tumors also frequently harbor *RAS* mutations, further contributing to oncogenesis.

CLINICAL PRESENTATION

The initial manifesting signs and symptoms of RMS are largely related to local mass effect. Tumors are often discovered as firm, nontender masses with localized lymphadenopathy. Although both subtypes can occur throughout the body, ERMS most commonly occurs in the head, neck, and urogenital tract, while ARMS frequently develops in extremities or head and neck. Orbital tumors can manifest with proptosis, periorbital swelling, and ptosis. Head and neck tumors can produce cranial nerve deficits. RMS of the extremities may resemble unresolving hematomas. Sarcoma botryoides is a form of vaginal RMS, classically described as a grapelike mass extending from the vaginal vault and often manifesting with vaginal bleeding (Fig. 129.1).

At the time of presentation, 15% to 25% of patients will have at least one site of metastasis, most commonly in the lungs but also frequently discovered in bone, bone marrow, and draining lymph nodes.

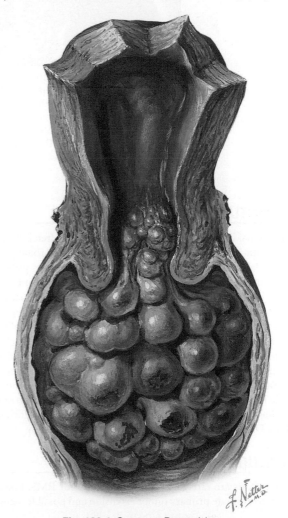

Fig. 129.1 Sarcoma Botryoides.

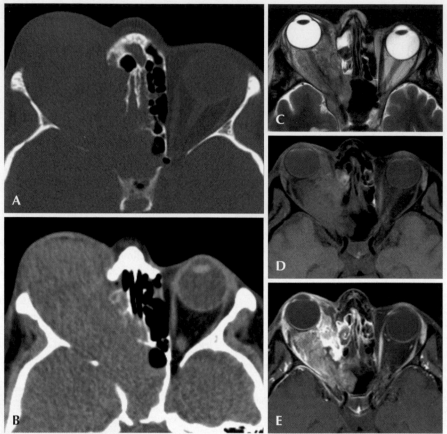

Fig. 129.2 Orbital Rhabdomyosarcoma. Axial bone window (A) and soft-tissue window (B) CT reconstructions demonstrate a large lesion centered on the right orbit extending into the ethmoid and sphenoid sinuses and the middle cranial fossa with extensive bony destruction. Axial T 2 (C), T 1 (D), and fat-saturated post gadolinium T 1 (E) MRI demonstrates avid enhancement of the lobulated mass and associated dural involvement overlying the right temporal lobe, as well as right-sided proptosis. (Reused with permission from Campion T, Miszkiel K, Davagnanam I. The orbit. In: Adrian K, Dixon AK, Schaefer-Prokop C. *Grainger & Allison's Diagnostic Radiology*. 7th ed. New York, NY: Elsevier; 2020:1562-1598, Fig. 60.34.)

DIFFERENTIAL DIAGNOSIS

The differential diagnosis for soft tissue masses in children is broad and includes both benign and malignant causes. Abscess, orbital cellulitis, or lymphadenitis should be considered in febrile patients with tender masses. A recent history of injury with subsequent development of soft tissue swelling and overlying bruising suggests possible hematoma. In contrast to malignant masses, which tend to invade underlying tissues, benign tumors such as neurofibromas and lipomas are generally freely mobile and relatively superficial. Malignant masses that can clinically resemble RMS include neuroblastoma, Ewing sarcoma, non-Hodgkin lymphoma, and leukemia manifesting with localized chloroma. Importantly, neuroblastoma, Ewing sarcoma, and lymphoma can resemble RMS under the microscope. All appear as collections of small, round blue cells, making immunohistochemistry critical for their differentiation. Diagnosis of RMS is confirmed with tumor biopsy.

EVALUATION

Laboratory tests are rarely useful in the workup for RMS. Imaging is necessary to evaluate primary tumor extension and possible metastases and is a critical part of the initial evaluation. Magnetic resonance imaging (MRI) of the primary tumor can help delineate local tissue invasion and provide essential information for possible surgical excision (Figs. 129.2 and 129.3). All patients should undergo computed tomography (CT) chest imaging to evaluate for pulmonary metastases. Positron emission tomography (PET)-CT or whole-body PET MRI are useful for detection of additional metastatic lesions. Complete blood count, liver function studies, and creatinine are useful for determining end organ dysfunction. Bilateral bone marrow biopsy is essential for assessing bone marrow infiltration.

Tissue biopsy is required for diagnosis with tumor cells staining positive for skeletal muscle–specific proteins including desmin, myosin, myoglobin, and MyoD. RMS tumors can be classified pathologically as alveolar or embryonal. ARMS is named for the spaces formed between clusters of small round blue tumor cells and fibrous strands, resembling pulmonary alveoli, and is often defined by the presence of a characteristic *FOXO1/PAX3/PAX7* fusion. ERMS in contrast, does not have these septations. Instead, ERMS comprises tumor cells spread along different stages of skeletal muscle differentiation, from small round blue cells to elongated, spindle-shaped cells expressing several skeletal muscle proteins (Table 129.1).

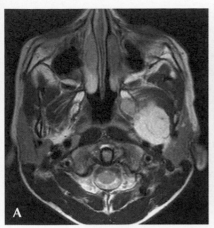
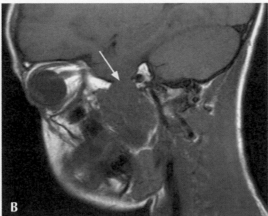
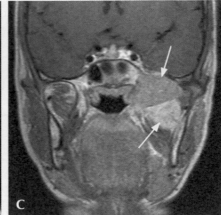

Fig. 129.3 Magnetic Resonance Imaging of Rhabdomyosarcoma of the Masticator Space. Axial T2-weighted magnetic resonance image (MRI) shows a hyperintense mass within the left masticator space. (B) Sagittal T1-weighted MRI reveals extension of the mass through an expanded foramen ovale *(arrow)*. (C) Coronal postcontrast T1-weighted image shows two different areas of enhancement *(arrows)* within the tumor, a relatively common finding with rhabdomyosarcoma. (Reused with permission from Day TA, Albergotti WG. Neoplasms of the neck. In: Flint PW, Haughey BH, Lund VJ, eds. *Cummings Otolaryngology: Head and Neck Surgery.* 7th ed. St. Louis, MO: Elsevier, 2020;1755-1772.e3, Fig. 115.8.)

TABLE 129.1 Pathologic Classification of Rhabdomyosarcoma

Pathologic Classification	Embryonal	Alveolar
Histologic features	Small, round or elongated cells with rich stroma, resembling skeletal muscle at varying stages of development	Tightly packed round cells with septations surrounding acellular regions, resembling pulmonary alveoli
Molecular characteristics	Loss of heterozygosity at 11p15	*FOXO1/PAX3* or *FOXO1/PAX7*
Clinical characteristics	Primary tumor: head, neck, and genitourinary tract Metastatic potential: moderate	Primary tumor: limbs and trunk Metastatic potential: high

TABLE 129.2 Rhabdomyosarcoma Staging

Stage	Tumor Location	Lymph Node	Distant Metastasis
1	Head, neck, genitourinary tract	Negative or Positive	None
2	All other sites and tumor ≤5 cm	Negative	None
3	All other sites and tumor >5 cm	Positive	None
4	All	All	Present

Risk Groups

Treatment of RMS often involves enrollment in clinical trials. The Children's Oncology Group stratifies treatment based on risk groups determined by a combination of histologic subtype, anatomic staging, and surgical group. As previously described, the majority of RMS cases can be histologically classified as embryonal or alveolar, but clinically are often classified as fusion positive or fusion negative. A minority of cases are neither and are classified as spindle cell/sclerosing RMS. Patients with ERMS tend to have a better prognosis than patients with ARMS, supporting the general classification of ERMS as lower risk than ARMS tumors. Staging for rhabdomyosarcoma is complex and combines tumor stage (Table 129.2) and group (Table 129.3) into risk group (Table 129.4). Risk groups take histology into account as well as factors involved in determining stage and group.

MANAGEMENT AND PROGNOSIS

Given the rarity of the condition, international clinical trials are critical to optimizing therapy for patients with RMS. For this reason, all patients should be offered participation in a clinical trial. Although the data are limited, previous clinical trials have helped to guide consensus treatment for most patients. Treatment regimens differ largely based on risk group but always require systemic chemotherapy. Surgical resection for local control is ideal when technically feasible. All patients except those with completely resected *FOXO1/PAX3/PAX7* fusion negative tumors should undergo adjuvant radiation therapy. For patients with intermediate-risk disease, chemotherapy generally includes a combination of vincristine, dactinomycin, and cyclophosphamide. Patients with low-risk disease require lower doses of chemotherapy. There is no clear consensus for optimal treatment of high-risk

TABLE 129.3   Rhabdomyosarcoma Grouping

Surgical Group

1	Complete resection
2	Resection with microscopic residual disease or lymph node involvement
3	Localized disease with gross residual disease after resection
4	Distant metastases

TABLE 129.4   Rhabdomyosarcoma Risk Stratification

	Low Risk	Intermediate Risk	High Risk
Surgical group	Groups I, II, and III when stage 1 Groups II and III when stage 2 and 3	ARMS: groups I, II, and III ERMS: group III if stage 2 or 3	Group IV
TNM staging	All stages when group I or II Stage 1 when group III	ARMS: stages 1, 2, and 3 ERMS: stages 2 and 3	Stage 4
Histology	ERMS	All	All
Treatment	Vincristine, dactinomycin, cyclophosphamide ± surgery, radiation	Same as low-risk treatment with higher dose cyclophosphamide	Combination chemotherapy through clinical trials
Prognosis	5-year OS 90%	4-year OS 70%	3-year OS 30%

ARMS, Alveolar rhabdomyosarcoma; *ERMS,* embryonal rhabdomyosarcoma; *OS,* overall survival; *TNM,* tumor, node, and metastasis.

disease, though several regimens of combination chemotherapy have been trialed. These patients should be enrolled in clinical trials whenever possible.

As risk grouping would suggest, prognosis for patients with RMS varies dramatically. In the most recent clinical trials, low-risk patients had 5-year overall survival rates near 90% with ongoing studies aimed at reducing long-term effects of therapy. Making up the majority of RMS patients, those with intermediate-risk disease have 4-year overall survival near 70% to 75%. Despite significant research, patients with high-risk disease continue to have a poor prognosis with overall survival at 3 years approaching 30%. Recent studies have shown that *FOXO1* fusion–positive tumors have worse prognosis than fusion-negative tumors. Current clinical trials are beginning to risk stratify treatment groups incorporating *FOXO1* fusion status with previously accepted risk groups.

FUTURE DIRECTIONS

The prominence of *FOXO1* fusion products in ARMS presents an attractive target for future therapeutics. Novel technologies aimed at disrupting *FOXO1* fusion protein activity or coregulators are currently in development and could represent the next generation of ARMS therapeutics.

SUGGESTED READINGS

Available online.

130

Histiocyte Disorders

Jeremy M. Grenier and Caroline Diorio

Histiocyte diseases are a group of rare conditions characterized by dysregulation of histiocytes (Table 130.1). Classically, the term *histiocyte* has been used to describe cells of monocyte-macrophage origin found within tissues. The underlying pathophysiology of these disorders is complex with characteristics of both malignancy and benign immune dysregulation. The most common histiocyte diseases are Langerhans cell histiocytosis (2 to 10 cases per million per year for children younger than 15 years of age), hemophagocytic lymphohistiocytosis (1 case per million per year), sinus histiocytosis with massive lymphadenopathy, and juvenile xanthogranuloma.

LANGERHANS CELL HISTIOCYTOSIS

Etiology and Pathogenesis

Langerhans cell histiocytosis (LCH), previously known as histiocytosis X, Hashimoto-Pritzker disease, and Hand-Schüller-Christian disease, is characterized by the accumulation of langerin+ CD1a+ dendritic cells (DCs) in various tissues, most commonly skin and bone. These pathologic cells are surrounded by an inflammatory infiltrate composed of lymphocytes, macrophages, and rare eosinophils. The origin of LCH cells is still obscure, with some evidence pointing to immune dysregulatory processes and other data suggesting a neoplastic origin. Pathologic DCs express high levels of proinflammatory molecules and are often greatly outnumbered by other inflammatory cells within individual lesions suggesting an element of immune dysregulation. In support of a neoplastic etiology, pathologic DCs are clonal within an individual patient suggesting that these cells arise from a common progenitor cell. In pathologic cells, the mitogen-activated protein kinase (MAPK) pathway is altered, with up to 60% of LCH patients harboring the activating *BRAFV600E* mutation.

Clinical Presentation

LCH can manifest with nonspecific signs and symptoms, often mimicking more common benign diseases, which frequently delays diagnosis (Fig. 130.1). Signs of LCH largely depend on the location of specific lesions. When skin is involved (approximately one-third of patients), a rash resembling cradle cap, candidiasis, or eczema can be seen. Painful or painless lytic bone lesions occur in up to 75% of patients and are easily visualized on plain film. Most lesions involve the skull, though they can occur throughout the skeletal system. Hepatosplenomegaly and cytopenias result when LCH lesions involve the liver, spleen, or bone marrow, respectively, and pulmonary lesions can rarely contribute to a pneumothorax. Importantly, LCH lesions are frequently discovered in the posterior pituitary, manifesting as diabetes insipidus, and require chronic management as discussed later. Although LCH lesions can occur almost anywhere, disease severity can be quite diverse, with the majority of patients experiencing single organ involvement.

Evaluation

Given the nonspecific clinical signs and rarity of the condition, LCH remains a challenging diagnosis for clinicians to recognize. In any patient with unexplained rash, lytic bone lesions, central diabetes insipidus, hepatosplenomegaly, or cytopenias, LCH should remain on the differential. Biopsy of a lesion showing langerin+ CD1a+ histiocytes is required for diagnosis. Additional workup should include evaluation of other potentially involved organs. Skeletal survey is a useful initial study to evaluate for skeletal lesions, though positron emission tomography imaging can also identify metabolically active skeletal lesions along with lesions within soft tissues. Complete blood count, liver function tests, coagulation studies, chest radiograph, and screening for diabetes insipidus should be performed in all suspected LCH patients. Magnetic resonance imaging (MRI) of the pituitary gland can identify lesions in patients with suspected central diabetes insipidus.

Management and Prognosis

Just as LCH clinical severity varies widely, so does management and prognosis. For LCH localized to the skin alone, lesions can resolve spontaneously, making close clinical observation a reasonable option. In cases of severe skin involvement, topical steroids, topical nitrogen mustard, systemic methotrexate, and thalidomide have been successfully used. For single bone lesions, observation, curettage, and intralesional steroid injection have equal efficacy. However, patients with lesions within orbital, temporal, sphenoid, mastoid, ethmoid, zygomatic, or maxilla bones (termed central nervous system [CNS] risk lesions) have increased risk for developing diabetes insipidus and require systemic treatment with vinblastine and prednisone. Patients with multiple osseous lesions also require systemic therapy to mitigate risk for reactivation. Multisystem disease can be stratified according to risk for more severe disease. High-risk disease is characterized by bone

TABLE 130.1 Histiocytic Disorders

	LCH	HLH	JXG
Clinical presentation	Rash, lytic bone lesions, hepatospleno-megaly, cytopenias	Fever, hepatosplenomegaly, cytopenias, altered mental status	Yellow skin nodules
Cause	Dysregulated Langerin+ histiocytes. *BRAFV600E* mutations in 60% of patients	Uncontrolled systemic inflammation secondary to overactive macrophages. Perforin mutations common in familial HLH	Accumulation of CD68⁺, CD163⁺ dermal histiocytes
Treatment	Varied based on disease severity: observation, local steroid injection, systemic chemotherapy	Etoposide, steroids, cyclosporine, methotrexate, HSCT	Observation or excision

HLH, Hemophagocytic lymphohistiocytosis; *HSCT,* hematopoietic stem cell transplantation; *JXG,* juvenile xanthogranuloma; *LCH,* Langerhans cell histiocytosis.

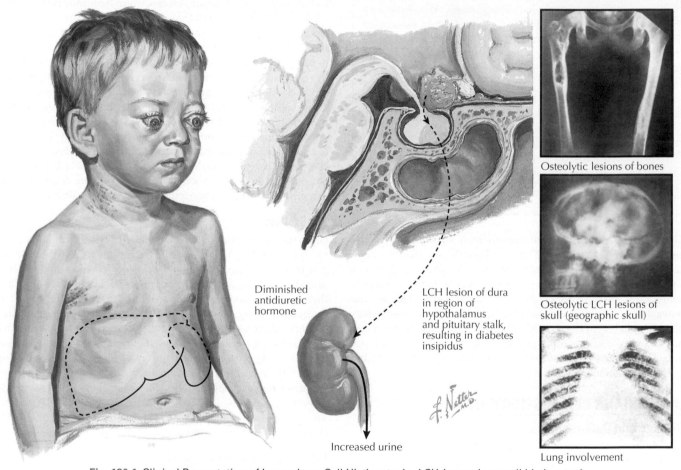

Diminished antidiuretic hormone

LCH lesion of dura in region of hypothalamus and pituitary stalk, resulting in diabetes insipidus

Increased urine

Osteolytic lesions of bones

Osteolytic LCH lesions of skull (geographic skull)

Lung involvement

Fig. 130.1 Clinical Presentation of Langerhans Cell Histiocytosis. *LCH,* Langerhans cell histiocytosis.

marrow or hepatic dysfunction. It is associated with worse prognosis and may require more intensive, longer treatment. Low risk multisystem disease generally responds well to therapy; however, some patients may experience relapse and require further treatment.

Future Directions

LCH-IV is an international clinical study evaluating several chemotherapy regimens for newly diagnosed and relapsed LCH which will likely impact the future standard of care. Given the high frequency of BRAF and MAPK pathway mutations in LCH, small molecule inhibitors targeting these pathways are promising therapies under investigation. If successful, these new therapies may allow some patients to avoid systemic chemotherapy.

HEMOPHAGOCYTIC LYMPHOHISTIOCYTOSIS

Etiology and Pathogenesis

Hemophagocytic lymphohistiocytosis (HLH) is a severe condition caused by unregulated activation of monocytes and macrophages, leading to systemic immune activation. Its name derives from the classic histologic description of hemophagocytosis, a finding in which tissue macrophages phagocytose cells of hematopoietic origin. A subgroup of patients has "primary" HLH associated with genetic mutations in granzyme production, processing, or delivery. The first described mutation associated with HLH was in perforin, a protein expressed by natural killer (NK) cells and cytotoxic T cells responsible for target cell lysis. The inadequate cytotoxic response resulting from this mutation is thought to trigger unregulated activation of macrophages and excessive production of inflammatory cytokines leading to clinical symptoms. "Secondary" HLH can also occur in individuals without known mutations, following an immunologic trigger such as infection, malignancy, or autoimmune disease. If "secondary" HLH is in the setting of rheumatologic disease, it is commonly referred to as macrophage activation syndrome.

Clinical Presentation

HLH is characterized by a profound inflammatory response to immunologic stimuli. Thus signs resemble those of systemic infections or severe inflammatory disease. Although severity of illness can vary, patients with HLH often present acutely ill and may progress to multiorgan failure without early intervention. Fever with concomitant elevation in inflammatory markers, particularly ferritin, is present in nearly all cases of HLH. Hepatosplenomegaly is also a common feature seen in more than 80% of cases and is often associated with hepatic dysfunction on further evaluation. Cytopenias are frequently observed with thrombocytopenia, normocytic anemia, and neutropenia, all common findings. When thrombocytopenia and hepatic dysfunction coexist, patients may show evidence of bleeding diathesis. Neurologic symptoms are common and can include altered mental status, seizures, neurologic deficits, or frank encephalitis.

Evaluation

HLH should remain on the differential for any child presenting acutely ill with unexplained systemic inflammation and multisystem dysfunction. In addition to a careful physical examination assessing for organomegaly, laboratory studies are helpful in confirming the diagnosis. Complete blood cell count, liver function tests, coagulation studies, inflammatory markers, ferritin, soluble interleukin 2R (IL-2R; soluble CD25), triglycerides, and functional testing of NK cell cytotoxicity, including expression of CD107a, should be ordered in all patients with suspected HLH. Bone marrow aspirate and biopsy may be necessary to rule out other malignant processes and to examine for hemophagocytosis, which is suggestive but not diagnostic of HLH. Patients with neurologic findings should undergo lumbar puncture and brain MRI for evaluation of CNS disease. The diagnostic criteria for HLH were most recently updated in 2004 and consist of either a known HLH-causing gene mutation or five of eight clinical and laboratory criteria as outlined in Box 130.1. For younger patients or patients with a family history of HLH, genetic testing for known mutations is recommended. For patients with suspected secondary HLH, studies should evaluate for bacterial infection, viral infections such as Epstein-Barr virus and cytomegalovirus, malignancy, and autoimmune disease.

Management and Prognosis

Untreated primary HLH has a poor prognosis with the majority of patients succumbing to their disease within 6 months of presentation. Clinical trials in the last 30 years have provided a framework for initial therapy of HLH. The combination of etoposide, systemic steroids, intrathecal methotrexate, and cyclosporine have improved early outcomes in these patients. However, hematopoietic stem cell transplant remains the only curative therapy with approximately 50% to 60% of

---

> ### BOX 130.1 Hemophagocytic Lymphohistiocytosis Diagnostic Criteria
>
> Known HLH-causing mutation or five of eight of the following:
> - Fever
> - Cytopenias of at least two lines
>   - Hemoglobin <9 g/dL
>   - ANC <1000/μL
>   - Platelets <100,000/μL
> - Splenomegaly
> - Hemophagocytosis noted in bone marrow, spleen, liver, or lymph node
> - Ferritin >500 ng/mL
> - Fibrinogen <150 mg/dL or triglycerides >265 mg/dL
> - Low or absent natural killer cell activity
> - Soluble IL-2R >2400 U/mL

ANC, Absolute neutrophil count; *HLH*, hemophagocytic lymphohistiocytosis.

children clinically cured. In secondary HLH, treatment of the underlying trigger should occur in conjunction with HLH-directed therapy of etoposide, corticosteroids, and cyclosporine. Despite these therapies, secondary HLH remains fatal in 20% of cases.

Future Directions

Novel biologic agents targeting inflammatory cytokines are currently under investigation for patients with HLH. Emapalumab, an antibody targeting interferon-γ, and anakinra, an IL-1β receptor antagonist are two promising agents that have demonstrated some clinical efficacy in small studies. Current studies are also investigating cytokine signatures that may help better diagnose or stratify HLH patients.

JUVENILE XANTHOGRANULOMA

Juvenile xanthogranuloma (JXG) is a histiocyte disorder consisting of red or yellow skin nodules. Although JXG can manifest at any age, most cases manifest before 2 years of age. Histologically, nodules consist of dermal histiocytes expressing CD68, CD163, and CD14. The cause for this condition is largely unknown. Reports have suggested an association among JXG, Noonan syndrome, neurofibromatosis, and juvenile chronic myelogenous leukemia. Most single lesions spontaneously resolve or are removed by excisional biopsy and carry an excellent prognosis. Rarely, patients can present with multiple lesions in different organ systems, requiring systemic chemotherapy.

SINUS HISTIOCYTOSIS WITH MASSIVE LYMPHADENOPATHY

Sinus histiocytosis with massive lymphadenopathy, formerly known as Rosai-Dorfman disease, manifests as significantly enlarged lymph nodes, usually within the cervical chain. The cause is unknown, but pathologic studies show CD1a⁻, CD163⁺, and CD68⁺ histiocytes within affected lymph nodes. Therapy is usually not necessary, and the majority of patients will experience slow resolution of lymphadenopathy over time.

SUGGESTED READINGS

Available online.

Pulmonology

Pelton A. Phinizy

131

Asthma

Kristin D. Maletsky and Jenny H. Lin

✳ CLINICAL VIGNETTE

A 2-year-old boy is brought to his pediatrician's office in January because of concerns of a persistent cough. Symptoms began in the fall when he started daycare and seemed to be getting "sick frequently." He coughs several times each week and has a nighttime cough several times a month. When he gets a viral respiratory illness, his cough lingers for 3 weeks. With exertion, he appears more tired than his peers.

He was born prematurely at 32 weeks gestation but did not require any respiratory support or supplemental oxygen in the postnatal period. He was hospitalized with respiratory syncytial virus (RSV) bronchiolitis at 10 months of age. Since then, he has been well aside from occasional viral respiratory illnesses (increased since starting daycare) and dry, itchy skin. His father has asthma and allergies.

Examination is notable for a dry cough and erythematous plaques on the extensor surfaces of his arms bilaterally. The rest of the examination, including the lungs, is unremarkable.

He is started on a trial of an inhaled corticosteroid twice daily and inhaled albuterol as needed for symptoms. When he is seen in clinic 6 weeks later, his nocturnal cough has resolved and he is able to keep up with his peers when he is playing. For the remainder of the winter, colds do not result in a prolonged cough. He is able to stop using the inhaled corticosteroid in the spring, which he then restarts the following fall/winter, and does well.

This scenario illustrates a common clinical presentation of asthma in preschoolers. His seasonal predilection and response to asthma medications in the absence of more worrisome symptoms are consistent with asthma, which is diagnosed clinically at his age. His risk factors include prematurity, RSV infection requiring hospitalization, atopic dermatitis, and parental asthma.

Asthma, a chronic inflammatory disorder of the airways, is the most common chronic pediatric pulmonary disorder and affects approximately 6 million American children. Prevalence in prepubescent children is higher in boys than girls; after puberty, girls are more commonly affected. As the third leading cause of hospitalization for children younger than 15 years of age, asthma is a significant source of morbidity and health care utilization in the United States. In addition to significant costs for asthma-related health care utilization, it is a leading cause of school absences. Disparities in asthma morbidity, mortality, and health care utilization are further evident based on race and socioeconomic status.

A multifaceted approach to asthma management, including environmental control, management of comorbid conditions, use of pharmacologic therapy, patient and family education, and frequent assessments of asthma control, severity, and response to therapy, is critical to help decrease both health care costs and asthma morbidity and mortality.

ETIOLOGY AND PATHOGENESIS

Asthma can be characterized by three key airway components: reversible obstruction, hyperresponsiveness, and inflammation. Mechanisms that contribute to airway obstruction include (1) acute bronchoconstriction of smooth muscles in the airway and mucus hypersecretion causing airway obstruction associated with an acute exacerbation and (2) airway edema and inflammation contributing to both acute and chronic obstruction (Fig. 131.1). Inciting triggers cause acute bronchoconstriction of hyperresponsive airways, leading to wheezing as air moves through narrowed airways. Key cellular components involved in the pathogenesis of asthma include mast cells, eosinophils, and to some degree, neutrophils, T-cells, macrophages, and epithelial cells (Figs. 131.1 and 131.2).

Both environmental and genetic factors contribute to the development of asthma in a susceptible individual. Environmental factors such as respiratory pathogens, allergens, and pollutants can cause airway inflammation/irritation and immune system dysregulation and lead to the development of asthma or worsening of existing disease. Exposure to tobacco smoke and childhood obesity have also been identified as modifiable risk factors. Nonmodifiable risk factors include gender and personal or family history of atopic disease.

CLINICAL PRESENTATION

History

The initial history obtained should detail symptoms including age of onset, frequency and duration of symptoms, triggers, alleviating/exacerbating factors, and seasonal pattern. Many children with asthma develop symptoms before the age of 5 years. In addition to recurrent episodes of wheezing or respiratory distress often in association with a viral respiratory illness, persistent dry cough, often occurring at night, is commonly reported. At times, this may be the *only* symptom. Nocturnal cough resulting from asthma usually occurs several hours into sleep, which differentiates it from cough associated with gastroesophageal reflux disease (GERD) or postnasal drip, which often occurs when a child reclines. Complete absence of nocturnal cough suggests an alternative diagnosis. Other symptoms may include shortness of breath and exertional cough.

There is often a history of prolonged cough with viral illnesses, sometimes misdiagnosed as "bronchiolitis/bronchitis" or "pneumonia," especially in the winter, with improvement in symptoms in warmer weather. The presence or absence of other symptoms, including atopy, and alleviating/exacerbating factors help differentiate the source of the cough. Of note, cough resulting from asthma is typically nonproductive and the presence of a productive cough should alert the clinician to other diagnoses. Sudden onset of wheezing, especially in a previously healthy toddler, should raise concern for the alternative diagnosis of foreign body aspiration.

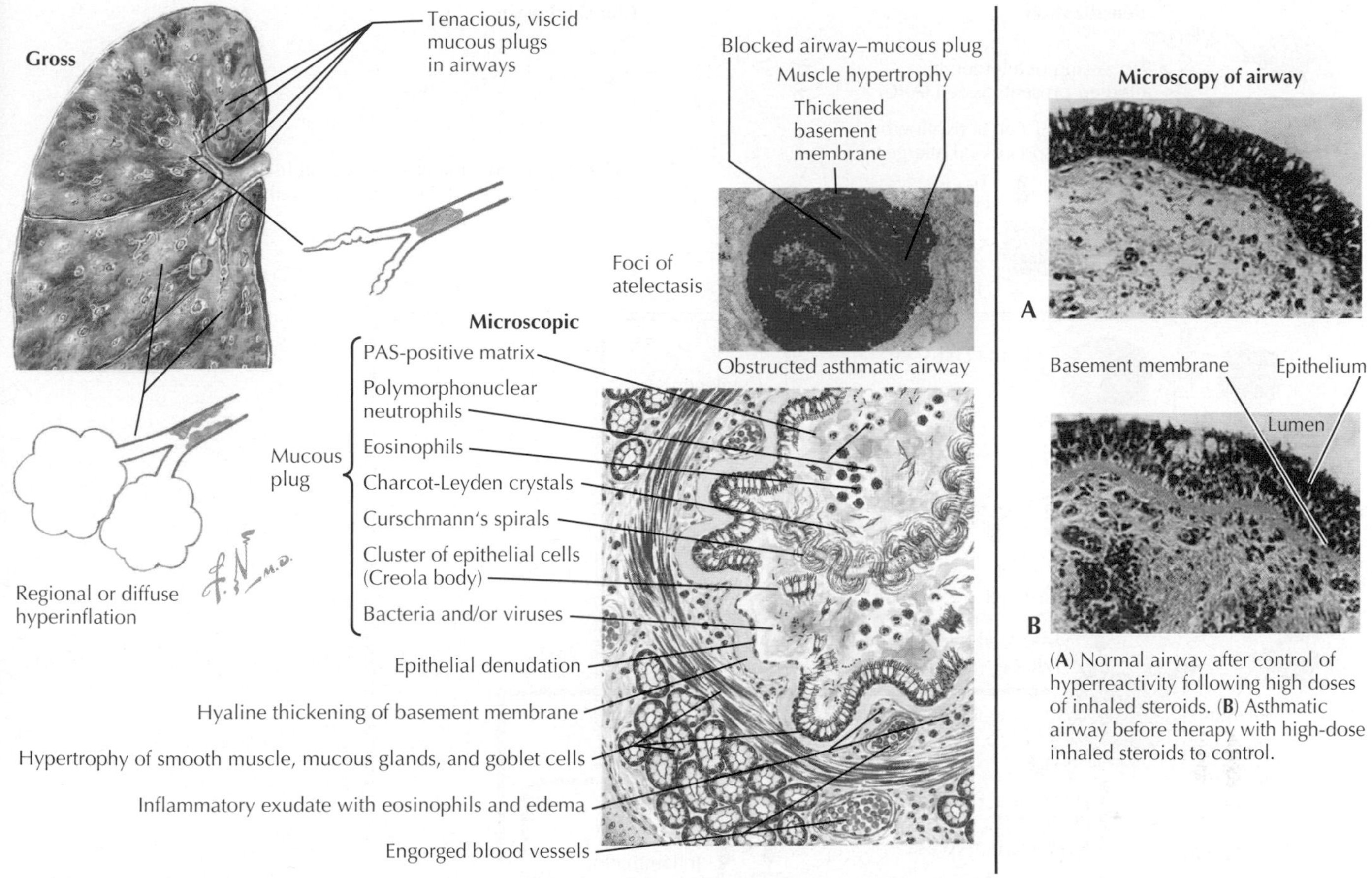

Gross

Tenacious, viscid mucous plugs in airways

Foci of atelectasis

Regional or diffuse hyperinflation

Mucous plug

Microscopic

PAS-positive matrix

Polymorphonuclear neutrophils

Eosinophils

Charcot-Leyden crystals

Curschmann's spirals

Cluster of epithelial cells (Creola body)

Bacteria and/or viruses

Epithelial denudation

Hyaline thickening of basement membrane

Hypertrophy of smooth muscle, mucous glands, and goblet cells

Inflammatory exudate with eosinophils and edema

Engorged blood vessels

Blocked airway–mucous plug

Muscle hypertrophy

Thickened basement membrane

Obstructed asthmatic airway

Microscopy of airway

A

Basement membrane   Epithelium

Lumen

B

(A) Normal airway after control of hyperreactivity following high doses of inhaled steroids. (B) Asthmatic airway before therapy with high-dose inhaled steroids to control.

Fig. 131.1 Pathology of an Acute Asthma Exacerbation.

A provider should also inquire about triggers for the asthma symptoms. These may include viral upper respiratory tract infections, environmental/seasonal allergens, airway irritants (smoke or strong scents), exercise, exposure to cold air, or changes in weather (Fig. 131.3). Symptoms associated with feeding should raise concern for another cause (e.g., GERD, aspiration, or a tracheoesophageal fistula).

Independent risk factors for developing asthma include a history of prematurity, severe respiratory syncytial virus (RSV) disease requiring hospitalization, and a history of atopy. Children with seasonal or environmental allergies, atopic dermatitis, food allergies, and a first-degree relative with asthma are at an increased risk for developing asthma.

A detailed history of exacerbations, prior hospitalizations (including need for intensive care unit [ICU] admission or endotracheal intubation), emergency department visits, systemic steroid use, rescue medication use, and frequency of daytime and nocturnal symptoms help to classify severity. A detailed review of systems may uncover symptoms suggesting another diagnosis. Patients should also be assessed for comorbid medical conditions that can exacerbate asthma, including GERD, allergic rhinitis, and sinusitis. Finally, it is essential to obtain a history of trialed medications—including inhaled β-2 adrenergic agonists and corticosteroids (inhaled or systemic)—and whether there was response to therapy.

Physical Examination

A child with an acute asthma exacerbation will most frequently demonstrate wheezing, which is classically described as a polyphonic, musical sound during exhalation, though it can also occur during inspiration with severe obstruction. This should be distinguished from monophonic wheezing caused by central airway obstruction, such as in tracheomalacia.

Because wheezing occurs as air moves through narrowed airways, absence of auscultated aeration in an asthmatic in respiratory distress could be an ominous sign signaling significant airflow obstruction.

Other notable signs of airway obstruction include decreased aeration, prolonged expiratory phase, and chest hyperinflation (a widened anteroposterior diameter). Signs of increased work of breathing or respiratory distress, including tachypnea, nasal flaring, and use of accessory muscles of respiration (e.g., sternocleidomastoid, intercostals, pectoralis major, and abdominal muscles), may be present. The patient also may be hypoxemic.

Skin should be examined closely for evidence of atopic disease, such as atopic dermatitis or allergic shiners, and the nose should be evaluated for signs of allergic rhinitis (e.g., swollen turbinates, transverse nasal crease due to the "allergic salute"). The presence of nasal polyps should trigger evaluation for cystic fibrosis, although they can also be seen in chronic allergic rhinitis. Digital clubbing is *never* a component of uncomplicated asthma and should prompt further evaluation.

DIFFERENTIAL DIAGNOSIS

One should remember that "not all that wheezes is asthma" (Table 131.1). Within the respiratory system, viral upper respiratory tract infections and allergic rhinitis are common causes of recurrent cough and wheezing. Other potential causes include foreign body aspiration, vocal cord dysfunction, tracheal/bronchial compression (by masses or vascular anomalies), dynamic airway collapse (e.g., tracheobronchomalacia), cystic fibrosis, and bronchopulmonary dysplasia. Key factors in the patient's history and physical examination will help guide a clinician's assessment of the correct cause of symptoms.

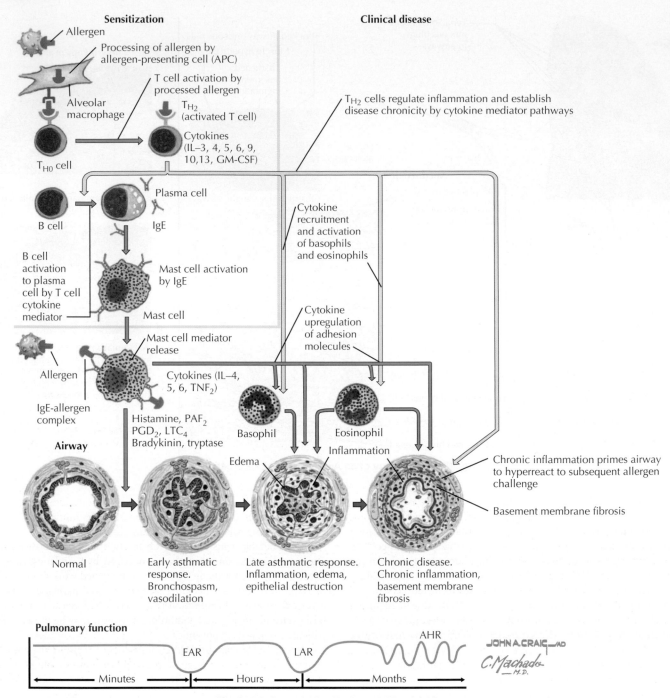

Fig. 131.2 Steps in the Pathogenesis of Asthma.

EVALUATION

History and physical examination are extremely important in the evaluation and diagnosis of asthma. Frequency of symptoms, activity limitation, and rescue medication use should be used to classify asthma severity and control and to guide management (Table 131.2).

Although spirometry is not required to diagnose asthma, in children 5 years and older it can help determine the degree of airway obstruction and confirm the presence of reversible obstruction. A post-bronchodilator improvement in forced expiratory volume in 1 second (FEV_1) of at least 12% compared with baseline is considered a positive bronchodilator response. The shape of the flow volume loops obtained on spirometry also offers helpful clues regarding other medical conditions such as vocal cord dysfunction, which can mimic asthma (Figs. 131.4 and 131.5).

In certain situations, additional testing with exercise pulmonary function tests or a methacholine challenge test may be useful. Other studies may be indicated to exclude another diagnosis in the presence of atypical or concerning symptoms (Table 131.1).

A patient experiencing an acute asthma exacerbation should be promptly evaluated and triaged based on symptom severity. Signs and symptoms including tachypnea, increased work of breathing, accessory muscle use, and pulse oximetry values should be used to guide management. Peak expiratory flow measurements (which correlate with FEV_1) may also be helpful in determining degree of airflow obstruction.

MANAGEMENT

Four hallmarks are essential in the successful management of a child with asthma: (1) assess and monitor asthma severity and control;

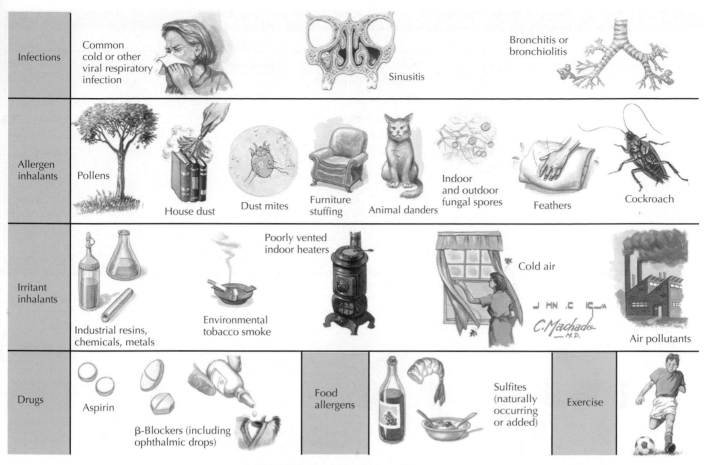

Fig. 131.3 Common Asthma Triggers.

TABLE 131.1	Differential Diagnosis of Wheezing in Infants and Children
Differential Diagnosis	**Potential Confirmatory Tests**
Obstruction of Large Airways	
Foreign body in trachea or bronchus	Chest radiography, bronchoscopy
Vocal cord dysfunction	Spirometry, laryngoscopy, or bronchoscopy
Vascular rings or laryngeal webs	Esophagram, chest CTA, laryngoscopy, or bronchoscopy
Tracheobronchomalacia, tracheal or bronchial stenosis	Bronchoscopy
Airway tumor or mass	Chest radiography, chest CT, bronchoscopy
Obstruction of Small Airways	
Viral bronchiolitis	Chest radiography, viral antigen or PCR testing
Bronchiolitis obliterans	Chest CT, lung biopsy
Cystic fibrosis	Sweat chloride test, CFTR genetic testing
Primary ciliary dyskinesia	Nasal nitric oxide, ciliary biopsy, genetic testing
Bronchopulmonary dysplasia	Perinatal history, chest radiography
Other Causes	
Gastroesophageal reflux	pH probe, upper gastrointestinal series, nuclear milk scan
Aspiration	Speech pathology evaluation, modified barium swallow
Tracheoesophageal fistula	Esophagram, bronchoscopy
Psychogenic cough	Diagnosis of exclusion

CFTR, Cystic fibrosis transmembrane conductance regulator; *CT,* computed tomography; *CTA,* computed tomography with angiography; *PCR,* polymerase chain reaction.

TABLE 131.2   Classifying Asthma Severity in Children 5 to 11 Years Old

Components of Severity	Intermittent	PERSISTENT		
		Mild	Moderate	Severe
Symptoms	<2 days/week	>2 days/week but not daily	Daily	Throughout the day
Nighttime awakenings	<2 times/month	3–4 times/month	>1 time/week but not nightly	Often several times/week
SABA use for symptom control	<2 days/week	>2 days/week but not daily	Daily	Several times per day
Interference with daily activity	None	Minor limitations	Some limitations	Severe limitations
Lung function	Normal FEV_1 between exacerbations			
FEV_1 (predicted or personal best)	>80%	>80%	60%–80%	<60%
FEV_1/FVC	>85%	>80%	75%–80%	<75%
Exacerbations requiring systemic corticosteroids	0–1/year	≥2/year	≥2/year	≥2/year
Recommended step for initiating therapy	Step 1	Step 2	Step 3	Step 3 or 4

FEV_1, Forced expiratory volume in 1 second; FVC, forced vital capacity; $SABA$, short-acting β2-agonist.
Adapted from National Asthma Education and Prevention Program, Third Expert Panel on the Diagnosis and Management of Asthma. Expert Panel Report 3 (EPR3). *Guidelines for the Diagnosis and Management of Asthma.* National Heart, Lung, and Blood Institute (US); 2007:73, Figure 3-4B. Available from *https://www.ncbi.nlm.nih.gov/books/NBK7232/.*

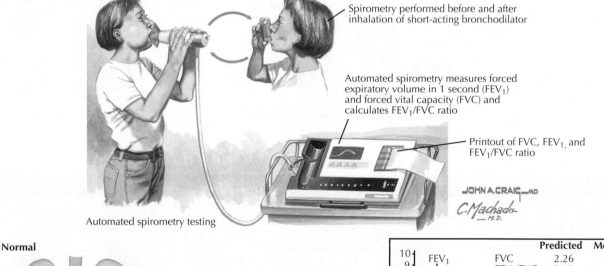

Spirometry performed before and after inhalation of short-acting bronchodilator

Automated spirometry measures forced expiratory volume in 1 second (FEV_1) and forced vital capacity (FVC) and calculates FEV_1/FVC ratio

Printout of FVC, FEV_1, and FEV_1/FVC ratio

JOHN A. CRAIG—MD
C. Machado —M.D.

Automated spirometry testing

Normal

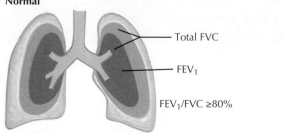

Total FVC

FEV_1

FEV_1/FVC ≥80%

	Predicted	Measured	%
FVC	2.26	2.63	116
FEV_1/FVC	2.13	2.30	108
FEV_1/FVC	94.5	87.5	93

In patients with normal function, FEV_1, FVC, and FEV_1/FVC are ≥80% of those predicted by age/sex/height. Bronchodilation does not increase values

Asthma

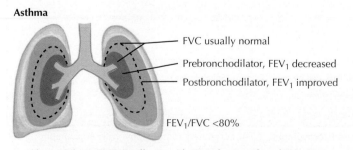

FVC usually normal

Prebronchodilator, FEV_1 decreased

Postbronchodilator, FEV_1 improved

FEV_1/FVC <80%

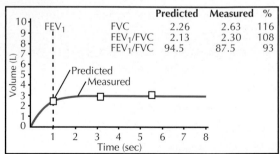
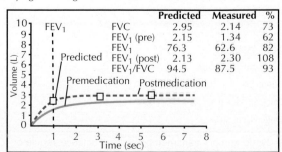

	Predicted	Measured	%
FVC	2.95	2.14	73
FEV_1 (pre)	2.15	1.34	62
FEV_1	76.3	62.6	82
FEV_1 (post)	2.13	2.30	108
FEV_1/FVC	94.5	87.5	93

In asthma patients, FVC usually normal, FEV_1 decreased, and FEV_1/FVC are <80%. Increase in absolute FEV_1 of >12% after bronchodilator suggests asthma

Fig. 131.4 Pulmonary Function Testing (Spirometry).

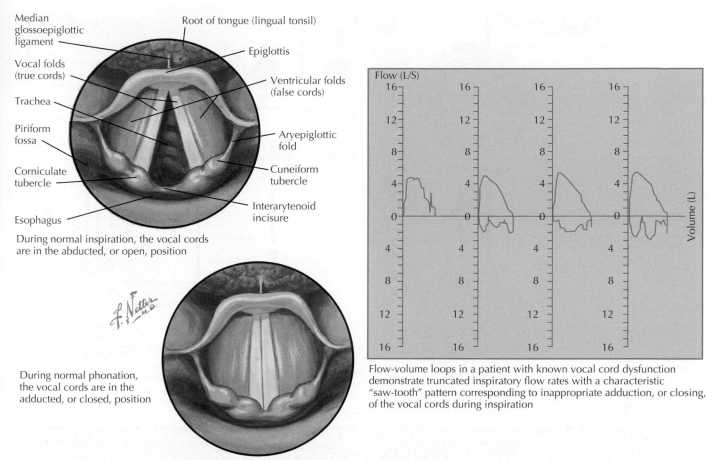

Median glossoepiglottic ligament

Vocal folds (true cords)

Trachea

Piriform fossa

Corniculate tubercle

Esophagus

Root of tongue (lingual tonsil)

Epiglottis

Ventricular folds (false cords)

Aryepiglottic fold

Cuneiform tubercle

Interarytenoid incisure

During normal inspiration, the vocal cords are in the abducted, or open, position

During normal phonation, the vocal cords are in the adducted, or closed, position

Flow (L/S)

Volume (L)

Flow-volume loops in a patient with known vocal cord dysfunction demonstrate truncated inspiratory flow rates with a characteristic "saw-tooth" pattern corresponding to inappropriate adduction, or closing, of the vocal cords during inspiration

Fig. 131.5 Vocal Cord Dysfunction.

(2) asthma education for the patient and caregivers; (3) control of environmental factors and comorbid conditions; and (4) pharmacologic therapy.

This chapter will focus primarily on pharmacologic therapy in asthma, of which the mainstays include inhaled bronchodilators and inhaled or systemic corticosteroids (Fig. 131.6). Medications can be classified as "rescue" or "preventive" (controller) based on their role in acute versus chronic management.

Acute Exacerbation

At the first signs of an asthma exacerbation, rescue inhaled or nebulized albuterol for acute bronchodilation should be started immediately and may be used as frequently as every 4 hours until symptom resolution. If there is no improvement, or a worsening in symptoms, a patient should be evaluated by a medical professional. A patient may require a short course of oral corticosteroid therapy (typically prednisolone or prednisone 2 mg/kg/day; maximum 60 mg/day, for 5 days).

For more severe exacerbations when patients present to the emergency department, immediate therapy typically consists of inhaled albuterol, inhaled ipratropium bromide (an anticholinergic bronchodilator), and supplemental oxygen if needed. Additionally, systemic corticosteroids should be used to assist in reducing airway inflammation. Although a typical steroid course is 5 days, some patients may require longer steroid courses and a steroid taper. If a patient does not show marked improvement within the first 2 hours or if there are ongoing signs of respiratory distress or hypoxemia, inpatient hospital admission is warranted.

In severe cases when the previously mentioned treatments fail to lead to significant improvement in symptoms, additional therapies are required. These can include continuous nebulized albuterol, subcutaneous epinephrine, subcutaneous terbutaline, and intravenous magnesium sulfate. Patients requiring these therapies are often admitted to the ICU for continued treatment and close monitoring. In some cases, intravenous β-agonists (such as terbutaline) are initiated in the ICU. Continuous electrocardiographic monitoring and frequent fluid and electrolyte assessments are essential in these patients because of increased myocardial stimulation and potential electrolyte shifts.

The use of supplemental oxygen with heated and humidified high-flow nasal cannula or the use of noninvasive positive pressure ventilation (NIPPV) with continuous positive airway pressure (CPAP) may be required to help improve work of breathing and ventilation-perfusion mismatch. When a patient is progressing toward respiratory failure, bilevel positive airway pressure (BiPAP) or endotracheal intubation may be indicated. Intubation and mechanical ventilation during an acute asthma exacerbation carry significant risks and should be avoided when possible.

Chronic Disease

Children with intermittent asthma may use an inhaled bronchodilator as needed, whereas those with persistent asthma require a daily controller medication, frequently an inhaled corticosteroid, for long-term control. Classification of asthma severity and control help guide initiation of treatment and when to step up or step down treatment (Table 131.3). As chronic use of inhaled corticosteroids is not without side effects (Fig. 131.7), patients require regular assessments throughout the year and should receive the minimum therapy required to achieve control. Comorbid medical conditions should also be treated. Discussion with families regarding avoidance and mitigation

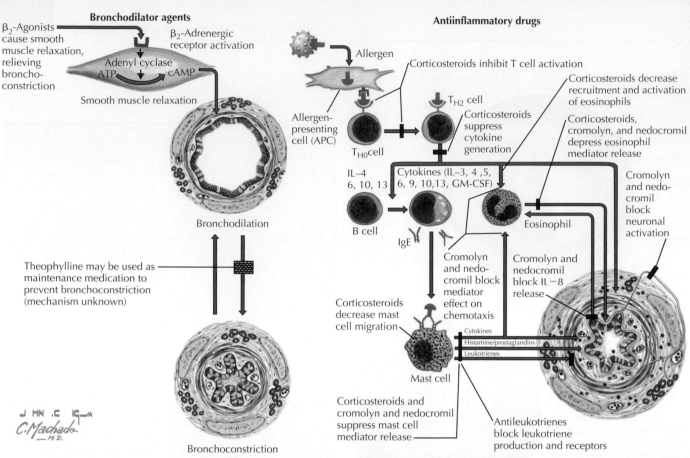

Fig. 131.6 Mechanisms of Action of Asthma Medications.

TABLE 131.3 Stepwise Approach for Long-Term Management of Asthma in Children 5 to 11 Years Old

	Step 1	Step 2	Step 3	Step 4	Step 5	Step 6
	Intermittent Asthma	**Persistent Asthma** (Consult With Asthma Specialist if Step 4 or Higher Care Required)				
Preferred treatment	PRN SABA	Daily low-dose ICS *and* PRN SABA	Daily and PRN combination low-dose ICS-formoterol	Daily and PRN combination medium-dose ICS-formoterol	Daily high-dose ICS-LABA and PRN SABA	Daily high-dose ICS-LABA and PRN SABA *and* oral corticosteroids
Alternative treatment	N/A	Daily LTRA,* *or* Cromolyn,* *or* Nedocromil,* *or* Theophylline,* *and* PRN SABA	Daily medium-dose ICS and PRN SABA *or* daily low-dose ICS-LABA *or* daily low-dose ICS *and* LTRA,* *or* daily low-dose ICS +Theophylline,* *and* PRN SABA	Daily medium-dose ICS-LABA *and* PRN SABA *or* daily medium-dose ICS *and* LTRA* *or* daily medium-dose ICS *and* Theophylline,* *and* PRN SABA	Daily high-dose ICS *and* LTRA* *or* daily high-dose ICS *and* Theophylline,* *and* PRN SABA	Daily high-dose ICS *and* LTRA* *and* oral corticosteroids *or* daily high-dose ICS *and* Theophylline* *and* oral corticosteroids, *and* PRN SABA
	Steps 2–4: Conditionally recommend the use of subcutaneous immunotherapy as an adjunct treatment to standard pharmacotherapy in individuals ≥5 years of age whose asthma is controlled at the initiation, build up, and maintenance phases of immunotherapy			Consider omalizumab **		
	Each step: Patient education, environmental control, and management of comorbidities					
Quick relief medication	Each step: SABA as needed for symptoms with intensity of treatment depending on severity of symptoms, up to 3 treatments every 20 minutes as needed. Note: Use of SABA >2 days/week for symptom relief other than exercise-induced bronchospasm generally indicates inadequate control and the need for step up in treatment.					

ICS, Inhaled corticosteroid; *LABA,* long-acting β2-agonist; *LTRA,* leukotriene receptor antagonist; *SABA,* short-acting β2-agonist.

*Cromolyn, Nedocromil, LTRAs including montelukast, and Theophylline were not considered in this update and/or have limited availability for use in the United States, and/or have an increased risk of adverse consequences and need for monitoring that make their use less desirable. The FDA issued a Boxed Warning for montelukast in March 2020.

**Omalizumab is the only asthma biologic currently FDA-approved for this age range.

Adapted from National Asthma Education and Prevention Program. 2020 Focused Updates to the Asthma Management Guidelines: A Report from the National Asthma Education and Prevention Program Coordinating Committee Expert Panel Working Group. National Heart, Lung, and Blood Institute (US); 2020, Figure I.c. Available from: https://www.nhlbi.nih.gov/health-topics/all-publications-and-resources/2020-focused-updates-asthma-management-guidelines.

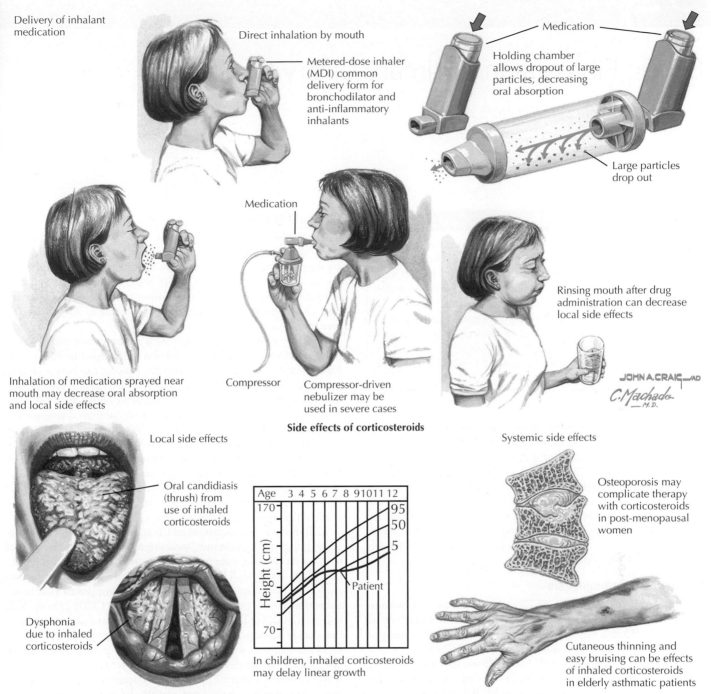

Delivery of inhalant medication

Direct inhalation by mouth

Metered-dose inhaler (MDI) common delivery form for bronchodilator and anti-inflammatory inhalants

Medication

Holding chamber allows dropout of large particles, decreasing oral absorption

Large particles drop out

Medication

Inhalation of medication sprayed near mouth may decrease oral absorption and local side effects

Compressor

Compressor-driven nebulizer may be used in severe cases

Rinsing mouth after drug administration can decrease local side effects

JOHN A. CRAIG—MD
C. Machado M.D.

Side effects of corticosteroids

Local side effects

Oral candidiasis (thrush) from use of inhaled corticosteroids

Dysphonia due to inhaled corticosteroids

In children, inhaled corticosteroids may delay linear growth

Systemic side effects

Osteoporosis may complicate therapy with corticosteroids in post-menopausal women

Cutaneous thinning and easy bruising can be effects of inhaled corticosteroids in elderly asthmatic patients

Fig. 131.7 Pharmacologic Management of Asthma, Including Side Effects of Corticosteroids.

of potential environmental triggers is essential, along with education regarding the importance of smoking cessation. Patients with asthma should receive annual influenza vaccination.

Regular follow-up with a clinician is essential for monitoring symptoms and assessing control so that appropriate adjustments can be made to prescribed therapy. An asthma action plan that outlines baseline management and escalation of treatment during an exacerbation should be updated and reviewed at every visit. Asthma education, assessment of spacer and inhaler technique (Fig. 131.7), and reinforcement of the necessity of adherence to treatment plans are also important.

Children and adolescents with persistent allergic or eosinophilic asthma who remain poorly controlled despite optimizing pharmacotherapy, mitigating environmental triggers, and improving adherence and technique may benefit from the use of biologics (e.g., omalizumab) or allergy immunotherapy (Chapter 22).

FUTURE DIRECTIONS

Although the genetics of asthma have been studied over the past several decades, recent advances in genome-wide association studies have identified several pertinent loci. There is potential to learn more about susceptibility, severity, and response to therapies as asthma genotype-phenotype associations are better elucidated.

SUGGESTED READINGS

Available online.

132

Cystic Fibrosis and Primary Ciliary Dyskinesia

Julianne McGlynn and Stamatia Alexiou

 CLINICAL VIGNETTE

A 5-year-old boy presents to the primary care clinic with runny nose, congestion, and wet cough. Symptoms are persistent, and his mother cannot recall him ever being completely asymptomatic. He was born full term, but required a brief hospital stay for unexplained tachypnea requiring oxygen. Newborn screen was normal. Examination shows frequent coughing and significant rhinorrhea. The heart's point of maximal impulse (PMI) is the right fourth intercostal space. Crackles are auscultated. Prior evaluation has shown normal sweat test, complete blood count, and immunoglobulins.

This presentation is concerning for a diagnosis of primary ciliary dyskinesia and warrants further diagnostic testing.

CYSTIC FIBROSIS

Cystic fibrosis (CF) is the most common fatal genetic disease of Whites. The disease is caused by a defect in the CF transmembrane conductance regulator (CFTR) gene, an epithelial chloride channel. Defective electrolyte transport in epithelial cells of several exocrine organs, including the lungs, pancreas, and gastrointestinal (GI) tract, leads to accumulation of viscid secretions. This multisystem disease, which most notably affects the lungs, typically presents as recurrent pulmonary infections and chronic airway inflammation ultimately resulting in respiratory failure.

Etiology and Pathogenesis

CF is caused by defects in the *CFTR* gene located on chromosome 7. This autosomal recessive disease has a significantly higher carrier frequency in Whites, with an incidence of 1 in 3200 and lower incidences in other races and ethnicities. Over 2000 *CFTR* gene mutations are currently described, with F508 deletion the most common. Defective *CFTR* structure, synthesis, processing, or function leads to abnormal electrolyte transport at epithelial surfaces, resulting in dehydration of luminal secretions, subsequent obstruction, and accompanying inflammation. In the airways, for example, excessive sodium and water resorption from the airway surface leads to dehydrated mucus, obstruction, and chronic bacterial colonization (Fig. 132.1). This process results in inflammation and progressive bronchiectasis, further impairing airway clearance (Fig. 132.2). In the GI system, obstruction of the pancreatic duct results in exocrine pancreatic insufficiency and intestinal fat malabsorption in 90% of patients (Fig. 132.3). Pancreatic endocrine function also can be impaired, resulting in CF-related diabetes (CFRD). Additionally, men are almost universally infertile because of congenital bilateral absence of the vas deferens. Thick cervical mucus is responsible for reduced fertility among women.

Clinical Presentation

In the United States, the newborn screen in all 50 states and Washington, DC will test for CF and a majority of affected individuals are diagnosed before symptom onset. Approximately 15% to 20% of infants with CF present in the first 48 hours of life because of inspissated meconium (meconium ileus) leading to small bowel obstruction (Fig. 132.3). Another early manifestation is failure to thrive caused by pancreatic exocrine insufficiency.

Children with CF will present with recurrent respiratory infections. Respiratory symptoms in children can be hard to differentiate from recurrent viral illnesses or asthma. Patients can have a chronic productive cough with yellow or green sputum. Physical examination may reveal increased anteroposterior diameter of the chest, wheezing from lower airway obstruction, crackles from peripheral airspace disease, and digital clubbing (Fig. 132.4). Patients with CF characteristically develop chronic lung infections with *Staphylococcus aureus, Haemophilus influenzae,* and *Pseudomonas aeruginosa.* Sinus disease can manifest as chronic nasal congestion and recurrent otitis media with physical examination revealing nasal polyps and sinus tenderness. Patients should be monitored for signs of obstructive sleep apnea as a result of this upper airway obstruction.

Common GI manifestations in CF are poor weight gain and frequent greasy or malodorous stools from fat malabsorption. Bowel obstruction can also occur in older children as a result of fecal impaction in the distal small bowel, known as distal intestinal obstruction syndrome. Intussusception can occur because inspissated fecal material acts as a "lead point" in the terminal ileum. CFRD presents with hyperglycemia, but ketoacidosis and microvascular diabetic complications rarely develop. CFRD is rare in the first decade of life, and then incidence increases with age. Liver disease, the most prominent type being focal biliary cirrhosis, which can progress to portal hypertension, is also common. Other GI problems may occur in CF, including gastroesophageal reflux, chronic pancreatitis, and rectal prolapse.

Diagnosis

Diagnosis is based on detecting physiologic evidence of altered epithelial electrolyte transport (a positive sweat test result), *CFTR* mutation, and clinical symptoms. On the newborn screen, blood is assayed for immunoreactive trypsin, a pancreatic proenzyme whose serum concentration is elevated in CF because of pancreatic duct obstruction. Children identified by newborn screening undergo further testing with a sweat chloride test. A positive result confirms the diagnosis, whereas a negative result makes CF unlikely. However, an intermediate result is indeterminate and additional workup is required, including repeating the sweat test and genetic testing. If the diagnosis remains in question, other tests of CFTR physiologic function can be pursued.

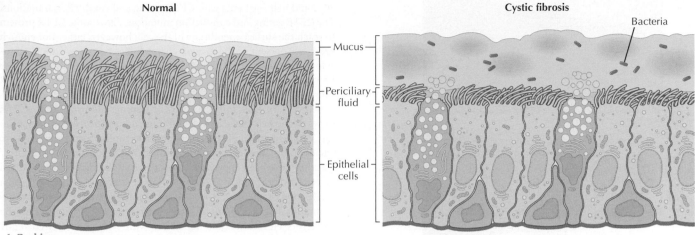

Normal   Cystic fibrosis

Mucus

Periciliary fluid

Epithelial cells

Bacteria

J. Perkins
MS, MFA, CMI

Abnormal electrolyte transport at the airway epithelium leads to a net absorption of sodium and water from the periciliary liquid (PCL) layer and airway mucus. The smaller PCL volume leads to trapping of cilia in tenacious mucus, impairing effective mucus clearance.

Fig. 132.1 Abnormal Electrolyte Transport.

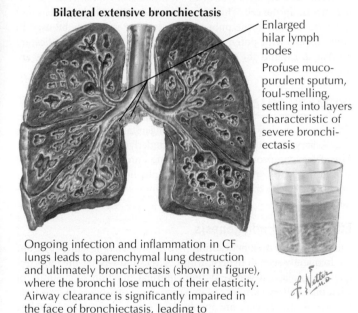

Bilateral extensive bronchiectasis

Enlarged hilar lymph nodes

Profuse mucopurulent sputum, foul-smelling, settling into layers characteristic of severe bronchiectasis

Ongoing infection and inflammation in CF lungs leads to parenchymal lung destruction and ultimately bronchiectasis (shown in figure), where the bronchi lose much of their elasticity. Airway clearance is significantly impaired in the face of bronchiectasis, leading to accumulation of mucus and facilitating the vicious cycle of infection and inflammation.

Fig. 132.2 Ongoing Infection and Inflammation in Cystic Fibrosis (CF) Lungs.

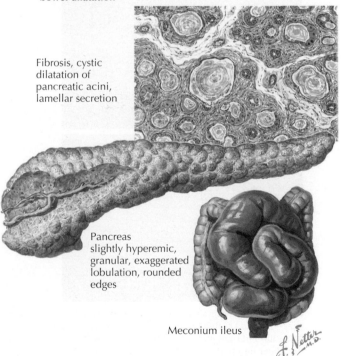

Cystic fibrosis of the pancreas (hence the name of the disease) and meconium ileus showing distal ileal obstruction and small bowel dilatation

Fibrosis, cystic dilatation of pancreatic acini, lamellar secretion

Pancreas slightly hyperemic, granular, exaggerated lobulation, rounded edges

Meconium ileus

Fig. 132.3 Common Gastrointestinal Pathologic Findings in Cystic Fibrosis.

Management

CF management centers on optimizing nutritional status, preventing or attenuating lung function decline, and aggressively treating CF exacerbations. Prophylactic airway clearance treatments, such as chest physical therapy (CPT) and high-frequency chest wall oscillation, aim to decrease viscidity and volume of secretions, facilitate mobilization, and aid expectoration. Regular exercise is an effective adjunct to airway clearance. Recombinant human DNAse is an enzyme that breaks down deoxyribonucleic acid (DNA) released from neutrophils in the airways. Its use has demonstrated improvement in sputum clearance and lung function. Hypertonic saline also improves mucociliary clearance and lung function by thinning mucus and stimulating coughing.

In patients with chronic airway colonization, intermittent use of inhaled antibiotics, such as tobramycin, can help reduce sputum

bacterial density and improve lung function. For acute lung exacerbations, intensive CPT and antibiotics are cornerstones of care. In patients with severely diminished lung function, evaluation for lung transplantation is considered.

Maintaining adequate nutritional status in CF is vital. In those with exocrine pancreatic insufficiency, oral supplemental pancreatic enzymes revolutionized CF nutritional management. Adequate intake of enzymes results in improvement in nutrition, GI symptoms,

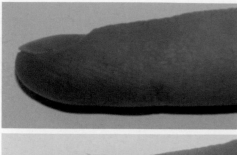

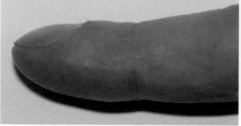

A. The angle between the nailbed and the nailfold (lovibond angle) should normally be <165 degrees as in the upper figure in A. Note the loss of this normal angle in the individual with clubbing (lower image).

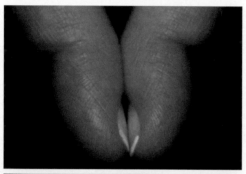

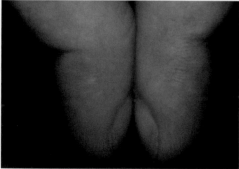

B. Schramroth's sign demonstrated. The diamond shaped space created by both lovibond angles during apposition of right and left index fingers (as seen in the upper figure) is lost in the individual with clubbing.

Fig. 132.4 Digital Clubbing.

and serum levels of fat-soluble vitamins A, D, E, and K. In the setting of cholestatic liver disease, ursodeoxycholic acid may slow disease progression.

The development of CFRD is associated with poorer lung function and worse nutritional status. Yearly glucose tolerance screening is recommended at age 10. Most patients with CFRD ultimately need insulin replacement.

CFTR modulators are emerging as promising therapies and have made significant advances in the treatment of CF. They target specific defects in the CFTR protein and are broken down into three groups: potentiators, correctors, and activators.

Ivacaftor, the first modulator to become available, was approved in 2012 and helps patients with CFTR gating and conduction mutations. The CFTR gating and conduction mutations allow some CFTR protein to reach the surface membrane of the cell; however, either not enough protein is present or the protein channel does not allow enough chloride to flow through. Potentiators, such as ivacaftor, allow chloride to flow through the channel by increasing the likelihood that the CFTR protein gate remains open.

Correctors help improve protein folding, allowing more CFTR to reach the cell surface. By combining a corrector with a potentiator, CFTR function at the cell membrane can be further augmented. Dual-combination drugs, such as lumacaftor/ivacaftor and tezacaftor/ivacaftor have been approved for those with two copies of the F508del mutation. Tezacaftor/ivacaftor also can be used to treat people with a single copy of one of 26 specified mutations, regardless of their other mutation. The newest modulator, approved in 2019, combines the correctors elexacaftor and tezacaftor with ivacaftor. It is currently approved for anyone with CF who is 12 years of age or older with at least one F508del mutation.

Future Directions

Activators are the third type of CFTR modulators that increase CFTR production in the cell. They are currently in clinical phase trials and not yet available to the public; however, they will likely be used in combination with potentiators and correctors. Further studies are needed to expand the population for whom these modulators are approved.

PRIMARY CILIARY DYSKINESIA

Primary ciliary dyskinesia (PCD) is a congenital condition of impaired mucociliary clearance resulting from underlying ciliary dysfunction. This defect compromises a critical innate immune defense leading to symptoms in the organ systems where cilia have an important functional role such as the respiratory tract, sinuses, middle ear, and reproductive system.

Etiology and Pathogenesis

Cilia in PCD are dyskinetic, immotile, or completely absent. Mutations are frequently seen in dynein, with *DNAH5* and *DNAI1* the most frequently implicated genes. Without normal function or quantity of cilia, mucociliary clearance is impaired and predisposes to infection. Embryonic nodal cilia are involved in controlling organ laterality. When these cilia are defective or absent, organ sidedness becomes random, leading to a 50% chance of situs inversus.

Clinical Presentation

The clinical manifestations of PCD are broad. At birth, respiratory distress is observed in the term neonate in 80% of PCD cases, albeit attributed to an alternative cause such as transient tachypnea of the newborn or pneumonia. Recurrent and/or persistent upper and lower respiratory tract infections are typical. A daily wet chronic cough is often present and, almost universally, children have rhinosinusitis. Nasal polyps may be visualized, and wheezes or crackles may be auscultated on examination. Recurrent acute otitis media and chronic serous otitis media are a result of dysfunctional cilia in eustachian tubes. Conductive hearing loss can result as a complication of recurrent ear infections. Common organisms cultured from sputum include *H. influenzae, Moraxella catarrhalis, S. aureus, Streptococcus pneumoniae,* and, usually at older ages, *P. aeruginosa.* Radiographic imaging demonstrates peribronchial thickening, atelectasis, hyperinflation, and bronchiectasis (preferentially in the middle lobe, lower lobes, or lingula). Spirometry testing may be normal at a young age but can evolve to show an obstructive pattern.

Laterality defects, such as situs inversus, are present in about 50% of patients with PCD and may be incidentally discovered on chest radiograph or physical examination. Kartagener syndrome is the classic triad of situs inversus, chronic sinusitis, and bronchiectasis seen in a subset of patients with PCD. From a reproductive standpoint, patients often experience fertility problems. Males commonly have immotile sperm. Females demonstrate lower fertility rates and are at higher risk for ectopic pregnancy as malfunctioning cilia impede the ovum's transit through the fallopian tube. Other clinical associations with PCD include cardiac defects, pectus excavatum, and scoliosis.

Diagnosis

PCD diagnosis is often delayed, with median age at diagnosis of approximately 5 years because ear infections and sinopulmonary symptoms are not uncommon in preschool-aged children. Diagnosis relies on high clinical suspicion coupled with a few diagnostic tests because there is no one gold standard diagnostic test. The four essential clinical characteristics to consider for PCD are daily, year-round wet cough; daily rhinosinusitis present since infancy; unexplained neonatal respiratory distress in a term baby; and situs inversus. Having at least two of the four key features gives a sensitivity of 80% and specificity of 72%. Nasal nitric oxide can serve as a screening test in patients over 5 years. High-speed video microscopy analyzes ciliary movement, and electron microscopy examines the ultrastructure of cilia taken from mucosal brushings or biopsies. Notably, 30% of PCD cases have a normal ciliary appearance, so lack of a structural defect does not exclude the diagnosis. Finally, genetic testing is available and is expanding. Given the overlap in symptoms, CF and immunodeficiency should be excluded.

Management

PCD therapies center around managing symptoms, and the treatment team should include pediatric pulmonology, otolaryngology, and audiology. Although there is no cure, life expectancy is normal. Respiratory treatment focuses on augmenting airway clearance. Antibiotics are used for upper and lower respiratory tract infections and bronchiectasis exacerbations. Recommendations include the pneumococcal and influenza immunizations and avoiding smoke exposure.

Future Directions

PCD therapies are not currently standardized, and many are extrapolated from similar pulmonary conditions, notably CF. Without a single gold standard diagnostic test, algorithms for diagnosis are being adjusted, as additional diagnostic modalities are being studied and refined.

SUGGESTED READINGS

Available online.

133

Sleep Medicine

Alisha George and Olufunke Afolabi-Brown

CLINICAL VIGNETTE

A 5-year-old girl with a history of trisomy 21 presents to her pediatrician for a well-child visit. Her mother reports a history of snoring. She also reports difficulty awakening in the morning and daytime hyperactivity. She has a history of hypothyroidism, treated with levothyroxine, and seasonal allergies but is otherwise healthy. On examination, she is well-appearing with facial features typical for Down syndrome. Her body mass index is at the 40th percentile for age. She has 2+ sized tonsils, macroglossia, and boggy nasal turbinates. Overnight polysomnography reveals severe obstructive sleep apnea (OSA) with an obstructive apnea-hypopnea index (AHI) of 22 events per hour and oxyhemoglobin saturation nadir of 87%. She undergoes adenotonsillectomy, after which a repeat polysomnogram shows improved, but ongoing OSA (AHI of 10 events per hour). Continuous positive airway pressure is initiated with dramatic improvement in her symptoms.

This patient has several risk factors for OSA: trisomy 21, tonsillar hypertrophy, and allergic rhinitis. The first-line treatment for pediatric OSA is adenotonsillectomy; however, children with risk factors, such as Down syndrome, should have a postoperative polysomnography to assess for residual OSA.

NORMAL SLEEP

Sleep is a naturally occurring state of decreased consciousness and inhibited motor and sensory activity. Sleep is a critical part of human existence, though the exact function remains unknown. It appears to play a role in energy conservation, tissue growth and repair, learning, and memory. It comprises distinct stages and patterns on electroencephalography (EEG), including rapid eye movement (REM) sleep and non-REM (NREM) sleep. Sleep in humans is regulated by two separate processes. The homeostatic process, also known as Process S, represents an increasing drive to sleep the longer the body remains awake. The circadian rhythm, or Process C, is a sleep-wake cycle that repeats approximately every 24 hours and is influenced by multiple environmental factors, the most prominent of which is light.

A multidisciplinary expert panel convened by the National Sleep Foundation made recommendations regarding sleep duration (Table 133.1). Many children cannot achieve the target sleep duration or have disrupted sleep because of bedtime problems and night awakenings. Of children under the age of 3 years, 20% to 30% experience difficulties with sleep onset or maintenance. These sleep issues are often amenable to behavioral modifications, including optimizing sleep hygiene, developing positive bedtime routines, and implementing graduated extinction techniques. Children may require pharmacologic interventions, particularly in special populations with neurodevelopmental delays.

SLEEP-DISORDERED BREATHING

Sleep-disordered breathing (SDB) is a group of conditions that represent abnormal breathing during sleep with sleep disruption and resultant daytime impairment. It encapsulates primary snoring, obstructive sleep apnea (OSA), central sleep apnea (CSA), sleep-related hypoxemia, and sleep-related hypoventilation.

Etiology and Pathogenesis

Primary snoring, the mildest form of SDB, results from relaxed upper airway tissue vibrations during breathing. OSA is characterized by repeated episodes of partial or complete upper airway obstruction resulting in diminished airflow and a disruption of normal ventilation and sleep architecture (Fig. 133.1). OSA is commonly found in children with tonsillar and adenoidal hypertrophy, allergic rhinitis, obesity, craniofacial syndromes, neurologic disorders, and other airway abnormalities (Table 133.2). When associated with daytime impairment, it is termed obstructive sleep apnea *syndrome* (OSAS).

CSA is transient cessation in airflow because of absent respiratory effort, associated with either gas exchange abnormalities, disrupted sleep architecture, or both. CSA and sleep-related hypoventilation, an elevation in carbon dioxide levels above 50 mm Hg for at least 25% of total sleep time, may be secondary to neuromuscular weakness or an impairment in respiratory drive (e.g., brainstem abnormalities, congenital central hypoventilation syndrome). Of note, elevated central apnea indices may be seen in newborns as a result of immaturity and resultant instability of the respiratory control centers.

Clinical Presentation

SDB occurs in children of all ages. Primary snoring is relatively common, occurring in 10% to 30% of children, while the prevalence of OSAS ranges from 1.2% to 5.7%. Some children, especially those with significant craniofacial and neurologic disorders, may present at birth or early infancy. Peak prevalence occurs between 2 and 8 years of age, which coincides with the peak of tonsillar and adenoidal hypertrophy. OSAS occurs equally in prepubertal males and females, though is more prevalent in males in the postpubertal population.

Caregivers may report a wide variety of nocturnal symptoms, notably snoring, gasping, and witnessed apneas (Box 133.1). Chronic congestion, nasal speech, morning headaches, and difficulty awakening also may be reported. It is critical to survey potential daytime impairment. Although excessive daytime sleepiness is more common in adults with SDB, affected children may present with hyperactivity, inattention, aggressive behaviors, moodiness, and poor school performance.

Long-standing, untreated sleep apnea can have cardiovascular and metabolic implications, including endothelial dysfunction, systemic hypertension, pulmonary hypertension, dyslipidemia, and obesity.

Evaluation and Management

Clinical examination may reveal obesity, midface hypoplasia, adenoidal facies, nasal turbinate hypertrophy, micrognathia/retrognathia,

TABLE 133.1 Recommended Hours of Sleep by Age

Age Group	Years	Hours of Sleep (per 24 Hours)
Newborns	0–3 months	14–17 hours
Infants	[a]4–12 months	12–15 hours
Toddlers	1–2 years	11–14 hours
Preschool-aged	3–5 years	10–13 hours
School-aged	6–12 years	9–11 hours
Adolescents	13–18 years	8–10 hours

[a]There is a large variability in the hours of sleep in infants younger than 3 months.

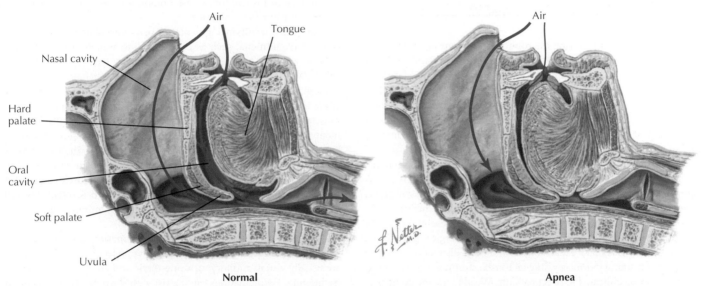

Fig. 133.1 Anatomic representation of upper airway obstruction resulting in diminished airflow and disrupted ventilation.

TABLE 133.2 Risk Factors for Pediatric Obstructive Sleep Apnea

Anatomic	Neurologic/Genetic	Environmental	Others
Adenoid and tonsil hypertrophy	Syndromes • Down syndrome	Tobacco smoke exposure	Family history
Rhinitis	Hypotonia • Cerebral palsy • Neuromuscular diseases	Reduced family income	Male sex
Craniofacial anomalies • Micrognathia • Retrognathia • Midface hypoplasia		Drugs • Benzodiazepines • Opioids • General anesthetics	Asthma
Obesity			

tonsillar hypertrophy, macroglossia, hypotonia, and other craniofacial or neurologic abnormalities. The oropharyngeal examination should include the Mallampati classification (Fig. 133.2A) and tonsil size assessment (Fig. 133.2B), independent OSA predictors. Imaging may be a useful adjunct, though not diagnostic in isolation. Lateral radiographs of the soft tissue neck may demonstrate adenotonsillar hypertrophy or other obstructive anatomy. Computed tomography and magnetic resonance imaging are considered in specific cases for surgical planning.

The American Academy of Pediatrics (AAP) recommends that all children be screened with a detailed history and physical examination for evidence of OSA. These clinical findings alone are, however, inadequate for the accurate diagnosis of OSA. The gold standard for diagnosis of sleep apnea and gas exchange abnormalities is an in-laboratory polysomnogram consisting of EEG, electrooculography, chin and leg electromyography, airflow signals (i.e., oronasal thermal flow and nasal pressure transducer), pulse oximetry, carbon dioxide monitoring (i.e., end-tidal or transcutaneous), thoracoabdominal inductance plethysmography, and snoring microphone. Polysomnography yields an apnea-hypopnea index (AHI) or the number of obstructive respiratory events per hour of sleep time, as well as gas exchange data (Fig. 133.3). The AHI informs the type and severity of sleep apnea. While commonplace in adult settings, home sleep apnea tests are not standard of care in the pediatric population. Additionally, pulse oximetry monitoring or audiovisual recordings are not diagnostic but may be used in settings with limited access to full polysomnography.

The first-line therapy for pediatric OSA is adenotonsillectomy, resulting in the resolution of symptoms in up to 80% of children. Risk factors associated with persistent OSA include obesity, Down syndrome, craniofacial abnormalities, hypotonia, and African American race. Postoperative polysomnography can help ensure the resolution of OSA or determine the need for further therapy. Other surgical procedures, including rapid maxillary expansion, mandibular distraction, midface advancement, supraglottoplasty, lingual tonsillectomy, and partial glossectomy, may be indicated in select patients. Weight loss, including bariatric surgery, also may be critical in children or adolescents with obesity.

In cases of significant residual OSA or when surgery is contraindicated or not feasible, continuous positive airway pressure (CPAP) or bilevel positive airway pressure (BLPAP) may be warranted. BLPAP is often the mainstay of management of significant CSA and sleep-related hypoventilation as well. Positive airway pressure (PAP) therapy serves as a pneumatic stent of the upper airway during sleep, decreasing respiratory events (Fig. 133.4). Adherence to positive airway pressure (PAP) therapy is challenging in the pediatric population and, when available, behavioral therapy should be implemented to aid with PAP desensitization. Patients requiring PAP should first be fitted with the appropriate mask interface. An in-laboratory PAP titration study should be completed around the time of PAP initiation to determine optimal pressures and then repeated annually.

Mild OSA may be treated with nasal corticosteroids and leukotriene receptor antagonists based on these medications' anti-inflammatory properties. In otherwise healthy children with mild OSA and without any comorbidities, watchful waiting with supportive care can be considered; these children should be re-evaluated within 6 months or sooner if symptoms worsen. Other treatments, including positional therapy, orthodontic appliance, and hypoglossal nerve stimulator, are not well-studied in the pediatric population and are not widely used at this time. In rare cases, in which noninvasive PAP is not tolerated or sufficient to treat life-threatening SDB, tracheostomy may be pursued.

NARCOLEPSY

Narcolepsy is a chronic neurologic disorder characterized by fragmented sleep, excessive daytime sleepiness, cataplexy, hallucinations, and sleep paralysis.

Etiology and Pathogenesis

Narcolepsy is caused by a deficiency of orexin-containing neurons in the lateral hypothalamus. The neurotransmitter, orexin, is vital for maintaining alertness and stabilizing sleep-wake states; its loss leads to chronic sleepiness and the intrusion of REM sleep into wakefulness.

Clinical Presentation

The prevalence of narcolepsy ranges from 20 to 50 per 100,000 in Western countries, with significantly higher rates in East Asian populations. Males and females are affected equally. The peak onset of narcolepsy occurs during adolescence, though some studies suggest a bimodal peak in the teens and thirties. Excessive daytime sleepiness, which must be present for at least 3 months, is the symptom that usually prompts further evaluation.

Narcolepsy results in fragmentation of nocturnal sleep and intrusion of REM phenomena, such as cataplexy, into wakefulness. Cataplexy is the key finding that differentiates narcolepsy type 1 (formerly, narcolepsy with cataplexy) from narcolepsy type 2 (formerly, narcolepsy without cataplexy). Occurring in up to 80% of pediatric narcolepsy cases, it is conventionally described as the partial or complete loss of muscle tone with potential for truncal, facial, and extremity involvement (e.g., ptosis, jaw weakness, tongue protrusion, slurred speech, knee buckling, total body collapse to the ground). Such symptoms may be misinterpreted as clumsiness, syncope, or attention-seeking behaviors. Cataplexy spares respiratory and ocular muscles and is not associated with loss of consciousness or amnesia. It is often triggered by strong emotions and typically lasts seconds to minutes before fully reversing.

Narcolepsy can be accompanied by hallucinations and sleep paralysis, both of which can be hypnagogic or hypnopompic. Hallucinations are usually visual, auditory, or somesthetic and are often described as frightening. Hallucinations can coexist with sleep paralysis, which is a complete weakness during sleep-wake transitions. Narcolepsy is also associated with weight gain and obesity, probably related to derangements in the secretion of leptin, a satiety hormone.

Evaluation and Management

The first step in evaluating narcolepsy is a comprehensive sleep history detailing sleep schedule, nocturnal awakenings and behaviors, and naps. Information must be obtained on caffeine, alcohol, and tobacco use because these may influence sleep patterns. A modified Epworth Sleepiness Scale (ESS), which rates the likelihood of falling asleep in various situations, is obtained at every clinic visit to establish the degree of sleepiness and monitor response to therapies. Total sleep time can be estimated with sleep logs or objective measures such as wrist actigraphy, in which a watch-like instrument records activity level. It is essential to exclude contributors to sleepiness related to underlying medical and psychiatric disorders, medication side effects, substance abuse, and insufficient sleep.

Evaluation of narcolepsy involves an overnight polysomnogram and multiple sleep latency test (MSLT). The overnight polysomnogram excludes confounding diagnoses (e.g., sleep apnea) that may contribute to excessive daytime sleepiness. In narcolepsy, the polysomnogram often reveals a short sleep latency, fragmented nocturnal sleep, and a REM period within 15 minutes of sleep onset (SOREMP). The following day, an MSLT is performed, consisting of five 20-minute nap opportunities, separated by 2-hour intervals. A narcolepsy diagnosis is established if a patient has an average sleep latency of less than 8 minutes on MSLT and at least 2 SOREMPs between the overnight polysomnogram and MSLT. A comprehensive drug screen is recommended before testing.

A. Friedman Classification: Palate Positions
(Modified Mallampati)

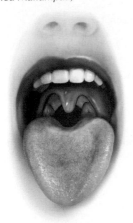 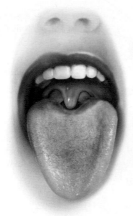 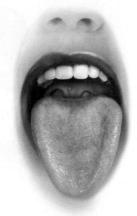 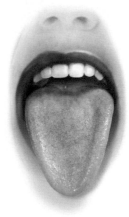

Position I
Allows visualization of the entire uvula and tonsils/pillars

Position II
Allows visualization of the uvula but not the tonsils

Position III
Allows visualization of the soft palate but not the uvula

Position IV
Allows visualization of the hard palate only

B. Tonsillar-Size Classification

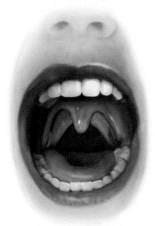 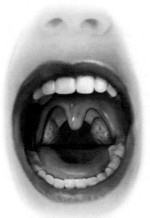 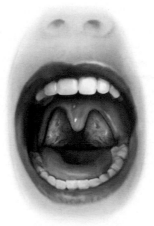 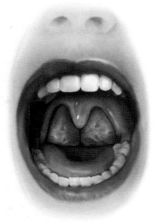

Grade 1
Within tonsillar fauces

Grade 2
Outside tonsillar fauces, up to 50% of airway to midline

Grade 3
Outside tonsillar fauces, up to 75% of the distance to the midline

Grade 4
Outside tonsillar fauces, >75% of the lateral airway dimension

Fig. 133.2 (A) The Modified Mallampati classification describes tongue size relative to oropharyngeal size. The test is conducted with the patient in the sitting position, the head held in a natural position, the mouth wide open and relaxed, and the tongue inside the mouth without any protrusion or phonation. The subsequent classification is assigned based upon the pharyngeal structures that are visible. Class I = visualization of the soft palate, fauces, uvula, anterior and posterior pillars. Class II = visualization of the soft palate, fauces, and uvula. Class III = visualization of the soft palate and the base of the uvula. Class IV = soft palate is not visible at all. If the patient phonates, this falsely improves the view. If the patient arches his or her tongue, the uvula is falsely obscured. The test was initially adapted to predict ease of intubation but can be used to predict the potential severity of obstructive sleep apnea. (B) Clinical evaluation of tonsillar size is based on the following scheme. Grade 1 = within tonsillar fauces; grade 2 = outside tonsillar fauces, up to 50% of the airway to the midline; grade 3 = outside tonsillar fauces and up to 75% of the distance to the midline; and grade 4 = 75% of the lateral airway dimension. (Reused with permission from Avidan AY. Sleep and Its Disorders, In: Jankovic J, ed. *Bradley and Daroff's Neurology in Clinical Practice.* 8th ed. Philadelphia, PA: Elsevier; 2022:1664-1744.e9, Figure 101.50; based on Mallampati SR, Gatt SP, Gugino LD, et al. 1985. A clinical sign to predict difficult tracheal intubation: a prospective study. *Can Anaesth Soc J.* 1985;32:429-434.)

Treatment of narcolepsy involves lifestyle modification, emphasizing a regular sleep schedule, and incorporating brief daytime nap(s) to alleviate daytime sleepiness. Wake-promoting medications, including methylphenidate, (dextro)amphetamine, (ar)modafinil, pitolisant, and solriamfetol can be prescribed. Certain antidepressants (e.g., venlafaxine, fluoxetine) can be used to treat significant cataplexy.

Oxybates (such as sodium oxybate) are agents used to target both sleepiness and cataplexy, but patients and families must be counseled on its abuse potential. Treatment response can be monitored using the ESS and maintenance of wakefulness test (MWT). Formal assessment with an MWT should be considered in affected adolescents before obtaining a driver's license. Notably, narcolepsy may be accompanied

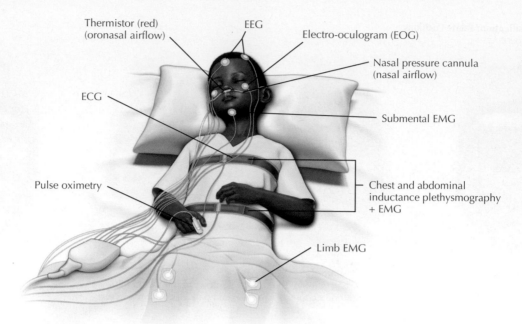

A. A child set up for a polysomnogram

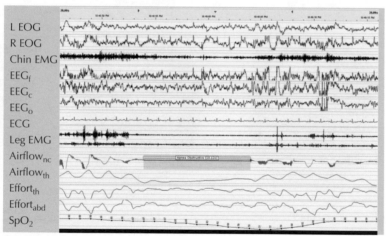

B. An epoch out of a PSG showing an obstructive apnea (pink highlight); the lower half shows the same patient now asleep on CPAP with resolution of apneic events.

Fig. 133.3 (A) Pediatric polysomnogram. (B) One epoch of a polysomnogram showing a respiratory event (obstructive apnea). Obstructive apneas are respiratory events with a 90% or greater decrease in airflow signal in the presence of ongoing respiratory effort for at least two breaths' duration. Other hypopneas (not shown) are respiratory events with a 30% or greater decrease in nasal pressure signal for at least two breaths' duration associated with a 3% or greater oxygen desaturation and/or arousal.

by symptoms of depression and anxiety. Practitioners should consider a referral to mental health services for the evaluation and treatment of comorbid mood disorders.

DISORDERS OF AROUSAL

The term *parasomnias* refers to a broad group of sleep disorders characterized by unwanted abnormal behaviors or experiences. Disorders of arousal are the most common parasomnias occurring in the pediatric population; the three main subtypes are confusional arousals, sleepwalking, and sleep terrors.

Etiology and Pathogenesis

Disorders of arousals represent dissociative-like states with features of both wakefulness and NREM sleep. Episodes most commonly

arise toward the end of the first sleep cycle and are characterized by the disrupted transition from slow-wave sleep to lighter sleep stages. Although the specific mechanism remains unknown, there appears to be a strong genetic link, with 60% of affected children having a first-degree relative with an arousal disorder. Disorders of arousal can be triggered or exacerbated by sleep deprivation, psychosocial stressors, sleep-disordered breathing, restless legs syndrome, and periodic limb movements.

Clinical Presentation

Disorders of arousal are characterized by a lack of awareness of the environment with varying degrees of motor activity and autonomic arousal. They can occur in very young children, though the prevalence decreases with age and often disappears by the adolescent years. Episodes have variable duration, ranging from a few seconds to

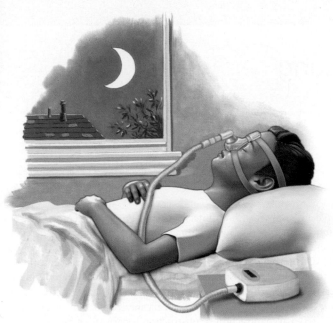

Fig. 133.4 Continuous Positive Airway Pressure With Nasal Interface.

minutes. Children commonly have one episode per night but may have multiple episodes. In most cases, the child will return to bed without fully awakening and have no recollection of the episode(s) the following day.
- During confusional arousals, children are often found confused, disoriented, and sitting up in bed. Although there is generally limited motor and autonomic activity, children may become somewhat agitated and thrash in bed. Confusional arousals can be precipitated by forced awakenings and have the potential to progress to sleepwalking.

- The key features of sleepwalking are prominent motor activity (i.e., walking, crawling) and automatic behavior. Similar to other disorders of arousal, children appear confused and disoriented.
- Sleep terrors are dramatic episodes characterized by intense crying or screaming, usually lasting less than 15 minutes (but may surpass 1 hour). They are common in infants and toddlers. Children may appear confused or distressed, which can be quite alarming to caregivers. However, attempts to calm the child often result in more significant confusion and aggression.

Evaluation and Management

Diagnosis is made based on history. Although polysomnography is not necessary for diagnosis, disorders of arousal may be incidentally identified.

Management involves caregiver reassurance and safety precautions to ensure no harm comes to the child during an episode. Examples of safety precautions include placing the child's mattress on the floor, having the child sleep in a sleeping bag, locking all windows and doors, using an alarm system, and securing all firearms. Triggers of these parasomnias should be addressed, including underlying sleep-disordered breathing, which can fragment sleep and increase the likelihood of these parasomnias. Increasing total sleep time to optimal levels may help. Caffeine should be eliminated or minimized from the child's diet.

FUTURE DIRECTIONS

Innovative diagnostic tools for pediatric OSA are needed, which can serve as alternative options for children whose sensory or neurocognitive challenges may limit their ability to undergo a successful polysomnogram. Additionally, future studies on the exact mechanism of disorders of arousal are needed to inform other therapeutic options.

SUGGESTED READINGS

Available online.

134

Congenital Anomalies of the Lung

Alyssa R. Thomas and Wai Wong

 CLINICAL VIGNETTE

An infant is born at 37 weeks by spontaneous vaginal delivery. Prenatal history was notable for polyhydramnios seen on third trimester ultrasonography. Shortly after birth, the infant is noted to be tachypneic with copious oral secretions and intercostal retractions. In the neonatal intensive care unit, nurses attempt to place a nasogastric tube but feel resistance after several centimeters. On chest radiograph, the nasogastric tube is coiled in a blind pouch. Endoscopic evaluation ultimately reveals esophageal atresia and tracheoesophageal fistula.

CONGENITAL ANOMALIES OF THE AIRWAY

Laryngeal and Subglottic Anomalies

Etiology and Pathogenesis

Laryngomalacia is both the most common extrathoracic congenital anomaly and the most common cause of stridor in infants. Poor tone of the laryngeal muscles causes the larynx to collapse on inspiration. Endoscopic findings include prolapse of arytenoids and an omega-shaped epiglottis. Congenital high airway obstruction syndrome (CHAOS) is a rare and life-threatening syndrome associated with complete upper airway obstruction, hyperechoic and dilated lungs and airways, flattened and inverted diaphragm, and fetal hydrops. CHAOS can be due to laryngeal or tracheal atresia. Laryngeal webs are due to failed resorption of tissue at the laryngeal inlet and is often associated with cardiac abnormalities and velocardiofacial syndromes. Laryngeal clefts result from failed fusion of the lateral growth plates of the posterior cricoid cartilage.

Congenital subglottic stenosis is narrowing of the airway lumen in the region of the cricoid cartilage. Subglottic hemangiomas are benign vascular neoplasms that can enlarge over the first months of life and cause airway compromise if untreated.

Presentation

Laryngomalacia presents with a staccato inspiratory stridor within the first month of life that is louder with feeding or activity and improves at rest and in the prone position. Anatomic upper airway narrowing such as laryngeal web, subglottic stenosis, or subglottic hemangiomas can present as stridor that worsens with agitation or recurrent croup. Subglottic hemangiomas should be considered in infants with facial hemangiomas in the beard distribution. Laryngeal clefts may present with noisy breathing, dysphagia, aspiration, or recurrent pneumonia.

Evaluation and Management

Diagnostic evaluation for upper airway lesions includes direct laryngoscopy, flexible and/or rigid bronchoscopy, and modified barium swallow if there is a concern for aspiration. Mild laryngomalacia typically resolves without intervention in the second year of life, but surgical intervention with supraglottoplasty can be considered in severe cases with failure to thrive, respiratory distress, or cyanosis. CHAOS or near-complete laryngeal webs require tracheostomy at birth to bypass the obstructed airway or an ex-utero intrapartum surgery (EXIT) if the lesion is detected prenatally. Laryngeal webs can be excised or ablated with lasers. Laryngeal clefts can be surgically repaired. Laryngotracheal reconstruction is performed for severe subglottic stenosis. Symptomatic subglottic hemangiomas are managed with systemic propranolol.

Tracheal and Bronchial Anomalies

Tracheoesophageal fistulas (TEFs), which may occur with or without esophageal atresia (EA), occur in approximately 1 to 2 per 3500 live births. These anomalies occur as a result of incomplete separation of the lung bud from the ventral foregut. There are five anatomic variants of TEF/EA; most common (85%) is a proximal EA with a distal fistula (Fig. 134.1). "H-type" TEF describes the bridging fistula between the otherwise intact trachea and esophagus. TEF/EA is usually sporadic but may be associated with trisomies 13, 18, or 21; CHARGE (*c*oloboma, *h*eart defect, *a*tresia choanae, *r*etarded growth and development, *g*enital hypoplasia, *e*ar anomalies/deafness) syndrome; and the VACTERL (*v*ertebral defects, *a*nal atresia, *c*ardiac defects, *t*racheoesophageal fistula, *r*enal anomalies, and *l*imb abnormalities) association.

Tracheomalacia is a condition in which there is dynamic collapse of the trachea during breathing. Primary tracheomalacia is an intrinsic weakness resulting from decreased cartilaginous support of the trachea (Fig. 134.1). Secondary tracheomalacia can occur in a variety of conditions, including extrinsic tracheal compression from vascular malformations such as vascular rings, bronchopulmonary dysplasia, TEF, or any condition with chronic irritation or inflammation of the airways. Tracheal stenosis is narrowing of the trachea and can be congenital, such as complete tracheal rings, or acquired after intubation injury, for example. Complete tracheal rings are associated with left pulmonary artery slings.

Bronchial abnormalities include bronchomalacia, which is dynamic narrowing of the bronchi caused by intrinsic airway properties (e.g., lack of cartilage), acquired postinflammatory narrowing after an infection, or extrinsic compression. Williams-Campbell syndrome is characterized as a congenital absence of the cartilage in the subsegmental bronchi that results in distal bronchiectasis. Mounier-Kuhn syndrome is congenital tracheobronchomegaly with dilation of the airways as a result of muscular and elastic tissue atrophy. Bronchial stenosis is narrowing of the bronchi. Tracheal bronchus is an abnormal bronchus that originates from the trachea above the level of the carina (Fig. 134.1).

A. Tracheoesophageal fistula

Most common form (90% to 95%) of tracheoesophageal fistula. Upper segment of esophagus ending in blind pouch; lower segment originating from trachea just above bifurcation. The two segments may be connected by a solid cord

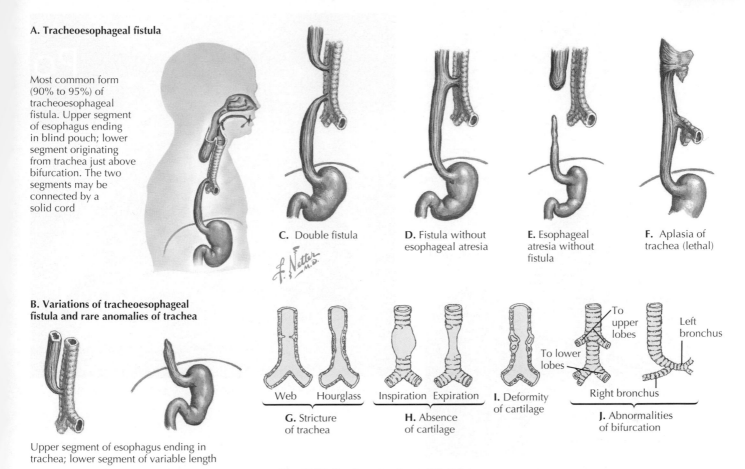

C. Double fistula

D. Fistula without esophageal atresia

E. Esophageal atresia without fistula

F. Aplasia of trachea (lethal)

B. Variations of tracheoesophageal fistula and rare anomalies of trachea

Upper segment of esophagus ending in trachea; lower segment of variable length

Web Hourglass

G. Stricture of trachea

Inspiration Expiration

H. Absence of cartilage

I. Deformity of cartilage

To upper lobes

To lower lobes

Right bronchus

Left bronchus

J. Abnormalities of bifurcation

Fig. 134.1 Tracheoesophageal Fistula.

Presentation

TEF/EA is suspected prenatally when there is polyhydramnios (resulting from impaired fetal swallowing of amniotic fluid) and absent or small fetal stomach on ultrasound. In the immediate postnatal period, infants with TEF/EA have drooling or frothing because of the inability to swallow oral secretions. Aspiration of the secretions into the lungs can lead to respiratory distress. H-type fistulas may have delayed diagnosis and present with a history of recurrent pneumonias or dysphagia.

Tracheal abnormalities typically present with noisy breathing, respiratory distress, and prolonged recovery from respiratory illness. The phase of breathing in which the adventitious sounds are auscultated depends on the location of the tracheal or bronchial narrowing or collapse: inspiratory stridor may be auscultated if the lesion is extrathoracic whereas intrathoracic lesions may have a "barking" cough or an expiratory wheeze. Symptoms may be mistaken for croup or refractory asthma.

Evaluation and Management

In cases of TEF/EA, a nasogastric or orogastric tube cannot be passed, with the tube seen coiled in the blind pouch on chest radiograph. For more subtle cases, diagnosis of TEF may be identified with bronchoscopy or by injecting water-soluble contrast or air under fluoroscopic guidance. Initial management involves suctioning secretions with a sump to prevent pneumonitis. Infants should undergo evaluation for other elements of VACTERL. Surgical repair is done to divide the fistula and anastomose the proximal and distal esophageal pouches. Even after surgical repair, many children will have wheeze, prolonged respiratory illnesses, dysphagia, esophageal strictures, and/or esophageal dysmotility.

If there is suspicion for a tracheal anomaly, the gold standard for diagnosis is flexible or rigid bronchoscopy. Other diagnostic studies such as airway fluoroscopy, esophagram, or computed tomography (CT) can sometimes be helpful to identify areas of malacia or stenosis as well as sources of external compression. Tracheomalacia often resolves spontaneously as the airway matures and grows, but depending on the severity, patients with tracheomalacia may benefit from treatment with inhaled anticholinergic medications, continuous positive airway pressure, tracheostomy with or without mechanical ventilation, aortopexy, or external splint. Surgery is necessary for symptomatic vascular rings or slings. But, similar to TEF/EA, children may continue to have symptoms of tracheomalacia after the repair because of abnormal cartilage development in the setting of the previous external compression.

CONGENITAL ANOMALIES OF THE LUNG PARENCHYMA

Etiology and Pathogenesis

Congenital lobar emphysema (CLE) is a condition characterized by hyperinflation of the affected lobe (Fig. 134.2). Although a specific cause is not always identified, a frequent cause is air trapping induced by obstruction with a ball-valve effect. Examples include meconium aspiration, bronchial cartilage dysplasia, and external bronchial compression. The left upper and right middle lobes are the most frequently affected.

Congenital pulmonary airway malformation (CPAM), previously known as cystic adenomatous malformation, is a broad term for hamartomatous lung lesions composed of a proliferation of bronchial tissue (Fig. 134.3). CPAM develops during the pseudoglandular phase of

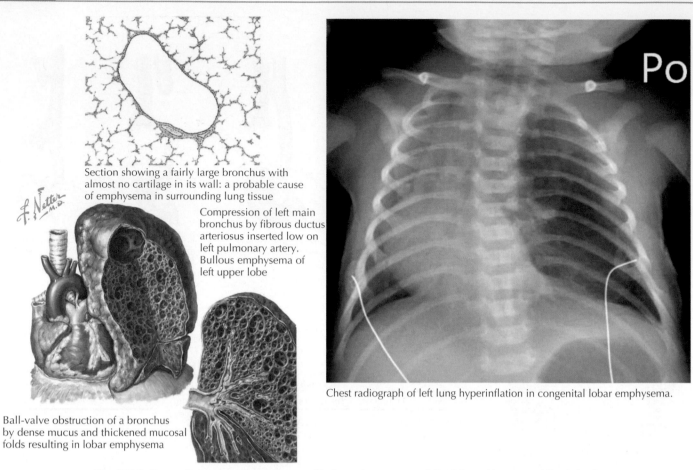

Section showing a fairly large bronchus with almost no cartilage in its wall: a probable cause of emphysema in surrounding lung tissue

Compression of left main bronchus by fibrous ductus arteriosus inserted low on left pulmonary artery. Bullous emphysema of left upper lobe

Ball-valve obstruction of a bronchus by dense mucus and thickened mucosal folds resulting in lobar emphysema

Chest radiograph of left lung hyperinflation in congenital lobar emphysema.

Fig. 134.2 Congenital Lobar Emphysema. (Radiograph courtesy of Dr. Misun Hwang and Dr. Luis O. Tierradentro-Garcia, Department of Radiology, Children's Hospital of Philadelphia.)

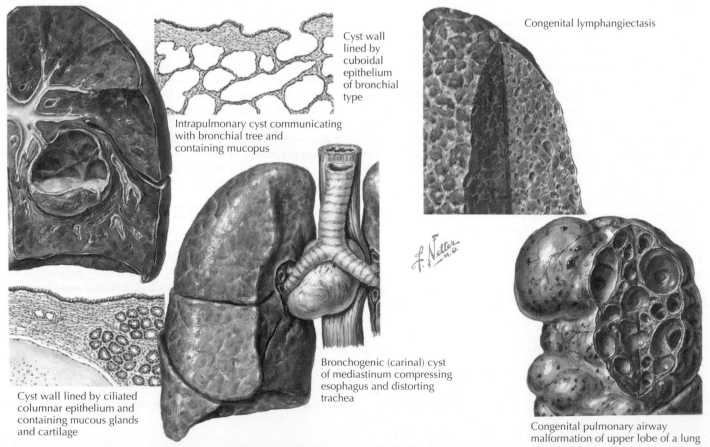

Cyst wall lined by cuboidal epithelium of bronchial type

Intrapulmonary cyst communicating with bronchial tree and containing mucopus

Congenital lymphangiectasis

Cyst wall lined by ciliated columnar epithelium and containing mucous glands and cartilage

Bronchogenic (carinal) cyst of mediastinum compressing esophagus and distorting trachea

Congenital pulmonary airway malformation of upper lobe of a lung

Fig. 134.3 Congenital Bronchogenic and Pulmonary Cysts.

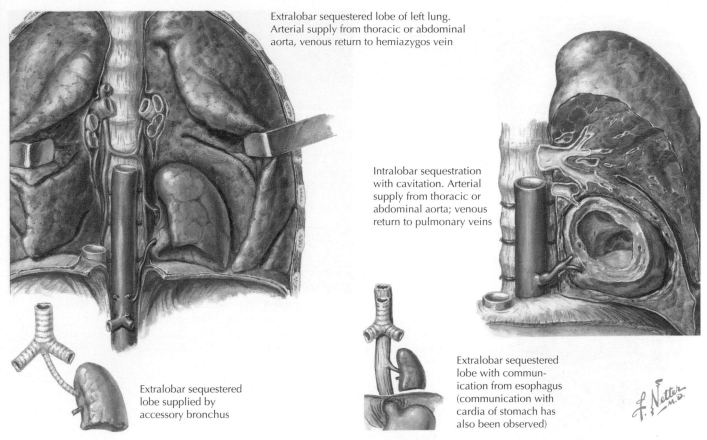

Extralobar sequestered lobe of left lung. Arterial supply from thoracic or abdominal aorta, venous return to hemiazygos vein

Intralobar sequestration with cavitation. Arterial supply from thoracic or abdominal aorta; venous return to pulmonary veins

Extralobar sequestered lobe supplied by accessory bronchus

Extralobar sequestered lobe with communication from esophagus (communication with cardia of stomach has also been observed)

Fig. 134.4 Bronchopulmonary Sequestration.

lung development (weeks 7 to 17 of gestation). The lesions maintain a tiny connection to the tracheobronchial tree and derive their blood supply from the normal pulmonary circulation. CPAM is the most common congenital cystic lung lesion, occurring in approximately 1:25,000 to 1:35,000 live births. The lesions are most frequently unilobar and are only rarely bilateral. The Stocker histologic classification system includes types 0 to 4. Type 0 is rare and usually fatal. Type 1 is the most common and prognostically favorable form of CPAM, occurring in about 50% of cases, and consisting of a small number of larger cysts lined by ciliated pseudostratified epithelium. Type 2 is the second most common, consisting of numerous small cysts and frequently associated with other congenital anomalies, including congenital diaphragmatic hernia (CDH). Importantly, types 1 and 4 have malignant potential, with type 4 associated with pleuropulmonary blastoma.

Bronchopulmonary sequestration (BPS) is a mass of microcystic, nonfunctioning lung tissue that is thought to be derived from the primitive foregut (Fig. 134.4). These lesions do not have a normal connection with the tracheobronchial tree and receive their blood supply from the systemic circulation by aberrant vessels, in comparison to CPAM. Intralobar BPS is contained within the normal lung and covered by the same pleura. Extralobar BPS is covered by their own pleura and can be located above or below the diaphragm. Extralobar BPS is associated with other congenital anomalies, including cardiac defects, TEF, esophageal duplication, and CDH. Notably, there are hybrid lesions with histologic features of CPAM but a systemic-derived blood supply.

Bronchogenic cysts are formed from a single bud off of the primitive foregut, which usually lack a connection with the main tracheobronchial tree (Fig. 134.3). The cysts are mainly located in the mediastinum near the carina and histologically contain elements of respiratory epithelium and cartilage.

Pulmonary hypoplasia can occur as a primary problem of lung development or can be secondary to another anomaly. Examples include pulmonary hypoplasia resulting from oligohydramnios in the setting of renal anomalies or premature rupture of membranes, compression in the setting of other lesions such as CPAM, visceral herniation in CDH, congenital pulmonary valve stenosis, or impaired fetal breathing movements. *Pulmonary agenesis* is usually unilateral and thought to be due to vascular disruption.

Congenital diaphragmatic hernia is a developmental defect of the diaphragm, which results in herniation of abdominal organs into the chest cavity (Fig. 134.5). CDH stems from failure of the pleuroperitoneal canal to close early in gestation. The majority of defects are posterolateral ("Bochdalek") and left-sided. There is also a reduced size of the vascular bed and remodeling of the pulmonary vessels, which leads to pulmonary hypertension. CDH is associated with congenital heart disease, neurologic defects, and chromosomal abnormalities.

Clinical Presentation

Many infants with a prenatal diagnosis of a lung parenchymal lesion are asymptomatic. Smaller lung lesions may be identified as a recurrent opacity on chest radiography or recurrent pneumonia. However, in severe cases, a large mass may cause mediastinal shift and impair pulmonary venous return, leading to compromised cardiac output and fetal hydrops. Likewise, at birth, infants with large lesions can display significant respiratory distress and cardiopulmonary decompensation. In CDH, examination can reveal a scaphoid-appearing abdomen caused by viscera migration into the chest, decreased breath sounds, and bowel sounds in the thorax. These patients may be critically ill because of pulmonary hypertension. CLE is symptomatic in the neonatal period, typically within the first 6 months after birth, with progressive respiratory

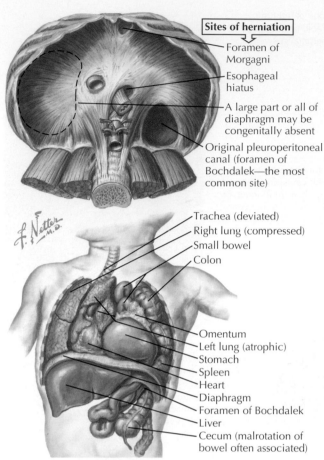

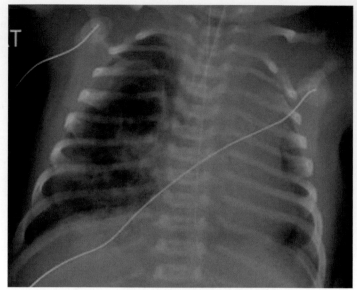

Chest radiograph of right-sided congenital diaphragmatic hernia.

Fig. 134.5 Congenital Diaphragmatic Hernia. (Radiograph courtesy of Dr. Misun Hwang and Dr. Luis O. Tierradentro-Garcia, Department of Radiology, Children's Hospital of Philadelphia.)

distress, decreased breath sounds over the affected lobe, and sometimes wheezing resulting from airway compression.

Evaluation and Management

Antenatal

The natural history of parenchymal lung lesions is highly variable. Improved sonographic techniques and an evolving understanding of the pathophysiology of these lesions has allowed detection at earlier stages of disease during antenatal screening. The sonographic appearance of the lesion and the origin of the blood supply on Doppler ultrasound, can help diagnose CPAM and BPS. If further imaging is required, fetal magnetic resonance imaging (MRI) can help differentiate these lesions. Of note, development of fetal hydrops is a very poor prognostic sign with near complete mortality in the absence of intervention.

The decision to perform a fetal intervention depends on the severity of the lesion by sonographic findings. Antenatal steroid administration in CPAM is associated with improved survival of high-risk fetuses, potentially as a result of growth arrest of the lesion. In utero treatments for CPAM include decompression of a dominant cyst by thoracoamniotic shunting or surgical resection for debulking. In severe cases of CDH, fetal intervention with fetal tracheal occlusion (FETO) is thought to improve lung growth by preventing escape of fetal lung fluid. Infants with significant cardiopulmonary compromise and mediastinal shift may undergo an EXIT procedure. This allows for surgical intervention such as lesion resection, ventilatory stabilization, or cannulation for extracorporeal membrane oxygenation (ECMO). Given the severity

of postnatal outcomes, infants with antenatally suspected lung lesions should be delivered at a specialized center with appropriate neonatal and surgical resources.

Postnatal

Chest radiography is often the initial evaluation. CPAM may visually appear as air-filled cysts, cysts with air-fluid levels, bubbly lucencies representing many smaller cysts, or a solid mass (Fig. 134.6). CLE may initially appear opaque because of retained fetal lung fluid, and later become hyperlucent, hyperexpanded lung. It is particularly important to distinguish CLE from pneumothorax; notably, lung markings can be visualized out to the periphery in CLE (Fig. 134.2). There may be air-filled bowel loops in the chest in CDH (Fig. 134.5). Because chest radiography may appear normal in the newborn period for CPAM and BPS, advanced thoracic imaging is recommended with MRI or contrast enhanced CT if there is high suspicion for a lung lesion.

Surgical excision of the affected lobe is the treatment for symptomatic CLE, whereas conservative management is reasonable for asymptomatic or mild cases. For most cases of CPAM and BPS, surgery is elective at 2 to 6 months of age unless the infant has respiratory distress at birth. Surgery is typically recommended for high-risk cases involving large lesions, pneumothorax, multifocal cysts, or a family history of pleuropulmonary blastoma-related conditions. In the case of watchful waiting, the lesion is followed with serial imaging because of the risk for infection and malignant transformation. Notably, after resection, young infants can have significant compensatory growth of

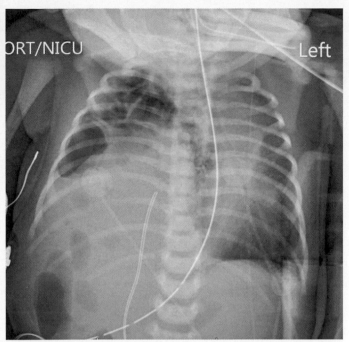

Fig. 134.6 Chest Radiograph of Right-Sided Large Air-Filled Cyst in Congenital Pulmonary Airway Malformation. (Courtesy Dr. Misun Hwang and Dr. Luis O. Tierradentro-Garcia, Department of Radiology, Children's Hospital of Philadelphia.)

the residual lung tissue and thus have an excellent prognosis for lung function.

Infants with CDH are rapidly intubated, and a sump is placed in the delivery room to decompress the bowels. If conventional mechanical ventilation fails, high-frequency oscillatory ventilation is often used. Inhaled nitric oxide may be used to lower pulmonary vascular resistance. ECMO is a rescue therapy for persistent severe hypoxemia or impaired ventilation. Genetic testing and echocardiography should be part of the evaluation. CDH is repaired surgically by reduction of the herniated viscera after clinical stabilization.

PULMONARY VASCULAR MALFORMATIONS

Etiology and Pathogenesis

Pulmonary vascular malformations, although rare, can be severe and result in significant morbidity. Arteriovenous malformations (AVMs) in the lungs allow blood to flow directly between small pulmonary arteries and veins without passing through pulmonary capillary beds; this shunting causes significant cyanosis unresponsive to supplemental oxygen administration. AVMs are most common in the setting of hereditary hemorrhagic telangiectasia (HHT). Anomalous pulmonary venous drainage results in aberrant return of pulmonary venous blood to the right side of the heart instead of the left. An example of this is scimitar syndrome. Alveolar capillary dysplasia with misalignment of the pulmonary veins (ACD-MPV) is a rare and lethal condition characterized histologically by pulmonary arteriolar remodeling, simplified alveoli, and congested pulmonary veins.

Congenital pulmonary lymphangiectasia (CPL) is a developmental disorder of the lymphatic system leading to lymphatic dilation. Primary CPL is localized to the lungs. Secondary CPL is due to obstructed venous return in congenital cardiac disease or diffuse lymphatic disease as in Noonan, Turner, or Down syndromes.

Clinical Presentation

Pulmonary AVMs and other vascular malformations may be asymptomatic or present with dyspnea, fatigue, cyanosis resulting from right-to-left shunting, digital clubbing, and hemoptysis. Because of the shunt, systemic "paradoxical" emboli can cause stroke or brain abscess. In HHT, there may be telangiectasias of the skin of the face, hands, lips and the oral mucosa as well as spontaneous, and sometimes difficult to control, epistaxis. Symptoms in scimitar syndrome relate to the degree of left-to-right shunting with a potential for heart failure, but may also include recurrent pneumonia and wheeze. Infants with ACD-MPV have uneventful deliveries, but within hours of birth experience progressive respiratory failure and severe, refractory pulmonary hypertension. CPL may manifest antenatally with nonimmune hydrops fetalis or postnatally with neonatal chylothorax. Chylothoraces can manifest in the first hours to weeks of life and can, in severe cases, lead to respiratory failure.

Evaluation and Management

Pulmonary AVMs may be treated with coil embolization or surgical resection. Patients with HHT should be evaluated for cerebral and hepatic AVMs. Other vascular malformations such as scimitar syndrome may need surgical care but also need management of associated congenital anomalies. Antenatal management of chylothoraces includes thoracoamniotic shunting to mitigate lung tissue compression and hypoplasia. Postnatally, infants may be medically managed using parenteral nutrition and medium-chain triglyceride oil to decrease output from the thoracic duct. Some are treated with somatostatin and octreotide. An emerging therapy for persistent lymphatic malformations is embolization.

A contrast echocardiogram using agitated saline may identify the presence of a shunt. Chest CT or pulmonary angiography are necessary for definitive diagnosis. ACD-MPV is diagnosed by lung biopsy, although some will have *FOXF1* gene deletion or mutation. ECMO should be considered to treat refractory pulmonary hypertension and progressive respiratory failure of these infants, but the condition is typically fatal without lung transplantation.

FUTURE DIRECTIONS

Advanced imaging modalities for parenchymal lung disease continue to progress to reduce radiation exposure with CT imaging. Although CT is still frequently the gold standard, MRI is seeing an increasing role. Fetal imaging and surgery such as FETO have provided improved survival in cases with poor prognoses. Advanced imaging techniques may also be helpful for characterizing even dynamic airway abnormalities. In terms of therapeutics, medications such as ipratropium and bethanechol are sometimes used to alter smooth muscle tone in tracheobronchomalacia but these may warrant further investigation in large clinical trials.

SUGGESTED READINGS

Available online.

135

Infections of the Lower Airway

Allison M. Blatz and Julie L. Fierro

 CLINICAL VIGNETTE

A previously healthy 4-year-old girl presents to the emergency department with cough, fever, and abdominal pain of 2 days' duration. Her vital signs are notable for a temperature of 104.1°F (40.1°C), a respiratory rate of 30 breaths/min, and a heart rate of 125 beats/min. Her oxyhemoglobin saturation on room air is 94%. On examination, she is tired appearing but well hydrated. She does not have retractions, grunting, or nasal flaring. Upon auscultation, there are crackles over the left lower lobe. Her abdomen is soft, nontender, and nondistended with normoactive bowel sounds. Her capillary refill is less than 2 seconds. A chest radiograph shows a left lower lobe infiltrate. She is diagnosed with a left lower lobe community acquired pneumonia and is prescribed high-dose amoxicillin. Because she has acceptable oxygen saturations, appears well on examination, has good fluid intake, and tolerates amoxicillin, she is discharged on a 7-day course of amoxicillin with instructions for close follow-up with her primary care doctor.

Lower respiratory tract infections (LRTIs) are infections of the lower airway, most commonly caused by viruses or bacteria, and include pneumonia, bronchiolitis, and tracheitis. These infections most commonly manifest with cough; however, the clinical presentation, diagnosis, and management differ for each disorder. The World Health Organization uses the clinical symptoms of cough and fast or difficult breathing relative to age to define pneumonia. In high-income countries, pneumonia is commonly defined as the presence of fever and signs of LRTI (e.g., cough, tachypnea, hypoxia) with or without abnormalities on chest radiograph. Bronchiolitis is an acute obstructive lower airway disease caused by a viral infection in infants younger than 24 months of age.

EPIDEMIOLOGY

The annual incidence of pneumonia is greatest among children younger than 1 year and decreases as children age. Community acquired pneumonia (CAP) causes almost 20% of deaths in children younger than 5 years in low- and middle-income countries but less than 1% of children hospitalized with pneumonia in the United States die. CAP remains a frequent cause of outpatient pediatric visits and hospitalization. Bacterial tracheitis, a rare acute LRTI, has an estimated incidence of 0.1 cases per 100,000 children per year. It is commonly diagnosed in children with an artificial airway. The peak incidence of severe bronchiolitis occurs in infants aged 2 to 6 months. Approximately 1% of infants younger than 12 months are hospitalized with bronchiolitis. Hospitalization rates are five times higher in high-risk groups, including premature infants with bronchopulmonary dysplasia (BPD) and patients with congenital heart disease.

MICROBIOLOGY

Pneumonia is caused by many different organisms, with viruses and bacteria being the most common causes (Table 135.1). Cause varies with age. Respiratory viruses such as respiratory syncytial virus (RSV); influenza A and B; parainfluenza 1, 2, and 3; adenovirus; and human metapneumovirus can be identified in up to half of patients admitted to the hospital for CAP. In 2019 the SARS coronavirus-2 emerged as a novel pathogen responsible for more than 5 million deaths worldwide in 2 years because of severe pneumonia in adults. The literature thus far shows that children usually have a milder, self-limited illness.

The most common bacterial cause of childhood CAP is *Streptococcus pneumoniae* (Fig. 135.1). *Staphylococcus aureus* is also a frequent cause of severe CAP even in previously healthy children without exposure to health care settings. *Mycoplasma pneumoniae* is a common pathogen in school-age children, adolescents, and young adults and tends to manifest with a longer, more indolent course.

Less common causes of CAP include nontypeable *Haemophilus influenzae*, enteric gram-negative pathogens (in cases of aspiration or neurologic compromise), *Mycobacterium tuberculosis*, *Legionella pneumophila*, herpes simplex virus (in newborns), varicella-zoster virus, and endemic mycoses such as *Histoplasma capsulatum*, *Coccidioides immitis*, and *Blastomyces dermatitidis*. Before the introduction of the conjugate *H. influenzae* type b (Hib) vaccine, Hib was a common cause of CAP. In areas where Hib vaccine uptake is low, Hib should still be considered a common cause of CAP.

Acute bacterial tracheitis is commonly caused by *S. pneumoniae*, nontypeable *H. influenzae*, *Moraxella catarrhalis*, and other respiratory colonizers. Enteric gram-negative organisms may also be causative, especially in patients with artificial airways.

Bronchiolitis is due to viral pathogens with specific tropism for bronchiolar epithelium. RSV accounts for half of bronchiolitis cases, though many infants infected with RSV only develop upper respiratory tract symptoms and not lower airway disease.

PATHOGENESIS

Pneumonia occurs when infection causes the alveoli to fill with pus. Viral illness alone can cause necrotizing pneumonia (Fig. 135.2). Preceding viral illness may play a role in the pathogenesis of bacterial pneumonia as viral-induced airway damage makes the respiratory tract more susceptible to bacterial superinfection.

Acute bacterial tracheitis typically occurs in a previously healthy child after a respiratory viral infection. In a child with an artificial airway, tracheitis may result from an organism that colonizes the artificial airway.

In bronchiolitis, viral infection of the lower airways affects the epithelial cells and mucosal surfaces of the human respiratory tract.

TABLE 135.1 Common Bacterial and Viral Causes of Community Acquired Pneumonia by Age in Healthy Children in the Developed World

≤3 Months	3 Months to 5 Years	≥5 Years
Bacterial		
Bordetella pertussis	Haemophilus influenzae (nontypeable)	Chlamydophila pneumoniae
Chlamydia trachomatis	Staphylococcus aureus	Mycoplasma pneumoniae
Enteric gram-negative organisms	Streptococcus pneumoniae	Staphylococcus aureus
Streptococcus agalactiae (GBS)	Streptococcus pyogenes	Streptococcus pneumoniae
Streptococcus pneumoniae		Streptococcus pyogenes
Viral		
Adenovirus	Adenovirus	Adenovirus
Coronaviruses	Coronaviruses	Coronaviruses
Human metapneumovirus	Human metapneumovirus	Influenza A and B
Influenza A and B	Influenza A and B	
Parainfluenza viruses 1, 2, 3	Parainfluenza viruses 1, 2, 3	
Rhinovirus	Rhinovirus	
RSV	RSV	

GBS, Group B streptococcus; *RSV,* respiratory syncytial virus.

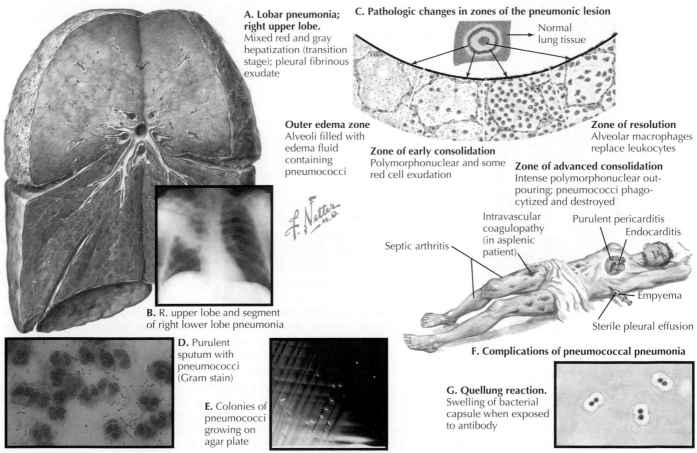

A. Lobar pneumonia; right upper lobe.
Mixed red and gray hepatization (transition stage); pleural fibrinous exudate

B. R. upper lobe and segment of right lower lobe pneumonia

C. Pathologic changes in zones of the pneumonic lesion

Normal lung tissue

Outer edema zone
Alveoli filled with edema fluid containing pneumococci

Zone of early consolidation
Polymorphonuclear and some red cell exudation

Zone of resolution
Alveolar macrophages replace leukocytes

Zone of advanced consolidation
Intense polymorphonuclear outpouring; pneumococci phagocytized and destroyed

D. Purulent sputum with pneumococci (Gram stain)

E. Colonies of pneumococci growing on agar plate

Septic arthritis
Intravascular coagulopathy (in asplenic patient)
Purulent pericarditis
Endocarditis
Empyema
Sterile pleural effusion

F. Complications of pneumococcal pneumonia

G. Quellung reaction.
Swelling of bacterial capsule when exposed to antibody

Fig. 135.1 Streptococcal Pneumonia.

Bronchiolar epithelial cell necrosis, ciliary disruption, and peribronchiolar lymphocytic infiltration are the earliest lesions. Edema of the small airways and mucus secretion mixed with denuded epithelial cells causes obstruction and narrowing of the airways (Fig. 135.3). Atelectasis can cause hypoxemia by ventilation-perfusion mismatch. Dynamic collapse of the airways during exhalation can lead to air trapping and hyperinflation. With severe obstructive lung disease and respiratory muscle fatigue, hypercapnia can develop. Infants with BPD have alveolar simplification and thus decreased small airways diameter because of reduced elastic recoil. Because airflow resistance is inversely

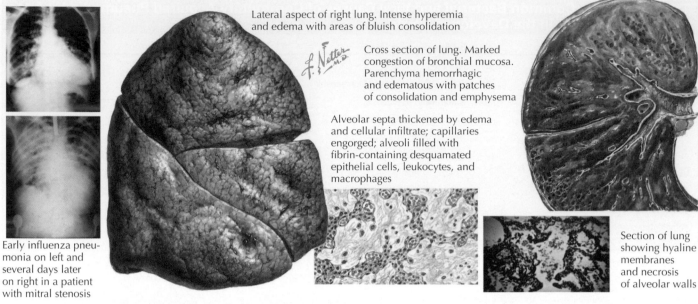

Lateral aspect of right lung. Intense hyperemia and edema with areas of bluish consolidation

Cross section of lung. Marked congestion of bronchial mucosa. Parenchyma hemorrhagic and edematous with patches of consolidation and emphysema

Alveolar septa thickened by edema and cellular infiltrate; capillaries engorged; alveoli filled with fibrin-containing desquamated epithelial cells, leukocytes, and macrophages

Early influenza pneumonia on left and several days later on right in a patient with mitral stenosis

Section of lung showing hyaline membranes and necrosis of alveolar walls

Fig. 135.2 Influenza Pneumonia.

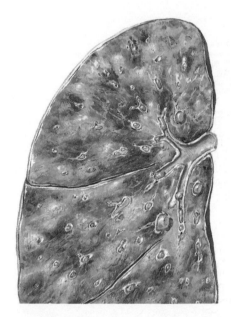

Small airways are partially or completely obstructed by edema, mucous secretions, denuded epithelial cells, and inflammatory infiltrates. These pathologic changes can lead to regional or diffuse air trapping, and nonuniform alveolar ventilation

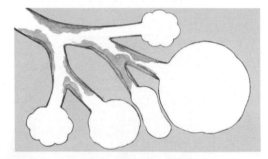

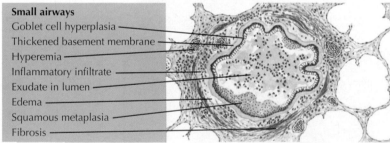

Small airways
Goblet cell hyperplasia
Thickened basement membrane
Hyperemia
Inflammatory infiltrate
Exudate in lumen
Edema
Squamous metaplasia
Fibrosis

Fig. 135.3 Bronchiolitis Pathogenesis.

related to the radius of the airway to the fourth power, airflow in infants with BPD can be compromised with minimal reduction in the bronchiolar lumen.

CLINICAL PRESENTATION

Children with LRTIs classically present with fever, cough, and tachypnea. The spectrum of illness is broad and ranges from mild, well-appearing children to those who require intubation and intensive care. The clinical manifestations of CAP are equally diverse, and few physical examination findings allow for distinction among viral, bacterial, and atypical causes. The differential diagnosis of pneumonia includes pulmonary anatomic abnormalities, foreign bodies, chemical irritants, autoimmune diseases, and malignancies.

Combinations of multiple physical examination findings, such as tachypnea, crackles, and increased respiratory effort, raise the specificity for a clinical diagnosis of pneumonia. Children with pneumonia may also have vomiting or abdominal pain. Abdominal pain occurs most commonly in patients with basilar pneumonia. Wheezing and exacerbation of underlying asthma are symptoms more typically encountered in patients with CAP caused by viruses and atypical bacteria (*M. pneumoniae* or *Chlamydophila pneumoniae*). Children with LRTIs caused by atypical bacteria often have mild and nonspecific symptoms such as headache, low-grade fever, pharyngitis, and cough for 5 to 7 days before their presentation with pneumonia.

Children with bacterial tracheitis present with barking cough, stridor, high fever, and respiratory distress that yields an overall "toxic" appearance. Patients can develop life-threatening, fulminant respiratory failure as a result of airway inflammation and obstruction from accumulation of mucopurulent secretions causing complete airway obstruction.

In RSV-induced bronchiolitis, non-specific upper respiratory tract symptoms (rhinorrhea and mild cough) begin about 3 to 5 days after viral exposure. The progression to the lower respiratory tract is

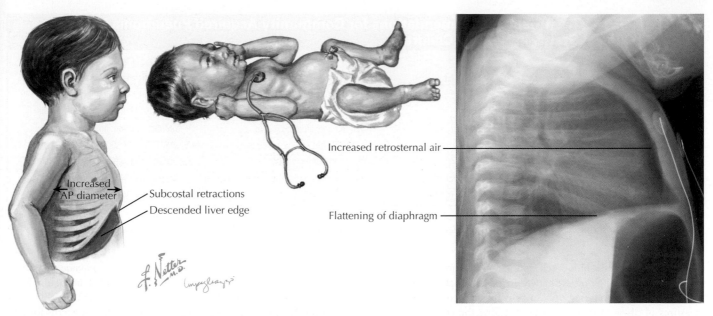

Fig. 135.4 Clinical Evaluation of Wheezing and Bronchiolitis.

characterized by the presence of tachypnea, hypoxemia, nasal flaring, and intercostal or subcostal retractions. Significant hypoxemia, grunting, and marked use of accessory muscles are signs of severe disease and impending respiratory failure (Fig. 135.4). Central apnea also can be an early manifestation of RSV infection, particularly in those with a history of prematurity.

Viral bronchiolitis is associated with obstruction of the intrathoracic small airways; thus the presence of expiratory heterophonous wheezing is a common but nonspecific sign. Wheezing in infants can be better appreciated on pulmonary auscultation when elicited by gentle chest compression (so-called "squeeze the wheeze") to induce forced expiratory flow. A marked reduction in amplitude of breathing sounds suggests very severe disease. Auscultation in bronchiolitis may also reveal inspiratory crackles as small airways reopen and prolongation of the expiratory phase. The other cardinal feature of small airway obstruction is pulmonary hyperinflation. Hyperinflation leads to an increase in anteroposterior diameter of the chest wall, the presence of subcostal retractions, and palpation of a normal-sized liver below the costal margin.

EVALUATION

Radiology

Chest radiographs are not necessary for diagnosis of a LRTI in a well-appearing patient in the outpatient setting. In the case of respiratory distress, hypoxemia, failed outpatient antibiotic management, or a patient requiring hospitalization, a chest radiograph should be obtained. A lobar pneumonia is typically seen with bacterial pneumonia. Interstitial infiltrates are more frequently seen with viral and atypical bacterial pathogens. Hilar lymphadenopathy and nodular disease suggest infection with *M. tuberculosis, Pneumocystis jiroveci,* and endemic mycoses such as *Histoplasma, Coccidioides,* or *Blastomyces* species. Pneumatoceles are air-filled cavities that can be visualized on chest radiography caused by alveolar rupture especially in *S. aureus* pneumonia. More detailed imaging with chest computed tomography (CT) should be sought if an underlying pulmonary malformation is being considered. Because follow-up chest radiograph results can remain abnormal long after complete clinical recovery, they are generally unwarranted in patients with uncomplicated recoveries.

The diagnosis of bronchiolitis is clinical but can be supported by radiographic imaging findings such as hyperinflation, increased peribronchial markings, and patchy subsegmental atelectasis. The absence of cystic lesions, pleural effusions, and focal densities suggestive of bacterial infection can be helpful diagnostically.

Microbiology

Rapid viral detection tests (i.e., immunofluorescence or polymerase chain reaction [PCR]) may be useful in the case of an LRTI, particularly if there is diagnostic uncertainty or for epidemiologic purposes. For example, a positive influenza test may decrease the need for additional diagnostic studies and antibiotic use.

A bacterial etiologic diagnosis is seldom made in cases of childhood CAP because invasive diagnostic procedures such as a direct lung specimen or a bronchoalveolar lavage would be required. Sputum cultures may be sent for culture in older children or in those with an artificial airway. Nasopharyngeal aspirates can provide good samples on which to perform PCR testing for both viral and bacterial CAP causes. PCR from a nasopharyngeal aspirate is the diagnostic method of choice for *Bordetella pertussis* and *M. pneumoniae. C. trachomatis* (in neonates) and *C. pneumoniae* also can be detected by PCR, although prolonged shedding can occur, causing PCR test results to remain positive after the initial period of active disease.

Tuberculin skin testing and/or a serum interferon-γ release assays should be considered for patients with tuberculosis risk factors, but these methods cannot distinguish latent from active disease. A urine antigen test for *L. pneumophila* can be considered in immunocompromised children and older adolescents. In patients with an appropriate travel history and chest radiography results, *Histoplasma* serology or urine antigen can be considered.

Blood culture results are seldom positive in outpatients with CAP and are therefore not recommended in well-appearing patients without hypoxia. Up to 10% of patients requiring admission may have a positive blood culture, and the rate of positive blood cultures may be even higher in those with pneumonia complicated by empyema. Blood cultures in these patient populations may provide useful microbiologic data, including antibiotic sensitivities. Gram stain and bacterial culture of pleural fluid should always be performed in patients with pneumonia with an associated pleural effusion or empyema that has been

TABLE 135.2   Treatment Recommendations for Community Acquired Pneumonia by Age and Clinical Status in Healthy Children

Age	Outpatient Treatment	Inpatient Treatment	Inpatient Treatment for Complicated Pneumonia[a]
≤3 months	Not recommended	Ampicillin + gentamicin IV[b]	Ampicillin + ceftriaxone IV[b]
3 months to 5 years	*Preferred*: oral amoxicillin	*Preferred*: ampicillin IV	*Preferred*: clindamycin + ceftriaxone IV
	Second line: oral clindamycin or amoxicillin-clavulanate[b]	*Second line*: clindamycin or ceftriaxone IV	*Second line*: vancomycin + ceftriaxone IV (for severe patients)
≥5 years	*Preferred*: oral amoxicillin[b]	*Preferred*: ampicillin IV[b]	*Preferred*: clindamycin + ceftriaxone IV[b]
	Second line: oral clindamycin, amoxicillin-clavulanate, or levofloxacin[b]	*Second line*: clindamycin, ceftriaxone, or levofloxacin IV	*Second line*: vancomycin + ceftriaxone IV (for severe patients)[b]

[a]Complicated pneumonia is defined as the presence of large pleural effusions, an empyema, or necrotizing pneumonia.
[b]Consider adding erythromycin or azithromycin if *Chlamydia trachomatis*, *Bordetella pertussis*, or *Mycoplasma pneumoniae* is suspected.
IV, Intravenous.

drained. Serum white blood cell count and inflammatory markers cannot be used to differentiate between viral and bacterial pneumonia reliably and should be used only to provide supplementary objective measures of disease resolution when tracking the course of a severe pneumonia.

TREATMENT

The decision to provide treatment for an LRTI in the outpatient or inpatient setting depends on the severity of the child's illness. For patients with hypoxemia, respiratory distress, or an inability to maintain hydration, hospitalization is required. Hospital admission should be considered for any patient 3 months of age or younger with pneumonia. Many patients with bacterial tracheitis will require emergent intubation for airway protection. For a child hospitalized with bronchiolitis, supportive care is the mainstay of therapy and involves appropriate fluid replacement and use of supplemental oxygen when necessary. Severe cases of bronchiolitis may require mechanical ventilatory support. Data do not support the routine use of nebulized hypertonic saline, racemic epinephrine, or albuterol. Monthly administration of monoclonal anti–F antibody (palivizumab) throughout the RSV season has become standard of care for infants at high risk for severe respiratory illness.

Because it is extremely difficult to distinguish between viral and bacterial pneumonia clinically, it is reasonable to provide empiric antimicrobial therapy to outpatients with a clinical diagnosis of CAP. Amoxicillin remains the initial drug of choice for outpatient pediatric pneumonia (Table 135.2). High-dose amoxicillin (80 to 90 mg/kg/day divided into two doses) or ampicillin (200 mg/kg/day divided into four doses) should have efficacy against resistant *S. pneumoniae*, whose resistance is mediated by alterations in penicillin-binding proteins and can be overcome at higher drug concentrations. Clindamycin is an appropriate alternative treatment in patients with penicillin allergies given its excellent pneumococcal coverage. Macrolides also can be considered but are not as effective as the aminopenicillins, and there is increasing macrolide resistance among pneumococcal strains. Levofloxacin is a fluoroquinolone effective against most resistant pneumococcal strains and has a broad-spectrum range of activity (including atypical

pathogens such as *Legionella* species and *M. pneumoniae*); it can be used in patients with multiple antibiotic allergies. Fluoroquinolones are not approved by the US Food and Drug Administration (FDA) for children 18 years of age or younger based on safety concerns for tendon rupture, but data support its safety in children.

The incidence of community-acquired methicillin-resistant *Staphylococcus aureus* (CA-MRSA) has increased in recent years and is a cause of severe, necrotizing pneumonia. Although local patterns vary, CA-MRSA is typically susceptible to clindamycin. Therefore clindamycin should be used in severe or necrotizing pneumonia in hospitalized patients unless local clindamycin resistance is high. In such cases, vancomycin or trimethoprim-sulfamethoxazole can be used. The duration of uncomplicated CAP treatment is typically 7 days but will be longer in patients with complicated courses.

Patients with persistent symptoms or failure to improve after 48 hours on appropriate empiric therapy should have chest radiography performed or repeated, partly to detect a new or evolving pleural effusion or empyema. Although some simple parapneumonic effusions require no intervention, large effusions or an empyema may require drainage to expedite recovery. Patients who fail treatment with oral amoxicillin and do not have an effusion, may receive inpatient treatment with ampicillin, with or without a macrolide. Those admitted to the hospital with an empyema or necrotizing pneumonia should receive broad-spectrum antibiotics that provide coverage against highly resistant *S. pneumoniae* (typically a third-generation cephalosporin) and MRSA isolates.

FUTURE DIRECTIONS

Prospective study is needed to identify the most appropriate duration of antibiotics for CAP and to identify new treatments for bronchiolitis. Little is known about the long-term pulmonary sequelae and residual lung function of those who have recovered from severe pneumonia.

SUGGESTED READINGS

Available online.

SECTION XX

Rheumatology

Pamela F. Weiss

136

Chronic Arthritis

Jessica Perfetto and Pamela F. Weiss

Juvenile idiopathic arthritis (JIA) is the most common rheumatologic disease among children. The term JIA describes a clinically heterogeneous group of diseases characterized by arthritis that begins before age 16 years, involves one or more joints, and lasts at least 6 weeks. Prevalence estimates for JIA range from 7 to 150 per 100,000; specific epidemiologic characteristics vary by JIA subtype.

ETIOLOGY AND PATHOGENESIS

Similar to many chronic illnesses, JIA is likely caused by genetic and environmental factors. Although discussion of the full extent of genetic associations identified to date is beyond the scope of this chapter, human leukocyte antigen (HLA) associations exist for each of the JIA subtypes, with the greatest number for oligoarticular disease. In addition to subtyping, these associations also play a role in determining disease course and clinical outcome. Among patients with enthesitis-related arthritis, the presence of HLA-B27 may contribute to disease pathogenesis. Non-HLA candidate genes, including *PTPN22, MIF, SLC11A6, WISP3, CTLA4,* and *TNFA,* have been independently confirmed to be associated with various JIA subtypes. Additionally, the presence of autoantibodies such as antinuclear antibody (ANA, found in about 40% of patients, with the highest positivity among patients with oligoarticular JIA) and rheumatoid factor (RF, present in approximately 5% to 10%) gives evidence for immune dysfunction in JIA. The presence of multilineage cells and associated cytokines in the synovium indicate involvement of all levels of the immune system in disease pathogenesis, including innate immunity (by inflammatory cells and cytokines), cell-mediated immunity (by activated T-lymphocytes), and humoral immunity (by autoantibodies).

CLINICAL PRESENTATION

The diagnosis of JIA is made from a detailed history, comprehensive physical examination, directed laboratory tests and imaging, and following the child over time. Distinct clinical features characterize each of the JIA subtypes during the first 6 months of disease. In all subtypes arthritis frequently manifests as pain and stiffness that is often worse in the morning and after prolonged inactivity ("gelling"). Stiffness and pain are often relieved by physical activity. Swelling is present in at least one or more joints for at least 6 weeks and is typically not episodic. Up to 25% of children have painless arthritis.

Oligoarticular Juvenile Idiopathic Arthritis

Oligoarticular JIA is defined by arthritis in four or fewer joints during the first 6 months of disease. Oligoarticular JIA is the most common form of JIA, typically occurs before age 4 years, and affects girls more often than boys at a ratio of 4:1. The knee is the most commonly affected joint followed by the ankles and small joints of the hand (Fig. 136.1). The temporomandibular joint (TMJ) is also commonly affected. Persistent oligoarthritis affects a maximum of four joints throughout the disease course, and extended oligoarthritis affects more than four joints after the first 6 months of disease. Extended disease is associated with a worse prognosis.

Although children with oligoarticular JIA have the greatest likelihood of remission among the JIA subtypes, complications can cause long-lasting morbidities. Asymmetric joint disease (particularly at the knee) can lead to leg length discrepancy caused by hyperemia from inflammation, leading to accelerated growth in the affected limb. Children with swollen and painful joints may hold them in a flexed guarding position to avoid active extension, which leads to weakening and shortening of the surrounding muscles, tendons, and ligaments. This can cause flexion contractures, or lack of passive extension range of motion of the affected joint. Severe disease of the TMJ can lead to difficulty chewing, malocclusion, or micrognathia (Fig. 136.2). Asymptomatic anterior uveitis is common in oligoarthritis, particularly among young girls who are ANA positive, and must be screened for at disease presentation and serially thereafter. Complications of uveitis include visual impairment, posterior synechiae, cataracts, band keratopathy, and glaucoma (Fig. 136.3).

Polyarticular Juvenile Idiopathic Arthritis

Polyarticular JIA, defined by arthritis in five or more joints during the first 6 months of disease, is the second most frequent subtype of JIA. It is divided into two subtypes: RF-negative and RF-positive disease. Seronegative disease affects girls more frequently than boys. Seropositive patients are often adolescent girls who experience an insidious disease onset involving primarily the large and small joints of

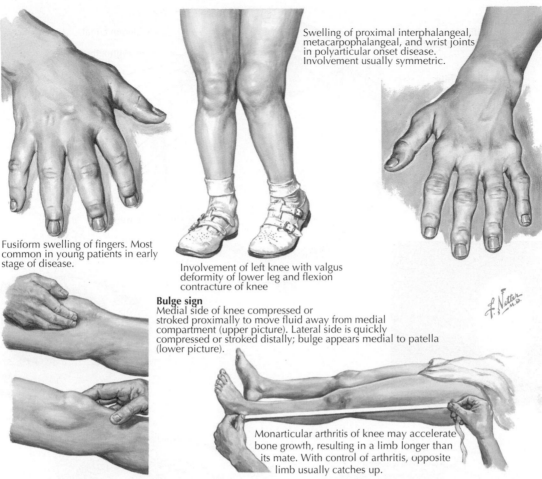

Swelling of proximal interphalangeal, metacarpophalangeal, and wrist joints in polyarticular onset disease. Involvement usually symmetric.

Fusiform swelling of fingers. Most common in young patients in early stage of disease.

Involvement of left knee with valgus deformity of lower leg and flexion contracture of knee

Bulge sign
Medial side of knee compressed or stroked proximally to move fluid away from medial compartment (upper picture). Lateral side is quickly compressed or stroked distally; bulge appears medial to patella (lower picture).

Monarticular arthritis of knee may accelerate bone growth, resulting in a limb longer than its mate. With control of arthritis, opposite limb usually catches up.

Fig. 136.1 Joint Involvement in Juvenile Arthritis.

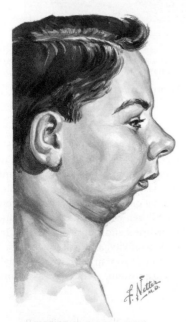

Receding chin results from early closure of mandibular ossification centers in progressive disease

Fig. 136.2 Micrognathia Due to Severe Disease of the TMJ.

the hands and feet, the cervical spine, and TMJ. Rheumatoid nodules, boutonniere deformities (proximal interphalangeal [PIP] joint flexion and distal interphalangeal [DIP] joint hyperextension), and swan-neck deformities (PIP joint hyperextension and DIP joint flexion) are frequently seen in seropositive patients, whose disease process most closely mimics that of adult rheumatoid arthritis. Systemic symptoms are uncommon.

Systemic Juvenile Idiopathic Arthritis

Systemic JIA is defined by arthritis; fever for at least 2 weeks with high quotidian spikes for at least 3 days and at least one of the following: evanescent and erythematous rash, generalized lymphadenopathy, hepatosplenomegaly, and serositis (often pericarditis or pleuritis). The disease affects boys and girls equally and can occur at any age but most commonly in early childhood. The fever does not always follow the classic quotidian pattern, particularly early in the disease. Children often appear ill during fevers and well when afebrile. Arthritis is generally symmetric and polyarticular but may be absent at onset. The rash consists of discrete, salmon-pink macules that are more pronounced during fever and may be associated with the Koebner phenomenon (linear streaks on the skin elicited by scratching) (Fig. 136.4).

Complications of systemic JIA include macrophage activation syndrome (MAS), systemic amyloidosis, infections caused by

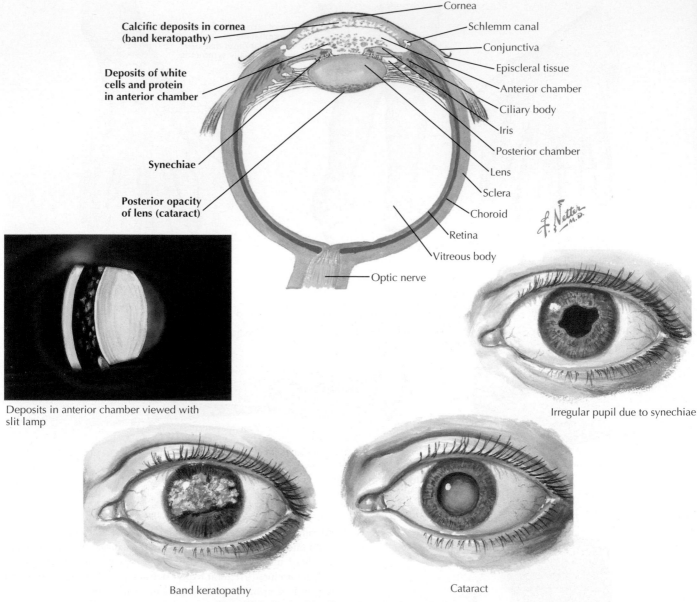

Fig. 136.3 Ocular Manifestations in Juvenile Arthritis.

immunosuppression, and the effects of chronic corticosteroids. Approximately 5% to 8% of children with systemic JIA develop MAS. This life-threatening complication is characterized by acute onset of sustained fever, hepatosplenomegaly, and lymphadenopathy. Associated laboratory abnormalities may include pancytopenia, elevated fibrin split products, transaminitis, hypertriglyceridemia, hyperferritinemia, *low* erythrocyte sedimentation rate (ESR), and elevated coagulation factors. Therefore a down-trending ESR in a patient with systemic JIA who is otherwise clinically worsening should prompt concern for MAS. Bone marrow examination reveals active phagocytosis of hematopoietic cells.

Psoriatic Arthritis

Psoriatic arthritis is defined by presence of arthritis and psoriasis, or if the rash is absent, arthritis and at least two of the following: dactylitis,

nail pitting or onycholysis, and psoriasis in a first-degree relative (Fig. 136.5). The arthritis is usually an asymmetric monoarthritis or polyarthritis affecting large and small joints and may develop several years before psoriasis. The disease affects girls slightly more than boys and has a bimodal onset, with peaks in the preschool years and early adolescence. Children with early-onset psoriatic arthritis share features with oligoarthritis and polyarticular JIA, including female predisposition, ANA positivity, and risk for uveitis. Late-onset psoriatic arthritis has more overlap with the spondyloarthropathies, including male predisposition, enthesitis, axial involvement, and HLA-B27 positivity.

Enthesitis-Related Arthritis

Enthesitis-related arthritis (ERA) is distinct from the other subtypes of JIA in that it may involve joints of the peripheral and

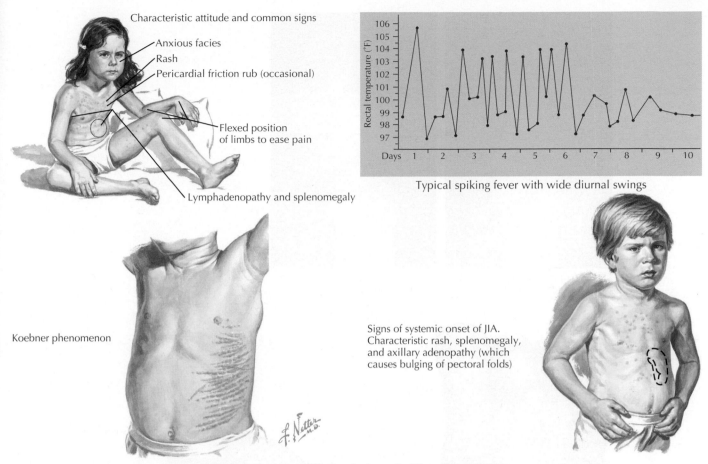

Characteristic attitude and common signs

Anxious facies

Rash

Pericardial friction rub (occasional)

Flexed position of limbs to ease pain

Lymphadenopathy and splenomegaly

Koebner phenomenon

Typical spiking fever with wide diurnal swings

Signs of systemic onset of JIA. Characteristic rash, splenomegaly, and axillary adenopathy (which causes bulging of pectoral folds)

Fig. 136.4 Features of Systemic Juvenile Idiopathic Arthritis.

axial (spine and sacroiliac joint) skeleton, inflammation at the attachments of tendons and ligaments to the bone (enthesitis), is male-predominant, and is associated with symptomatic eye inflammation. This disease spectrum is defined by arthritis and enthesitis *or* either arthritis or enthesitis with at least two of the following: the presence or a history of sacroiliac tenderness or lumbosacral pain; HLA-B27 antigen positivity; onset of arthritis in males after age 6 years; acute anterior uveitis; and a first-degree relative with ankylosing spondylitis, ERA, sacroiliitis with inflammatory bowel disease (IBD), reactive arthritis, or acute anterior uveitis. As with the other JIA subtypes, arthritis manifests as stiffness and pain in the morning that is relieved by activity whereas enthesitis is associated with pain mostly after activity.

On physical examination, enthesitis is identified by tenderness where the tendons insert into the bones. Some common enthesitis sites include the inferior pole of the patella, Achilles tendon insertion, plantar fascia insertion, and sacroiliac joints. Approximately 20% of children with ERA develop arthritis of the sacroiliac joint. Extraarticular manifestations of ERA may include symptomatic anterior uveitis (red, painful, photophobic eye) and gastrointestinal inflammation. Aortic insufficiency, aortitis, muscle weakness, and low-grade fever are rarely reported. ERA also can be the initial manifestation of IBD; extraintestinal manifestations occur in about 17% to 28% of pediatric patients, with these manifestations preceding the diagnosis of IBD in about 6% to 27% of patients (Chapter 57). Thus it is important to think about IBD in a patient with ERA who has gastrointestinal symptoms, growth failure, anemia, erythema nodosum, or recurrent aphthous stomatitis.

Undifferentiated Arthritis

Undifferentiated arthritis includes patients who do not fulfill criteria for any category or who meet criteria for more than one.

DIFFERENTIAL DIAGNOSIS

The differential diagnosis of children with suspected JIA is broad, given the heterogeneity of disease subsets. The most common classes of disorders that must be considered in the differential diagnosis of JIA include other rheumatologic diseases such as sarcoidosis or systemic lupus erythematosus, infection or postinfectious phenomena, malignancies, orthopedic conditions, and other inflammatory arthropathies (Box 136.1). The differential diagnosis of JIA is influenced by whether the presentation is acute, subacute, or chronic; the number of affected joints; and the presence of systemic features.

EVALUATION AND MANAGEMENT

Laboratory Analysis

There are no diagnostic laboratory tests confirmatory for JIA. When evaluating a child with suspected arthritis, a complete blood count with differential, a complete metabolic panel, C-reactive protein (CRP), and

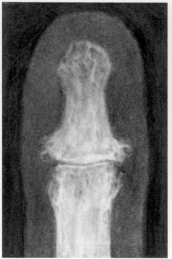

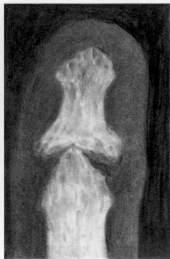

Erosion of cartilage and marginal erosion and osteophytes

Marked erosion joint with "pencil point-in-cup" appearance

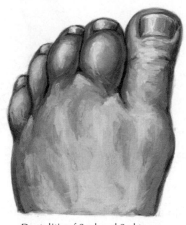

Dactylitis of 2nd and 3rd toes

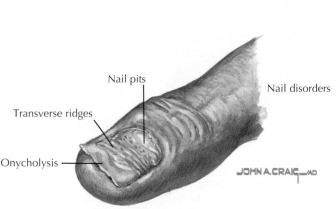

Nail pits

Transverse ridges

Nail disorders

Onycholysis

JOHN A. CRAIG—AD

Fig. 136.5 Psoriatic Juvenile Idiopathic Arthritis.

ESR should be part of the initial evaluation. These tests will document the presence or absence of systemic inflammation, identify hematologic abnormalities that may raise suspicion of malignancy, and detect hypoalbuminemia and/or anemia that may raise suspicion of IBD. In the setting of infection, ESR may continue to increase despite antibiotics, but CRP often rapidly declines with appropriate therapy because of its short half-life. In Lyme disease endemic areas, serologic testing for Lyme disease is recommended in children with oligoarthritis, particularly involving the knee.

Among children with JIA, ANA positivity represents an increased risk for anterior uveitis, earlier age of disease onset, and asymmetric arthritis. ANA can be positive in up to 20% to 30% of the normal population; thus an elevated ANA is *not* diagnostic of JIA. RF is infrequent in JIA; therefore it is not a good screening test for diagnosis. However, RF positivity in polyarticular JIA is associated with erosive synovitis, more aggressive disease, and poorer prognosis and therefore may influence the decision to treat more aggressively. Many children with RF-positive polyarticular JIA also have anti–citrullinated protein antibodies (ACPAs), which also lead to greater risk for aggressive and erosive disease. HLA-B27 is not diagnostic but is associated with risk for axial disease in ERA.

Synovial Fluid Analysis

Synovial fluid analysis and culture should be performed in children with acute joint swelling that is accompanied by fever or for whom the diagnosis is uncertain. In JIA, the synovial fluid is usually yellow and cloudy. Synovial fluid leukocyte counts are elevated (typically between 15,000 and 20,000 cells/mm^3 but can be higher) with neutrophil predominance.

Imaging

Plain radiographs are useful as part of the initial evaluation of arthritis to evaluate for periarticular osteopenia, erosions, fractures, or other bony abnormalities. Radiographic features of JIA include soft tissue swelling, widening or narrowing of the joint space, osteoporosis,

Infectious or Postinfectious
- Viral arthritis (rubella, parvovirus B19, hepatitis B)
- Bacterial infections (Lyme disease, tuberculosis, gonorrhea)
- Toxic synovitis
- Rheumatic fever
- Poststreptococcal arthritis
- Serum sickness
- Osteomyelitis

Oncologic
- Leukemia
- Osteosarcoma
- Ewing sarcoma
- Metastatic neuroblastoma

Orthopedic
- Legg-Calvé-Perthes disease
- Avascular necrosis from chronic corticosteroids
- Slipped capital femoral epiphysis

Rheumatologic
- Juvenile idiopathic arthritis
- Systemic lupus erythematosus
- Sarcoidosis
- Sjögren syndrome
- Dermatomyositis
- Vasculitis

Other
- Hemarthrosis
- Avascular necrosis
- Cystic fibrosis–associated arthritis
- Foreign body synovitis
- Pigmented villonodular synovitis

erosions, subluxation, or ankylosis. Erosive changes are uncommon before 2 years of active disease. Children with JIA are at risk for atlantoaxial instability, particularly in the setting of active cervical disease. If instability is suspected, flexion and extension films of the cervical spine should be obtained before anesthesia.

Other imaging modalities that may be useful in the evaluation of JIA include ultrasonography, bone scans, and magnetic resonance imaging (MRI). Ultrasonography is a noninvasive and inexpensive method to confirm a joint effusion and guide intraarticular corticosteroid injections. Bone scans are helpful to evaluate for osteomyelitis, malignancy, and joints with subclinical inflammation. MRI is the most sensitive technique to identify synovitis, early erosions, TMJ arthritis, and sacroiliitis.

Clinical Management

Treatment of JIA depends on disease subtype, severity of disease, prior response to therapy, and unique patient circumstances. The treatment goals are to reduce pain and inflammation, prevent permanent joint destruction, avoid comorbidities and medication toxicities, and optimize linear growth, quality of life, and overall function. Recently, a "treat-to-target" approach was recommended in which a treatment target is selected together with caregiver(s) and—when appropriate—the patient, with frequent therapeutic adjustments based on quantitative measures of disease activity aimed to achieve this target, regardless of the medication being used. The primary target for most patients with JIA is clinical remission; in some patients, particularly those with chronic disease, minimal disease activity may be an acceptable alternative target. This is usually achieved by early aggressive therapy with the goal of achieving the target within 6 months. This approach has shown improved long-term clinical outcomes in adult rheumatologic diseases, including systemic lupus erythematosus, rheumatoid arthritis, and gout. All patients with JIA should be routinely screened for uveitis, growth impairment or limb asymmetry, and TMJ involvement.

Pharmacologic Interventions

Nonsteroidal antiinflammatory drugs (NSAIDs), which have both analgesic and antiinflammatory properties, can be used while awaiting rheumatology evaluation or while definitive therapy is being determined; however, is not typically recommended as monotherapy for established disease. Intraarticular corticosteroid injections are often used to control disease locally, particularly in the setting of oligoarthritis. In children with polyarticular disease or oligoarticular disease that requires repeated intraarticular injections, conventional disease-modifying antirheumatic (cDMARD) or biologic DMARD (bDMARDs) agents are used. The most common cDMARDs include methotrexate, leflunomide, and sulfasalazine. Common bDMARDs include etanercept, adalimumab, infliximab, tocilizumab, and abatacept. Short corticosteroid courses can be used to quickly control inflammation until DMARD therapies take full effect; however, long-term use should be avoided. Biologic DMARDs that block interleukin-1 or interleukin-6, with or without systemic corticosteroids, are the mainstay of systemic JIA therapy.

Surgical Management

Orthopedic surgery has a limited role in the management plan for most children with JIA. However, in cases of refractory disease or persistent leg length discrepancy, an experienced orthopedic surgeon can help design an individualized surgical intervention. Possible interventions include arthroscopic synovectomy, soft tissue release, epiphysiodesis (growth plate fusion), total arthroplasty (joint replacement), and arthrodesis (joint fusion).

Physical and Occupational Therapy

Physical and occupational therapy play an important role in helping to maximize musculoskeletal health and function and to treat flexion contractures. Regular exercise programs will not exacerbate the disease and may even reduce disease symptoms. In cases of active joint disease in the upper extremities, occupational therapy can improve the capacity to perform activities of daily living and academic responsibilities.

FUTURE DIRECTIONS

Further research is necessary to correlate genetic variants associated with JIA, presumed genetic susceptibility, and translation of these findings to disease incidence and clinical care of patients. These genetic variants may also play a role in classification of disease; for instance, gene expression profiles differ between children with early (<6 years) and late (≥6 years) presentations, suggesting that age of onset may be a helpful criterion used for classification. In particular, immune checkpoint regulators have the potential to serve as biomarkers of disease activity and as directed therapeutic targets for personalized medicine. In addition, more randomized clinical trials are needed to better understand how advanced therapies used in adults with rheumatologic disease can be safely and effectively used in children with JIA. Finally, head-to-head trials comparing the efficacy and safety of newer and established agents would be beneficial in optimizing therapy and outcomes.

ACKNOWLEDGMENT

The authors would like to acknowledge Julie M. Linton, MD, for her contribution to the previous edition chapter.

SUGGESTED READINGS

Available online.

137

Juvenile Dermatomyositis

Adam S. Mayer and Pamela F. Weiss

 CLINICAL VIGNETTE

A 9-year-old girl is brought by her mother for evaluation of weakness that has been worsening over the past several weeks, most notably with activities such as climbing stairs and combing her hair. On examination, erythematous, scaling plaques on the dorsal surfaces of her metacarpophalangeal joints, as well as a faint violaceous rash over her upper eyelids are noted. When asked to stand, the patient uses the arms of her chair for assistance. Laboratory findings are notable for a moderately elevated creatine kinase and aspartate aminotransferase. The patient is diagnosed with juvenile dermatomyositis and started on a prolonged steroid taper along with weekly methotrexate and daily hydroxychloroquine. On her return visit in a few weeks, the patient's rash has mostly faded and her mother reports improvement in strength with everyday activities.

Juvenile dermatomyositis (JDM) is the most common inflammatory myositis during childhood, characterized by endothelial injury of the small vessels of the muscle, skin, and gastrointestinal tract. It is distinguished from adult-onset dermatomyositis (DM) by its prominent vasculopathic features and lack of association with malignancy.

ETIOLOGY AND PATHOGENESIS

The cause of JDM is unclear; however, roles for genetics, environmental exposures, and infections have been postulated. Certain human leukocyte antigen (HLA) alleles and genetic polymorphisms have been found to either be protective or to place individuals at risk for more severe disease. It has been suggested that infections, particularly viral, may trigger an unusual immune response in a genetically susceptible host. One retrospective study showed that between one-third and one-half of children diagnosed with JDM had a preceding infection, particularly a respiratory illness.

CLINICAL PRESENTATION

JDM is a rare inflammatory myopathy with an incidence of 2 to 4 cases per million per year. The peak incidence is in children 5 to 10 years of age. It is more common in girls than in boys, with reported ratios ranging between 2:1 and 5:1. There is no racial predominance in terms of diagnosis, but certain clinical features may predominate in different populations as described in the following sections.

Musculoskeletal Features

Classic JDM is manifested by symmetric, proximal muscle weakness, including muscles in the neck, shoulders, core, and hip flexors. Affected children may report problems with brushing or washing their hair, climbing stairs, and standing from a seated position (Gower sign). Dysphonia and dysphagia may be present because of weakness of the palate, cricopharyngeal muscles, and upper esophagus. Over time, joint contractures can develop as a result of muscle shortening and/or uncontrolled arthritis. Muscle tenderness also may be a prominent feature.

Amyopathic JDM is a subset characterized by predominant cutaneous features without apparent musculoskeletal involvement; however, subclinical myositis can often be detected in these cases through careful examination or magnetic resonance imaging (MRI).

Cutaneous Features

Dermatomyositis has several classic cutaneous findings (Fig. 137.1). Gottron papules are erythematous, raised, scaling plaques on the extensor surfaces of the knuckles, elbows, and knees that are present in over 90% of children at the time of diagnosis. The heliotrope rash is a violaceous discoloration of the eyelids often with associated edema; this is present in approximately 80% of children at diagnosis. About 40% of children also can have an erythematous malar or other facial rash. This rash can be ulcerative, cross the nasolabial folds (distinguishing it from the malar rash of systemic lupus erythematosus [SLE]), and extend onto the forehead. Patients can similarly develop erythematous, macular rashes in photodistributed areas such as the posterior neck and shoulders ("shawl sign") or the anterior neck and chest ("V sign"). Raynaud's phenomenon and associated nailfold capillary changes (proximal nailfold erythema, capillary dilatation, tortuosity, or dropout) are seen in up to 80% of patients. Skin ulceration reflects significant vasculopathy of the skin and may be a sign of internal organ vasculopathy. These lesions are associated with more severe disease and worse prognosis. Lipodystrophy is often underappreciated and can be associated with insulin resistance and dyslipidemia.

Calcinosis, or calcium deposition in the skin and subcutaneous tissues, can occur within a few years of diagnosis. These lesions can be painful and lead to significant morbidity and functional limitation. Risk factors for the development of calcinosis include delayed diagnosis or treatment, chronic disease course, tumor necrosis factor-α (TNF-α)-308a genotype, anti-p140 myositis antibody, age younger than 5 years at the time of diagnosis, and African descent. Calcinosis may regress after disease remission and there are no known efficacious targeted treatments.

Other less common skin manifestations associated with JDM are "mechanic's hands" (thickening of the margins of the palms and radial surfaces of the hands) and "inverse Gottron papules." These papules are similar to the traditional Gottron papules, but can be found on the palmar aspect of the hand, frequently overlying the ventral surface of the proximal or distal interphalangeal joints. Their presence has been largely associated with anti-MDA5 antibody positivity and an increased risk for pulmonary disease.

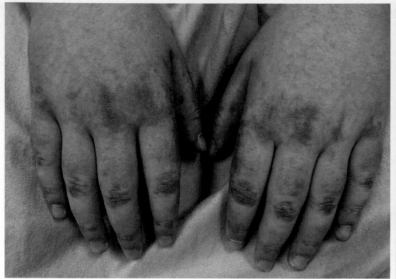

A. Gottron papules on extensor surfaces of phalangeal joints

B. Gottron papules on extensor surfaces of elbow

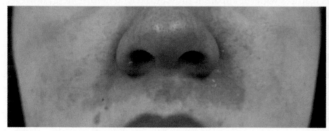

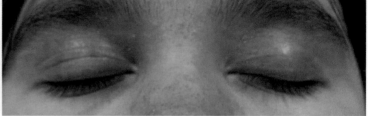

C. Malar rash crossing the nasolabial folds

D. Heliotrope rash

Fig. 137.1 Common Cutaneous Findings in Juvenile Dermatomyositis.

Other Disease Manifestations

Pulmonary involvement is less common in children than in adults. Despite this, interstitial lung disease (ILD) has been an increasingly recognized comorbidity of JDM, particularly in patients who are anti–aminoacyl tRNA synthetase antibody (anti-ARS) or anti–MDA5 antibody positive. Patients with anti-ARS antibodies are often found to have antisynthetase syndrome, which includes features of myositis, arthritis, ILD, Raynaud's phenomenon, and mechanic's hands. The ILD associated with anti-MDA5 positivity can be rapidly progressive, especially in patients of East Asian background. Gastrointestinal vasculopathy is also a rare but potentially life-threatening complication.

DIFFERENTIAL DIAGNOSIS

The diagnosis of JDM is primarily clinical, characterized by the presence of proximal muscle weakness and associated cutaneous findings, along with supportive laboratory, imaging, and occasionally more invasive studies. The 2017 European League Against Rheumatism/American College of Rheumatology (EULAR/ACR) classification criteria for JDM provide a standardized approach to diagnosis. Patients are classified as having true JDM if they meet "probable" criteria and have any characteristic cutaneous manifestation.

Although the diagnosis of JDM may seem straightforward, the common rashes of JDM can mimic other diseases. Gottron papules can be mistaken for psoriasis, eczema or seborrheic dermatitis. SLE, pityriasis rubra pilaris, sunburn, and other sun-induced eruptions may also mimic the photosensitive rashes of JDM. Nailfold capillary changes and Raynaud's phenomenon can be seen with systemic sclerosis, mixed connective tissue disease (MCTD), and SLE.

In the absence of cutaneous manifestations, JDM can be difficult to distinguish from other causes of proximal muscle weakness. Polymyositis manifests with similar proximal muscle weakness but lacks the cutaneous manifestations. Myositis can also be a manifestation of viral infections (e.g. influenza) or other connective tissue diseases such as SLE, scleroderma, and MCTD. Metabolic myopathies and genetic muscular dystrophies tend to have muscle pain and cramps primarily with exercise and may also have affected distal muscles. Lesions of the nervous system also may manifest with muscle weakness.

EVALUATION AND MANAGEMENT

When considering a diagnosis of JDM, the following muscle enzymes should be measured: alanine aminotransferase (ALT), aspartate aminotransferase (AST), lactate dehydrogenase (LDH), aldolase and creatine kinase (CK). All five enzymes should be checked because it is common for only a few to be elevated. CK levels are typically the first to increase but also the first to normalize; if CK levels are very high, then alternative diagnoses, such as rhabdomyolysis and muscular dystrophy, should be considered. ANA titers should be sent to evaluate for JDM mimickers, such as SLE and MCTD. Tests for myositis-specific and myositis-associated antibodies should be ordered at the time of diagnosis because they may help predict the clinical course and direct therapy (Table 137.1). EMG and muscle biopsy are invasive diagnostic procedures reserved for the cases that are diagnostic dilemmas. A swallowing study should be performed if dysphagia or neck flexor weakness is present. If weakness is absent on examination and/or muscle enzymes are normal, MRI and ultrasonography are methods to detect subclinical myositis.

TABLE 137.1 Myositis-Specific and Myositis-Associated Autoantibodies in Juvenile Dermatomyositis and Their Associations[a]

Autoantibody	Biologic Target	Prevalence (%)	Clinical Associations
Myositis-Specific Antibodies			
Anti–Mi-2	Nucleosome Remodeling Deacetylase complex	3–4	"Classic" JDM, favorable prognosis with good response to standard treatment
Anti-p140 (MJ)	Nuclear matrix protein 2	15–22	More severe musculoskeletal and gastrointestinal involvement Calcinosis Joint contractures
Anti-synthetases (e.g., anti-Jo-1)	Various aminoacyl t-RNA synthetase subgroups	1–3	Antisynthetase syndrome, increased mortality
Anti-SRP	Signal recognition peptide	1–3	Severe, refractory disease; proximal and distal weakness
Anti-HMGCR	HMG-CoA reductase	1	More severe, refractory muscular disease with less cutaneous involvement Necrotizing autoimmune myositis
Myositis-Associated Antibodies			
Anti-TIFγ (p155/140)	Transcriptional intermediary factor 1-γ	18–35	Severe cutaneous involvement, chronic disease course
Anti-MDA5	Melanoma differentiation-associated gene 5	6%	ILD, skin and oral ulcerations, arthritis, mild muscle disease

[a]MSAs are only seen in dermatomyositis whereas MAAs can be seen in other conditions, such as connective tissue disease.

HMG-CoA, β-Hydroxy β-methylglutaryl coenzyme A; *ILD,* interstitial lung disease.

Adapted from Pachman L, Khojah A. Advances in juvenile dermatomyositis: Myositis specific antibodies aid in understanding disease heterogeneity. *J Pediatr.* 2018;195:16-27. Table 1, pp. 22-23.

Treatment with systemic corticosteroids is the mainstay of early therapy. Typically, corticosteroids are started at high doses and weaned slowly over several months. Steroid-sparing agents, such as methotrexate, are typically initiated at the time of diagnosis. Intravenous immunoglobulin (IVIG) is particularly helpful for severe myositis or ulcerative skin lesions. Hydroxychloroquine is often helpful in overall disease control and photosensitive rashes. Cyclophosphamide is reserved for patients with severe, life- or organ-threatening disease.

Studies have begun assessing the role of biologics in JDM. The RIM trial (2013), a study evaluating rituximab (an anti–B cell biologic therapy) in both adult and pediatric DM patients, did not meet its primary or secondary endpoints, but did show a positive steroid-sparing effect. A follow-up study in 2017 showed improved cutaneous disease scores with the use of rituximab in both adult and juvenile DM. Several case reports and a phase II trial have demonstrated the efficacy of abatacept for refractory myositis and JDM-associated calcinosis.

Adjunctive therapies play a major role in the treatment of JDM as well. Sunscreen use and the avoidance of direct sun exposure is critical because ultraviolet light can trigger JDM flares. Calcium and vitamin D supplementation are advised given the increased risk for osteoporosis with prolonged corticosteroid use. Early participation in occupational and physical therapy is helpful for maintaining functional status and adapting to new limitations. Behavioral health therapy can be crucial for coping with symptoms and psychosocial challenges associated with the disease.

Serial examination of muscle strength, the skin, nailfold capillaries, and muscle enzymes are used to gauge response to medication and maintenance of remission. The Childhood Myositis Assessment Score (CMAS) provides an objective approach to testing muscle strength and endurance, and also can be trended over time as a correlate of disease activity.

FUTURE DIRECTIONS

As our understanding of autoantibodies and genomics continues to expand, we can begin developing individualized disease profiles for patients that can better predict their clinical presentation and optimal treatment regimen. Additionally, the continued study of newer biologic therapies will provide more robust data on the safety and efficacy of these steroid-sparing regimens for the various JDM clinical phenotypes.

ACKNOWLEDGMENT

The authors would like to acknowledge Naomi Brown, MD, for her contribution on the previous edition chapter.

SUGGESTED READINGS

Available online.

138

Vasculitis and Vasculopathy

Roberto Alejandro Valdovinos and Pamela F. Weiss

✳ CLINICAL VIGNETTE

A 12-year-old boy presented to the hospital after 2 days of persistent fevers, emesis, and significant abdominal pain. He was in good health before the onset of his fevers, and he did not recall any sick contacts. Over the past 2 days, he also noticed a rash that "came and went," and complained of headache and red eyes. His vital signs were significant for a blood pressure of 70/40 mm Hg, pulse of 140 beats/min, and a temperature of 104°F (40°C), and on examination he was encephalopathic, with bilateral, limbic-sparing conjunctivitis, cracked lips, edematous hands and feet, and a maculopapular rash over his chest. Laboratory tests revealed severe coagulopathy with elevated D-dimer and fibrinogen, hyponatremia, lymphopenia, drastically elevated inflammatory markers, pancytopenia with burr cells on peripheral smear, and evidence of cardiac dysfunction with elevated troponins and brain natriuretic peptide. An echocardiogram revealed left ventricular dysfunction, and he had a negative SARS-CoV-2 polymerase chain reaction with positive SARS-CoV-2 antibodies, consistent with a diagnosis of multisystem inflammatory syndrome in children. The patient required fluid resuscitation and vasopressors for blood pressure support and was treated with intravenous immunoglobulin 2 g/kg and intravenous corticosteroids (2 mg/kg/day). He rapidly recovered with immunomodulatory therapy, and echocardiogram before discharge revealed near-normal left ventricular function, for which he had outpatient cardiology follow-up.

Vasculitis and vasculopathy are distinct entities with differing pathophysiologies that inform presentation, diagnosis, and treatment. Vasculitis refers to inflammation of the blood vessel wall itself by immune cell infiltration, whereas vasculopathy describes the process by which injury originating outside a vessel's wall leads to compromised blood flow. Fibromuscular dysplasia is a key example of vasculopathy, characterized by a "string-of-beads" on angiography, and thought to be reactive hyperplasia and fibrosis secondary to repeated "pulsation-induced mechanical trauma." Multisystem inflammatory syndrome in children (MIS-C), a relatively new entity, is also thought to be an example of vasculopathy. Vasculitis can occur as a primary process, as in Behçet disease, or may be secondary to another process, such as systemic lupus erythematosus (Chapter 139). Overall, the primary childhood vasculitides are rare disorders, and the prevalence of diseases may be different based on the population studied. The incidence of vasculitis in patients younger than 17 years ranges from 12 to 53 cases per 100,000 children.

This chapter focuses on the primary vasculitides and a novel vasculopathy. A general overview is presented followed by a more detailed discussion of immunoglobulin A (IgA) vasculitis (IgAV; formerly Henoch-Schönlein purpura), Kawasaki disease (KD), and MIS-C.

ETIOLOGY AND PATHOGENESIS

The underlying cause of vasculitis has yet to be elucidated; however, like many chronic diseases, there is likely a complex interplay of genetic and environmental factors. Some theories suggest that the inflammation is attributable to the involvement of humoral factors, as seen in the antineutrophil cytoplasmic antibodies (ANCA)–associated vasculitides. Others suggest abnormal regulation of immune complex formation is contributory, as in IgAV. Lymphocyte involvement also has been implicated, specifically T-regulatory cell dysfunction. Additionally, antecedent infections, particularly streptococcal infections, have been suggested as a cause in many of the vasculitides such as IgAV, granulomatosis with polyangiitis (GPA), and polyarteritis nodosa (PAN).

Classification

Vasculitis can be classified based on the involvement of primarily large, medium, or small vessels (Fig. 138.1). In addition, certain vasculitides have a predilection for arteries, veins, or both. The vasculitides can be further classified histologically as granulomatous or nongranulomatous. The granulomatous diseases include Takayasu arteritis, GPA, and eosinophilic granulomatosis with polyangiitis (Chapter 140). The nongranulomatous vasculitides include PAN, KD, microscopic polyangiitis (MPA), IgAV, cutaneous leukocytoclastic vasculitis, and cryoglobulinemic vasculitis.

CLINICAL PRESENTATION

Vasculitis often manifests with vague symptoms and multiorgan involvement. Nonspecific systemic features may include prolonged fever without a clear source, unexplained hypertension, fatigue, malaise, weight loss, and rash. Therefore the diagnosis is often delayed and requires a high index of suspicion. Definitive diagnosis often relies on imaging (angiography) and tissue biopsy. The history should include questions about recent infections, medication exposures, and a detailed family history.

Certain patterns of clinical symptoms and organ involvement may be suggestive of a specific vasculitis. For example, whereas palpable purpura, arthralgias, abdominal pain, and renal disease suggest IgAV (Box 138.1); persistent fever, conjunctivitis, cervical lymphadenopathy, extremity swelling, mucocutaneous changes, and rash suggest KD. Microscopic polyangiitis is associated with high titers of protoplasmic-staining antineutrophil cytoplasmic antibodies (pANCAs) and typically manifests as pulmonary capillaritis and necrotizing glomerulonephritis. Hypersensitivity vasculitis is a necrotizing vasculitis that manifests with a papular rash that may be red or blistering and is often associated with infection or medication exposure. Hypocomplementemic

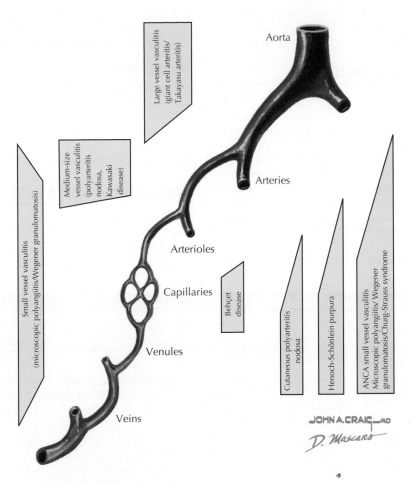

Fig. 138.1 Distribution of Specific Vasculitis Syndromes.

BOX 138.1 European League Against Rheumatism/Paediatric Rheumatology International Trials Organisation/Paediatric Rheumatology European Society Classification Criteria for Immunoglobulin A Vasculitis

Must have purpura or petechiae with lower limb predominance and *at least one* of the following:

- Acute-onset, diffuse abdominal pain
- Acute-onset arthritis or arthralgia
- Hematuria or proteinuria
- Leukocytoclastic vasculitis or proliferative glomerulonephritis on histology with predominant immunoglobulin A deposition

---

urticarial vasculitis manifests with urticarial skin lesions that last longer than 24 hours, often with lingering hyperpigmentation, and low serum complement levels of C4 and C3. Behçet disease is a unique systemic vasculitis that affects both arteries and veins of any size. The classic triad of Behçet disease includes oral ulcers, uveitis, and genital ulcers; however, any organ system can be affected.

PAN is a necrotizing vasculitis affecting the medium-sized arteries and can present with systemic disease or in a limited form that only involves the skin and joints. It occurs in school-aged children, and there is typically a history of a preceding upper respiratory tract infection or streptococcal pharyngitis. In unvaccinated children, hepatitis B can be causative. Symptoms include prolonged fevers, malaise, calf pain, testicular pain, and weight loss. Physical examination findings include painful nodules (particularly on the soles of the feet), livedo reticularis, myalgias, and arthritis of large joints. In the systemic form, any organ system can be affected; thus hypertension, renal abnormalities, gastrointestinal involvement, and coronary disease can be seen. Of the large-vessel diseases, temporal arteritis is not seen in childhood. Takayasu arteritis, the third most common childhood vasculitis, preferentially affects the large branches of the aorta. Examination may reveal bruits, hypertension, and absent pulses.

Physical Examination

Hypertension is common. Furthermore, Takayasu arteritis classically presents with a blood pressure (BP) difference of greater than 10 mm Hg between arms. Thus the physical examination should include evaluation of BP in all four extremities. Careful auscultation for bruits (carotid, aortic, and abdominal vessels) and palpation of all peripheral pulses is vital; absent peripheral pulses or symptoms of claudication (extremity pain with activity caused by decreased blood flow) may help narrow the differential diagnosis and areas of vessel involvement. A thorough skin examination is warranted, because the presence of vasculitic rashes (purpura), nodules, ulcerations, microinfarctions, or livedo reticularis may aid in diagnosis. A neurologic examination should focus on evidence of neuropathy; some of the vasculitides, such as PAN, are associated with mononeuritis multiplex. Two specific areas where blood vessels can be directly visualized are the eyes and the nailfold capillaries. As disease progresses, more specific signs may develop, but morbidity also increases. Therefore a high clinical suspicion for vasculitis is important.

EVALUATION AND MANAGEMENT

Laboratory Evaluation

The laboratory evaluation for vasculitis should include inflammatory markers, such as erythrocyte sedimentation rate (ESR) and C-reactive protein (CRP), which can be markedly elevated, and a complete blood count (CBC). Liver enzymes, blood urea nitrogen, creatinine, and urinalysis help to evaluate liver and renal involvement. Antibody tests, such as ANA and ANCA, and complement levels should be ordered depending on the type of vasculitis being considered. When clinical suspicion is high, imaging examinations, such as computed tomography angiography, magnetic resonance angiography, or conventional angiography, may help identify blood vessel abnormalities or reveal certain patterns of vessel involvement, such as "beading" seen in PAN

and aneurysms found in Takayasu arteritis. Typically, these examinations are especially useful when there is concern for large vessel disease. The diagnostic gold standard is tissue biopsy.

Management

Management depends on the specific type of vasculitis and should be done in consultation with a rheumatologist (Table 138.1). Induction with immunosuppressive agents with or without corticosteroids, followed by immunomodulatory maintenance therapy, is the cornerstone of treatment for almost all the vasculitides. In immune complex–mediated disease, plasmapheresis may have a role.

IMMUNOGLOBULIN A VASCULITIS

IgAV is the most common vasculitis in childhood, with an incidence of 3 to 27 cases per 100,000 children (Fig. 138.2). It is a leukocytoclastic vasculitis predominantly affecting the small blood vessels. The classic triad is described as nonthrombocytopenic palpable purpura, arthritis,

TABLE 138.1   Vasculitides in Childhood

	Histopathology	Clinical Findings	Associated Laboratory Findings	Treatment
Small Vessel				
MPA	Nongranulomatous necrotizing, pauci-immune vasculitis	Fever, fatigue, weight loss, purpura, lower respiratory tract symptoms, nonspecific abdominal pain, mononeuritis multiplex	pANCA (anti-MPO), hematuria, proteinuria, ↑ creatinine, diffuse ground-glass opacities on chest CT	Induction with rituximab or cyclophosphamide AND corticosteroids (1–2 mg/kg/day), followed by maintenance with induction agent
GPA	Granulomatous inflammation of the respiratory tract; necrotizing, pauci-immune vasculitis of small and medium vessels; renal: extracapillary proliferation and crescent formation (renal granulomata are rare)	Fever, fatigue, weight loss, purpura, upper respiratory tract signs (epistaxis, destructive sinusitis, nasal ulceration, saddle nose deformity, hoarseness), lower respiratory tract disease (hemoptysis); hearing loss	cANCA (anti-PR3), ↑↑ ESR, ↑↑ CRP, ↑ platelets, leukocytosis, anemia, hematuria, proteinuria, nodules and/or cavitated lesions on chest CT	Identical to MPA
IgAV	IgA and C3 deposition in vessel walls (IgA may be absent)	Hypertension, palpable purpura with lower limb predominance, arthritis, abdominal pain, testicular swelling	↑ ESR, ↑ CRP, mild leukocytosis, hematuria, proteinuria	NSAIDs, corticosteroids (1–2 mg/kg) with slow taper over 4–8 weeks
Medium Vessel				
PAN	Necrotizing vasculitis with aneurysm formation	Hypertension, painful skin nodules (especially soles of feet), arthritis, testicular pain, calf pain, livedo reticularis, maculopapular rash, mononeuritis multiplex	↑↑ ESR, ↑ platelets, mild leukocytosis, anemia, hematuria proteinuria, ↑ creatinine	Induction with cyclophosphamide AND corticosteroids (1–2 mg/kg/day), followed by maintenance with methotrexate or azathioprine
KD	Necrotizing vasculitis with fibrinoid necrosis; coronary artery aneurysms	Fever, nonpurulent, limbic-sparing conjunctivitis, cervical lymphadenopathy, extremity changes, strawberry tongue, skin exanthem	↑ ESR, ↑ CRP, ↑ platelets, ↑ ferritin, sterile pyuria, transaminitis, aseptic meningitis	IVIG (2 g/kg), aspirin (80–100 mg/kg/day) until afebrile for 48 hours; then 3–5 mg/kg/day
Large Vessel				
Takayasu arteritis	Spotty granulomatous inflammation of the vessel walls; aneurysms; vessel dissection	Hypertension, blood pressure difference of >10 mm Hg between arms, subclavian bruit, decreased peripheral pulses, claudication, headache	↑ ESR, anemia, mild leukocytosis, hypergammaglobulinemia	Induction with cyclophosphamide and/or methotrexate AND corticosteroids (1–2 mg/kg), followed by maintenance with methotrexate, azathioprine, or mycophenolate mofetil; revascularization in severe cases

anti-MPA, Anti-myeloperoxidase antibodies; *anti-PR3*, anti-proteinase 3; *cANCA*, cytoplasmic antineutrophil cytoplasmic antibodies; *CRP*, C-reactive protein; *ESR*, erythrocyte sedimentation rate; *GPA*, granulomatosis with polyangiitis; *IgAV*, IgA vasculitis; *IVIG*, intravenous immunoglobulin; *KD*, Kawasaki disease; *MPA*, microscopic polyangiitis; *NSAID*, nonsteroidal antiinflammatory drug; *PAN*, polyarteritis nodosa; *pANCA*, perinuclear antineutrophil cytoplasmic antibodies.

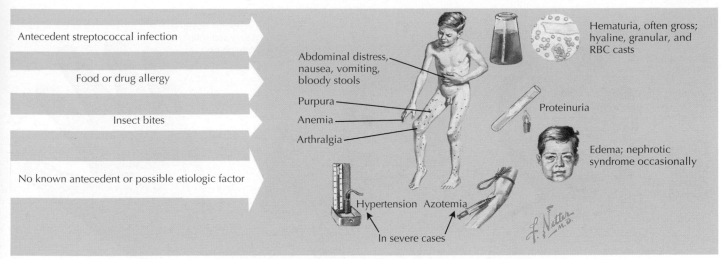

Fig. 138.2 Signs and Symptoms of Immunoglobulin A Vasculitis.

and abdominal pain. The most feared long-term morbidity of IgAV is chronic renal disease. It has a slight predilection for males at a 1.5:1 ratio, and most cases occur in winter and spring. Although IgAV can affect adults, the peak age of onset is between 4 and 6 years.

The pathophysiology of IgAV begins with abnormal glycosylation of IgA, against which self-antibodies form. Subsequently, IgA immune complexes form, which are then deposited in affected organs and small vessels, resulting in inflammation. Many cases involve a history of preceding upper respiratory tract illness. It was previously thought that vaccination was associated with development of IgAV; however, studies have presented strong evidence against such an association.

The most widely used criteria to guide the diagnosis of pediatric IgAV is the European League Against Rheumatism/Paediatric Rheumatology International Trials Organisation/Paediatric Rheumatology European Society (EULAR/PRINTO/PRES) classification criteria (Box 138.1). The purpuric rash has raised, nontender, nonpruritic, symmetric deep red-to-purple lesions that are most often found in dependent areas such as the buttocks and lower extremities, especially the feet and ankles. However, they also can be on the face, trunk, and upper extremities, and, although rarer, lesions may be bullous or necrotic. Edema of the skin can also be seen and can be easily confused for arthritis when it surrounds joints. Abdominal pain occurs in over 70% of patients and is characterized as colicky because it is secondary to bowel angina. More severe gastrointestinal symptoms include hemorrhage, intussusception (notably ileo-ileal), and pancreatitis. Up to 25% of children may have abdominal symptoms of IgAV before the onset of rash, making the diagnosis challenging. Up to 90% of patients also present with arthralgias or nonerosive arthritis, usually affecting large joints, such as the knee or ankle, but small joints also can be involved. The arthritis of IgAV is usually transient, lasting a few days to 1 week. Renal manifestations are seen in about 50% of patients with IgAV and tend to be asymptomatic. Findings range from microscopic hematuria or proteinuria to acute renal failure. Of the children who develop renal involvement, most do so within the first 6 months of disease. Finally, about 14% of boys with IgAV also experience orchitis.

Laboratory findings in IgAV are typically nonspecific. Evaluation should include a CBC (thrombocytopenia indicates an alternative diagnosis), chemistry (to assess for renal insufficiency), and a urinalysis (to check for blood or protein). BP is also important to monitor both at diagnosis and throughout the acute phase of illness; along with urinalysis, BP should be followed by primary care physicians for

6 months to identify late-onset renal disease. Renal biopsy may be warranted to determine the severity of renal disease.

The prognosis for patients with mild manifestations is very good. In general, NSAIDs are used for mild to moderate abdominal pain and the arthralgia of IgAV. Corticosteroids are indicated in patients with severe abdominal pain because they have been shown to shorten the duration of symptoms. Corticosteroids also may be beneficial in ameliorating bullous and necrotic skin lesions and are the mainstay in treating IgAV nephritis. Corticosteroids do not, however, prevent development of nephritis. Recurrences are seen in up to one-third of children, usually within 4 to 6 months of initial diagnosis and more often in older children and patients with renal involvement. Long-term morbidity usually depends on the severity of renal disease, with worse disease predicting worse outcome.

KAWASAKI DISEASE

KD is the second most common vasculitis in children (Fig. 138.3). It is considered an acute vasculitis of medium-sized arteries, most notably the coronary arteries. The peak age of onset is 2 years old, with most cases occurring in children between 6 months and 5 years of age. KD is also more common in boys than girls (1.5:1), and it has a higher incidence in Japanese and Korean populations. Although the cause of KD is unknown, studies have suggested that exposure to certain infectious agents, such as parvovirus, Epstein-Barr virus, and respiratory syncytial virus (RSV), may elicit a cytokine storm in genetically predisposed children.

Diagnosis is based on clinical criteria, which require the presence of persistent fever of at least 5 days and at least 4 of 5 clinical features (Table 138.2). The fever is typically minimally responsive to antipyretic medications. In some cases, patients can develop anterior uveitis, so a slit-lamp examination may be helpful if the diagnosis is unclear. A transient arthritis is noted in about one-third of patients and can involve any joint. The rash of KD is nonspecific and ranges from erythema at the perineal area to a morbilliform exanthem on the trunk or extremities. Vesicular or pustular lesions are not typical. Cervical lymphadenopathy is usually the least common finding of KD.

It should be noted that a certain subset of patients do not demonstrate enough clinical features to meet criteria for KD. Coronary abnormalities are the major cause of morbidity and mortality in patients, occurring in about 50% of untreated infants younger than 6 months of age and 25% of untreated children. Considering these

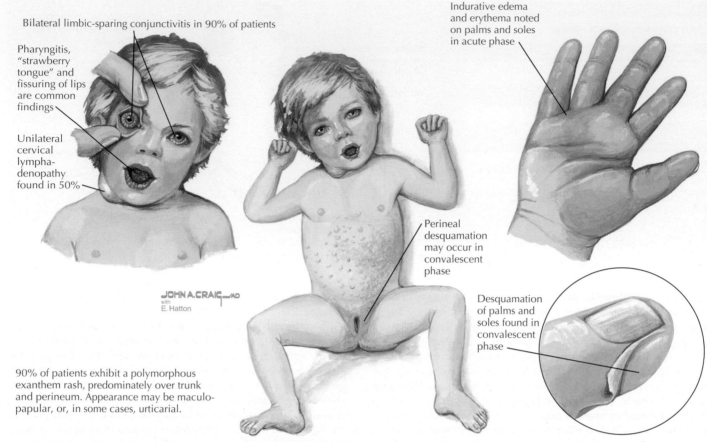

Bilateral limbic-sparing conjunctivitis in 90% of patients

Pharyngitis, "strawberry tongue" and fissuring of lips are common findings

Unilateral cervical lympha-denopathy found in 50%

Indurative edema and erythema noted on palms and soles in acute phase

Perineal desquamation may occur in convalescent phase

Desquamation of palms and soles found in convalescent phase

JOHN A. CRAIG—AD
with
E. Hatton

90% of patients exhibit a polymorphous exanthem rash, predominately over trunk and perineum. Appearance may be maculo-papular, or, in some cases, urticarial.

Fig. 138.3 Clinical Features of Kawasaki Disease.

TABLE 138.2 Diagnostic Criteria of Kawasaki Disease

Fever of 5 days or longer duration with *at least four* of the following clinical signs:

Sign	Children With Kawasaki Disease (%)
1. Bilateral limbic-sparing conjunctivitis	80–90
2. Oral mucosal membrane changes (e.g., injected or fissured lips, strawberry tongue, pharyngitis)	90
3. Peripheral extremity changes (e.g., erythema or edema of hands and feet in the acute phase or desquamation in the convalescent phase)	50–85
4. Polymorphous, nonvesicular exanthem, usually on the trunk	70–90
5. Cervical lymphadenopathy with anterior cervical lymph node ≥1.5 cm in diameter	25–70

The laboratory evaluation for KD should include a CBC (there is often marked thrombocytosis, as well as anemia for age), inflammatory markers, complete metabolic panel (elevated ALT), and urinalysis (assessing for sterile pyuria). A concurrent infection is common in children presenting with KD, so diagnostic suspicion should remain high in patients with an identified infectious pathogen.

After a diagnosis is made, treatment must be initiated because early intervention (within 10 days of onset of fever) has been shown to decrease the occurrence of coronary artery aneurysms by fivefold. Treatment consists of intravenous immunoglobulin (2 g/kg) and high-dose aspirin (80 to 100 mg/kg/day). Low-dose aspirin is started when the patient has been afebrile for 48 hours. Aspirin therapy is discontinued after inflammatory markers and platelet count have normalized unless there is evidence of coronary artery disease. An echocardiogram is repeated 6 to 8 weeks after diagnosis to monitor the patient's response to treatment.

The overall outcome for KD is excellent in most patients without cardiac involvement. Because of the monocyclic nature of the disease, most patients have a full recovery. Of patients who develop coronary artery abnormalities, lifelong cardiology monitoring is needed because of the increased risk for heart disease.

MULTISYSTEM INFLAMMATORY SYNDROME IN CHILDREN

Initially thought to be KD-like, MIS-C has now been recognized as a distinct entity characterized by a dysregulated, hyperinflammatory response to the novel SARS-CoV-2 virus with vasculopathy. Whereas COVID-19 and MIS-C are both severe consequences of SARS-CoV-2

startling numbers, supplemental criteria have been developed to identify patients with "incomplete KD." Infants under 6 months need only persistent fevers for 7 or more days and an abnormal echocardiogram to meet criteria, while those older than 6 months require 5 or more days of fever, two to three clinical criteria, elevated inflammatory markers, and three or more supplemental laboratory criteria or an abnormal echocardiogram.

infection, MIS-C is a postinfectious process occurring 2 to 6 weeks after initial exposure, invariably affecting children and adolescents. Patients with MIS-C often present in hyperinflammatory shock, requiring fluid resuscitation and/or vasopressors and ICU-level care. Most common presenting symptoms include fever, severe abdominal pain, emesis, diarrhea, rash, and bilateral, nonexudative conjunctivitis.

Laboratory analyses in MIS-C are notable for a relative thrombocytopenia and lymphopenia on CBC, neutrophilia, hypoalbuminemia on chemistry, markedly increased inflammatory markers (notably CRP, ferritin, and procalcitonin), coagulopathy characterized by elevated D-dimer and fibrinogen, and cardiac dysfunction made evident by exceedingly high troponin and brain natriuretic peptide. Burr cells and schistocytes are often present on blood smear. Many, but not all, have negative PCR testing for SARS-CoV-2, whereas most have positive antibodies to SARS-CoV-2. Echocardiography is recommended in all patients, because over 50% demonstrate cardiac dysfunction; diminished left ventricular ejection fraction is most commonly seen. Although abnormalities visualized on echocardiography appear to rapidly resolve with treatment in these patients, the long-term sequelae of cardiac inflammation are not yet known, so repeat imaging 4 to 6 weeks after presentation is recommended. If available, cytokine panels can be used to distinguish MIS-C from COVID-19 and KD if the presentation is ambiguous, because MIS-C demonstrates a unique signature of elevated interleukin 10 (IL-10), IL-6, IL-8, and tumor necrosis factor-α.

Treatment guidelines for MIS-C are in their early stages, and the current recommendation is early stabilization of patients followed by intravenous immunoglobulin and/or moderate- to high-dose glucocorticoids. For those whose disease is refractory to initial therapies, anakinra (IL-1 receptor antagonist) may be beneficial. Low-dose aspirin is recommended for patients with coagulopathies and coronary aneurysms.

Initial data suggest that the prognosis of patients with MIS-C who receive prompt care is very good, in part because most are previously healthy children. However, early estimates suggest that the death rate is close to 2%, thereby necessitating further insights regarding the disease's pathophysiology and high clinical suspicion.

FUTURE DIRECTIONS

Vasculitis and vasculopathy are rare childhood conditions but should be considered in any child with unexplained constitutional symptoms, significant inflammation, and multiorgan involvement. Given the rarity of these conditions, large clinical trials are extremely challenging to conduct. Instead, the development of patient registries is likely the key to being able to study these diseases in children in a systematic fashion.

SUGGESTED READINGS

Available online.

139

Systemic Lupus Erythematosus

Roberto Alejandro Valdovinos and Pamela F. Weiss

✳ CLINICAL VIGNETTE

A 17-year-old African American female adolescent sought medical attention for progressive, bilateral lower extremity edema. She first noted her edema about a month ago when she started having difficulty putting her shoes on, with swelling that steadily increased to involve her shins. She was fatigued, had missed several deadlines at school because she "could not focus," had developed bilateral knee and wrist swelling, and diffuse thinning of her hair. She had no significant medical history. Her vital signs were significant for a blood pressure of 155/90 mm Hg, and her examination demonstrated significant alopecia, swelling, and tenderness at the wrists and knees, and 2+ pitting edema of the lower extremities. Urine protein-to-creatine demonstrated significant proteinuria, and subsequent kidney biopsy revealed diffuse glomerulonephritis involving more than 50% of all glomeruli. Laboratory test results revealed low complement 3 (C3) and C4, as well as a high titer anti-dsDNA antibody, positive anti-Smith antibody, and homogeneous patterned antinuclear antibody positive at 1:1280, overall consistent with a diagnosis of systemic lupus erythematosus with lupus nephritis class IV. Her lupus nephritis was treated with a course of pulse steroids and cyclophosphamide induction therapy for 6 months, followed by transition to mycophenolate mofetil and initiation of hydroxychloroquine for her general disease. Her lower extremity edema resolved after induction therapy, and follow-up laboratory studies revealed normal complement levels and a normal anti-dsDNA level. Her alopecia and synovitis were greatly improved, and her first semester of college went very well.

Systemic lupus erythematosus (SLE) is a chronic autoimmune disease that has the potential to affect any organ system, with its most severe phenotypes leading to life-threatening renal and central nervous system (CNS) disease. The overall prevalence of SLE is 1 in 4000, and it is higher in women, those who live in urban areas, Asians, African Americans, African Caribbeans, and Hispanic Americans. Twenty percent of patients are diagnosed before age 16 years, with the average age of pediatric onset being 12. The primary treatment goal is reducing long-term, life-limiting complications, especially in children, who typically face a more severe disease course than adults.

ETIOLOGY AND PATHOGENESIS

The cause of SLE is multifactorial, involving genetic, environmental, hormonal, and immunologic factors, ultimately resulting in loss of self-tolerance, complement activation, and immune complex deposition in various organs. Several genes have been identified that confer susceptibility to SLE, including human leukocyte antigen haplotypes, complement-related genes (e.g., *C1q*), Fc receptors, polymorphisms in cytokines, B-cell activation factor (BAFF), and T-cell receptors.

Familial clustering has been reported, and the concordance rates among monozygotic and dizygotic twins are 11% to 50% and 7.7%, respectively.

The pathogenesis of SLE involves immune dysregulation characterized by abnormal clearance of apoptotic debris, B- and T-cell abnormalities, and autoantibody and immune complex formation. In SLE, the system of apoptotic debris removal is dysfunctional, allowing for the presentation of autoantigens, commonly nucleic acids, driven in part by interferon type 1 (IFN-1), to T-cells. These T-cells stimulate B-cells to produce autoantibodies that bind directly to cells in end organs leading to direct injury or formation of immune complexes in the circulation that deposit in tissues and cause inflammation. Additionally, early classic complement deficiencies are associated with SLE.

Other factors hypothesized to play a role in the cause of SLE include hormones (e.g., estrogen is theorized to contribute to B-cell autoreactivity), Epstein-Barr virus and other infections, exposure to ultraviolet light (resulting in apoptosis), and childhood psychological stress. Together, genetic susceptibility, immunologic dysregulation, and environmental influences likely act to trigger SLE.

CLINICAL PRESENTATION

SLE in children largely presents during adolescence and is rare in those under the age of 5, with girls being affected approximately two times more often than boys until puberty, at which point the female-to-male ratio is 13:1. Constitutional signs and symptoms, including fever, fatigue, lymphadenopathy, hepatosplenomegaly, and weight loss, are common. The most frequently involved sites are the skin, joints, and kidneys. Manifestation may be insidious, with symptoms preceding the diagnosis by several months, or patients may present acutely with severe symptoms, such as with pleural or pericardial effusions, acute nephritic syndrome, or macrophage activation syndrome (MAS). The European League Against Rheumatism/American College of Rheumatology (EULAR/ACR) and the Systemic Lupus International Collaborating Clinics (SLICC) provide classification criteria that are used clinically to aid in the diagnosis of SLE (Table 139.1, Fig. 139.1). The SLICC criteria require that patients have at least four of the listed criteria, including at least one clinical criterion and one immunologic criterion, or that the patient have biopsy-proven lupus nephritis with a positive antinuclear antibody (ANA) or anti–double stranded DNA (anti-dsDNA) antibody. The EULAR/ACR (2019), in comparison, requires a positive ANA as an entry criterion, followed by additive, weighted criteria with a threshold of 10 or more points. The ANA is not a useful general screening test for rheumatologic disease and should not be ordered routinely in the absence of other criteria for SLE.

TABLE 139.1 European League Against Rheumatism and American College of Rheumatology (2019) and Systemic Lupus International Collaborating Clinics (2012) Classification Criteria for Systemic Lupus Erythematosus

Domain	EULAR/ACR Criteria (Points)	SLICC Criteria
Clinical		
Constitutional	Fever (2)	—
Hematologic	Leukopenia (3) Thrombocytopenia (4) Autoimmune hemolysis (4)	Leukopenia Thrombocytopenia Hemolytic anemia Direct Coombs
Neuropsychiatric	Delirium (2) Psychosis (3) Seizure (5)	Acute confusional state Psychosis Seizure Mononeuritis multiplex Myelitis
Mucocutaneous	Alopecia (2) Oral ulcers (2) SCLE/DLE (4) ACLE (6)	Nonscarring alopecia Oral or nasal ulcers Acute cutaneous lupus (e.g., malar rash) Chronic cutaneous lupus (e.g., discoid rash)
Serosal	Effusion (5) Acute pericarditis (6)	Effusion Pericarditis Rub
Musculoskeletal	Joint involvement (6)	Synovitis
Renal	Proteinuria (4) Class II/V nephritis (8) Class III/IV nephritis (10)	Urine protein/creatine >0.5 g protein/24 h Red blood cell casts
Immunologic		
Antiphospholipid antibodies	Anticardiolipin or anti-β glycoprotein antibodies, or lupus anticoagulant (2)	Anticardiolipin or anti-β glycoprotein antibodies, or lupus anticoagulant, or false-positive rapid plasma reagin
Complements	C3 or C4 low (3) C3 and C4 low (4)	Low C3 Low C4 Low CH50
SLE-specific antibodies	Anti-Sm (6) Anti-dsDNA (6) ANA	Anti-Sm Anti-dsDNA ANA

ACLE, Acute cutaneous lupus erythematosus; *ACR,* American College of Radiology; *ANA,* anti-nuclear antibody; *anti-dsDNA,* anti–double stranded DNA; *anti-Sm,* anti-Smith antibody; *DLE,* discoid lupus erythematosus; *EULAR,* European League Against Rheumatism; *SCLE,* subacute cutaneous lupus erythematosus; *SLE,* systemic lupus erythematosus; *SLICC,* Systemic Lupus International Collaborating Clinics.
Adapted from Aringer M, Costenbader K, Daikh D, et al. 2019 European League Against Rheumatism/American College of Rheumatology classification criteria for systemic lupus erythematosus. *Arthritis Rheum.* 2019;71(9):1400–1412; and Petri M, Orbai A-M, Alarcòn GS, Gordon C, et al. Derivation and validation of systemic lupus international collaborating clinics classification criteria for systemic lupus erythematosus. *Arthritis Rheum.* 2012;64(8):2677–2686.

Mucocutaneous Manifestations

There are four skin and mucocutaneous criteria: acute cutaneous lupus (including malar rash), chronic cutaneous lupus (including discoid rash), oral or nasal ulcers, and nonscarring alopecia. The malar rash, or classic "butterfly rash," is typically maculopapular and photosensitive, classically extending across the nasal bridge, sparing the nasolabial folds, and nonscarring. Depending on the race of the child, it may be either hyperpigmented or hypopigmented. In contrast, the less common discoid rash is inflammatory and lesions are coin-shaped, raised, erythematous, and typically located on the face (notably the ears), scalp, and extremities. Discoid lesions are scarring and lead to permanent alopecia when they occur on the scalp. The oral and nasal ulcers associated with SLE are usually painless; oral ulcers are classically located on the hard palate. Other common skin manifestations include livedo reticularis, Raynaud's phenomenon, and digital ulcerations (Fig. 139.2).

Musculoskeletal Manifestations

Nonerosive, symmetric polyarthritis affecting both the small and large joints is common. Frequently affected joints include the knees, wrists, and fingers. Although the joint effusions are often minimal, the arthritis is painful with substantial joint-line tenderness and impaired range of motion. As in juvenile idiopathic arthritis, morning stiffness is common.

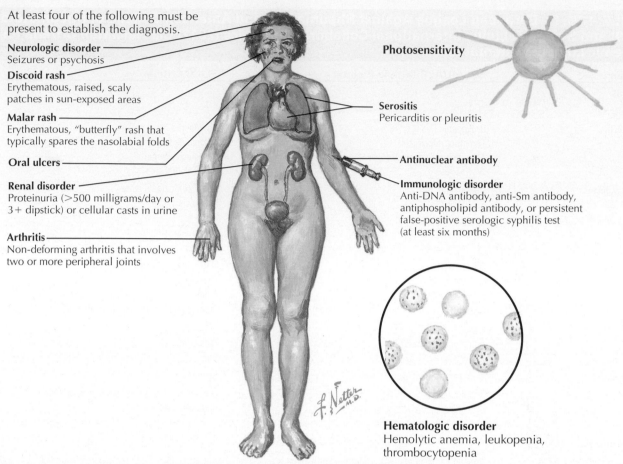

At least four of the following must be present to establish the diagnosis.

Neurologic disorder
Seizures or psychosis

Discoid rash
Erythematous, raised, scaly patches in sun-exposed areas

Malar rash
Erythematous, "butterfly" rash that typically spares the nasolabial folds

Oral ulcers

Renal disorder
Proteinuria (>500 milligrams/day or 3+ dipstick) or cellular casts in urine

Arthritis
Non-deforming arthritis that involves two or more peripheral joints

Photosensitivity

Serositis
Pericarditis or pleuritis

Antinuclear antibody

Immunologic disorder
Anti-DNA antibody, anti-Sm antibody, antiphospholipid antibody, or persistent false-positive serologic syphilis test (at least six months)

Hematologic disorder
Hemolytic anemia, leukopenia, thrombocytopenia

Fig. 139.1 Criteria Used for the Diagnosis of SLE.

Renal Manifestations

Renal disease is present in 50% to 75% of pediatric SLE and is a strong determinant of prognosis. Its severity ranges from microscopic hematuria to chronic renal disease. Lupus nephritis usually develops within 2 years of diagnosis and has a strong predilection for African American, Asian, and Hispanic American patients. SLE patients with significant proteinuria or abnormal renal function should undergo renal biopsy to classify their degree of renal involvement to aid in treatment decision making. The classification of lupus nephritis includes six classes, ranging from minimal mesangial involvement to diffuse involvement and glomerulosclerosis (Fig. 139.3).

Neuropsychiatric Manifestations

The most common neuropsychiatric manifestations of SLE are headache, cognitive dysfunction, psychosis, and seizures. Headache occurs frequently and may result in presentation to the emergency department because of difficulty with managing the pain. Cognitive dysfunction in SLE patients may be subtle and should be screened for carefully. Because SLE patients often present during adolescence, deteriorating school performance, concentration difficulties, and changes in mood secondary to SLE may be wrongfully attributed to teenage behavior. Children with psychosis may experience hallucinations, confusion, and suicidal ideation. Seizures may occur and are usually generalized. Acute causes of severe headache, seizure, psychosis, and behavioral changes in lupus patients should be considered, including CNS vasculitis, increased intracranial pressure, CNS infection, posterior reversible encephalopathy syndrome (PRES), and cerebral vein thrombosis.

Other less common neuropsychiatric manifestations of SLE include movement disorders such as unilateral chorea and parkinsonism, cranial neuropathies, and stroke.

Hematologic Manifestations

Cytopenias seen in patients with SLE include Coombs-positive hemolytic anemia, leukopenia, lymphopenia, and thrombocytopenia. Coagulation abnormalities are also frequently present, often associated with antiphospholipid syndrome. The presence of lupus anticoagulant predisposes patients to the development of cerebral and deep vein thromboses, which may lead to thromboemboli and recurrent miscarriage later in life.

Cardiopulmonary Manifestations

Pleuritis and pericarditis, forms of serositis, are common manifestations of SLE in children. These patients often complain of pleuritic chest pain, and friction rub may be auscultated on examination. Cardiac issues that may arise less commonly are valvular heart disease, Libman-Sacks endocarditis, and myocarditis. Pulmonary involvement may also include pneumonitis, pneumothorax, and pulmonary hemorrhage.

DIFFERENTIAL DIAGNOSIS

The differential diagnosis of SLE is broad and includes acute and chronic diseases that affect many organ systems (Box 139.1). Broad categories most important to consider include infectious, oncologic, rheumatic, and drug-induced causes.

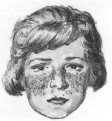

Malar rash

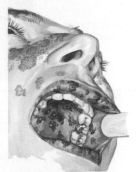

Painless oral ulcers

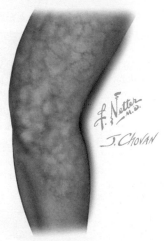

Livedo reticularis

Fig. 139.2 Skin and Mucous Membrane Manifestations of SLE.

Morbidity and Mortality

A diagnosis of SLE carries a 2.4 times increased risk in all-cause mortality compared to the general population, with the most common cause of death being cardiovascular disease later in life, followed by renal and respiratory complications of the disease itself. The long-term survival of children with SLE has improved significantly over the years with earlier diagnosis, the use of immunosuppressant therapies early in the disease course, and better understanding of the appropriate management of end-stage renal disease. However, combined with the leukopenia and hypocomplementemia inherent to SLE, an unfortunate consequence of immunosuppressive therapies is that they leave patients at-risk for invasive infection, which is the most common cause of death early in the disease course. Five-year survival rates are now near 100%, and 10-year survival rates are greater than 85%.

The morbidity and mortality attributed to renal disease is related to the histologic findings of lupus nephritis on kidney biopsy (Fig. 139.3). End-stage renal disease is most strongly associated with proliferative

subtypes, including focal lupus nephritis (class III) and diffuse lupus nephritis (class IV). Over the long-term, renal disease, vasculitis, a hypercoagulable state, lipid abnormalities, and steroid therapy can all contribute to life-limiting, accelerated cardiovascular disease, including atherosclerosis, stroke, and myocardial infarction during adolescence and young adulthood.

EVALUATION AND MANAGEMENT

The diagnosis of SLE is established using classification criteria (see Table 139.1). Inflammatory markers (C-reactive protein [CRP] and erythrocyte sedimentation rate [ESR]) are helpful as a general screen of the degree of inflammation present. Classically, the ESR is markedly elevated, and the CRP is normal or mildly elevated in patients with SLE. Hypocomplementemia, particularly low C3 and C4, is associated with active disease, especially in patients with lupus nephritis. The partial thromboplastin time (PTT) is prolonged when the lupus anticoagulant is present; however, despite PTT prolongation, the lupus anticoagulant leads to a hypercoagulable state clinically as described earlier. A complete urinalysis should be performed in all SLE patients. If proteinuria is present, a first-morning urine protein-to-creatinine ratio or 24-hour urine collection should follow. If proteinuria is significant (>500 mg/24 hr) a renal biopsy is warranted before therapy initiation to stage the lupus nephritis and aid in treatment decision making. It is also recommended that children with a new diagnosis have a baseline electrocardiogram, echocardiogram, and chest radiograph.

Management

The chronicity, waxing and waning course, and multisystem effects of SLE make it challenging to treat. The benefits of therapies must be weighed against the side effects, risks, and impact on quality of life for adolescents who are already experiencing psychosocial stressors. Long-term adherence to therapies is key to improving survival. Optimizing disease management requires placing safeguards in patients' lives by educating family members about the disease, offering psychologic support, developing patient-centered school plans, and providing robust support systems for families with low socioeconomic status.

General recommendations for all children with SLE include sun protection (use of sunscreen, hats, and light clothing in the summer), a healthy diet and exercise regimen to decrease cardiovascular risk factors, avoidance of tobacco, multivitamin therapy (especially vitamin D and calcium to prevent osteoporosis), and vaccination (inactivated vaccines only for patients with active disease or those receiving immunosuppressive therapy).

The approach to pharmacologic therapy depends on disease severity and the organ systems affected. The overall model of treatment is similar to the approach used in treating patients with oncologic disease, with induction treatment initially to induce remission followed by maintenance therapy to sustain remission.

Mild Disease

For disease that is limited to arthralgias and myalgias, treatment with nonsteroidal anti-inflammatory drugs (NSAIDs) or the antimalarial drug hydroxychloroquine (HCQ), a disease-modifying agent (DMARD), may be sufficient. HCQ also can be used to address rash and alopecia. Hydroxychloroquine's benefits also include SLE flare prevention, improved renal and mortality outcomes, and a damping of the thrombotic effects of antiphospholipid syndrome. Although exceedingly rare, HCQ retinopathy can result in permanent changes in color and peripheral vision, thereby warranting routine ophthalmologic screens.

A. Mesangial type

Glomerulus showing increased mesangial material (PAS stain)

Fluorescence slide*: mesangial deposits of immune complexes

B. Focal proliferative type

Glomerulus showing focal proliferative change and adhesions of glomerular tufts (H and E)

Fluorescence slide: granular deposits of immune complexes in capillary walls

C. Diffuse proliferative type

Glomerulus showing proliferative change, fibrinoid necrosis and hematoxylin body (arrow) (H and E)

Fluorescence slide: massive deposits of immune complexes

Electron microscopic diagram: massive subendothelial deposits of immune complexes

D. Membranous type

Diffuse thickening of basement membrane (PAS stain)

Fluorescence slide: diffuse homogeneous granular deposits along capillary walls

Electron microscopic diagram: diffuse subepithelial deposits

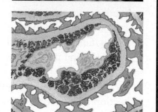

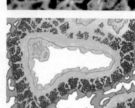

* All fluorescence slides stained with fluorescein-labeled rabbit antihuman gamma globulin

Fig. 139.3 Renal Manifestations of SLE.

BOX 139.1   Differential Diagnosis of Systemic Lupus Erythematosus

Infectious
- Human immunodeficiency virus
- Epstein-Barr virus
- Parvovirus B19
- Cytomegalovirus
- Tuberculosis
- Sepsis
- Acute rheumatic fever

Oncologic
- Leukemia
- Lymphoma

Rheumatologic
- Systemic-onset juvenile idiopathic arthritis
- Sarcoidosis
- Mixed connective tissue disease
- Other systemic vasculitis

Drug Induced
- Hydralazine
- Procainamide
- Penicillamine
- Quinidine
- Isoniazid
- Minocycline
- Anti–tumor necrosis factor (TNF) therapy

Miscellaneous
- Kikuchi-Fujimoto disease
- Castleman disease

Moderate to Severe Disease

Patients with refractory arthritis, organ involvement, or acute flares are treated with a short course of corticosteroids and initiation of a specific corticosteroid-sparing agent tailored to the specific disease manifestation. Examples include cytotoxic-immunosuppressants such as methotrexate, azathioprine, cyclophosphamide, and mycophenolate mofetil, as well as synthetic biologics like belimumab and rituximab. Cyclophosphamide or rituximab are typically used for organ-threatening disease. Rituximab can be beneficial for severe Coombs-positive anemia. Although the DMARDs and biologics reduce inflammation and the need for long-term corticosteroid use, they may introduce other toxicities, including immunosuppression, infertility, and risk for future malignancy.

In addition to medication used to modify the course of the disease, management of comorbidities is also very important in SLE. Aggressive treatment of hypertension and early consultation with a pediatric nephrologist are critical in preserving renal function. Consultation with a pediatric neurologist is recommended if neuropsychiatric manifestations are present. Psychiatric evaluation may be necessary to aid in the decision to treat with antidepressant or antipsychotic medications.

FUTURE DIRECTIONS

Breakthroughs in elucidating the pathophysiology in SLE have allowed for targeted therapies that more specifically address abnormalities in the disease mechanisms implicated, thereby reducing exposure to cytotoxic drugs. New biologics and synthetic small protein inhibitors that target proinflammatory interferon, interleukin, and JAK-STAT pathways are being tested in clinical trials. Ongoing research is being performed to illuminate disease phenotype on a molecular level, with the goal of more precisely characterizing patient disease at presentation and providing individualized therapies.

SUGGESTED READINGS

Available online.

140

Granulomatous Disease

Sarah E. Capponi and Pamela F. Weiss

Noninfectious granulomatous disease is rare in children, with the exception of Crohn's disease (see Chapter 57). This group of diseases includes sarcoidosis, familial juvenile systemic granulomatosis (Blau syndrome), granulomatous and lymphocytic interstitial lung disease (GLILD), and granulomatous vasculitides (granulomatosis with polyangiitis [GPA, formerly Wegener's granulomatosis] and eosinophilic granulomatosis with polyangiitis [eGPA, formerly Churg-Strauss syndrome]).

SARCOIDOSIS

Sarcoidosis is an uncommon multisystem disorder involving granulomatous infiltrates in affected organs. Sarcoidosis occurs in children worldwide without gender predominance. The incidence ranges from 0.29 to 0.80 per 100,000 children and varies across countries. Sarcoidosis is exceedingly rare in children younger than 5 years, with the average age of onset between 11 and 13 years. Globally, a race predilection has not been reported; however, there is a higher prevalence in 8- to 15-year-old Black children of the southeastern United States.

Etiology and Pathogenesis

Despite considerable research, the cause of sarcoidosis is unknown. Inheritance is multigenic with relatively weak human leukocyte antigen associations varying with populations studied. An infectious cause has been postulated, with *Mycobacterium tuberculosis* and *Propionibacterium acnes* suggested as triggers. Mycobacterial DNA has been detected by polymerase chain reaction in sarcoidosis lesions, and a candidate mycobacterial antigen, *M. tuberculosis* catalase-peroxidase

protein (mKatG), has been proposed as a trigger for an adaptive immune response that leads to granuloma formation. Exposure to other inorganic matter such as silica also has been postulated as a trigger for disease development.

Sarcoidosis is characterized by nonnecrotizing granulomas consisting of tightly packed epithelioid cells and macrophages surrounded by lymphocytes (Fig. 140.1). In the lung, CD4+ T cell–mediated alveolitis occurs early followed by granuloma formation. Granulomas may resolve without sequelae or may heal with residual fibrosis.

Clinical Presentation

Sarcoidosis in children occurs in two distinct forms. Older children (age 8 to 15 years) typically present with symptoms resembling the adult form of disease, including lymphadenopathy, lung involvement, systemic signs (fever, weight loss), and hypercalcemia. Joint involvement is rare in the adolescent patient population. In children younger than 5 years, the onset typically consists of the triad of rash, arthritis, and uveitis. Pulmonary involvement is rare in sarcoidosis with very early onset. Löfgren syndrome (the triad of ankle arthritis, erythema nodosum, and bilateral hilar lymphadenopathy, which is pathognomonic for sarcoidosis in adult patients) is uncommon in children. Sarcoidosis commonly manifests with lymphadenopathy and may affect a wide range of organs (Fig. 140.2), with an average of three to five organs involved at time of diagnosis.

Lymphadenopathy is the most common manifesting sign in childhood sarcoidosis. Enlarged nodes are generally nontender, firm, and mobile. Hepatosplenomegaly occurs in 30% to 50% of patients. Chronic dry cough, shortness of breath, and chest pain are the most common pulmonary symptoms. Radiographic pulmonary involvement most commonly presents as hilar adenopathy and pulmonary infiltrates. Children may be asymptomatic from a pulmonary standpoint despite having restrictive disease on pulmonary function testing (PFT) and positive radiographic findings.

Uveitis (anterior, posterior, or panuveitis) is the most common ocular manifestation. Uveitis is typically asymptomatic and must be evaluated for by slit-lamp examination. The incidence of uveitis is reported as high as 70% in some patient cohorts, but other cohorts report uveitis in 20% to 40% of patients. Keratic precipitates (tightly packed lymphocytic accumulations) are characteristic and occur at the corneal edge or pupil-iris junction. Synechiae may occur from longstanding inflammation, typically between the lens and iris, resulting in irregular pupils. Conjunctival granulomas (small, pale yellow, translucent nodules), keratitis, glaucoma, or retinitis may also occur.

Typical rashes include yellow-brown erythematous papules on the face or larger violaceous plaques on the trunk, extremities, and buttocks. Other skin involvement includes nodular (e.g., erythema nodosum), papular, macular, or ichthyosiform lesions; hypopigmentation; hyperpigmentation; or ulceration.

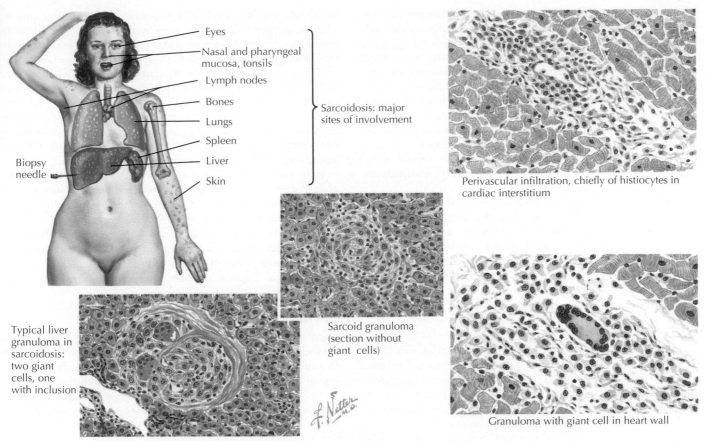

Eyes

Nasal and pharyngeal mucosa, tonsils

Lymph nodes

Bones

Lungs

Spleen

Liver

Skin

Sarcoidosis: major sites of involvement

Biopsy needle

Perivascular infiltration, chiefly of histiocytes in cardiac interstitium

Typical liver granuloma in sarcoidosis: two giant cells, one with inclusion

Sarcoid granuloma (section without giant cells)

Granuloma with giant cell in heart wall

Fig. 140.1 Granulomatous Disease in Sarcoidosis.

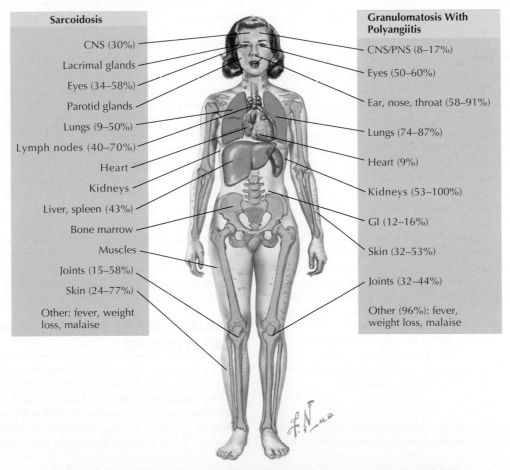

Sarcoidosis

CNS (30%)

Lacrimal glands

Eyes (34–58%)

Parotid glands

Lungs (9–50%)

Lymph nodes (40–70%)

Heart

Kidneys

Liver, spleen (43%)

Bone marrow

Muscles

Joints (15–58%)

Skin (24–77%)

Other: fever, weight loss, malaise

Granulomatosis With Polyangiitis

CNS/PNS (8–17%)

Eyes (50–60%)

Ear, nose, throat (58–91%)

Lungs (74–87%)

Heart (9%)

Kidneys (53–100%)

GI (12–16%)

Skin (32–53%)

Joints (32–44%)

Other (96%): fever, weight loss, malaise

Fig. 140.2 Clinical Features in Sarcoidosis and Granulomatosis With Polyangiitis.

Joint manifestations are characterized by boggy tenosynovitis with effusion that is minimally painful or painless. Joint involvement may be oligoarticular (four or fewer joints) initially but frequently progresses to polyarthritis over time. Associated stiffness and limited range of motion, typical in other forms of chronic arthritis, are generally minimal at diagnosis; however, with increased duration of disease, they become more apparent. Bony involvement is rare, but in the right setting, vertebral sarcoidosis should be considered in a child with back pain. Additionally, the small bones of the hands and feet may be involved. Nodular or inflammatory muscle lesions are rare.

Central nervous system (CNS) disease includes cranial nerve abnormalities (e.g., optic neuritis or facial nerve palsy), encephalopathy, seizures, and mass lesions.

Salivary or lacrimal gland involvement may present similarly to Sjögren syndrome (recurrent parotitis, sicca syndrome, or lacrimal gland enlargement). Pancreatitis is very rare. Renal involvement is usually the result of nephrocalcinosis and nephrolithiasis rather than direct granulomatous inflammation. Heart block, cardiomyopathy, or ventricular arrhythmias may occur but are less common in children than adults. Cytopenias may result from granulomatous infiltrates in bone marrow. Vasculitis affecting any size of vessel has been reported rarely.

Differential Diagnosis

Sarcoidosis should be considered in any child presenting with fever, weight loss, and lymphadenopathy, especially if accompanied by rash, arthritis, or hilar adenopathy, or in any child with fever of unknown origin (see Chapter 83). Other conditions that must be considered in a child suspected of having sarcoidosis include infection, malignancy, immunodeficiency, and other rheumatic illnesses.

Evaluation and Management

Sarcoidosis is a diagnosis of exclusion. Diagnosis rests on the presence of typical clinical symptoms, imaging findings, and biopsy-confirmed noncaseating granulomas.

Blood and Urine Studies

There are no diagnostic tests for sarcoidosis. Elevated angiotensin-converting enzyme (ACE) levels, elevated 1,25 dihydroxyvitamin D levels, calciuria, cytopenias, and elevated inflammatory markers are supportive of a diagnosis in the right clinical setting. Many children have increased inflammatory markers (e.g., erythrocyte sedimentation rate [ESR], C-reactive protein [CRP], and platelets.) Macrophages in sarcoid granulomas synthesize ACE, and these levels can be trended in patients with confirmed disease and correlate with disease activity. Macrophages in granulomas express the enzyme α1-hydroxylase, and thus are able to independently convert inactive vitamin D to active 1,25-dihydroxyvitamin D (calcitriol). This results in increased intestinal calcium absorption and bone resorption and is largely unregulated by parathyroid hormone levels. Calciuria (as measured by the ratio of urine calcium to creatinine) is present in many children with sarcoidosis and may occur with or without overt hypercalcemia. Other common nonspecific findings include leukopenia, anemia, eosinophilia, hypergammaglobulinemia, and positive rheumatoid factor (RF). Immunoglobulins should be checked to evaluate for common variable immunodeficiency and testing for CTAL4 deficiency should be considered. In early-onset sarcoidosis, genetic tests for *NOD2/CARD15* mutations should be performed (see later section on Blau syndrome). It is also imperative to rule out *M. tuberculosis* infection.

Imaging

Imaging is helpful to evaluate for findings suggestive of sarcoidosis and other causes as well as for ascertaining potential sites for biopsy. Chest radiographs should be performed to evaluate for hilar adenopathy or other pulmonary involvement. Lung involvement in sarcoidosis is grouped into stage I (hilar adenopathy alone), stage II (hilar adenopathy and lung granulomas), stage III (lung granulomas alone), and stage IV (lung fibrosis), with stage IV being most severe and less reversible. Most children with sarcoidosis present with stage I, II, or III lung disease; no children studied have presented with stage IV pulmonary involvement. High-resolution chest computed tomography (CT) should be performed to further characterize abnormalities found on chest radiographs suggestive of sarcoidosis. Lung parenchymal findings on CT may include reticular or ground glass opacities, cysts, or nodules.

Plain radiographs of the hands and vertebrae may demonstrate lytic bone lesions in up to 19% of children. A gallium scan or ^{18}F-fluorodesoxyglucose–positron emission tomographic (FDG-PET) scan is useful in determining extent of pulmonary and extrapulmonary involvement. Lacrimal and parotid gland involvement results in the so-called "panda" pattern, in which gallium uptake in the nasopharynx and lacrimal and parotid glands results in a PET image resembling the face of a panda. Magnetic resonance imaging is preferred for evaluation of suspected CNS or bone involvement.

Histology

Biopsy-proven granulomatous inflammation is key to the diagnosis of sarcoidosis. Tissue should be sampled from the most accessible site, which may be determined by imaging if not clinically apparent. Typical histologic findings include noncaseating epithelioid cell granulomas; however, this is not specific and does not distinguish sarcoidosis from other granulomatous diseases, including infection and immunodeficiency.

Pulmonary Function Testing

PFTs should be performed to evaluate for subclinical pulmonary involvement and often reveal a restrictive lung disease pattern.

Ophthalmologic Evaluation

Ophthalmologic evaluation, including a slit-lamp examination, should be sought early in the diagnostic workup because ocular lesions typical of sarcoidosis are often asymptomatic and are not common in infections or malignancy.

Management

Patients with sarcoidosis benefit from management at a tertiary care center with multiple specialists. Sarcoidosis may be responsive to corticosteroid monotherapy and may be controlled on low to moderate daily doses. For cases in which low-dose corticosteroids are not adequately effective because of persistent disease or side effects, immunomodulatory therapies, such as methotrexate or tumor necrosis factor-α monoclonal antibodies (infliximab or adalimumab), may be used. Other immunomodulatory agents that have been used include azathioprine, cyclophosphamide, mycophenolate mofetil, tacrolimus, and cyclosporine. No studies have been conducted in children to assess efficacy of any particular immunosuppressive regimen.

FAMILIAL JUVENILE SYSTEMIC GRANULOMATOSIS (BLAU SYNDROME)

Blau syndrome is an autosomal dominant disease characterized by the triad of arthritis, uveitis, and dermatitis along with evidence of noncaseating granulomas and mutations in *NOD2/CARD15*. The *NOD2/CARD15* gene encodes for a gain of function mutation causing the formation of granulomas. There is evidence to suggest that early-onset sarcoidosis is the sporadically inherited form of Blau syndrome, and the clinical manifestations of early-onset sarcoidosis and Blau syndrome are indistinguishable. This disease is rare, typically occurs in infants and young children (median age, 2 years; range, 2 months to 14 years), and is more common among Whites. Arthritis is most commonly polyarticular and is nonerosive. Tenosynovitis is also common. Dermatitis consists of nonerythematous, scaly, ichthyosiform rash. Erythema nodosum, liver granulomas, and large vessel vasculitis have also been reported. The lungs are typically not affected.

Diagnostic and management considerations for Blau syndrome are similar to those for sarcoidosis, with the addition of genetic testing for the NOD2/CARD15 mutation. There are no evidence-based treatment guidelines. As with sarcoidosis, children must be routinely evaluated by ophthalmology. Ocular outcomes in children with Blau syndrome are frequently worse than in sarcoidosis because of uveitis that is often difficult to control.

GRANULOMATOUS AND LYMPHOCYTIC INTERSTITIAL LUNG DISEASE

GLILD is increasingly recognized as a complication of common variable immunodeficiency (CVID). The lung is involved in 50% of the granulomatous diseases associated with CVID. It is important to distinguish GLILD from sarcoidosis.

Etiology and Pathogenesis

The cause of GLILD is unknown. With long-standing disease, granulomatous involvement in multiple organs has been described in 10% to 15% of patients with CVID.

Clinical Presentation

GLILD should be considered only in patients with CVID. The median age at diagnosis is between 30 and 40 years old, but it has been reported in the adolescent patient population. Pulmonary findings are present in 50% of patients and include bibasilar inspiratory crackles on examination. Extrapulmonary manifestations are common, with hepatosplenomegaly and lymphadenopathy frequently reported. This is in contrast to sarcoidosis, where eye and joint involvement is much more common than hepatic and splenic involvement. GLILD also has not been reported to have significant skin involvement, unlike sarcoidosis. The natural history of GLILD has not been completely characterized, but it seems to be more clinically aggressive.

Histology

Patients with GLILD will have nonnecrotizing granulomas when biopsied. Two other histologic features present include follicular bronchiolitis and lymphocytic interstitial pneumonia, a subtype of organizing pneumonia.

Evaluation and Management

If GLILD is suspected, laboratory and radiographic information can be helpful to distinguish this entity from sarcoidosis. Immunoglobulin A, G, and M levels should be evaluated and will be low in patients with CVID. A markedly suppressed IgG level is common in CVID. Imaging of the chest with high-resolution CT should be obtained. GLILD has a radiographic pattern of large, randomly distributed pulmonary nodules, some of which display ground glass surrounding them ("halo sign"). Lower lobe lung involvement is more common in GLILD, and perihilar involvement is uncommon, in contrast with sarcoidosis. Bronchiectasis often develops in these patients. Pulmonary function testing should be performed regularly, because both obstructive and restrictive lung disease patterns have been reported.

Treatment relies on immunosuppression. There have been no randomized control trials of therapeutic options in GLILD to date. Although corticosteroids are often used as first-line agents, case reports suggest that steroid-sparing immunosuppression, such as azathioprine and rituximab, may be more effective.

GRANULOMATOSIS WITH POLYANGIITIS

Granulomatosis with polyangiitis (GPA, formerly Wegener's granulomatosis) is a systemic disease characterized by granulomatous inflammation and necrotizing vasculitis predominantly involving small vessels. A rare disease, the incidence is approximately 0.1 in 100,000 children, with a female predominance (4:1) and a median pediatric age at onset of 14.5 years (range, 9 to 17 years).

Etiology and Pathogenesis

The cause of GPA is unknown, but a pathogenic role for antineutrophil cytoplasmic antibodies (ANCAs), specifically anti–proteinase 3 (anti-PR3), has been proposed in the mechanism of initial endothelial cell damage. A correlation with Staphylococcus aureus infections and GPA flares suggests that extrinsic factors play a role.

Clinical Presentation

The triad of pulmonary, renal, and sinus involvement characterizes classic GPA; however, the most common manifestation is nonspecific constitutional symptoms (fever, weight loss) and arthralgias. Limited GPA involves the upper airway and spares the lungs and kidneys.

Pulmonary involvement ranges from asymptomatic pulmonary nodules to hemorrhage and respiratory failure. Common symptoms include cough, dyspnea, and hemoptysis.

Renal involvement includes necrotizing glomerulonephritis, which is an organ-threatening manifestation and may initially be asymptomatic with progression to renal failure necessitating hemodialysis or transplantation.

Upper airway manifestations typically involve sinusitis or recurrent epistaxis but may also include oral or nasal ulcers, recurrent otitis media, hearing loss (conductive or sensorineural), subglottic stenosis, or granulomatous inflammation of nasal cartilage resulting in nasal septal perforation or saddle nose deformity.

Ocular involvement includes scleritis, episcleritis, conjunctivitis, or uveitis and may manifest as blurry vision, eye pain, or without symptoms. Before establishment of the diagnosis, the eye involvement is frequently misdiagnosed as allergic conjunctivitis.

Arthritis may occur with active disease but is usually not chronic or destructive. Myalgias and arthralgias are common.

The rash of GPA most commonly manifests as palpable purpura (often misdiagnosed as Henoch-Schönlein purpura) or erythematous nodules, but necrotizing vasculitic lesions and ulcerations may occur.

Less common manifestations include involvement of the CNS (seizures, optic neuritis, and cranial nerve palsies), heart (infarction, arrhythmia, or valvulitis), gastrointestinal tract (nausea, vomiting, or pain), and venous thromboembolism.

Differential Diagnosis

The differential diagnosis depends on manifestation and often requires evaluation for other causes of nonspecific systemic symptoms or fever of unknown origin (see Chapter 83). Infectious causes of granulomatous vasculitis must be considered (Box 140.1). Other rheumatologic illnesses and chronic granulomatous disease (especially in young children) should be considered.

Evaluation and Management

The diagnostic criteria for childhood GPA put forth by the European League Against Rheumatism (EULAR) can be found in Box 140.2.

Blood and Urine Studies

No diagnostic laboratory tests exist for GPA, although 90% to 95% of children are ANCA positive, with cANCA (cytoplasmic antineutrophil cytoplasmic antibodies) occurring more frequently than pANCA (perinuclear antineutrophil cytoplasmic antibodies) (87% versus 13%, respectively). Anti-PR3 and myeloperoxidase antibodies also should be evaluated. RF is positive in up to 63% of children with GPA. ESR and CRP and other acute-phase reactants (e.g., platelets) are typically elevated, and a mild anemia is often present. Elevated serum creatinine occurs in up to 44% and abnormal urinalysis (proteinuria, microscopic hematuria, and red blood cell casts) in up to 50%.

Imaging

Chest radiograph abnormalities, typically nodular infiltrates, are present in up to two-thirds of children, half of whom are asymptomatic. Pleural effusions and pneumothoraces may occur. Chest and sinus CTs should be obtained to characterize the extent of pulmonary and sinus involvement. FDG-PET scan may help characterize the extent of extrapulmonary involvement and to determine the least invasive biopsy site.

Pulmonary Function Tests

Decreased diffusion capacity of the lung for carbon monoxide (DLCO) suggests early pulmonary hemorrhage.

Ophthalmologic Evaluation

Because ophthalmologic manifestations are common in GPA, ophthalmologic evaluation, including a slit-lamp examination, should be sought early in the diagnostic workup.

Histology

Classic granulomas in GPA include central necrosis, histiocytes, lymphocytes, and giant cells. The pathologic findings vary by biopsy site. Typical kidney lesions include pauci-immune crescentic necrotizing glomerulonephritis, with granulomas or vasculitis rarely noted. Biopsies from the upper respiratory tract (sinus or nasal septum) may reveal granulomas with giant cells or necrotizing vasculitis. Whereas lung nodules typically show granulomas, other air-space disease may reveal vasculitis or posthemorrhagic changes.

Management

Corticosteroids are a mainstay of early GPA management. Immunomodulatory therapy choices depend on the extent of organ involvement. For life-threatening disease, cyclophosphamide or rituximab is warranted. Rituximab has fewer systemic toxicities in children and may be preferred as first-line induction therapy. Plasmapheresis is also used for severe, life-threatening disease and has been shown to speed renal recovery but has not been shown to decrease overall rates of renal disease or prevent relapses. For more limited disease, azathioprine, methotrexate, or mycophenolate mofetil have been used. Trimethoprim-sulfamethoxazole is often used as adjunct treatment; whether the benefit is attributable to antimicrobial properties (i.e., in limiting *S. aureus*–associated GPA flares or opportunistic infections with *Pneumocystis*) or to other antiinflammatory properties is unclear. GPA is generally well controlled with therapy; however, relapse is common in up to 50% of patients, especially as medication is weaned or discontinued. Notably, approximately one-third of children with GPA develop irreversible renal insufficiency.

EOSINOPHILIC GRANULOMATOSIS WITH POLYANGIITIS

Also known as allergic granulomatosis, eGPA, is a granulomatous small vessel vasculitis associated with asthma, eosinophilia, and allergic rhinitis. Classification criteria include asthma, eosinophilia (>10% of white blood cells), allergies, peripheral neuropathies (mononeuritis, polyneuritis, or mononeuritis multiplex), transient pulmonary infiltrates, paranasal sinus abnormalities, and extravascular eosinophils. The 2012 Revised International Chapel Hill Consensus Conference Nomenclature of Vasculitides defines eGPA in adults as an "Eosinophil-rich and necrotizing granulomatous inflammation often involving the respiratory tract, and necrotizing vasculitis predominantly affecting the small and medium vessels and associated with asthma and eosinophilia. ANCA is more frequently positive when glomerulonephritis is present." There are no specific criteria for children because eGPA is rare. The mean age of onset is 12 years, ranging from 2 to 18 years, with a slight female predominance (1.4:1). The cause and pathogenesis are currently unknown.

Clinical Presentation

At diagnosis, the majority of children report a history of asthma, atopy, and sinusitis. Nonfixed pulmonary infiltrates on chest radiography occur in the majority of patients. Skin involvement is often present. Typical findings are leukocytoclastic vasculitis manifesting as purpura, but other rashes (maculopapular, cutaneous nodules, livedo reticularis, ulcers, and bullae) occur as well. Other manifestations include peripheral neuropathy; gastrointestinal, musculoskeletal, cardiac inflammation (myocarditis, pericarditis); and mild nonprogressive renal disease. Involvement of the lymph nodes, mammary glands, orbits, salivary glands, testes, and thymus also has been noted.

Evaluation and Management

No tests are diagnostic, but eosinophilia, high IgE, and elevated inflammatory markers are common. ANCAs are detected in 25%, with one-third having cANCA and two-thirds having pANCA. On histologic examination, affected tissues demonstrate vasculitis of small arteries, veins, or both with associated extravascular eosinophilic infiltrates and necrotizing granulomas. High-dose corticosteroids in combination with other immunomodulatory therapies, such as cyclophosphamide or azathioprine, are the mainstays of treatment. Overall prognosis is guarded, with relapses being common and mortality from disease manifestations (intestinal perforation, cardiac failure, and respiratory insufficiency) occurring in 18% within 1 to 2 years of diagnosis.

FUTURE DIRECTIONS

Newer immunomodulatory agents are promising in the treatment of patients with these diseases. The greatest hurdle in determining optimal therapy for noninfectious granulomatous disease in children is the lack of systematic evaluation owing to the low incidence of these diseases. Establishment of registries for these rare conditions will allow for a more systematic and comprehensive evaluation of their characteristics, pathogenesis, genetics, and outcomes, which are prerequisites for improving therapeutic management.

SUGGESTED READINGS

Available online.

Page number followed by *f* indicates figure, by *t* table, and by *b* box.